AF540743

Endodontics:

Biological Concepts and Technological Resources

Endodontics:
Biological Concepts and Technological Resources

Mario Roberto Leonardo
Full Professor of the Restorative Dentistry Department (Endodontic Course) –
Araraquara School of Dentistry – UNESP, SP, Brazil.
Collaborator Professor (Pediatric Dentistry Course) at the Ribeirão Preto
School of Dentistry-USP, SP, Brazil.
Visiting Professor (Sabbatical Professor) – Connecticut University – U.S.A. (1983/1985).

Renato de Toledo Leonardo
Assistant Professor Doctor of the Restorative Dentistry Department (Endodontic Course) – Araraquara School of Dentistry – UNESP, SP, Brazil.

Translation Reviewer
Cornelis H. Pameijer, DMD, DSc, PhD
Professor Emeritus, University of Connecticut

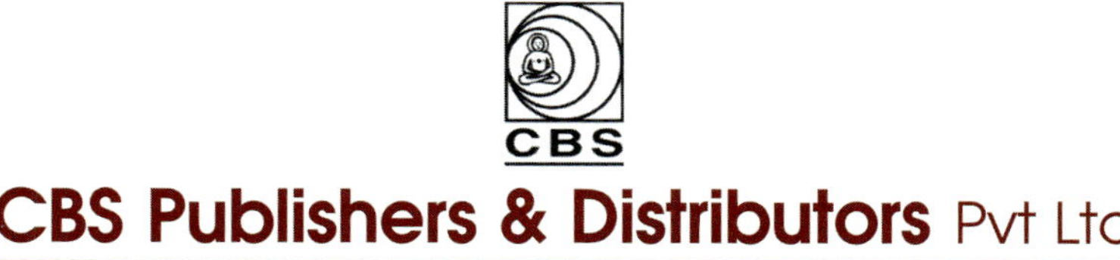

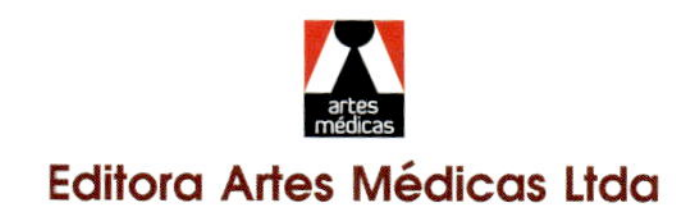

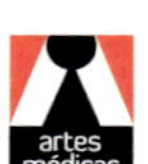

Artes Médicas is an imprint of Grupo A.

Editora Artes Médicas Ltda
Rua Dr Cesário Mota Jr 63 – Vila Buarque
01221-020 SÃO PAULO SP
B R A Z I L

Ph: 55 11 3221-9033 Fax: 55 11 3223-6635

This Edition has been published by special arrangement with Editora Artes Médicas Ltda
CBS ISBN: 978-81-239-2234-8

Special Indian Edition: 2012

Published by Satish Kumar Jain and produced by Vinod K. Jain for
CBS Publishers & Distributors Pvt Ltd
4819/XI Prahlad Street, 24 Ansari Road, Daryaganj, New Delhi 110 002, India.
Ph: 23289259, 23266861, 23266867 Fax: 011-23243014 Website: www.cbspd.com
e-mail: delhi@cbspd.com; cbspubs@airtelmail.in

Corporate Office: 204 FIE, Industrial Area, Patparganj, Delhi 110 092
Ph: 4934 4934 Fax: 4934 4935 e-mail: publishing@cbspd.com; publicity@cbspd.com

Branches

- **Bengaluru:** Seema House 2975, 17th Cross, K.R. Road, Banasankari 2nd Stage, Bengaluru 560 070, Karnataka
  Ph: +91-80-26771678/79 Fax: +91-80-26771680 e-mail: bangalore@cbspd.com
- **Pune:** Bhuruk Prestige, Sr. No. 52/12/2+1+3/2 Narhe, Haveli (Near Katraj-Dehu Road Bypass), Pune 411 041, Maharashtra
  Ph: +91-20-64704058, 64704059, 32342277 Fax: +91-20-24300160 e-mail: pune@cbspd.com
- **Kochi:** 36/14 Kalluvilakam, Lissie Hospital Road, Kochi 682 018, Kerala
  Ph: +91-484-4059061-65 Fax: +91-484-4059065 e-mail: cochin@cbspd.com
- **Chennai:** 20, West Park Road, Shenoy Nagar, Chennai 600 030, Tamil Nadu
  Ph: +91-44-26260666, 26208620 Fax: +91-44-45530020 e-mail: chennai@cbspd.com

Representatives

- **Mumbai** 0-9833017933
- **Kolkata** 0-9831437309
- **Hyderabad** 0-9885175004
- **Patna** 0-9334159340
- **Manipal** 0-9742022075

Printed at RP Printers, Noida

Presentation

Publication of a book by two authors, father and son, is an important task, and can only result in work in which respect, impartiality, honesty and seriousness preponderate. In order to emphasize this, a brief analysis of the academic lives of both writers is appropriate.

Prof. Mario Roberto Leonardo has trailed the paths of Endodontics since the 1960s. His commitment to and thoughtful regard for the root canal system, apical and periapical tissues and endodontic biological aspects have led him to the most distant places to disseminate this knowledge, divulged in hundreds of articles published in magazines of impact, and in his text book Endodontics: root canal treatment. Technical and Biological Principles, now in its 5th edition. His stay in the United States of America also helped him to consolidate his own philosophy, concerned with the difficult task of performing and teaching how to perform an ideal root canal treatment.

Prof. Renato de Toledo Leonardo, has followed the same school since the early 1990s, continuously gained scientific knowledge, and obtained his doctor's degree in pathology. With the impetuosity and restlessness inherent to youth, he sought to add the advantages offered by contemporary technology to the scenario. After spending a period in Spain, he accepted invitations that took him to over 50 countries to give courses in Endodontics. Thus, he also learned and consolidated the concept of the association between biology and technique.

From these two life experiences, and with the main goal of improving endodontic post-treatment success rates, the idea of writing a book came to mind. The two authors took advantage of the things they had gained from endodontic world and allowed friends and specialist colleagues to contribute to the undertaking.

The result was the book Endodontics: *Biological concepts and technological resources,* which represents the sum of 65 years of knowledge, dedication and passion for the specialty we have embraced, with the inestimable help of collaborators. With the dissemination of this information we seek to improve the quality of oral health in the world.

The Authors

Preface

The more time goes by, the more we appreciate professionals who do not "speak only for the sake of speaking", but lay out pathways. Furthermore, we are fortunate and blessed by a selected group of professors who bring teachings and skills, both to the clinic and research in dentistry. These esteemed professionals, especially those with great communication skills, stimulate our minds, motivate us to be the best clinicians. Professors Mario and Renato Leonardo are part of this rare group and greatly contribute to the improvement in our careers.

What makes them so special, is perhaps the influence exerted on them by the environment in which they work. Professor Renato's maternal grandfather was one of the pioneers of the Araraquara School of Pharmacy and Dentistry – UNESP, one of the most important schools of Dentistry in Brazil. In addition to his father-in-law's support, Professor Mario also counted on the extraordinary cooperation of his wife and lifetime companion, Marisa Barbosa de Toledo Leonardo, for the histological processing of his researches, when he worked as a professor at the University of Connecticut – EUA.

If there were genetic or environmental influences, what matters is that they were endowed with capabilities that resulted in knowledge and working lives entirely devoted to Endodontics, for which we are eternally grateful.

If we were professionals who wished to progress and offer excellent treatment to our patients, with whom we are truly concerned, we would always wish to acquire the most correct, profound and valuable knowledge. This book contains information that exceeds the highest expectations, both for clinic and with respect to the scientific field.

Its contents certainly meet all our needs. The valuable teachings it contains lead us to better knowledge, not only of the complex endodontic world, but also of the procedures necessary for restoring patients' oral and general health, based on a humanistic approach. I feel certain that this book will remind us, especially in the field of Endodontics, that "what really matters is the patient in the chair".

Sincerely,

Dr. Dan Fischer

Collaborators

ADRIANA DE JESUS SOARES

Doctor in Endodontics from the Dentistry School of Piracicaba – UNICAMP, SP, Brazil.

ALEJANDRO JAIME

Specialist in Endodontics; Head, Endodontics Dept. School of Dentistry, Universidade Maimónides – Buenos Aires, Argentina.

Professor, Endodontics Dept. Instituto de Saúde Bucal – Santa Fé, Argentina.

ALEXANDRE SILVA BRAMANTE

Doctor in Endodontics from the Dentistry School of Bauru – USP, SP, Brazil.

ANDRÉA GONÇALVES

Assistant Professor Doctor of the Radiology Course at the Dentistry School of Araraquara – UNESP, SP, Brazil.

CAMILLA NICOLE PECORA

Dental surgeon graduated from the University of Chieti – Italy

Clinical Instructor of the course of "Technical Advancements and Biological Bases in Implant Dentistry", at the University of New Jersey – USA and at the University of Guarulhos.

CARLOS ALBERTO FERREIRA MURGEL

Professor of Operative Microscopy at E.A.P. – A.P.C.D. – Central, SP, Brazil. Professor of Operative Microscopy and Endodontics – Pacific Endodontics Research – San Diego, Ca, USA.

Resident in Endodontics at the University of Iowa, USA

Member of the Editorial Board of the Journal of Endodontics.

CARLOS ALBERTO SPIRONELLI RAMOS

Professor Doctor of the Endodontics Course at the Dentistry School of the State University of Londrina, Paraná, Brazil.

CARLOS GARCIA PUENTE

Professor of Endodontics at the Dentistry School of the University of Maimonides, Buenos Aires, Argentina.

CLÓVIS MONTEIRO BRAMANTE

Full Professor of the Department of Dentistry, Endodontics and Materials at the Dentistry School of Bauru – USP, SP, Brazil.

CORNELIS PAMEIJER

Emeritus Professor at the University of Connecticut – USA.

DANIEL SILVA HERZOG FLORES

Professor of Endodontics at the Dentistry School of the University of San Luis Potosi, Mexico.

FÁBIO LUIZ CAMARGO VILLELA BERBERT

Assistant Professor Doctor of the Restorative Dentistry Department (Endodontic Course) – Dentistry School of Araraquara – UNESP, SP, Brazil.

FERNANDO DURÁN-SINDREU TEROL

Coordinator of the Masterís Course in Endodontics at the International University of Catalunya.

FRANCISCO JOSÉ DE SOUZA FILHO

Full Professor Doctor of the Endodontics Course at the Dentistry School of Piracicaba – UNICAMP, SP, Brazil.

GABRIELE EDOARDO PECORA

Ex-Associate Professor of the Surgery Department and Co-Director of the Advanced Implant Dentistry Program – Cunny University, Buffalo – USA.

Ex-Adjunct Professor of Endodontics and of the Microsurgery and Endodontics Center at the University of Pennsylvania – USA.

Adjunct Professor of Operative Dentistry and Director of the "Advanced Techniques and Biological Aspects in Implant Dentistry" program UDMNJ – New Jersey.

Professor of Implant Dentistry and Co-Director of the Implant Dentistry Course "Basic and Advanced Techniques in patients" at the University of Guarulhos, SP, Brazil.

IDOMEO BONETTI FILHO

Adjunct Professor of the Restorative Dentistry Department (Endodontics Course) at the Dentistry School of Araraquara – UNESP, SP, Brazil.

IVALDO GOMES DE MORAES

Adjunct Professor of the Department of Dentistry, Endodontics and Materials at the Dentistry School of Bauru – USP, SP, Brazil.

JAMIL AWAD SHIBLI

Head of the Oral Implant Dentistry Clinic and Assistant Professor of the Periodontal Department – Research Division in Dentistry at the University of Guarulhos, SP, Brazil.

JUAN SAAVEDRA

Professor of Endodontics at the Dentistry School of the Universidade Central da Venezuela (UVC), Venezuela.

LÉA ASSED BEZERRA DA SILVA

Full Professor of the Childrenís Clinic, Preventive and Social Dentistry Department (Pediatric Dentistry Course) at the Dentistry School of Ribeirão Preto– USP, SP, Brazil.

MARCELO GONÇALVES

Assistant Professor Doctor of the Radiology Course at the Dentistry School of Araraquara – UNESP, SP, Brazil.

MARCO AURÉLIO GAGLIARDI BORGES

Master in Endodontics from the Dentistry School of Araraquara –UNESP, SP, Brazil.

MARIA GUIOMAR AZEVEDO BAHIA

Adjunct Professor of Endodontics at the Restorative Dentistry Department at the Dentistry School of the Federal University of Minas Gerais (UFMG), MG, Brazil.

MÁRIO TANOMARU FILHO

Adjunct Professor of the Restorative Dentistry Department (Endodontics Course) at the Dentistry School of Araraquara – UNESP, SP, Brazil.

MIGUEL ROIG CAYÓN

Head of the Dental Restorative Area at the International University of Catalunya.

PAULO NELSON-FILHO

Full Professor of the Childrenís Clinic, Preventive and Social Dentistry Department (Pediatric Dentistry Course) at the Dentistry School of Ribeirão Preto– USP, SP, Brazil.

RAQUEL ASSED BEZERRA DA SILVA

Assistant Professor of the Childrenís Clinic, Preventive and Social Dentistry Department (Pediatric Dentistry Course) at the Dentistry School of Ribeirão Preto – USP, SP, Brazil.

RENATO MIOTTO PALO

Voluntary Professor, Endodontics, Dentistry School of São José dos Campos-UNESP.

RICARDO M. OLIVEIRA-FILHO

Professor of the Pharmacological Department of the Biomedical Science Institute of Brazil – USP, SP, Brazil.

RICHARD D. TUTTLE

Private Practice at Layton, Utah-USA

Research and Development, Clinical Lab Division Manager and Clinical Appications Advisor – Ultradent, Inc.

RICHARD MOUNCE

Specialist in Endodontics in Vancouver, WA, USA.

TATIANA RAMIREZ MORA

Master in Endodontics at the Dentistry School of the Universidade de San Luis Potosi – Mexico.

Present Professor of Endodontics at the Dentistry School at the Universidade de Costa Rica – Costa Rica.

Summary

1

Introduction

Demystifying root canal treatment

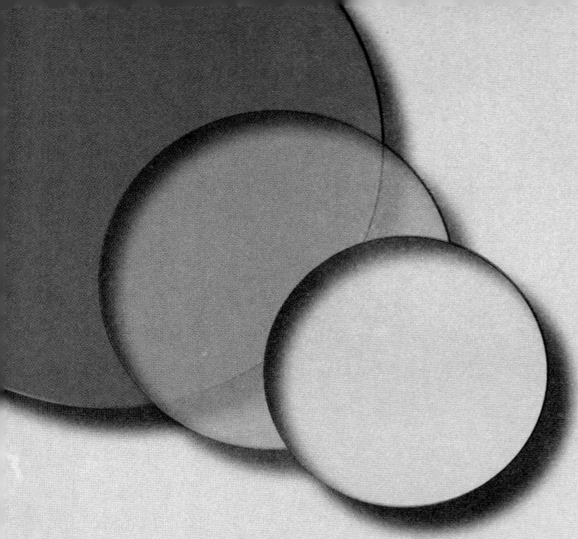

Mario Roberto Leonardo
Léa Assed Bezerra da Silva

The technological development involving treatment of root canals has elevated the endodontic specialty over the last few years to a level of **technical uniqueness** not seen in its entire history. According to Spångberg[133] in an editorial published in 2003 in the Journal *Oral Surgery, Oral Medicine, Oral Pathology, Oral Radiology, Oral Medicine, Oral Pathology, Oral Radiology and Endodontics*, 300 to 350 scientific articles in this area alone have been published annually in the U.S.A. over the last few years. These publications appeared in high impact American and international journals, while taking advantage of advanced research methodologies, both *in vivo* and *in vitro* and/or *ex vivo*.

The above-mentioned factors have lead to two distinct philosophies in clinical conduct, representing two schools of thought that disseminate and teach this specialty. The first one uses the technological advances and incorporate them into the daily practice of modern Endodontics, and is represented by professionals and endodontists who are more interested in the **how** to perform root canal treatment as quickly as possible, generally in **a single session**. **The other school of thought** is concerned more about **how, when, why,** and in **which** manner to perform root canal treatment. Thus, we can reason that the first operate on the basis of the technical principles of the treatment, whereas the latter adopt the same principles, but base them on biological ideology.

Therefore, at present there are two categories of educators and endodontists. The first are considered disciples of the strictly technical school and can be referred to as Technologists*. These professionals and educators disseminate information and operate using modern techniques, new equipment, innovative materials and new treatment methods, with the goal to perform a root canal treatment much faster than could be done some years ago. For the disciples of the technical development in endodontics, the apical limit of instrumentation and root canal filling is not always respected, and the majority of them appreciate a little extrusion of the filling material, which the North Americans call **"*apical puff*"**.

* Webster's new Collegiate Dictionary 1979, Springfield, MA USA.

For the Technologists the main support for therapeutic decision-making is based on clinical and radiographic evaluations of the results of treatment, performed at different post-treatment observation periods, and mainly a reliance on long professional experience. These results therefore generate data that are based on non-controlled studies, mostly without the support of comparative data, (histopathological results), which must be retrieved from clinical observations during and after treatment.

In root canal treatment of teeth with pulp necrosis (gangrene) and with evident radiographically chronic periapical lesions (apical periodontitis), microscopic (histological) findings compared with radiographs are frequently different.

Considering that after endodontic treatment the histopathological findings[69] do not always coincide with the clinical/radiographic results, the latter alone **should not be considered a parameter** for determining the success of this therapy. Charts 1.1, 1.2, 1.3 and 1.4 and the Figs. 1.1A-D, Figs. 1.2A-F, 1.3A-C and 1.4A-C, confirm the above statement.

Our findings[69] confirm that in many cases the chronic periapical reaction (apical periodontitis) can persist for years after the root canal has been filled, even in the absence of clinical signs and symptoms and/or with radiographic repair. This is in agreement with Katebzadeh et al.[60], 1999; Katebzadeh et al.[61], 2000 and Nair et al.[95], 2005.

"SHOULD THE ENDODONTIC CONCEPT OF SUCCESS BE RECONSIDERED?"

CHART 1.1 – Case 5A[69]

EVALUATORS	RADIOGRAPHIC INTERPRETATION			CLINICAL EVALUATION**	FILLING MATERIAL	FOLLOW-UP TIME**
	SUCCESS	FAILURE	APICAL LIMIT OF FILLING			
I	SUCCESS	-	1 mm short of the apex* (arrow)	SUCCESS	ZINC OXIDE AND EUGENOL AND GUTTA-PERCHA CONES	FIVE YEARS AND SIX MONTHS
II	SUCCESS	-	1 mm short of the apex* (arrow)			
III	SUCCESS	-	1 mm short of the apex* (arrow)			
IV	SUCCESS	-	1 mm short of the apex* (arrow)			
V	SUCCESS	-	1 mm short of the apex* (arrow)			
VI	SUCCESS	-	1 mm short of the apex* (arrow)			

* Radiographic apical limit, considered ideal by the authors in this case of pulp necrosis and periapical lesion.
** Post-treatment Clinical and Radiographic Control.

CASE 5A[69]

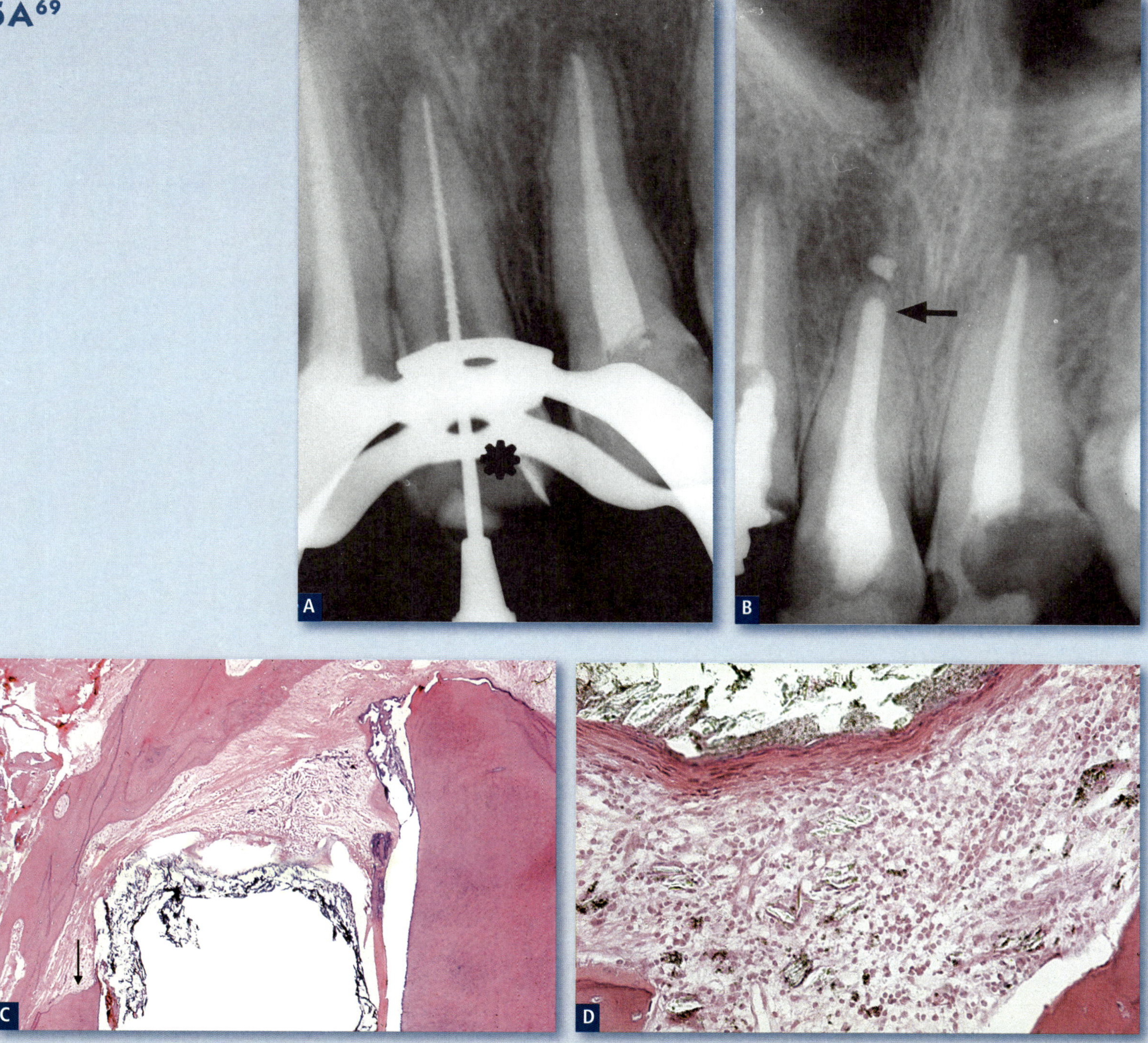

FIGS. 1.1A-D

A – Periapical radiograph, with file No.40 being used to determine the root canal working length in a human tooth (1.1), showing evidence of chronic periapical lesion (apical periodontitis) (03.05.67). Case 5A[69].

B – Post-treatment radiograph (follow-up) obtained five years and six months after root canal filling (10/31/1972), showing evidence of biologically ideal limit of the filling (arrow), complete radiographic periapical repair of the pre-existing lesion and a small amount of extrusion of filling cement.

C – Histological section (panoramic view) of the apical and periapical regions of the tooth shown in Fig. 1.1B, showing evidence of connective tissue with inflammatory infiltrate of the chronic type, determining cement resorption of one of the root canal walls (arrow), to the point of allowing the filling material to come into contact with the periodontal ligament. Also note that the apical filling limit on one of the sides of the foramen (histological) did not correspond to that observed radiographically (arrow) by the evaluators. H&E.40X.

D – Histological section showing evidence of filling cement fragment (zinc oxide and eugenol), distant from the foramen and enveloped by a thin layer of fibrous tissue and by moderate to intense inflammatory infiltrate of the chronic type. H&E.200X.

CHART 1.2 – Case $8H_1$[69]

EVALUATORS	RADIOGRAPHIC INTERPRETATION			CLINICAL EVALUATION	FILLING MATERIAL	FOLLOW-UP TIME
	SUCCESS	FAILURE	APICAL LIMIT OF FILLING			
I	SUCCESS	-	1 to 2 mm short of the apex* (arrow)	SUCCESS	KERR PULP CANAL SEALER** AND GUTTA-PERCHA CONES	ONE YEAR AND TWO MONTHS
II	SUCCESS	-	1 to 2 mm short of the apex* (arrow)			
III	SUCCESS	-	1 to 2 mm short of the apex* (arrow)			
IV	SUCCESS	-	1 to 2 mm short of the apex* (arrow)			
V	SUCCESS	-	1 to 2 mm short of the apex* (arrow)			
VI	SUCCESS	-	1 to 2 mm short of the apex* (arrow)			

* The apical limit of filling was from 1 to 2 mm short of the radiographic apex, considered ideal by the authors, in this case of a vital pulp.
** Kerr Mg. Co. USA.

CASE $8H_1$[69]

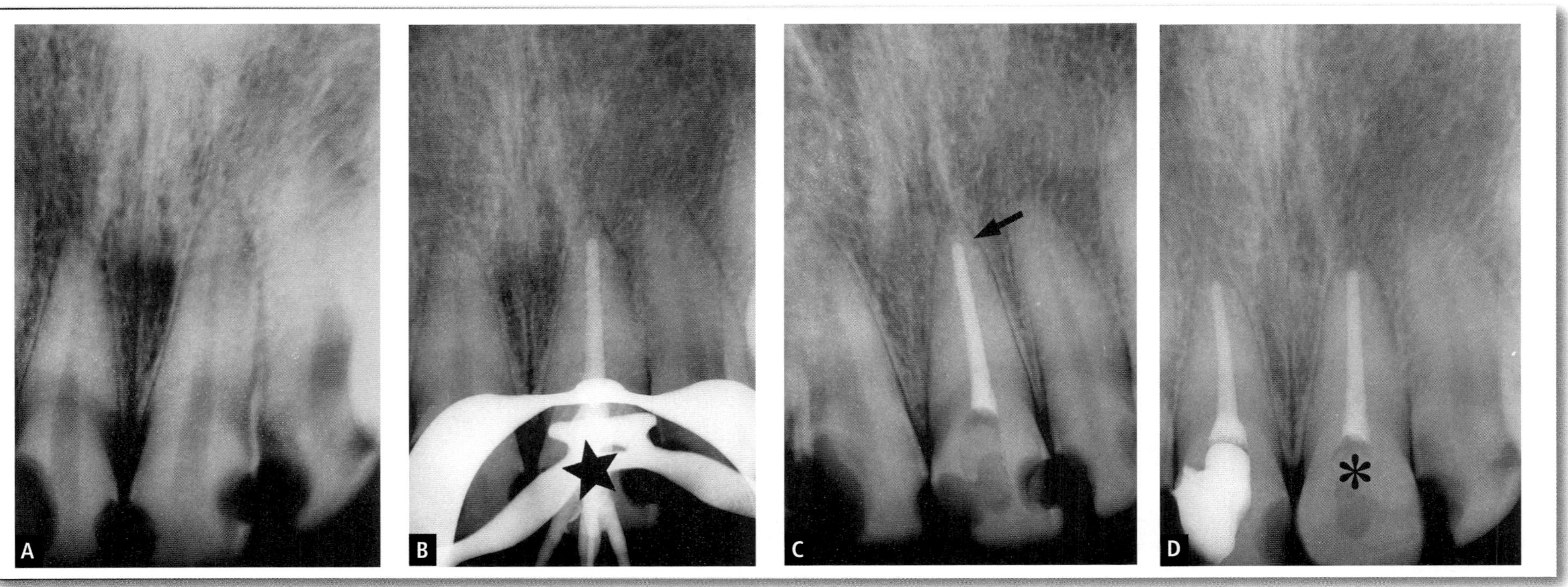

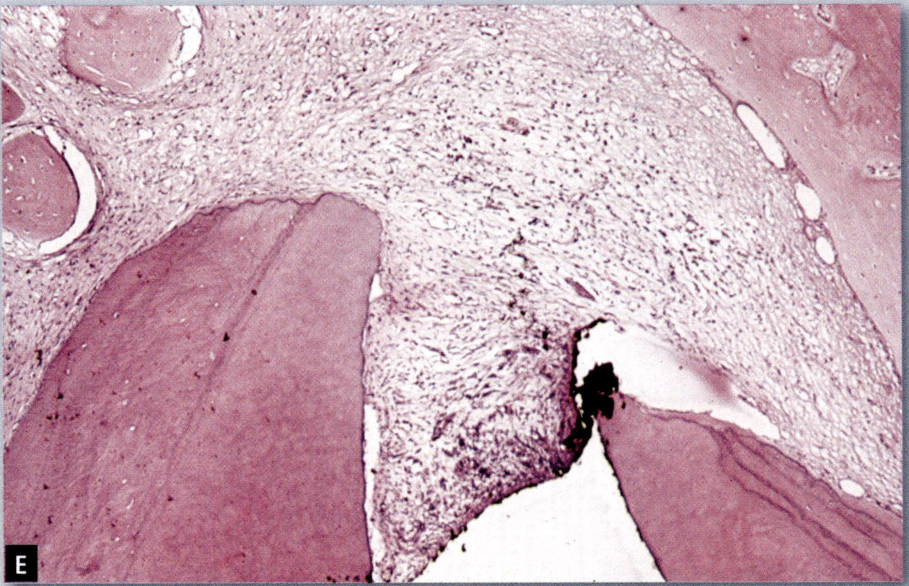

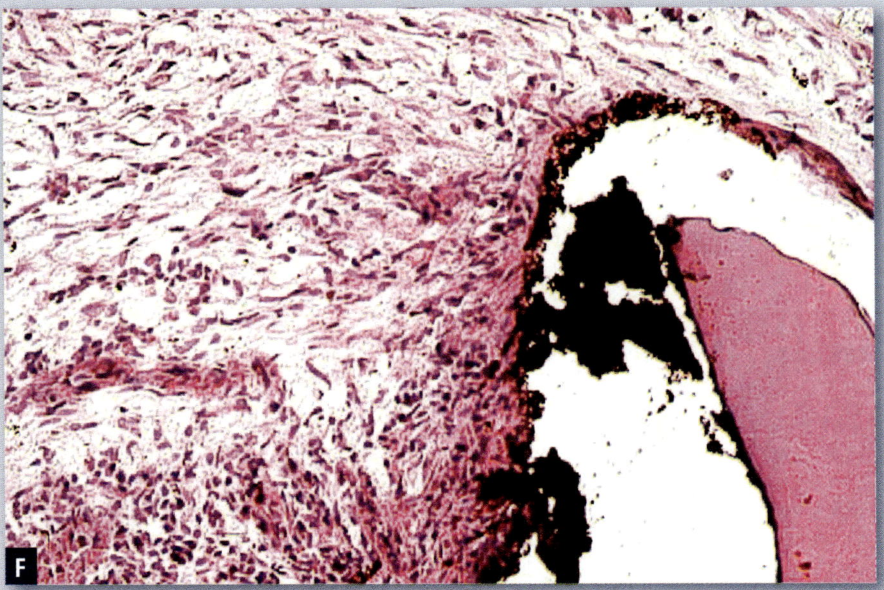

FIGS. 1.2A-F

A – Periapical radiograph for diagnosis of human maxillary left central incisor (2.1), with clinical diagnosis of irreversible acute pulpitis (8/23/1971). Case $8H_1$[69].

B – Radiograph obtained after active lateral condensation of the filling in the case shown in Fig. 1.2A, with gutta-percha cones and Kerr Pulp Canal Sealer cement.

C – Final periapical radiograph, obtained after root canal filling. Note the apical filling limit (arrow) 1.5 mm short of the radiographic apex.

D – Post-operative periapical radiograph (follow-up) (10/20/1972), one year and two months after root canal filling, showing evidence of success. Note presence of lamina dura.

E – Histological section (panoramic view) of the case in Fig. 1.2D, showing evidence of the apical (pulp stump) and periapical regions, with inflammatory infiltrate of the chronic type. There are particles of filling material (Kerr Pulp Canal Sealer) located between the pulp stump and the root canal wall. H&E.40X.

F – Magnification of the previous figure, showing the filling material next to the pulp stump, which presents inflammatory infiltrate of the chronic type. H&E.200X.

CHART 1.3 – Case 4A[69]

EVALUATORS	RADIOGRAPHIC INTERPRETATION			CLINICAL EVALUATION**	FILLING MATERIAL**	FOLLOW-UP TIME
	SUCCESS	FAILURE	APICAL LIMIT OF FILLING			
I	SUCCESS	-	1 mm short of the radiographic apex*	SUCCESS	ZINC OXIDE AND EUGENOL AND GUTTA-PERCHA CONES	FIVE YEARS AND EIGHT MONTHS
II	SUCCESS	-	1 mm short of the radiographic apex*			
III	SUCCESS	-	1 mm short of the radiographic apex*			
IV	SUCCESS	-	1 mm short of the radiographic apex*			
V	SUCCESS	-	1 mm short of the radiographic apex*			
VI	SUCCESS	-	1 mm short of the radiographic apex*			

• Apical limit from 1 mm short of the radiographic apex, considered ideal by the authors in this case of pulp necrosis and periapical lesion.

CASE 4A[69]

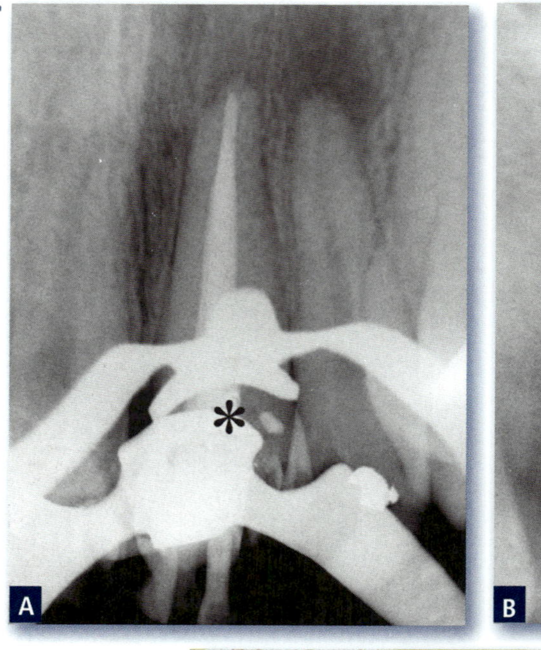

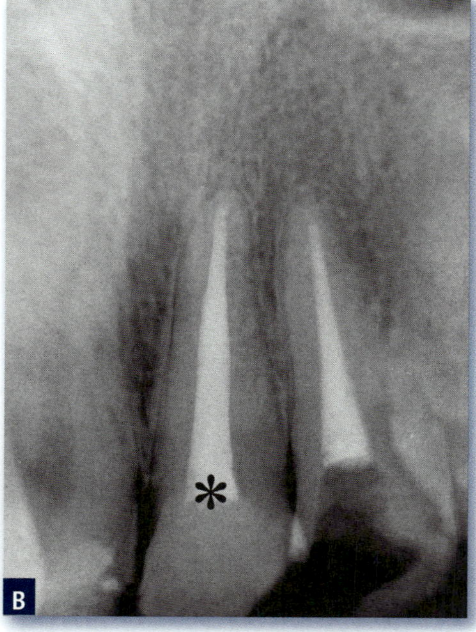

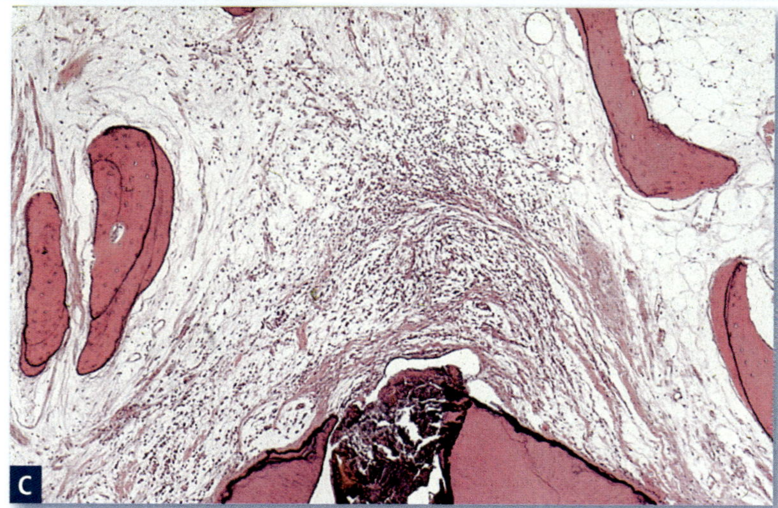

FIGS. 1.3A-C

A – Periapical radiograph obtained after performing active lateral condensation of the root canal filling of human tooth (2.1) with zinc oxide and eugenol cement/gutta-percha cones. Note the presence of chronic periapical lesion (02.02.67). Case 4A[69].

B – Post operative radiograph (follow-up) obtained five years and eight months after root canal filling. Note the radiographic repair of the previous periapical lesion (10.09.1972).

C – Panoramic view of histological section of the apical and periapical region of tooth (21) showing radiographic evidence in Fig. 1.3B, with intense inflammatory infiltrate of the chronic type, as a result of the presence of basophilic amorphous tissue, with numerous fragments of contaminated dentin obliterating the foramen. H.E.40X.

Note: When the endodontic treatment of the present case was performed, (4A), the dominant concept at the time (1960s/1970s) determined that the apical limit of instrumentation and filling should be 1 mm short of the radiographic apex. At present, for cases like this, with a treatment denominated NECROPULPECTOMY II, (cases with apical periodontitis) foraminal debridement is indicated, that is, the removal of the contaminated contents at the foramen level, with a Foraminal Apical Instrument (FAI.).

CHART 1.4 – Case 9D[69]

EVALUATORS	RADIOGRAPHIC INTERPRETATION			CLINICAL EVALUATION	FILLING MATERIAL	FOLLOW-UP TIME
	SUCCESS	FAILURE	APICAL LIMIT OF FILLING			
I	SUCCESS	-	1 mm short of the radiographic apex*	SUCCESS	ZINC OXIDE AND EUGENOL AND GUTTA-PERCHA CONES	SIX YEARS AND TWO MONTHS
II	SUCCESS	-	1 mm short of the radiographic apex*			
III	SUCCESS	-	1 mm short of the radiographic apex*			
IV	SUCCESS	-	1 mm short of the radiographic apex*			
V	SUCCESS	-	1 mm short of the radiographic apex*			
VI	SUCCESS	-	1 mm short of the radiographic apex*			

• Apical limit of 1 mm short of the radiographic apex, considered ideal by the authors in this case of pulp necrosis and periapical lesion.

CASE 9D[69]

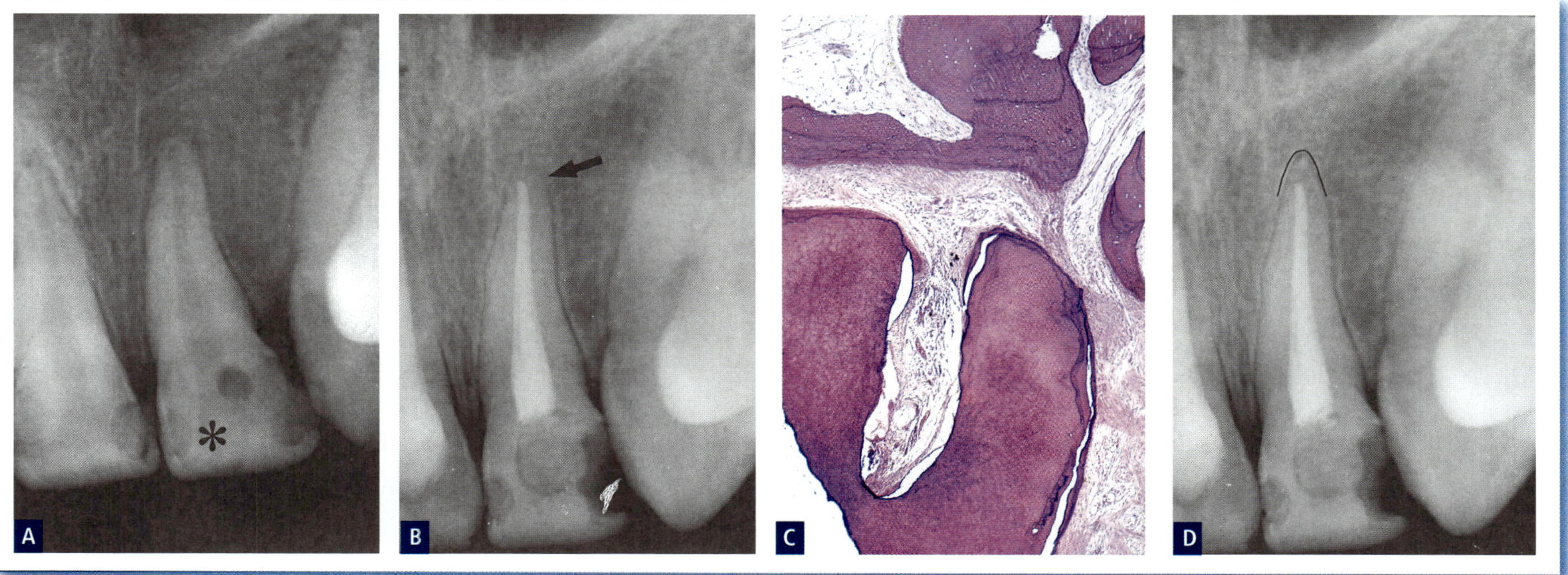

FIGS. 1.4A-D

A – Periapical radiograph for diagnosis of human tooth (2.1) (08.16.66), showing a coronal restoration without pulp protection and a circumscribed periapical rarefaction osteitis, suggesting a clinical/radiographic diagnosis of apical granuloma. Case 9D[69].

B – Post operative periapical radiograph (10/16/1972), six years and two months after root canal filling using the technique of active lateral condensation of gutta-percha cones and zinc oxide and eugenol cement. **Note**: Six university professors who evaluated the radiograph considered the apical limit of filling ideal at 1 mm short of the radiographic apex (arrow).

C – Panoramic view of histological section of the apex and periapical area of the tooth shown in Fig. 1.4B. Note that the apical portion of the canal was not filled and that granulomatous tissue with inflammatory infiltrate of the chronic type is present. Histologically it could be shown that the canal was partially filled, and did not confirm the limit of 1 mm short of the apex according to the radiographic evaluation of the six professors.

D – After the histological confirmation that the root canal was partially filled, a more accurate evaluation allowed the radiographic apex, now outlined by a continuous line, to be better observed.

All the human clinical/surgical cases mentioned where done during the 70`s, according to the Protocol of Helsinki (Finland) of 1964.

TECHNOLOGIST PRINCIPLES OF ROOT CANAL TREATMENT

"Technologist" School
Objectives

- Make use of the technical advances in Endodontics,
- Make use of many years of clinical experience.
- Perform root canal treatment in one single session in all cases.
- As a general rule do not use temporary dressings; that is, do not use calcium hydroxide as intra-canal topical medication between sessions.
- Shorten the time of root canal filling as much as possible.
- Perform treatment as fast as possible, with greater comfort for the patient and less professional stress.
- Use irrigation solutions and filling materials, without considering biocompatibility issues.
- Determine SUCCESS of treatment based only on clinical and radiographical evidence.

"Bio-Technologist" School

The school in which the professors and professionals apply the technology, but respect the biological principles and concepts, we call "BIO-TECHNOLOGISTS". This school subscribes to the notion that in an era of full fledged health promotion, clinical procedures should not be carried out without scientific histopathological evidence. For these professionals, clinical guidance must always be backed by knowledge from laboratory, clinical, radiographic, tomographic and microscopic histological research, that provide scientific evidence.

According to Spångberg[134], Kaare Langeland of the University of Connecticut (USA), a recognized teacher and researcher who passed away recently (09/07/2007), used to emphasize:

> *"The majority of therapeutic procedures in Endodontics are based on philosophical considerations, and what is worse, on personal opinions and/or on clinical experience of different authors, instead of on scientific evidence" (1995).*

* **TECNICIST:** That is technical; Who applies technics.
** **TECNOLOGIST:** Expert in technology. (Scientific knowledge applied to production).
Michaelis – Moderno Dicionário da Língua Portuguesa. Companhia Melhoramentos. São Paulo, 1998.

Again, according to Langeland:

> *"Endodontic therapy is influenced to a high degree by propaganda and personal opinions, instead of scientific investigations" (1995).*

According to this school of thought, the success of root canal treatment is defined not only by post-treatment clinical and radiographic evaluation, but also by correlating clinical treatment observations with histological findings from experimental research.

Without any doubt, this approach will contribute to a quiet painless post-operative treatment, and particularly, to a larger percentage of clinical, radiographic and histological success, and to post-treatment apical and periapical repair. Histological success, compared to clinical conditions of treatment, is the best possible success one can obtain from *in vivo* conducted experiments.

BIO-TECHNOLOGICAL PRINCIPLES OF ROOT CANAL TREATMENT

- Make use of the technical advances in Endodontics.
- Attempt to attain the biologically ideal apical limit of instrumentation and filling, using 3rd generation electronic apex locators.
- After tooth length determination, verify the anatomical diameter of the root canal at the level of the Real Working Length of instrumentation.
- Make an Apical Safe Stop.
- Preserve the vitality of the pulp stump (endoperiodontal stump) in cases of treatment of teeth with vital pulp, since this tissue is coded by nature itself to become mineralized, provided it is kept vital and free of inflammatory cells.
- Use biologically compatible irrigation solutions (with the aim of preserving the vitality of the remaining pulp, including the pulp stump in cases of vital pulp).
- Detoxify the toxic/septic content of the root canal in a crown/down direction, without pressure, in cases of pulp necrosis without or with evident radiographically periapical lesion (apical periodontitis).
- Inactivate the endotoxins (Bacterial LPS) in a crown/down direction, in cases of treatment of teeth with pulp necrosis.
- After working length determination and detoxifying of the toxic/septic contents of the root canal in a crown/down direction, determine the anatomic foramen diameter in cases of teeth with pulp necrosis and evident periapical lesion (apical periodontitis).
- Control infection throughout the root canal system (ramifications, isthmus, dentinal tubules, extra-radicular infection, apical biofilm) in cases of pulp necrosis and periapical lesion (apical periodontitis).

- Promote cleaning, shaping and disinfection (when necessary) and the most hermetic three-dimensional filling, particularly of the **apical five millimeters** of the root canal.
- Combat the microorganisms that cause apical bacterial biofilm.
- Use bactericidal, but biocompatible irrigation solutions, in cases of teeth with pulp necrosis and periapical lesion.
- Use temporary dressing that is a topical medication between sessions, when indicated.
- Attempt to limit canal filling to the dentinal root canal (C-D-C Limit).
- Use biologically compatible root canal filling materials.

BIOLOGICAL PRINCIPLES ASSOCIATED WITH THE NEW ENDODONTIC TECHNOLOGY

"Bio-Technological School"
Objectives

- Silent trans- and post-operative stages (painless).
- Greater comfort for the patient.
- Less professional stress.
- Biological sealing of the apical foramen by mineralized tissue and/or fibrous tissue repair.
- Higher percentage of clinical, radiographic and histological post-treatment success.
- Transform the conventional perception that root canal treatment is synonymous with pain, by replacing it with a concept of being painless.
- Raise the prestige of the professional.
- Raise the prestige of the specialty itself.

Currently, in view of the fact that there are two schools of thought that teach Endodontics, the teachers of each school assume a responsibility of fundamental importance, as an educator's major mission is to be an opinion leader and to teach disciples. This is being done by means of lectures, courses and conferences, during which theoretical, philosophical and technical principles and/or their clinical experience with respect to root canal treatment are transmitted to young students, recently graduated students, clinicians, and particularly endodontists.

In this sharing of knowledge, the educator's own professional education is very important. If his/her education is based solely on his/her long clinical/professional experience and/or acquisition through personal opinions, the teacher will be educating new professionals with his/her own profile, that is, of a **technologist**. In order for his/her conduct to be considered a science, the educator should, in addition to the technical principles acquired through his/her (extremely valid) professional experience, apply the biological principles that govern the treatment, thus transmitting a **bio-technologist** profile.

In the latter case, as in any branch of science in which health is involved, root canal treatment should be instituted only after a diagnosis has been made, since endodontic treatment is directly related to the pathological alterations of the pulp and periapical area.

To make a diagnosis, the practitioner must understand the signs and symptoms of the pathological changes of the pulp and periapex at the time of the start of the endodontic therapy.

Thus, as in all medical specialties, when a patient's health is involved, a diagnosis must be based on the knowledge of Semiology, Histology, Pathology, Microbiology, among other basic disciplines. In conjunction with clinical experience, a diagnosis will establish the fundamental basis for the therapy, enabling a more precise prognosis, and consequently a higher percentage of clinical, radiographic and histological success (Fig.1.5).

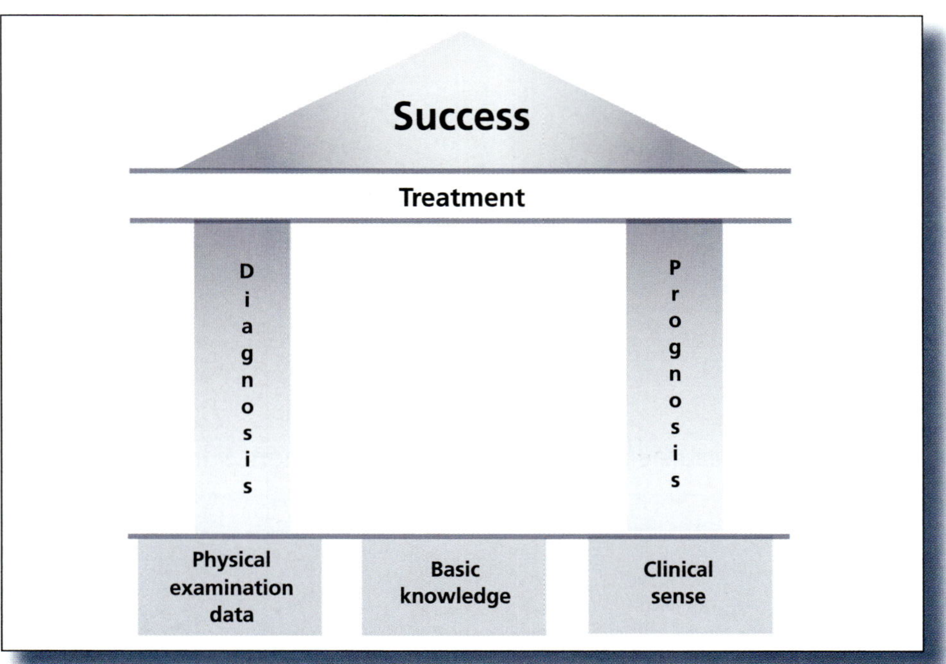

FIG. 1.5

According to the text.

Thus, based on the symptoms of the pulp (that has been removed), which represent its physiopathological and bacteriological state, with in addition macroscopic signs after its exposure, and a periapical radiograph, the practitioner can perform different types of root canal treatment, which **according to our terminology**[70], can didactically be denominated as:

VITAL PULPECTOMY (BIOPULPECTOMY) – Root canal treatment of teeth with pulp vitality, indicated in cases diagnosed as:

- Irreversible acute pulpitis.
- Chronic pulpitis.
- Internal resorptions.
- Root canal treatment of normal teeth for prosthetic and/or surgical purposes (Figs. 1.6A-D).

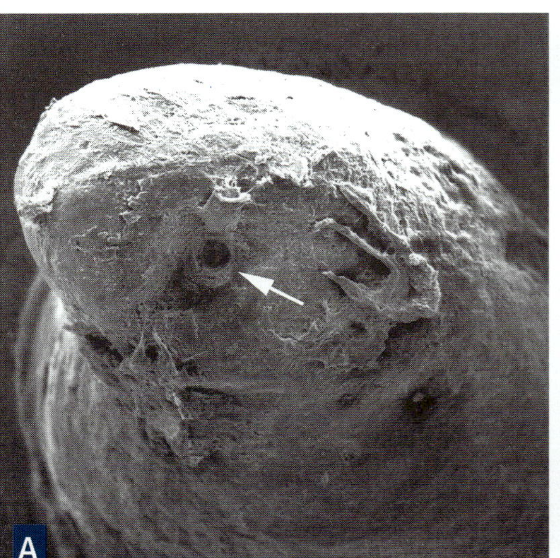

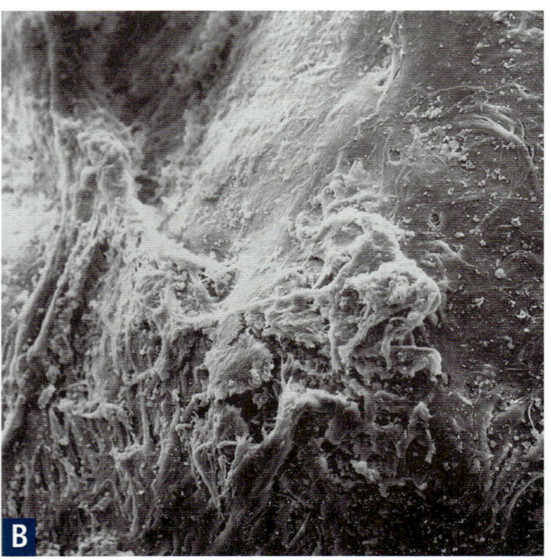

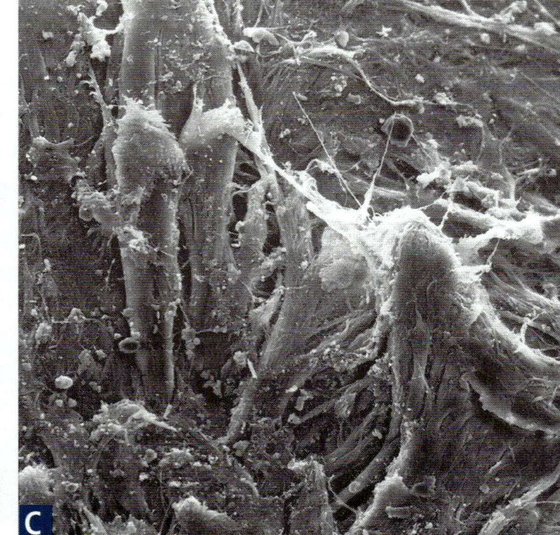

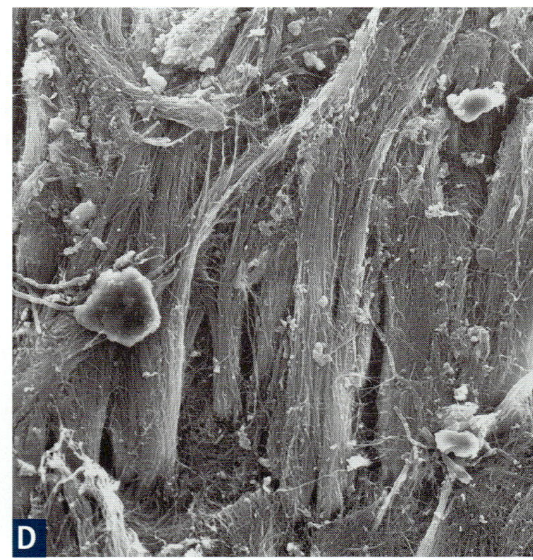

FIGS. 1.6A-D[75]

Scanning electron micrograph of the root apex of a human tooth with a vital pulp.
A – The normal morphological structure of the apex. Note the main foramen opening short of the root apex (arrow). (Original magnification 30X)
B – Higher magnification of the root apex. The cementum is covered with collagen fibers, with live tissue at the foramen level. (Original magnification 100X)
C – Higher magnification of the previous figure, showing evidence of cells and collagen fibers that are present as interlaced strands. (Original magnification 200X).
D – Higher magnification of C, showing evidence of interlaced collagen fibers, without areas of cement exposure and without microorganisms. (Original magnification 1000X)

NECROPULPECTOMY I – Root canal treatment of teeth without pulp vitality and without **RADIOGRAPHICALLY PERIAPICAL LESION**. Considered a recent infectious process, or at a stage of equilibrium (**primary infection**). This periapical reaction is still intraosseous (alveolar bone) and has not had sufficient time to affect the cortical bone, whether buccal and/or lingual. The predominant microbiota in these cases consist of Gram-Positive Aerobes. Therefore, the treatment called by us as NECROPULPECTOMY I is indicated in cases diagnosed as:

- Pulp necroses.
- Pulp gangrene.
- Acute apical periodontitis of bacterial origin.
- Acute dento-alveolar abscesses (Figs.1.7A-D).

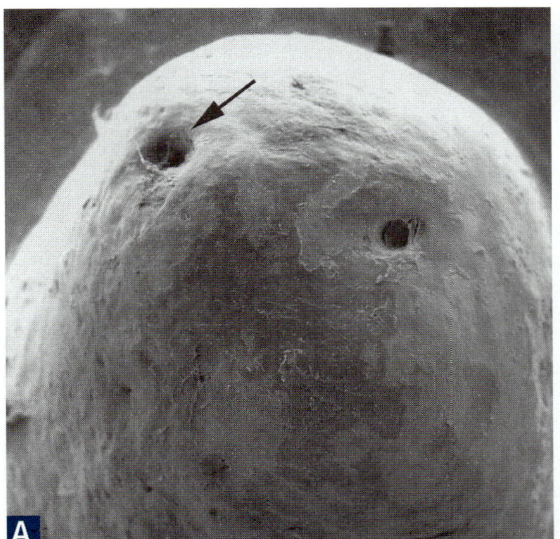
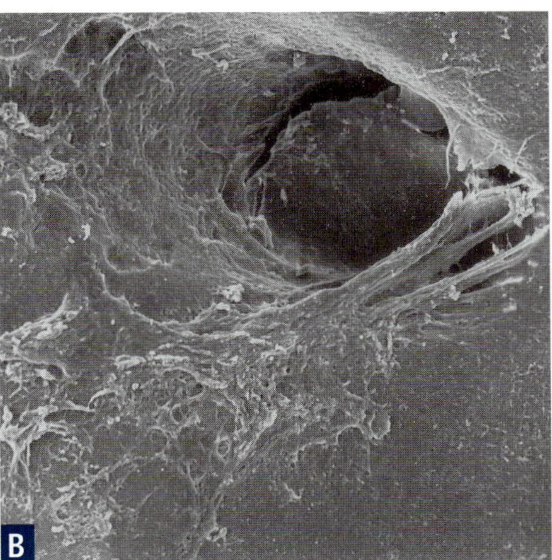
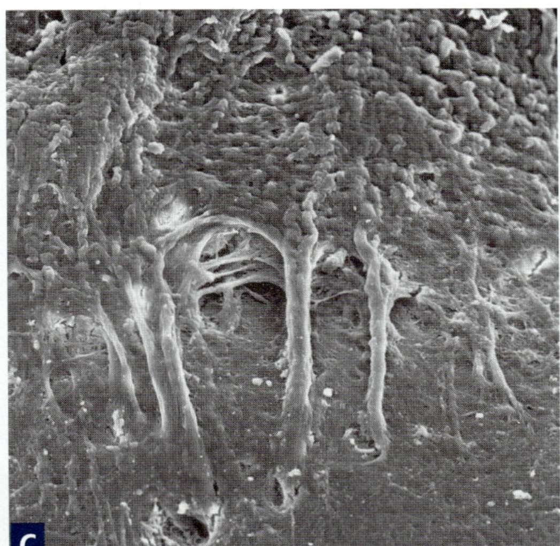
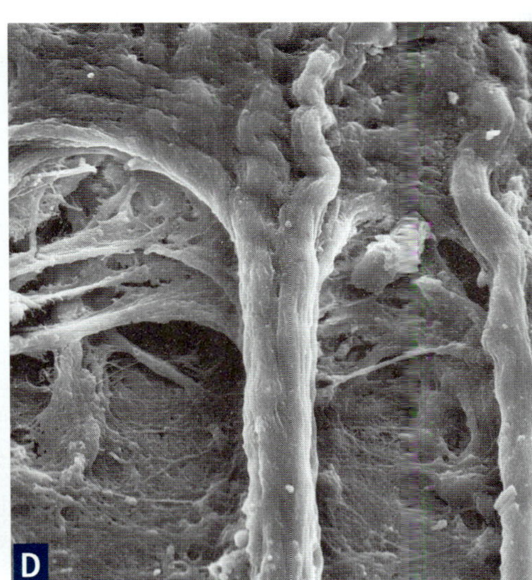

FIGS. 1.7A-D[75]

Scanning electron micrograph of the root apex of a human tooth with pulp necrosis (gangrene) without radiographically visible periapical lesion.
A – Normal structure of the apex. Note the main foramen (arrow) and adjacent foramina. (Original magnification 30X).
B – Main foramen with collagen fibers along its opening. (Original magnification 100X)
C and D – Higher magnifications of the apical structure showing evidence of cementum covered with collagen fibers and connective tissue at the level of the main foramen. There is an absence of microorganisms. C – Original magnification 200X. D – Original magnification 1000X.

NECROPULPECTOMY II – Root canal treatment of teeth with necrosis (gangrene) and with evident, **chronic radiographically visible periapical lesion (apical periodontitis).** These cases are considered infectious processes of long duration (2, 3 or more years) (**primary infection**), in which the periapical reaction affects the cortical bone, whether buccal or lingual, showing radiographic evidence of the lesion. The predominant microbiota in these cases consists of Gram-negative anaerobes[5,138,147]. Therefore, the treatment, designated by us as NECROPULPECTOMY II is indicated in cases that are clinically and radiographically diagnosed as apical periodontitis:

- Chronic dento-alveolar abscesses.
- Apical granulomas.
- Radiographic images suggestive of apical cysts.
- Phoenix abscess (*flare-up*) (Figs. 1.8A-D and Figs. 1.9A-I).

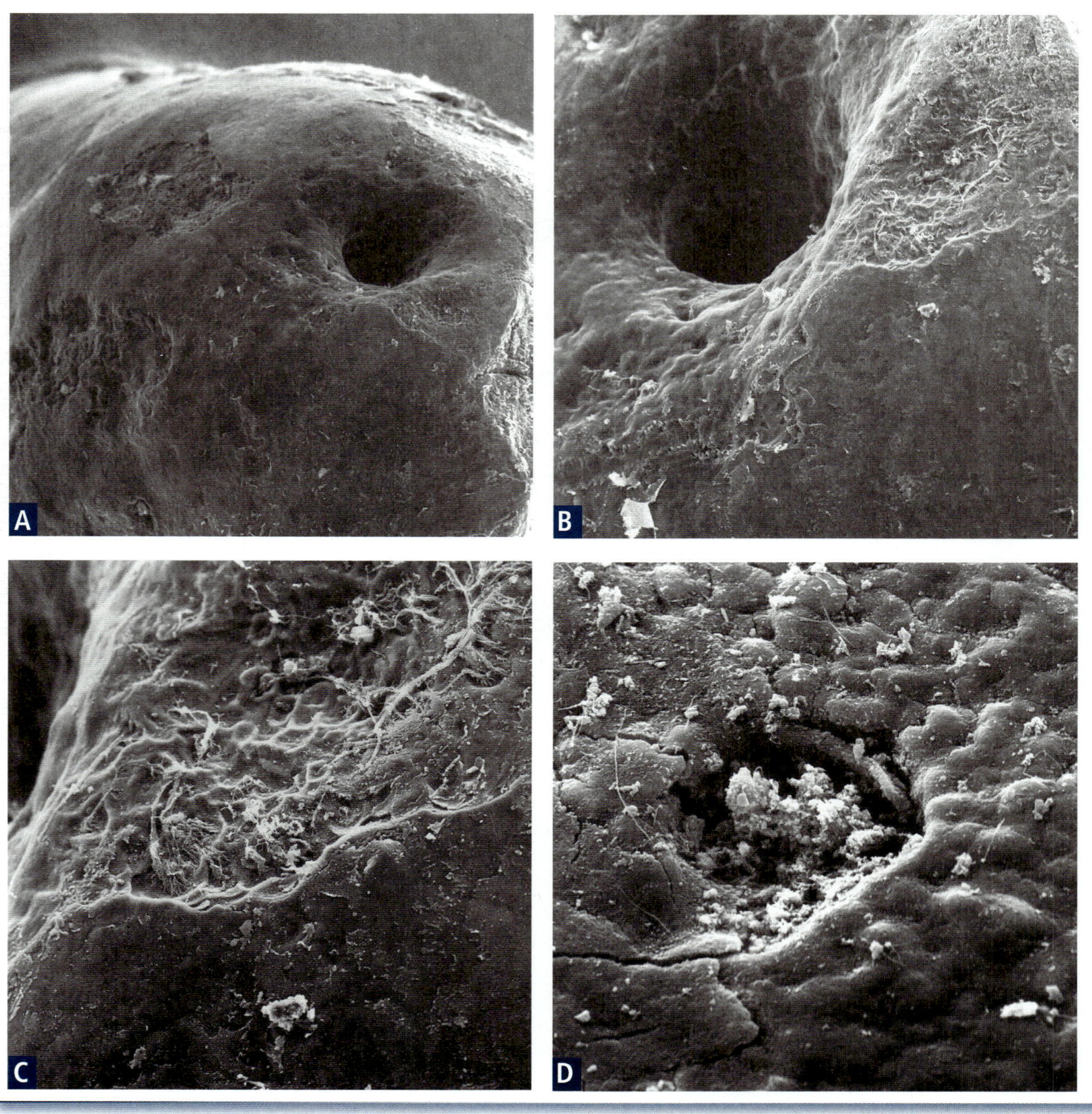

FIGS. 1.8A-D[75]

Scanning electron micrograph of the root apex of a human tooth with pulp necrosis (gangrene) with radiographically visible periapical lesion (apical periodontitis).
A – Morphological alterations in the apical cement, close to the main foramen, with areas of cement resorption and intact areas. (Original magnification 80X)
B – Higher magnification of Fig. 1.8A, showing evidence of cement resorption (Original magnification 200X)
C – Higher magnification of the cement resorption observed in B, showing microorganisms and apical bacterial biofilm. (Original magnification 500X)
D – Microorganisms in the cement resorption area and presence of biofilm. (Original magnification 2000X)

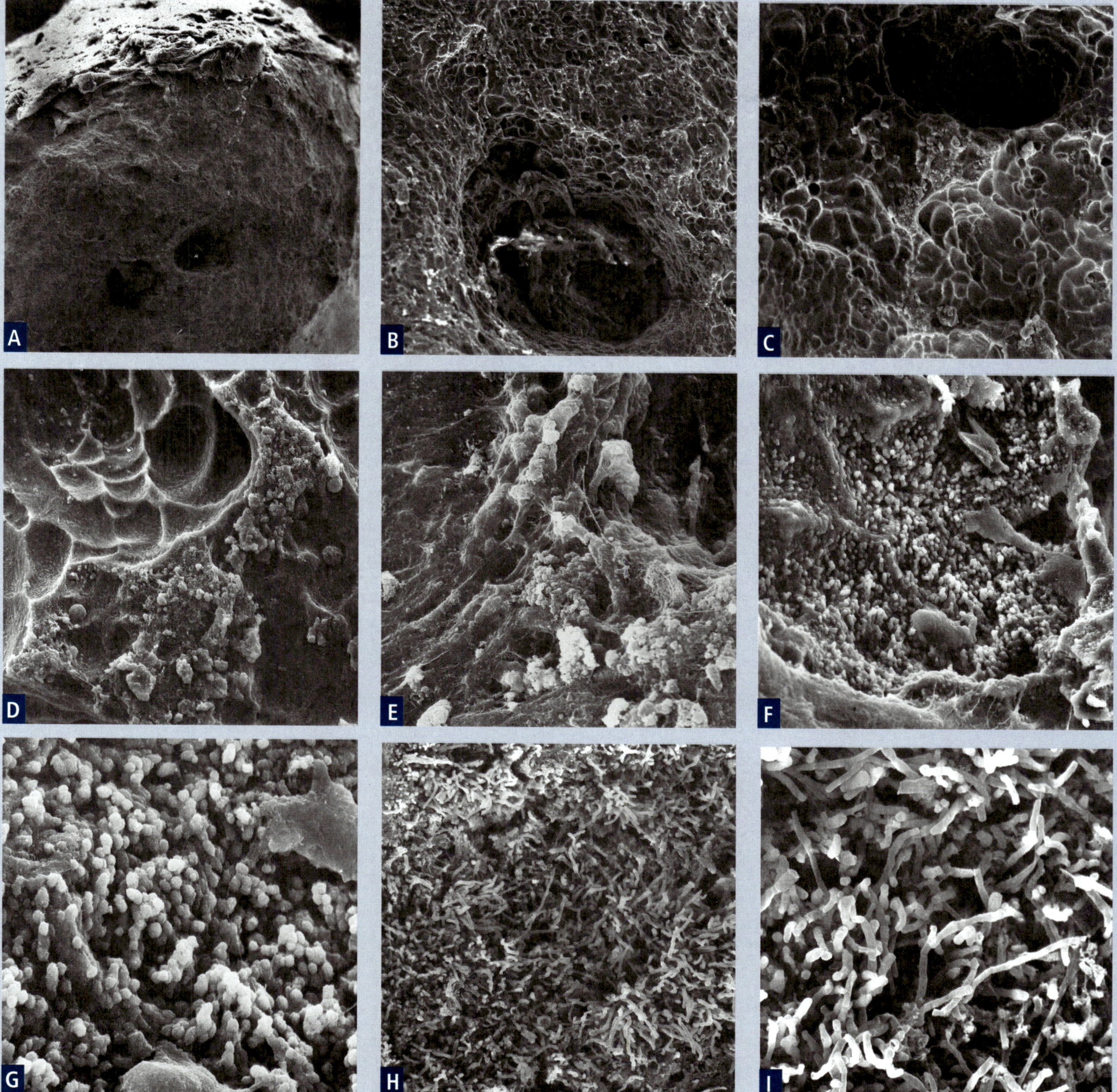

FIGS. 1.9A-I[80]

Scanning electron micrograph of the root apex of a human tooth with pulp necrosis (gangrene) and evident periapical lesion, radiographically visible (apical periodontitis).

A – Considerable morphological alterations in the apical root cement, close to the main foramen. (Original magnification 50X)

B – Higher magnification of the previous figure, showing evidence of areas of resorption of different severity and depths. (Original magnification 200X)

C – Higher magnification of Fig. 1.9B showing evidence of extensive cement resorption. (Original magnification 300X)

D – Extensive areas of cement resorption with microorganisms and apical bacterial biofilm. (Original magnification 1000X)

E – Higher magnification of the Fig. 1.9D, highlighting the presence of apical bacterial biofilm. 200X,

F – Presence of different bacterial morphotypes in apical cement resorption. Presence of cocci. (Original magnification 1150X)-

G – Higher magnification of Fig 1.9F. Note the presence of cocci. (Original magnification 3000X)

H – Presence of bacillus and filamentous bacteria. (Original magnification 1150X)

I – Higher magnification of previous figure. Filamentous form bacteria. (Original magnification 3000X)

RE-TREATMENT – Root canal treatments performed more than 2 years ago and frequently have chronic periapical lesions (**Secondary Infection**).

According to the literature [74,83,131], VITAL PULPECTOMIES and NECROPULPECTOMIES I, with respect to both technical and conceptual aspects, have been founded on solid concepts that have repeatedly proven to be sound, even in randomized clinical studies[44]. They can be biologically performed in a single session, depending on the practitioner's technical skills.

The literature reveals a high percentage of success in these cases, >90% on average, observed through clinical and radiographic evaluations over a period of 20 years (Chart 1.5).

However, with respect to NECROPULPECTOMIES II and RE-TREATMENTS, there are still many unanswered questions and the best clinical treatment for these cases has not been firmly established. As shown by surveys evaluating clinical/radiographic success/failure, these cases have a very low percentage of success whether treated by general clinicians (Chart 1.7) or specialists (Charts 1.5, 1.6 and 1.10). How do dental students do under these circumstances? Evaluations of clinical/radiographic success/failure of root canal treatments performed by students under the supervision of dental school faculty have shown promising results (Chart 1.8).

Recently, Molander et al.[91], in a randomized clinical/radiographic trial evaluated endodontic treatment performed by 4 specialists, either in a single session or in two sessions and obtained 65% and 75% success for NECROPULPECTOMIES II (apical periodontitis) and RE-TREATMENTS, subsequently. It is surprising that these authors considered these low percentages of success as satisfactory.

CHART 1.5 – Evaluation of clinical/radiographic post-treatment success of root canals performed by specialists (last 20 years) – Longitudinal/Prospective Studies.

YEAR	AUTHORS	PERCENTAGES OF SUCCESS	FOLLOW-UP TIME
1987	Byström *et al.*[16]	85%	2 – 5 years
1987	Matsumoto *et al.*[89]	88%	–
1987	Ørstavik *et al.*[100]	95%	1 – 4 years
1988	Akerblom & Hasselgreen[2]	89% (necropulpectomy) 97.9% (vital pulpectomy)	2 – 12 years
1988	Shah[120]	84%	0.5 – 2 years
1990	Sjögren *et al.*[130]	96% (vital pulpectomy) 86% (necropulpectomy)	–
1993	Smith *et al.*[131]	88% (vital pulpectomy) 82% (necropulpectomy)	5 years
1993	Yoshimura *et al.*[149]	83% (vital pulpectomy) 76% (necropulpectomy)	6 months – 1 year
1995	Friedman *et al.*[42]	90.2% (vital pulpectomy) 73% (necropulpectomy)	0.5 – 1.5 years
1996	Ørstavik[99]	94%	–
1999	Trope *et al.*[145]	74% (calcium hydroxide) 64% (single session)	1 year
2002	Peters & Wesselink[107]	81% (two sessions) 71% (single session)	4-5 years
2003	Rodrigues Araújo Filho[115]	89.8% (single session)	–
2004	Field *et al.*[40]	endodontist I – 82.7% endodontist II – 81.8% endodontist III – 90.6% endodontist IV – 95.2% (single session)	6 months – 4 years
2004	Kojima *et al.*[66]	82.8% (vital pulpectomy) 78.9% (necropulpectomy)	–
2004	Imura *et al.*[56]	93.7% (vital pulpectomy) 88.4% (necropulpectomy) (single session)	18 months
2004	Bussey[15]	82% (single session) 80% (two sessions)	8.1 months
2004	Shipp *et al.*[122]	91.5% (diabetics) 85.5% (non diabetics)	–
2006	Debelian[25]	98.5% (vital pulpectomy) (single session) 94.3% (necropulpectomy) (two sessions) $Ca(OH)_2$ (calcium hydroxide)	6 – 18 months
2006	Gesi *et al.*[44]	93% (vital pulpectomy)	3 years
2007	Conner *et al.*[23]	90% (vital pulpectomy) 73% (necropulpectomy)	1 year
2007	Imura *et al.*[57]	91% (GENERAL) 94.9% (vital pulpectomy) 91.9% (necropulpectomy I) 85.4% (necropulpectomy II)	18 – 24 years
2007	Molander *et al.*[91]	necropulpectomy II 65% (single session) 75% (two sessions)	2 years
	OVERALL MEAN SUCCESS	**83.75%**	

CHART 1.6 – Evaluation of clinical/radiographic post-treatment success of root canals of teeth with previous chronic periapical lesion (NECROPULPECTOMY II – apical periodontitis) performed by specialists – Longitudinal/Prospective Studies.

YEAR	AUTHORS	PERCENTAGES OF SUCCESS	FOLLOW-UP TIME
1987	Byström *et al.*[16]	85%	2 – 5 years
1987	Matsumoto *et al.*[89]	67%	–
1988	Eriksen *et al.*[37]	82%	3 years
1988	Molven & Halse[92]	65%	10 – 17 years
1988	Akerblom & Hasselgren[2]	63%	–
1988	Shah[120]	84%	2 years
1990	Sjögren *et al.*[130]	86%	8 – 10 years
1991	Murphy *et al.*[93]	70%	12 months
1993	Smith *et al.*[131]	81%	5 years
1995	Friedman *et al.*[42]	69%	6 – 18 years
1996	Caliskan & Sen[17]	80%	2 – 5 years
1996	Ørstavik[99]	75%	4 years
1997	Sjögren *et al.*[129]	68%	–
2004	Kojima *et al.*[66]	78,9%	13 years
2004	Ørstavik *et al.*[101]	79%	6 months – 4 years
2006	Marquis *et al.*[88]	80%	4 – 6 years
2007	Imura *et al.*[57]	85.4%	18 – 24 years
2007	Conner *et al.*[23]	50%	1 year
2007	Molander *et al.*[91]	70%	2 years
	OVERALL MEAN SUCCESS	**74.63%**	

CHART 1.7 – Evaluation of clinical/radiographic post-treatment success of root canals performed by general clinicians in patients in different countries, cities and/or communities – Population Studies.

YEAR	AUTHORS	CITY/ COUNTRY		PERCENTAGE OF SUCCESS	FILLING QUALITY% (POOR)	PERIAPICAL LESION (%) (%)	FOLLOW-UP TIME
1983	Laurell *et al.*[67]	Switzerland		75%	–	–	–
1983/93	Cantarini *et al.*[18]	Argentina		–	69.7%	–	10 years
1986	Hugoson *et al.*[53]	Jömköping/Sweden		70%	–	–	–
1986	Allard & Palmqvist[3]	Sweden (rural area)		73%	–	27%	–
1986	Petersson *et al.*[110]	Sweden (hospital attendance)		74%	–	31%	–
1987	Bergström *et al.*[10]	Sweden (general clinics)		71%	36.6%	28.8%	–
1987	Eckerbom *et al.*[31]	Sweden (general clinics)		77%	–	26%	–
1988	Eriksen *et al.*[35]	Norway (urban area)		64%	–	34%	11 years
1989	Petersson *et al.*[109]	Sweden (urban area)		–	15.9%	26.5%	–
1990	Ödesjö *et al.*[98]	Sweden (general population)		75%	70%	24.5%	–
1991	Imfeld[55]	Switzerland (elderly patients)		69%	64%	31%	–
1991	Eriksen & Bjertness[35]	Norway (elderly patients)		84%	67%	36.6%	–
1991	Hülsmann *et al.*[54]	Germany		–	–	60%	–
1992	Acetoze *et al.*[1]	Araraquara/Brazil (Araraquara School of Dentistry)		–	60.30%	42.86%	–
1993	De Cleen *et al.*[28]	Amsterdam/Holland (adults)		61%	49.4%	44.6%	–
1993	Grieve & McAndrew[47]	England		53%	–	77%	–
1993	Peterson[108]	Sweden (retrospective study)		50%	31%	–	20-60 months
1995	Buckley & Spangberg[14]	USA (university patients)		42%	58%	31.3%	–
1995	Buckley % Spangberg[14]	USA		–	–	31%	20-80 months
1995	Eriksen *et al.*[34]	Norway (urban population – 35 years)		84%	14%	38.1%	9 years
1995	Soikkonen[132]	Helsinki/Finland (patients between 45 and 86 years of age)		–	75%	18%	–
1995	Ray & Trope[113]	USA		61%	82%	39%	–
1997	Saunders *et al.*[119]	Scotland (subpopulation)		55.3%	46%	58.1%	2 years
1997	Weiger *et al.*[148]	Stuttgart/Germany (urban population)		41.4%	49%	61%	–
1998	Marques *et al.*[87]	Porto/Portugal (urban population between 30-39 years)		78%	54%	21.7%	8 years
1999	Sidaravicius *et al.*[125]	Vilnius/Lithuania (urban population between 35-44 years)		65%	61%	39.4%	–
2000	De Moor *et al.*[29]	Belgium (patients from the Ghent Univ. Hospital)		40.7%	40.7%	40.4%	3 years
2000	Kirkevang *et al.*[65]	Denmark (urban population)		–	32.4%	67.6%	–
2001	Kirkevang *et al.*[64]	Denmark (urban population)		–	–	52.2%	–
2002	Boucher *et al.*[13]	France (subpopulation)		–	49.3%	26.7%	–
2002	Lupi-Pegurier *et al.*[85]	Nice/France		–	68.8%	31.5%	–
2003	Chueh *et al.*[21]	Taiwan/Taipei (urban population)		34.8%	62%	–	–
2003	Dugas *et al.*[30]	Canada	population-Toronto population-Saskatoon	60.1% 58.0%	44.0% 51.0%	–	–
2004	Kojima *et al.*[66]	(Meta analysis) – Japanese patients		82.8% (bio) 78.9% (necro)	–	–	13 years
2004	Jiménez-Pinzón *et al.*[58]	Seville/Span		–	–	64.5%	–
	OVERALL MEAN SUCCESS			**65%**	**52.96%**	**39.57%**	

CHART 1.8 – Evaluation of clinical/radiographic post-treatment success of root canals performed by graduate and post-graduation students (last 20 years). (Cross–sectional studies in a convenience sample).

YEAR	AUTHORS	PERCENTAGES OF SUCCESS	FOLLOW-UP TIME
1983	Swartz *et al.*[140]	87.79%	20 years
1985	Besse *et al.*[11]	73.23%	1 year
1988	Molven & Halse[92]	93% (vital pulpectomy) 85% (necropulpectomy)	10 – 17 years
1990	Sjögren *et al.*[130]	91%	8 – 10 years
1991	Berger[9]	88.8% (single session) 91.6% (two sessions)	1 year
1991	Fritz & Wichmann[43]	96%	3 – 7 years
1996	Orth[102]	69%	–
1998	Kane *et al.*[59]	71.62%	–
2002	Benenati & Khajotia[7]	91.05%	–
2003	Cheung & Chan[20]	48% (prospective study*)	20 years
2003	Dammaschke *et al.*[24]	85.1%	10 years
2004	Ørstavik *et al.*[101]	94% (necropulpectomy I) 79% (necropulpectomy II)	6 months – 4 years
2006	Marquis *et al.*[88]	93% (necropulpectomy I) 80% (necropulpectomy II)	4 – 6 years
	OVERALL MEAN SUCCESS	**85.37%**	

* Because it is a prospective study, the percentage of 48% success, after 20 years of evaluation, was not included in the general mean.

CHART 1.9 – Evaluation of clinical/radiographic post-treatment success of root canals partially filled (re-treatments) in teeth with periapical lesions, performed by specialists (last 20 years) – Longitudinal/Prospective Studies.

YEAR	AUTHORS	PERCENTAGES OF SUCCESS	FOLLOW-UP TIME
1979	Bergenholtz *et al.*[8]	48%	20 years
1988	Åkerblom & Hasselgren[2]	62.5%	2 – 12 years
1988	Molven & Halse[92]	71%	10 – 17 years
1990	Sjögren *et al.*[130]	62%	–
1995	Friedman *et al.*[42]	56%	–
1998	Sundqvist *et al.*[139]	74%	–
2007	Imura *et al.*[57]	85%*	18 – 24 months
	OVERALL MEAN SUCCESS	**66%**	

* Because no reference is made in the study to the percentage of success in cases of re-treatment of root canals in teeth with previous periapical lesion, it was not included in the final mean.

CHART 1.10 – General percentages of clinical/radiographic post-treatment success of root canals of teeth with evident chronic periapical lesion (NECROPULPECTOMIES II – apical periodontitis), in cases of RE-TREATMENTS AND PERSISTENCE OF CHRONIC PERIAPICAL LESION obtained by specialists and general practitioners.

	SPECIALISTS	GENERAL CLINICIANS
NECROPULPECTOMY II	74.8%	65%
RETREATMENTS	66%	–
PERSISTENCE OF CHRONIC PERIAPICAL LESION	–	39.57%

WHAT COULD BE THE POSSIBLE REASONS FOR THE LOW PERCENTAGE OF SUCCESS IN THE ROOT CANAL TREATMENT OF TEETH WITH PULP NECROSIS WITH EVIDENT RADIOGRAPHICALLY PERIAPICAL LESION (APICAL PERIODONTITIS) CALLED BY US AS NECROPULPECTOMIES II AND CASES OF RE-TREATMENTS?

Some of the justifications on which the bio-technological school bases *Necropulpectomies II*

Leonardo et al.[71] (1994), evaluated radiographically and histo-microbiologically, post-operative apical and periapical repair in root canals of dog teeth after experimentally induced periapical lesions. They observed that, as in humans[69], the cementum of the apical third is of a cellular type, that is, it contains cementocytes and is therefore permeable. This is different from the middle and cervical thirds, which are acellular and are impermeable. The permeability of the apical cementum in the **apical five millimeters**, in cases of pulp necrosis and periapical lesion (apical periodontitis), enables bacterial invasion, which originates from the root canal and destroys the cementocytes and invades the cementoplasts. The latter have star-shaped spaces that are connected and allow the spreading of microorganisms throughout the entire apical cementum, which is already has undergone resorbtion due to the periapical inflammatory process, and now represent the so-called "**extra-radicular infection**" (Figs. 1.10A-B, 1.11A-B and 1.12A-B).

According to the above, from a biological point of view, one may infer that the **apical five millimeters** of the radicular root canal should be recognized as a **critical zone** in the treatment of teeth with pulp necrosis (gangrene) and evident radiographically chronic periapical lesion (apical periodontitis). This therefore represents one of the major endodontic challenges[128].

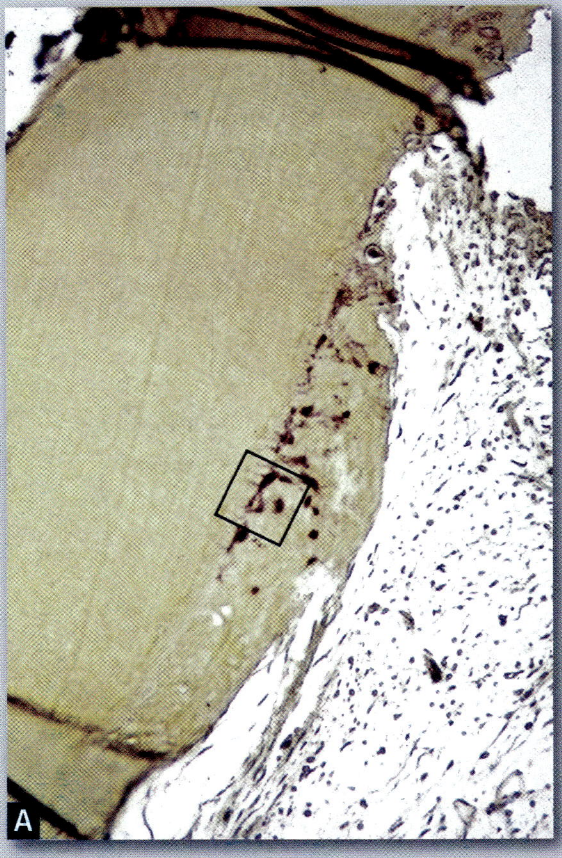

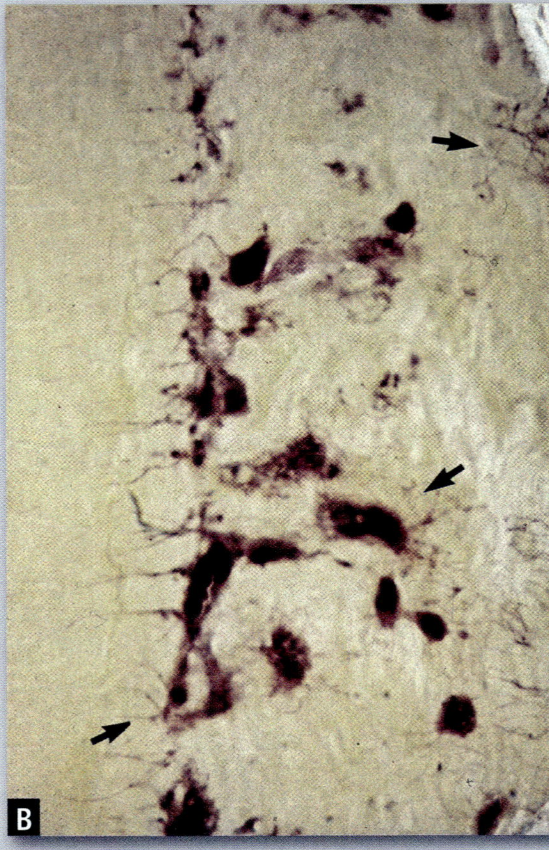

FIGS. 1-10A-B[71]

A – Histological section of the root apex of a dog tooth, with evident periapical lesion (apical periodontitis), experimentally induced. Note the presence of microorganisms in the cementoplasts of the resorbed apical cement, constituting extra-radicular infection. (Brown & Brenn stain, Original magnification 80X)

B – Higher magnification of Fig. 1.10A, showing evidence of cementoplasts replete with microorganisms (arrows). (Brown & Brenn stain, Original magnification 200X)

FIGS. 1.11A-B[71]

Histological section of the root apex of a dog tooth, with evident periapical lesion (apical periodontitis), experimentally induced.

Note in 1.11A, the presence of microorganisms throughout the resorbed cementum.

In 1.11B, higher magnification of Fig. A, showing evidence of star-shaped cementoplasts that are interconnected, determining extra-radicular infection. (Brown & Brenn, Original magnification 80X and 200X)

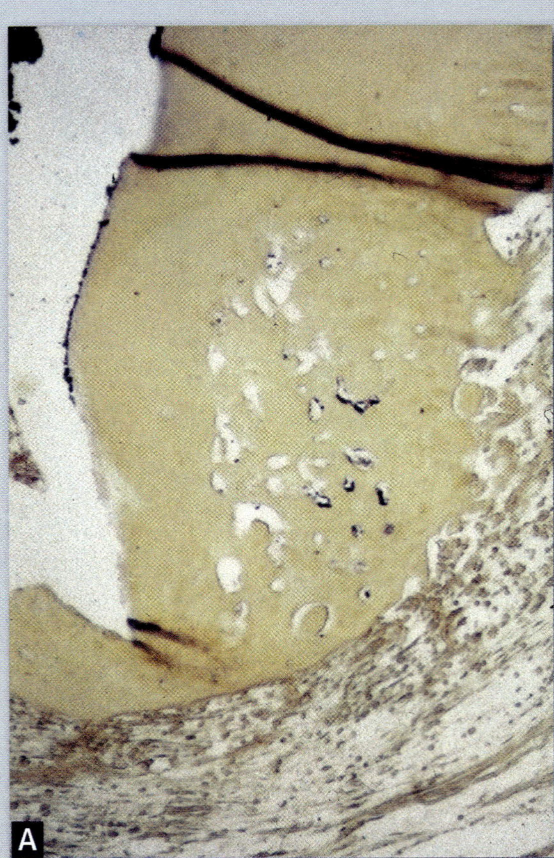

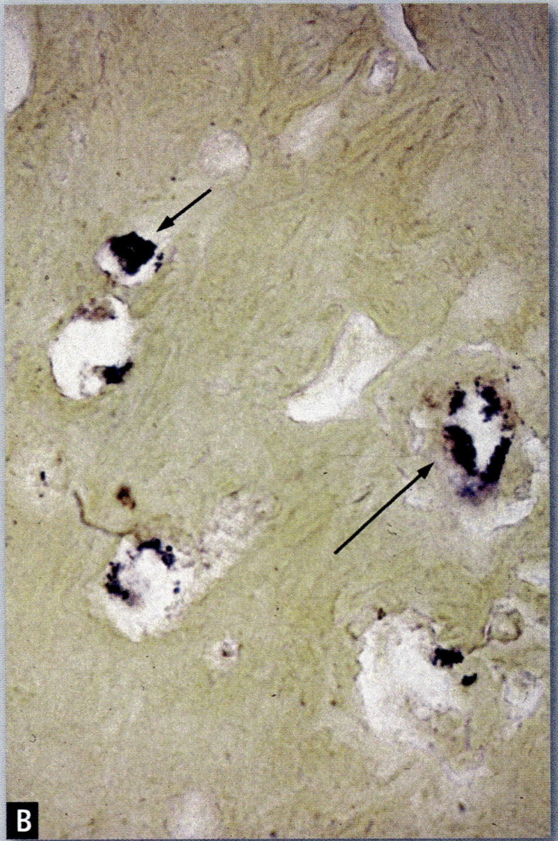

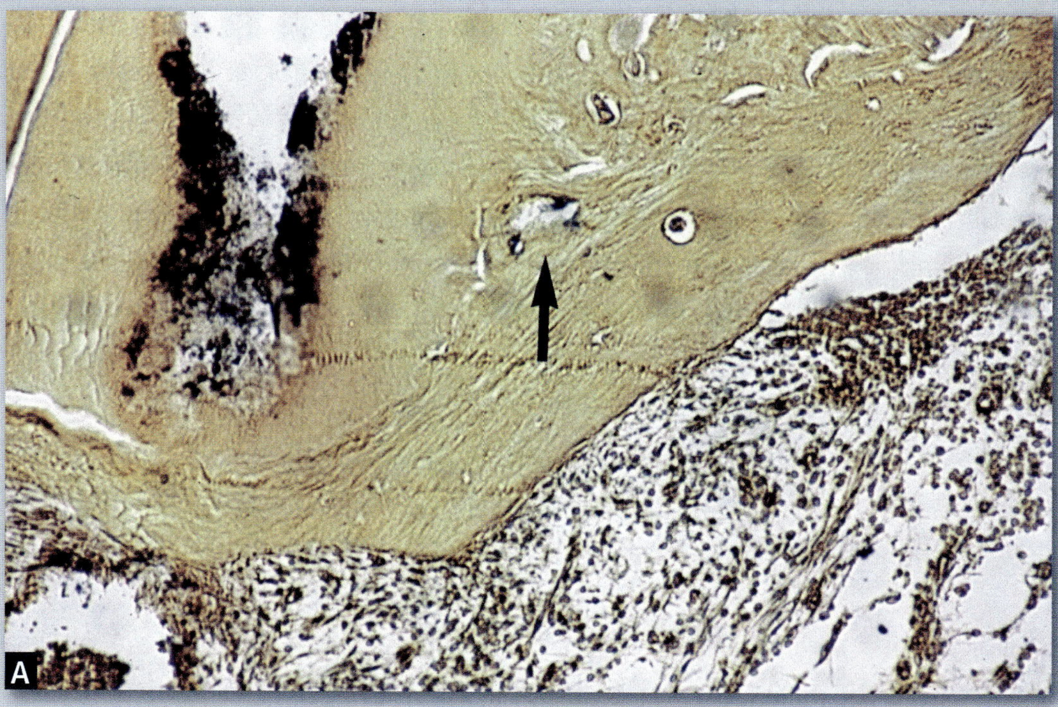

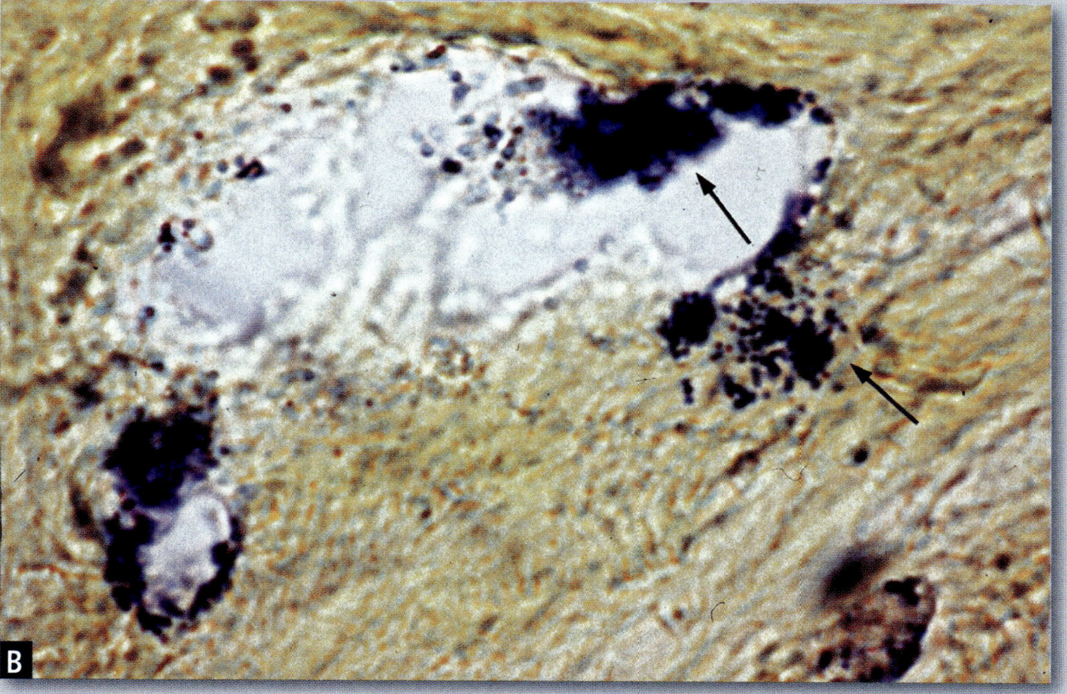

FIGS. 1.12A-B[71]

A – Histological section of the root apex of a dog tooth, with evident periapical lesion (apical periodontitis), experimentally induced. Note the presence of microorganisms in the cementoplasts (arrow) that are star-shaped, indicating extra-radicular infection. (Brown & Brenn, Original magnification 80X)

B – Higher magnification of the previous figure, showing evidence of cementoplasts containing microorganisms. (Brown & Brenn, Original magnification 200X)

Studies have shown that this infection is induced by an accumulation of inflammatory and immune cells that are located in the periapical regions of the tooth, in other words, a host defense response. These cells cause biochemical alterations such as pH, and attract immunoglobulin and cytokines, and initiate and perpetuate progressive bone and cement resorption, frequently reaching the dentin.

Therefore, from a clinical point of view, especially the **apical five millimeters** of a root canal of teeth with evident periapical lesion should be subjected to perfect cleaning and shaping, effective disinfection, and should be complemented with the most hermetic three-dimensional filling, which then can lead to an excellent post-operative prognosis.

As Simon[128] acknowledges, to accomplish these objectives is one of the greatest challenges in endodontics.

Even if the **apical five millimeters** are properly shaped and disinfected, in the absence of an adequate root filling, radiographic repair may occur, but nevertheless an invagination of granulomatous tissue, rich in blood vessels, chronic inflammatory cells, phagocytes (macrophages) and constituents of the adaptive immune response, will occur (Figs. 1.4A-C).

At present, special attention is being paid to the cellular mechanisms and molecules involved in the body's response so that repair of the periapical lesion (endodontic success) occurs. Cytokines, Interleukin-1β (IL-1β), Interleukin-1α (IL-1α), the Tumor Necrosis Factor-1α (IL-1α) and the Lymphotoxins (TNF-β), are considered the main factors involved in periapical bone resorption by acting on the activation of osteoclastogenesis (Stashenko et al.[135], 1987; Stashenko et al.[137], 1992; Tronstad[144], 1992; Stashenko et al.[136], 1994). In humans, IL-1β is possibly the most important and most powerful mediator (Lim et al.[82], 1994; Shimauchi et al.[121], 1998). The production and activity of IL-1 is potentially modulated by a cascade of pro- and anti-inflammatory cytokines, produced by lymphocytes of the T-helper type 1 (Th 1) and T-helper type 2 (Th 2), types respectively (Rossi[116], 2008).

The most recent progress in molecular biology techniques has enabled the study of immunopathogeny diseases, such as periapical lesions, at a molecular level (Rossi[116], 2008). **The lack of therapeutic consensus in the endodontic literature, and particularly among endodontists, with regard to root canal treatment in teeth with necrosis (pulp gangrene) and with evident periapical lesions (apical periodontitis), is possibly the result of a lack of profound knowledge of their immunopathogeny (Rossi[116], 2008).**

On the other hand, the **old concept** that a perfect filling of the root canal will entomb the microorganisms of the root canal system because of the impermeability of the cement, is currently considered correct, but only for the cervical and middle thirds, in regions in which the cement is acellular, meaning impermeable. For the **apical five millimeters**, however, this concept is not valid, because of the permeability of the cement, which is cellular in this region.

Various investigations, in dog teeth with induced chronic periapical reaction[72], or in humans[95] in cases of pulp necrosis (gangrene) with radiographic suggestion of periapical lesion[68], have proven that biomechanical preparation alone does not conquer these microorganisms, even when the most bactericidal irrigation solutions are used as a complement in root canal instrumentation. These microorganisms are inaccessible to this important endodontic operative step: biomechanical preparation[51,72,141].

Therefore, in NECROPULPECTOMIES II (apical periodontitis), the use of a topical medication between sessions as a temporary dressing, generally a calcium hydroxide-based material, would be justified. This product, through its ionic dissociation, mainly hydroxyl ions, will reach the **extra-radicular infection**, making the environment alkaline (pH=9 to 12), which unsuitable for bacterial development and proliferation.

On the other hand, studies have also shown that microorganisms located in the apical resorbed cementum protect themselves against the action of organic defense mechanisms and systemic antibiotic medication, when initiated. This auto-protection takes place through a veritable mechanical barrier, the extracellular (Polysaccharide) protein (PEC), which characterizes the so-called **apical bacterial biofilm**. The microorganisms present in biofilm are protected from other competitive bacterial species, from the host immunological system, and from systemic antibiotics. This pathological entity is observed in 100% of the cases of teeth with evident chronic periapical lesion (apical periodontitis), whether permanent[75] or primary teeth[114] (Figs. 1.13A-B). The etiology of biofilm itself proves its existence in 100% of the cases with evident radiographically periapical lesion; that is: presence of moisture, microorganisms and resorbed mineralized tissue.

In summary, we can confirm that today the **apical five millimeters** are considered the **critical zone of Biological Endodontics**, particularly in cases of root canal treatment of teeth with pulp necrosis and evident chronic periapical lesion (apical periodontitis), because of the following situations:

- Permeability of the apical cement (**apical five millimeters**), promoting the bacterial invasion originating from the lumen of the root canal, reaching the cementoplasts and determining **extra-radicular infection**.
- Resorption of the apical cementum, creating veritable craters and exposing the dentinal tubules in which the microorganisms proliferate and protect themselves.
- Apical bacterial biofilm, formed by microorganisms that live in a veritable community, and protect themselves by means of ECP (Extracellular Polysaccharide), from the action of organic defenses and systemic antibiotic medication, when initiated.
- Apical foramen, replete with necrotic debris, microorganisms, and toxins that need to be removed by the action of the **Foraminal Apical Instrument** (FAI)*, before the initiation of biomechanical preparation.

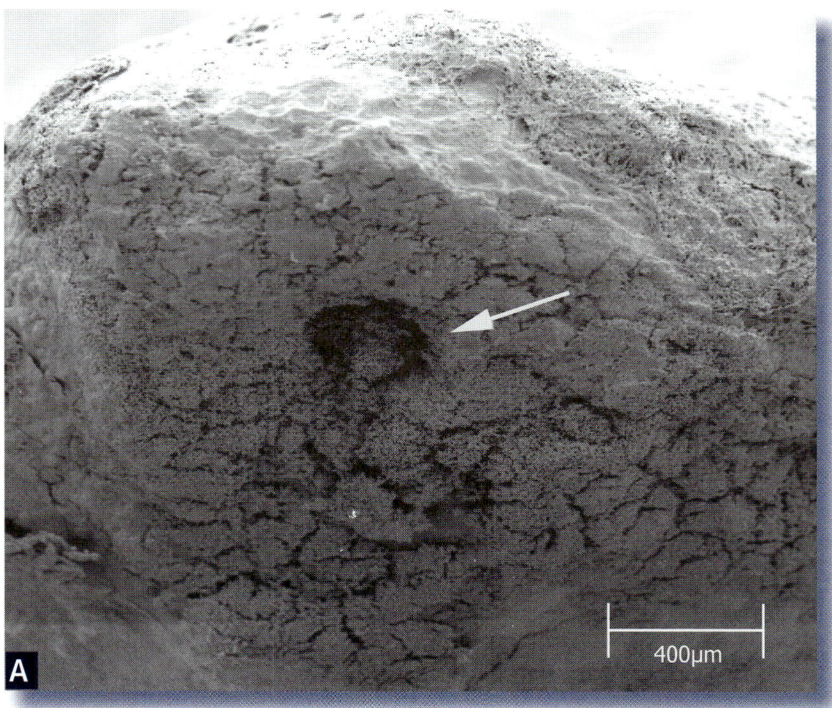

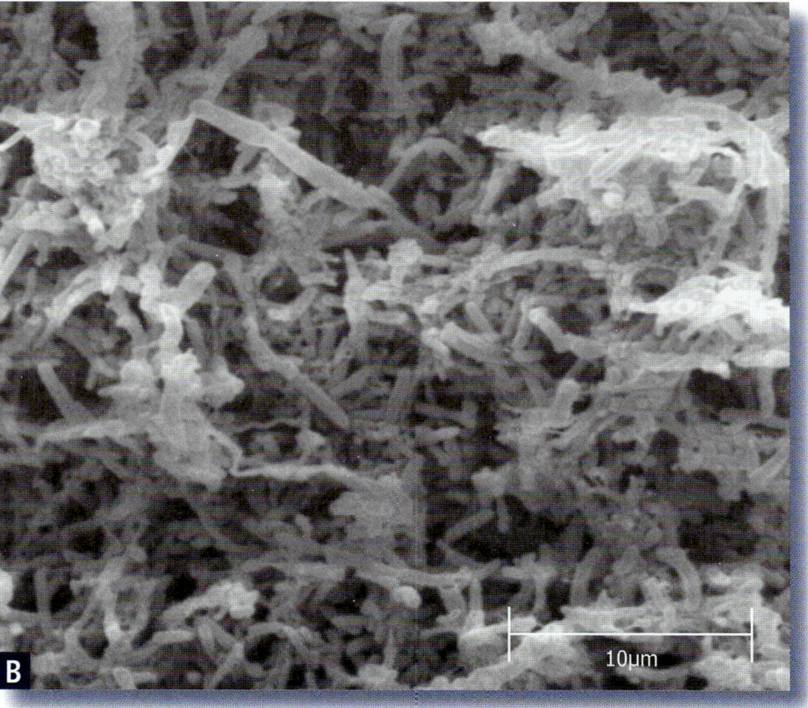

FIGS. 1.13A-B[114]

A – Scanning electron micrograph of the root apex of a human primary tooth, showing evidence of large morphological alterations in the cementum close to the apical foramen (arrow). (Original magnification 50X)

B – Higher magnification of the previous figure, showing evidence of the presence of bacterial biofilm and microorganisms. (Original magnification 1000X)

* FAI. The largest file that fits the anatomic diameter of the apical foramen, at the determined tooth length.

- The **apical five millimeters** present an area that because of the difficulty of access is not conducive for perfect cleaning and shaping, effective disinfection and a three-dimensional hermetical filling is considered the **critical area** of the bio-technologist concept. For these reasons the objectives of endodontic treatment are frequently not achieved.
- PERIAPICAL REACTION – the tissues here are rich in blood vessels and inflammatory and immune cells (defense) that determine biochemical changes, which will perpetuate the inflammation and bone and cement resorption in a progressive and permanent manner, as long as the cause is not removed.

CALCIUM HYDROXIDE

The use of calcium hydroxide, as a topical medication between sessions (temporary dressing), has been shown to be highly effective in apical and periapical histological post-treatment repair of root canals; that is in treatment of teeth with evident chronic periapical lesion (apical periodontitis)[51,72,141]. The microorganisms located in the ramifications, dentinal tubules, isthmus, apical cementum craters (cementum resorptions) and in the apical biofilm, which escaped the action of biomechanical preparation, are attacked by the hydroxyl ions, generated by ionic dissociation of the calcium hydroxide. The action mechanism of calcium hydroxide on microorganisms located inside the apical bacterial biofilm has not entirely been proven yet. As biofilms facilitate the absorption of nutrients, the action mechanism has been attributed to the hydroxyl ions from ionic dissociation, penetrating into the biofilm nutrition canaliculi, attacking the microorganisms in it, and making the environment alkaline, thus combating the cause; that is, its etiologic factor.

The predominant microbiota in cases of pulp necrosis and periapical lesion (apical periodontitis) is represented by Gram-negative anaerobes. **Endotoxins (bacterial LPS)** are components of the cell walls of these bacteria, which are released during bacterial reproduction and/or proliferation, or also through aggression resulting from mechanical agents or medication.

At present **biological endodontics** scientifically comprises and accepts the importance of **bacterial LPS (endotoxins)** in cases of pulp necrosis and periapical lesion (apical periodontitis), either because of their etiology, the persistence of periapical reactions, or as the main cause of intensifying chronic periapical acuteness, the so called Phoenix abscesses ("*Flare-ups*") caused by the treatment itself and/or spontaneously[78].

Endotoxins are substances that have been proven to[96]:

- Be powerful cytotoxic agents.
- Act as antigens (immunologic reaction).
- Stimulate the release of enzymes from lysosomes.
- Activate osteoclasts.
- Activate the Schwartzman reaction.
- Activate the Hageman factor (activate the pain-potentiating mediators).
- Activate the complement system via C3 (release of vasoactive products, accentuating inflammation)
- Cause degranulation of mastocytes (histamine release).
- Cause the release of collagenase from macrophages.

The only biological substance capable of detoxifying (inactivating) **endotoxins**, is calcium hydroxide[72,97,126,141], as a temporary dressing.

In Re-Treatments

With respect to **re-treatments**, it is now known that the predominant microbiota located in the un-filled part of the root canal (**secondary infection**), although mixed, is predominantly composed of aerobic bacteria, which are considered the most resistant to endodontic treatment, for example *Enterococcus faecalis* and *Pseudomonas aeruginosa*.

According to Love (2001)[84] the capacity of *Enterococcus faecalis* to cause periapical pathology as determined from cases that failed, is based on their ability to invade the dentinal tubules and remain viable in situ (Figs. 1.14A-B).

The difficulty in eliminating *Enterococcus faecalis* from root canal systems may be in part related to their ability to penetrate into the dentinal tubules, with in addition their considerable resistance to the action of anti-septic solutions and medications, more so than any other microorganism found in endodontic infections[49].

Pinheiro et al.[111], in 2003, studied root canals of teeth that required re-treatment. They verified that the bacterial strain most frequently isolated was *Enterococcus faecalis,* which was present in 52 cases with microbial growth in the canals in 94% of the cases.

Gomes et al.[45], in 2006, by means of culture and polymerase chain reaction (PCR) analysis, showed evidence by means of PCR detection that in cases of re-treatments, *Enterococcus faecalis* was responsible for 76% of the **secondary infection**.

At the University of Brescia – Italy (2006), after performing an apicoectomy in a partially filled right maxillary 2nd premolar, Luciano Giardino, showed evidence of the presence of *Enterococcus faecalis,* considered a **secondary infection,** by means of Scanning Electronic Microscopy (SEM) (Figs.1-15A-B).

In these cases, considering that *Enterococcus faecalis*, together with *Pseudomonas aeruginosa*, are considered bacteria that are most resistant to endodontic treatment[49], the use of a topical medication between sessions is justified, for instance calcium hydroxide with chlorhexidine or camphorated chlorophenol (*see* chapter 2.IX). While $CaOH_2$ alone is not very effective against these bacteria, the latters are considered highly effective bactericides[79,127].

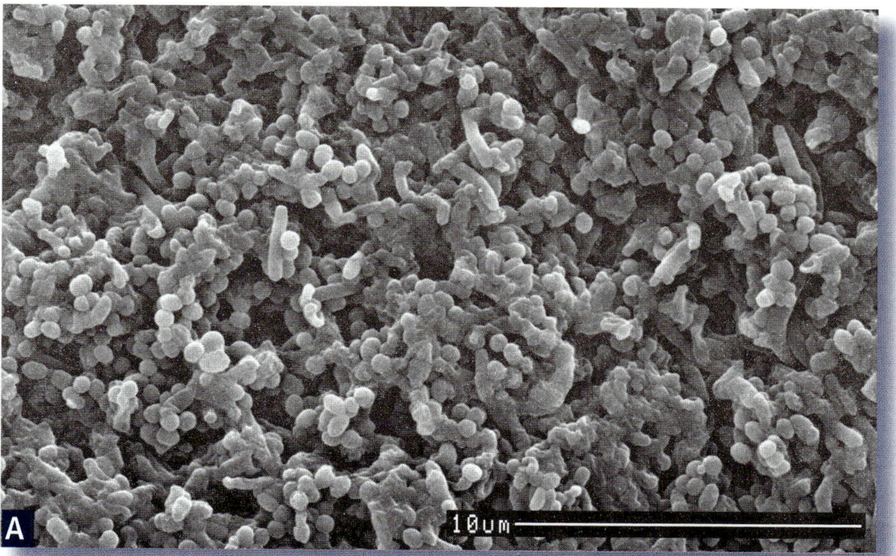

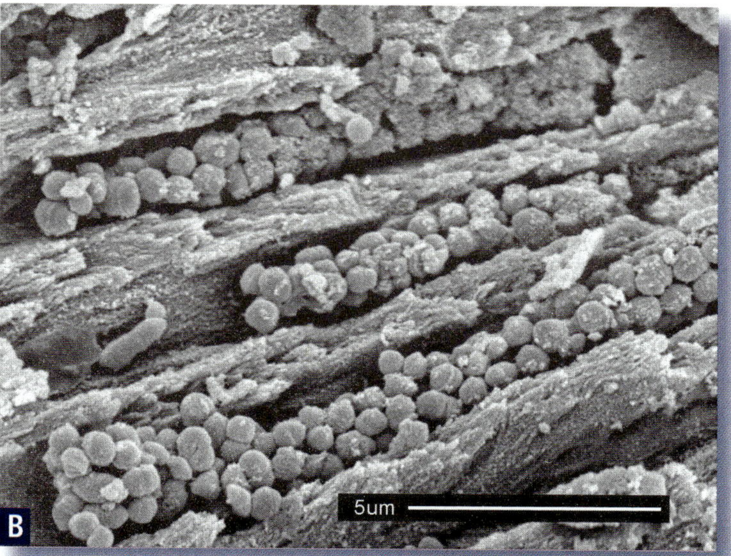

FIGS. 1.14A-B

A – Scanning electron micrograph showing evidence of artificially induced bacterial biofilm on dentin.

B – Scanning electron micrograph showing evidence of artificially induced bacterial biofilm, with *enterococcus faecalis* within the dentinal tubules.

(Courtesy of Fernanda Geraldes Pappen, Post-Graduate student in Endodontics (Doctorate) – Dentistry Faculty of Araraquara, SP, Brazil – UNESP (2008) and Prof. Markus Haapasalo, University of British Columbia, Vancouver, BC, Canada)

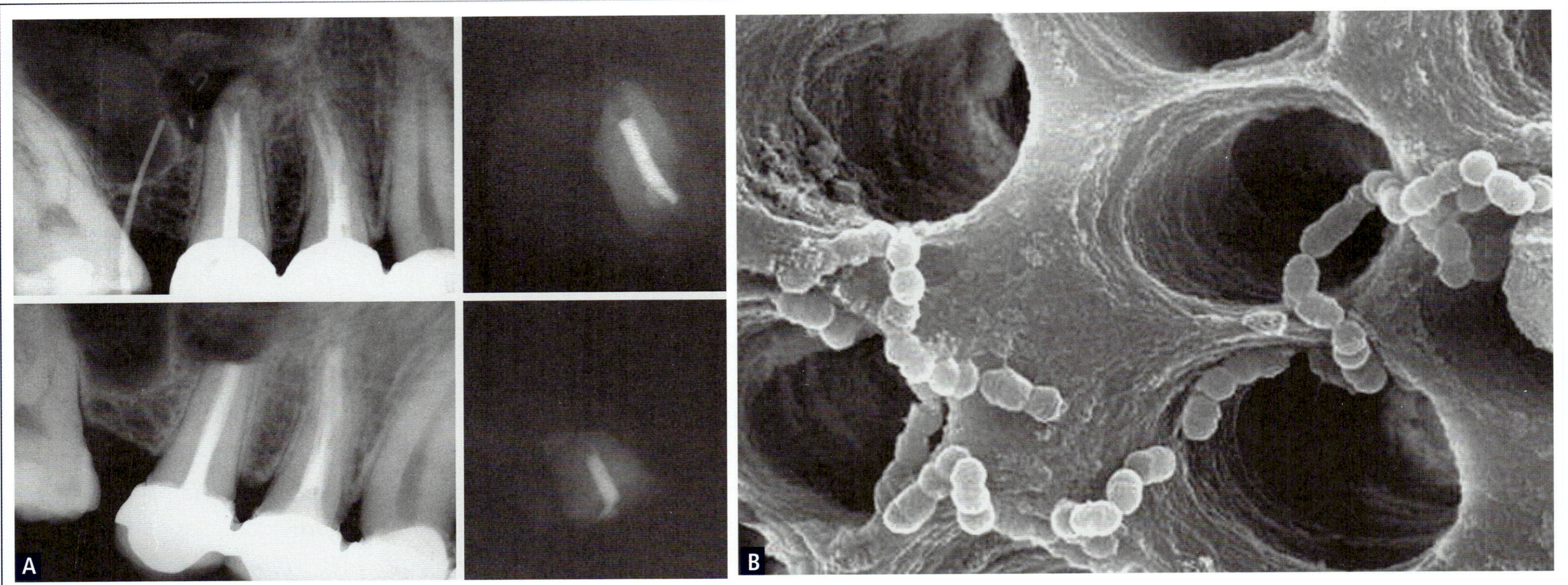

FIGS. 1.15A-B[104]

A – Radiographs of a maxillary second premolar with the apical five millimeters without filling, before and after apicoectomy as well as radiographs of the resected apical fragment.
B – Scanning electron micrograph of the un-filled resected fragment of the root canal after apicoectomy, showing the presence of *Enterococcus faecalis*.
(Courtesy of Luciano Giardino, University of Brescia (Italy), 2006)

These facts provide evidence that re-treatment in one single session is not possible. The low percentages of success reported in clinical/radiographic surveys, regardless whether the treatment is performed by endodontists or general practitioners, justify two sessions with these medications as temporary dressings (Chart 1-9).

Finally, if we consider that today the large majority of cases that are diagnosed for root canal treatment are frequently teeth with pulp necrosis (gangrene) and obvious evident chronic periapical lesions (NECROPULPECTOMIES II – apical periodontitis), as well as RE-TREATMENTS, one can conclude that this situation is reason for concern and deserves discussion with regard to the quality of treatments offered at the present time.

According to Charts 1.5, 1.6, 1.7, 1.9 and 1.10, the **low percentages** of success reported in a large variety of clinical/radiographic evaluations, justify the above-mentioned concern.

Chart 1.11 also shows evidence that as a result of this poor endodontic success rate, the incidence and/or persistence of **post-treatment periapical lesions** is relatively high, with a mean ranging from 7 to 67%.

The above-mentioned evaluations (Charts 1.4, 1.5, 1.6 and 1.10) explain the high number of cases of RE-TREATMENT that demand new endodontic intervention. This number can be higher, once the number of cases of clinically quiet and painless cases is not included.

CHART 1.11 – Post-treatment persistence or appearance of chronic periapical lesion of root canals (last 20 years).

YEAR	AUTHORS	CITY/ COUNTRY	PERCENTAGES OF CHRONIC PERIAPICAL LESION
1986	Petersson *et al.*[110]	Sweden	31%
1987	Bergström *et al.*[10]	Sweden	29%
1987	Eckerbon *et al.*[31]	Sweden	26%
1988	Eriksen *et al.*[36]	Norway	26%
1989	Petersson *et al.*[109]	Sweden	65%
1989	Eckerbom *et al.*[32]	Sweden	22%
1990	Odesjö *et al.*[98]	Sweden	25%
1991	Eriksen & Bjertness[35]	Norway	37%
1991	Imfeld[55]	Sweden	31%
1991	Eckerbon *et al.*[33]	Sweden	26%
1993	De Cleen *et al.*[28]	Germany	39%
1993	Petersson[108]	Sweden	31%
1995	Ray & Trope[113]	USA	39%
1995	Buckley & Spängberg[14]	USA	31%
1995	Eriksen *et al.*[34]	Norway	38%
1997	Saunders *et al.*[119]	Scotland	58%
1997	Weiger *et al.*[148]	Germany	61%
1998	Marques *et al.*[87]	Portugal	22%
1999	Sidaravicius *et al.*[125]	Lithuania	39%
2000	De Moor *et al.*[29]	Belgium	40%
2001	Kirkevang *et al.*[65]	Denmark	67%
2001	Kirkevang *et al.*[64]	Denmark	52%
2002	Boucher *et al.*[13]	France	26%
2002	Lupi-Pegurier[85]	France	31%
2004	Jiménez-Pinzón *et al.*[58]	Spain	64%
2006	Gesi *et al.*[44]	Italy	7%
2006	Marquis *et al.*[88]	Canada	14%
OVERALL MEAN PERSISTENCE OF ENDODONTIC POST-TREATMENT PERIAPICAL LESION		**35.8%**	

THIS SITUATION UNDOUBTEDLY INTERFERES WITH THE CONCEPT OF THE ENDODONTIC SPECIALTY

Currently a great deal of importance is being given to the quality of **three-dimensional hermetical sealing** of the root canal system, which must be offered by the filling materials and by the post-treatment **coronal restoration**, which should act as an effective mechanical barrier to bacterial leakage in a crown/apex direction[123,124], this being a preponderant etiologic factor for the prevention of post-treatment periapical pathosis[52,63,113,118].

We know that more than 900 bacterial species have been identified in the oral cavity. Therefore, the root canal is exposed to bacterial invasion from the oral cavity, as well as from the products of their metabolism.

Due to the fact that traditional zinc oxide and eugenol-based cements associated with gutta-percha cones do not bond to dentin, they do not prevent leakage of bacteria and their by-products in an apical direction[41,86,112,143]. The bacteria coming from the oral cavity have transformed the clinical practice of endodontics that has been in use for over 60 years. Because of this, present-day concepts in Endodontics are challenging the established techniques.

Cheung & Chan[20] (2003), in a prospective study evaluating success/failure over a period of 10 to 20 years, reported that after 15 and 20 years, 50% of the endodontic treatments failed. The authors concluded that the location of the tooth, periapical conditions before treatment, type of root filling material, type of posts and the coronal restoration had a significant influence on the long-term success.

It is accepted that filling the root canals with these traditional cements, complemented with gutta-percha cones is results with clinical in radiographic success of the treatment, as long as an effective coronal restoration is present that prevents microleakage at the conclusion of the endodontic treatment[52,86,113]. They also attributed this relative success to restorations with amalgam up to the 1980s.

We can confirm that a root canal filling, from a physical/chemical point of view, must meet the following three demands[73]:

1º) "Entomb" the bacteria that remain behind after the treatment within the root canal system (dentinal tubules, isthmus, ramifications), which is a reality for the cervical and middle thirds; (that are acellular and impermeable cementum areas). The cementum of the apical third (**apical five millimeters**) is cellular and therefore permeable.

2º) Prevent the leakage of fluids from the periapical tissues into the root canal system and reaching the bacteria that survived endodontic treatment.

3º) Act as a mechanical barrier, thus preventing re-infection of the root canal system through the oral cavity.

Apparently, the above-mentioned conventional materials do not fulfill these three requirements.

On the other hand, Patel et al.[106], using a confocal microscope, recently observed that the sealer (RealSeal System), penetrated deep into the dentinal tubules. Their data showed that in each third of the root canal, penetration of Real Seal (adhesive filling technique) into the dentinal tubules was significantly greater than that of Tubliseal, a zinc oxide and eugenol-based cement ($p<0.05$).

Therefore, the search for root canal filling materials has focused on materials that bond to dentin as well as to the solid cones to prevent crown-apex bacterial leakage. In the present day endodontic literature these systems are referred to as "monobloc", when bonding technology is employed[90].

The potential of root canal filling materials to form a homogeneous unit, bond to dentin and to solid cones, served as the hypothesis for a study conducted by Moisiadis et al.[90] at the Biomaterial Research Center of the University of Leuven in Belgium. After biomechanical preparation of the root canal with the oscillating system Endo-Eze AET (Advanced Endodontic Technology) (Ultradent Products Inc. USA) the root canals were irrigated with Concepsis (Ultradent Products Inc. USA) followed by 4 minutes of irrigation and flooding with 18% EDTA solution and finally rinsed with distilled water. After drying, the root canals were filled with a methacrylate-based resin sealer (Endo-Rez – Ultradent Products Inc. USA) and kept in an incubator at 95% humidity, at 37° Celsius for 7 days. At the end of this period, the teeth were immersed in a solution of 30% hydrochloric acid for complete dissolution of the dentin. Only the filling material remained (Figs. 1.16A-C).

The images in Figs. 1.16A, B and C, show how the filling material penetrated into the dentinal tubules up to 1000 µm.

Real Seal System (SybronEndo Sds, Glendora, CA USA) and the methacrylate-based EndoRez System in conjunction with resin coated gutta-percha cones at present represent the monobloc concept of bonded root canal fillings. (Real Seal was previously known as Resilon/Epiphany)

A root canal filling sealer based on an epoxy-amine resin, marketed by Dentsply/DeTrey as AH- Plus (Dentsply/De Trey Gmbh, Konstanz Germany) and by Dentsply/Maillefer under the name TopSeal (Dentsply Maillefer, Baillaigues Switzerland), has excellent sealing properties, as demonstrated by Almeida et al.[4] in an ex-vivo dye penetration study, who found statistically significant better results for this material, compared to Procosol (zinc oxide and eugenol-based) and Ketac-Endo (glass ionomer-based).

With regard to biocompatibility, a study by Leonardo et al.[76] in dog`s teeth, in which pulpectomies and root canal filling with AH Plus were performed over an experimental period of 90 days, reported excellent histological results. The apical and periapical repair tissues were free of inflammatory cells, with biological sealing of the foramen by mineralized tissue, either partially in (75%) or complete in (12.5%) of the cases. These histopathological results with respect the biocompatibility of AH Plus sealer were considered excellent, particularly if we consider an experimental period of only 90 days (Figs.1.17, 1.18, 1.19, 1.20, 1.21A-B, 1.22, 1.23A-B and 1.24A-C).

* Ultradent Products Inc. South Jordan, Utah, USA.
** Clorexidina 2% Ultradent – South Jordain UT, USA.
*** Ultradent Products Inc. South Jordan, Utah, USA.
**** Penntron Clinical Technologies, LLC, Wallingford, CT, USA.
***** SybronEndo – SDS-Kerr, USA.

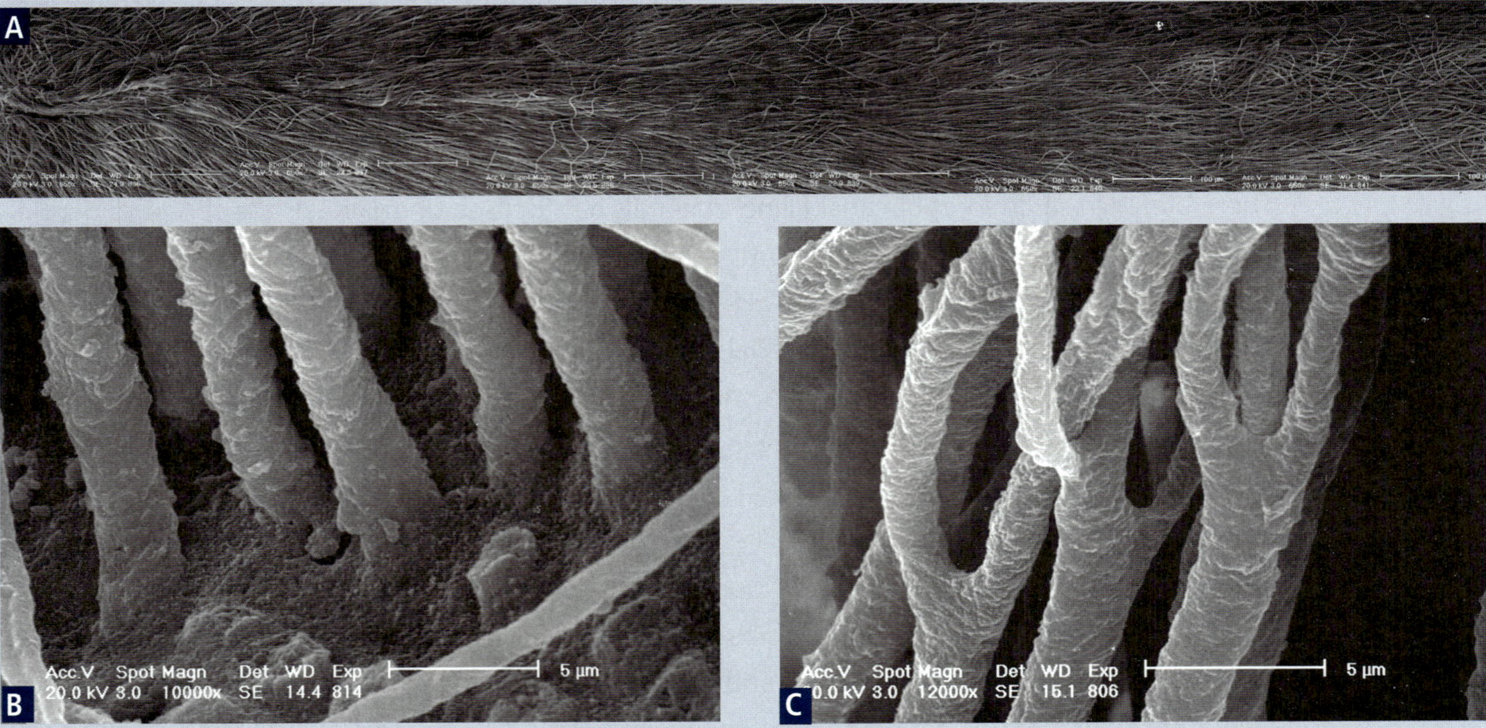

FIGS. 1.16A-C

A – EndoREZ inside dentinal tubules.

B and C– High magnification of the filling material penetrating into the dentinal tubules and branching of the resin tags after dissolving of the dentin.

Lambrechts P, Van Meerbeek B. Bergmans L. Moisiadis P. *Environmental and normal FESEM evaluation of EndoREZ leakage inside dentinal tubules*. Catholic University of Leuven, Belgium. U.Z. St. Rafael. BIOMAT Research Cluster.

(Courtesy of the authors[90])

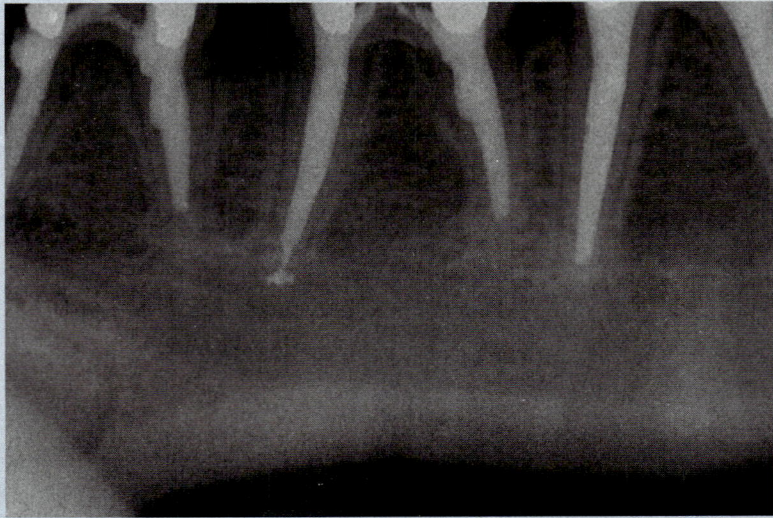

FIG. 1.17[76]

Periapical radiograph of dog teeth, showing root canal fillings of the 2nd, 3rd and 4th mandibular left premolars with AH Plus sealer (Dentsply/De Trey). Note the small amount of extrusion of the filling material in the mesial root of the mandibular left 3rd premolar.

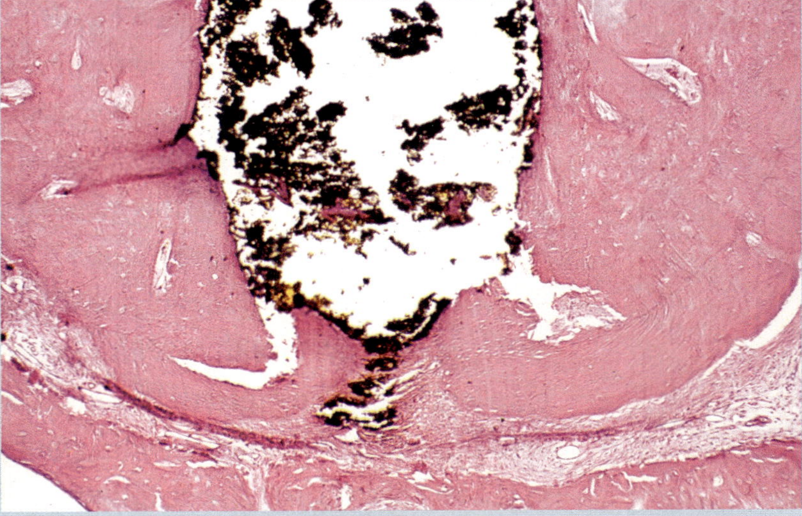

FIG. 1.18[76]

Histological section of the apical and periapical region of a dog tooth; mesial root of the mandibular 4th molar Fig. 1.17, showing evidence of complete sealing of the foraminal opening by newly formed mineralized tissue, 90 days after vital pulpectomy and root canal filling with AH Plus (Dentsply/DeTrey). Normal apical periodontal ligament and alveolar bone is present with active osteoblasts. (Magnification 24X, H&E stain).

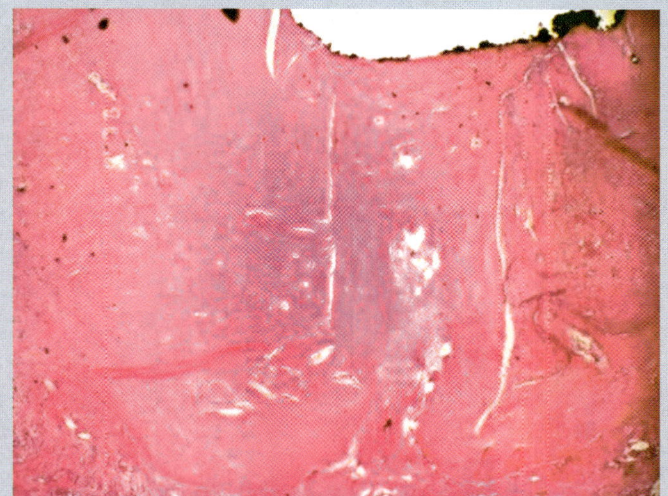

FIG. 1.19[76]

Histological section of the apical region of a dog tooth – distal root of the mandibular left 3rd premolar in Fig. 1.17, showing evidence of complete sealing of the foraminal opening by a considerable amount of newly formed mineralized tissue, in direct contact with the AH Plus filling material, 90 days after vital pulpectomy. Note the apical stop, determining the apical filling limit of the root canal. (Magnification 80X, H&E stain).

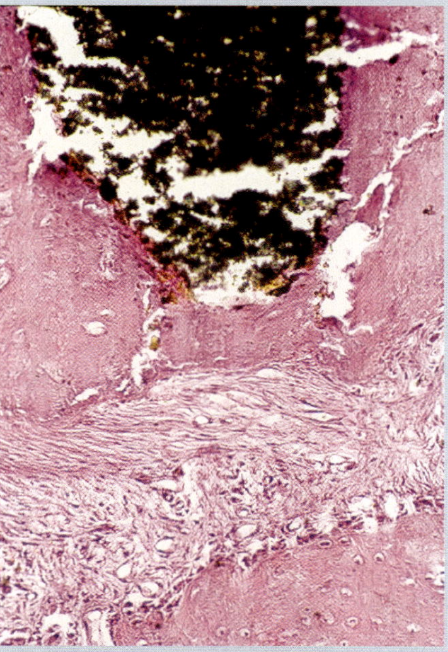

FIG. 1.20[76]

Histological section of the apical and periapical region of a dog tooth – mesial root of the mandibular left 2nd premolar in Fig. 1.17. Partial sealing of the foraminal opening by newly formed mineralized tissue in direct contact with the filling material (AH Plus) after 90 days can be seen. Thickening of the apical periodontal ligament and normal alveolar bone, with active osteoblasts (lamina dura) can be observed. (Magnification 40X, H&E stain).

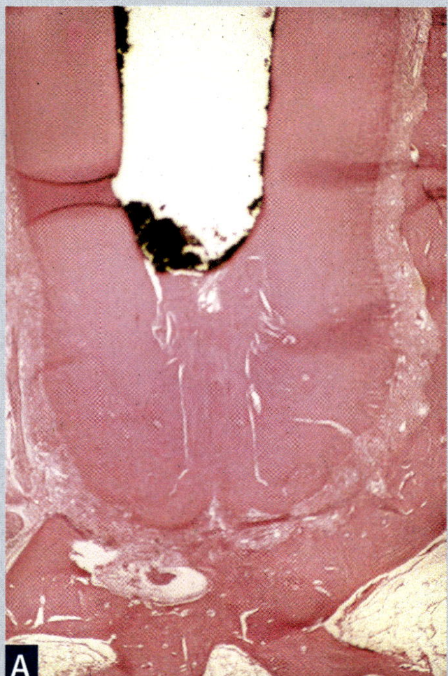

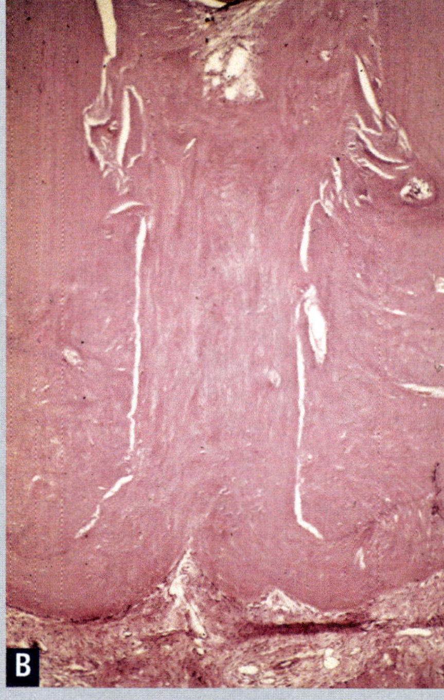

FIGS. 1.21A-B[76]

A – Histological section of the apical and periapical region of a dog tooth – distal root of the mandibular left 2nd premolar in Fig. 1.17. Presence of extensive newly formed mineralized tissue, partial sealing the foraminal opening and in direct contact with the filling material (AH Plus), 90 days after vital pulpectomy can be seen. Normal apical periodontal ligament and normal alveolar bone (lamina dura) is present. (Magnification 24X, H&E stain).

B – Higher magnification of the previous figure, showing evidence of partial sealing of the foraminal opening and normal apical periodontal ligament. (Magnification 40X, H&E stain).

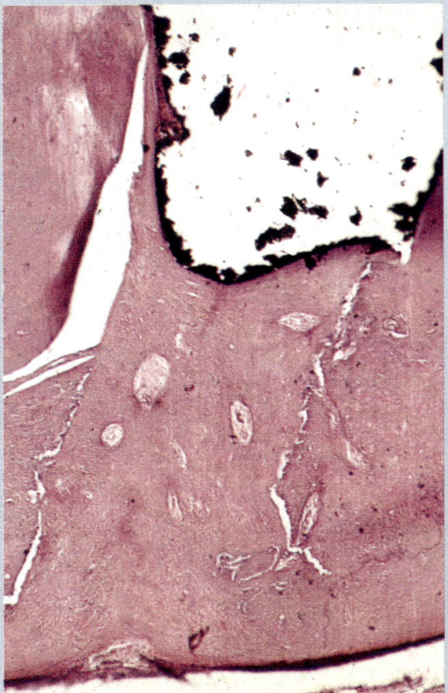

FIG. 1.22[76]

Histological section of the apical region of a dog tooth, 90 days after vital pulpectomy, showing evidence of partial sealing of the foraminal opening by newly formed mineral tissue, in direct contact with the filling material (AH Plus). Note presence of interstitial tissue with a large number of cementoblasts. (Magnification 40X, H&E stain).

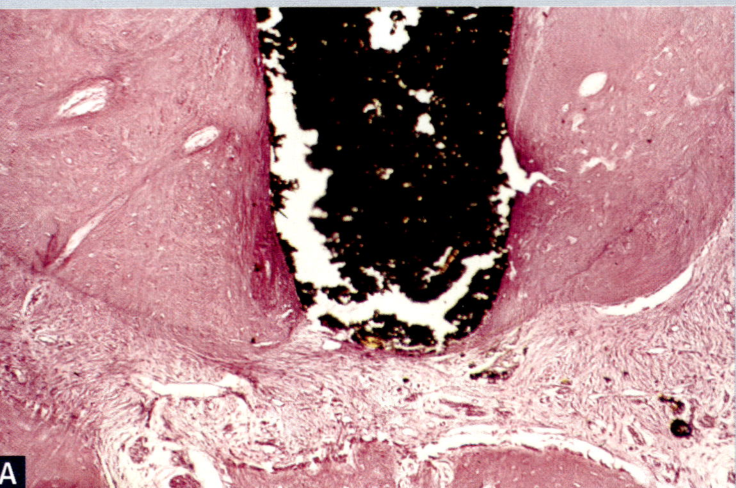

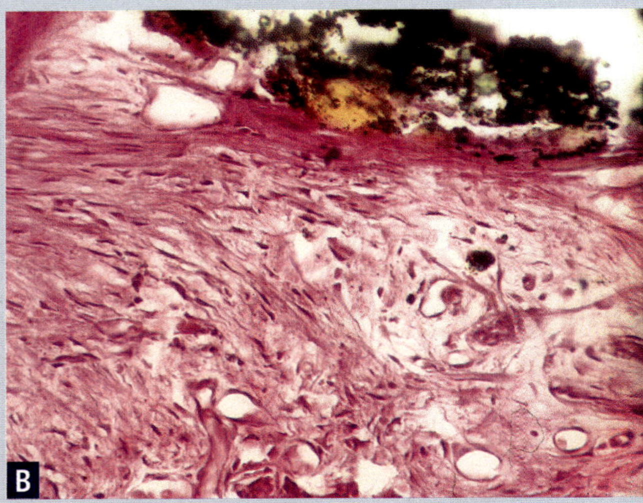

FIGS. 1.23A-B[76]

A – Histological section of a dog's tooth, showing root canal filling (AH Plus) extending exactly to the foramen level 90 days post operatively. Note the formation of mineralized tissue and continuous and regular fibrous lining–the filling material. Apical periodontal ligament is slightly thickened, with absence of inflammatory cells. (Magnification 40X, H&E stain)

B – Higher magnification of the previous figure, showing continuous, regular fibrous lining adjacent to the filling material. Presence of fibroblasts and collagen fibers running in various directions. There are numerous active osteoblasts in the alveolar bone. Absence of inflammatory cells. (Magnification 100X, H&E stain).

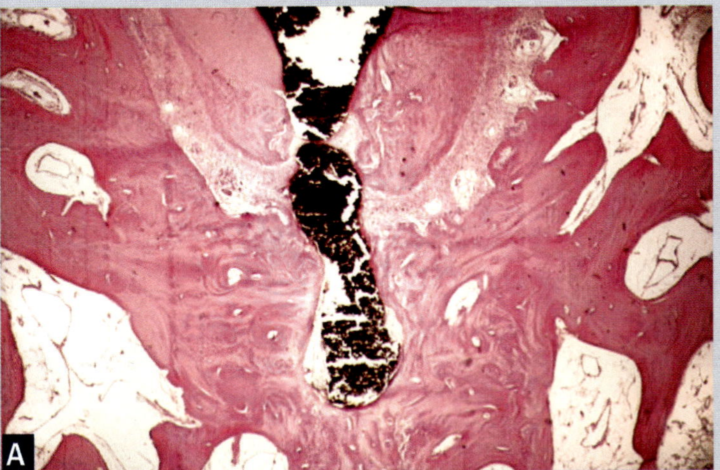

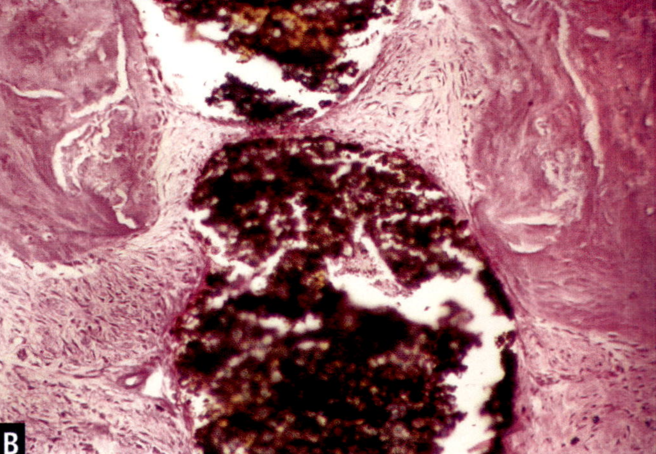

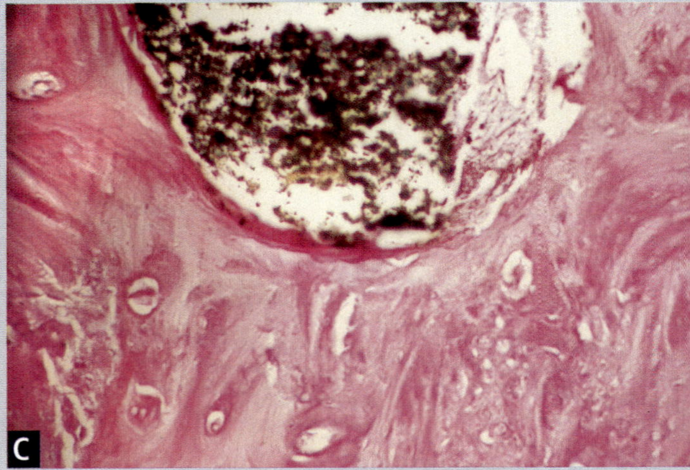

FIGS. 1.24A-C[76]

A – Low-power view of the apical and periapical regions of a dog tooth – mesial root of the mandibular left 3rd premolar (Fig. 1.17). Extruded filling material (AH Plus) into the periapical region can be seen. 90-day postoperative view after vital pulpectomy. Note the excellent relationship between the filling material and connective tissue and newly formed bone. (Magnification 24X, H&E stain).

B – Magnification of Fig. 1.24A of the region at the apical foramen showing apical periodontal ligament with connective tissue. Absence of inflammatory cells. (Magnification 40X, H&E stain)

C – Enlargement of Fig. 1.22A, showing newly formed bone tissue adjacent to the extruded AH Plus cement. (Magnification 64X, H&E stain).

In another study by Leonardo et al.[73], the *in vivo* response of the apical and periapical tissues of dog teeth after root canal filling with the Epiphany/Resilon System was evaluated and compared to root canals filled with a new formulation of Sealapex, (SybronEndo sds Kerr) cement, with or without coronal restorations. The authors concluded that the Epiphany/Resilon System was tolerated significantly better than Sealapex cement (new formulation), whether with or without coronal restoration. The aim of leaving the teeth without coronal restorations was to evaluate the influence of coronal leakage and the effect it had on the success of the root canal treatment after 90 days (Figs. 1.25A-B, 1.26A-D, 1.27A-B, 1-28A-B, 1-29A-C).

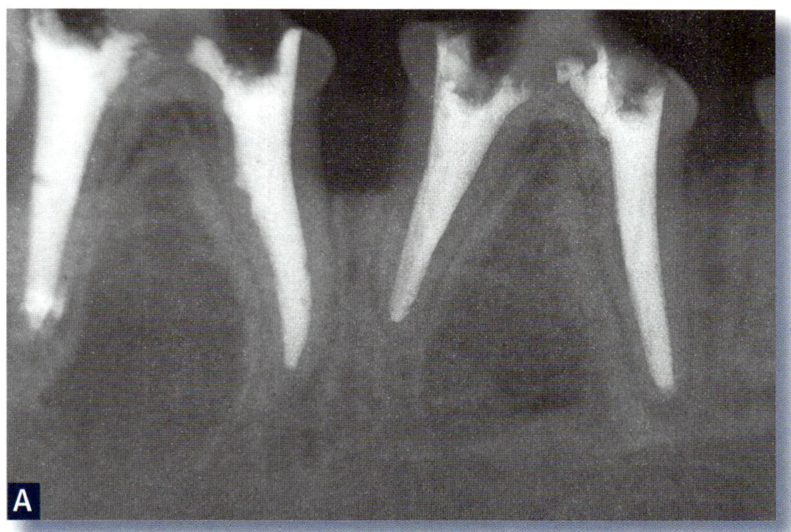

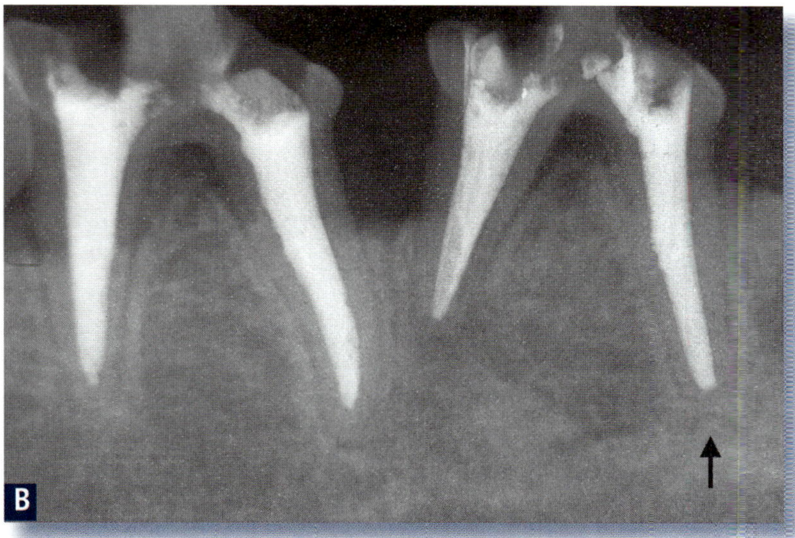

FIGS. 1.25A-B

A – Post operative periapical radiograph of root canals fillings of the right mandibular 3rd and 4th premolars. Note the absence of coronal restorations and apical limit of filling at the level of the apical stop. Note also slight extrusion of the filling material (Epiphany/Resilon System), in the distal root of the 4th premolar.

B – Post-operative control radiograph (follow-up) 90 days after filling root canals without coronal restorations. Note the reabsorption of the filling material (Epiphany/Resilon System), in the distal root of the mandibular right 4th premolar.

* Penntron Clinical Technologies, LLC, Wallingford, CT, USA.
** SybronEndo – SDS-Kerr, USA.

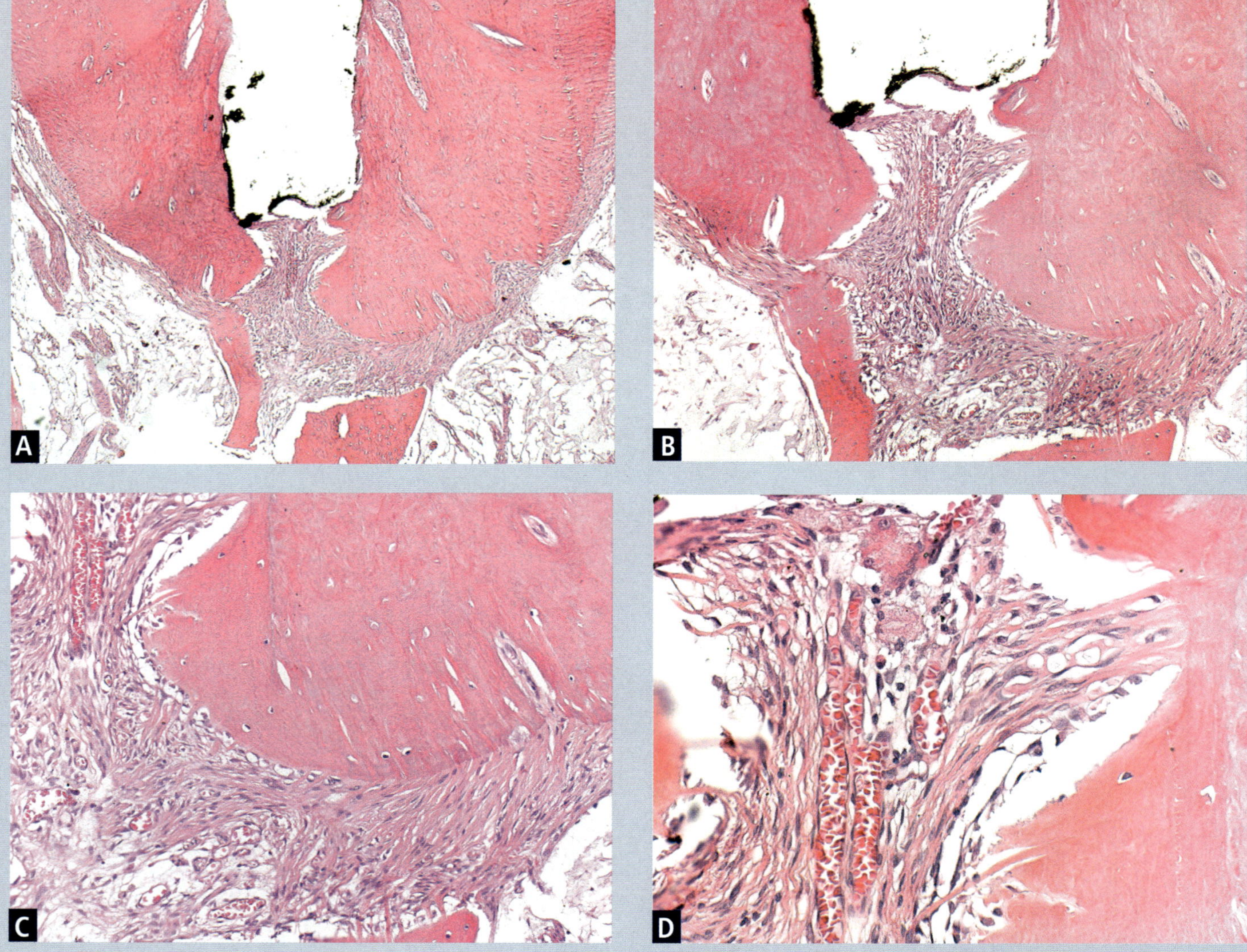

FIGS. 1.26A-D[73]

A – Low power view of a histological section of the apical and periapical regions of the mesial root of the mandibular right 3rd premolar in Fig. 1.25B (arrow), 90 days after vital pulpectomy and root canal filling with the Epiphany/Resilon system. No coronal restoration was made with the object to evaluate the effect of crown/apex leakage on the periapical tissues. Note the filling limit at the level of the apical Stop and filling material/ repair tissue interface. Apical periodontal ligament slightly thickened. (Magnification 24X, H&E stain)

B – Higher magnification of previous figure. Invagination of interstitial tissue at the foraminal opening with large number of fibers. (Magnification 40X, H&E stain)

C – Higher magnification of previous figure, showing interstitial tissue rich in fibers, vessels and cells. Active cementoblasts. Note the Sharpey fibers along the apical periodontal ligament. (Magnification 60X, H&E stain).

D – Magnification of previous figure, showing abundant presence of Sharpey fibers, blood vessels, while there is an absence of microorganisms. (Magnification100X, H&E stain).

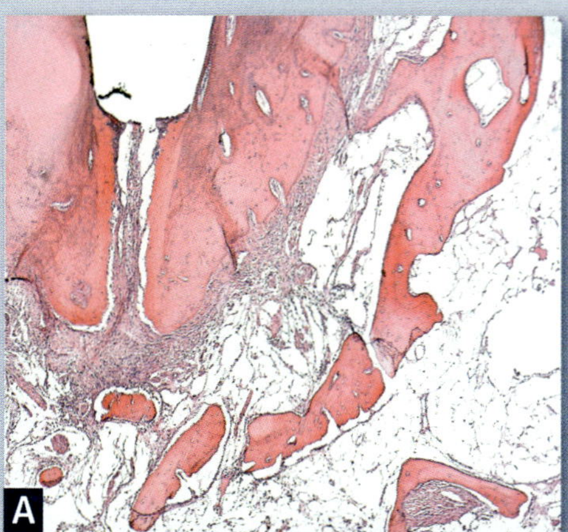

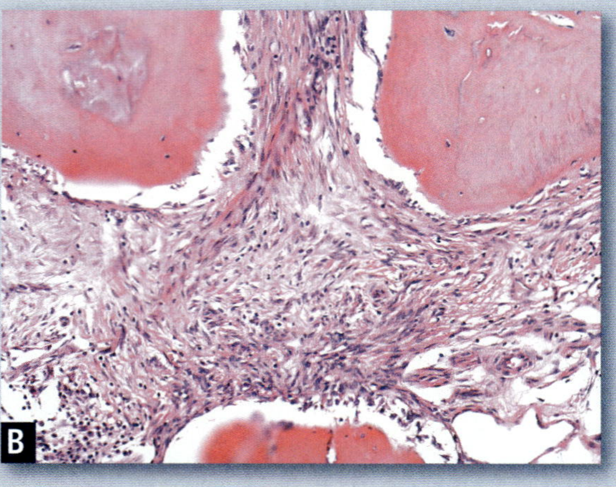

FIGS. 1.27A-B[73]

A – Low power view of the apical and periapical region of the mesial root of the right mandibular 4th premolar of a dog tooth, 90 days after vital pulpectomy. Root canal filling with Epiphany/Resilon system, without coronal restoration. Note the apical limit of filling at the level of the apical stop and interface of the filling material and fibrous repair tissue, as well as newly formed mineralized tissue adjacent to the cement canal walls. Apical periodontal ligament is slightly thickened. (Magnification 24X, H&E stain).

B – Higher magnification of the previous figure, showing repair tissue penetrating the entrance of the foraminal opening. This tissue is rich in fibers, vessels and cells. Note active repair by osteoblasts and cementoblasts and absence of microorganisms. (Magnification 60X, H&E stain).

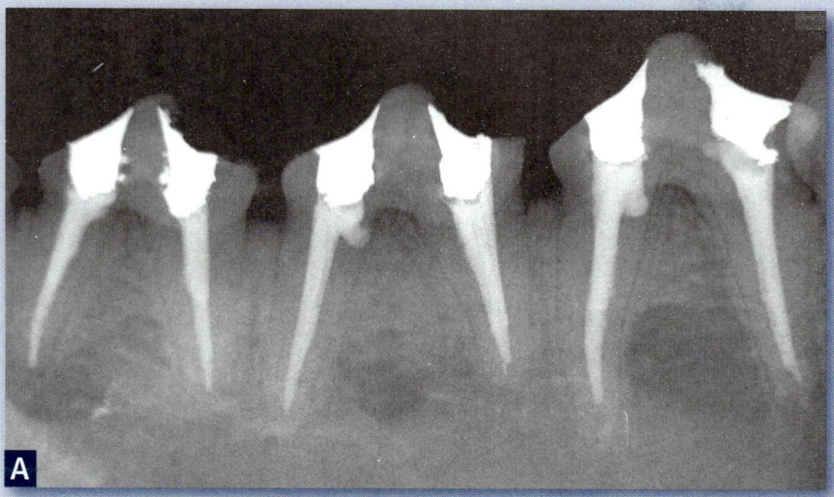

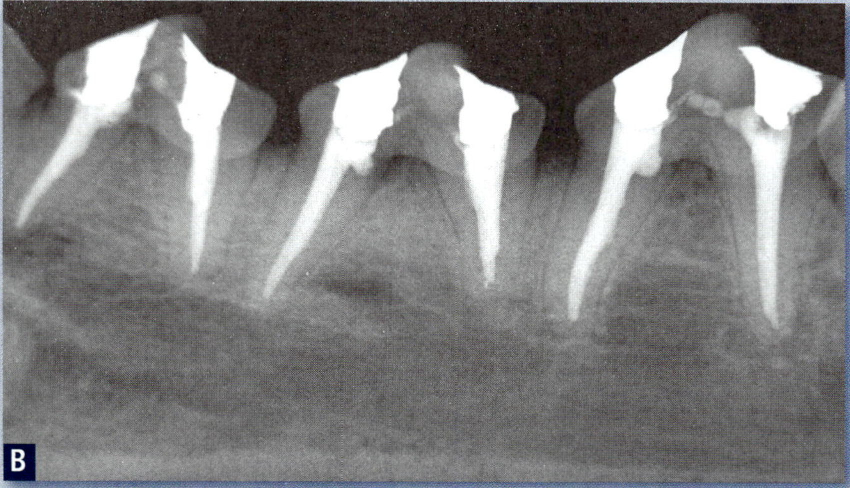

FIGS. 1.28A-B

A – Periapical radiograph obtained immediately after root canal treatment of the mandibular left 2nd, 3rd and 4th premolars in a dog. The coronal restorations were done in glass ionomer cement and amalgam and the root canals filled with the Epiphany/Resilon system. Note the apical limits of filling, all at the level of the apical stop.

B – Follow-up radiograph after 90 days. Note the presence of lamina dura in all the roots.

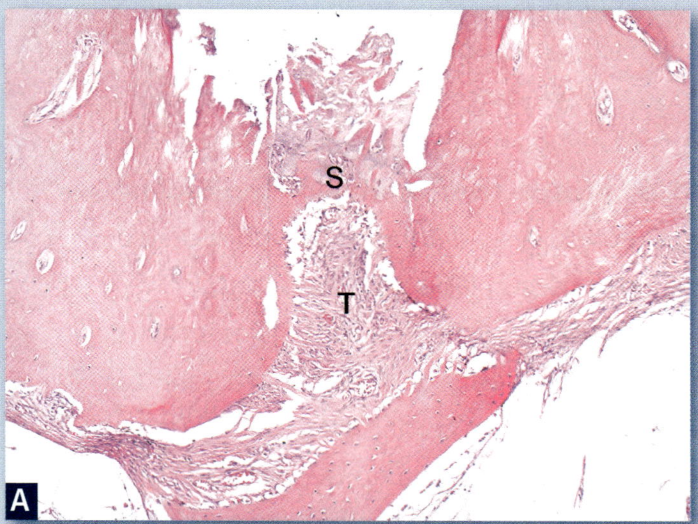

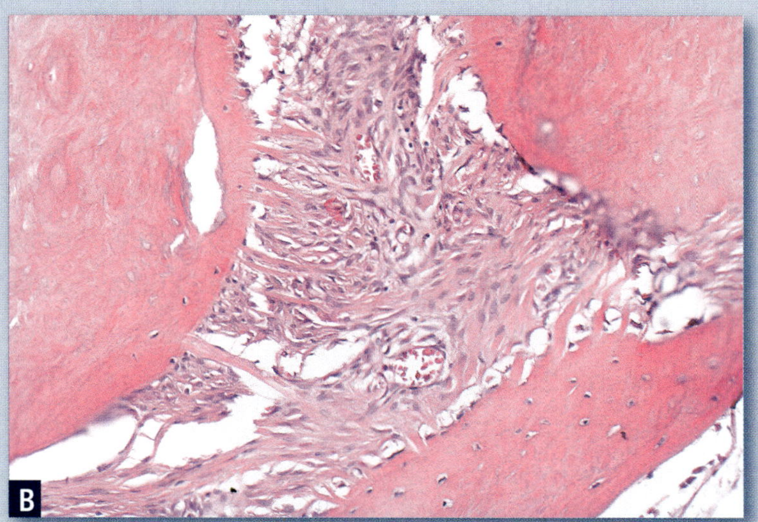

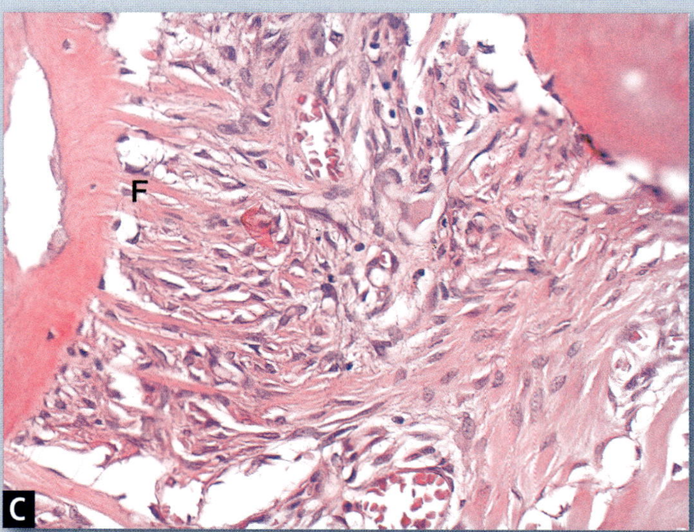

FIGS. 1.29A-C[73]

A – Histological section of the apical region of the mesial root of the mandibular left 3rd premolar of a dog tooth. After vital pulpectomy and root canal filling with the Epiphany/Resilon system, coronal restorations were carried out in glass ionomer cement and amalgam. Note the biological sealing of the apical foramen by newly formed mineralized tissue (S). Penetration into the foraminal space of interstitial tissue (T). The apical periodontal ligament is normal. (Magnification 24X, H&E stain)

B – Higher magnification of the previous figure, showing a large number of fibers, including Sharpey fibers, normal cells and vessels. Normal apical periodontal ligament with active osteoblasts can be seen. (Magnification 40X, H&E stain)

C – Higher magnification of the previous figure of interstitial tissue at the entrance of the foraminal opening, rich in fibers (highlighting the Sharpey fibers (F)), blood vessels and absence of microorganisms and inflammatory cells. (Magnification 80X, H&E stain)

Correlation of the possible systemic risks, as a result of infectious accidents during endodontic treatment of teeth with evident radiographic chronic periapical lesions (Apical periodontitis) and/or as a consequence of persistent chronic periapical lesion post-treatment

In view of the previously described facts, mainly based on the low percentage of post-treatment success, the present endodontic literature, although still very controversial, shows that during root canal treatment of teeth with evident chronic periapical lesions as a consequence of pulp necrosis (gangrene) or poorly filled root canals (endodontic failures), a relationship to systemic problems, such as arthritis, myocardial infarction, cerebral stroke, endocarditis, etc. can be made.

Murray & Saunders[94] in 2000, in a review of the literature, confirmed that a relationship between root canal treatment and general health exists and that some research suggested a possible correlation between dental health and cardiovascular diseases. The perfection of more sophisticated methods, such as molecular biology and techniques of improved culture methods, have enabled researchers to confirm that bacteria are present in peripheral blood as a result of endodontic treatment in cases of teeth with evident chronic periapical lesions (apical periodontitis). Furthermore, the authors established a potential correlation between bacteremia or bacterial endotoxins subsequent to root canal treatment of teeth with evident periapical lesion, and severe systemic complications. The authors concluded that further research is necessary to confirm systemic complications as a result of root canal treatment, and suggested that scientifically controlled **prospective/controlled longitudinal studies** should be conducted in groups of the population, to conclusively determine the indisputable correlation between general health and chronic periapical inflammation (apical periodontitis).

The endodontic literature[12,26,38,146,150] is rife with citations of severe systemic accidents as a result of oral infections and/or unsuccessful root canal treatments. The majority of these reports refer to acute infectious processes, however, there is controversy with respect to chronic periapical lesions. There are, however, few **controlled/prospective longitudinal studies** that prove this actually occurs. Among the few articles published, a **controlled/prospective longitudinal study** in 708 male patients by Caplan et al.[19] (2006), investigated whether the presence of a evident chronic periapical lesion of endodontic (bacterial origin) was or was not related to the development of cardiovascular disease. Every 3 years, up to *32 years*, the participants underwent medical and dental examinations. The authors concluded that among the patients of up to 40 years of age, the presence of an **evident chronic periapical lesion of endodontic origin was significantly associated with the diagnosis of cardiovascular disease ($p<0.05$)**. For patients over the age of 40 years, no statistical significance was observed.

The findings of this research are consistent when correlating the relationship between a chronic periapical inflammation of bacterial origin and the development of cardiovascular disease, especially among young male patients.

Though subjective (Leonardo & Leonardo, unpublished data), by means of hundreds of courses in Brazil and many Latin American, Asian and European countries, information was collected on many cases of bacteremias associated with a high incidence of cardiovascular disease, including endocarditis, related to root canal treatment of teeth with evident chronic periapical lesion. Nevertheless, as previously mentioned, there are few (**controlled/prospective**) longitudinal studies.

Goymerac & Wollard[46], in 2004, in a pertinent review of the theory of focal infection and its possible relationship with systemic diseases, confirmed that teeth that were well treated endodontically have not been related to systemic diseases. They also confirmed that the treatment of periodontal disease reduces the occurrence of systemic disease.

Nevertheless, the lack of knowledge of recent studies on the part of the practitioner, for example about the incidence of bacteremias and fungemias that occur during root canal treatment of teeth with evident periapical lesion, is unacceptable. The latest studies have shown that this is as high as 50% [27].

Debelian et al.[27], (1997) collected microorganisms in cases of bacteremia and fungemia in patients undergoing to root canal treatment in teeth with evident periapical lesions, and isolated bacteria and fungi in 50% of the patients, the Gram-negative anaerobes being the predominant microorganism.

The presence of 50% bacteremias justifies a change in paradigm with respect to treatment of root canals of teeth with **evident periapical lesions and cases of retreatment**, that is the necessity to detoxify the toxic content of the root canal in a crown-down method (See Chapter 2-XVII). It should be emphasized that bacteremia occurring in healthy patients are of no systemic consequence. Nevertheless, in patients with pre-existing pathologies, for example leukemia or immunodepressed patients, there is greater risk of generalized septicemia, which could be fatal if antibiotic prophylaxis were not instituted (*see* Chapter 2-XXI).

FINAL CONSIDERATIONS

The above-mentioned facts and references, and in view of the fact that currently in endodontics worldwide technologists prevail, rather than bio-technologists, lead us to a moment of deep reflection.

Based on GROSSMAN[48] (1951) who quoted: ***"Presumption should not be substituted for precision where health is concerned"***, our reflection leads us to propose that modern Endodontics should demand that a new approach be taken in clinical practice with respect to cases with evident chronic periapical lesions (apical periodontitis) that require treatment, as well as in all cases of re-treatment. Furthermore, a new method must be established with respect to the criteria used for evaluating success/failure of this treatment. Increased emphasis should be directed on the requirement to attend Continuing Endodontic Education Courses by universities and dental associations for general clinicians as well as endodontic specialists, with the purpose to provide the participants with up-to-date knowledge that will allow them to stay current in their field of interest.

We should also realize that skepticism with respect to the use of a "temporary dressing" in NECROPULPECTOMIES II and RE-TREATMENTS still persists. In part this is due to the lack of practitioners carefully informing themselves of the latest development in scientific research and being aware of the historical development in endodontics. Technological advances, new research methodologies, the perfection of more sophisticated techniques such as molecular biology and new cell or tissue culture techniques, have elucidated the presence of the dominant microbiota in teeth with evident periapical lesions (Gram-negative anaerobes), and in cases of re-treatment, a mixed microbiota. The latter, however, contains predominantly aerobic bacterial strains such as the *Enterococcus faecalis* and *Pseudomonas aeruginosa*. Technological advances such histological and histomicrobiological studies, as well as scanning electronic microscopy (SEM), have enabled us to recognize that in teeth with evident periapical lesions (apical periodontitis), due to the complex anatomy of the root canal system with ten thousands of dentinal tubules, uncountable ramifications, isthmuses, cement erosions and apical bacterial biofilm, are invaded by microorganisms. Furthermore, current biological Endodontics has led to an understanding of the importance of **bacterial LPS (endotoxins)**, substances proven to be cytotoxic, which, if not "neutralized", will be responsible for sustaining periapical lesions. Their irreversible adherence to resorbed mineralized tissues, such as the periapical alveolar bone, cement and dentin, particularly at the **apical five millimeters,** regions inaccessible by biomechanical preparation, have led us to accept the use of the "temporary dressing", with the goal of producing a degradation and inactivation of this important detrimental cytotoxic agents.

Temporary dressing is regarded with a certain amount of skepticism leading its proponents to be careful in expressing that they are skilled in the use of this technique. Nevertheless, greater emphasis is currently being attached to systemic manifestations arising from chronic pathological changes in the oral cavity, such as bacterial endocarditis, myocardial infarction, atherosclerosis, fever of unknown origin, urticaria, and uveitis, meningitis and cerebral abscesses[62,81,103].

Since the apical and periapical tissues are in direct contact with the entire body by means of microcirculation, a scientifically up-to-date approach would treat these NECROPULPECTOMIES II with the understanding that he/she is faced with an LPS-dependant disease. Therefore the most important objective is to inactivate it, even though it may be located at a small distance from the lumen of the root canal.

Based on the facts that have been presented in this chapter, we can conclude that biologically only the calcium hydroxide-based compounds that are used as **temporary dressing** are capable of inactivating bacterial LPS, and therefore, they are the material of choice for these cases. Among the calcium hydroxide-based compounds, the aqueous vehicle (physiological solution, anesthetic, etc.) and the viscous medium (polyethylenoglycol "400") allow the release of hydroxyl ions determining the inactivation of LPS. Since the aqueous vehicle of calcium hydroxide used as an intracanal dressing is rapidly dissolved, particularly in teeth with excessive exudates we recommend viscous vehicles (Calen-SS White. Artigos Dentários Ltda, Rio de Janeiro, Brazil), because they are less soluble, and thus do not require frequent replacement as they last up to 14 days. Adequate time is of the essence as these ions take at least 14 days to penetrate through the dentin of the **apical five millimeters (critical zone for biological endodontics)** to reach the extra-radicular infection and the microorganisms that are contained inside the biofilm.

In cases of RE-TREATMENTS as described in this chapter, the association of calcium hydroxide and chlorhexidine or camphorated chlorophenol, is highly efficient in combating the anaerobic and aerobic bacterial strains, such as *Enterococcus faecalis* and *Pseudomonas aeruginosa*. Finally, the scientific advances in microbiology, pathology, immunology and molecular biology, and the technical advances in Endodontics are to be commended. In a relative short period of just years advances have been achieved not seen over the course of its entire history. In particular, rotary and oscillatory systems, the reappearance of ultrasound, third generation electronic apex locators, operating microscopes and advanced root canal filling methods. These advances (**technical and biologica**l) provide for a much faster treatment with more comfort to the patient compared to a few years ago. In addition, a lack of post-operative discomfort and a high percentage of clinical, radiographic and histological success can be attributed to these recent advances. They must continue to go forward leading to treatment in a single session in cases with a microbiota, pathosis and anatomy that will allow it. In NECROPULPECTOMIES II (apical periodontitis) and RE-TREATMENTS, the **temporary dressing** therapy should continue to be indicated, as it certainly is the most prudent course of action to control an endodontic infection of the root canal system.

Considering the transition Endodontics is experiencing, and after considerable introspection, we can state:

> *"The educational leaders responsible for the scientific aspect of endodontics should have a strong ethical and moral commitment to improve a patient's health and should endeavor* ***to seek the link that is lost between biology and the technical development of this specialty****".*

Mario Roberto Leonardo – 2003

References

1. Acetoze P. et al. Incidência de dentes com canais radiculares parcialmente obturados. RGO. 1992;40(2):107-109.
2. Äkerblom A, Hasselgreen G. The prognosis for endodontic treatment of obliterated root canals. J Endod. 1988;14:565-567.
3. Allard V, Palmqvist S. A radiographic survey of periapical conditions in elderly people in a Swedish population. Endod Dent Traumatol. 1986;2:103-108.
4. Almeida WA, Leonardo MR, Tanomaru Filho M, Silva LAB. Evaluation of apical sealing of three endodontic sealers. Int Endod J. 2000;33:25-27.
5. Assed S. et al. Anaerobic microorganisms in root canal of human teeth with chronic apical periodontitis by indirect immunofluorescence. Endod Dent Traumat. 1996;12(2):66-69.
6. Barthel CR, Zimmer S, Trope M. Relationship of radiologic and histologic signs of inflammation in human root filled teeth. J Endod. 2004;2:75-79.
7. Benenati FW, Khajotia SS. A radiographic recall evaluation of 894 endodontic cases treated in a dental school setting. J Endod. 2002;28(5):391-395.
8. Bergenholtz G, Lekholm V, Milthon R, Engström B. Influence of apical overinstrumentation and overfilling on re-treated root canals. J Endod. 1979;5:310-314.
9. Berger CR. Tratamento endodôntico em sessão única ou múltipla. Rev. Gaúcha Odont. 1991;39(2):93-97.
10. Bergström J, Eliasson S, Ahlbery KF. Periapical status in subjects with regular care habits. Comm. Dent. Oral Epidem. 1987;15:.236-239.
11. Besse H, Woda A, Clavel J. Études statistiques des résultats médiats des traitements endodontiques réalisés à la Faculté de Clermont-Ferrand. Rev Fr Endod. 1985;4:41-51.
12. Boscolo-Rizzo P, Marchiori C, Montolli F, Vaglia A, Da Mosto MC. Deep neck infections: a constant challenge. ORL J Otorhinolaryngol Relet Spec. 2006;68(6):259-265.
13. Boucher Y, Matonian L, Rillard F, Machtou P. Radiographic evaluation of the prevalence in a French sub population. Int. Endod. J. 2002;35:229-238.
14. Buckley M, Spängberg LSW. The prevalence and technical quality of endodontic treatment in an American subpopulation. Oral Surg Oral Med Oral Pathol. 1995;79:92-100.
15. Bussey KL. A comparison of success with 1-appointment and 2-appointments molar root canal therapy. J. Endod. 2004;30:274 (Abst. PR4).
16. Byström A, Happonen RR, Sjögren V, Sundqvist G. Healing of periapical lesions of pulpless teeth after endodontic treatment with controlled asepsis. Endod Dent Traumatol. 1987;3:58-63.
17. Caliskan MK, Sen BH. Endodontic treatment of teeth with apical periodontitis using calcium hydroxide: a long-term study. Endod Dent Traumatol. 1996;12:215-221.
18. Cantarini C, Massone EJ, Goldberg F, Fraglik SR, Artaze LP. Evaluación radiográfica de 600 tratamientos endodonticos efectivados en el periodo de 1983-1993. Rev Asoc Odontol Argent. 1996;84:256-259.
19. Caplan DJ. et al. Lesions of endodontic origin and risk of coronary heart disease. J. Dent. Res. 2006;85(11):996-1000.
20. Cheung GSP, Chan TK. Long-term survival of primary root canal treatment carried out in a dental teaching hospital. Int Endod J. 2003;36:117-128.
21. Chueh LH. et al. Technical quality of root canal treatment in Taiwan. Int. Endod. J. 2003;36(6):416-422.
22. Citrome GP, Kaminski EJ, Heuer MA. A comparative study of tooth apexification in the dog. J Endod. 1979;5(10):290-297.
23. Conner DA, Caplan DJ, Teixeira FB, Trope M. Clinical outcome of teeth treated endodontically with a nonstandardized Protocol and root filled with Resilon. J Endod. 2007;53(11):1290-1292.
24. Dammaschke T. et al. Long-term survival of root-canal-treated teeth: A retrospective study over 10 years. J Endod. 2003;29(10):638-643.
25. Debelian GJ. Treatment outcome of teeth treated with an evidenced based disinfection Protocol and filled with Resilon™. J Endod. 2006 (Abst.);3:251.
26. Debelian GJ, Olsen I, Tronstad L. Systemic diseases caused by oral microorganisms. Endod Dent Traumatol. 1994;10(2):57-65.
27. Debelian GJ, Olsen I, Tronstad L. Characterization and tracing of microorganisms from bacteremia and fungemie of patients undergoing endodontic therapy. Division of Endodontic and Department of Oral Biology, UIO, 1997.
28. De Cleen MJH, Schuurs AHB, Wesselink PR, Wu MK. Periapical status and prevalence of endodontic treatment in an adult dutch population. Int Endod J. 1993;26:112-114.
29. De Moor RJG. et al. Periapical health related to the quality of root canal treatment in a Belgian population. Int Endod J. 2000;33:113-120.
30. Dugas NN. et al. Periapical health and treatment quality assessment of root-filled teeth in two Canadian populations. Int Endod J. 2003;36:181-192.
31. Eckerbon M, Anderson JE, Magnusson T. Frequency and technical standard of endodontic treatment in a Swedish population. Endod Dent Traumatol. 1987;3:245-248.
32. Eckerbon M, Anderson JE, Magnusson T. A longitudinal study of changes in frequency and technical standard of endodontics treatment in a Swedish population. Endod Dent Traumatol. 1989;5:27-31.
33. Eckerbon M, Magnusson T, Martinsson T. Prevalence of apical periodontitis crowned teeth and teeth with posts in a Swedish population. Endod Dent Traumatol. 1991;7:214-220.
34. Eriksen HM, Berset GP, Hansen BF, Bjertness E. Changes in endodontic status 1973-1993, among 35-year-olds in Oslo Norway. Int Endod J. 1995;28:129-132.
35. Eriksen HM, Bjertness E. Prevalence of apical periodontitis and results of endodontic treatment in niddle-aged adults in Norway. Endod Dent Traumatol. 1991;7:1-4.
36. Eriksen HM, Bjertness E, Ørstavik D. Prevalence and quality of endodontic treatment in an urban adult population in Norway. Endod Dent Traumatol. 1988;4:122-126.
37. Eriksen HM, Ørstavik D, Keretes K. Healing of apical periodontitis after endodontic treatment

using three different root canal sealers. Endod Dental Traumatol. 1988;4:114-117.

38. Ewald C, Kuhn S, Kalff R. Pyogenic infections of the central nervous system secondary to dental affections – a report of six cases. Neurosurg Rev. 2006;29(2):163-167.

39. Ferraresi A, Yoko Ito, I. Avaliação da concentração inibitória mínima (CIM) e concentração bactericida mínima (CBM) de pasta de hidróxido de calico com p-monoclorofenol canforado e de p-monoclorofenol canforado. Faculdade de Odontologia de Barretos, SP. (Bolsa de Iniciação Científica – Fapesp), 1990.

40. Field JW, Gutmann JL, Solomon ES, Rakusin H. A clinical radiographic retrospective assessment of success rate of single-visit root canal treatment. Int Endod J. 2004;37:70-82.

41. Friedman S, Komorowski R, Mallet W. et al. In vivo resistance of coronally induced bacterial imgress by an experimental glass ionomer cement root canal sealer. J Endod. 2000;26:1-5.

42. Friedman S, Löst C, Zarrabian M, Trope M. Evaluation of success and failure after endodontic therapy using glass ionomer cement sealer. J. Endod. 1995;21:384-390.

43. Fritz V, Wichmenn M. Nachuntersuchieng von wirzel kanalfüllugen aus dens studentischen kursbetrilb. Dtsch Zahnörztiz.1991;96:33-35.

44. Gesi A, Hakeberg M, Warfvinge J, Bergenholtz G. Incidence of periapical lesions and clinical symptoms after pulpectomy – A clinical and radiographic evaluation of 1-versus 2-session treatment. Oral Surg. Oral Méd. Oral Pathol. Oral Radiol. Endod. 2006;101:379-388.

45. Gomes BPFA. et al. Enterococcus faecalis in dental root canals detected by culture and by polymerase chain reaction analysis. Oral Surg. Oral Med. Oral Pathol. Orfal Radiol. Endod. 2006;102:247-253.

46. Goymerac B, Wollard G. Focal infection: a new perspective on an old theory. Gen Dent. 2004;52(4):357-361.

47. Grieve AR, McAndrew RA. A radiographic study of post-retained crowns in patients attending a dental hospital. Br Dent J. 1993;174:197-201.

48. Grossman LI. Endodontic Practice 5ª ed. Lea & Febiger. 1960:341.

49. Haapasalo M, Örstavik D. In vitro infection and disinfection of dentinal tubules. J Dent Res. 1987;66(8):1375-1379.

50. Holland R, Souza V. Ability of a new calcium hydroxide root canal filling material to induce hard tissue formation. J Endod. 1985;12:535-543.

51. Holland R. et al. A comparison of one versus two appointment endodontic therapy in dog's teeth with apical periodontitis. J Endod. 2003;29(3):121-124.

52. Hommez GM, Coppeus CR, De Moor RJ. Periapical health related to the quality of coronal restorations and root filling. Int Endod J. 2002;35:608-609.

53. Hugoson A. et al. Oral health of individuals aged 30-80m years in Jonköping, Sweden, in 1973 and 1983 II. A review of clinical and radiographic findings. Swedish Dental J. 1986;10:175-194.

54. Hülsmann M, Lorch V, Franz B. Untersuching zur Häufigkeit and quality von wurzel füllungen: line. Auswertung UM ortopantomogrammen. Deustsche Zahmarztliche Zeitung. 1991;46:296-299.

55. Imfeld TN. Prevalence and quality of endodontic treatment in an elderly urban population of switzerland. J Endod. 1991;17:604-607.

56. Imura N. et al. Fatores de sucesso em Endodontia: análise retrospectiva de 2.000 casos clínicos. Rev Assoc Paul Cir Dent. 2004;1:29-34.

57. Imura N, Pinheiro ET, Gomes BPFA, Zaia AA, Ferraz CCR, Souza Filho F.J. The outcome of endodontic treatment. A retrospective study of 2000 cases performed by a specialist. J Endod. 2007;33(11):1278-1282.

58. Jiménez-Pinzón JJ. et al. Prevalence of apical periodontitis and frequency of root-filled teeth in adult spanish population. Int Endod J. 2004;37:167-173.

59. Kane AW, Sarr M, Faye B, Wadju N. Long term evaluation of results of endodontic treatments of dental pulp necrosis (74 cases obturated by the monocanal technique). Dakar Med, 1998;43(2):216-219.

60. Katebzadeh N, Hupp J, Trope M. Histological periapical repair after obturation of infected root canal in dogs. J Endod. 1999;25:364-368.

61. Katebzadeh N, Sigurdsson A, Trope M. Radiographic evaluation of periapical healing after obturation of infected root canals: an in vivo study. Int Endod J. 2000;33:60-66.

62. Kazor CE, Mitchell PM, Lee AM, Stoches LN, Loesche WJ, Dewhirst FE, Paster BJ. Diversity of bacterial population on the tongue dorsa of patients with halitosis and healty patients. J Clin Microbiol. 2003;41(2):558-63.

63. Kerblon A, Hasselgren G. The prognosis for endodontic treatment of obliterated root canals. J Endod. 1988;14:565-567.

64. Kirkevang LL, Hörsted-Bindslev P, Ørstavik D, Wenzel A. A frequency and distribution of endodontically treated teeth and apical periodontitis in urban Danish population. Int Endod J. 2001;34:198-205.

65. Kirkevang LL, Ørstavik D, Hörsted-Bindslev P, Wenzel A. Periapical status and quality of root fillings and coronal restoration in a Danish population. Int Endod J. 2000;33:509-515.

66. Kojima K. et al. Success rate of endodontic treatment of teeth with vital and nonvital pulps. A meta-analysis. Oral Surg. Oral Med. Oral Pathol. Oral Radiol. Endod. 2004;97:95-99.

67. Laurell L, Holm G, Hedin M. Tandhälsan vukana i Gävieborgs län. Tandäkartindningen. 1983;75:759-777.

68. Leonardo MR. Contribuição para o estudo dos efeitos da biomecânica e da medicação tópica na desinfecção dos canais radiculares (Tese-Doutorado). Faculdade de Farmácia e Odontologia de Araraquara; 1965.

69. Leonardo MR. Contribuição para o estudo da reparação apical e periapical pós-tratamento de canais radiculares. (Tese-Livre Docência). Faculdade de Odontologia de Araraquara; 1973.

70. Leonardo MR. Endodontia: tratamento de canais radiculares – princípios técnicos e biológicos. São Paulo: Artes Médicas (Divisão Odontológica); 2008.

71. Leonardo MR, Almeida WA, Ito IY, Silva LAB. Radiographic and microbiologic evaluation of post treatment and apical and periapical repair of root canals of dog's teeth with experimentally induced lesion. Oral Surg. Oral Med. Oral Pathol. 1994;78:232-238.

72. Leonardo MR, Almeida WA, Silva LAB, Utrilla LS. Histopathological observations of periapical repair in teeth with radiolucent areas submitted to two different methods of root canal treatment. J Endod. 1995;21(3):137-141.

73. Leonardo MR, Barnett F, Debelian GJ, Pontes Lima RE, Silva LAB. Root canal adhesive filling in dogs' teeth with or without coronal restoration: a histopathological evaluation. J Endod. 2007;33(11):1200-1303.

74. Leonardo MR, Leal JM, Simões Filho AP. Pulpectomy: immediate root canal filling with calcium hydroxide (concept and procedures). Oral Surg. Oral Med. Oral Pathol. 1980;49(5):441-450.

75. Leonardo MR, Rossi MA, Silva LAB, Ito IY, Bonifácio KC. EM evaluation of bacterial biofilm and microorganisms on the apical external root surface of human teeth. J Endod. 2002;28(12):815-818.

76. Leonardo MR, Silva LAB, Almeida WA, Utrilla LS. Tissue response to an epoxy resin-based root canal sealer. Endod Dent Traumatol. 1999;15:28-32.

77. Leonardo MR, Silva LAB, Leonardo RT, Utrilla LS, Assed S. Histological evaluation of therapy using a calcium hydroxide dressing for teeth with incompletely formed apical and periapical lesions. J Endod. 1993;19(7):348-352.

78. Leonardo MR, Silva RAB, Assed S, Nelson Filho P. Importance of bacterial endotoxin (LPS) in Endodontics. J Applied Oral Science. 2004;12(2):93-98.

79. Leonardo MR, Tanomaru Filho M, Silva LAB, Nelson Filho P, Bonifácio KC, Ito IY. In vivo antimicrobial activity of 2% chlorhexidine used as a root canal irrigant solution. J Endod. 1999;25:167-171.

80. Leonardo MR. et al. Scanning electron microscopy of the apical structure of human teeth. Ultra-structural Pathology. 2007;31:321-325.

81. Li X, Kolltveit KM, Tronstad L, Olsen I. Systemic diseases caused by oral infection. Clin Microbiol Rev. 2000;13(4):547-558.

82. Lim GC, Torabinejad M, Kettering J, Limkhardt TA, Finkelman RD. Interleukin 1-beta in symptometric and asymptomatic human periradicular lesions. J Endod. 1994;20(5):225-227.

83. Lin L, Shovlin F, Skribrer J, Langeland K. Pulp biopsies from the teeth associated with periapical radiolucency. J Endod. 1984;10:431-448.

84. Love RM. Enterococcus faecalis – a mechanism for its role in endodontic failure. Int Endod J. 2001;34:399-405.

85. Lupi-Pegurien L. et al. Periapical status prevalence and quality of endodontic treatment in an adult trench population. Int Endod J. 2002;35:690-697.

86. Madison S, Swenson K, Chiles SA. An evaluation of coronal microleakage in endodontically treated teeth. Part II. Sealer types. J Endod. 1987;13:109-112.

87. Marques MD, Morura B, Eriksen HM. Prevalence of apical periodontitis and results of endodontic treatment in an adult, portuguese population. Int Endod J. 1998;31:161-165.

88. Marquis VI, Dao T, Farzaneb M, Abitbol S, Friedman S. Treatment outcome in endodontics: the Toronto study. Phase III: Initial treatment. J. Endod. 2006;32(4):299-306.

89. Matsumoto T, Nagai T, Ida K, Ito M, Kawai Y, Horiba N, Sato R, Nakamura H. Factors affecting successful prognosis of root canal treatment. J Endod. 1987;13:239-242.

90. Moisiadis P. et al. Environmental and normal Fe-SEM evaluation of Endo-Rez leakage inside dentinal tubules MS (Thesis) Catholic University of Leuven Belgiun U.Z. St. Rafael BIOMAT Research Cluster.

91. Molander A, Warfvinge J, Reit C, Kuist T. Clinical and radiographic evaluation of one and two-visit endodontic treatment of asymptomatic necrotic teeth with apical periodontitis: A randomized clinical trial. J Endod. 2007;33(10):1145-1148.

92. Molven O, Halse A. Success rates for gutta-percha and kloroperka N-Ø root fillings made by undergraduate students: radiographic findings after 10-17 years. Int Endod J. 1988;21:243-250.

93. Murphy WK, Kaugars GE, Collett WK, Dodds RN. Healing of periapical radiolucencies after nonsurgical endodontic therapy. Oral Surg. Oral Med. Oral Pathol. 1991;71:620-624.

94. Murray CA, Saunders WP. Root canal treatment and general health: a review of the literature. Int Endod J. 2000;23:1-18.

95. Nair PNR, Henry S, Cano V, Vera J. Microbial status of apical root canal system of human mandibular first molars with primary apical periodontitis after "one visit" endodontic treatment. Oral Surg. Oral Med. Oral Pathol. Oral Radiol. Endod. 2005;99:231-252.

96. Nelson Filho P. Efeito de endotoxina (LPS), associada ou não ao hidróxido de calico, sobre os tecidos apicais e periapicais de dentes de case: avaliação histopatológica. (Tese-Doutorado). Faculdade de Odontologia de Araraquara-UNESP; 2000.

97. Nelson Filho P, Leonardo MR, Silva LAB, Assed S. Radiographic evaluation of the effect of endotoxin (LPS) plus calcium hydroxide on apical and periapical tissues of dogs. J Endod. 2002;28:694-696.

98. Odesjö B, Helldén L, Salonen L, Langeland K. Prevalence of previous endodontic treatment technical standard and occurrence of periapical lesions in a randomly selected adult general population. Endod Dent Traumatol. 1990;6:265-272.

99. Ørstavik D. Time-course and risk analyses of the development and healing of chronic apical periodontitis in man. Int Endod J. 1996;29:150-155.

100. Ørstavik D, Kerekes K, Eriksen HM. Clinical performance of three endodontic sealers. Endod Dent Traumatol. 1987;3:178-186.

101. Ørstavik D, Qvist V, Stoltze K. A multivariate analysis of the outcome of endodontic treatment. Eur J Oral Sci. 2004;112:224-230.

102. Orth K. Der postendodontische therapieerfolg. Eine klinisch röntgenologische nachuntersuchieng von 239 wurzelkanalbebondlugen des studentischen kursbetribles der Universität Mainz (Marter's thesis) – Mainz Germany; 1996.

103. Papa ED. Diseminación de la infección odontogênica: revision de la literatura. Acta Odontol Venez. 2000;28:1.

104. Pappen FG, Souza EM, Giardino L, Leonardo RT, Leonardo MR, Ito IY. Antimicrobial activity of new solutions used in endodontic therapy. G Italiano Endo. 2006;20:211-214.

105. Pashley EL, Myers DR, Pashley DH, Whitford GM. Systemic distribuition of C14 formaldehyde from formocresol treated pulpotomy sites. J Dent Res. 1980;59:503-608.

106. Patel DV, Sherriff M, Ford TRP, Watson TF, Mannocci F. The penetration of Real Seal primer and tubliseal into root canal dentine tubules: a confocal microscopic study. J Endod. 2007;40:67-71.

107. Peters LB, Wesselink PR. Periapical healing of endodontically treated teeth in one and two visits obturated in the presence or absence of detectable microorganisms. Int Endod J. 2002;35:660-667.

108. Petersson K. Endodontic status of mandibular premolars and molars in swedish adults. A reperted cross-sectional study in 1974 and in 1985. Endod Dent Traumatol. 1993;9:185-190.

109. Petersson K, Lewin B, Hakansson J, Olsson B, Wennbery A. Endodontic status and suggested treatment in a population requiring substantial dental care. Endod Dent Traumatol. 1989;5:153-158.

110. Petersson K. et al. Technical quality of root fillings in an adult swedish population. Endod Dent Traumatol. 1986;2:99-102.

111. Pinheiro ET, Gomes BPFA, Ferraz CCR, Sousa ELR, Souza-Filho FJ. Microorganisms from canals of root-filled teeth with periapical lesions. Int Endod J. 2003;36:1-11.

112. Pisano DM, Difiore PM, Mcclanahan SB, Lauterischlager EP, Duncan JI. Intraorifice sealing of gutta-percha obturated root canals to prevent coronal microleakage. J Endod. 1998;24:659-662.

113. Ray HA, Trope M. Periapical status of endodontically treated teeth in relation to the technical quality of the root filling and the coronal restoration. Int Endod J. 1995;28:12-18.

114. Rocha CT, Rossi MA, Leonardo MR, Rocha IB, Nelson Filho P, Silva LAB. Biofilm on the apical region of roots in primary teeth with vital and necrotic pulpar with vital and necrotic pulps with or without radiographically evident apical pathosis. Int Endod J. In press 2008.

115. Rodrigues Araujo Filho W. Tratamento de canais radiculares de dentes desvitalizados realizado em sessão única: avaliação clínica e radiográfi-

ca. (Tese-Doutorado) Faculdade de Odontologia da Universidade de São Paulo; 2003.

116. Rossi A. Interferon-gama, interleucina-10, molécula de adesão celular-1 e receptor de quimiocinas-5 desempenham papel protetor enquanto interleucina-4 não altera o desenvolvimento da lesão periapical experimentalmente induzida em camundongos. Ribeirão Preto, SP: (Tese-Doutorado) – Faculdade de Medicina de Ribeirão Preto-USP (Departamento de Patologia); 2008.
117. Rowe AHR. Problem of intracanal testing of endodontic materials. Int Endod J. 1980;13(2):96-103.
118. Safavi KE, Dowden WE, Langeland E. Influence of delayed coronal permanent restoration on endodontic prognosis. Endod Dent Traumatol; 1987;3:187-191.
119. Saunders WR, Saunders EM, Sadiq J, Cruickshank E. Technical standard of root canal treatment in an adult Scottish sub-population. Brit Dent D. 1997;182:382-386.
120. Shah N. Nonsurgical management of periapical lesions: a prospective study. Oral Surg. Oral Med. Oral Pathol. 1988;66(sup.):365-371.
121. Shimauchi H, Takayama S, Imai-Tanaka T, Okada H. Balance of interleukin-1 beta and interleukin-1 receptor antagonist in human periapical lesions. J. Endod. 1998;24(2):116-119.
122. Shipp AJ, Glick B, Sheetz J, Clark S. Comparison of root canal therapy success rate in patients reporting diabetes with patients denyng diabetes. J Endod. 2004;4:257(Abst. OR-9).
123. Shipper G, Ørstavik D, Teixeira FB, Trope M. An evaluation of microbial leakage in roots filled with a thermoplastic synthetic polymer-based root canal filling material (Resilon). J Endod. 2004;30:342-347.
124. Shipper G, Teixeira FB, Arnold RR, Trope M. Periapical inflammation after coronal microbial inoculation of dog roots filled with gutta-percha or Resilon. J Endod. 2005;31:91-96.
125. Sidaravicius B, Aleksejuniene J, Eriksen HM. Endodontic treatment and prevalence of apical periodontitis in an adult population of vinius, Lithuania. Endod Dent Traumatol. 1999;15:210-215.
126. Silva LAB, Nelson Filho P, Leonardo MR, Rossi MA, Pansani CA. Effect of calcium hydroxide on bacterial endotoxin in vivo. J Endod. 2002;28:94-98.
127. Silva RAB. Hidróxido de cálcio e clorexidina – estudo em cultura de células e em tecido subcutâneo de camundongos. Avaliação da atividade antimicrobiana. (Dissertação-Mestrado) – Universidade de São Paulo-Ribeirão Preto; 2007.
128. Simon JHS. The apex: how critical is it? Gen Dent. 1994;42(4):330-334
129. Sjögren U, Figdor D, Persson S, Sundqvist G. Influence of infection at the time of root filling on the outcome of endodontic treatment of teeth with apical periodontitis. Int Endod J. 1997;30:247-306.
130. Sjögren U, Hägglund B, Sundqvist G, Wing K. Factors affecting the long-term results of endodontic treatment. J Endod. 1990;16:498-504.
131. Smith CS, Setchell DJ, Harty FJ. Factors influencing the success of conventional root canal therapy – a five years retrospective study. Int Endod J. 1993;26:321-332.
132. Soikkonen KT. Endodontically treated teeth and periapical findings in the elderly. Int Endod J. 1995;28:200-203.
133. Spångberg L. Editorial: Endodontics in the era of evidence-based practice. Oral Surg. Oral Med. Oral Pathol. Oral Radiol. Endod. 2003;5:517-518.
134. Spangberg LW. Dr. Kaare Langeland (In Memoriam). Oral Surg, Oral Méd, Oral Pathol, Oral Radiol Endod. 2007;104(3).
135. Stashenko P, Dewhirst FE, Pêros WJ, Kent RL, Ago JM. Synergistic interactions between interleukin 1, tumor necrosis factor, and lymphotoxin in bone resorption. J Immunol. 1987;138(5):1464-1468.
136. Stashenko P, Wang CY, Tani-Ishii N, Yu SM. Pathogenesis of induced rat periapical lesions. Oral Surg. Oral Méd. Oral Pathol. 1994;78(4):494-502.
137. Stashenko P, Yu SM, Wang LY. Kinectics of immune cell and bone resorptive responses to endodontic infections. J Endod. 1992;18:422-426.
138. Sundqvist G. Bacteriological studies of necrotic dental pulps (PhD Thesis) – Uméa University Odontological Dissertation nº 7 – University of Uméa – Suécia; 1976.
139. Sundqvist G, Figdor D, Persson S, Sjögren V. Microbiologic analysis of teeth with failed endodontic treatment and the outcome of conservative retreatment. Oral Surg, Oral Med, Oral Pathol. 1998;85:86-93.
140. Swartz DB, Skidmore AE, Griffin Jr J.A. Twenty years of endodontic success and failure. J Endod. 1983;9(5):198-202.
141. Tanomaru JMG, Leonardo MR, Tanomaru Filho M, Bonetti Filho I, Silva LAB. Effect of different irrigation solution and calcium hydroxide on baterial LPS. Int Endod J. 2003;36:733-739.
142. Tanomaru Filho M, Leonardo MR, Silva LAB. Effect of irrigating solution and calcium hydroxide root canal dressing on the repair of apical and periapical tissues of teeth with periapical lesion. J Endod. 2002;28(4):295-299.
143. Timpawat S, Amonchat C, Trisuwan W. Bacterial coronal leakage after obturation with three root canal sealers. J Endod. 2001;27:36-39.
144. Tronstad L. Recent development in endodontic research. Scand. J Dent Res. 1992;100:52-59.
145. Trope M, Delano EO, Ørstavik D. Endodontic treatment of teeth with apical periodontitis: single vs. multivisit treatment. J Endod. 1999;25:345-350.
146. Wagner KW, Schon R, Schumacher M, Schmelzeisen R, Schulze D. Case report: brain and liver abscesses caused by oral infection with Streptococcus intermedius. Oral Surg, Oral Med, Oral Pathol, Oral Radiol Endod. 2006:102(4):21-23.
147. Wayman BE, et al. A bacteriological and histological evaluation of 58 periapical lesions. J. Endod. 1992;4:152-155.
148. Weiger R, Hitzler S, Hermle C, Löst C. Periapical status quality of root canal fillings and estimated endodontic treatment needs in an urban German population. Endod Dent Traumatol. 1997:13:64-74.
149. Yoshimura et al. 1993. Apud: Kojima K. et al. Success rate of endodontic treatment of teeth with vital and nonvital pulps. A meta-analysis. Oral Surg, Oral Med, Oral Pathol. 2004;47:95-99.
150. Younessi OJ, Walker DM, Ellis P, Dwyer DE. Fatal Staphylococcus aureus infective endocarditis: the dental implications. Oral Surg, Oral Med, Oral Pathol, Oral Radiol Endod. 1998;85(2):168-172.

2

Technological development observed in Endodontics

Mario Roberto Leonardo

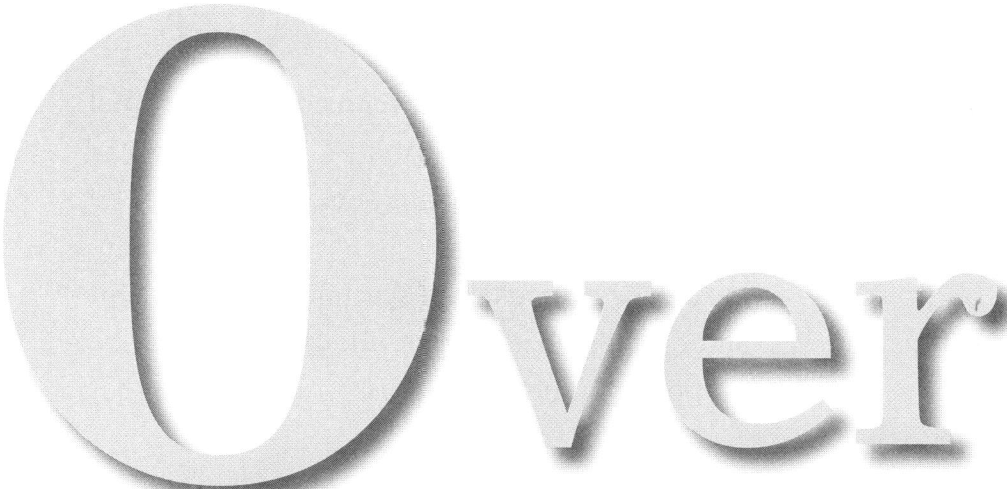

the past few years, **Endodontics** has lived through technological advancements that have reached **technical improvements** never before observed in the history of the specialty. It is important to point out that the majority of these technical developments have been incorporated into the daily activities of endodontists, because they are considered:

RELIABLE*

Most endodontists have already incorporated these technological developments into their daily clinical activities, and having better mastery of them, began to rely on using them and proving their efficiency.

APPLICABLE*

As time went by, the presentation of the new appliances was improved and simplified: electronic foramen locators, re-use of ultrasound, mechanized instrumentation systems (rotary or oscillatory), new root canal filling methods and surgical devices, including the operating microscope. Thus, their application on daily endodontic clinic has become easier and safer.

PREDICTABLE*

With the use of technological development, professionals may hope for a much more favorable prognosis, with painless (silent) post-operative periods and particularly, a higher percentage of post-treatment clinical, radiographic and histologic success.

* Kim S. – Modern endodontic practice: instruments and techniques. Dent Clin IV Amer 48:1-9,2004.

PROFITABLE

Technological development has enabled root canal treatment to become a painless, faster and safer procedure than it was before, providing patients with a greater satisfaction and comfort, translated into economic advantage for the patient as well as the endodontist, who is under less professional stress, and has thus also improved his/her quality of life.

In this chapter, the endodontic technological developments **the authors consider** fundamental for the professional's technical improvement, will be discussed and illustrated in chronological order and also **based on pioneering**, with the aim of raising the status of the professionals in the eyes of their patients and the community.

These goals will be reached by professionals who endeavor to follow this technical development in the correlated literature, in courses to recycle and/or update knowledge, and by those who are able to acquire the technology, and consequently apply it in the difficult task of performing root canal treatment in an ideal manner.

Each of these new technological developments will be described and illustrated in this chapter, which will be sub-divided into sub-chapters written by their respective authors.

TECHNOLOGICAL DEVELOPMENTS IN ENDODONTICS*

1980	Marshall FJ, Pappin J. A crown-down pressureless preparation root canal enlargement technique. (Instrumentação do canal radicular, no sentido coroa/ápice, sem pressão). Oregon Health University. Portland, Oregon USA; 1980. **PREPARATION (DEBRIDEMENT) OF ROOT CANALS IN THE CROWN/APEX DIRECTION (CROWN-DOWN) WITHOUT PRESSURE MODIFIED OREGON TECHNIQUE** *Written by Mario Roberto Leonardo and Marco Aurelio Gagliardi Borges*	**CHAPTER 2-I**
1980	Abou-Rass M, Frank AL, Glick DH. The anticurvature filing method to prepare the curved root canal. (Limagem anticurvatura, no preparo de canais radiculares curvos). J Amer Dent Ass. 1980;101:792-794. **WEARING OR ANTICURVATURE FILING IN THE PREPARATION (DEBRIDEMENT) OF CURVED ROOT CANALS IN MOLARS** *Written by Mario Roberto Leonardo*	**CHAPTER 2-II**

* In the opinion of the authors

1980	Mcspadden JT. Ranson & Randolph – McSpadden compactor: self study course for the thermatic condensation of gutta-percha. (O uso do compactador na condensação termomecânica de guta-percha). Toledo, Ohio, EUA Ranson & Randolph 1980. **GUTTA PERCHA THERMO-PLASTICIZATION TECHNIQUES IN THE FILLING OF ROOT CANAL SYSTEMS** *Written by Miguel Roig Cayón and Fernando Durán-Sindreu Terol*	**CHAPTER 2-III**
1982	Goerig AC, Michelich RJ, Schultz HH. Instrumentation of root canals in molar using the step down technique. (Instrumentação de canais radiculares de molares, usando a técnica step down). J Endod. 1982;12:550-557. **DEBRIDEMENT TECHNIQUE FOR MOLAR ROOT CANAL PREPARATION IN THE CROWN/APEX DIRECTION (STEP-DOWN) MODIFIED GOERIG et al.TECHNIQUE** *Written by Mario Roberto Leonardo and Mario Tanomaru Filho*	**CHAPTER 2-IV**
1989 1994 1998	Yamaoka M, Yamashita Y, Saito T. Electrical root canal measuring instrument based on a new principle – makes measurements possible in wet root canals. Osada Product Information. 1989;6:12(June). Kobayashi C, Suda H. New electronic canal measuring device based on the ratio method. J Endod. 1994;20(3):111-114. Marsreliez CJ. Method and apparatus for apical detection with complex impedance measurement. United States Patent. No 5759159, current U.S. class. 600/547-1998. **ELECTRONIC FORAMEN LOCATORS (THIRD GENERATION)** *Written by Carlos Alberto Spironelli Ramos and Clóvis Monteiro Bramante*	**CHAPTER 2-V**
1989	Buchanan LS. Management of the curved root canal. (Como manejar (vencer as dificuldades) em canais radiculares curvos). J Calif Dent Ass. 1989;17:18-27. **BUCHANAN – PATENCY FILE CONCEPT (1989)** *Written by Mario Roberto Leonardo*	**CHAPTER 2-VI**
1991	Leonardo MR, Leonardo RT. Progressive Neutralization (crown/apex) of the septic-toxic content on the root canal. Chapter 14:214. In: Leonardo MR, Leonardo RT. Endodontics: root canal treatment. (Endodontia: tratamento de canais radiculares) 2nd ed. Ed, Médica Panamericana; 1991. **FORAMINAL DEBRIDEMENT CONCEPTION AND ITS CLINICAL IMPORTANCE** *Written by Mario Roberto Leonardo*	**CHAPTER 2-VII**

1990 Pecora, G. First presentation in the use of the (SOM) Surgical Operating Microscope in surgical endodontics. Annual session of the American Association of Endodontics. Las Vegas, Nevada, EUA; 1990.

1991 Rubinstein RA. New horizons in endodontic surgery. Part I. The operating microscope. Dent Rev. 1991;30:7-19.

1992 Rubinstein RA. New horizon in endodontic surgery. Part II – Periapical ultra sonics and more. Dent Rev. 1992;30:4-10.

1992 Carr GB. Microscopes in endodontics. (O uso do microscópio (cirúrgico) na endodontia). J Calif Dent. Ass. 1992;11:55-61.

PARAENDODONTIC SURGERY WITH A MICROSCOPE **CHAPTER 2-VIII**
Written By Gabrieli Edoardo Pecora, Camila Nicole Pecora and Jamil A. Thibli

1993 Leonardo MR. Safe and easy way to use calcium hydroxide as a temporary dressing. (Maneira fácil e segura para usar o hidróxido de cálcio como curativo de demora). J Endod. 1993;6:319-320.

USE OF CALCIUM HYDROXIDE (CALEN PASTE) AS A TOPICAL MEDICATION BETWEEN SESSIONS (TEMPORARY DRESSING) **CHAPTER 2-IX**
Written by Raquel A. Bezerra da Silva, Léa Assed Bezerra da Silva and Paulo Nelson Filho

1993 McSpadden JT. Une nouvelle approache pour la préparation et l´obturation canalaire: les instruments mecanisés en nickel-titane et la gutta-percha multiphases. (A new technique for root canal preparation and filling: Motor-driven nickel-titanium instruments and gutta-percha thermo-plasticization). Rev France Endod. 1993;1:9-19.

ROTARY SYSTEMS IN ENDODONTICS **CHAPTER 2-X**
Written by Renato de Toledo Leonardo, Carlos Garcia Puente and Maria Guiomar Azevedo Bahia

ENDO-SEQUENCE AND ACTV-GP SYSTEMS **CHAPTER 2-X-1**
Written by Daniel Silva Herzog Flores and Tatiana Ramirez Mora

UNIVERSAL PROTAPER SYSTEM **CHAPTER 2-X-2**
Written by Idomeo Bonetti Filho

TWISTED FILE SYSTEM **CHAPTER 2-X-3**
Written by Richard Mounce and Renato de Toledo Leonardo

1993 Lee SJ, Monsef M, Torabinejad M. Sealing ability of a mineral trioxide for repair of lateral perforations. J Endod. 1993;19:541-544.

USE OF MINERAL TRIOXIDE AGGREGATE (MTA) IN ENDODONTICS **CHAPTER 2-XI**
Written by Clóvis Monteiro Bramante, Ivaldo Gomes de Moraes and Alexandre Silva Bramante

1996	Tyrrel BC. et al. Interpretation of chemically created lesions using direct digital imaging. O uso do sistema de imagem digital na interpretação de lesões induzidas quimicamente. J Endod. 1996;2:74-78. **DIGITAL RADIOGRAPHY IN ENDODONTICS** *Written by Andréa Gonçalves and Marcelo Gonçalves*	**CHAPTER 2-XII**
1997	Carr GB. Ultrasonic root end preparation. (O ultra-som no preparo da retro-obturação). Dent Clin North A Am. 1997;41(3):541-543. **THE REAPPEARANCE OF ULTRASOUND IN ENDODONTICS** *Written By Carlos Alberto Ferreira Murgel*	**CHAPTER 2-XIII**
1998	Mozzo P, Procacci C, Tacconi A, Martini PT, Andreis IA. A new volumetric CT machine for dental imaging based on the cone-beam technique: preliminary results. Eur Radiol. Berlin, v.8(9):1558-64,1998. **COMPUTERIZED TOMOGRAPHY IN ENDODONTICS** *Written By Marco Aurélio Gagliardi Borges*	**CHAPTER 2-XIV**
1998 1999	Khayat BG. The operating microscope. (O microscópio operatório: o emprego da magnificação no tratamento endodôntico). Pract Periodont Aesthet. 1998;1:137. Souza Filho FJ, Teixeira FB. Uso do microscópio em Endodontia (The use of the microscope in Endodontics) In: Pereira Lopes H, Siqueira JR JF. Endodontia (Biologia e Técnica), MEDSI: Rio de Janeiro; 1999:633-650. **THE CLINICAL MICROSCOPE IN CONTEMPORARY ENDODONTICS: WHY KEEP ON SEEING WITH ONE'S FINGERS?** *Written by Francisco J. Souza Filho and Adriana de Jesus Soares*	**CHAPTER 2-XV**
2000	Malamed SF, Gagnon S, Leblanc D. Efficacy of articaine: a new amide local anesthetic. J Am Dent Assoc. 2000;131:635-642. **PAIN CONTROL IN ENDODONTICS (ANESTHETICS)** *Written by Ricardo M. Oliveira-Filho*	**CHAPTER 2-XVI**
2004	Silva LAB, Leonardo MR, Assed S, Tanomaru Filho M. Histological study of the effect of some irrigant solution on bacterial endotoxin in dogs. (Avaliação histologica do efeito de detoxificação (neutralização) de algumas soluções irrigadoras sobre endotoxinas bacterianas). Braz Dent J. 2004;2:104-114. **DETOXIFICATION (NEUTRALIZATION) OF SEPTIC/TOXIC CONTENT (ENDOTOXINS) IN THE TREATMENT OF ROOT CANALS WITH PULP NECROSIS AND EVIDENT PERIAPICAL LESION** *Written by Mario Roberto Leonardo and Léa Assed Bezerra da Silva*	**CHAPTER 2-XVII**

2005	Garcia Puente C, Saavedra J. Microscópio em Endodontia (Microscope in Endodontics). In: Leonardo MR. Endodontics: tratamento de canais radiculares – princípios técnicos e biológicos. 4ª ed. Artes Médicas: São Paulo; 2005:1451-1491. **ERGONOMICS IN THE USE OF THE OPERATING AND SURGICAL MICROSCOPE IN ENDODONTICS** *Written by Carlos Garcia Puente and Juan Saavedra*	**CHAPTER 2-XVIII**
2005	Fisher D. Root canal preparation with Endo-Eze AET: changes in root canal shape assessed by microcomputed tomography. (Preparo do canal radicular com Endo-Eze AET: alterações na forma do canal, avaliadas pela tomografia microcomputadorizada). Int Endod J. 2005;38(7):456-464. **OSCILLATORY DEBRIDEMENT – AET SYSTEM (ANATOMIC ENDODONTIC TECHNOLOGY) – ENDO-EZE** *Written by Renato de Toledo Leonardo and Fábio Luiz Camargo Villela Berbert*	**CHAPTER 2-XIX**
2007	Tay FR, Pashley DH. Monoblocks in root canals: a hypothetical or a tangible goal. (Monobloco nos canais radiculares: uma meta hipotética ou real). J Endod. 2007 Apr;33(4):391-8. Leonardo MR, Barnett F, Debelian GJ, Pontes Lima RF, Silva LAB. Root canal adhesive filling in dog´s teeth with or without coronal restorations: a histopathological evaluation. (Técnicas adesivas de obturação do canal radicular de dentes de cães, com ou sem restauração coronária: avaliação histopatológica). J Endod. 2007;33(11):1299-1303. **ADHESIVE TECHNIQUES FOR ROOT CANAL FILLING** **A.D.O. System ("Apical Delivered Obturation") – Endo-Rez** *Written by Renato de Toledo Leonardo, Cornelius Palmeijer and Marco Aurélio Gagliardi Borges*	**CHAPTER 2-XX**
2007	AMERICAN COLLEGE OF CARDIOLOGY AND AMERICAN HEART ASSOCIATION TASK FORCE ON PRACTICE GUIDELINES. Manual for ACC/AHD guideline writing committees: Methodologies and policies from ACC/AHD. Task Force on Practice Guidelines; 2007. **Bacterial Endocarditis Prevention** *Written by Ricardo M. Oliveira-Filho* **Pain control in Endodontics (ANALGESICS AND ANTI-INFLAMMATORY medications)** *Written by Ricardo M. Oliveira-Filho*	**CHAPTER 2-XXI** **CHAPTER 2-XXII**

2.1

Preparation (debridement) of root canals in crown/apex direction (Crown-Down) without pressure

Oregon Technique[5] (Modified)

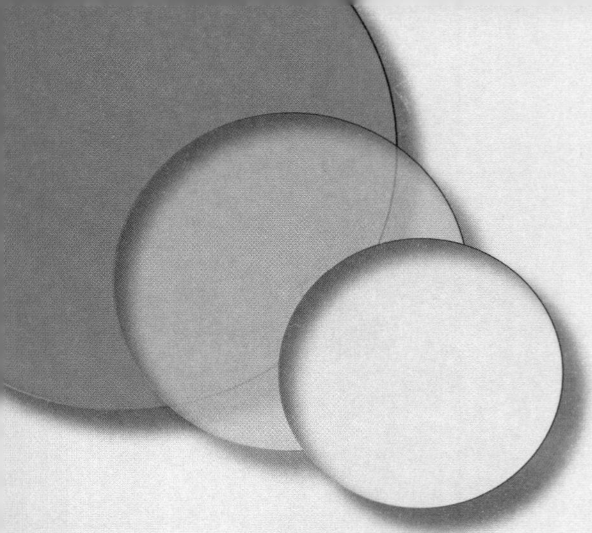

Mario Roberto Leonardo
Marco Aurélio Gagliardi Borges

The pioneers Marshall & Pappin[5] caused a veritable impact on endodontists when they published a **new concept in root canal instrumentation** (debridement). The authors changed an established technique used for ± 160 years, the apex/crown principle, which has been responsible for post-operative sequelae such as "acute apical periodontitis", particularly in cases of pulp necrosis (gangrene).

Their new principle of crown/apex root canal instrumentation without pressure, was offered by means of the **pioneering** OREGON techniques in 1980[5], and shortly thereafter described by Goerig et al.[4], in 1982. While initially these techniques only had an impact on endodontists, currently they are included in the curriculum of all Dental Schools in the world, instead of the obsolete preparation technique using the apex/crown principle.

This new preparation principle, which begins in the cervical and middle thirds of the root canal with large diameter files (D_1), is complemented with Gates Glidden drills. After this it advances with files in an apical direction, gradually and sequentially diminishing their diameters (D_1) until the temporary working length (TWL) is achieved. After that the working length is determined, in cases called by us as NECROPULPECTOMIES I (root canal treatment of teeth with pulp necroses without radiographically periapical lesions) up to the real working length (RWL), and in cases called by us as NECROPULPECTOMIES II (root canal treatment of teeth with pulp necroses with evident radiographically periapical lesion – APICAL PERIODONTITIS) up to the real tooth lenght (RTL). With this technique, root canals are practically clean and conform in taper throughout their full extent.

The crown/down principle without pressure is based on previous studies, by Brilliant & Christie[1] and Coffae & Brilliant[2], published in 1975, and Mullaney[7], in 1979. In subsequent years it was also mentioned by other authors such as De Deus[3], in 1982, Morgan & Montgomery[6], in 1984, Ruiz-Hubard et al.[8], in 1987 and Valdrighi et al.[9], in 1991. This new concept was incorporated into debridement techniques mainly because it avoids extrusion of infected residues, microorganisms and their by-products, such as **endotoxins**, into the periapical area, thus considerably reducing painful post-operative complications (acute apical periodontitis) as well as avoiding the causing Fenix abscesses (flare-up), which can seriously affect the image and perception of the patient towards the practitioner.

As mentioned before, these techniques are included in the endodontic curriculum in all Dental Schools that use the mechanical/manual technique alone, or as a prerequisite for later use of rotary and/or oscillatory systems in cases of Necropulpectomy I and II.

We use the technique with slight modifications, but we have kept the names of the authors out of respect for their pioneering work. The modifications we have made refer to the terminology used today as well as to the fact that originally, the OREGON technique was only used for straight root canals, while we indicate it for curved molar root canals as well, by altering the kinetics of instrument use. Thus, when we use pre-curved files in the curved portion of the root canal, we do not apply rotational movements; but rather when we feel resistance, we apply "tentative rotation", followed by lateral friction against the canal walls, and afterwards, small-amplitude, repetitive back and forth movements. In the curved portion of the root canal, a pre-curved instrument used with rotational movements, such as used for straight canals according to the original technique, can cause changes in its anatomic configuration.

OREGON TECHNIQUE[5] (MODIFIED)
(Technical Sequence)

Main indication: Necropulpectomy II

Other indications: Necropulpectomy I

Action principle: Crown/apex without pressure ("Crown-Down Pressureless Technique")

Original recommendation: Straight and wide or relatively wide root canals

Modified technique: Straight and/or curved atresic root canals of molars

Recommendations: To remove and "neutralize" the toxic/septic content of the root canals before biomechanical preparation and/or use of rotary systems which do not offer radial land.

Technical sequence – Necropulpectomy II in the mandibular second pre-molar with a single canal

Note: When mandibular pre-molars with pulp necrosis (gangrene) and evident periapical lesion have a single canal, they have a larger volume of endodontic space, and consequently, a higher concentration of endotoxins which, in addition to the action of gravity, make them teeth with the greatest possibility of developing acute chronic periapical lesions (Fenix abscess/Flare-up).

1st Session

1. Organization of the clinical working tray (Figs. 2.I-1A-B), including:

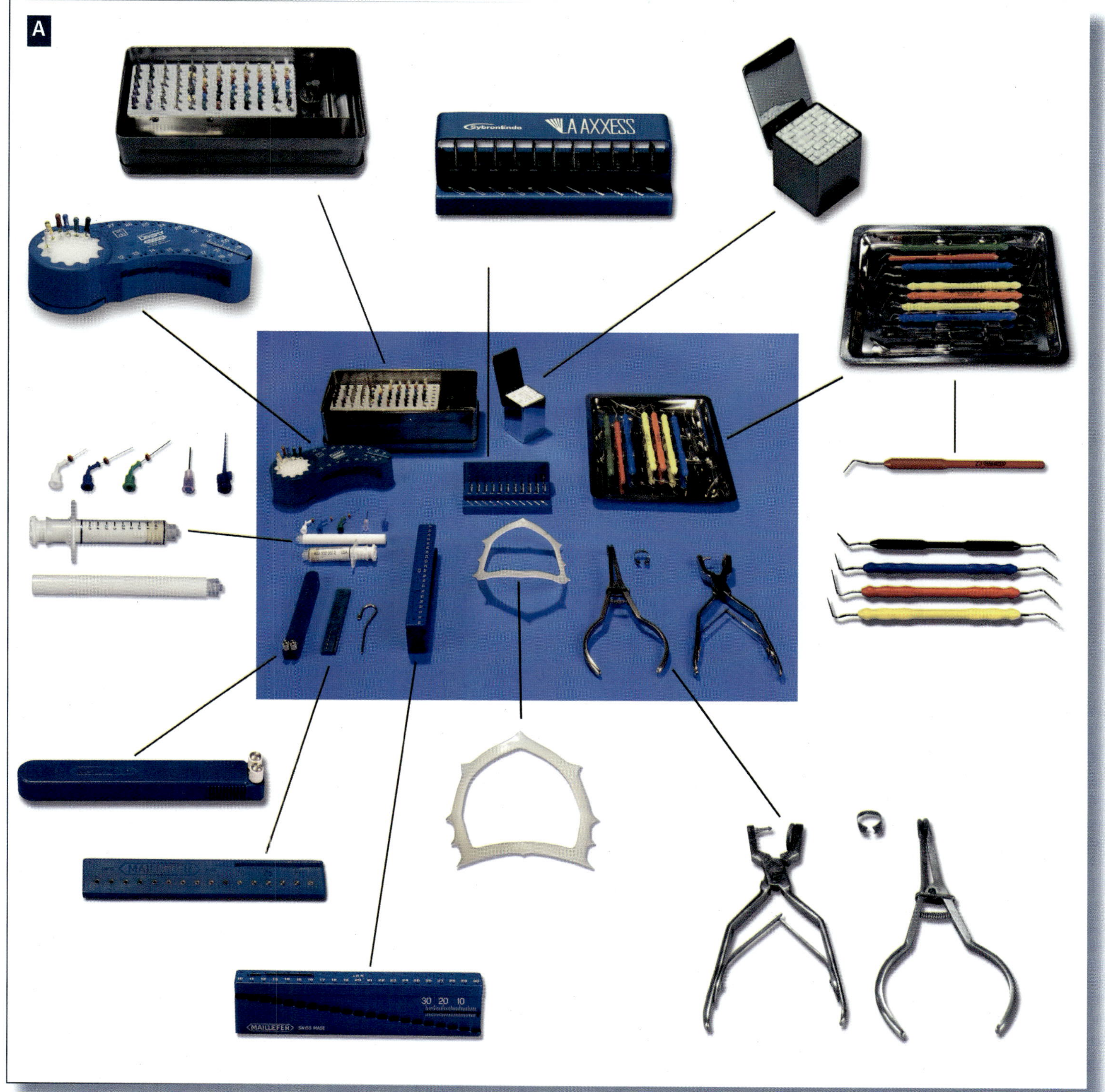

FIG. 2.I-1A

Clinical set up (Sterilized instruments and materials).

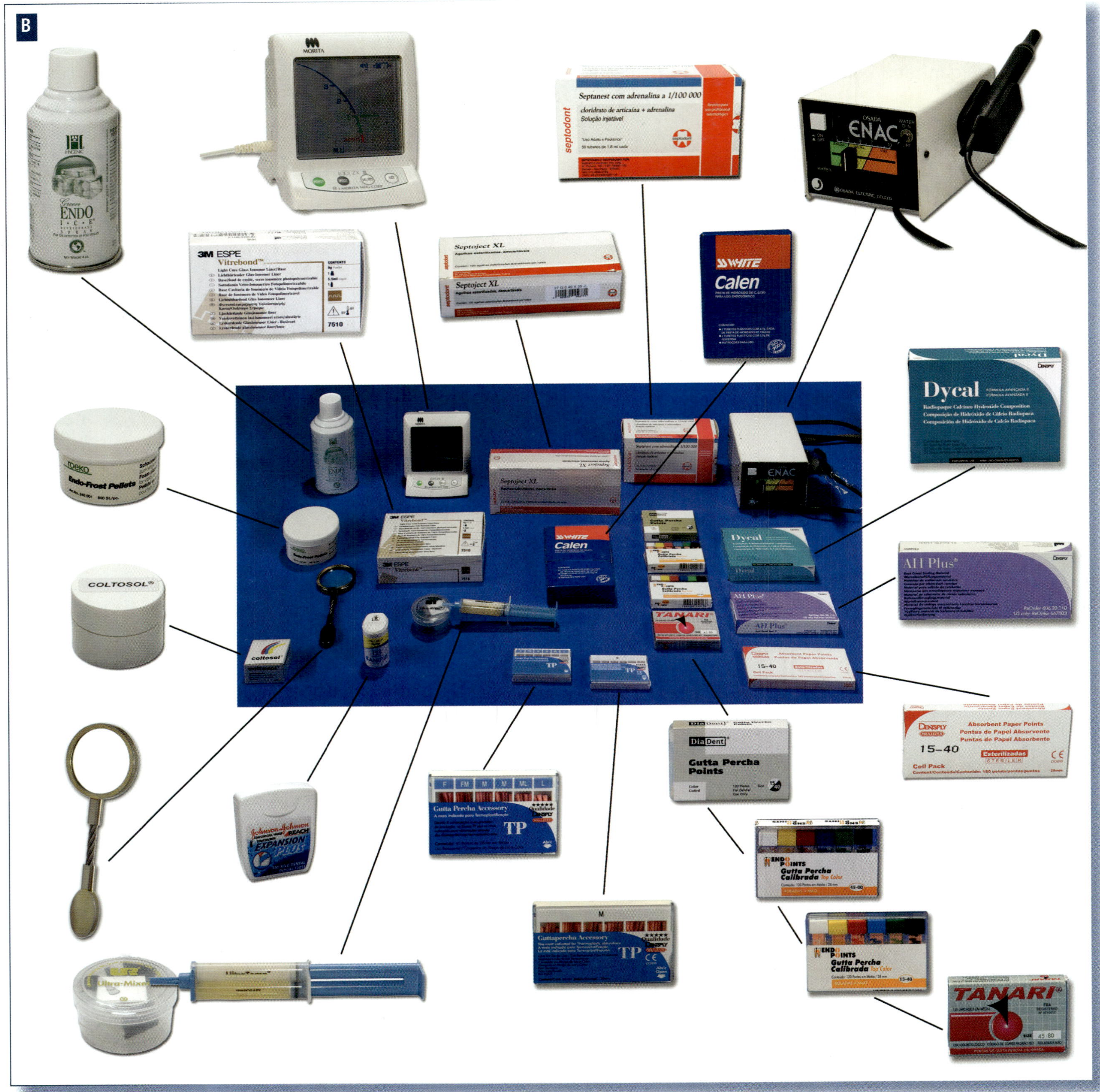

FIG. 2.I-1B

Auxiliary set up (equipment and non-sterilized material).

1.1 Radiograph for diagnosis (Fig. 2.I-2).

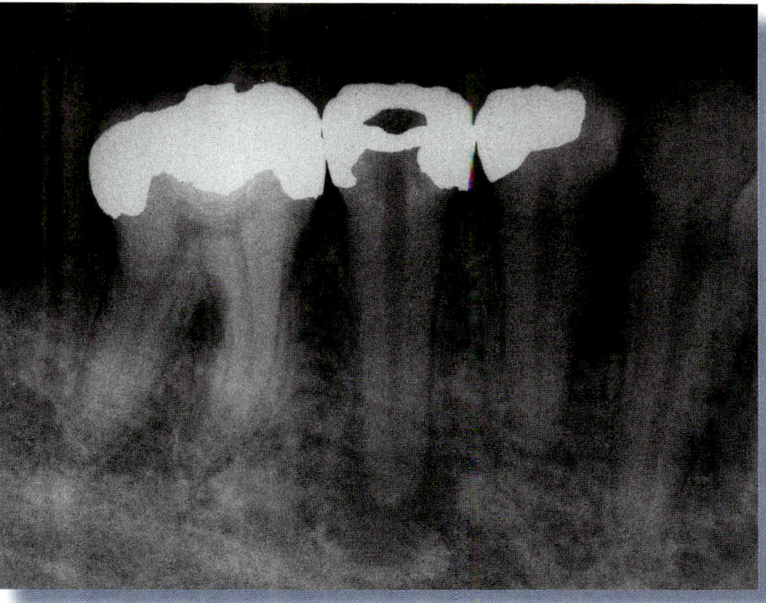

FIG. 2.I-2
Radiograph for diagnosis.

1.2 Selection and organization of stainless steel Type K files (Colorinox – Dentsply/Maillefer) with numbers compatible for the cervical, middle and apical thirds of the root canal, from the largest diameter (L.K. No 80) to the smallest diameter (L.K. No 15). In addition, Gates Glidden drills No 2, 3, 4 and 5 (Fig. 2.I-3).

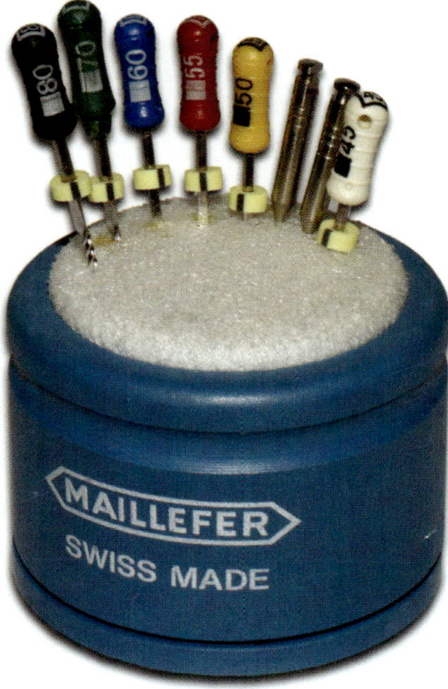

FIG. 2.I-3
"Clean – Stand"* with type K files and Gates Glidden drills.

2. Mouth rinse for the oral cavity with antiseptic.

3. Clinical Examination (Fig. 2.I-4).

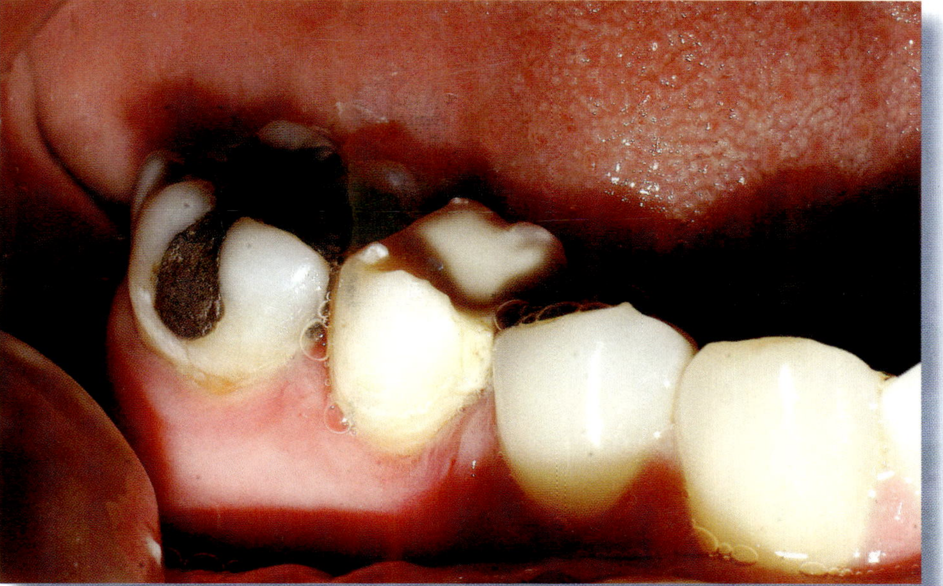

FIG. 2.I-4
Clinical examination.

4. Radiographic diagnosis of the case: Circumscribed rarefaction osteitis with diagnosis suggesting apical granuloma.

5. Indication: Necropulpectomy II.

6. Endodontic treatment planning.
   6.1 Determining the apparent tooth length (ATL) measured on the radiograph used for diagnosis (Fig. 2.I-5).
      6.2.1 Determining temporary working length (TWL). ATL = 22 mm - 2 mm = TWL (20 mm).
   6.3 The files should be sequentially organized from the largest to the smallest diameter. The Gates Glidden drills Nos. 2, 3, 4 and 5 in the TWL. e.g.: ATL = (22 mm) - 2 mm (safety measurement) = TWL (20 mm) (Fig. 2.I-6).

* Dentsply/Maillefer – Ballaigues – Switzerland.

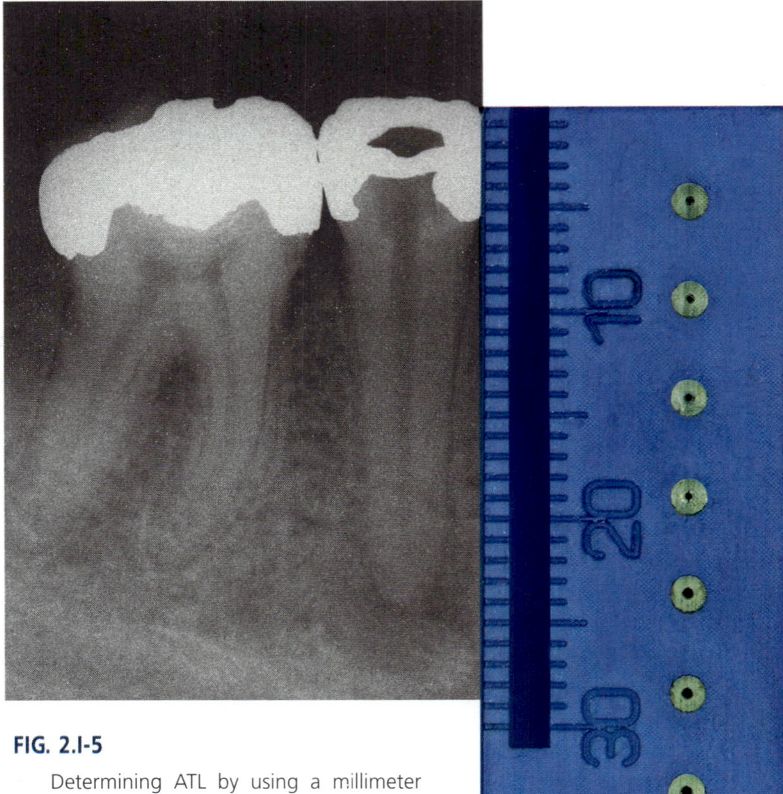

FIG. 2.I-5
Determining ATL by using a millimeter ruler on the radiograph for diagnosis.

6.4 Observe the radiograph for diagnosis and estimate the approximate diameter of the access to the root canal.

7. Placement of the rubber dam clamp (Fig. 2.I-7).

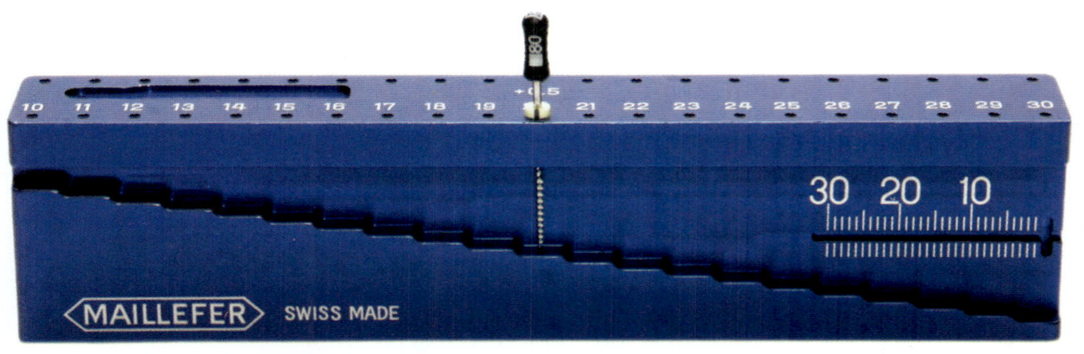

FIG. 2.I-6
Adjusting the type K file at the TWL.

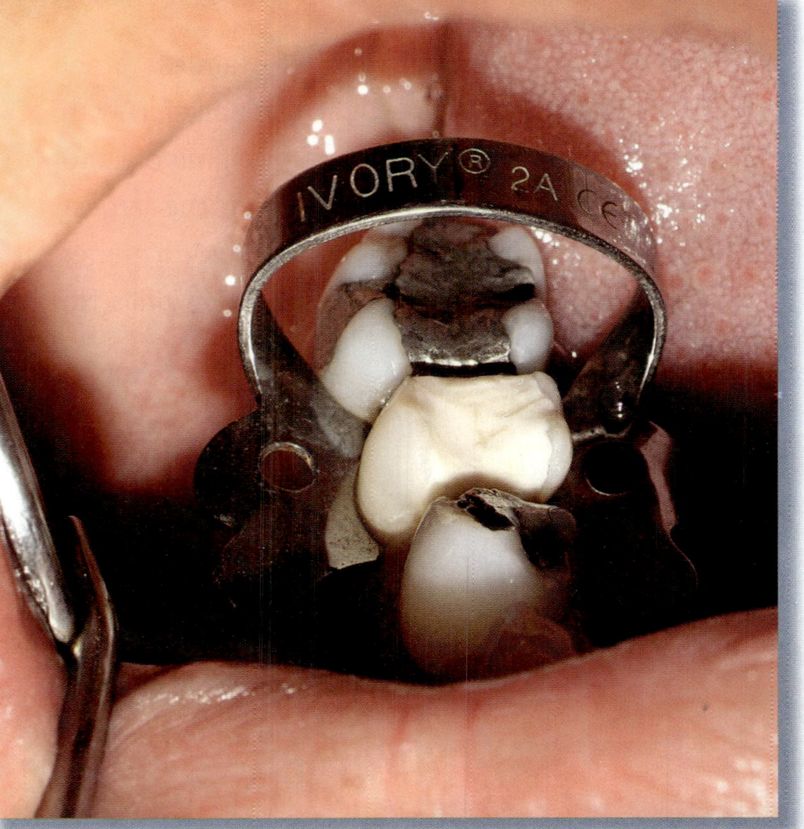

FIG. 2.I-7
Placing the rubber dam clamp.

8. Isolation of tooth with rubber dam.

8. Disinfection of the operative area with 2% chlorhexidine gluconate after placement of rubber dam (Fig. 2.I-8).

9. Gaining access through the glass ionomer filling (VIDRION-R)* using a high speed round bur (Figs. 2.1-9 and 2.1-10A).

10. Acccessing the pulp chamber (2.I-10B).

    10.1. Additional widening of the access cavity. Fig. 2.1-11 shows the access opening to the pulp.

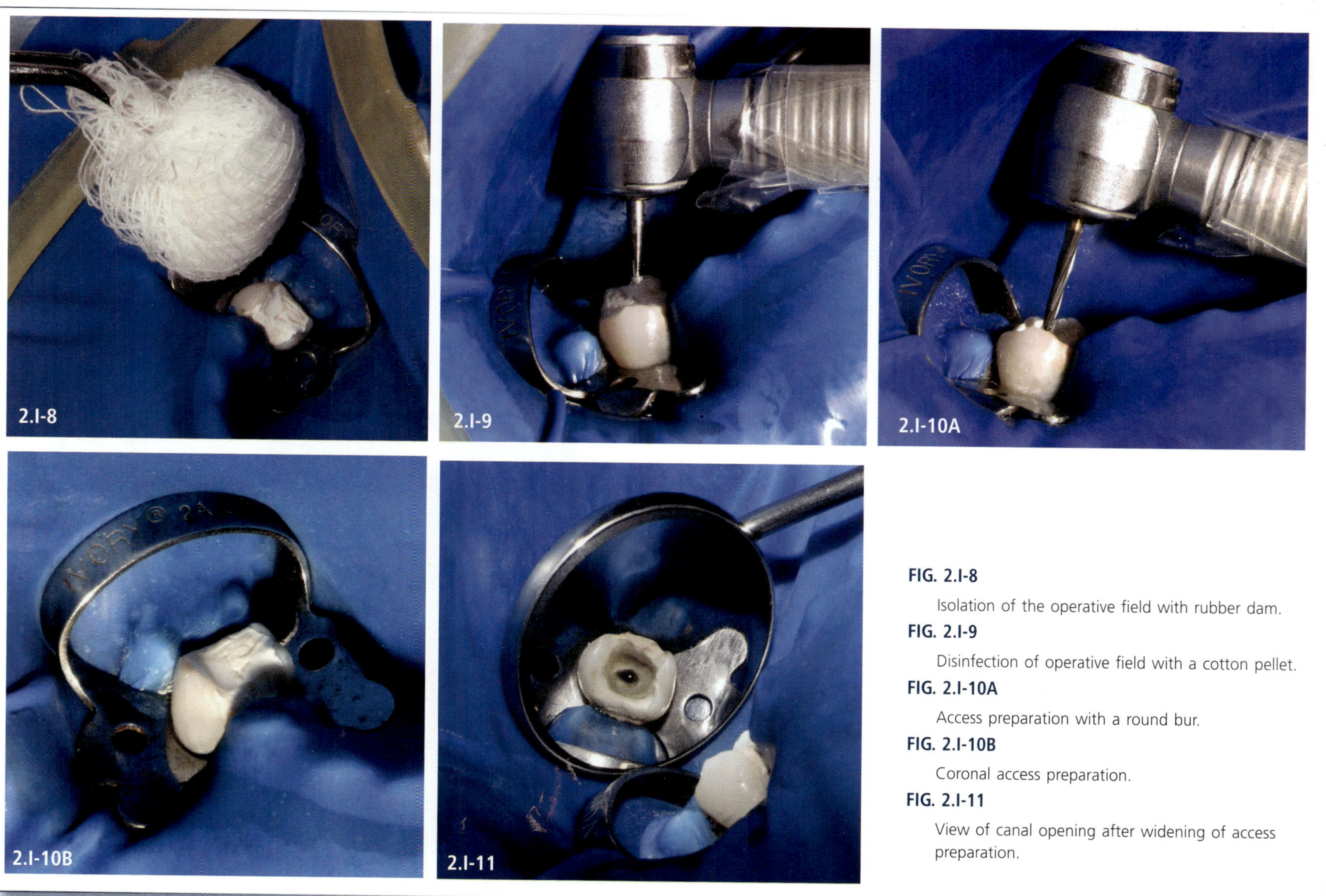

FIG. 2.I-8
Isolation of the operative field with rubber dam.

FIG. 2.I-9
Disinfection of operative field with a cotton pellet.

FIG. 2.I-10A
Access preparation with a round bur.

FIG. 2.I-10B
Coronal access preparation.

FIG. 2.I-11
View of canal opening after widening of access preparation.

*S.S.White – Artigos Dentários Ltda. Rio de Janeiro, RJ, Brazil.

11. Copious irrigation of the pulp chamber and root canal with a concentrated solution of 5.25% sodium hypochlorite (USP) or double-strength chlorinated soda (4-6%) (Fig. 2.I-12).

12. Examination of the root canal entrance with an endodontic explorer (12F Dentsply/Maillefer). (Confirm and remember the location and diameter of the root canal entrance) (Figs. 2.I-12A-B).

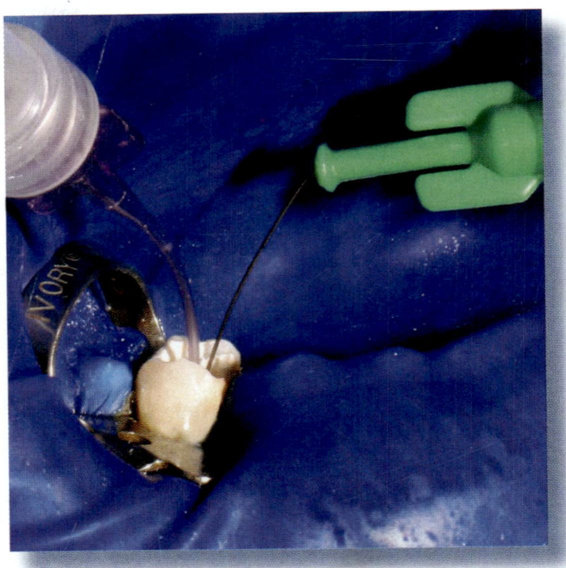

FIG. 2.I-12

Abundant irrigation with Irrigation needles (Ultradent* NaviTips).

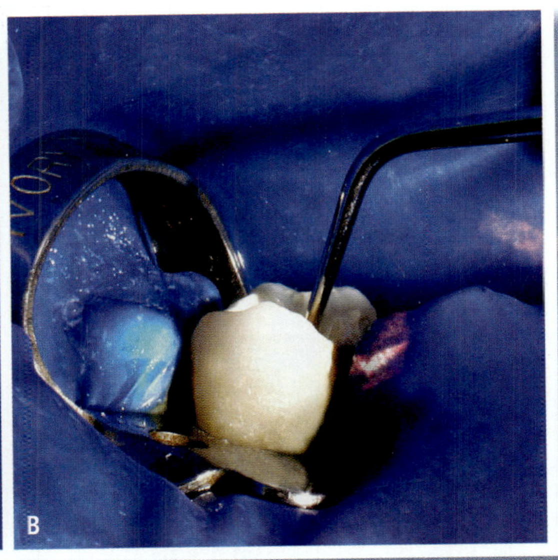

FIGS. 2-I-13A-B

A – Exploration of the access opening.
B – Exploration of the canal entrance.

13. Passive placemen of the Type K file, number 80 (compatible with the diameter of the root canal entrance), until resistance is felt (Fig. 2.I-14).

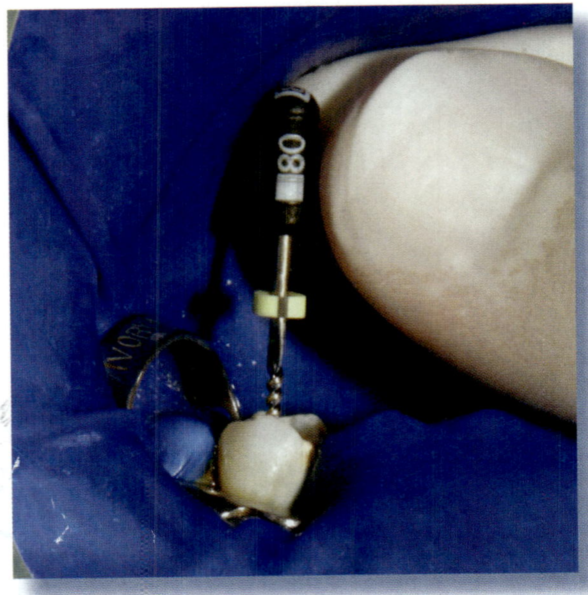

FIG. 2.I-14

Passive insertion of the type K file No 80.

* Ultradent Products, Inc. South Jordan, UTAH, USA.

13.1 Turn the No. 80 file clockwise without pressure until it locks in place.

13.2 Apply lateral pressure to the root canal walls with continuous small-amplitude up-and down motion.

13.3 Repeat the previous maneuver (item 13.2) until a complete turn can be made without the type K file No. 80 getting locking in.

14. Repeat previous procedures with files of subsequently smaller diameters (= smaller numbers) (Nos. 70, 60, 55, 50), progressing in a crown/apex direction, without pressure, up to the TWL. (Figs. 2.I-15, 16, 17, 18).

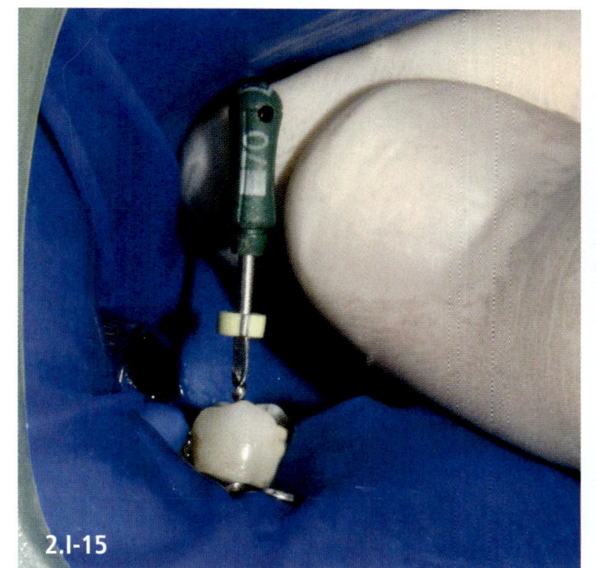

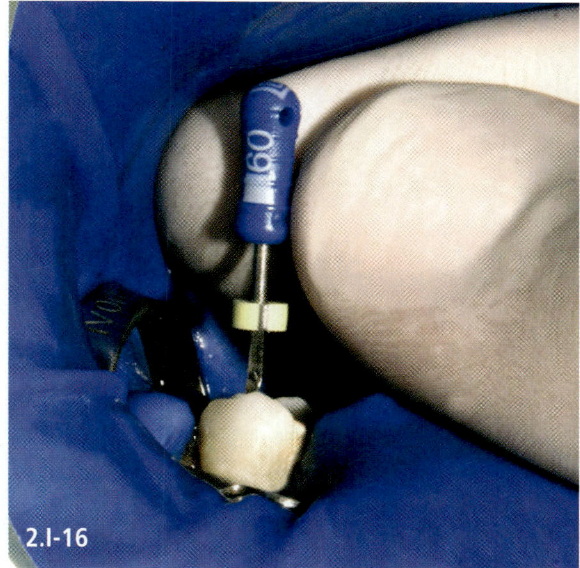

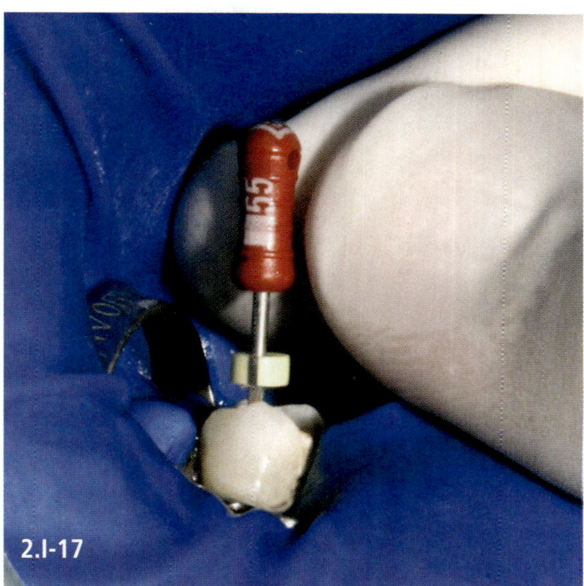

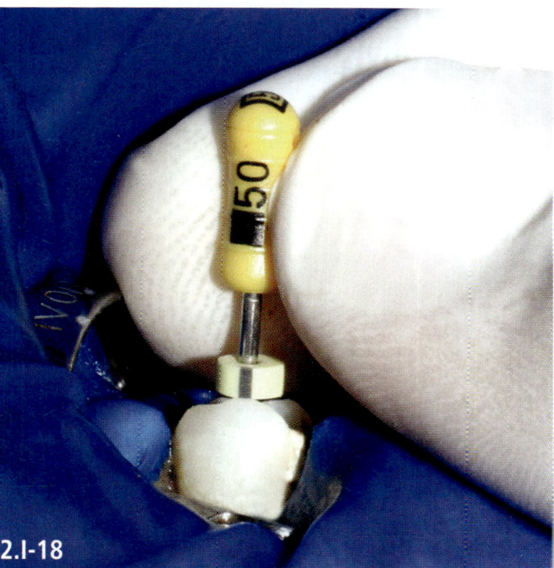

FIG. 2.I-15
Passive insertion of the type K file No 70.

FIG. 2.I-16
Passive insertion of the type K file No 60.

FIG. 2.I-17
Passive insertion of the type K file No 55.

FIG. 2.I-18
Passive insertion of the type K file No 50, attaining the TWL.

15. After use of the type K file No 50 or when the TWL is reached, use Gates Glidden drills No 2, 3 and 4 and, if possible (depending on the canal diameter) a No. 5 (Figs. 2.I-19 and 20).

16. Irrigate the root canal abundantly after using the Gates Glidden drills. **From now on** use Labarraque solution (2.5% sodium hypochlorite solution) (Fig. 2.I-21).

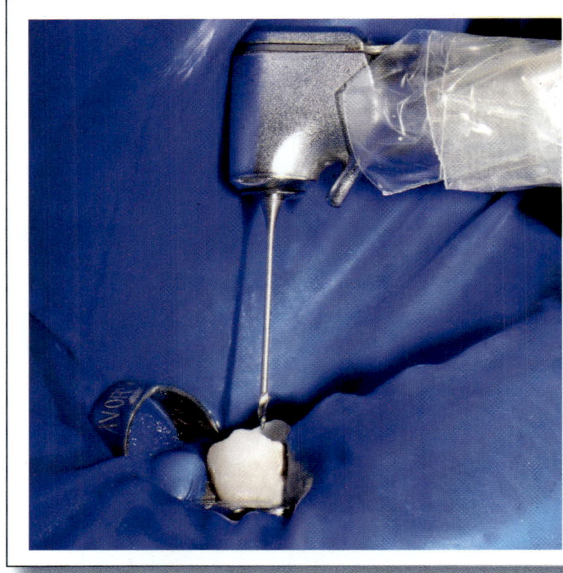

FIG. 2.I-19
Use of Gates Glidden No 3.

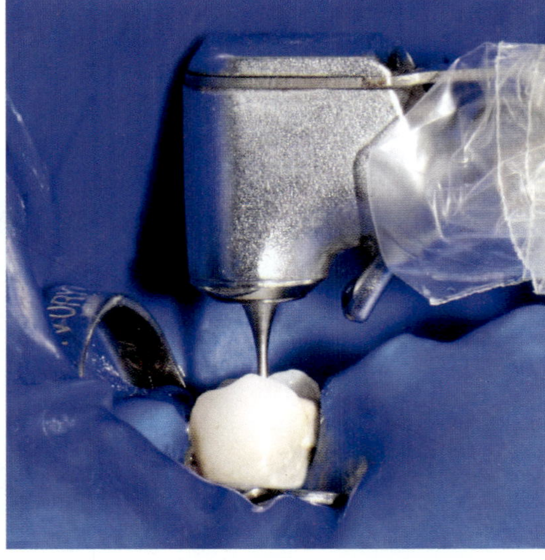

FIG. 2.I-20
Use of Gates Glidden No 4.

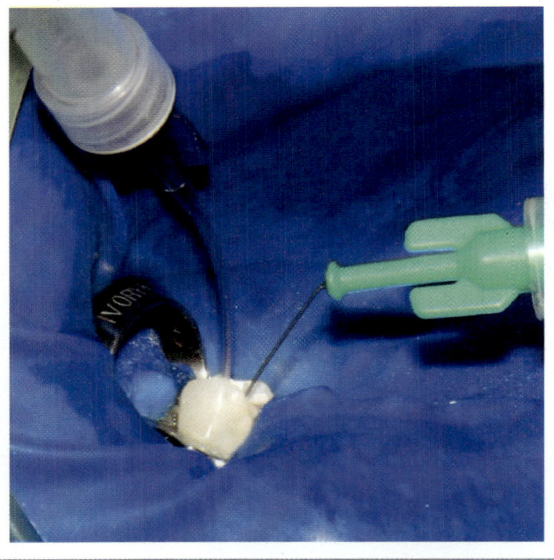

FIG. 2.I-21
Abundant irrigation with Ultradent NaviTip.

Note: In cases of short roots that are wide with straight canals, always use the Gates Glidden drills with a stop (made of silicone) and determine the TWL.

Irrigate/aspirate/flood the root canal after use of each file.

Always pay attention to the working length of the root; that is, the TWL.

Note: The possibility of a sudden reduction in the root canal diameter, which frequently occurs in mandibular premolars, does not always allow the sequential use of these files, and one may go from No. 45, for example, to No. 20 or even 15.

17. Working length determination – to obtain the real tooth length (RTL) and after this, the real working length (RWL) (Figs. 2.I-22 and 23A-C).

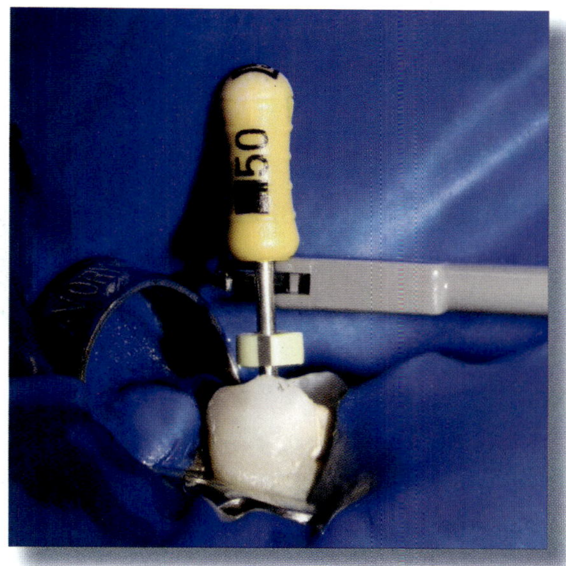

FIG. 2.I-22
Working length determination with electronic apex locator.

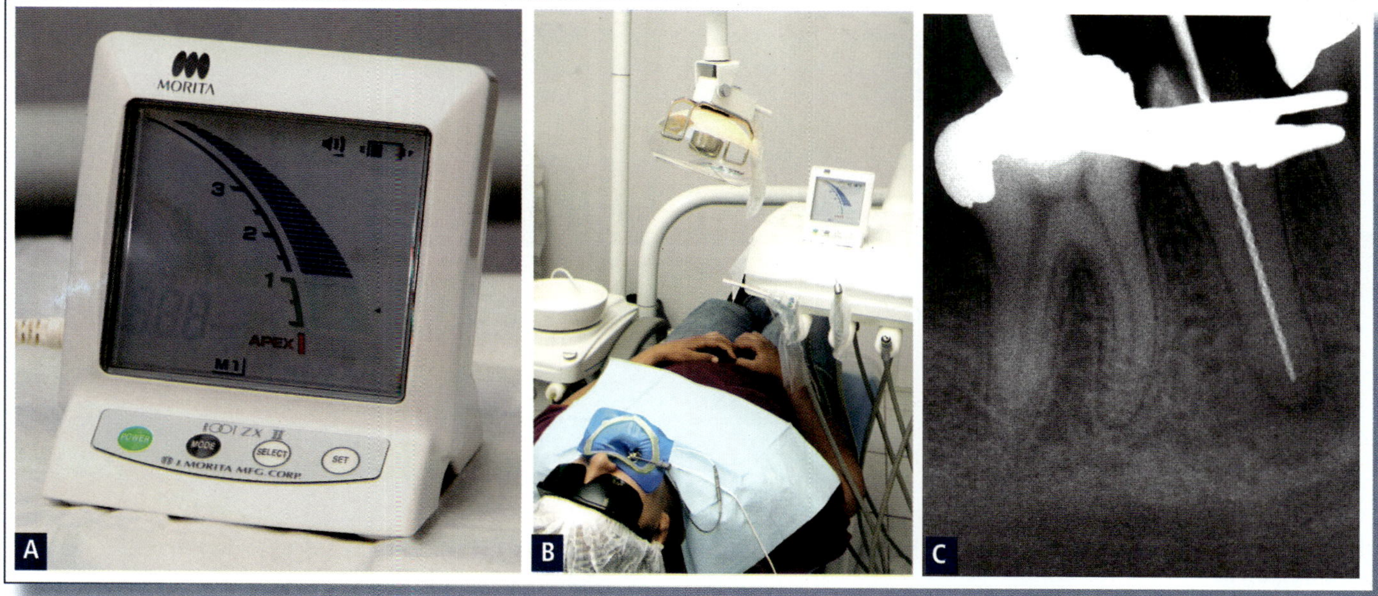

FIGS. 2.I-23A-C
A – Root ZX II* electronic apex locator.
B – Root ZX II loop placed in patient's mouth.
C – Radiograph to confirm working length.

* J. Morita MFG. Corp – Japan.

18. Irrigation/aspiration/flooding (copious amounts).

19. Continue with disinfecting in a crown/apex direction, up to RTL.

Note: In the curved portion of a root canal, pre-curve the files but do not use rotary movements. In these cases, one must only make tentative rotations and lateral friction against the root canal walls, followed by small-amplitude repetitive back and forth movements on all the root canal walls.

20. To reach TWL, identify the Foramen Apical Instrument (FAI) (Figs. 2.I-24A-B).

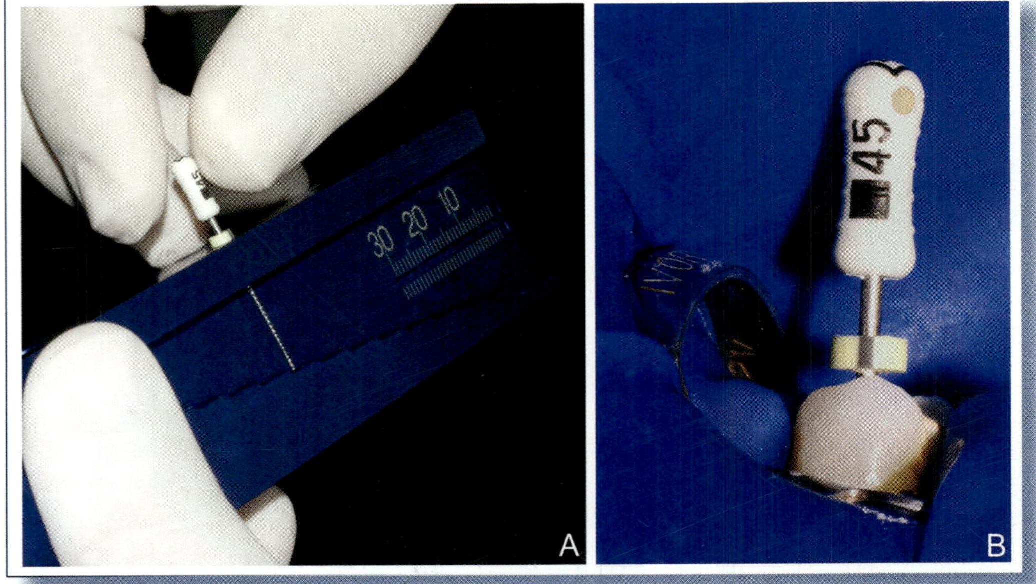

FIGS. 2.I-24A-B

A – Adjustment of file for the working length.
B – Foraminal Apical Instrument for debridement.

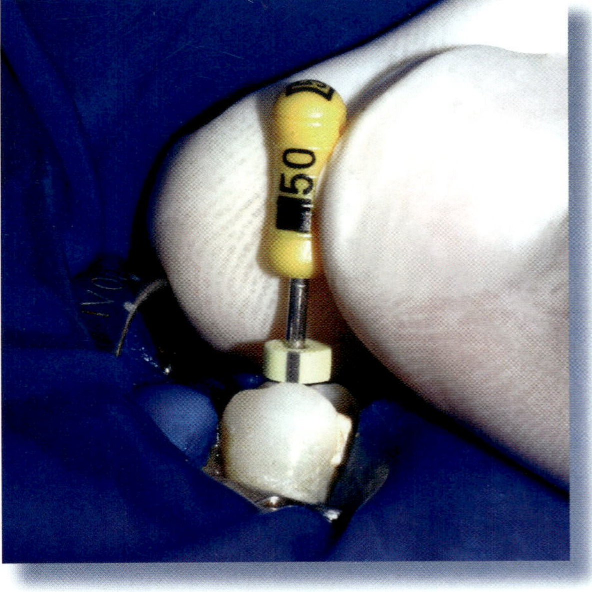

FIG. 2.I-25

Determining the apical stop, starting with type K file No 50.

21. Foramen debridement.

22. Identification of the Initial Apical Instrument (IAI) (Fig. 2.I-25).
    22.1 Make the apical stop, 1 mm short of the RTL.

23. Complement the apical stop with 2 or 3 instruments above IAI, at the RWL, reaching the memory instrument (MI), type K file No 60 (Figs. 2.I-26 and 27).

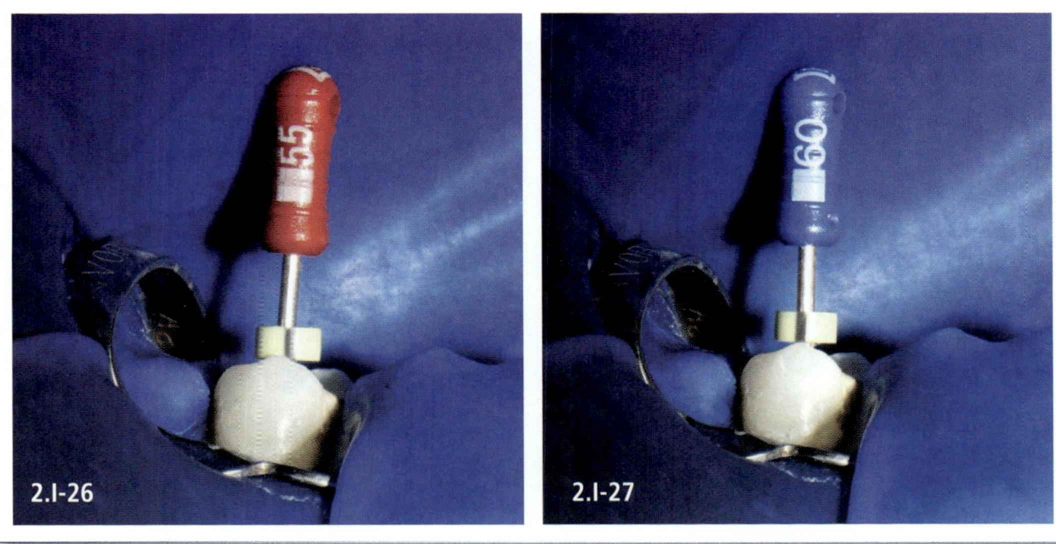

2.I-26
2.I-27

FIG. 2.I-26

Verification of apical stop with a type K file No 55.

FIG. 2.I-27

Finalizing apical stop. Type K file No 60 (memory instrument).

23.1 Use the FAI during this step (Fig. 2.I-28).

Note: Irrigate the root canal abundantly after use of each file.

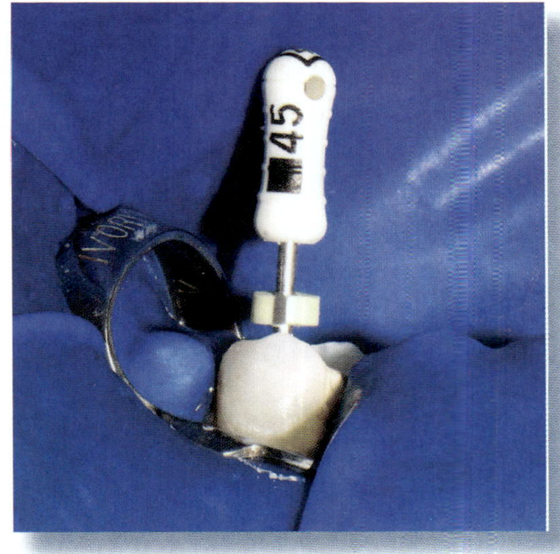

FIG. 2.I-28

Repeating with Foraminal Apical Instrument (FAI).

24. Use the step-back technique (from the apical stop up to the root canal diameter obtained by Gates Glidden drill) with type K files No 70 and 80. Reuse FAI during this procedure (Figs. 2.I-29A-B).

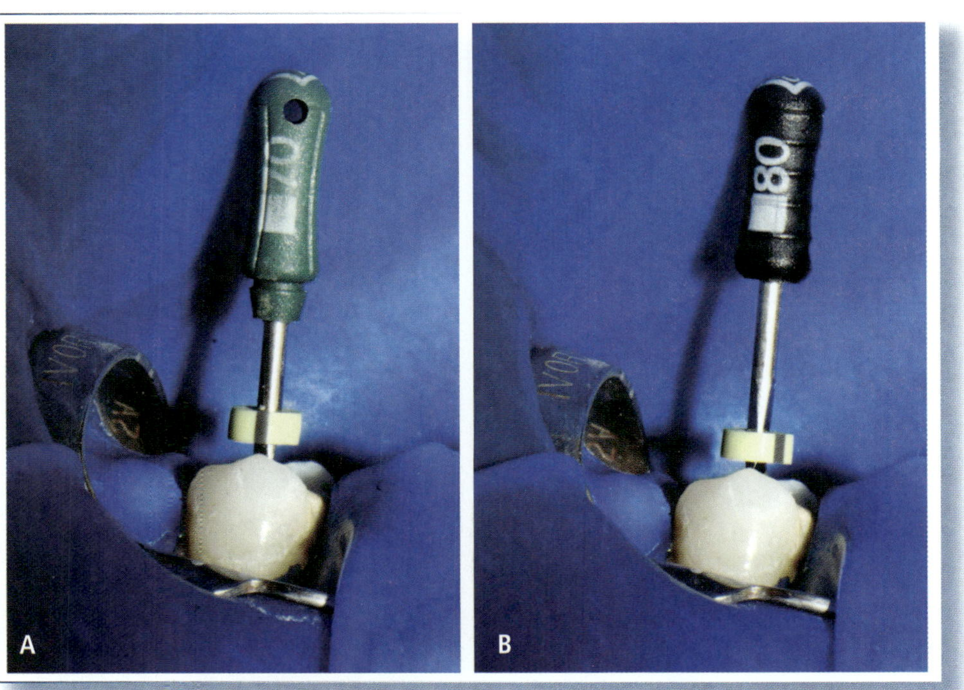

A
B

FIGS. 2.I-29A-B

A – Step-back with type K file No 70.
B – Step-back with type K file No 80.

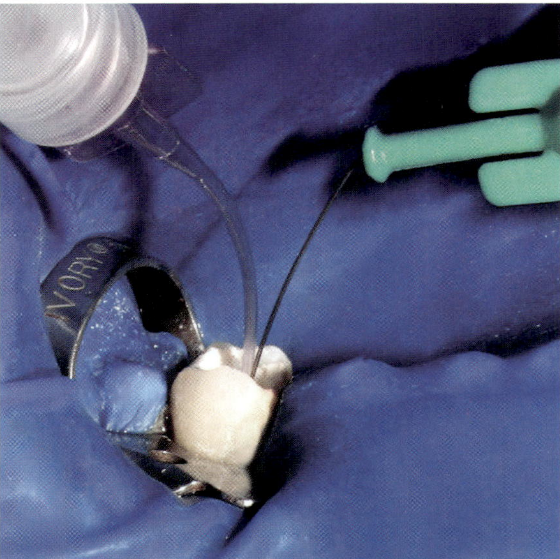

FIG. 2.I-30
Abundant irrigation with Ultradent NaviTip.

25. Irrigation/aspiration/drying of root canal with 2.5% sodium hypochlorite solution (Labarraque solution) (Fig. 2.I-30).

26. Apply ultrasound to remove smear layer (Figs. 2.I-31A-B).

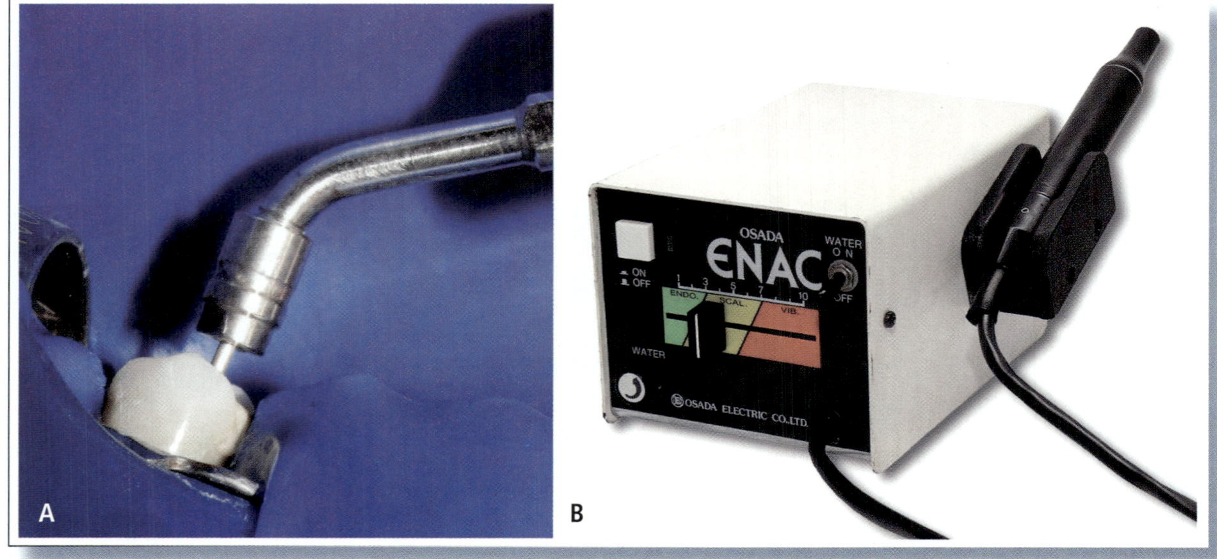

FIGS. 2.I-31A-B
A – Irrigation with ultrasound.
B – Enac* ultrasound unit.

27. Aspiration/drying with a capillary tip (Fig. 2.I-32) and sterile paper points.

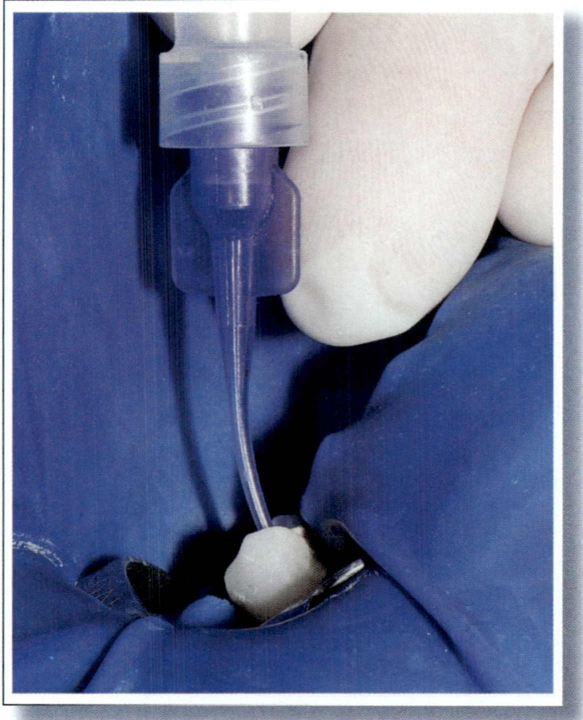

FIG. 2.I-32
Aspiration with Capillary Tip (Ultradent).

* Osada Eletric Co. Ltda., Japan.

28. Placement of the temporary dressing (Calen/PMCC) (Figs. 2.I-33A-H).

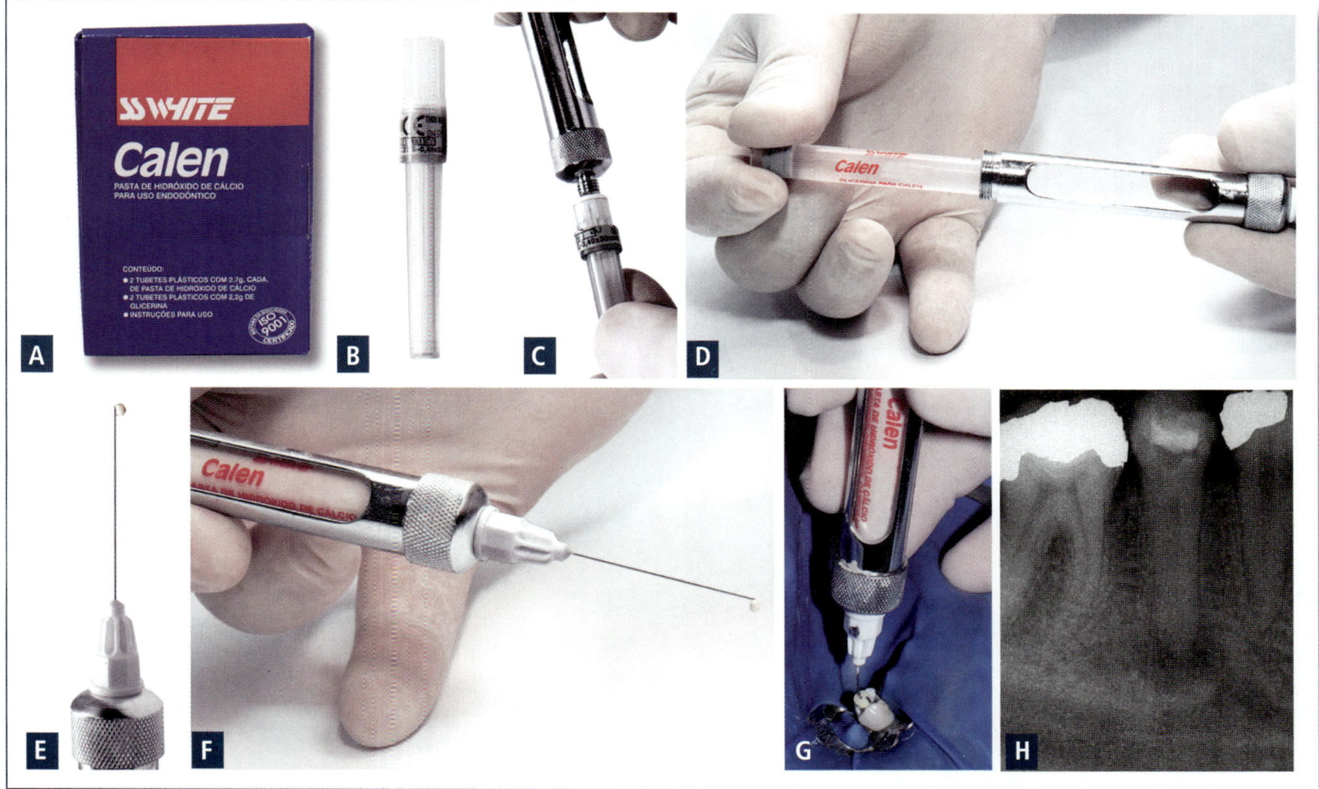

FIGS. 2.I-33A-H

A – Calen*.
B – Septojet XL 27G long needle (Septodont**).
C – Septoject syringe ML with long needle.
D – Placing the glycerin tube in ML syringe.
E – Drop of glycerin at the tip of the needle.
F – Drop of Calen at tip of needle.
G – Filling the root canal with Calen.
H – Periapical radiograph, showing the canal filled with Calen.

29. After placement of a sterile cotton pellet in the pulp chamber a temporary sealing is placed (Fig. 2.I-34).

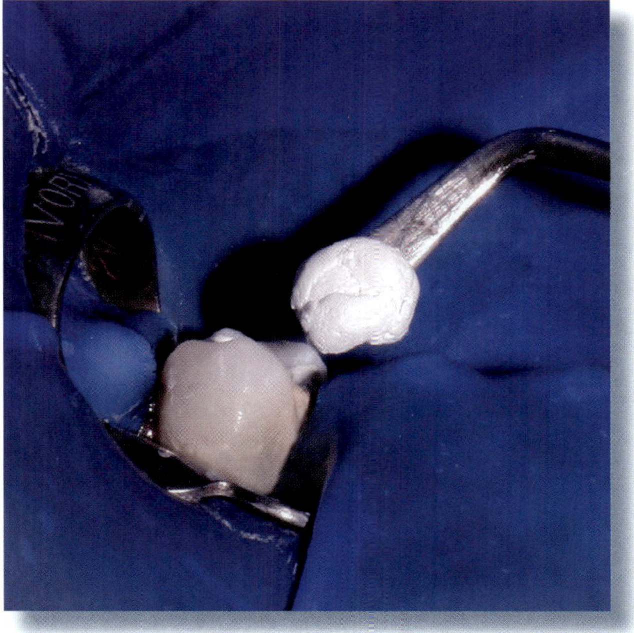

FIG. 2.I-34

Placement of temporary sealing.

* Calen – S.S. White. Artigos Dentários Ltda. Rio de Janeiro, RJ – Brazil.
** Septodont – Saint-Maur-des-Fossés, Cedex, France.

30. The temporary sealing is covered by a glass ionomer restoration (Fig. 2.I-35).

30.1 Cimpat or
30.2 Cotosol or
30.3 Lumicon

Periapical radiograph, showing extravasation of CALEN/PMCC (Fig. 2.I-36), only for academic purpose.

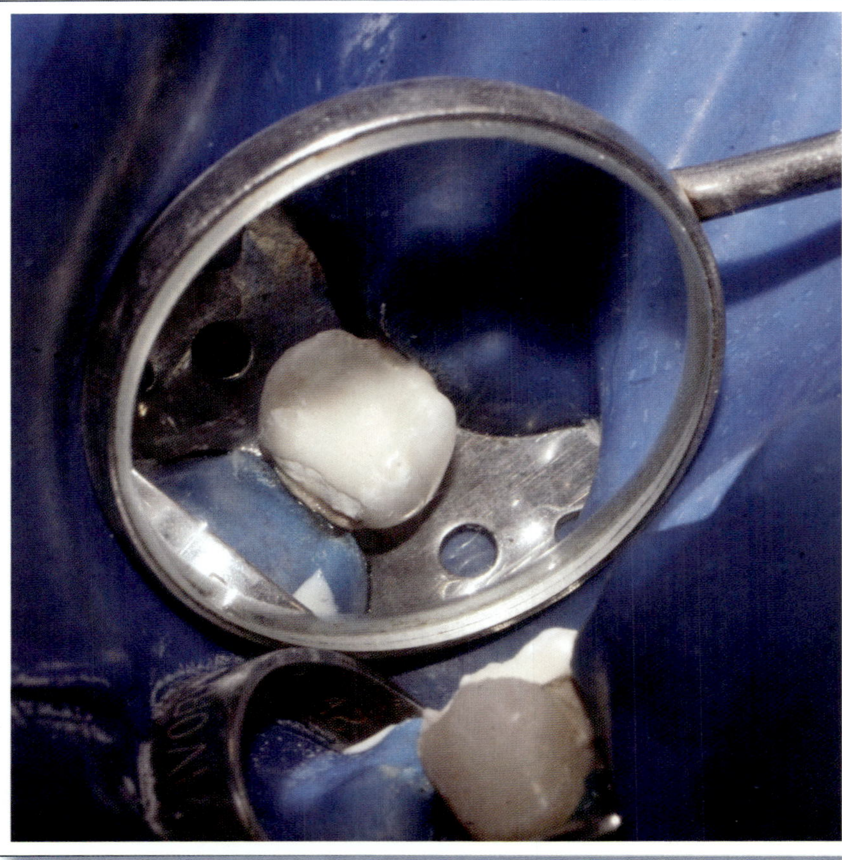

FIG. 2.I-35
Temporary restoration with glass ionomer.

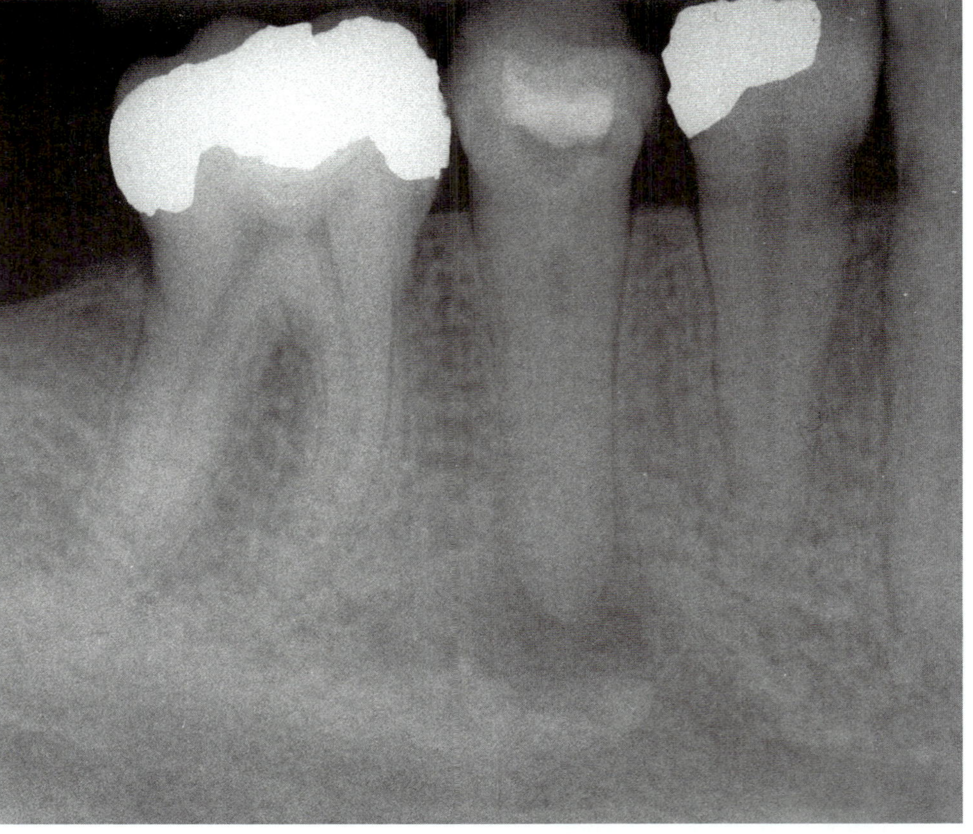

FIG. 2.I-36
Periapical radiograph of the canal filled with Calen/PMCC.

2nd Session: Minimum: 14 days
Maximum: 60 days

First rubberdam is placed, followed by antisepsis of the operative field and removal of the provisional restoration. Subsequently:

1. Removal of the temporary dressing (Calen/PMCC).
   1.1 Irrigation with 2.5% sodium hypochlorite solution (Labarraque solution).
   1.2 Stir with MI and FAI.

2. Dry root canal with aspiration, followed by sterile paper points.

3. Apply ultrasound (Fig. 2.I-37) or flood the root canal with EDTA solution (agitating for 3 minutes with MI and FAI).

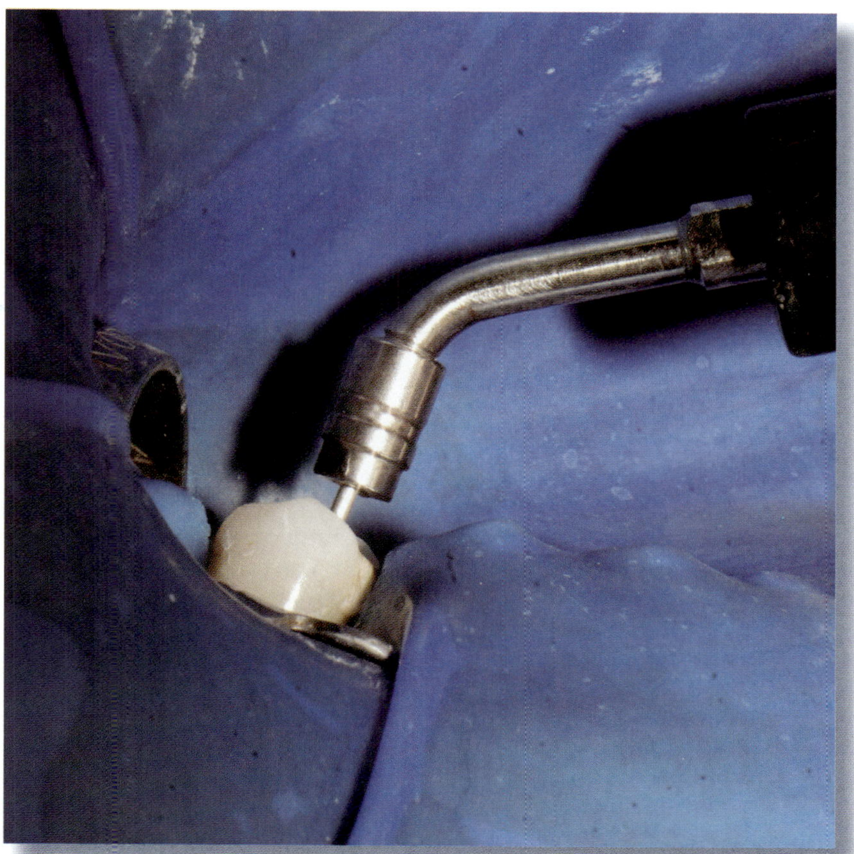

FIG. 2.I-37
Application of ultrasound.

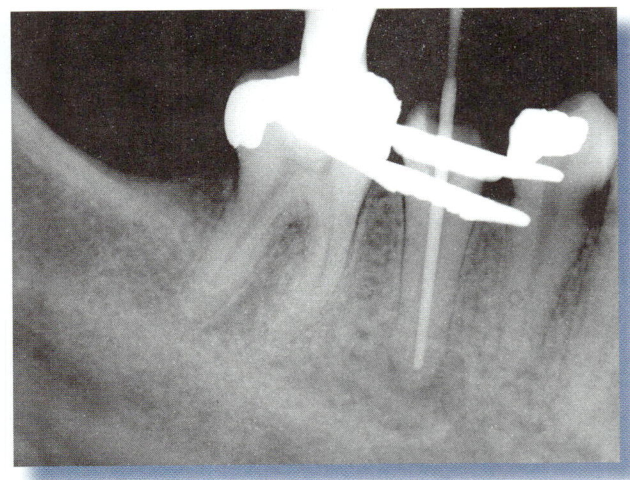

FIG. 2.I-38

Periapical radiograph of fitting gutta percha cone.

4. Root canal filling: gutta-percha cone thermo-plasticized technique (Tagger's hybrid technique, modified).

   Periapical radiograph of gutta percha cone fit. (Fig. 2.I-38).

   4.1 Indicated sealers:

   4.1.1 AH Plus (Dentsply/DeTrey) or Topseal (Dentsply/Maillefer) (Figs. 2.I-39A-J).

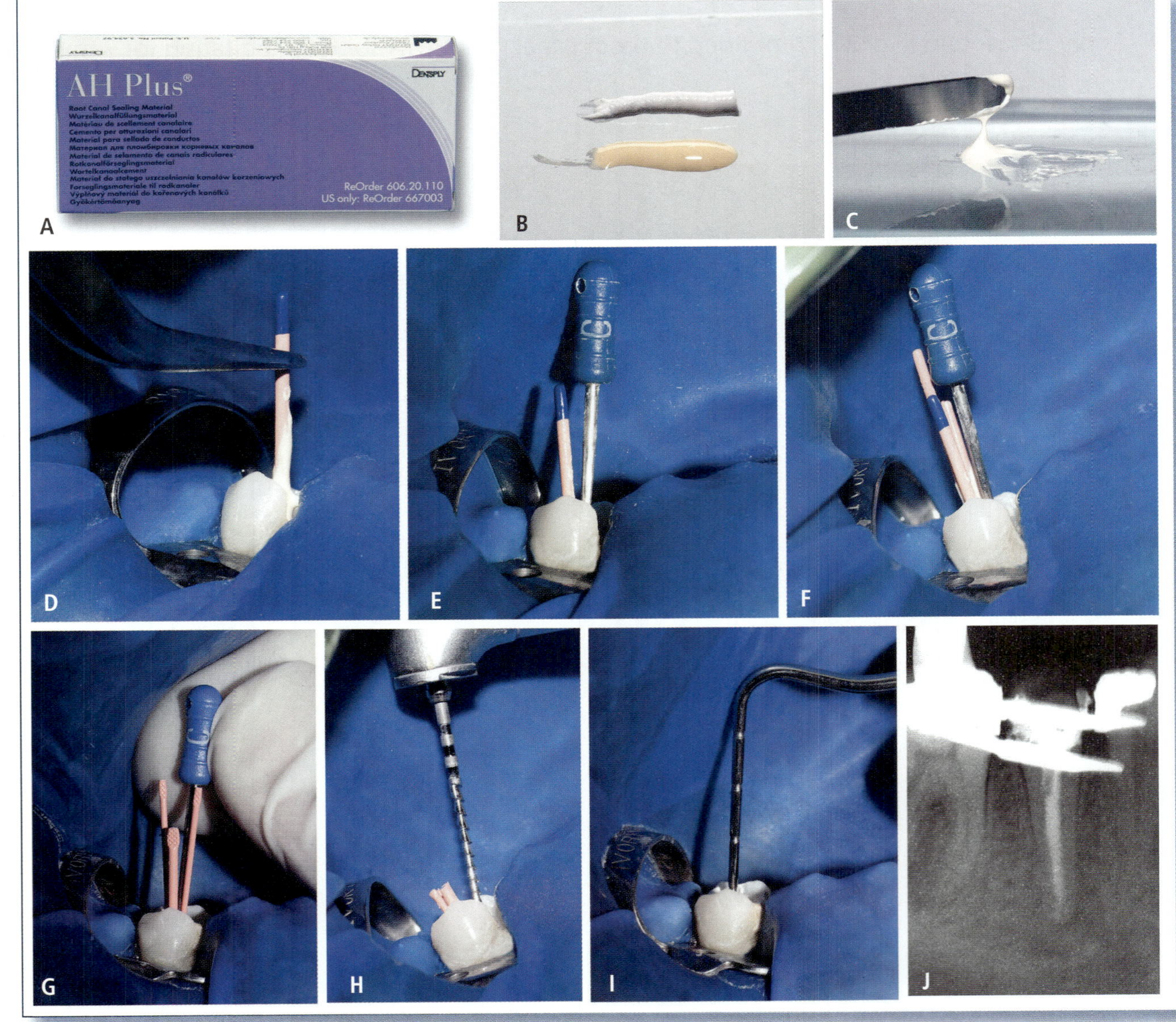

FIGS. 2.I-39A-J

A – AH-Plus* cement.
B–C – Equal lengths of AH-Plus paste. (B) and final mix (C).
D – Placing the master cone coated with cement in the root canal.
E – Opening lateral space with finger spreader.
F – Lateral condensation.
G – Creating space for Gutta Condenser.
H – Thermoplasticizing gutta-percha.
I – Vertical condensation.
J – Periapical radiograph after filling the root canal (Final)

* AH-Plus-Dentsply-DeTrey – Switzerland.

5. Removal of root canal filling in cervical third, placement of calcium hydroxide cement (Dycal-Dentsply/Caulk Div.) and filling of the pulp chamber with a glass ionomer cement until later restoration with complete crown (Fig. 2.I-40).

6. Final radiograph of root fill and glass ionomer temporary restoration (Fig. 2.I-41).

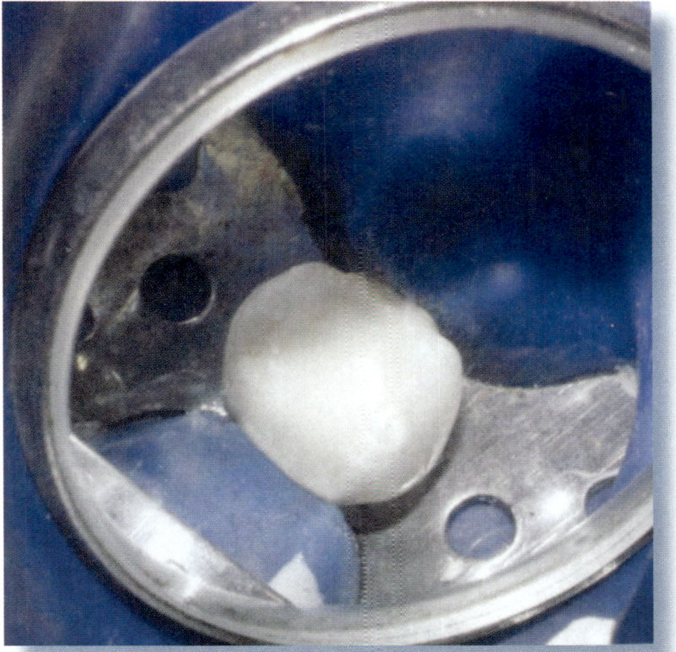

FIG. 2.I-40
Restoration of coronal structure.

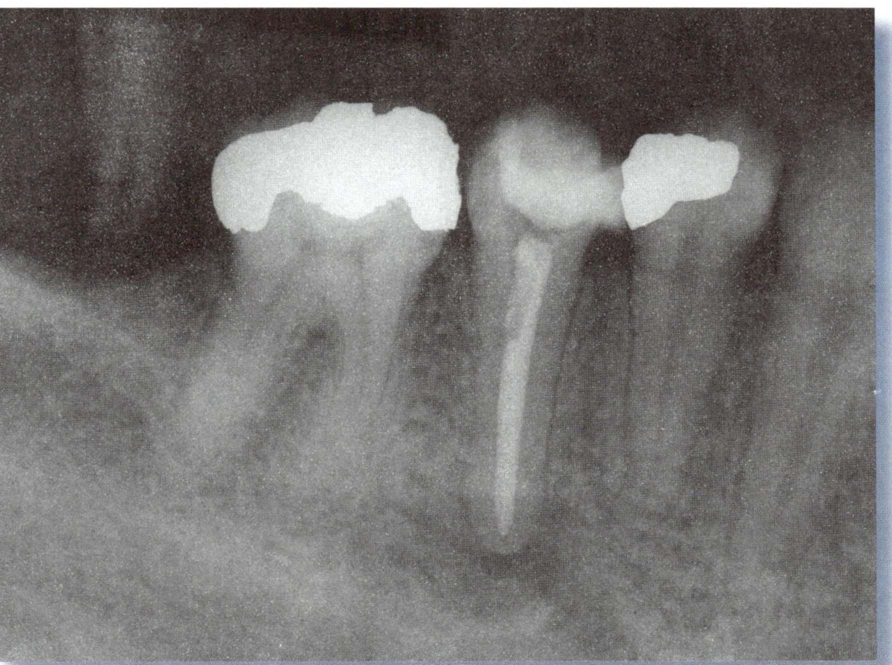

FIG. 2.I-41
Postoperative radiograph.

CASES OF NECROPULPECTOMY I

The steps of this technique are similar, with the exception of:

1. **Irrigation solution** – Use of diluted 1% sodium hypochlorite solution.
   1.1 Milton solution.
2. **Foramen debridement** – This must not be done, except in cases of drainage via the canal that was performed in acute dento-alveolar abscesses.
3. **Apical limit of debridement** – (1.5 mm short of the RTL).
4. **Temporary dressing** – not necessary to use.
5. **Root canal filling** – Whenever possible, fill the root canal in the same session.
6. **Filling material** – AH Plus (Dentsply/DeTrey) or Topseal (Dentsply /Maillefer).

References

1. Brilliant JD, Christie WH. A test of endodontics. J Acad Gener Dent, v. 23, p.29-36, 1975.
2. Coffae KP, Brilliant JD. The effect of serial preparation versus nonserial preparation of tissue removal in the root canals of extracted mandibular molars. J Endod, v.1, p.211-214, 1975.
3. De Deus QD. Endodontia. 3.ª ed. Medsi: Rio de Janeiro, 1982, p.344-362.
4. Goerig AC, Michelich RJ, Schultz HH. Instrumentation of root canals in molar using the step down technique. J Endod, v.8, n.12, p.550-557, 1982.
5. Marshall FJ, Pappin JA. A crown-down pressureless preparation root canal enlargement technique. Manual técnico da Universidade de Oregon (Oregon Health Sciences University). Portland – Oregon, USA, 1980.
6. Morgan LF, Montgomery S. An evaluation of the crown-down pressureless technique. J Endod, v.10, n.10, p.491-498, 1984.
7. Mullaney TP. Instrumentation of finely curved canals. D Clin N Amer, v.23, p.575-592, 1979.
8. Ruiz-Hubard EE, Gutmann JL, Wagner MJ. A quantitative assessment of canal debris forced periapically during root canal instrumentation using two different techniques. J Endod, v.13, p.554-558, 1987.
9. Valdrighi L, Biral RR, Pupo J, Souza Filho FJ. Técnicas de instrumentação que incluem instrumentos rotatórios no preparo biomecânico dos canais radiculares. In: Leonardo MR, Leal JM. Endodontia: tratamento de canais radiculares. 2.ª ed. Ed. Médica Panamericana: São Paulo, 1991, p.290-299.

2.11

Anticurvature filing when preparing curved root canals in molars

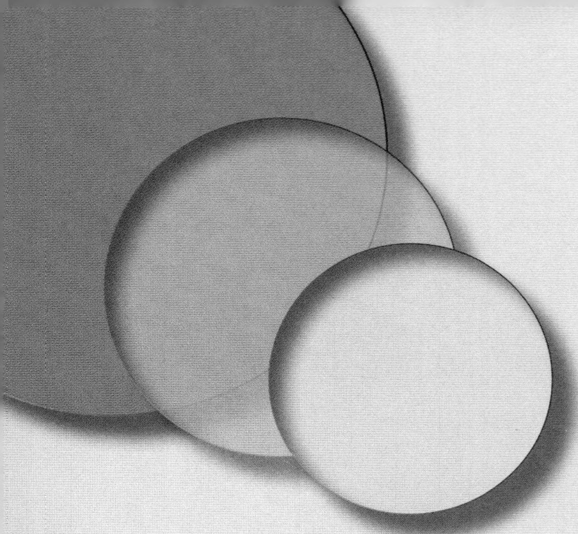

Mario Roberto Leonardo

The mesio-buccal and mesio-lingual root canals of mandibular molars, particularly of the first molar, as well as the mesio-buccal root canal of maxillary molars possess the so-called **double curvature**, which makes it very difficult to perfectly debride, especially in the **apical five millimeters**. The first curvature, with an initial trajectory in a disto-mesial direction, located at the level of the coronal two-thirds of the roots, and the second curvature, at the level of the apical third (in the mesial root of mandibular molars and mesio-buccal root of maxillary molars), their trajectory is reversed; that is, in a mesial to distal direction (Fig. 2.II-1). The second curvature has a trajectory that has an accentuated curve in a distal direction, which occurs in 79% of cases in mandibular molars and in 78% in maxillary molars[3]. When this **double curvature** is added to the **marked convexity** of the mesial wall of the pulp chamber, the practitioner must be knowledgeable and have the technical resources and skills to overcome anatomic difficulties when performing endodontic treatment. This will allow him/her to easily reach the **apical five millimeters**, considered to be the critical zone in biological endodontics and a challenge to endodontist[4], especially in cases of necropulpectomy II. Once these anatomic difficulties have been overcome, the practitioner can clean and model the region adequately, as well as disinfect it, if necessary, and perform the most hermetic and three dimensional filling possible, resulting in a much more favorable prognosis.

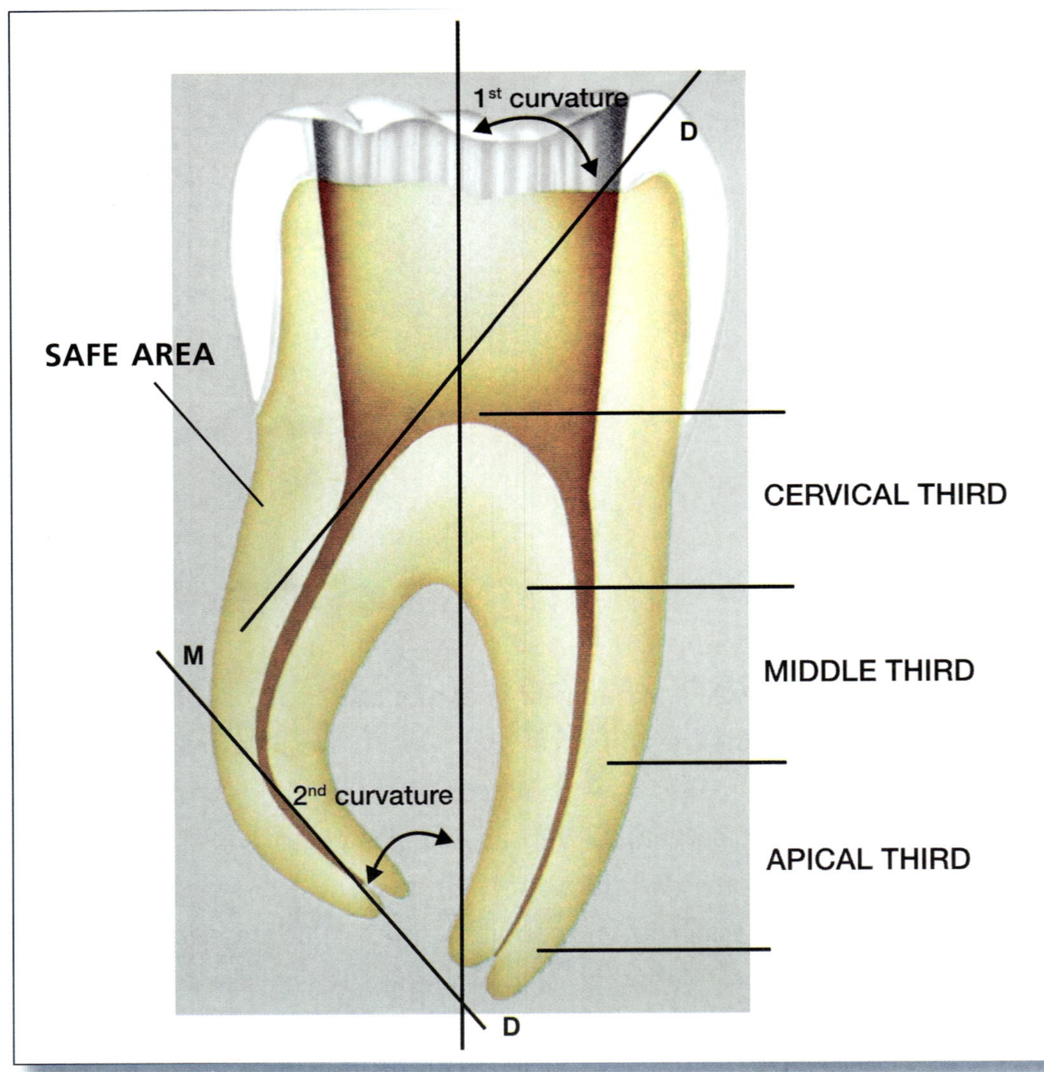

FIG. 2.II-1
Diagrammatic illustration of the so-called double curvature.

In order to overcome this challenge, the compensatory wearing, in the the pulp chamber, as well as the anti-curvature filing, at the coronal two-thirds of the root canal, idealized by Abou-Rass et al[1], are operating procedures of fundamental importance.

Compensatory wearing is performed by removing the convexity of the pulp chamber walls, particularly of the mesial wall, which generally covers the entrances of the mesial root canals.

For this operating procedure, the use of stainless steel burs are recommended; such as Endo-Z burs (Dentsply/Maillefer) or diamond no cutting tips burs, such as Nos. 3080, 3081 and 3082 (MSK); Button burs(Ultradent), "Endo Axxess" and Diamendo (Dentsply/Maillefer) diamond points activated by ultrasound.

ANTICURVATURE OR FILLING

Anti-curvature filing is the operating procedure performed in maxillary or mandibular molars, for the purpose of rectifying the first root canal curvature at the level of the cervical and middle thirds (safe area)[1] to gain direct and straight access to the apical curvature (second curvature), observed in the large majority of cases.

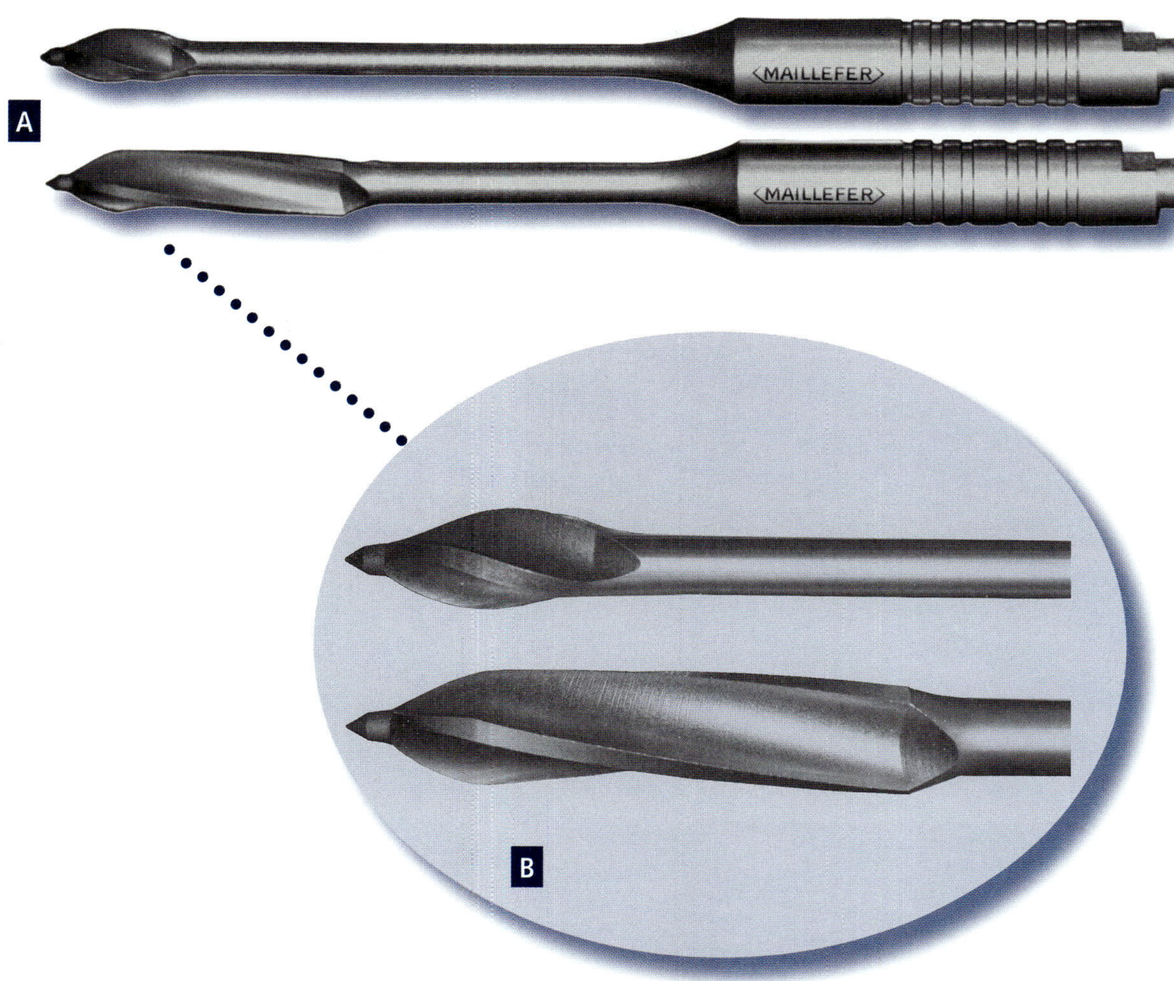

FIGS. 2.II-2A-B

A – Gates Glidden and Largo (Peeso Reamer) Burs.
B – Higher magnification of Fig. 2.II-2A.

Means used:

- Gates-Glidden and Largo (Peeso Reamer) Burs (Figs. 2.II-2A-B)
- Manual Anti-curvature files:
  Hedströen files
  Ergoflex* files (Figs. 2.II-3A-C)
- LA Axxess (SybronEndo)** (Figs. 2.II-4A-C).
- Access kit (Dentsply/Maillefer) (Fig. 2.II-5)
- Access kit (Ultradent Products Inc***) (Fig. 2.II-6)
- Nickel-titanium instruments with large tapers, motor-driven type (rotary systems):
  Orifice Shapers (Profile System – Dentsply/Maillefer)
  Orifice Openers (K_3 √ENDO)
  S_X (Protaper – Dentsply/Maillefer) (Fig. 2.II-7)
  Endoflare (Hero/Hero Shapers – Micromega)
  Pre-Race (Race-FKG-Dentaire)
  Ultrasound (diamond points)

* FKG Dentaire – Suiss.
** SybronEndo (seds) – Glendora, CA, USA.
*** Ultradent Products Inc.– South Jordan, Utah, USA

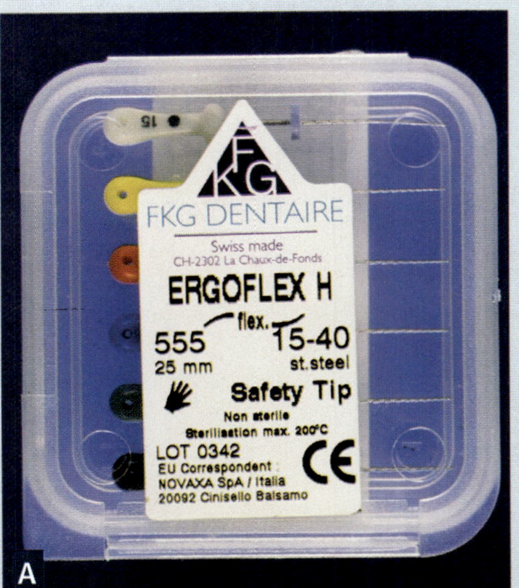

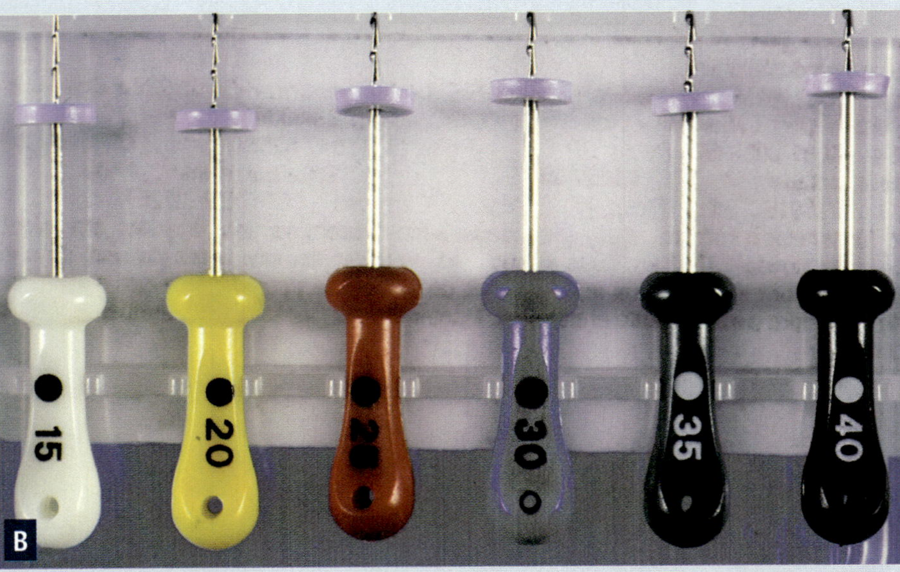

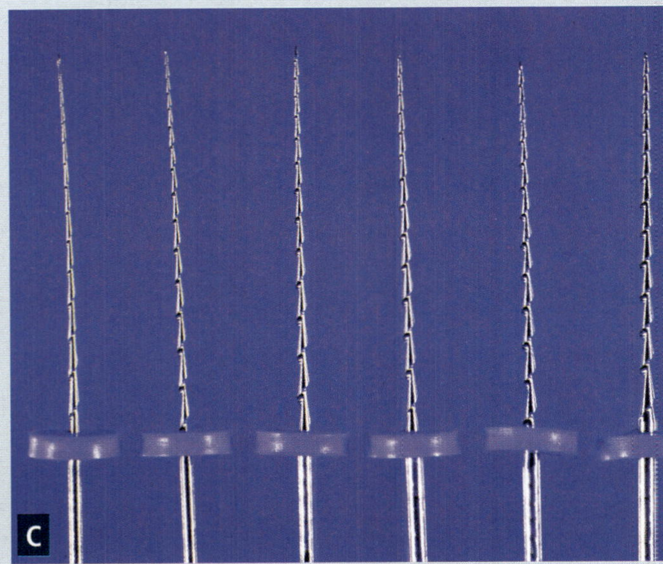

FIGS. 2.II-3A-C

A – Manual anti-curvature files – Ergoflex – (FKG Dentaire).
B – Note the conformation of the handle, which promotes the operating procedure.
C – Active part of the Ergoflex files (15 to 40).

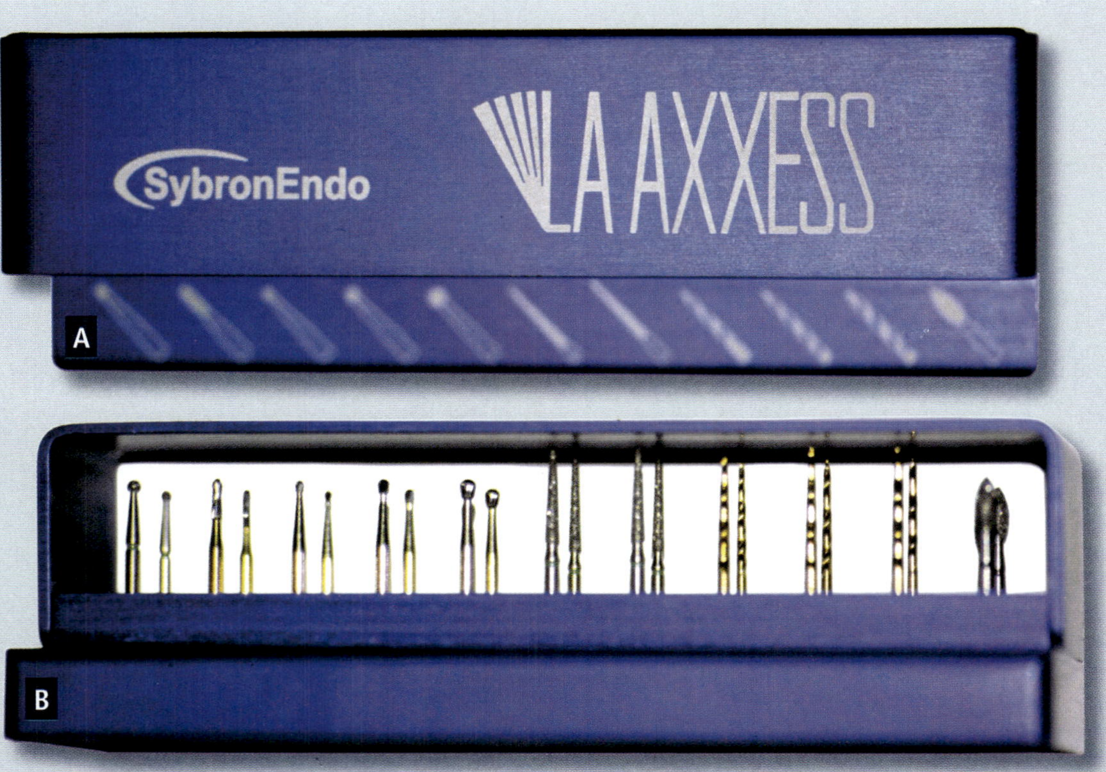

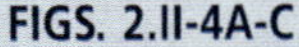

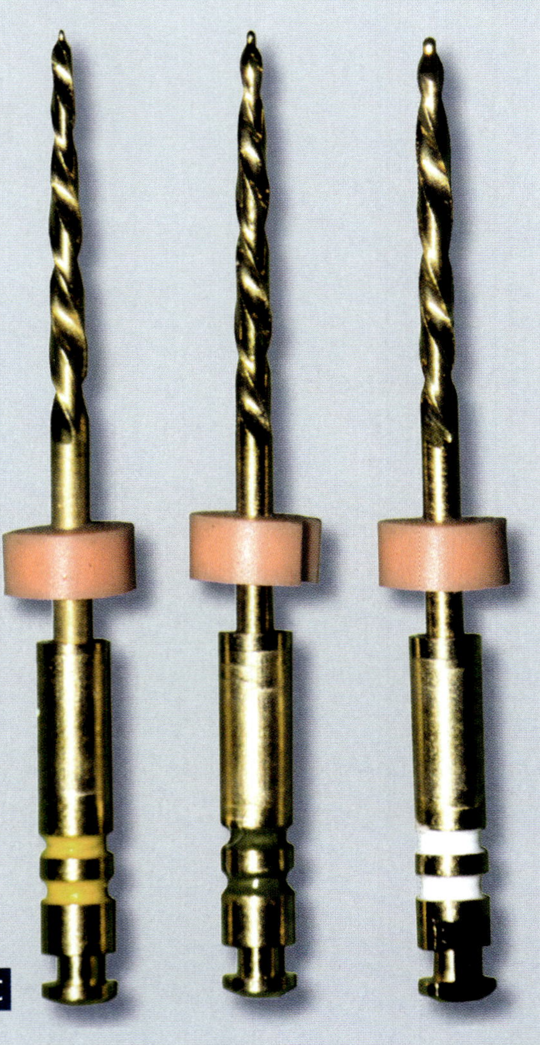

FIGS. 2.II-4A-C

A and B – Kit – SybronEndo – LA AXXESS, which comes with anticurvature files instruments.
C – LA AXXESS – No. 1 – two yellow rings (0.20), for small diameter root canals.
LA AXXESS – No. 2 – two green rings (0.35), for medium diameter root canals.
LA AXXESS – No. 3 – two white rings (0.45), for wide root canals.

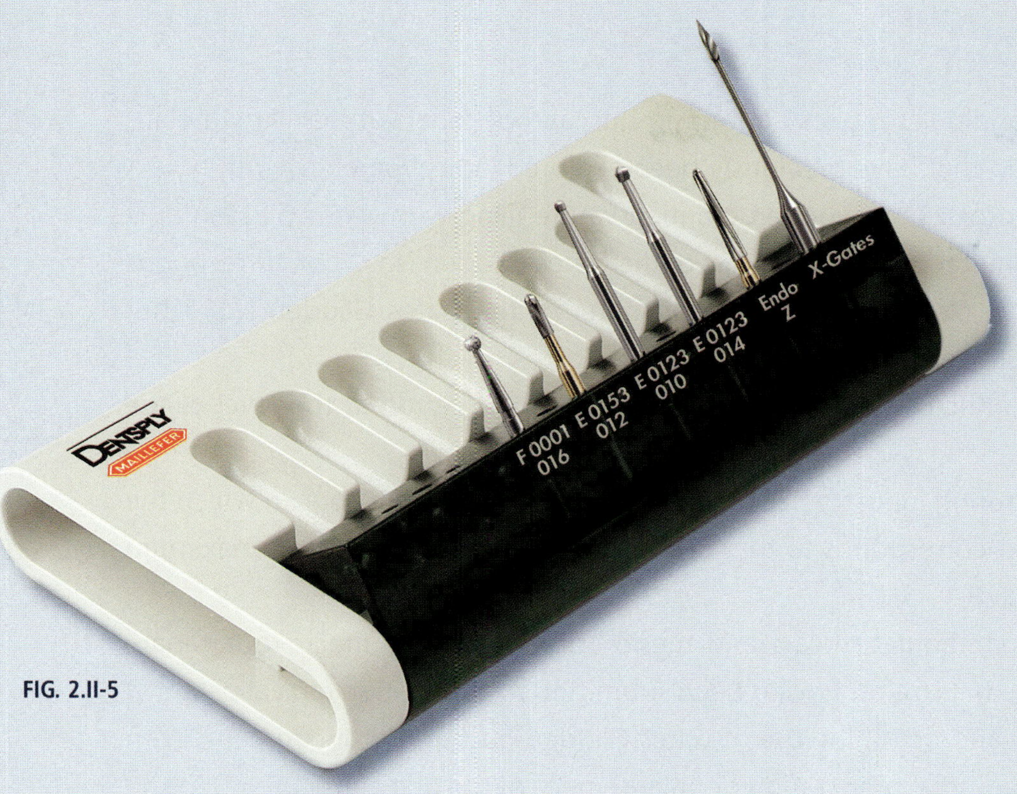

FIG. 2.II-5

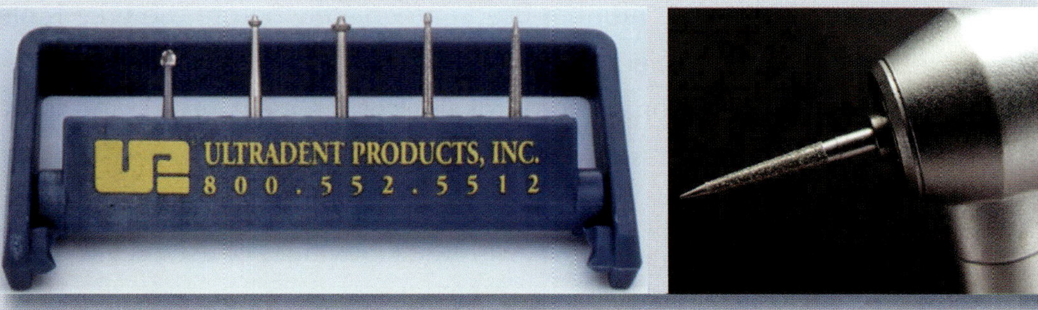

FIG. 2.II-6

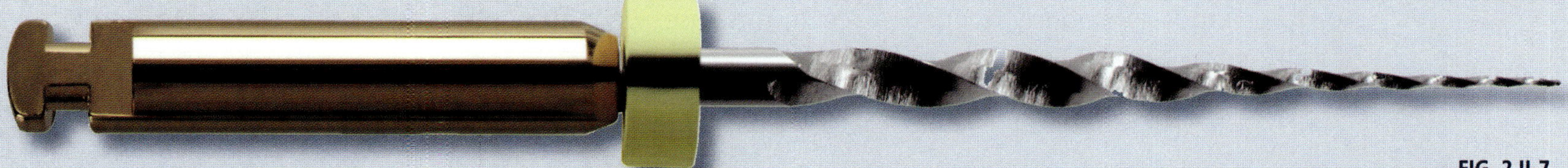

FIG. 2.II-7

FIG. 2.II-5

Kit – Dentsply/Maillefer, which contains anti-curvature files instruments.

FIG. 2.II-6

Kit – Ultradent Button Burs, with non-cutting tip, for a compensatory wearing.

FIG. 2.II-7

Sx Instrument of Protaper Universal System for anti-curvature filing.

The mesial root canal of mandibular molars and mesio-buccal root canals of maxillary molars, when wide or relatively wide and that have previously been explored (apical patency) with type K files (stainless steel), Nos. 20 and/or 25, may undergo anticurvature filing with Gates Glidden burs (GG) Nos. 2 and 3. The larger diameter of the active part of the Gates Glidden No. 2 bur corresponds to the diameter (D_1) of a type K file No. 70, and the diameter of the Gates Glidden No. 3 bur corresponds to the D_1 of a type K file No. 90.

GG Bur Nos. 2 and 3 allow anticurvature wear without risking perforation at the level of the furcation[2].

Dentsply/Maillefer manufacturing industry has recently launched the X-Gates bur, in which the point diameter of the active part corresponds to that of the Gates Glidden No.1 and its maximum diameter to that of No. 4 (Fig. 2.II-8).

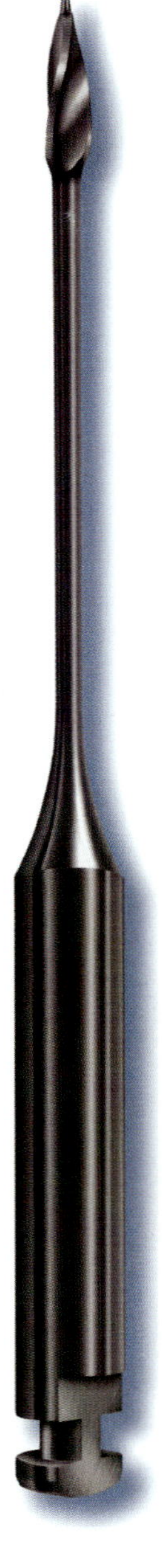

FIG. 2.II-8
X-Gates Burs (Dentsply/Maillefer).

For mesial root canals of mandibular molars and mesio-buccal maxillary molar root canals, when they are extremely atresic; that is, after having been submitted to exploration (apical patency) with regular type K files Nos. 10 and/or 15, the use of Gates Glidden burs and/or instruments with large taper is recommended after initial preparation or enlargement of the first curvature up to the length that corresponds to the safe area. This type of preparation is performed with Hedströen type files of the number used immediately before the type K file used for the exploration, with brush-stroke movements (lateral friction) on the safe area. Therefore, if the exploration/catheterization of the coronal two-thirds (half of the root) was performed with a type K file No. 10, it is advisable to initially use a Hedströen type file No. 08. If type K file No. 15 is used, a Hedströen No. 10 will be indicated.

In this sequence, with the kinematics of use previously described, when Hedströen type file No. 20 is used, the root canal will be now sufficiently prepared to receive Gates Glidden burs and/or rotary instruments of larger diameters and tapers.

We do not recommend the use of Gates Glidden bur No. 1, especially for beginners, due to the high risk of fracture, as has been proven in the endodontic literature. We also do not recommend its direct use in atresic molar root canals, because the function of the Gates Glidden bur is to widen or to enlarge a previously opened space. In this case, we initially open the space with Hedströen or Ergoflex type files.

References

1. Abou-Rass M, Frank AL, Glick DH. The anticurvature filing method to prepare the curved root canal. J Amer Dent Ass. 1980;101:792-794.
2. Carneiro Leão E. Avaliação do preparo biomecânico dos canais radiculares utilizando técnicas escalonadas, associadas ou não às brocas Gates Glidden em raízes mesiais de molares inferiores. Estudo in vitro. Tese (Doutorado) – Faculdade de Odontologia de Pernambuco (FOP), Camaragibe, Pe; 1991.
3. Pucci FM, Reig R. Conductos radiculares. Montevideo: A. Barreiro y Ramos. 1945:216-230.
4. Simon JHS. The apex: how critical is it? Gen. Dent. 1994;42(4):330-334.

2.III

Thermoplasticized Gutta-percha techniques for filling the root canal system

Miguel Roig Cayón

Fernando Durán-Sindreu Terol

According to the American Association of Endodontists (AAE), an adequate root filling is defined as and characterized by three-dimensional filling of the entire root canal system, as closely as possible to the cemento-dentinal junction.

Filling is the last operative stage of root canal treatment, and is of fundamental importance for medium and long-term success.

It is recognized that the majority of authors consider cleaning and shaping of the root canal system the stage of treatment that resolves pulpo-periapical problems[30,49]. That is why it is considered the most critical stage for the clinical/radiographic success of endodontic treatment. However, if this critical step initially leads to success, it should be prolonged by the necessity of a hermetic/three-dimensional filling of the root canal system. In other words, if root canal cleaning and shaping lead to success, filling maintains it by preventing the recurrence of periapical pathosis.

For a better understanding of the importance of filling we must know its goals, which are:

- To eliminate bacterial leakage from the oral cavity or periapical tissue into the interior of the root canal system;
- To seal all the irritating factors that could not be eliminated during the cleaning and shaping stages inside the endodontic system[15]. Non-elimination of these etiologic factors and continued periapical irritation from the persistent infection of the root canal system, are some of the main causes of failure[40]. Therefore, the long-term stability of the filling must be maintained, since solubilization of the filling material at an apical level will lead to loss of the seal, and consequently loss of the established objectives. An inadequate, or poor three-dimensional filling of the root canal system will also be a cause of endodontic treatment failure.

From the above, we can conclude that the final objective of any endodontic treatment should be the complete three-dimensional filling of the root canal system with a biocompatible material, in order to achieve preservation of the tooth as a sound, functional unit.

Hermetic three-dimensional filling of the root canal system is clearly important to attain the treatment goals, at all times starting from the premise that achieving adequate prior cleaning and shaping depends on the clinician's capability.

Having accepted the need for filling the root canal system, we must consider how to implement this.

By its morphological configuration, the root canal is not just a single and simple tubular space, located inside the root. It also has ramifications, accessory and lateral canals, anastomoses and bifurcations (Fig. 2.III-1), which modify the configuration of this space, making it difficult to perform a three dimensional filling and meet the final treatment objective, which is clinical/radiographic success. Filling the root canal system is therefore not a simple task and it will be necessary to use suitable techniques and materials to meet the treatment objectives.

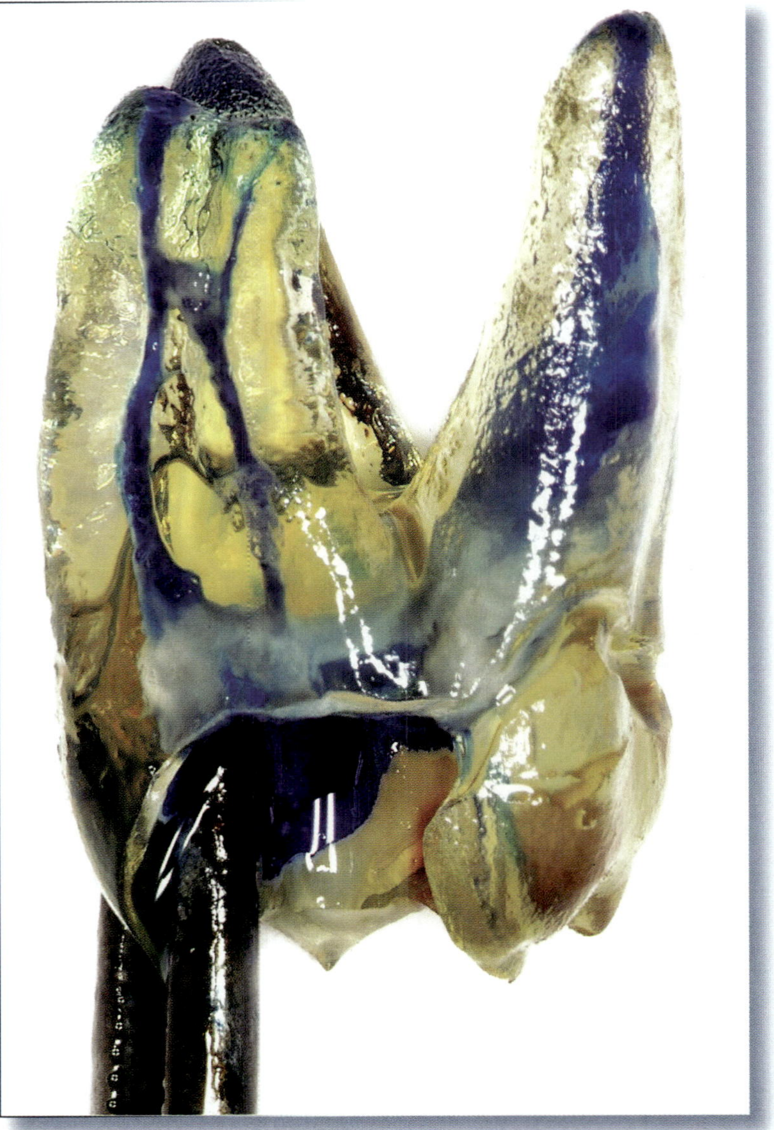

FIG. 2.III-1
From the diaphanization of this maxillary first molar we can note the anatomic complexity of the root canal system, with special mention of the mesiovestibular root, with two main canals, a central anastomosis, and a new bifurcation in the apical portion. Courtesy of Dr. Guillermo Topham.

REQUISITES FOR FILLING THE ROOT CANAL SYSTEM

As root canal filling is essential to a good prognosis, it is important to determine when and/or how this must be done. At a minimum three requisites must be observed:

- **The root canal must be disinfected**;
- **The root canal must be debrided and shaped**;
- **The root canal must be dry*.**

* Except for methacrylate based resin sealers, in which case the dentin needs to be moist.

To the above-mentioned requisites, some authors have added a fourth condition: the absence of spontaneous or provoked pain. The latter condition is questionable. For instance, in cases of patients who present with acute symptoms as a result of a treatment and in cases of pulp necrosis (gangrene) and/or acute dento-alveolar abscess. In these cases final treatment is postponed to make sure the symptoms are resolved before completion of the case[26,56]. In these complex situations, the systemic therapeutic procedures that are required (*see* chapter 2.XXII) make it difficult to complete the treatment in one single session.

- **Disinfected root canal**

In order to determine whether a root canal had been disinfected, the lumen of root canals used to be cultured for the presence of bacteria. This technique was used almost universally for many years. Only when a negative culture was obtained, filling of the root canal was recommended. Today we know that a negative culture is not necessarily synonymous with disinfection or sterility of the root canal system, as there are multiple anaerobic species capable of causing disorders, which cannot be identified by conventional cultures. To decide whether or not the root canal is disinfected, we have to use other criteria. In the absence of options, we can consider that a root canal is sufficiently clean when irrigation is performed by means of an adequate protocol. After having achieved a sufficient diameter for root canal cleaning by debridement, that is five instruments in addition to the initial apical instrument, or anatomic instrument. Insufficient instrumentation prevents the diffusion of the irrigation solution through the root canal system, making it difficult to disinfect it[50].

It is difficult to establish what the ideal irrigation protocol is. Mostly irrigation is carried out with sodium hypochlorite solution of an adequate concentration (over 2.5%), preferably at a temperature of over 40ºC, combined with a calcium chelating agent in the final stage, and alternated with a surfactant solution, such as alcohol. This allows for good results. Some authors consider that this combination is adequate for root canal treatment of teeth with a radiographic periapical lesion. Others indicate the use of a temporary dressing for these cases.

- **Debrided and shaped root canal**

In order to fill the main root canal adequately, it is necessary to perform sufficient root canal preparation. With the filling materials at our disposal today, preparation consists of shaping the root canal so that it has a tapered configuration, with the narrowest portion at the apical end of the canal. Thus it is possible to compact the filling material against this narrower point and achieve three-dimensional filling of the root canal system. If the narrowest point is at the level of the coronal thirds and not at the end of the apical preparation, compaction of the material will be insufficient at the most apical point **(apical five millimeters),** leaving empty spaces that will allow bacteria to develop and thus compromise the prognosis of the treatment.

Instrumentation demands not only a tapered shape, but also sufficient widening of the root canal, which will allow it to have a circular or oval shape, which is much easier to fill than an irregular shape. Insufficient widening will not only make it more difficult to introduce the filling material, but the instruments for compaction as well.

At present the use of files with tapers larger than the 0.02 mm/mm increase established by the ISO allows the morphology of the main canal treated to be evaluated. Although it is not a precise evaluation, we should not forget that in many cases, the cross section of the root canal is not circular, therefore, we are only evaluating the smaller diameter at each point.

- **Dry root canal**

With the filling materials at our disposal today, it is convenient for the root canal to be dry in order to fill it adequately. To do this, we can use different techniques and products, ranging from sterile paper points and irrigation with isopropyl alcohol or ethanol, and proceed with heated instruments. A wet or moist root canal affects the physical-chemical properties of the thermoplastized filling materials. The presence of a periapical inflammatory process may prevent adequate drying of the canal, as the exudates from the periapex into the root canal system will not allow for it. Under these conditions, it is inadvisable to perform the filling in the same session and should be postponed, while a temporary dressing inside the root canal system between sessions should be placed.

APICAL LIMIT OF FILLING

It is important to establish up to which point to fill root canals; that is, what is the apical limit. The literature indicates that it is necessary to fill the entire portion of the canal that has been prepared. Relatively short preparations, up to 2 mm short of the apical foramen[72] and filling at this level, offer a better prognosis than cases that are overfilled[48,49,53,54,58]. This is not contradictory, since the root canal preparation must limited to the tooth, without going beyond it. Furthermore, it is important that it is not excessively short, because a filling more than 2 mm short of the apex will severely compromise the prognosis[16]. In general, a filling limit to one millimeter short of the radiographic apex is accepted as adequate. This is a general rule, however, and serves only as a guideline, since the clinician must make adjustments according to the conditions of each case, which are based on pathological and anatomical knowledge, tactile sense, radiographic interpretation, and mostly on the values of the electronic apex locators.

The explanation in the previous paragraph indicates that extrusion of the filling material into the periapex is an undesirable effect in filling. Extrusion of the filling material leads us to differentiate two clinical situations: Overextension of the material and overfilling.

Overextension: Overextension occurs, in the absence of good apical preparation (apical stop), when the material extrudes into the periapex. In this case, the material flows out due to the lack of apical preparation (apical stop) preventing good apical sealing.

Overfilling: When there is good apical preparation (apical stop) it does not prevent the existence of passage-ways for the material to penetrated into the periapex, especially when an apical patency file is used. In principle, the preparation retains the gutta-percha when we compact it against the preparation, but part of the filling material, primarily sealer cement, and in some thermoplastic techniques the gutta-percha, can also be extruded.

Overfilling with filling material is always undesirable, as apical sealing is usually not good. When the apical preparation (apical stop) is not adequate, the material will be extruded without adequately sealing the apical end of the preparation. This promotes marginal leakage into this empty zone, causing a recurrence of periapical pathologies over the medium and long term. Overfilling, by definition, implies that there is a space in the apical preparation against which the filling material is compacted (apical stop). In these cases, the main objective of filling is achieved (hermetic apical sealing), and provided that the filling material is inert (non irritant) towards the periapical tissues, all that may occur would be a delayed or absence of apical repair.

ROOT CANAL FILLING MATERIALS

For adequate filling of the root canal system, whatever the chosen technique or system may be, we must depend on a material in a solid or semi-solid state, and a sealing material called a sealer (filling cement). Sealers are necessary for filling the spaces between the dentinal walls and the material in solid state. It must also fill the empty spaces, lateral and accessory canals, or gaps between auxiliary cones, in cases of active lateral condensation. Furthermore, they will facilitate entry of the material in a solid state, with an effect similar to that of a lubricant.

None of the sealers (cements) possess all the ideal properties proposed by Grossman[21]. Most sealers (cements) are based on zinc oxide-eugenol, calcium hydroxide, glass ionomer and resins. All offer a certain amount of toxicity until they are completely set or polymerized, this being the reason why we should avoid their extrusion into the periapical tissues. Of all the mentioned groups, any one that is chosen must be capable of providing the desired sealing with few or minimal risks. Perhaps the most discussed are the calcium hydroxide-based cements, indicated because of their therapeutic activity and inducing mineralization, an activity that must not occur, because for this to take place, they need to be soluble, and solubility is a property absolutely undesirable for a sealer. The glass ionomer-based cements have the disadvantage of being outstandingly difficult to remove in cases of retreatments, and there are doubts about their solubility in comparison with other cements.

To take a sealing cement (any of the chosen ones) into the root canal, different systems are proposed. No difference has been found between delivering the sealer with paper points, gutta-percha cones, a file turning in an counter clockwise direction or with a Lentulo spiral[68], which is why we can choose any of these systems, although all leave significant spaces without filling[23]. The only systems that has shown the greatest efficacy in distributing the sealer throughout the entire root canals, is ultrasound[1,57] and the use of a Navitip (Ultradent Products Inc), although other authors have found no differences[68].

Over the last 150 years, numerous solid-state materials have been recommended for root canal filling. Historically, gutta-percha has been shown to be the material of choice, from the crown to the apical portion. Although it may not be ideal, it is the material that best meets the desirable properties of an ideal filling material as stated by Grossman[21], which are:

- Be easy to introduce into the root canal.
- Does not undergo shrinkage.
- Seals the root canal laterally and apically.
- Must not be an irritant to the periapical tissues.
- Must be impermeable and non-porous.
- Must be chemically stable in periapical tissue fluids.
- Must be bacteriostatic.
- Radiopaque.
- Must not alter the natural color of teeth.
- Must be sterile or capable of being sterilized.
- When liquid or semi-solid, should convert into a solid.
- Must be easily removed from the root canal in cases of retreatment.

Gutta-Percha Cones: Its disadvantages, such as lack of rigidity and adhesiveness, or easily becoming debonded when submitted to pressure, does not diminish the advantages. Various alternatives to gutta-percha have been investigated, but up to the time of the writing of this text, only a few other material have shown to be a suitable substitute, and therefore gutta-percha remains one of the standards for quality fillings.

It has been clinically shown that gutta-percha together with a sealing cement, fulfills the necessary requirements of biocompatibility and sealing[15], which have made it the most widely used filling material in the world. This is possible thanks to one of the main properties of gutta-percha in the endodontic field: its capacity to plasticize under heat and allowing to being compacted under pressure inside the root canal[5].

Recently, resin-based filling materials have been proposed, notably Resilon® (Pentron Clinical Technologies, Wallingford, CT, USA), an industrial polyurethane adapted for endodontic use, as an alternative to gutta-percha. (Note: Pentron Clinical Technologies was acquired by SybronEndo and all Resilon based materials marketed by several commercial companies are now called RealSeal.)

In its physical properties, Resilon resembles gutta-percha, and allows the root canal system to be filled with the same techniques (active vertical or lateral condensation with heat and thermoplastic injection. The Resilon-based systems incorporate filling resin (equivalent to gutta-percha), a sealing cement, under the label of Epiphany® (Pentron Clinical Technologies, Wallingford, CT, USA), capable of bonding to dentin and to the core resin (Resilon). This same system under the label of RealSeal is distributed by SybronEndo (Glendora,

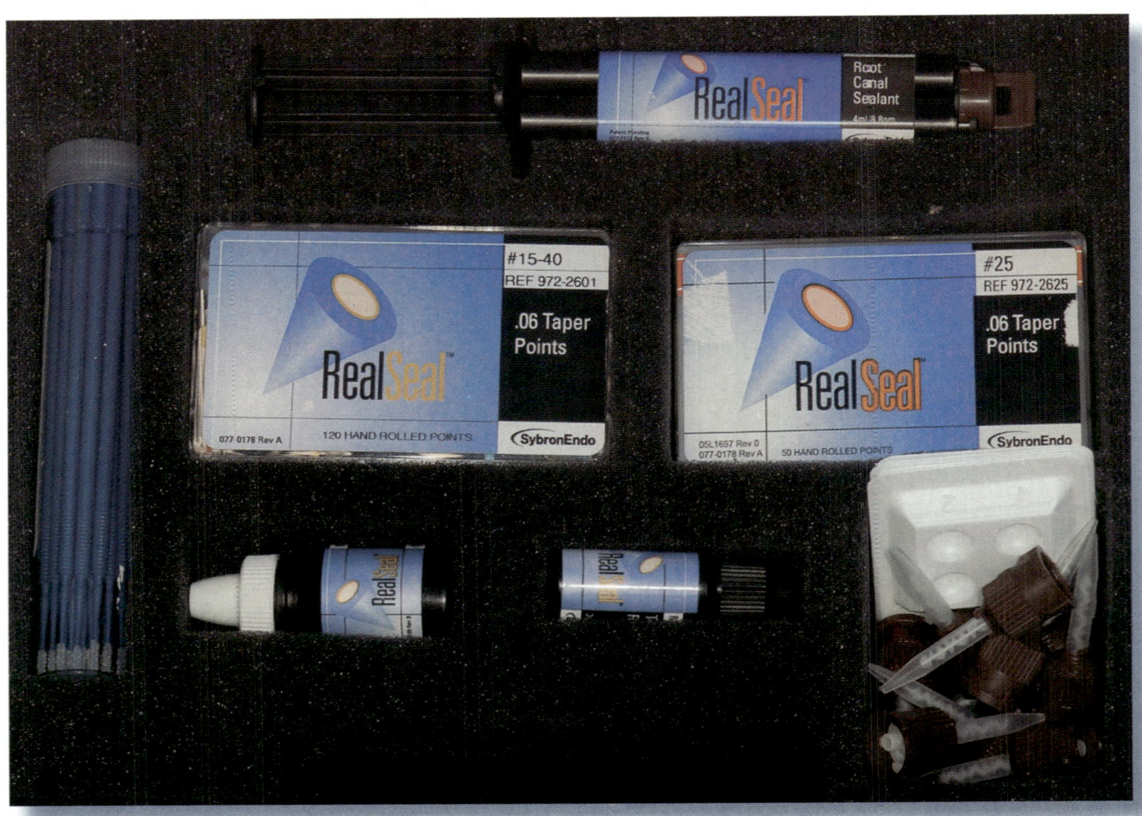

FIG. 2.III-2
RealSeal Introduction Pack. Includes the filling points, sealer and adhesive.

CA, USA) (Fig. 2.III-2). The main characteristic of these materials, according to its proponents, is that the resin sealer bonds to the canal walls and the filling material, thus forming a "monobloc", which, in principle, would result in less marginal leakage and greater strength of the tooth, as shown in some articles[33,51,52,62]. Furthermore, the handling characteristics are very similar to that of gutta-percha, with exception of the plasticization temperature, which must be lower than that used in thermoplastic techniques, making it relatively simple to use (Fig. 2.III-3).

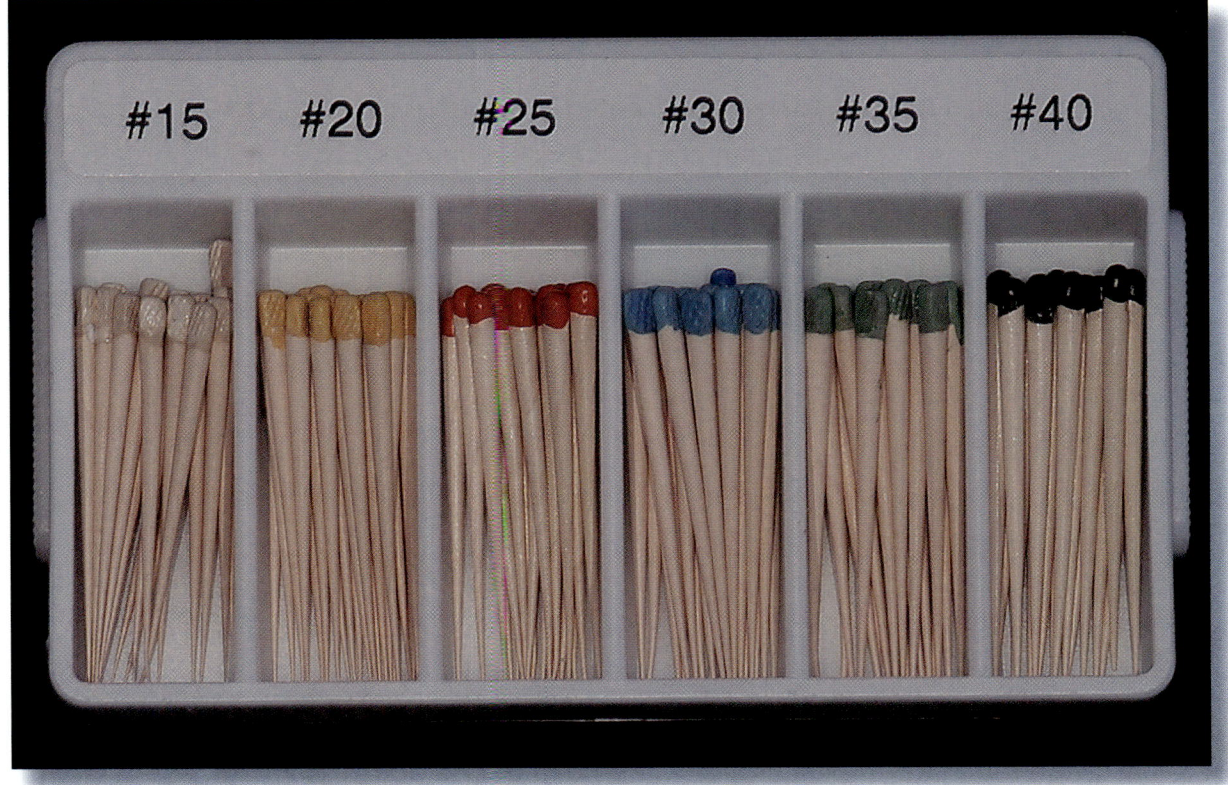

FIG.2.III-3

RealSeal filling points.
Note the similarity to conventional gutta-percha points.

Moreover, biologically, it presents excellent results when microscopically evaluated in the periapical region of dog teeth (Leonardo et al.[33], 2007).

Another resin-based system is the ADO (Apical Delivered Obturation) EndoRez System is described separately in Chapter 2-XX.

With respect to the most suitable method for three-dimensional root canal filling, there is no general agreement at present. Nevertheless, it would seem that the thermoplastic techniques allow better three-dimensional filling of the root canal system because of the property of gutta-percha to become plasticized.

FILLING TECHNIQUES

The techniques available to us at present for filling the root canal system vary according to the direction in which the gutta-percha is compacted (laterally or vertically) and the temperature that is applied, either cold or heated (plasticized). There are many methods but among them five stand out:

- Active lateral condensation;
- Vertical condensation (heated gutta-percha);
- Injectable thermoplasticized gutta-percha;
- Thermo mechanical or thermo compaction of gutta-percha;
- Core or solid center conductors covered with alpha phase gutta-percha.

All the above-mentioned techniques, except active lateral condensation, belong to the group of heated or thermoplasticized gutta-percha filling techniques. This group of techniques takes advantage of the changes in the phase of the gutta-percha and the changes that are produced in its physical properties by the increase in temperature. Heating, or thermoplasticizing gutta-percha to a temperature higher than 42°C, makes changes from a solid to a sticky mass that is not ductile or malleable. In the past it was believed that it had an adhesive capacity, because of adhesion to the root canal without requiring a sealer (cement). Temperatures between 42°C and 49°C produce a change in gutta-percha to the alpha phase, the properties of which have previously been described. When gutta-percha is heated to a temperature between 56°C and 62°C it reaches the gamma phase, the properties of which are not well known, since they appear to be similar to those of the alpha phase. Afterwards, it was observed that the material that was at phase α or γ, by the action of the body temperature went back to phase β, which has no bonding capability by itself, as the gutta-percha did not remain adhered to the root canal walls. It formed an interface between the materials and the root canal walls; therefore the use of a sealer cement in these techniques was necessary.

The importance of these phases, apart from the changes in physical properties, lies in the fact that gutta-percha expands on being heated, going from the beta to the alpha or gamma phase. However, when it cools it goes reverts to the beta phase and undergoes slight shrinkage, which seems to be greater than the initial expansion. This shrinkage needs to be compensated for, which is accomplished by compaction of the material during the process, to maintain a good fit of gutta-percha and prevent the creation of spaces between the root canal walls and the material itself.

The thermal plasticity of gutta-percha is the factor that allows it to be used in thermoplastic root canal filling techniques.

In the literature, there are numerous articles advocating a particular technique. Some authors proclaim that the technique they propose or advocate is the best. Others point out that no study has been capable of demonstrating that one technique is better than the other. Amongst these, we believe it is important to pay attention to a recent prospective study by the Toronto group, which evaluated the success and failure at 4 and 6 years after treatment[17]. The results showed a higher percentage of success in teeth treated with a more flared preparation, and filled with vertical condensation (heated gutta-percha) than the group with step-back preparation, filled with active lateral condensation. Furthermore, they found greater success in the group of teeth in which the limit of filling was at the correct working length. This perhaps can be explained in that the filling techniques that use thermoplasticized gutta-percha are capable of filling the anatomical complication of the root canal system[63], and appear to be the most suitable to enable us to achieve the desired three-dimensional filling.

ACTIVE LATERAL CONDENSATION

The conventional active lateral condensation technique consists of adjusting the main gutta-percha cone at the level of the apical stop, followed by the use of the tapered condenser to create the necessary space for the successive introduction of auxiliary gutta-percha cones. It is a universally accepted and widespread technique[11], in addition to being considered the standard among the filling techniques.

The technique is applicable in the majority of cases, and requires a root canal preparation of a progressively tapered shape and an apical stop made in sound dentin, allowing good apical control of the filling material[19] thus avoiding extrusion.

The gutta-percha cones are standardized in shapes and sizes and correspond to the shapes and sizes of the standardized instruments. They are color coded matching the instruments, and are selected according to the diameter of the apical stop. When standardized type K or Hedström files are used for root canal preparation, and there are no residues remaining at the level of the apical stop, the main cone fits to the real working length. The ISO standards allow gutta-percha cone manufacturers a tolerance of ±0.05 millimeters, which implies that a cone labeled with number 20, and therefore has a theoretical apical diameter of 0.20 mm, could in reality be a 15 (0.20-0.05), or a 25 (0.20+0.05). Therefore, it is advisable to calibrate the gutta-percha points with a calibrated ruler at the time of filling.

After it has been calibrated, the cone should fit to the real working length, and is inserted with pliers. Once it has been inserted, the cone will come into contact with the root canal walls at 1-3 mm from the apex, where it should be adjusted to the desired length. It should resist going beyond the apical stop when submitted to apical pressure and should be slightly resistant to removal, which is called "tug-back". The final position of the gutta-percha cone inside the root canal can be determined by marking it on an incisal or occlusal reference point with a sharp instrument or pliers. After this, proof that the proper cone has been chosen, is verified radiographically. If the cone reaches the real working length, or is 0.5 mm short and if it fits and radiographically there is a lateral space visible between the master cone and the root canal wall, from the junction of the apical and middle thirds of the root canal up to the coronal third, one may proceed with compaction.

The three methods used for evaluating adequacy of fit of the master cone, as explained in the previous paragraph, can be assessed by visual testing, tactile sense and radiographic proof.

After the choice and radiographic confirmation of the master gutta-percha cone, we now select a digital spreader with the largest diameter capable of penetrating up to 1 to 2 mm short of the real working length. The spreaders can be of the finger/palm or digital type. The latter provide better tactile control and reduce the risk of vertical fractures from lateral pressure in comparison with the manual type[34]. There are special nickel-titanium digital spreaders on the market, that are more flexible, reduce the lateral forces against the walls, and better penetrate the curvatures of the root canal, in comparison to the usual stainless steel spreaders[8,27,47].

Once the master gutta-percha cone has been adjusted and removed the smear layer must be removed using and EDTA or citric acid solution.

After selecting the master cone and spreader and removal of the smear layer followed by drying, the endodontic sealer/cement is inserted. It has been suggested that it is essential to distribute the sealer throughout the root canal, in order to obtain the best possible sealing. In cold lateral compaction, it is acceptable to use the master gutta-percha cone itself, a file or Lentulo spiral for placing the sealer material[23,68]. However, to obtain the best distribution of the sealer, we recommend the use of an ultrasound activated instrument[1]. Whatever the vehicle of choice, it should be covered with a small quantity of sealer (cement). Once introduced into the canal, it will distribute the sealer uniformly on the prepared walls. The sealer must extend to the real working length of the canal, however care should be exercised to avoid completely filling it.

One the sealer has been inserted the selected master cone is introduced into the root canal, followed by placing the spreader in the most apical position possible. It is necessary to insert the gutta-percha cone slowly to achieve careful distribution of the sealer, thus eliminating trapping air and minimizing sealer extrusion through the apical foramen. It is important for the cone to be at most two millimeters short of the real working length[3]. The digital spreader should not be used with a great deal of pressure, as this does not improve the fit of the material while it can cause vertical fracture of the tooth. After placing the spreader so that the gutta-percha cone is suitably compacted, it is removed with clockwise/anti-clockwise rotation followed by placing an auxiliary gutta-percha cone is quickly as possible into the open space. The size of the auxiliary gutta-percha cone should correspond to that of the digital spreader that was used. This step is repeated until the point is reached when the spreader cannot penetrate beyond one third of the initial working length.

Subsequently, a heated instrument is used (condenser Glick No.1 or Thermal Condenser) to remove the excess of the auxiliary cones, and at the same time to plasticize the gutta-percha in the coronal portion of the root canal. We then proceed with vertical compaction using pluggers to improve the gutta-percha adaptation to the canal walls, promoting coronal sealing of the root canal. The pluggers used should not be wedged in the canals; this requires the careful placement of a pluggers in the coronal portion of the canal before filling. Once the gutta-percha has been compacted in the coronal portion, the pulp chamber must be cleaned with cotton pellets soaked in alcohol, to remove unhardened sealer and gutta-percha remnants. After placement of a temporary restoration, a postoperative radiograph is made.

The active lateral condensation technique is relatively simple. It provides sufficient filling of the root canal system, allows good control of the filling limit, avoids extrusion of the material into the periapex[19], and is applicable to the majority of clinical situations.

The main problem is related to the difficulty of filling irregularities in the root canal system, which is different for the thermoplastic techniques[70,71] and largely determined by the canal morphology. In addition there is a greater risk of causing vertical root fractures should pressure on the spacer be exceeded. Lastly, the final filling is not always homogeneous and voids may be present.

VERTICAL CONDENSATION

In the 1960s, Schilder[46] proposed vertical condensation of heated gutta-percha as a technique for filling the root canal system. The goal of this technique was the filling of the root canal in three dimensions with a homogeneous mass of gutta-percha and a minimum quantity of sealer. The technique was based on the premise that by compacting heated gutta-percha, one can obtain better adaptation of the material to the irregularities of root canals, while at the same time lateral canals, ramifications and isthmus are filled in a more predictable manner.

As in all the filling techniques, in order to perform it efficiently, the cleaning and shaping of root canals is fundamental. For this technique, as in almost all, a progressive tapered shaping of the root canal in a crown apex direction without apical deformation, is necessary. In contrast to active lateral condensation, non standardized gutta-percha cones are used, taking into account the shape of the root canal. The master cone must reach to within1 mm of the preparation length and must be adjusted to the apical stop, that is, offer resistance to removing the gutta-percha cone (tug-back). In general, a gutta-percha cone slightly less tapered than the canal preparation is used, as this assures that a gutta-percha cone adjustment is established at the apical stop, and not in other parts of the root canal.

The technique is based on heating the gutta-percha cone and compacting it afterwards in successive applications. Therefore, various pluggers of different diameters must be selected, so that they act in the different portions of the canal. The larger diameter plugger should be used in the coronal part and the smaller diameter, in the more apical portion of the root. When selecting a plugger, it is important that it does not bind with the canal walls, because when apical pressure is exerted to condense the gutta-percha root fracture may occur, in addition to not condensing the gutta-percha. But the plugger can also not be too loose inside the canal. This will prevent condensing of the gutta-percha, preventing it to adapt well to the anatomy of the root canal system.

Once the gutta-percha cone and pluggers have been selected, the filling can start. The master gutta-percha cone covered with a sealing cement, is placed in the root canal. The portion of the gutta-percha cone that protrudes from the canal is removed with a plugger heated in a flame or by using a Touch N' Heat device (SybronEndo, Orange, CA, USA). Subsequently the more coronal gutta-percha is heated, part of which is also removed when heated, and pressure is exerted on the gutta-percha in an apical direction, using an unheated plugger. This step is subsequently repeated, but now with narrower pluggers, because we are working progressively closer to the apical part of the preparation. Once we are to within four millimeters of the real working length, the first part of filling is considered complete. To fill the remainder of the canal, techniques such as thermoplastic gutta-percha injection, Tagger's hybrid technique, active lateral condensation or the Thermafil system can be used.

In vertical condensation, one obtains the best results when the plugger reaches the apical part of the preparation[9,28,70]. This is a problem when this technique is used in canals with excessive curvatures, as they do not allow the plugger to reach to within 4 millimeters of the apical limit.

CONTINUOUS WAVE CONDENSATION

In the 1990s, Buchanan[10] introduced System B (SybronEndo, Orange, CA, USA), which simplified the vertical condensation technique. This technique represents a number of differences compared to the classical vertical condensation technique. In System B, the same instrument heats and condenses the gutta-percha. With the classical technique, the gutta-percha is heated with one instrument and a separate condenser is used for compaction (Fig. 2.III-4). In the various steps of the classical technique, pluggers of progressively narrower size were used as we approach the apex. But in the continuous wave technique, the entire vertical condensation is performed in one single step.

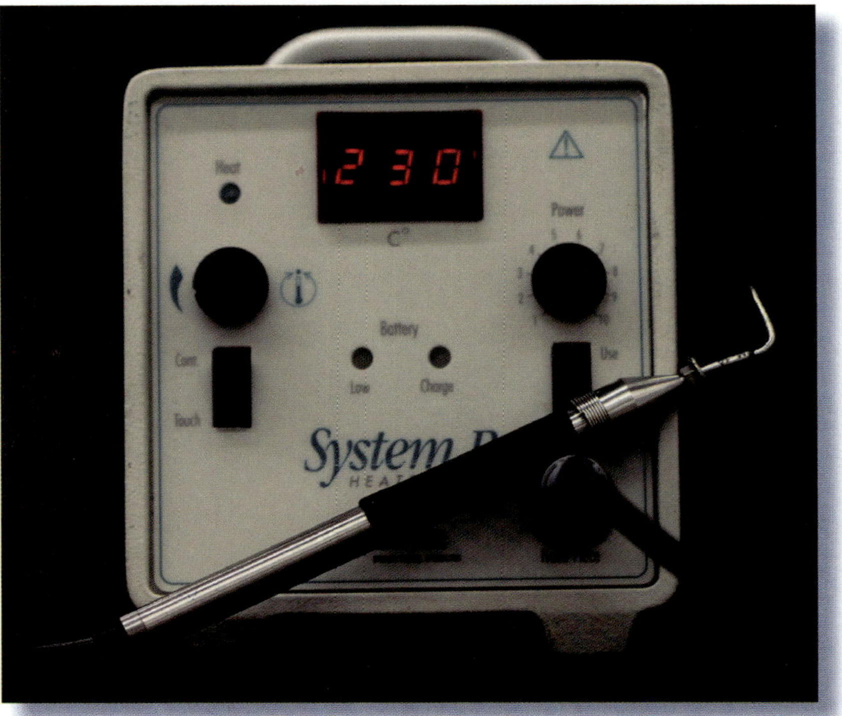

FIG. 2.III-4

System B device for filling with continuous wave of heat.
The temperature for use with gutta-percha ranges from 200 to 250ºC.

System B consist of five pluggers with different tapers, 4%, 6%, 8%, 10%, 12% and one with an apical diameter of 0.5 mm (Fig. 2.III-5). The first step of the technique consists of selecting the plugger to be used. One should select the plugger with the largest taper that reaches less than 5-7 mm of the real working length. According to the authors, the best results are obtained when the plugger reaches 3-5 mm short of the real working length[22,32,55,67].

A gutta-percha cone will be selected based on the root canal preparation. In wider preparations, we will use cones with larger tapers. In general, if we use a plugger with a 6% taper and we will select a thin cone. A thin-medium cone will be selected if the plugger chosen has an 8% taper. A medium cone, if the plugger has a 10% taper and a medium-large cone if the plugger taper is 12%. Analytic Endodontics, Glendora, CA, USA offers gutta-percha cones with different tapers (4%, 6%, 8%, 10% and 12%) for filling with System B (Fig. 2.III-6). The gutta-percha cone must reach the real working length and be submitted to the tug-back test.

After drying the root canal, the gutta-percha cone, covered with cement, is introduced to the real working length. The System B is programmed for a temperature of 200ºC and the plugger

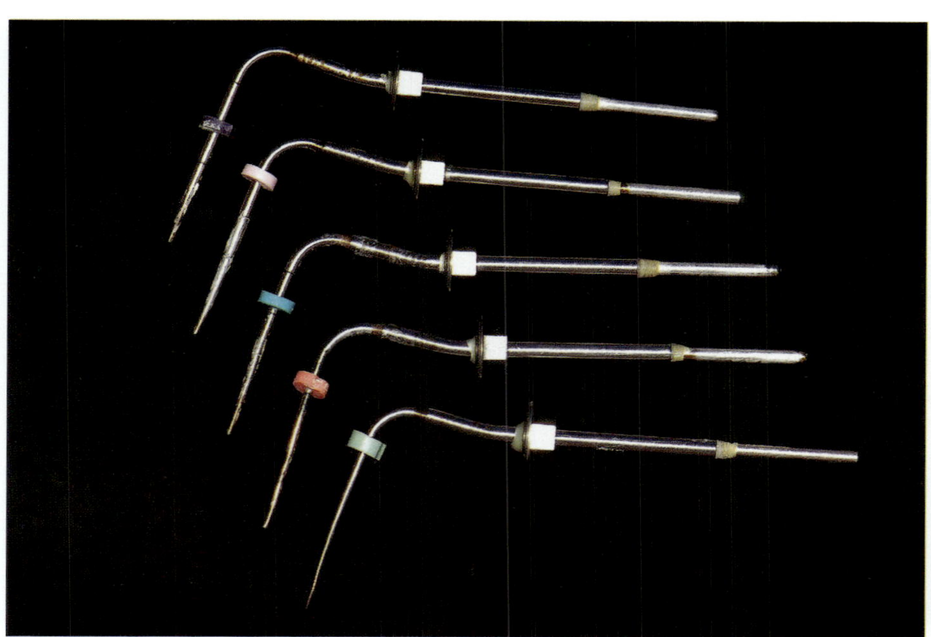

FIG. 2.III-5

Filling points for the System B (conventional or for Elements) with different tapers.

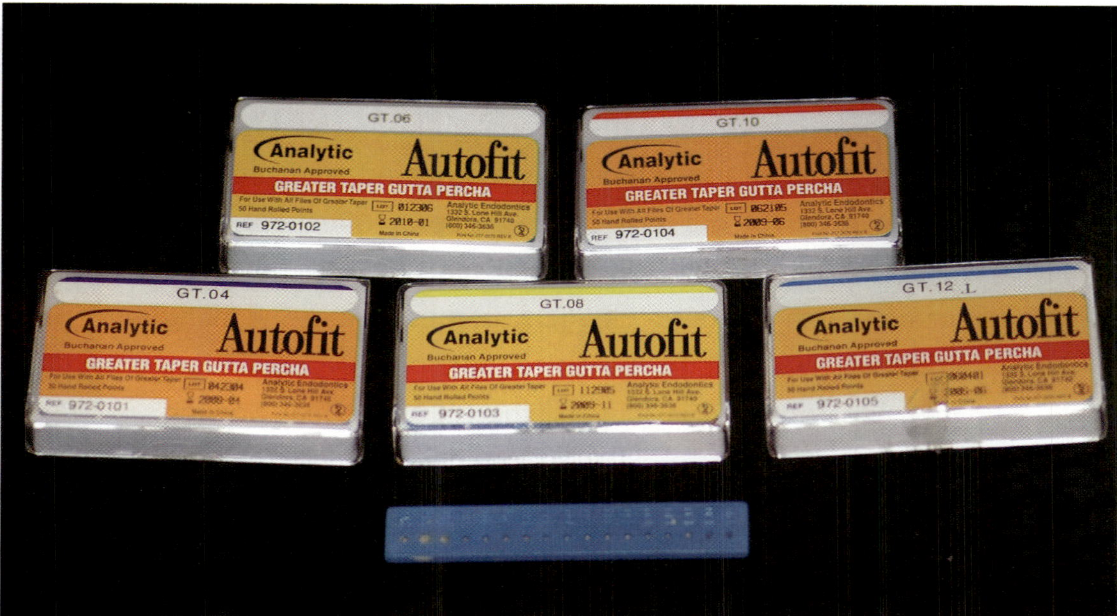

FIG. 2.III-6

The Analytic company markets points with different tapers; very practical for the System B. It is necessary to calibrate the apical diameter by means of a calibration ruler.

is heated to cut the gutta-percha that protrudes from the canal. Subsequently, in a single movement, the gutta-percha is heated and condensed in an apical direction, with the plugger heated to 200ºC. When the plugger reaches a distance 3 mm from the point it should penetrate, one stops applying heat and exerts apical pressure until the plugger reaches a distance approximately one millimeter from the predetermined maximum point of penetration, maintaining pressure in an apical direction for about ten seconds. The plugger must be at a distance of 1 mm from where it will bind with the root canal walls, otherwise it will not condense the gutta-percha and may cause a vertical fracture when force is applied on the root canal walls. To remove the plugger after condensing the gutta-percha, heat it for a second and remove it in a coronal direction (Fig. 2.III-7). In oval canals, one can place an auxiliary cone adjacent to the main cone to increase the quantity of gutta-percha inside the canal, and allow hydraulic forces to generate.

Once the apical third filling is concluded, the rest of the canal can be filled with thermoplasticized gutta-percha injection, either with Tagger's technique or active lateral condensation, or Thermafil.

THERMOPLASTIC GUTTA-PERCHA INJECTION TECHNIQUES

The difference between the thermoplastic gutta-percha injection techniques and the previous one is heating the gutta-percha, which is done outside the root canal. Thermoplastic gutta-percha injection techniques are indicated in cases in which a canal is very wide, such as in teeth with incomplete root formation, in which the apical part is first filled with MTA, in C-shaped root canals, or in teeth with internal resorption. The system is also very useful for filling the middle and coronal thirds of canals in which the apical third was filled by vertical condensation[9,66] and for completely filling the root canal. A problem with the thermoplastic gutta-percha injection techniques is the lack of apical control[2]. Therefore, in many cases, they are used to complement other filling techniques used for filling the apical portion of the root canal.

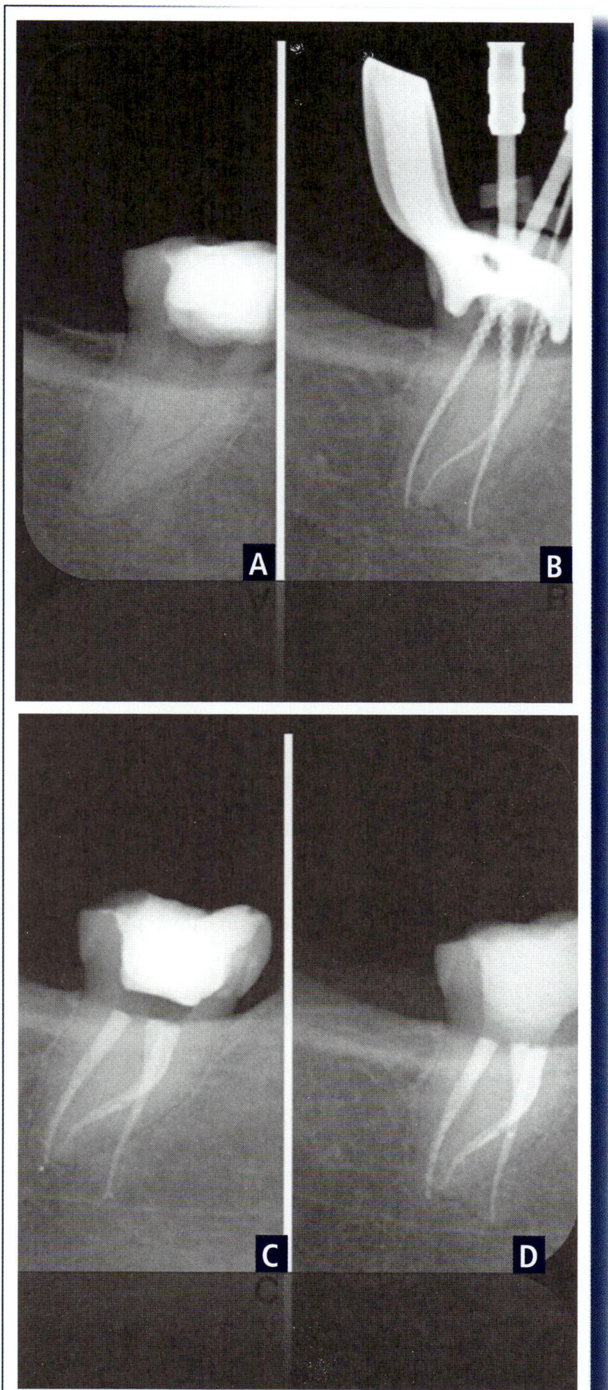

FIGS. 2.III-7A-D

Mandibular molar root canal treatment according to the descending wave technique. Follow-up of 5 years. Courtesy of Dr. Joan de Ribot.

- **Obtura II**

The Obtura II system (Obtura Spartan, Fenton MO, USA) uses a gun loaded with a gutta-percha cartridge, which is heated to a temperature of up to 170ºC (Fig. 2-III.8). To inject gutta-percha into the canal, we use silver needles connected to the gun. The silver needle size is chosen considering the root canal anatomy, with the larger diameter being used in the wider canals. To fill the canal with thermoplastic gutta-percha, the segmented technique, or another technique requiring several steps can be used, taking quantities of gutta-percha into the root canal sequentially, and afterwards proceeding with condensation, or a technique in which gutta-percha is introduced into the full extent of the canal in a single step. When using the segmented technique, we must choose different pluggers that fit the part of the canal where they will act. The smaller pluggers will work in the more apical parts and the larger ones in the more coronal parts. One chooses a silver needle that reaches within 3-5 mm of the apical preparation (apical stop). Sealing cement is inserted inside the canal with any of the previously mentioned techniques. In the segmented technique the silver needle is introduced 3-5 mm short of the apical stop, and 3-4 mm of gutta-percha is injected by pressing the trigger of the gun. After this, the gutta-percha is compacted in an apical direction with a single previously selected plugger. It is important to perform correct compaction, as thermoplastic gutta-percha contracts when it cools. Once compaction has been concluded, another 3-4 mm of gutta-percha is applied, and compaction continues, using a plugger with a smaller diameter. These steps must be repeated until the canal is completely filled. In the single step canal filling technique, we inject gutta-percha into 3-5 mm of the apical preparation (apical stop) and the silver needle will retract as the canal is filled. Once the filling has been completed, we exert pressure in the apical direction with a plugger, until the gutta-percha cools, thus partially compensating the gutta-percha shrinkage, which can be up to a volume of 2%[20].

An alternative to the Obtura II gun is the Elements system (SybronEndo, Orange, CA, USA). This system offers the cable of System B and a gutta-percha gun in a single device (Fig. 2.III-9). Cartridges that incorporate a tip are loaded into the gutta-percha gun (Fig. 2.III-10). This allows the use of both gutta-percha and RealSeal. It is cleaner and easier to manage than the Obtura gun, and has the ergonomic advantage of offering two unified devices.

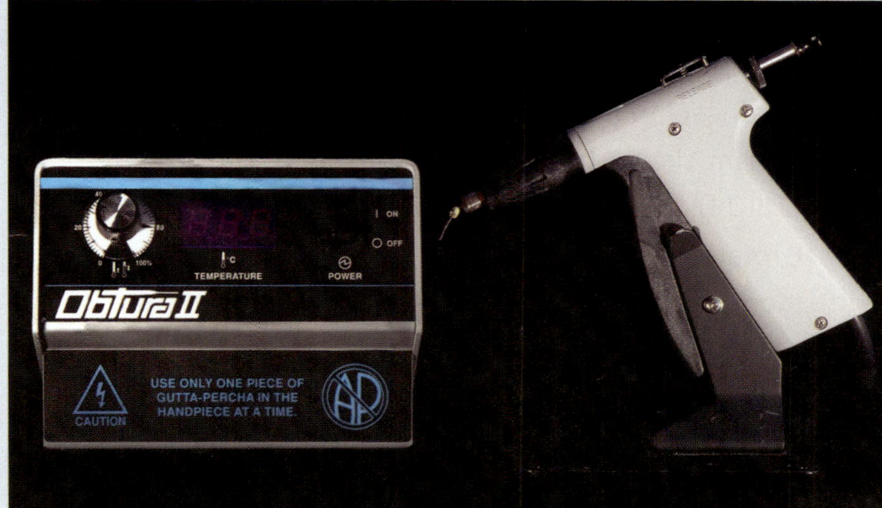

FIG. 2.III-8

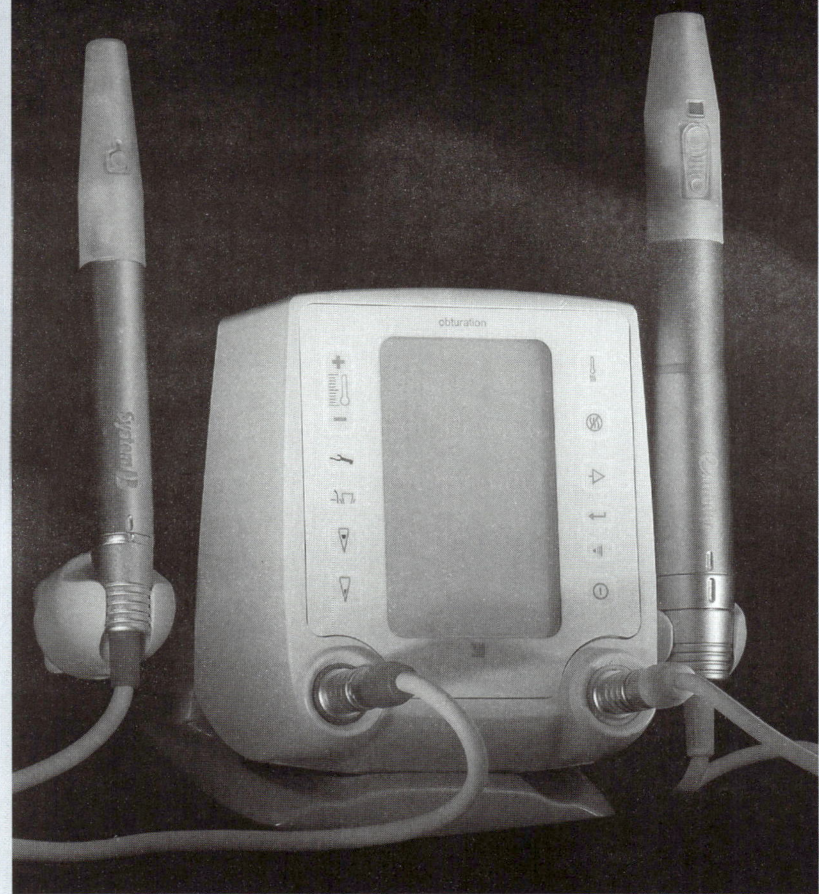

FIG. 2.III-9

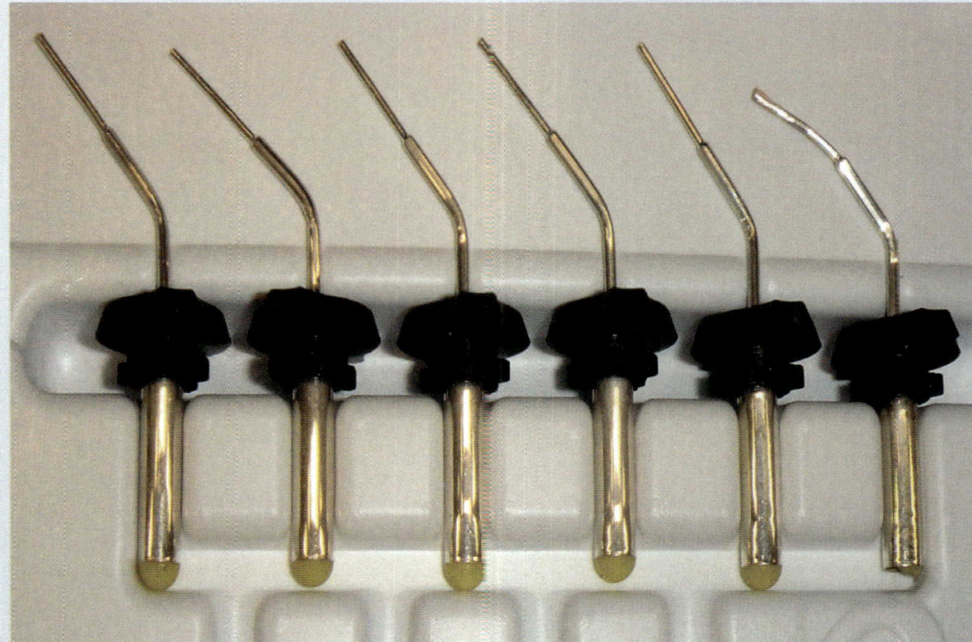

FIG. 2.III-10

FIG. 2.III-8

Obtura II gutta-percha injection gun.

FIG. 2.III-9

The Elements filling system combines a System B with a gutta-percha Extruder gun.

FIG. 2.III-10

Points for the Extruder system of Elements. Each point takes its corresponding load of gutta-percha or RedSeal.

THERMOCOMPACTORS

John McSpadden, in 1979, introduced the new concept of thermoplasticization of gutta-percha. Initially, the McSpadden condenser was an instrument similar to a type of an inverted Hedström file, or with the design of an inverted screw (Fig. 2.III-11). The instrument was mounted in a contra-angle hand piece and when used in a root canal, rotates between 8,000 – 10,000 rpm.

At these speeds, the heat generated by friction plasticizes the gutta-percha, and due to the design of the blades, compacts the material in an apical direction, while the condenser moves in a coronal direction. An experienced professional can feel the pressure in the opposite direction, allowing the instrument to exit the canal by its own action. With a certain amount of experience, canals can be filled in seconds.

However, the fragility and fracture potential of the instruments, as well as the possibility of overfilling, in addition to the difficulty of mastering the technique, resulted in reluctance on the part of endodontists to use this technique. Nevertheless, over time, with the appearance of different configurations in instruments and methods of application, it has become a more generally accepted technique.

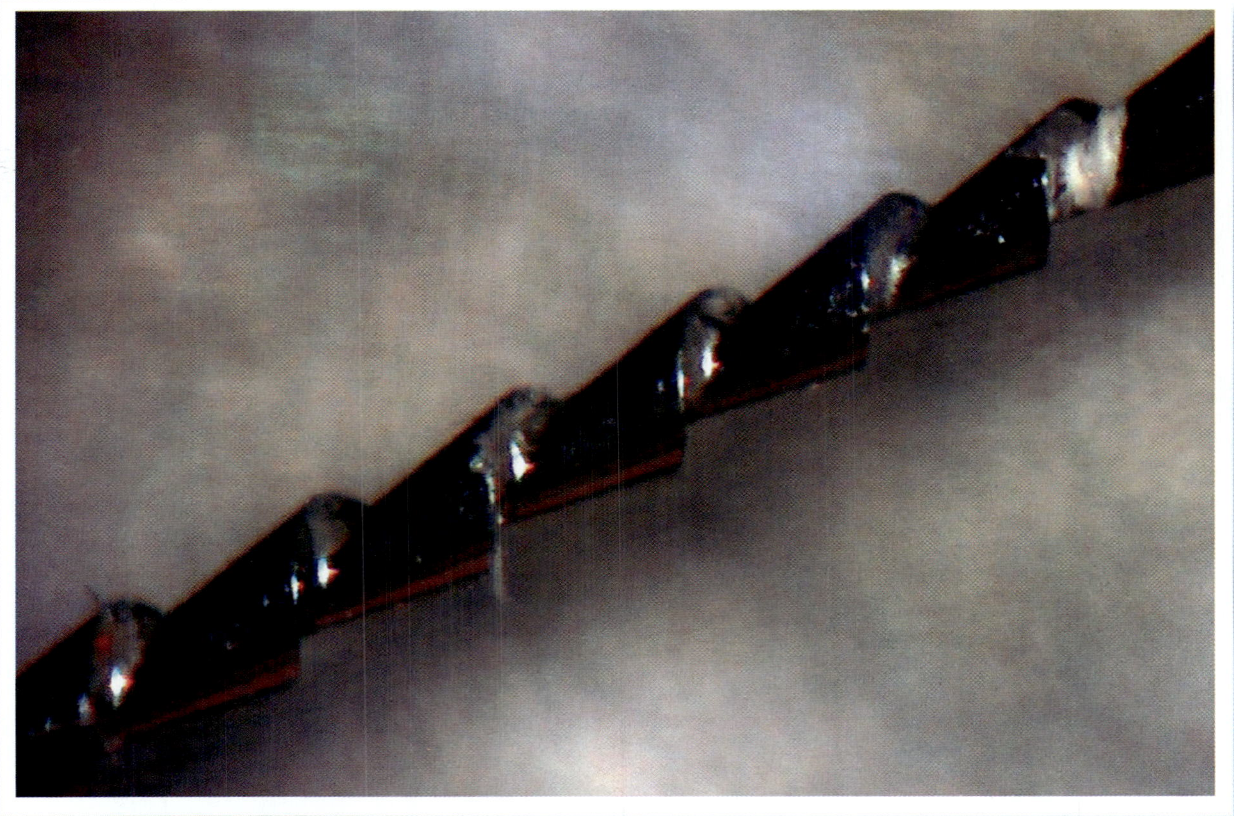

FIG. 2.III-11
Details of the spirals of a thermo-compaction instrument. Note the similarity to the spirals of a Hedström type file, but in an opposite direction.

In Europe, Maillefer modified the inverted Hedström type file and called it the Gutta-Condenser, and Zipperer called it the Engine Plugger, the latter resembling an inverted type K file. More recently, variations have been introduced, and these instruments are now made of a nickel-titanium alloy offering greater flexibility; for instance the Pac Mac condensers (Analytic-Endodontics, Glendora, CA, USA).

Numerous studies evaluated the efficacy of this root canal filling technique. The findings vary greatly, but appear to be positive. The technique is fast and saves gutta-percha cones. The root canal system sealing appeared to be adequate and radiographically there appeared to be good adaptation to the anatomic irregularities according to some publications[25,29].

The problems revolve around extrusion of the filling material, excavations of the root canal walls, fracture of the thermo condenser, possibilities of vertical fractures and dentin destruction[41].

The potential of this technique to produce excessive and harmful heat was also identified, thus increasing the external root temperature[4,18,24,36,39,44,45], capable of causing lesions in the periodontal supporting tissues due to overheating, leading to resorption and ankylosis. However, if the heat transmitted to the supporting tissues is sufficiently intense, the damage produced in these tissues may also occur with other techniques in which heated gutta-percha is used[37,38].

Lower speeds and placement of gutta-percha at a lower temperature were necessary to minimize the high temperatures and stress in the root canal system during rotary compaction. Furthermore, the use of higher speeds than what was recommended produced inferior sealing.

Nevertheless, careful root canal preparation and penetration depth of the rotary condenser will help to avoid possible operative accidents with the use of this technique. Familiarization of these techniques by means of *in vitro* practice is strongly recommended.

Tagger et al.[61] recommended a hybrid technique, in which the apical third of the canal is filled using cold active lateral condensation while the remainder is completed with a thermo condenser. The approach resolves control at the apical limit of filling, which is inherent to thermo condensation, accelerates filling and reduces the quantity of gutta-percha. Homogeneous and efficient filling can be obtained, and although the results are variable[43], it is a valid technique that complements lateral condensation very well[59,60].

THERMAFIL

In 1978, Johnson proposed a remarkable and at the same time easy method to fill a root canal with the use of alpha phase gutta-percha, thermoplasticized and applied in the canal by means of an endodontic file. Of interest is that his proposal became a commercial reality ten years later.

It was this technique that lead to the development of Thermafil (Dentsply Maillefer, Ballaigues, Switzerland) and similar methods, which is having a great impact on present-day endodontics. Thermafil is a patented endodontic filler that consists of a flexible central transporting rod, in sizes and tapers equivalent to those of endodontic files, uniformly lined with a layer of refined alpha phase gutta-percha. Initially the transporter was made of steel (in reality, a file) but later, due to the need for biocompatibility, they were made of titanium. The difficulty of taking it into the canal promoted another modification. Currently, these rods are made of radiopaque plastic (Fig. 2.III-12). The fillers are sold in different ISO sizes, and there are also Thermafil fillers adapted to specific instrumentation techniques, such as GT Profile or Protaper Universal (Dentsply Maillefer, Ballaigues, Switzerland) denominated F_1, F_2, F_3, F_4 and F_5. The plastic rods, apart from being equal in appearance and efficiency, do not have the same composition. The larger diameters of 40 to 90 are made of polysulphone polymer; that is why they can dissolve in chloroform, which is very useful in cases of retreatments.

As with all filling techniques, this one requires the use of a sealer cement. Not all cements appear to be suitable, and it is inadvisable to use zinc oxide and eugenol-based cements, such as Tubliseal or Wach paste, whereas resin-based sealers, such as AHPlus, AH 26 or similar ones, are recommended[26]. The smear layer must be removed with a chelating agent or low concentration acid (such as 10% citric acid), to promote flow of the material into the opened dentinal tubules to facilitate sealing[6]. It has been demonstrated that elimination of the smear layer, followed by filling with the Thermafil system, significantly diminishes bacterial penetration via the coronal aspect.

The technical advantages include easy placement (Fig. 2.III-13), the possibility of the thermoplasticized gutta-percha flowing into the irregularities of the canal, as well as into the lateral and accessory canals [69] and homogeneity of the filling[14].

The disadvantages are: Inability to control the density of filling in canals with an irregular shape; difficulty in removing the transporter and gutta-percha during retreatments and preparation of a space for prosthetic posts. In addition there is a greater risk of extrusion of material into the periapical tissues[13,14,31].

The use of these devices begins with the selection of a suitable transporter. Therefore, one has to select a transporter with a diameter equal to or slightly larger than the largest instrument that was used to the working length. To prove whether this is correct, since it is not possible to take a radiograph for proof, there is a type of transporter on the market, without gutta-percha, which is radiopaque and corresponds to the transporter size. This is called a verifier. When placed in the

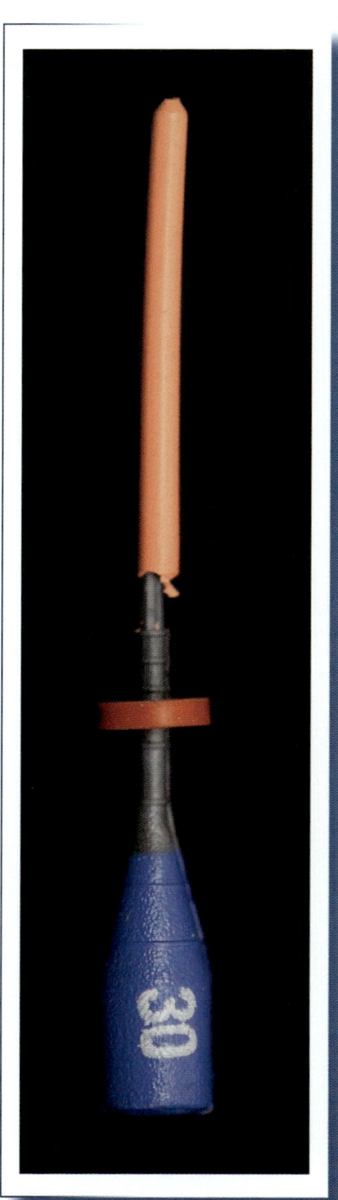

FIG. 2.III-12
Thermafil Filler with a 30 A diameter. Calibration is in accordance with the ISO standard and requires a preparation with a minimum taper of 0.04 mm/mm.

canal, a radiograph will show whether it reaches the desired location. Bear in mind that transporters can have different tapers, but they are almost always equal to or larger than 4%. Non-telescopic manual instrumentation can make it impossible to perform adequate filling with this system.

Once the canal has been dried the transporter is heated in a specific Thermaprep Plus oven, (Dentsply Maillefer, Ballaigues, Switzerland), provided by the system. First a small amount of sealer has to be placed inside the canal with for instance a paper point or a file coated with cement while turning the file in a counter-clockwise direction. Heating of the Thermofil takes only a few seconds and when it reaches the correct temperature, it is removed from the oven and immediately placed in the canal. Be aware of the fact that the length to which the transporter must be taken has to be determined beforehand, in order to take advantage of the marks of 18, 19, 20, 22, 24, 27 and 29 mm on the filler handle. The filling length and filling of the irregularities in the canal improves when placement is done quickly. Fast insertion also improves the filling[35].

After having placed the transporter in the canal, rapid cooling causes shrinkage of the material. Thus it is necessary to maintain firm apical pressure on the transporter for approximately 10 seconds, to compensate for shrinkage,

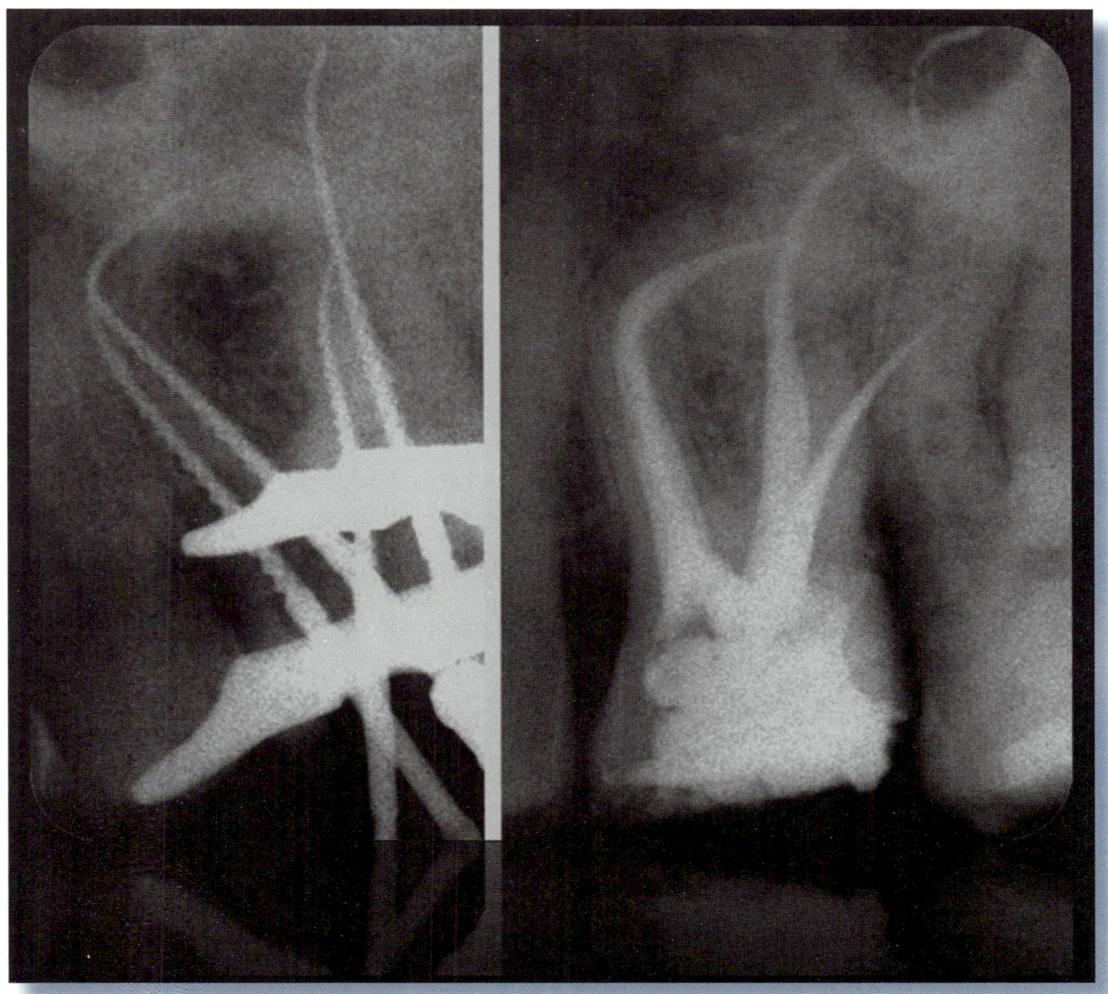

FIG. 2.III-13

The Thermafil technique is useful for filling curved and long canals. Courtesy of Dr. Silvia Caudet.

avoiding spaces between the gutta-percha and root canal walls.

Finally, the rod at the canal opening is cut. This can be done with use any high-speed bur, but it is preferable to use a smooth round bur without cutting edges, so that the rod is separated by heat. This avoids the risk of distortion occurring on the floor of the pulp chamber.

Finally, the gutta-percha is condensed with a manual compactor, particularly at the entrance of the canals, followed by a postoperative radiograph.

If the root canal is wide in a bucco-lingual direction, we can use a finger spreader next to the rod, creating space for auxiliary cones with simultaneous lateral or vertical condensation. If there is sufficient space, we can also use an injectable technique. Cold cones easily adhere to the softened mass.

It is not necessary to precurve the Thermafil condensers, provided that the canal has been correctly prepared, since the flexible transporter will easily accommodate the length of the curves. With this technique, the gutta-percha will flow into the irregularities of the canal, such as anastomoses, lateral canals and resorptions.

- **Successfil**

There are systems similar to Thermafil on the market, sold by other companies. Among them, there is Successfil (Coltène Hygienic, Akron, OH, USA), which is also a solid center transporter covered with alpha phase. But in this case the gutta-percha is kept in a syringe, and once heated, it is taken to the transporter before being inserted into the canal. The Successfil transporters, made of titanium or radiopaque plastic, are placed to the depth corresponding to the gutta-percha in the syringe, and dispensed by pressing the plunger. The technique for using it has similar advantages and disadvantages to those of Thermafil.

- **Simplifill**

A filling system with a rigid and slightly different transporter is Simplifill (Lightspeed Technologies, San Antonio, TX, USA), specifically designed for the Lightspeed instrumentation system. It consists of a rod covered with gutta-percha on its last 5 mm. A rod is selected that corresponds to the memory-file (largest diameter instrument that reached the real working length), and after a sealer has been in the canal the rod is inserted in the canal with firm pressure. When the real working length is reached, the rod is remove with a quick counter-clockwise turn of up to four turns. According to the manufacturer, the remainder of the filling should be completed with a resin-based cement only, or with another filling technique (vertical compaction, thermo injected gutta-percha, thermo compaction, active lateral condensation or whatever is considered most appropriate). It is a filling system with sealing efficacy similar to that of any other system[42].

CORONAL SEALING

We cannot overemphasize the importance of optimum coronal sealing. The absence of a good coronal restoration will inevitably cause coronal leakage[64,65], considered one of the main causes of endodontic treatment failure. Brief exposure of the filling material to the oral environment, between a week and a month, according to some authors, can lead to treatment failure. It is essential to prevent any possible contamination from occurring, and therefore, it is important to perform the definitive restoration as soon as possible. However, when a definitive restoration cannot be performed, we must proceed with temporary sealing, as hermetically as possible using a glass ionomer or composite resin, the latter with an adhesive system)[7,12].

References

1. Aguirre AM, El-Deeb ME, Aguirre R. The effect of ultrasonics on sealer distribution and sealing of root canals. J Endod, v.23, n.12, p.759-764, 1997.
2. Al-Dewani N, Hayes SJ, Dummer PM. Comparison of laterally condensed and low-temperature thermoplasticized gutta-percha root fillings. J Endod, v.26, n.12, p.733-738, 2000.
3. Allison DA, Michelich RJ, Walton RE. The influence of master cone adaptation on the quality of the apical seal. J Endod, v.7, n.2, p.61-65, 1981.
4. Beatty RG, Vertucci FJ, Hojjatie B. Thermomechanical compaction of gutta-percha: effect of speed and duration. Int Endod J, v.21, n.6, p.367-375, 1988.
5. Beatty RG, Zakariasen KL. Apical leakage associated with three obturation techniques in large and small root canals. Int Endod J, v.17, n.2, p.67-72, 1984.
6. Behrend GD, Cutler CW, Gutmann JL. An in-vitro study of smear layer removal and microbial leakage along root-canal fillings. Int Endod J, v.29, n.2, p.99-107, 1996.
7. Belli S, Zhang Y, Pereira PN, Pashley DH. Adhesive sealing of the pulp chamber. J Endod, v.27, n.8, p.521-526, 2001.
8. Berry KA, Loushine RJ, Primack PD, Runyan DA. Nickel-titanium versus stainless-steel finger spreaders in curved canals. J Endod, v.24, n.11, p.752-754, 1998.
9. Bowman CJ, Baumgartner JC. Gutta-percha obturation of lateral grooves and depressions. J Endod, v.28, n.3, p.220-223, 2002.
10. Buchanan LS. Continuous wave of condensation technique. Endod Prac v.1, n.4, p.7-10, 13-15, 18 passim, 1998.
11. Cailleteau JG, Mullaney TP. Prevalence of teaching apical patency and various instrumentation and obturation techniques in United States dental schools. J Endod, v.23, n.6, p.394-396, 1997.
12. Chailertvanitkul P, Saunders WP, MacKenzie D. The effect of smear layer on microbial coronal leakage of gutta-percha root fillings. Int Endod J, v.29, n.4, p.242-248, 1996.
13. Clinton K, Van Himel T. Comparison of a warm gutta-percha obturation technique and lateral condensation. J Endod, v.27, n.11, p.692-695, 2001.
14. Da Silva D, Endal U, Reynaud A, Portenier I, Orstavik D, Haapasalo M. A comparative study of lateral condensation, heat-softened gutta-percha, and a modified master cone heat-softened backfilling technique. Int Endod J, v.35, n.12, p.1005-1011, 2002.
15. Delivanis PD, Mattison GD, Mendel RW. The survivability of F43 strain of Streptococcus sanguis in root canals filled with gutta-percha and Procosol cement. J Endod, v.9, n.10, p.407-410, 1983.
16. Farzaneh M, Abitbol S, Friedman S. Treatment outcome in endodontics: the Toronto study. Phases I and II: Orthograde retreatment. J Endod, v.30, n.9, p.627-633, 2004.
17. Farzaneh M, Abitbol S, Lawrence HP, Friedman S. Treatment outcome in endodontics: the Toronto Study. Phase II: initial treatment. J Endod, v.30, n.5, p.302-309, 2004.
18. Fors U, Jonasson E, Berquist A, Berg JO. Measurements of the root surface temperature during thermo-mechanical root canal filling in vitro. Int Endod J, v.18, n.3, p.199-202, 1985.
19. Gilhooly RM, Hayes SJ, Bryant ST, Dummer PM. Comparison of lateral condensation and thermomechanically compacted warm alpha-phase gutta-percha with a single cone for obturating curved root canals. Oral Surg, Oral Méd, Oral Pathol, Oral Radiol Endod, v.91, n.1, p.89-94, 2001.
20. Grassi MD, Plazek DJ, Michanowicz AE, Chay IC. Changes in the physical properties of the Ultrafil low-temperature (70 degrees C) thermoplasticized gutta-percha system. J Endod, v.15, n.11, p.517-521, 1989.
21. Grossman L. Endodontics. 11 ed. Philadelphia: Lea & Febiger, 1988.
22. Guess GM, Edwards KR, Yang ML, Iqbal MK, Kim S. Analysis of continuous-wave obturation using a single-cone and hybrid technique. J Endod, v.29, n.8, p.509-512, 2003.
23. Hall MC, Clement DJ, Dove SB, Walker WA. 3rd. A comparison of sealer placement techniques in curved canals. J Endod, v.22, n.12, p.638-642, 1996.
24. Hardie EM. Further studies on heat generation during obturation techniques involving thermally softened gutta-percha. Int Endod J, v.20, n.3, p.122-127, 1987.
25. Harris GZ, Dickey DJ, Lemon RR, Luebke RG. Apical seal: McSpadden vs lateral condensation. J Endod, v.8, n.6, p.273-276, 1982.
26. Johnson WT, Gutmann JL. Obturation of the cleaned and shaped root canal system. In: Cohen, S.; Hargreaves, K., editors. Pathways of the pulp. 9th ed. St Louis: Mosby Elsevier, p.358-398, 2006.
27. Joyce AP, Loushine RJ, West LA, Runyan DA, Cameron SM. Photoelastic comparison of stress induced by using stainless-steel versus nickel-titanium spreaders in vitro. J Endod, v.24, n.11, p.714-715, 1998.
28. Jung IY, Lee SB, Kim ES, Lee CY, Lee SJ. Effect of different temperatures and penetration depths of a System B plugger in the filling of artificially created oval canals. Oral Surg, Oral Méd, Oral Pathol, Oral Radiol Endod, v.96, n.4, p.453-457, 2003.
29. Kersten HW, Fransman R, Thoden van Velzen SK. Thermomechanical compaction of gutta-percha. II. A comparison with lateral condensation in curved root canals. Int Endod J, v.19, n.3, p.134-140, 1986.
30. Klevant FJ, Eggink CO. The effect of canal preparation on periapical disease. Int Endod J, v.16, n.2, p.68-75, 1983.
31. Kytridou V, Gutmann JL, Nunn MH. Adaptation and sealability of two contemporary obturation techniques in the absence of the dentinal smear layer. Int Endod J, v.32, n.6, p.464-474, 1999.
32. Lea CS, Apicella MJ, Mines P, Yancich PP, Parker MH. Comparison of the obturation density of cold lateral compaction versus warm vertical compaction using the continuous wave of condensation technique. J Endod, v.31, n.1, p.37-39, 2005.
33. Leonardo MR, Barnett F, Debelian GJ, Pontes Lima RE, Silva LAB. Root canal adhesive filling in dogs' teeth with or without coronal restoration: a histopathological evaluation. J Endod, v.33, n.11, p.1200-1303, 2007.
34. Lertchirakarn V, Palamara JE, Messer HH. Load and strain during lateral condensation and vertical root fracture. J Endod, v.25, n.2, p.99-104, 1999.
35. Levitan ME, Himel VT, Luckey JB. The effect of insertion rates on fill length and adaptation of a thermoplasticized gutta-percha technique. J Endod, v.29, n.8, p.505-508, 2003.

36. Lipski M. Root surface temperature rises in vitro during root canal obturation using hybrid and microseal techniques. J Endod, v.31, n.4, p.297-300, 2005.

37. Lipski M. In vitro infrared thermographic assessment of root surface temperatures generated by high-temperature thermoplasticized injectable gutta-percha obturation technique. J Endod, v.32, n.5, p.438-441, 2006.

38. Lipski M, Wozniak K. In vitro infrared thermographic assessment of root surface temperature rises during thermafil retreatment using system B. J Endod, v.29, n.6, p.413-415, 2003.

39. McCullagh JJ, Biagioni PA, Lamey PJ, Hussey DL. Thermographic assessment of root canal obturation using thermomechanical compaction. Int Endod J, v.30, n.3, p.191-195, 1997.

40. Nair PN. On the causes of persistent apical periodontitis: a review. Int Endod J, v.39, n.4, p.249-281, 2006.

41. O'Neill KJ, Pitts DL, Harrington GW. Evaluation of the apical seal produced by the McSpadden compactor and the lateral condensation with a chloroform-softened primary cone. J Endod, v.9, n.5, p.190-197, 1983.

42. Santos MD, Walker WA, 3rd Carnes DL Jr. Evaluation of apical seal in straight canals after obturation using the Lightspeed sectional method. J Endod, v.25, n.9, p.609-612, 1999.

43. Saunders EM. The effect of variation in thermomechanical compaction techniques upon the quality of the apical seal. Int Endod J, v.22, n.4, p.163-168, 1989.

44. Saunders EM. In vivo findings associated with heat generation during thermomechanical compaction of gutta-percha. 1. Temperature levels at the external surface of the root. Int Endod J, v.23, n.5, p.263-267, 1990.

45. Saunders EM. In vivo findings associated with heat generation during thermomechanical compaction of gutta-percha. 2. Histological response to temperature elevation on the external surface of the root. Int Endod J, v.23, n.5, p.268-274, 1990.

46. Schilder, H. Filling root canals in three dimensions. Dent Clin North Am, p.723-744, 1967.

47. Schmidt KJ, Walker TL, Johnson JD, Nicoll BK. Comparison of nickel-titanium and stainless-steel spreader penetration and accessory cone fit in curved canals. J Endod, v.26, n.1, p.42-44, 2000.

48. Seltzer S. Long-term radiographic and histological observations of endodontically treated teeth. J Endod, v.25, n.12, p.818-822, 1999.

49. Seltzer S, Soltanoff W, Smith J. Biologic aspects of endodontics. V. Periapical tissue reactions to root canal instrumentation beyond the apex and root canal fillings short of and beyond the apex. Oral Surg, Oral Méd, Oral Pathol, v.36, n.5, p.725-737, 1973.

50. Senia ES, Marshall FJ, Rosen S. The solvent action of sodium hypochlorite on pulp tissue of extracted teeth. Oral Surg, Oral Méd, Oral Pathol, v.31, n.1, p.96-103, 1971.

51. Shipper G, Orstavik D, Teixeira FB, Trope M. An evaluation of microbial leakage in roots filled with a thermoplastic synthetic polymer-based root canal filling material (Resilon). J Endod, v.30, n.5, p.342-347, 2004.

52. Shipper G, Teixeira FB, Arnold RR, Trope M. Periapical inflammation after coronal microbial inoculation of dog roots filled with gutta-percha or resilon. J Endod, v.31, n.2, p.91-96, 2005.

53. Sjogren U, Hagglund B, Sundqvist G, Wing K. Factors affecting the long-term results of endodontic treatment. J Endod, v.16, n.10, p.498-504, 1990.

54. Smith CS, Setchell DJ, Harty FJ. Factors influencing the success of conventional root canal therapy – a five-year retrospective study. Int Endod J, v.26, n.6, p.321-333, 1993.

55. Smith RS, Weller RN, Loushine RJ, Kimbrough WF. Effect of varying the depth of heat application on the adaptability of gutta-percha during warm vertical compaction. J Endod, v.26, n.11, p.668-672, 2000.

56. Southard DW, Rooney TP. Effective one-visit therapy for the acute periapical abscess. J Endod, v.10, n.12, p.580-583, 1984.

57. Stamos DE, Gutmann JL, Gettleman BH. In vivo evaluation of root canal sealer distribution. J Endod, v.21, n.4, p.177-179, 1995.

58. Swartz DB, Skidmore AE, Griffin JA Jr. Twenty years of endodontic success and failure. J Endod., v.9, n5, p.198-202, 1983.

59. Tagger M, Gold A. Flow of various brands of Gutta-percha cones under in vitro thermomechanical compaction. J Endod, v.14, n.3, p.115-120, 1988.

60. Tagger M, Tamse A, Katz A. Efficacy of apical seal of Engine Plugger condensed root canal fillings – leakage to dyes. Oral Surg, Oral Med., Oral Pathol, v.56, n.6, p.641-646, 1983.

61. Tagger M, Tamse A, Katz A, Korzen BH. Evaluation of the apical seal produced by a hybrid root canal filling method, combining lateral condensation and thermatic compaction. J Endod, v.10, n.7, p.299-303, 1984.

62. Teixeira FB, Teixeira EC, Thompson JY, Trope M. Fracture resistance of roots endodontically treated with a new resin filling material. J. Am. Dent. Assoc., v.135, n.5, p.646-652, 2004.

63. Torabinejad M, Skobe Z, Trombly PL, Krakow AA, Gron P, Marlin J. Scanning electron microscopic study of root canal obturation using thermoplasticized gutta-percha. J Endod, v.4, n.8, p.245-250, 1978.

64. Torabinejad M, Ung B, Kettering JD. In vitro bacterial penetration of coronally unsealed endodontically treated teeth. J Endod, v.16, n.12, p.566-569, 1990.

65. Trope M, Chow E, Nissan R. In vitro endotoxin penetration of coronally unsealed endodontically treated teeth. Endod. Dent. Traumatol., v.11, n.2, p.90-94, 1995.

66. Villegas JC, Yoshioka T, Kobayashi C, Suda H. Obturation of accessory canals after four different final irrigation regimes. J Endod, v.28, n.7, p.534-536, 2002.

67. Villegas JC, Yoshioka T, Kobayashi C, Suda H. Three-step versus single-step use of system B: evaluation of gutta-percha root canal fillings and their adaptation to the canal walls. J Endod, v.30, n.10, p.719-721, 2004.

68. Wiemann AH, Wilcox LR. In vitro evaluation of four methods of sealer placement. J Endod, v.17, n.9, p.444-447, 1991.

69. Wolcott J, Himel VT, Powell W, Penney J. Effect of two obturation techniques on the filling of lateral canals and the main canal. J Endod, v.23, n.10, p.632-635, 1997.

70. Wu MK, Van Der Sluis LW, Wesselink PR. A preliminary study of the percentage of gutta-percha-filled area in the apical canal filled with vertically compacted warm gutta-percha. Int Endod J, v.35, n.6, p.527-535, 2002.

71. Wu MK, Wesselink PR. A primary observation on the preparation and obturation of oval canals. Int Endod J, v.34, n.2, p.137-141, 2001.

72. Wu MK, Wesselink PR, Walton RE. Apical terminus location of root canal treatment procedures. Oral Surg, Oral Med., Oral Pathol, Oral Radiol. Endod., v.89, n.1, p.99-103, 2000.

2.IV

Technique of molar root canal debridement in a crown/apex direction

Goerig et al.[2] Technique (Modified)

Mario Roberto Leonardo
Mário Tanomaru Filho

Applying the same crown/apex principle without pressure as the Oregon technique, which was originally indicated only for straight root canals, Goerig et al.[2] made some modifications and indicated it for the debridement of curved molar root canals.

The original technique recommended by Goerig et al.[2] is sequentially performed in three operative stages:

1. Coronal Access
2. Root access
3. Apical preparation

Although this sequence is performed with manual and mechanical procedures, it is based on biological principles. Applied in a crown/apex direction in cases of Necropulpectomy, it will promote mechanical removal and subsequent detoxyfication of the septic/toxic content of the root canal with irrigant solutions, consequently avoiding extrusion of these necrotic and infected remnants into the periapical region. This considerably reduces unwanted acute apical periodontites (post-operative pain), as well as cases of Flare-up, or according to Samuel Seltzer, Fenix abscesses, which effects the patient's perception of the endodontic profession.

At that time, root canal debridement (step-down) according to Goerig et al.[2], and the OREGON technique (crown-down), which applied the crown/apex principle without pressure, that is, beginning the preparation from the cervical third and gradually advancing towards the apical direction (in accordance with a sequential diminishing of the file diameter (D_1)), caused great impact because for 160 years canal preparation was performed in the opposite way, that is, applying the apex/crown principle, which is greatly responsible for acute apical periodontitis.

With the passage of time and the clinical experience gained by practitioners (mastery of the technique), the techniques that used the preparation principle of the crown/apex direction offered many advantageous, and were incorporated in the present technique of manual/mechanical root canal debridement. It should be noted that the faculties of dental schools in the United States of America decided not to teach the apex/crown principle (step-back) treatment technique in their undergraduate and postgraduate curriculum, but rather the crown-down tehnique.

Based on the original technique of Goerig et al.[2], we refined the same technique with modifications, particularly with the use of updated terms that differ from the terminology of the original technique. In addition some technical details were included to improve the application of the fundamental principles.

GOERIG ET AL.[2] TECHNIQUE (MODIFIED)

NOTE: This technique is recommended for conservative followers of manual/mechanical debridement, who have not yet incorporated the new oscillatory and/or rotary root canal preparation systems in their daily clinical practice, particularly with respect to atresic and curved roots of molars.

Operative stages

1. Coronal opening (access preparation), which Goerig et al.[2] originally called **coronal access**.
2. Reaming or anti-curvature filing, previously called **root access**.
3. Perform apical stop, originally called **apical preparation**.

Stage 1 – Coronal opening

Coronal opening is the operative act that opens (exposes) the pulp chamber. The initial objective of coronal opening (access preparation) is to access the internal anatomy of the pulp chamber on the occlusal (posterior teeth) and/or lingual (anterior teeth) surfaces. Thus, with this operative stage nothing more than the removal of the roof of the pulp chamber is accomplished, that is, to expose the size and shape of the pulp chamber for direct vision and access.

It has the aim of obtaining unobstructed, direct and broad access to the entrance or entrances of the root canals and this initial operative step must be complemented with **radicular access** preparation creating a **convenience shape**.

- Proper **radicular access** is performed at the level just coronal to the root canal orifices. Typically, the mesial wall of mandibular molars have a cervical bulge that may prevent the clinician from obtaining straight line access into the root canals (radicular access). This cervical convexity needs to be straightened in order to have proper radicular access into the root canals. The BATT burs and preferably the Endo-Z burs (Dentsply/Maillefer) are used for this purpose. SybronEndo (sds) Glendona, CA, USA, offers a kit, LA-AXXESS, that includes burs to prepare the radicular access:
    - Long tapered diamond tips
    - Extra-long tapered diamond tips

Dentsply/Maillefer (Ballaigues, Switzerland) also offers an Endodontic access kit composed of a spherical diamond tip (for access opening), transmetal bur (for metal restorations), long shank spherical tips, Endo Z and X-Gates burs. Ultradent Products Inc, USA, offers the Access Kit for the same purposes.

- **Convenience form** is the operative step in which the final contour of the coronal opening is prepared and it is performed by means of cutting with high speed burs, for example the Endo-Z bur, or cylindrical/tapered diamond tips without an active tip, with the aim of determining a divergence in an occlusal direction of the pulp chamber walls and coronal opening itself. This greater divergence, particularly of the mesial walls of the pulp chamber of molars, will make endodontic treatment much easier because. According to Paiva & Antoniazzi[3], light (illumination) and instruments (direction) always takes place in a mesio-distal direction. Convenience shaping of the coronal opening also consists of including the inclined slope of the buccal cusp of mandibular pre-molars and mesio-buccal cusps in mandibular and maxillary molars, with the aim of obtaining direct access to the root canals.

NOTE: The statement by Paiva & Antoniazzi[3], with regard to illumination of the operative field, is not applicable when the operating microscope is used.

ADVANTAGES OF RADICULAR ACCESS PREPARATION AND CONVENIENCE FORM

a. To allow broad visualization of the floor of the pulp chamber in molars, while facilitating the location and making a mental assessment of the root canal openings.
b. To facilitate direct access in a straight line and exploration (apical patency) of the canal or root canals.
c. To promote maintaining the original direction in which root canals run, particularly in the apical third (**apical five millimeters**).
d. To diminish the acuteness of the curvature at the cervical third, reducing the possibility of operative errors such as steps, trepanations, perforations, etc.
e. To allow and facilitate faster debridement of curved root canals of molars.

Stage 2 – Filing and anticurvature preparation

The direction of the mesial root canals of mandibular molars and mesio-buccal canals of maxillary molars, at the cervical thirds (coronal and middle), is from distal to mesial. At the level where the middle third joins with the apical third, the curvature runs in an opposite direction, with their trajectories in a distal direction, referred to as double curvature, which greatly contributes to successful debridement of the root canals in these cases. The first curvature (at the cervical level) can be overcome with reaming or anticurvature filing (*see* Chapter 2.II).

For this operative stage, according to the original technique described by Goerig et al.[2], the authors recommended direct and sequential use of Hedström type files No 15 and 25, creating space for later use of Gates Glidden drills Nos. 2 and 3. In this stage, which is a modification of the original technique, we prefer to first open a space with type K files that match with the anatomy of the two coronal thirds of the root canal, for the purpose of examination. This is followed with a Hedström file of an immediate previous number to that of the last type K file, and then continued with larger

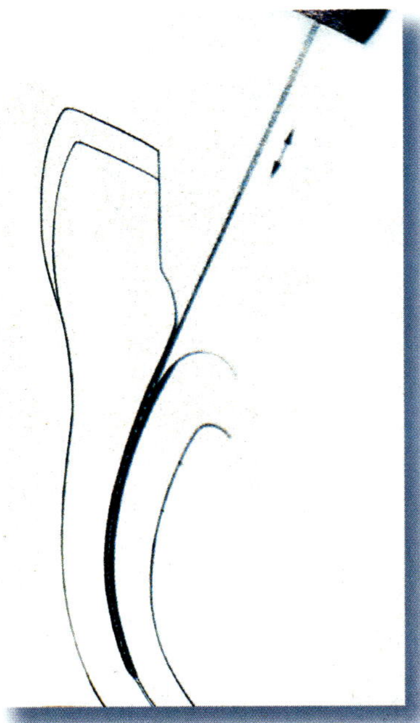

FIG. 2.IV-1

Diagrammatic drawing, showing exploration (catheterization) of the atresic and curved root canal of the mandibular molar with a type K file No 20, indicating the use of a Hedströen type file No 15 to begin anticurvature filing in accordance with the modified Goerig et al.[2] technique.

diameters (Fig. 2.IV-1). During this sequence, any operative risk with the use of the Hedström type files must be avoided and they must never be used with rotary movements.

The action with the use of Hedström type files is as follows:

1. Introduction of the Hedström type file of an immediately previous number to that of the last type K file used make space.
2. Lateral traction (removal) with successive small excursions against the root canal walls, particularly on the safe area.
3. Continue using only the Hedström type files with larger diameters sequentially, until reaching No 20 and/or 25 files using the same action.

After the anticurvature filing stage, with initial use of type K file followed only then with the Hedström type files, up to No 20 and/or 25, the use of Gates Glidden burs (GG) is indicated for the mesial root canals of molars using only No 2 and 3 files. For the distal root canal of mandibular molars and lingual canals of maxillary molars, the Gates Glidden sequence can go up to No 4 (Fig. 2.IV-2).

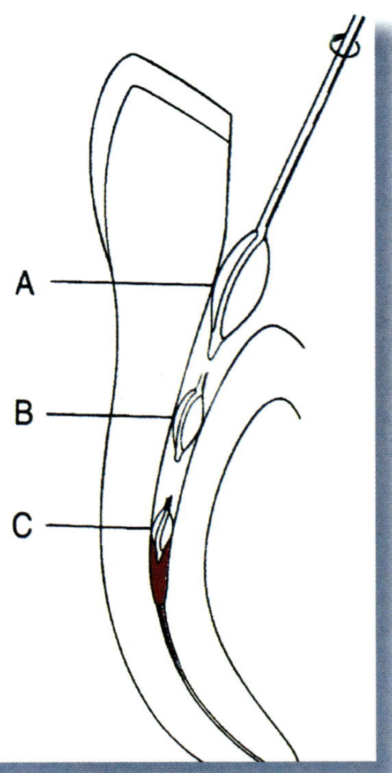

FIG. 2.IV-2

Diagrammatic drawing, showing the use of the Gates Glidden burs No 2, 3 and 4 to complement the anticurvature filing performed in the single distal root canal of the mandibular molar.

ADVANTAGES OF RADICULAR ACCESS PREPARATION AND ANTICURVATURE FILING

- To remove dentin interferences that correspond to the safe area, according to Abou-Rass et al.[1] and overcome obstacles offered by the cervical curvature (first curvature so-called double curvature, seen in the mesial roots of mandibular molars and mesio-buccal roots of maxillary molars).
- With the initial use of type K files, and then with the Hedström type, before using the GG burs, the possibility of perforations (trepanations) at furcation level is significantly reduced.
- Provide better abundant irrigation and at greater depth in atresic and curved root canals.
- In cases of necropulpectomies, to allow removal of the largest concentration of necrotic remnants, microorganisms, their products, byproducts and endotoxins before debridement of the apical five millimeters (3rd stage of the technique).
- To provide a more stable and reliable working length which, in this technique, is done after the operative step (access preparation or anticurvature filing).
- To allow free and direct access to the **apical five millimeters**.
- To facilitate establishing an **apical stop**, the reason for obtaining clinical, radiographic and histologic success of root canal treatment when the biological principles are adhered to.
- To promote maintaining of the original direction of root canals in their **apical five millimeters**.
- To promote reducing the effect of root canal curvatures, diminishing the possibility of operative errors such as steps, trepanations, etc.
- To allow for and promote faster and safer debridement of curved root canals of molars.
- To enable treatment of cases of biopulpectomies and particularly of necropulpectomies.

Stage 3 – Establishing the apical stop

With the modified technique of Goerig et al.[2], the **apical stop**, which involves the **apical five millimeters** and constitutes the critical zone of biological endodontics, is easy to make, thanks to the previous steps. Coronal opening (Stage 1), including radicular access preparation and convenience form, followed by reaming or anticurvature filing (Stage 2) allow free, full and direct access to the apical limit of debridement (real working length) making it easy to perform the apical stop.

GOERIG ET AL.[2] TECHNIQUE (MODIFIED)
(Hypothetical technical sequence)

Main indication: Necropulpectomy II.

Other indications: Necropulpectomy I and biopulpectomy.

Recommendation: for practitioners who still prefer to use mechanical/manual debridement techniques for straight atresic and/or curved root canals.

Action principle: Crown/apex without pressure (step-down pressureless technique).

Recommendation: maxillary molars (buccal canals) and mandibular molars (mesial canals) with accentuated cervical curvatures.

Technical sequence in the case of biopulpectomy in molars

1st Session:

1. Organization of the clinical tray.
2. Mouth wash for the oral cavity with antiseptic solutions.
3. Clinical examination.

4. Radiography for diagnosis (Fig. 2.IV-3).
5. Clinical and radiographic diagnosis: Irreversible acute pulpitis submitted to emergency treatment.
6. Indication: biopulpectomy.
7. Endodontic treatment planning.
   - 7.1. Determining the temporary working length (TWL).
     - 7.1.1. Apparent tooth length – ATL – 2 mm = TWL.
   - 7.2. In the radiograph for diagnosis, note the approximate diameter of the root canal openings.
   - 7.3. In the radiograph for diagnosis, note the apparent length that corresponds to the safe area (to perform anticurvature filing).
8. Anesthesia.
9. Tooth preparation to receive a rubber dam.
10. Placement of the rubber dam.
11. Antisepsis of the operative field with 2% chlorhexidine gluconate.
12. Coronal opening (surgical access) (Fig. 2.IV-4).
    - 12.1. Radicular access preparation (Fig. 2.IV-5).
    - 12.2. Convenience form (removal of inclined slope of the mesio-buccal cusp) (Figs. 2.IV-6 and 2.IV-7).
13. Copious irrigation of the pulp chamber and root canal opening only, with concentrated solution of 5.25% sodium hypochlorite and 10 cc of oxygenated water (biopulpectomy).

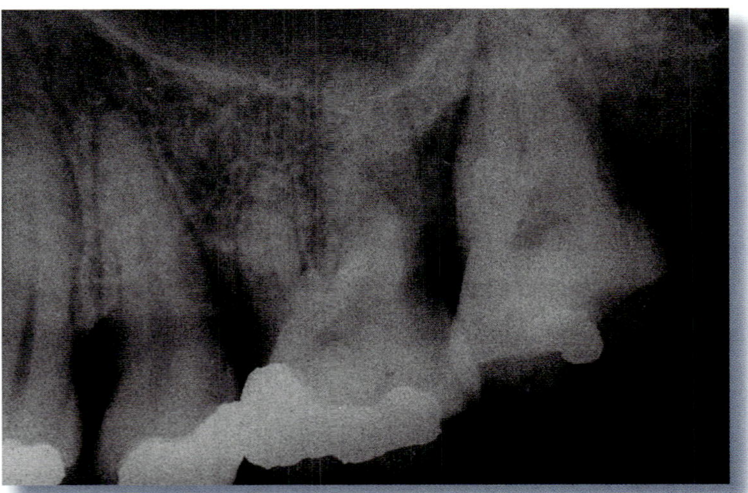

FIG. 2.IV-3

Periapical radiograph for diagnosis of the maxillary left first molar (26) previously submitted to emergency endodontic treatment. Note double curvature of vestibular root canals, reason for greater indication of the Goerig et al.[2] technique (modified), even as previous preparation for the use of rotary systems.

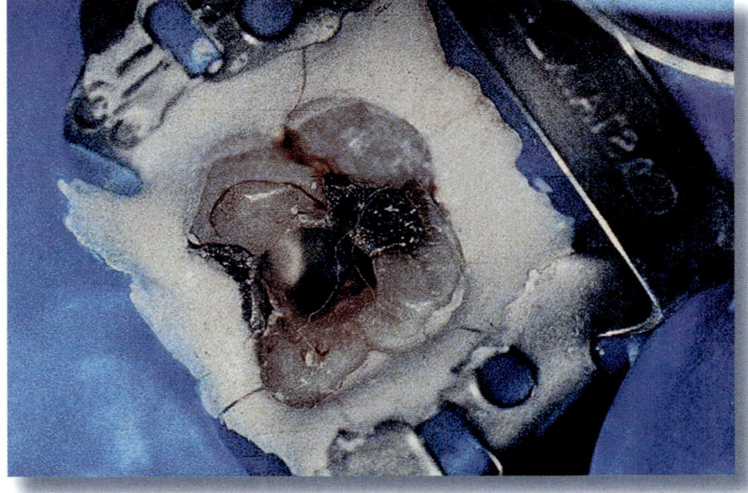

FIG. 2.IV-4

Clinical aspect showing the pulp chamber after removal of the temporary coronal sealing and a piece of cotton used as dressing during emergency attendance.

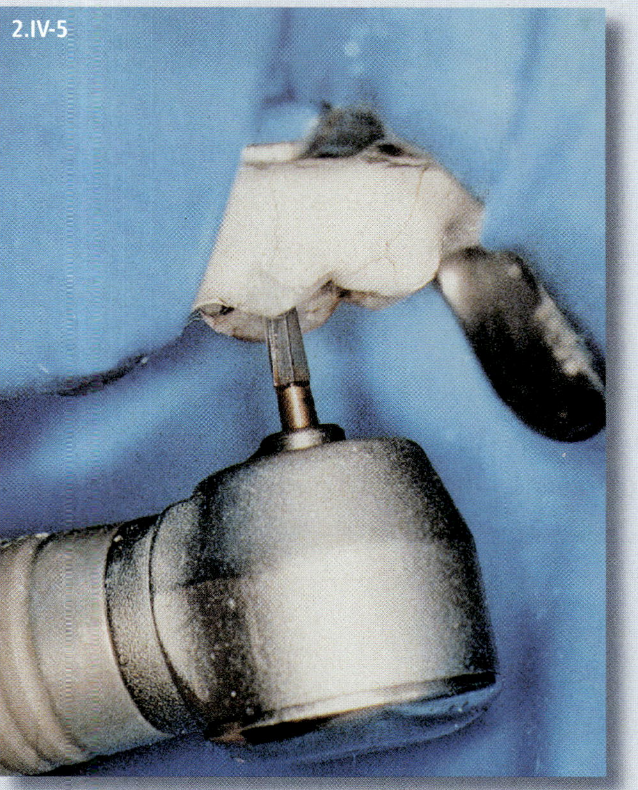

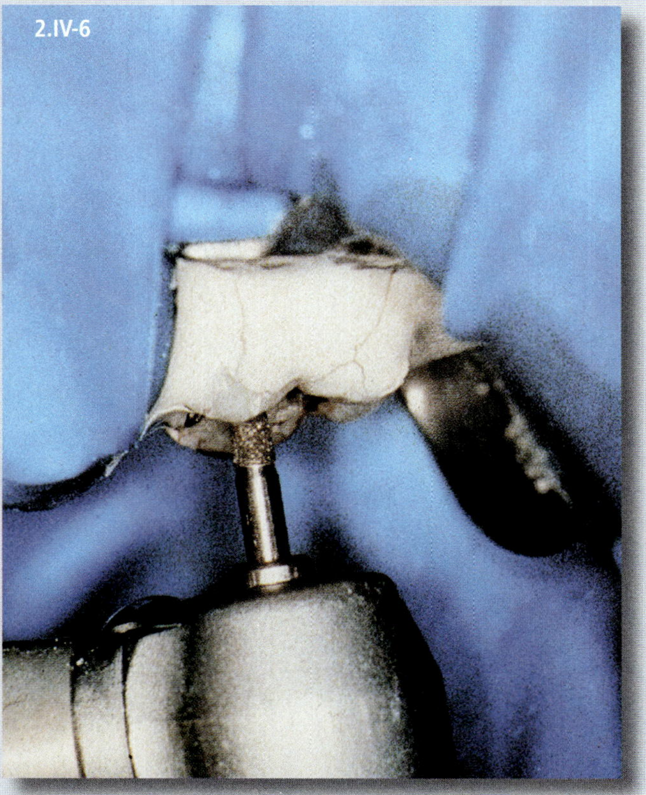

FIG. 2.IV-5

Clinical aspect showing compensatory wear performed with the Endo-Z cutter (bur) (Dentsply/ Maillefer).

FIG. 2.IV-6

Clinical aspect showing convenient shaping performed with a cylindrical/tapered diamond tip No 3.082 (MKS).

FIG. 2.IV-7

Periapical radiograph, for academic purposes, showing the maxillary left first molar after coronal opening, compensatory wear and convenient shaping, visualizing the direct, straight line to the root canal entrances.

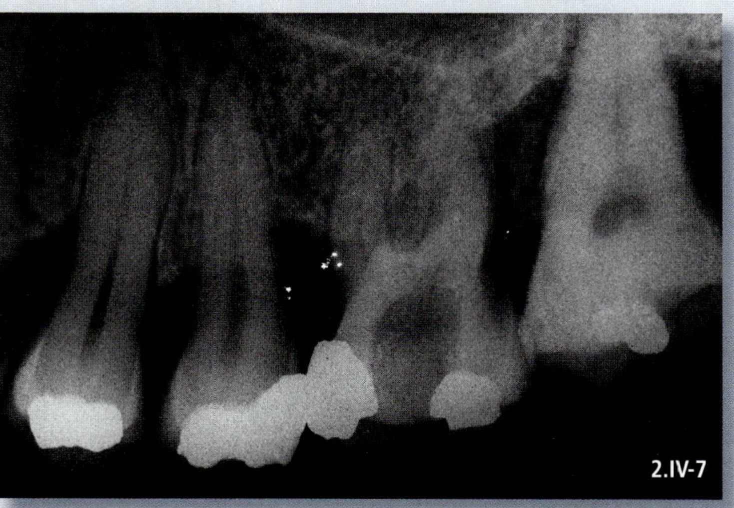

14. Location of the root canal opening with an endodontic explorer (12F Dentsply/Maillefer) (mental assessment of the location and diameter of the root canal entrances).

15. Exploration (catheterization) of root canals with a stainless steel type K file (Colorinox – Dentsply/Maillefer), of a number (diameter D_1) that matches the diameter (openings) of the root canals, up to the length that corresponds to the safe area or up to half of the roots.

16. Anticurvature Filing. Begin anticurvature filing with a Hedström* type file of a number immediately previous to the type K file used for root canal exploration, taken up to the length that corresponds to the safe area or up to half the root (Fig. 2.IV-8).

16.1. If the type K file used for root canal exploration (item No 15) was a number 10, begin anticurvature filing with Hedström type file number 8. If the type K file was number 15, begin anticurvature filing with the Hedström type file number 10.

17. Continue anticurvature filing only with the Hedström type files up to number 20.
For example: H.F. No 10 (irrigation/aspiration/flooding).
H.F. No 15 (irrigation/aspiration/flooding).
H.F. No 20 (irrigation/aspiration/flooding) (Figs. 2.IV-9 and 2.IV-10).

18. Copious aspiration/flooding/irrigation with 1% sodium hypochlorite solution (biopulpectomy).

19. Complement with anticurvature preparation with Gates Glidden (GG) drills.

19.1. Buccal root canals of maxillary molars – GG No 2 and 3 (Figs. 2.IV-11 and 2.IV-12).

19.2. Lingual root canals (maxillary molars – GG No 2, 3 and 4).

NOTE:
The Gates Glidden drills are used in the root canal while rotating using small back and forth movements until resistance is met. Repeat this operative step twice, going to the next drill with a higher number.

* Proper files for anticurvature filing named hand master file, are suggested – Endo Technic Corporation – EUA or Ergoflex – FKG-Dentaire – Switzerland.

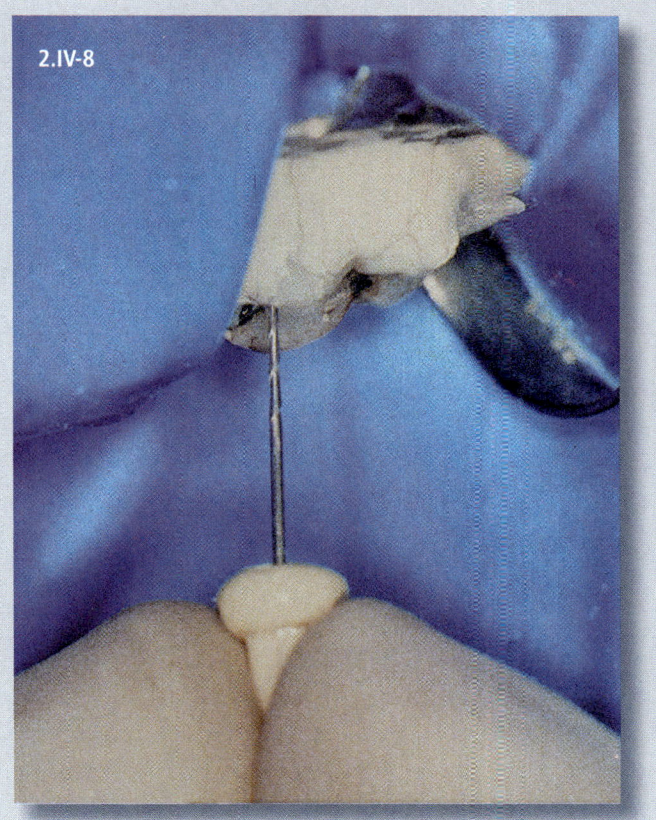

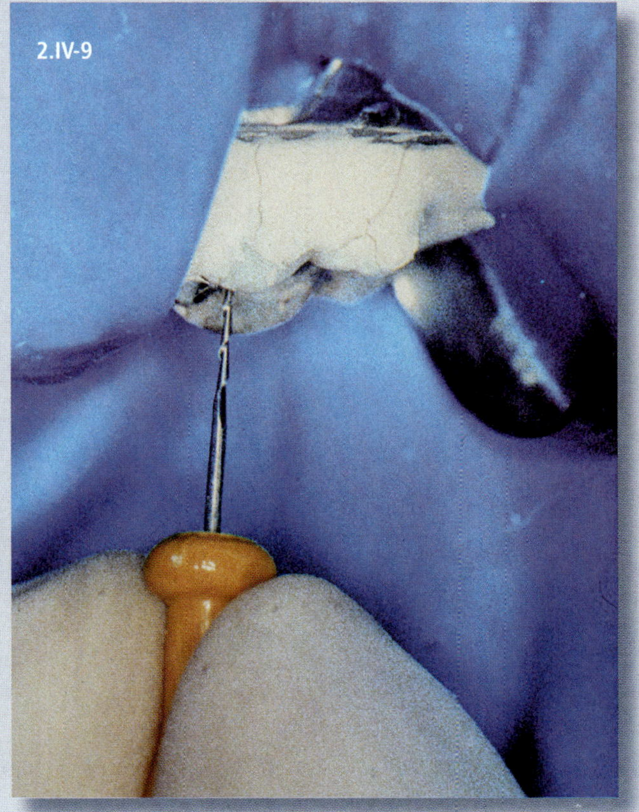

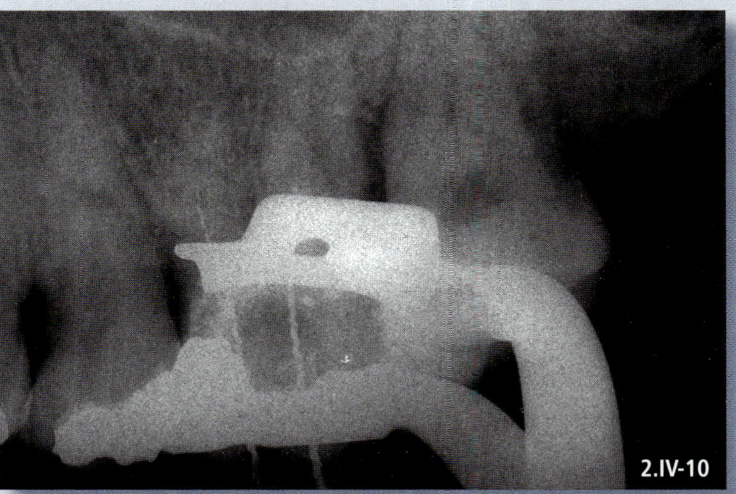

FIG. 2.IV-8

Clinical aspect of the anticurvature filing performed with the Hand Master File No 15 (Endo Technic Corporation – USA).

FIG. 2.IV-9

Clinical aspect of the anticurvature filing performed with the Hand Master File No 20 (Endo Technic Corporation – USA), leaving the root canals prepared to receive the Gates-Glidden burs.

FIG. 2.IV-10

Periapical radiograph, for academic purposes, showing the anticurvature filing performed with the Hand Master File No 15 in the mesiovestibular root canal and No 20 in the distovestibular root canal of the maxillary left first molar. Note that the length reached by these files corresponds to length of the safety area.

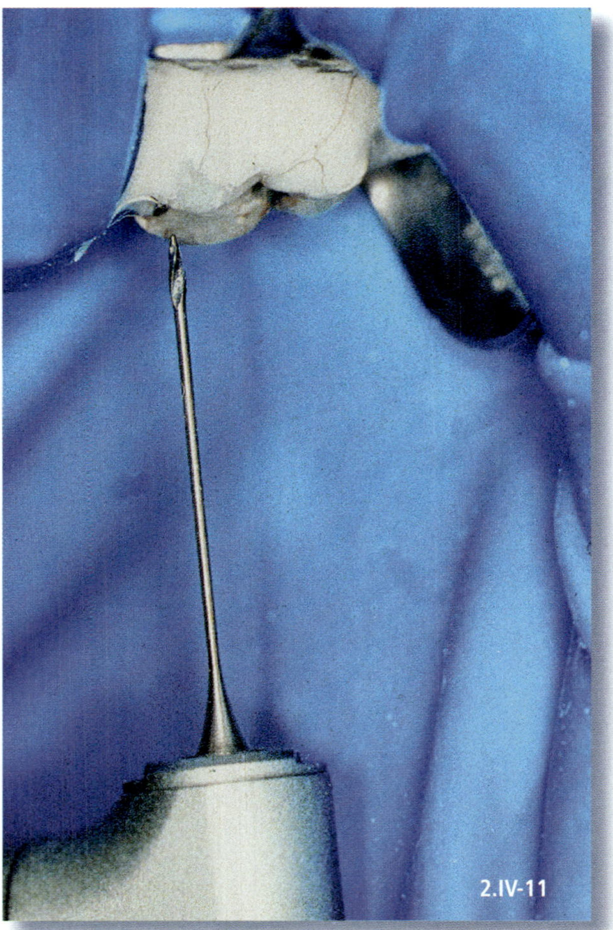

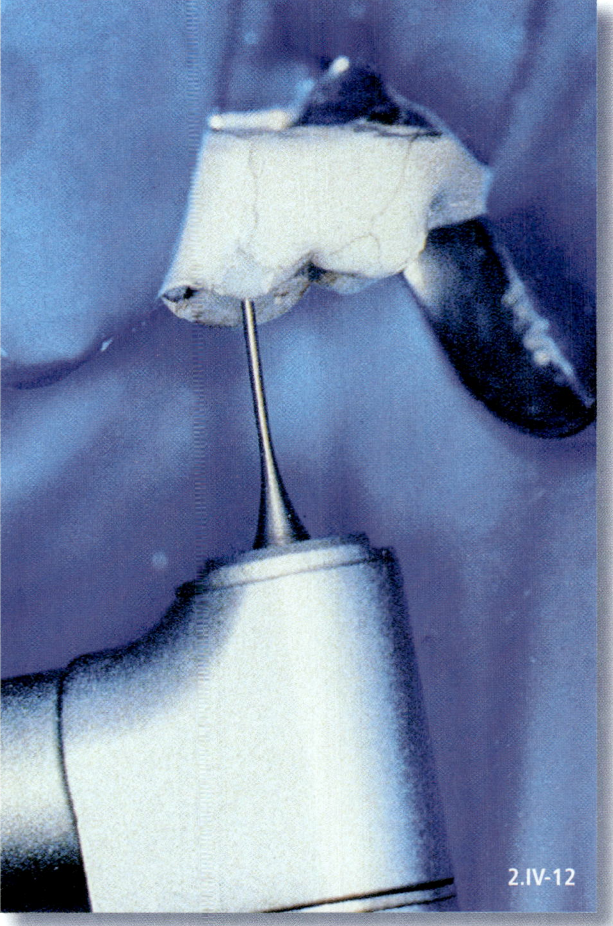

FIG. 2.IV-11

Clinical aspect showing Gates Glidden bur (cutter) No 2 prepared to be taken to the mesiovestibular root canal of the maxillary left first molar.

FIG. 2.IV-12

Clinical aspect showing the use of the Gates Glidden bur (cutter) No 2 complementing anticurvature wear performed in the mesiovestibular root canal of the maxillary left first molar.

20. Copious irrigation/aspiration/flooding with a 1% sodium hypochlorite solution.

21. After anticurvature wear, determine working length.

22. Obtaining the real tooth length (RTL) and the real working length (RWL) (Fig. 2.IV-13).

23. Establishing the apical stop (1.5 mm short of the RTL).

23.1. Identification of the Initial Apical Instrument (IAI) (anatomical diameter) at the RWL (RTL – 1.5 mm = RWL).

24. Complementing the apical stop.

24.1. Two or three instruments above the IAI at the RWL until the memory instrument is reached (MI).

25. Step-back from apical stop until the diameter of the root canal, obtained with the Gates Glidden drills, is reached.
26. Irrigation/aspiration/drying of the root canal.
27. Flooding with EDTA solution, stirring it with the MI for 3 minutes.
28. Irrigation with 1% sodium hypochlorite solution (EDTA neutralization) aspiration/drying of the root canal.
29. Filling of root canals (Fig. 2.IV-14).
    - **29.1.** Tagger hybrid technique.
        - **29.1.1.** Filling cement – AH Plus (Dentsply/DeTrey) or Topseal (Dentsply /Maillefer).
        - **29.1.2.** Epiphany/Resilon system (Pentron Clinical Technologies – USA).
          Real Seal system (SybronEndo – USA).
    - **29.2.** Active lateral condensation technique.
30. Removal of root canal filling at the coronal third, placement of calcium hydroxide-based cement (Dycal-Caulk/Dentsply) and filling of the pulp chamber with glass ionomer cement for later restoration of the tooth.

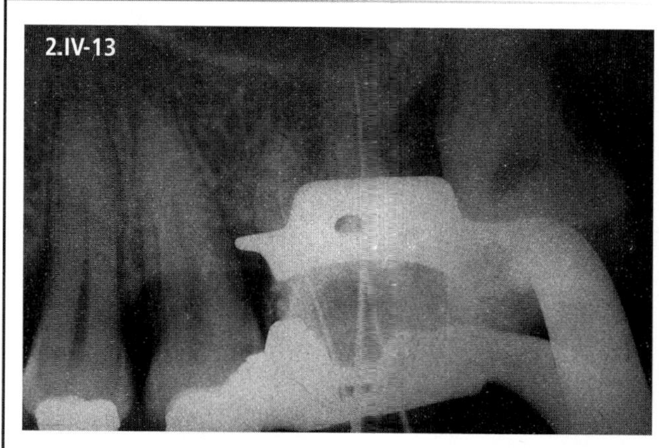

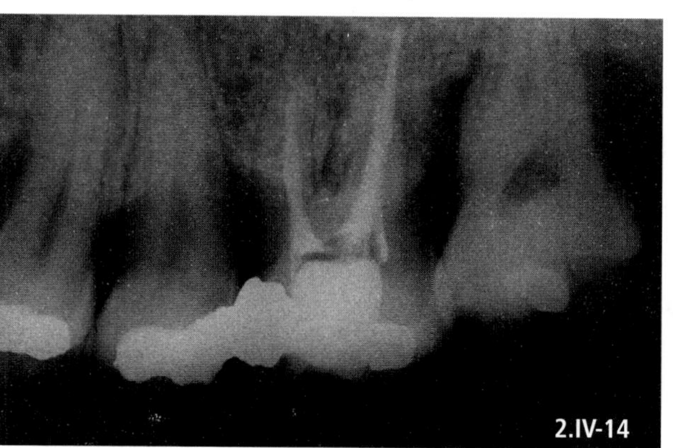

FIG. 2.IV-13

Periapical radiograph to confirm the real working length.

FIG. 2.IV-14

Final periapical radiograph showing the root canal filling. In comparison with the radiograph for diagnosis, note the rectification of the double curvature of the mesiovestibular root canal.

CASES OF NECROPULPECTOMY I

The steps of the technique are similar, with the following exceptions:

1. **Irrigant solution** – Use of diluted 1% sodium hypochlorite solutions.
2. **Foraminal Debridement** – Must not be performed, except in cases already submitted to drainage, via canal, in cases of acute dentoalveolar abscesses.
3. **Apical limit of debridement** – (1.5 mm short from the RTL).
4. **Delayed dressing** – Need not necessarily be used.
5. **Root Canal Filling** – Whenever possible, fill the root canal in the same session.
   - **5.1.** Tagger hybrid technique (when indicated)
   - **5.2.** Filling material.
     - **5.2.1.** AH Plus (Dentsply De Trey)
     - **5.2.2.** Top Seal (Dentsply/Maillefer)
     - **5.2.3.** Epiphany/Resilon system (Pentron Clinical Technologies)
     - **5.2.4.** Real Seal system (SybronEndo – USA)
6. **Follow-up** – For a period of 2 years.

CASES OF NECROPULPECTOMIES II

Differences

1. **Irrigant Solutions** – During mechanical/manual preparation, in the crown/apex direction, until the temporary working length is reached (TWL), to establish working length, use the concentrated 5.25% sodium hypochlorite solution (USP). After obtaining the real tooth length (RTL), use the diluted 2.5% sodium hypochlorite solution.
2. **Foraminal debridement** – Identifying the foraminal apical instrument (FAI) (anatomical diameter of the apical foramen) and promoting cleaning, unobstructing and slightly widening the apical foramen.
3. **Apical limit of debridement** – 1.0 mm short of the RTL.
4. **Delayed dressing** – Use Calen® for a minimum period of 14 days and maximum of 60 days.
5. **Root canal filling** – Fill the root canal after placing the dressing, but in a second treatment session.
   - **5.1.** Tagger hybrid technique (when indicated).
   - **5.2.** Active lateral condensation.
6. **Filling material**
   - **6.1.** AH Plus (Dentsply/De Trey – Switzerland)
     Top Seal (Dentsply/Maillefer – Switzerland)
     Epiphany/Resilon system (Pentron Clinical Technologies – USA)
     Real Seal system (SybronEndo – USA)
7. **Follow up** – Every year for at most 4 years.

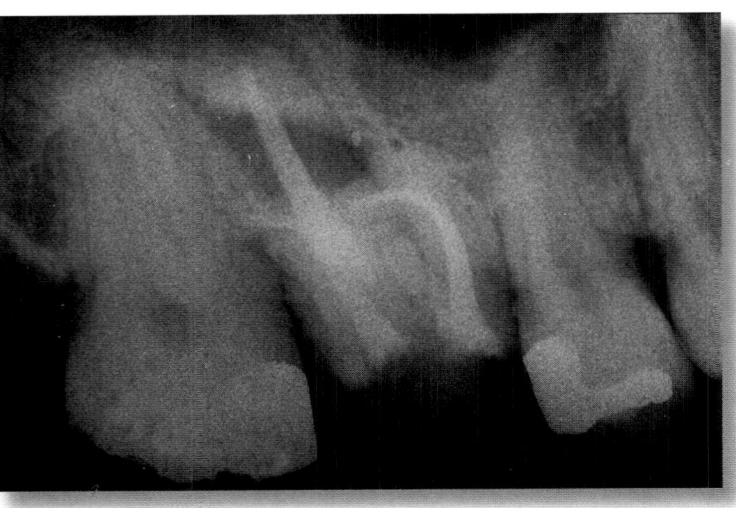

FIG. 2.IV-15

Periapical radiograph of the maxillary right second molar (17) submitted to mechanical/manual debridement by the modified GOERIG et al.[2] technique. Note the rectification of accentuated curvature of the mesiovestibular canal that has become accessible as a result of the technique used.

References

1. Abou-Rass M, Frank AL, Glick DH. The anticurvature filing method to prepare the curved root canal. J Amer Dent Ass. 1980;101:792-794.
2. Goerig AC, Michelich RJ, Schultz HH. Instrumentation of root canals in molars using the step-down technique. J Endod. 1982;12:550-557.
3. Paiva JG, Antoniazzi JH. Endodontia. Bases para a prática clínica. 2ª ed. Artes Médicas: São Paulo; 1988:501.

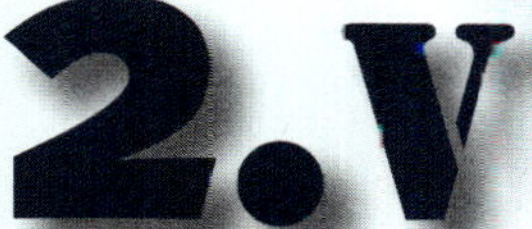

Electronic Apex Locators

"... it seems to be a paradox that Endodontics depends on precise measurements, but does not have adequate devices for measuring"[57]

Paiva & Antoniazzi[57], 1988, one year before publication[77] of the electronic working length method by frequency-dependent impedance.

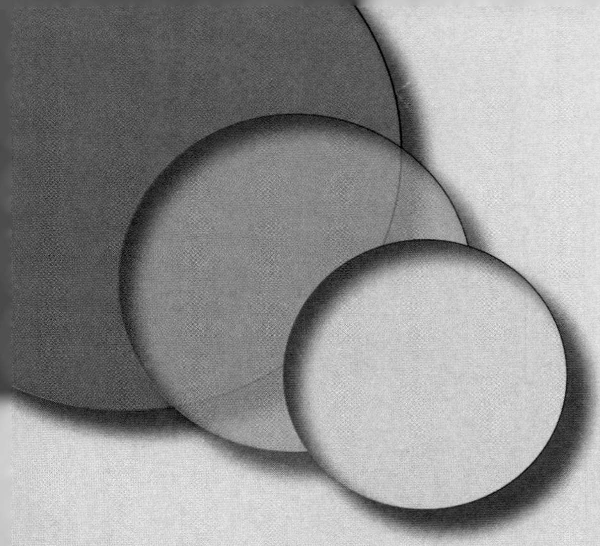

Carlos Alberto Spironelli Ramos
Clovis Monteiro Bramante

Among

the many aspects concerning endodontic treatment, one interesting statement appears to adequately summarize the reality that surrounds the clinical performance of endodontic treatment: "The most important stage of Endodontics is the one we are performing"[2]. In a clear and succinct manner, this author explains the reality of clinical practice, since all the steps are important, and depend on each other, and if performed correctly, result in successful treatment. In spite of being in complete agreement with this statement, daily experience with this specialty and its relationship with general clinical practice, have shown a different trend of professional attitude, which at the very least, asks for simplification of the manner in which the final result of meticulous and complex endodontic treatment is evaluated. When faced with a radiograph to examine an endodontically treated tooth, the operator almost invariably first analyzes the length of the filling, and relates this point with the presumed position of the location of the apical foramen. The diagnosis, treatment plan and prognosis are continually based on this analysis and define the intervention that would be most adequate for each case.

The above-mentioned situation is not a rule without exceptions. A clinical understanding and knowledge of the biological principles on which endodontic treatment is based, are not restricted to analysis of the length of the filling only. More realistic and cautious operators assess the collected information, presented in part by the radiographic image, clinical data and prior history of the case. Nevertheless, at least at first, critical observation of the apical limit of filling occurs, demonstrating the importance of this operative step in endodontic treatment.

Endodontic clinical practice is subjected to some paradoxes. One of these discusses the apical extend of root canal debridement/filling. Using a conventional assessment, the result of endodontic treatment is first evaluated by the apical position of its filling. This, in spite of the general knowledge that the location of the apical foramen does not invariably show the radiographical apex.[8] However, the majority of practitioners routinely resort to this location to determine the final quality of the treatment. Thus, the operator focuses his/her attention on the apical region, with the certainty that he/she will obtain pertinent information with respect to the status of the periapical tissues. This in turn supports his/her diagnostic assessment and determines his/her treatment plan. In summary, in daily practice it is the conventional belief that the success of endodontic treatment is linked to the apical location of its filling. Although partially true, this position indirectly contributes to establishing the importance of the correct identification and maintenance of the real working length (RWL) in endodontic treatment.

Determining the real working length is one of the earliest steps in endodontic therapy and refers to the measurement of tooth length, thus making it possible to identify the necessary references to establish the apical limit of debridement[63].

This procedure determines the distance to which the instruments may penetrate into the root canal, to what distance to work, and consequently, to which level of depth, tissues, impurities, metabolites and material(s) remain and to what distance other undesirable components need to be removed. The apical limit identifies the depth the canal filling may reach in obturation, and among other factors, affects the level of post-operative (dis)comfort[28].

It has been shown that debridement up to the limit of the radiographic apex, or beyond it, may compromise the success of endodontic therapy[69]. Swartz et al.[73] analyzed 1007 treated teeth, with a total of 1770 root canals, at intervals of six months, one year, two years, five years and ten years, with clinical and radiographic assessment. The authors concluded that overfilled root canals showed a four times higher failure rate, indicating the importance of determining and maintaining an apical limit of debridement and filling confined to the inside of the root canal (Chart 2.V-1).

CHART 2.V-1 – Success and Failure Analysis Apical limit of debridement and filling – (Swartz et al.[73]**)**

LEVEL OF FILLING	NO. OF CANALS	% OF SUCCESS	% OF FAILURES
More than 1 mm short of the radiographic apex	1432	91.90	8.10
1 mm short of the radiographic apex at the radiographic limit	215	89.77	10.23
Overfilling of cement and/or gutta percha	123	63.41	36.59
Total	1770	89.66 (mean)	10.34 (mean)

Sometimes the denomination **root apex** has erroneously been used to mean the **apical limit**. Although it is usually used to refer to the location to which the debridement and filling procedures need to be limited, the term apex does not clearly delineate the apical limit of debridement, one of the imperative references in the correct indication of the real working length[68].

The most precise definition conceives the **apex** as being the anatomic point most distant from the incisal edge or occlusal surface of the tooth[21], and the term **real working length** as being the distance between a point of reference located on the coronal aspect, and the other, at the terminal limit of preparation and root canal filling. The ideal point, unanimously agreed upon by authors since Grove's[25] studies, is located at the cemento-dentinal junction (or CDC, abbreviation of cemento-dentin-canal). Also by definition, this junction could be the point where dentin and cement meet in the root canal. The root canal – largest component of the pulp cavity and main scope of Endodontics – may be didactically divided into two conical-shaped canals, juxtaposed by their apices (Fig. 2.V-1). The longest, the dentinal canal, begins in the pulp chamber. Its walls are lined with dentin and converge into a minimum diameter in an apical direction. From then on, the dentinal canal establishes continuity with the other shorter canal with divergent walls, lined with cement, and therefore called the cement canal, which increases in diameter, and opens in the larger apical foramen. It presents a peculiar topography, more frequently shown to be lateral to the root apex, and not in continuity along the axis of the main canal, as one might imagine[20].

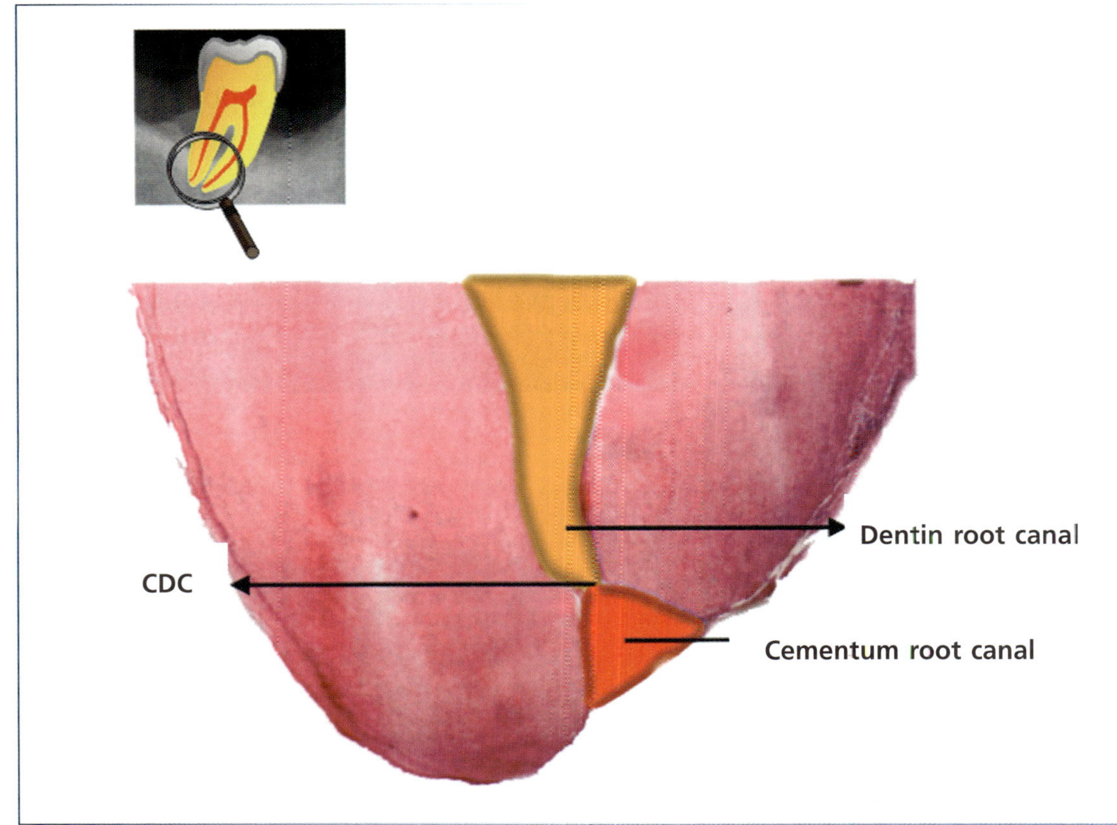

FIG. 2.V-1
Image of the apical terminus of the root canal, which can be described as two cones juxtaposed by their apexes (CDC = Cemento-Dentin Canal).

It is an established fact that root canal preparation and filling must be limited to the dentinal canal – the area occupied by pulp tissue, and at its apical extremity, restricted to the CDC limit – leaving the cement canal free of any intervention. Following the biological principles of preservation of apical periodontal tissues during endodontic treatment[41], some authors point out the need for determining an apical limit that does not cause tissue damage, and promotes regeneration of the area after treatment[8]. Seltzer et al.[66] showed that a canal filling must be limited to the **apical constriction** region, thus increasing endodontic treatment success rates. Ketterl[37] presented a clinical and radiographic study that followed up on 560 root canals, all of them with vital pulps, which received endodontic treatment. The author showed that the cases considered successful (90%), were those in which the apical limit was from 1 mm to 2 mm short of the radiographic apex. Sjögren et al.[69] studied teeth with periapical lesions, that were treated endodontically. In a clinical-radiographic follow-up for up to 10 years, they observed that the best results were found in those cases in which the apical limit of filling was up to 2 mm short of the radiographic apex (94% of success).

Therefore, special attention needs to be focused when determining the real working length, because in the light of the results of research on this subject, the apical constriction, and not the root apex, constitutes the most desirable point for establishing the apical limit of debridement.

MORPHOLOGICAL LOCATION OF THE APICAL FORAMEN

In a broad study concerning the different locations of the apical foramen in different teeth, in relation to the root apex, Morfis et al.[53] reported a great disparity, as shown in Chart 2.V-2.

CHART 2.V-2 – Location of main foramen in relation to the root apex (Morfis et al.)[53]

GROUP OF TEETH	PERCENTAGE OF FORAMENS LOCATED IN THE ROOT APEX (ORTHO-RADIAL POSITION)	MEAN DISTANCE FROM THE MAIN FORAMEN TO THE ROOT APEX (IN MM)
Maxillary incisors	40.5	0.472
Mandibular incisors	11.4	0.977
Maxillary premolars	15.36	0.816
Mandibular premolars	37.64	0.610
Maxillary molars (lingual root)	25	0.429
Maxillary molars (mesio-buccal root)	57.9	0.665
Maxillary molars (disto-buccal root)	25	0.418
Mandibular molars (mesial root)	61.5	0.818
Mandibular molars (distal root)	9.52	0.530

Analyzing the results of the study by Morfis et al.[53], particularly the positions related to the foramen of distal roots of mandibular molars (9.5% in straight apical position) and mandibular molars (11.5% in straight apical position) are outstanding, and this data resulted in the recommendation, by these authors, not to use the radiographic apex as a reference for all working length measures (Figs. 2.V-2 and 2.V-3).

The location and anatomic confirmation of the apical constriction were reported by Green[24], indicating that the apical foramen is funnel-shaped, with its widest portion starting in the external portion of the root, and ending with its narrowest portion from 0.52 mm to 0.66 mm inside the canal, which determines the apical constriction. Dummer et al.[17] examined incisors, canines and pre-molars using an optical microscope, and found a mean distance of 0.89 mm

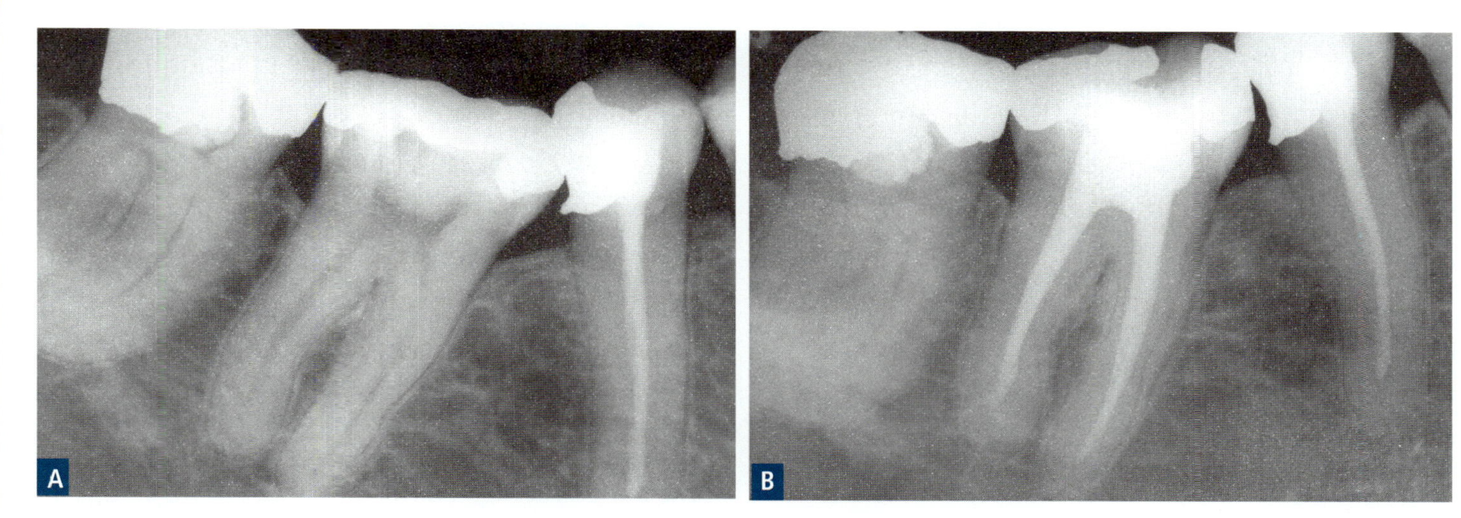

FIGS. 2.V-2A-E

A – Pre-operative radiograph of a right mandibular second molar. Note that it is not possible to visualize the foramen exit of the distal canal.
B – The same case, after filling the root canals, showing the foramen exit of the distal canal.

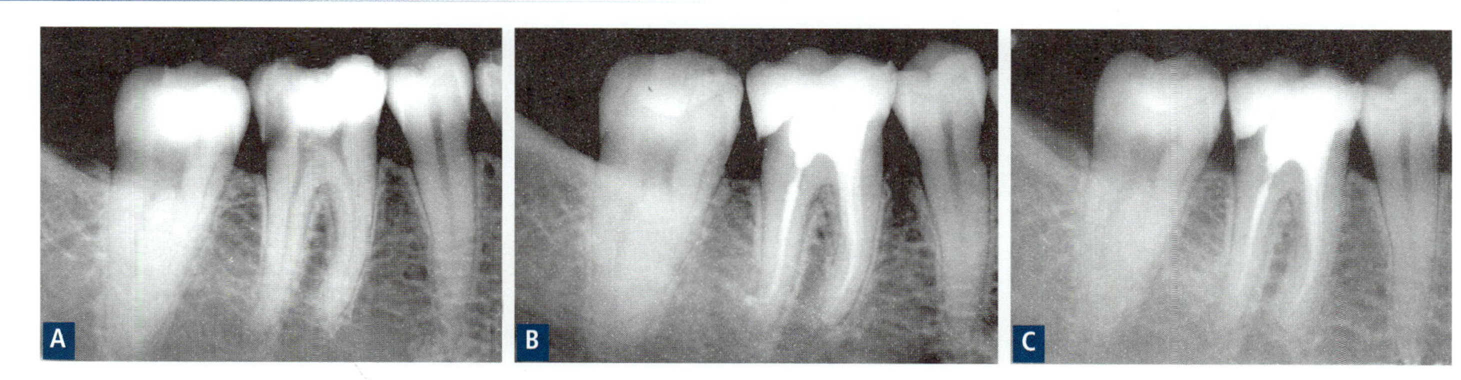

FIGS. 2.V-3A-C

Clinical sequence in the right mandibular first molar.
A – Pre-operative radiographic image, for the purpose of diagnosis and planning the treatment.
B – Radiographic image immediately after filling, with extrusion of the sealer cement indicating a lateral foramen exit of the distal canal, away from the anatomic root apex.
C – Radiographic image 30 days post treatment, showing resorption of the extruded cement. An analysis of the follow-up radiograph, might lead one to criticize the filling as being "short".

between the foramen and the apical constriction, ranging from 0.07 mm to 2.69 mm. The values found were similar to those studies by Kuttler[37], who reports mean distances of 0.524 mm, for patients between the ages of 18 and 25, and of 0.659 mm, for patients aged 55 years of age or above. The author reported that in 32% of the cases of young patients, the position of the apical foramen coincides with the anatomic apex and in 20% of cases, for patients over 55 years old.

Gutmann[27] confirmed that it is clinically impossible to establish the real location of the foramen and apical constriction until filling of the root canal has been completed (Fig. 2. V-4). Furthermore, he emphasized that the radiographic method for determining the apical limit does not consider anatomical variables, and in the cases of teeth with vital pulps, it frequently leads to over-debridement, traumatic injury of apical periodontal tissue, and consequently to postoperative pain.

APICAL RESORPTIONS

According to Leonardo[40], apical cemento-dentin resorptions are largely responsible for the failures observed in endodontic treatments of teeth with chronic periapical lesions, and they are difficult to see in the periapical radiographs that are usually taken. When examining 87 teeth that presented with pulp necrosis, Ferlini Filho[20] found that in only 63.88%, the radiographic examination showed any type of apical resorption, while in the microscopic examination the resorption process was present in 94.44% of the cases. The results of the radiographic and microscopic analysis revealed that some type of root resorption was present in the majority of the teeth with a chronic periapical process (Fig. 2. V-5). It was concluded that conventional radiographs are not reliable resources for diagnosing root resorptions in the initial stages.

A study by Ferlini Filho[20] is directly applicable to the concept of working length, approaching the question of resorption and its deleterious effects with regard to endodontic treatment. From the author's perspectives, one notes the relevance of the process of disruption of the apical tissues, apical cemento-dentin resorption and their close relationship with the placement of the apical limit of debridement, and consequently filling. The indication of this limit, in the majority of cases, has been done by the so-called radiographic methods of working length determination. However, it is difficult to establish this important anatomic reference point

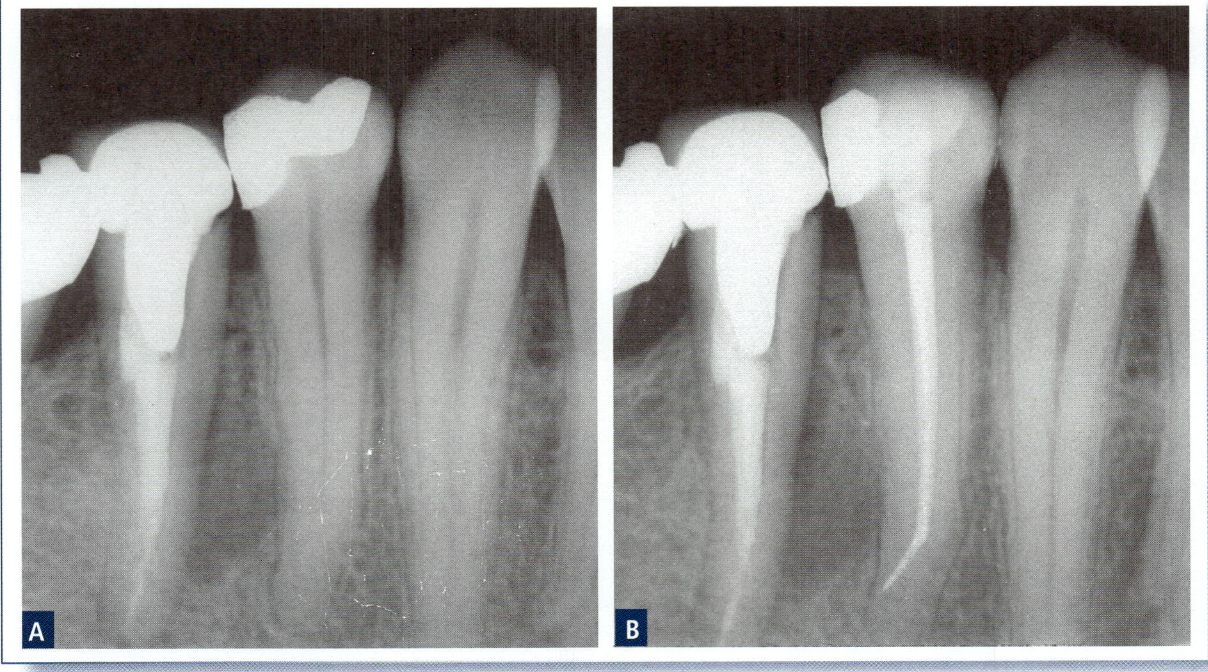

FIGS. 2.V-4A-B

A – Pre-operative radiograph of a right mandibular first molar, before endodontic treatment. Note again that it is not possible to see the foramen exit of the canal.

B – The same patient, after filling, showing the distal foramen exit of the root canal away from the anatomic root apex.

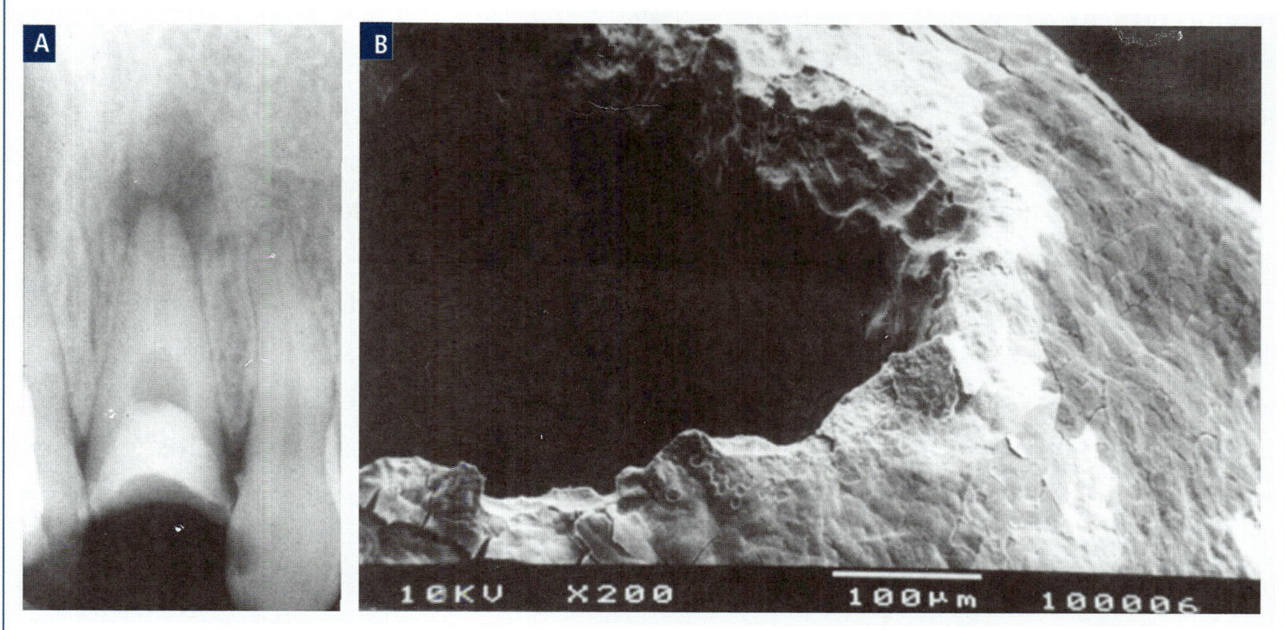

FIGS. 2.V-5A-B

A – Radiograph of a left maxillary central incisor diagnosed as endodontically compromised and with a periapical lesion.
B – Scanning Electron Microscopic image of root resorption which partially destroyed the root apex – apical resorption. Original magnification 200X[20] (image courtesy of Prof. Dr. João Ferlini Filho, UFRGS, Porto Alegre).

radiographically in a tooth with apical erosion as a result of resorption (Fig. 2.V-6), and therefore the radiographic limits are imprecise. This causes risks to debridement, because when the periapical tissues are accidentally reached, it will result in iatrogenicity that has well known manifestations with painful postoperative symptoms. The problem is aggravated when resorption is located on the buccal or lingual surfaces of the roots involved. This is considerably aggravated when one notes that the radiographic image of hard tissue resorptions do not interpret the full extent of the destructive process – which in its initial stages goes unnoticed during diagnostic assessment. We should add to this the fact that radiography is a limited resource, providing a two dimensional image of a process that has three dimensions[20].

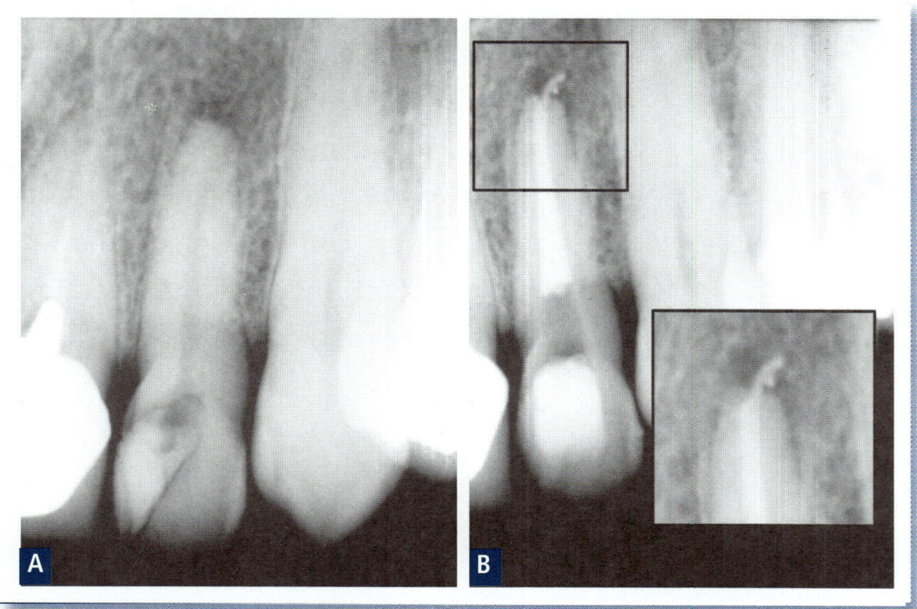

FIGS. 2.V-6A-B

A – Radiographic image of a left maxillary lateral incisor, diagnosed for endodontic treatment. Note apical lesion and apical resorption.
B – After filling the canal, note the extrusion of the filling material (*see* detail).

DETERMINING THE REAL WORKING LENGTH (RWL)

To determine the real working length several techniques have been scientifically described and assessed, among them digital tactile sense, radiographic methods[3,5,32] and electronic methods, each used alone or in combined, which according to some authors[55,56,67] would provide more reliability in determining an apical limit of debridement.

The variations in shape and position of an apical constriction make it difficult to detect by digital tactile sense[45]. The methods that use radiographic image interpretations also have limitations due to factors such as distortions[16], anatomic interferences and objects pertinent to endodontic treatment. There are also restrictions with respect the fact that they are two-dimensional images of three-dimensional objects[74], making it impossible to visualize the apical foramen and apical constriction[58], thus leading to subjective interpretation by the operator[38].

RADIOGRAPHIC METHODS

Indication of the real working length, based on radiographic interpretation, has been the method most used by clinicians and specialists in endodontic therapy[12]. The methods based on taking radiographs include those by Best[3], Bregman[6], and Ingle[32].

Of the techniques based on the interpretation of radiographic images, the one proposed by Ingle[32] has shown acceptable rates of accuracy. Bramante & Berbert[5] assessed several techniques to determine the tooth length, concluding that the methods by Best[3] and Bregman[6] showed the greatest variability in results, with only a small percentage that was correct. According to the authors, the method that resulted in measurements closest to the real length of the tooth, was the one proposed by Ingle[32].

Although it is the most widely used working length technique with a reasonable precision for locating the apical limit of debridement, the radiographic method by Ingle[32] has several limitations that tend to diminish its precision and reliability. The primary problem is to obtain a good radiographic image of the tooth being treated. The final quality of the radiograph is linked to several variables, involving the correct positioning of the film with regard to the object to be radiographed, correct angle of the X-ray beam, interferences of anatomic structures or the equipment used to isolate the operating field, exposure time to radiation and adequate radiographic processing[27] (Fig. 2. V-7).

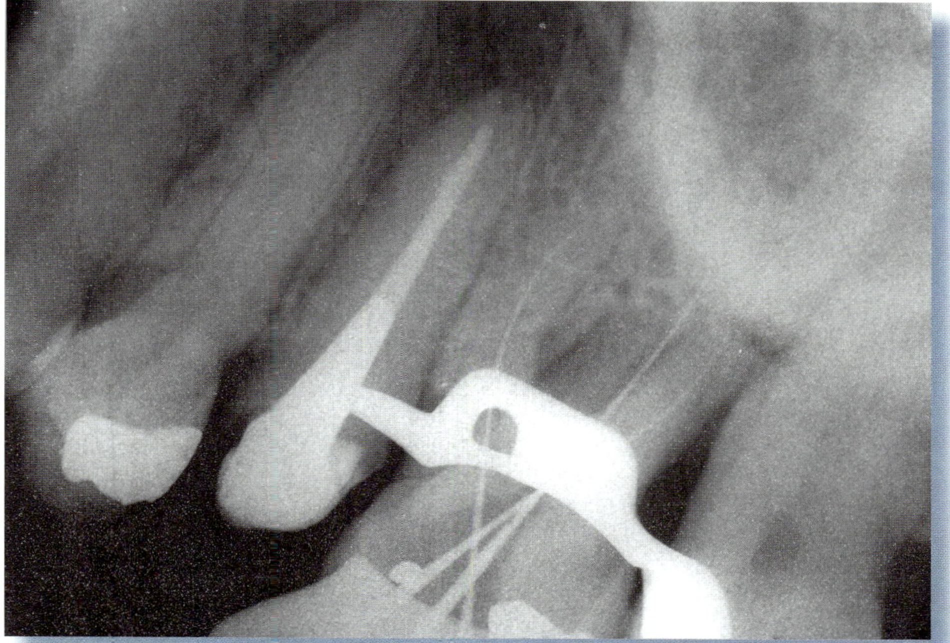

FIG. 2.V-7

Radiographic image of left upper quadrant, showing a common problem when radiographs are made to establish working length. The zygomatic process is superimposing the apexes of the maxillary molars making interpretation difficult or worse, preventing interpretation of the working apical limit by Ingle's technique[32].

Another difficulty related to the method by Ingle[32], which influences its precision, concerns the fact that interpretation of the acquired image is a subjective exercise, so that the result may vary from operator to operator[15,22]. Attempts to obtain the image from the position of the tip of the instrument and its relationship with the apical foramen, which is necessary to determine the real working length, may also be affected by the morphological details of the apex, which are not always visible on a radiograph[10]. Interpretation of the position of the instrument inside the root canal does not correspond to reality, since the image of the file outside the canal can be superimposed on the image of the root [27,64] (Fig. 2. V-8).

Principles of electronic measurement and its development

The electronic method has been studied and improved since the last half of the 20th century[71], aiming at adding precision to the technique. Since the first experiments by Susuki[72] and Sunada[71], (Fig. 2.V-9), the electronic method has shown appreciable technological advances, overcoming the initial problems, particularly with respect to the inability of taking readings in root canals containing irrigation solutions with electrical conductivity. During the last few years, studies assessing the electronic method have resulted in satisfactory accurate data, indicating that electronic apex locators have found a prominent place in clinical endodontics and endodontic research.

The early devices showed success rates that were lower than or comparable to radiographic techniques. However, when the third generation electronic apex locators were introduced, it was possible to establish the real working length with an accuracy of ± 0.5 mm under different clinical conditions in more over 80% of the cases (Ramos et al.[63]; Gordon[23]; Welk[79]; Pratten[59]; Dunlap[18]; Lucena et al.[43]). In addition to being more exact, the electronic method is safer for the patient and more convenient to the operator because it diminishes a patient's exposure to ionizing radiation, reduces treatment time, and is easier to use with patients who have difficulty opening their mouth. Furthermore they can be used

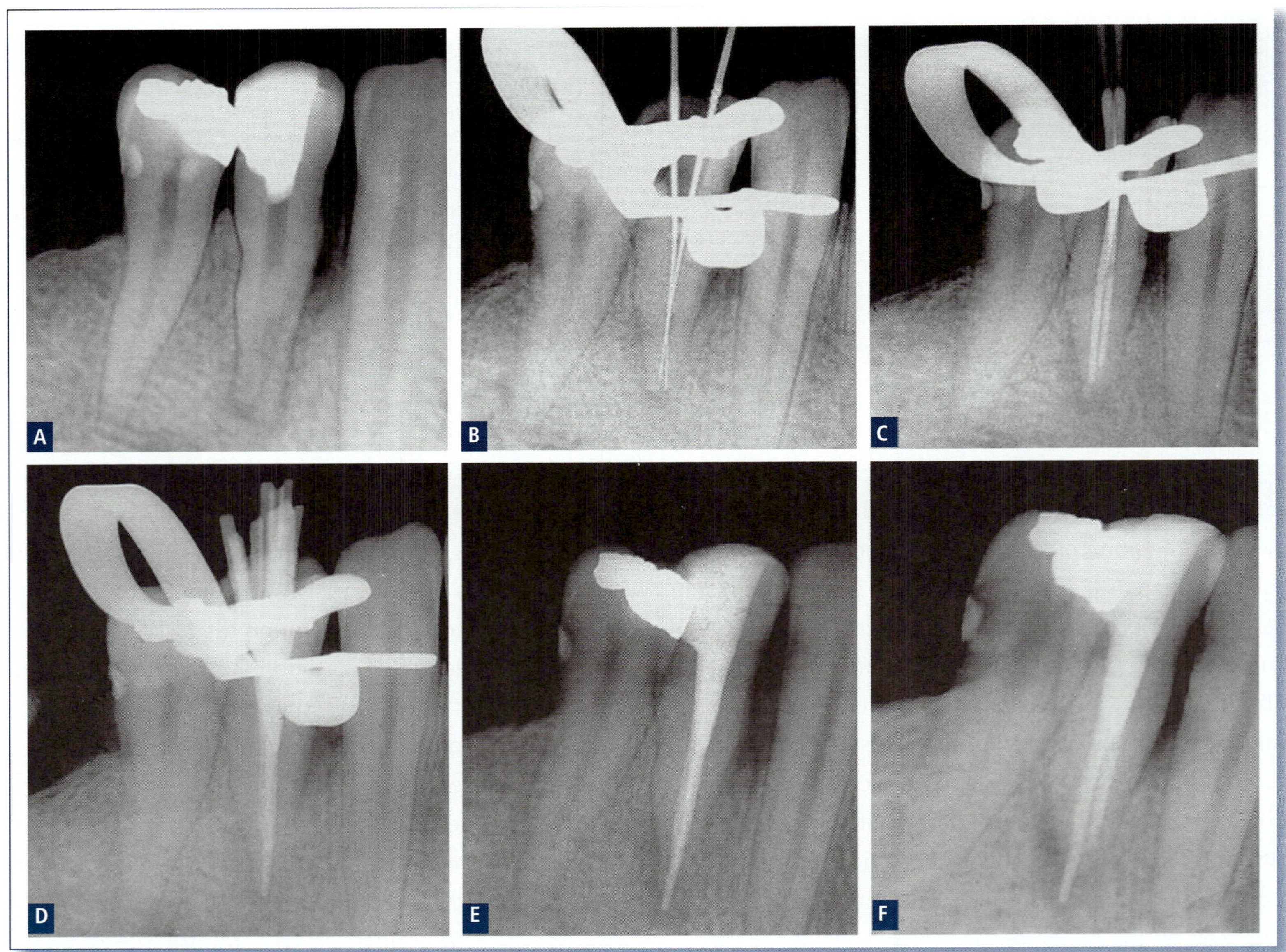

FIGS. 2.V-8A-F

Sequence of radiographic images illustrating endodontic treatment of the right mandibular first premolar. The pre-operative image suggested two roots, buccal and lingual.

A – Pre-operative radiograph for diagnosis.
B – Radiograph to determine working length, taken from a mesial angle.
C – Radiographic proof of try-in of gutta-percha cones.
D – Radiograph to verify correct filling before cutting the cones.
E – Radiographic image after filling and temporary restoration.
F – Another radiograph from a more mesial angle showing the overlap of filling material in the buccal root.

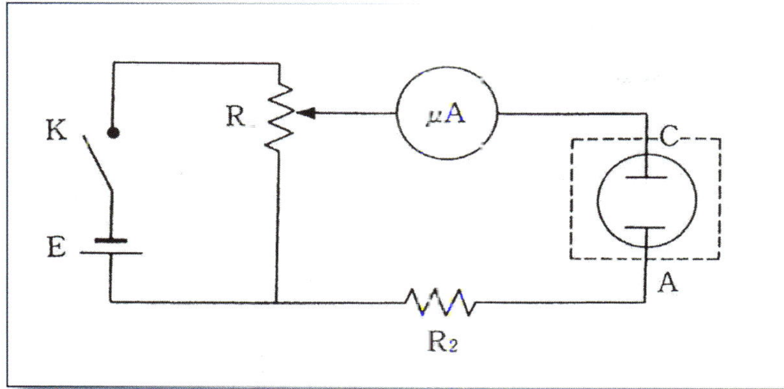

FIG. 2.V-9

Diagram of the circuit proposed by SUNADA to determine the apical foramen. A, anode or endodontic file and C, cathode or mucosa electrode.

in pregnant women. Because they are less subjective than the radiographic and tactile sense methods, the third generation electronic apex locators also present greater reproducibility of measurements when used correctly. In *in vivo* tests, Lucena et al.[43] demonstrated a reproducibility of three models of commercial brands, used by two operators, and obtained a mean reproducibility of 90 to 95%.

The electronic models determine the real working length by measuring electrical resistance when a direct current is applied, or by measuring electric impedance of signals with only one spectral component, or multi-frequency signals between an electrode inserted inside the root canal and another supported normally by the angle of the lower lip. Based on the type of signal used to measure impedance, McDonald[59] classified the devices as first generation (resistance method), second generation (impedance method), and third generation (the frequency-dependent method).

To diminish the variability of electronic apex locators using direct current, methods that used senoidal alternating current were developed. They represented an appropriate advance, because they were not subject to polarization problems. Yet they were still very imprecise in determining the position of the apical foramen when the root canal was filled with conductive material. Due to the fact that it is impossible to dry the root canal completely and the difficulty of completely removing pulp tissues, clinical application of the senoidal alternating current models is hardly feasible (Ramos & Bramante[64]).

In 1983, Ushiyama[75] proposed the stress gradient method, in which a source of alternating current was applied on the coronal portion of the canal and the difference in potential, due to the electrical field between the two tips of a bipolar electrode, was measured. The enamel, dentin and cement acted as electrical insulators and made the density of the electric current greater in the narrowest part of the canal. During the measurement, the difference in potential increases as the electrode is inserted into the canal and reaches its maximum value in the apical constriction. From this point onwards, the difference in potential decreases until it reaches the foramen (Fig. 2. V-10). Therefore, the relative diameter of the root canal can be estimated by measuring the electric field produced by the constant amplitude current. Since the root canal filled with isotonic NaCl has moderate resistance, Ushiyama[75] showed that the difference in potential produced in this electrolyte by an electric current in the order of 10μA, can easily be detected without disturbances caused by noise.

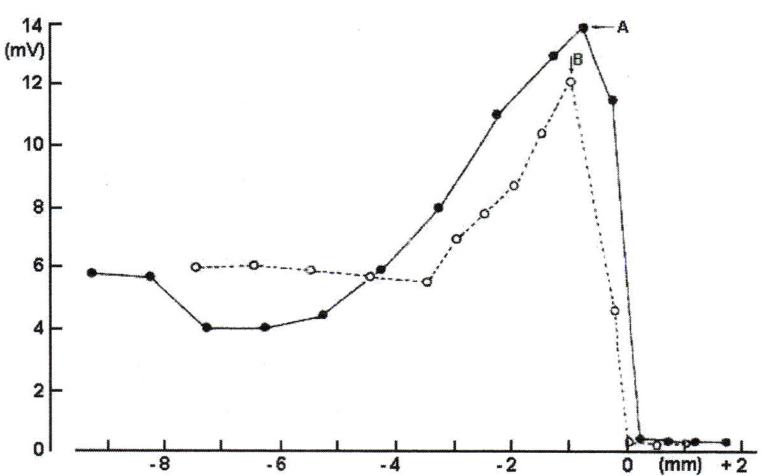

FIG. 2.V-10

Variation of the stress gradient in the root canal. Two different types of electrodes were used: Simple bipolar (curve A) and bipolar of the combined type (curve B). The ordinate and abscissa provide a difference in potential between the poles of the bipolar electrode and the distance of the electrode for AF (Apical Foramen), respectively. Positive distances indicate that the electrode tip is beyond the foramen, while for negative distances it is inside the canal.

Yamaoka et al.[77] suggested the first third generation electronic method, according to the classification of McDonald. It was based on the calculation of the difference between the basic and harmonic amplitudes of 5 kHz, of the difference in potential charge on the root canal, when a current with a square wavelength shape and basic frequency of 1 kHz were applied. Apit (Osada Elect. Co., Japan) implemented a modification of this method, applying a signal composed of the sum of two senoids. The device showed precision when determining the electronic position of the apical foramen, even in the presence of electrolytic solutions, but it needed to be calibrated for each root canal.

With the aim of determining the real working length irrespective of the root canal content and of proposing methods that did not need to be calibrated for each measurement, Kobayashi & Suda[34] suggested the calculation of a ratio, and Masreliez[48] presented a method that calculated the ratios among five sinus waves of different frequencies. Other methods were also proposed, such as the fourth generation of electronic apex locators, but none of them were shown to be more precise than the ratio method of Kobayashi[33].

RATIO METHOD

Kobayashi & Suda[34] presented a method based on simultaneously measuring two impedances of the canal using current sources with two different frequencies. Then the ratio between the two electric potentials proportional to each impedance is calculated. The quotient is shown on the device's meter and represents the position of a file tip in the canal. When the tip of the file is located at a certain distance from the apical foramen and since resistance of the root canal is negligible, the quotient is approximately equal to 1. When the endodontic file gets close to the apical foramen, resistance suddenly increases and there is a significant change in the quotient. Therefore, one can estimate the location of the file by the ratio between the impedances for different frequencies.

Figure 2.V-11(a) shows the values of quotients for different values of frequency between two spectral components. It should be noted that the value of the quotient remains practically constant up to point of –1 mm. From –1 mm to 0 mm, there is a significant variation in its value. From 0 mm, that is from the apical foramen, the quotient becomes stable again, because from this point the instrument has reached the apical periodontal tissues and adjacent structures.

Meares & Steiman[50] investigated the influence of the presence of sodium hypochlorite solution at different concentrations in the electronic determination of the apical foramen position. They showed that the instrument maintained precision in the measurements irrespective of the root canal content. They concluded that the discrepancy among the success rates, from 82% to 96.2%, obtained in other studies, resulted from the experimental protocol used and the inherent difficulty of reproducibility of the measurements of the canal length of the tooth from a common reference point.

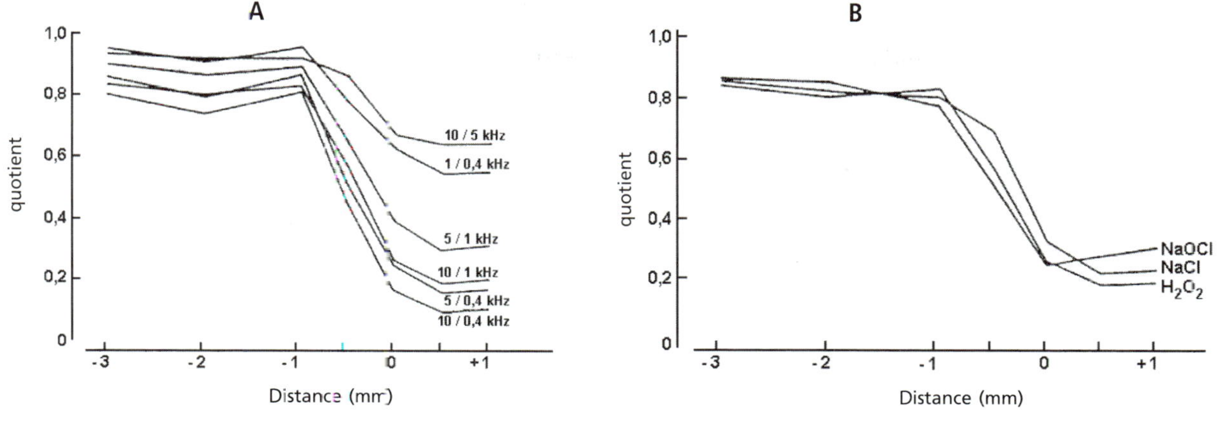

FIGS. 2.V-11A-B

A – Quotient of impedances for currents with different spectral components.
B – Variation of quotient of impedances for different solutions inside a canal. In both graphs, the negative distances are used for measurements short of, and positive distances for measurements beyond the apical foramen (modified by Kobayashi and Suda[34]).

MASRELIEZ'S METHOD

Masreliez's[48] method consists of the application of a current resulting from the combination of five senoids waves with selected frequencies, f1 to f5, for f1 to f5 equal 500 Hz, 1 kHz, 2 kHz, 4 kHz and 8 kHz, respectively. The shape of the stress wave on the load is measured, and the amplitude and phase of each of the spectral components are monitored. Then the position of the endodontic file inside the canal is determined by (Fig. 2. V-12):

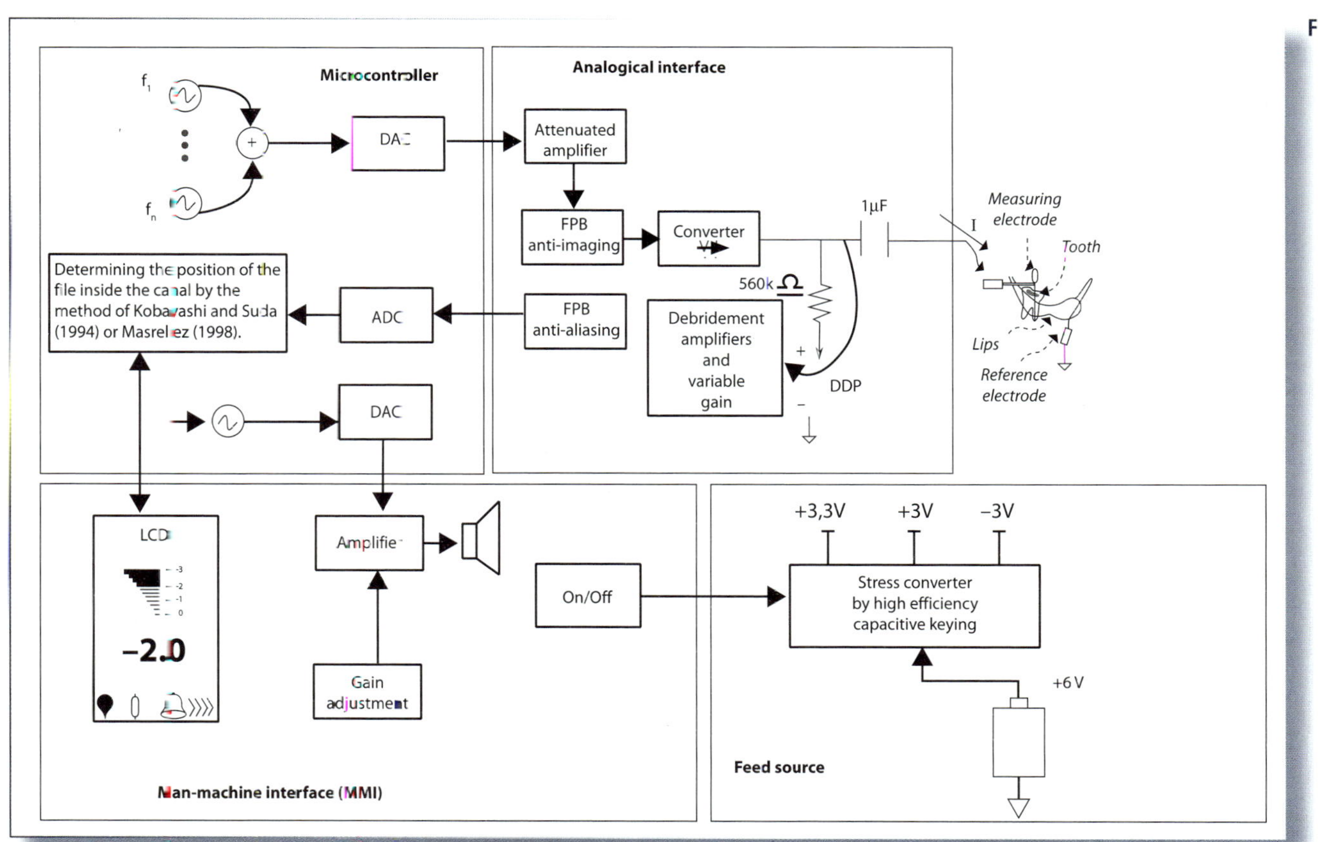

FIG. 2.V-12

Block Diagram of an experimental prototype. The diagram shows the main blocks and flow of data or signals from the instrument during the measuring process. The senoid generators of frequency f1 to fn represent the spectral components of signals generated for the methods of both Kobayashi & Suda and Masreliez.

$$P = \frac{\left\{\left[3*\left(\frac{A_1}{A_2}\right)*\left(\frac{A_1}{A_3}\right)*\left(\frac{A_1}{A_4}\right)*\left(\frac{A_1}{A_5}\right)\right]-\left[\frac{(-\phi_1-\phi_2-\phi_3-\phi_4)}{4}\right]\right\}}{36}$$

Where the value of P is used as a reference to determine the position of the file inside the canal, A1 to A5 are the amplitude modules of components f1 to f5, and φ1 to φ4 are the differences among the phases of components f2 to f5 and the phase of component f1.

Masreliez confirms that the phases of the spectral components significantly change when the endodontic instrument reaches the periapical tissues. For this reason he suggested that the combination of ratios of amplitudes and differences in phase, favor determination of the RWL with greater precision, irrespective of the root canal contents. This method was applied in the commercial appliances Apex Finder AFA Model 7005, Endo Analyser Model 8005 and Elements Diagnostic Unit and Apex Locator (Sybron Dental Specialties Inc.).

In studies comparing the electronic method with the radiographic method, different results were observed, because the apex locator devices of the frequency type indicated the position of constriction and exit of the apical foramen, while the radiographic analysis purports to interpret only the position of the radiographic apex,[11] which in fewer than 50% of the cases coincides with the real position of the apical foramen[52]. The majority of experiments that reported average success when using the electronic method compared the results with a radiographic analysis. This methodology is inadequate since it can lead to a false interpretation of the real position of the instrument tip in relation to the apical foramen, which is not always located at the radiographic apex[68].

Although with different features (appearance of the equipment, operating interface, marking points on the screen, types of batteries and accessories), the models of third generation devices that are commercially available (Endex Plus*, Ipex**, Root ZX II***, Bingo and Novapex****, Romiapex D-30 and Romiapex A-15*****, Mini and Elements Diagnostic Unit and Apex Locator******) operate on essentially the same principle.

* Osada, Japan.

** NSK, Japan.

*** J. Morita, Japan.

**** Forum, Israel.

***** Romidan-Romibras, Israel/Brazil.

****** SybronEndo, USA.

THE INFLUENCE OF THE PULP CONDITION ON THE PRECISION OF THE METHOD

The influence of the pulp condition on the precision and reliability of electronic measurement by the frequency-dependent impedance method was an object of in vivo verifications[1,18,49]. Arora & Gulabilava[1], Dunlap et al.[18] and Mayeda et al.[49] clinically observed electronic readings of the apical limit, which the authors defined by marking the apex position on the screen, in cases of teeth with pulp vitality and/or necrosis, and then assessing the real position of the instruments in relation to the apical foramen. Analysis of the results indicated that there was no statistically significant difference between the readings in vital or necrotic pulps.

The presence of an **inflamed** pulp in the path of the root canal to be measured makes it difficult to perform electronic measurements. Clinically, one notes that these electronic measurements are easier when measuring a root canal with necrotic pulp contents, or even in cases of re-treatments. Therefore, a partial pulpectomy is recommended (Fig. 2.V-13), followed by abundant irrigation with sodium hypochlorite solution to allow the canal to be measured without interference from the inflamed pulp in the root canal.

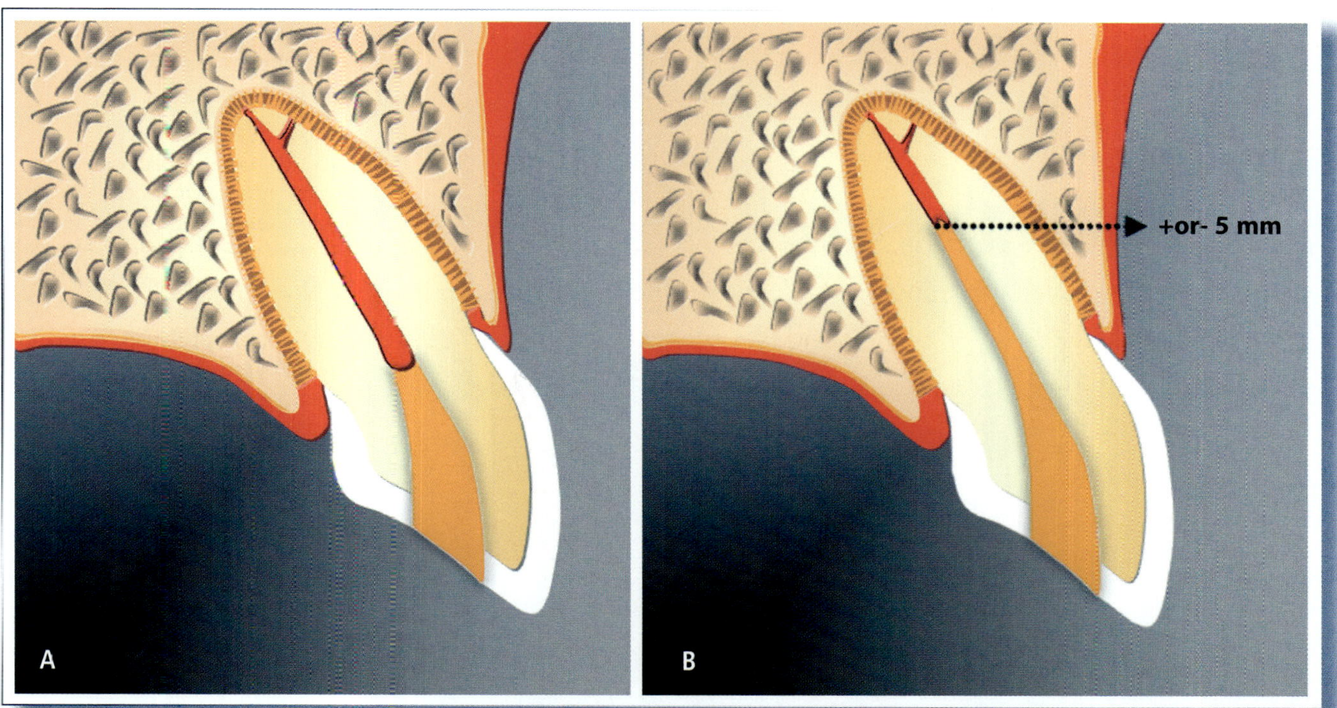

FIGS. 2.V-13A-B

Diagrammatic illustration of partial pulpectomy, according to the text.

This condition is explained by research on the concentration of cations in the human pulp, which revealed that pathologic alterations of this tissue indicate changes in its ionic concentration. Consequently, its electrophysiological characteristics are altered, indicating interferences in the measurements when using an electronic apex locator. Kovačević & Tamarut[36] have shown that the presence of a pulp with an acute inflammatory condition tends to alter the measurements, as this tissue underwent a change in its electrical conductivity. Higher values are recorded than for the calibrated device, giving unreliable readings. Clinically, it is noted that in these cases, placement of the instrument in the cervical third sometimes produces a measurement relative to the location of the foramen exit or beyond it. After partial removal of pulp tissues, followed by abundant irrigation and aspirating excess irrigation fluid, the measurement tends to return to normal. Ibarrola et al.[30] conducted a study on the precision of Root ZX readings, with variations in the methodology of measurements. In the first group, they measured immediately, without first progressively enlarging the canal. In the second group, they progressively enlarged the canal and then made a measurement. The values of the second group, after progressive enlargement, produced measurements that were closer to the real working length.

In cases of an incomplete apex, advanced apical resorption[9,51], or over- debridement[29], apical constriction can be compromised or absent, thus changing the electronic measurement of the root canal. The variation in impedance of the dentinal wall of the apical third will be reduced[31], resulting in shorter readings (Fig. 2. V-14). The flow of current in that location is altered, providing voltage gradient values closer to the values of the apical periodontal ligament. This interferes in the reading of variation in impedance, calculated from the application of two or more frequencies of alternating current.

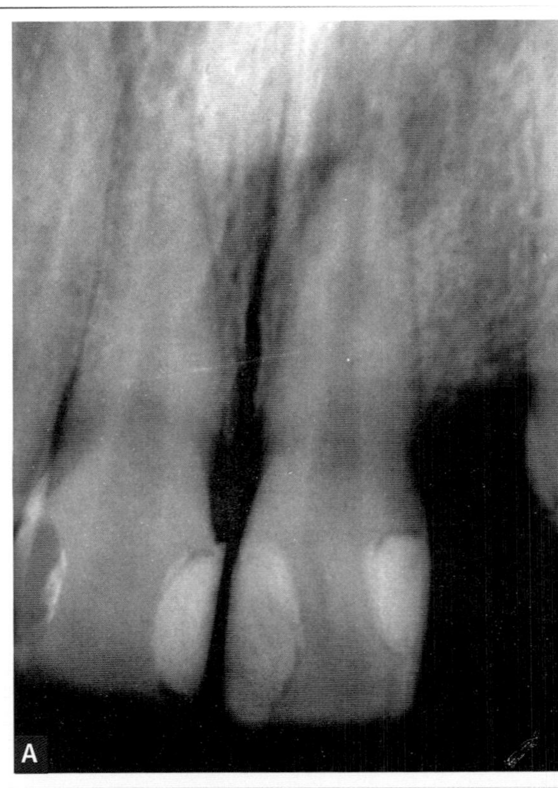

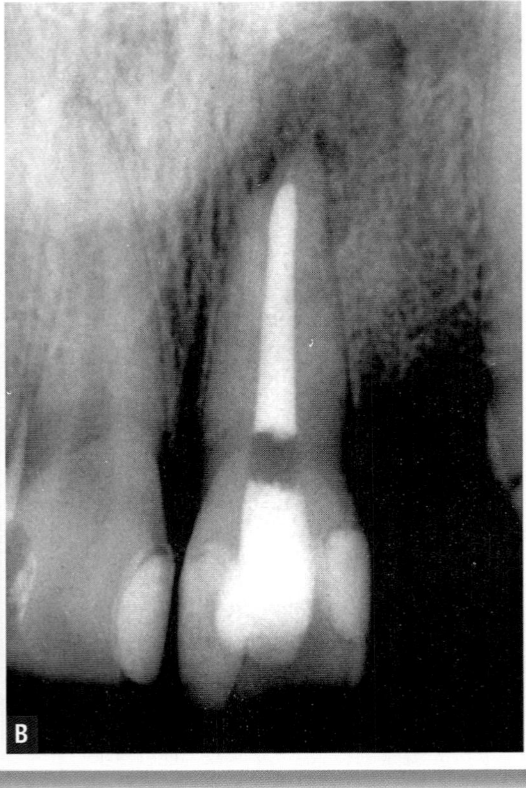

FIGS. 2.V-14A-B

Clinical Case.

A – Pre-operative radiograph of a left maxillary central incisor, with periapical lesion and suggestive of root resorption.

B – Post-operative radiograph. Note that the real working length determination, performed with an electronic apex locator (Root ZX), promoted the establishment of the apical stop for debridement thus allowing the filling material to remain at an adequate length.

HYBRIDIZATION OF EQUIPMENT

In 1997, Kobayashi et al.[35] introduced an electrical micromotor designed for root canal debridement, using nickel-titanium files in continuous rotation at low speed (240 to 280 rpm). Tri Auto ZX* (Fig. 2.V-15) has an internal module that allows electronic measurement of the canal, in a manner similar to that of Root ZX, and only requires minor adjustments. Proper training, imperative for learning any technical skill, is important to enable one to take full advantage of the device.

Dentaport ZX* (Fig. 2.V-16) is an electrical micrometer coupled to the apex locator Root ZX. In a manner analogous to that of Root ZX, the equipment screen displays scales for working length measurements, as well as providing speed and torque adjusted for rotary debridement. Another representative of this type of equipment is Siroendo Pocket, Sirona** (Fig. 2. V-34).

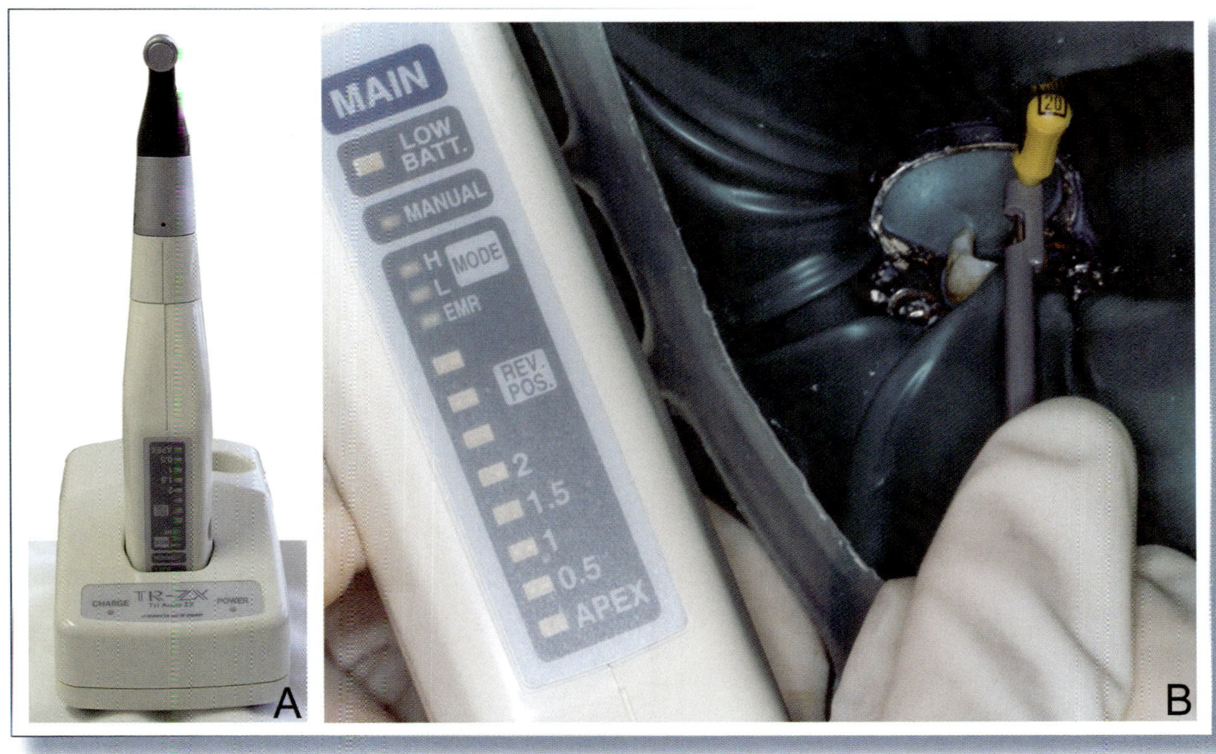

FIGS. 2.V-15A-B

A – The Tri Auto ZX Appliance, JMorita, on its base.
B – Measurement with the locator function of Tri Auto ZX.

* JMorita, Japan.
** Sirona, Germany.

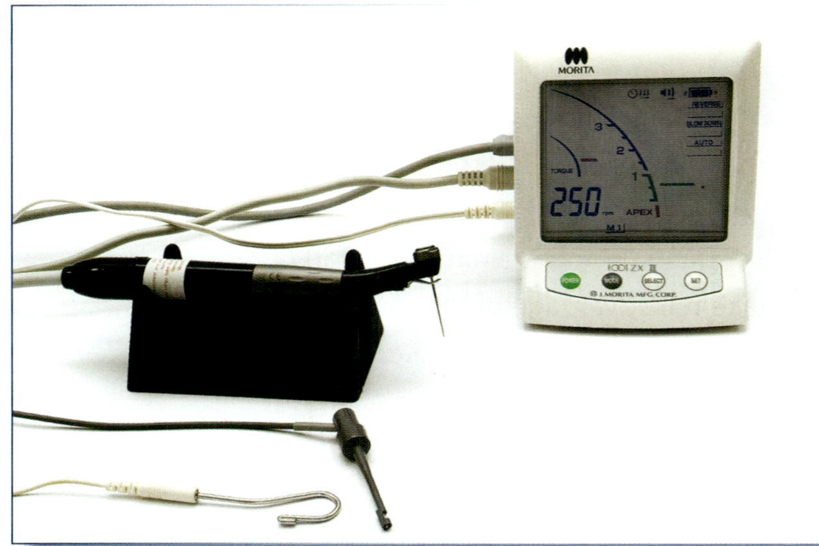

FIG. 2.V-16
Dentaport ZX, JMorita.

WORKING LENGTH MEASUREMENT TECHNIQUES

Radiographic (Ingle[32]) and electronic (frequency principle, third generation devices) working length measurement techniques will now be described. In the case of the electronic method, the basic use pertinent to all devices will be discussed. In these cases, the devices differ mainly in interface of use, accessories, batteries and interpretation on the monitor of the position of the apical constriction.

Ingle's Technique

Of the techniques that use radiography, the one proposed by Ingle is the most used. It is simple to perform and does not require anything more than basic clinical equipment to perform endodontic treatment. The operative stages are described below:

- an initial radiograph is taken to view the anatomy and view restorative materials in order to obtain a diagnosis; it is also used to establish a temporary radiographic length of the tooth (Fig. 2. V-17). This initial radiograph must be taken with a technique that allows the smallest distortion possible, which means the use of a parallel technique (long cone or indicator cone).

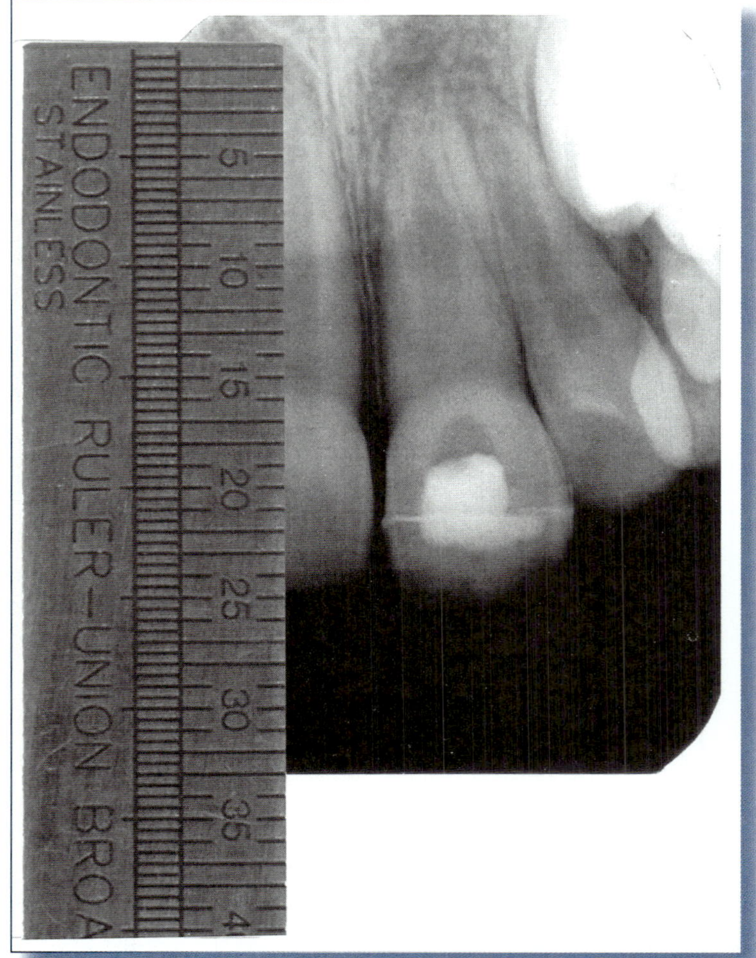

FIG. 2.V-17
Pre-operative radiograph for diagnosis and used to measure the tooth length with an appropriate millimeter ruler. A reading of 24.5 mm of tooth length was recorded. The use of an endodontic ruler is not recommended, because its thickness makes it difficult to visualize the scale in relation to the radiographic image.

- deduct 2 to 3 mm of the measurement determined from the radiograph, taking into account possible distortion of the radiographic image, which also serves as a safety measure against accidental trauma of the periapical tissues.
- transfer the length to an endodontic instrument, that has a rubber/silicone stop.
- introduce the instrument into the canal, so that that the stop touches the incisal edge or a cusp of a tooth at a tangent, which is now used as a point of reference: one of the points that will define the working length.
- proceed with taking a radiographic film.
- on the radiograph, measure the difference between the end of the instrument and the root apex, adding this value to or subtracting it from the length of the instrument. Thus, the length of the tooth is obtained (Fig. 2. V-18).
- in cases in which this difference is equal to or higher than **4 mm**, the instrument must be repositioned, and a new radiograph must be taken.
- thus, the length of the tooth is obtained. The real working length will be established by subtracting 1 mm (more or less, depending on the case) from the value found.

GROSSMAN's technique

This method resorts to the mean length of the teeth (Chart 2.V-3) for initial insertion of the instrument, and after this, a radiograph is taken and corrections are made, in a similar way to the one used with Ingle's technique.

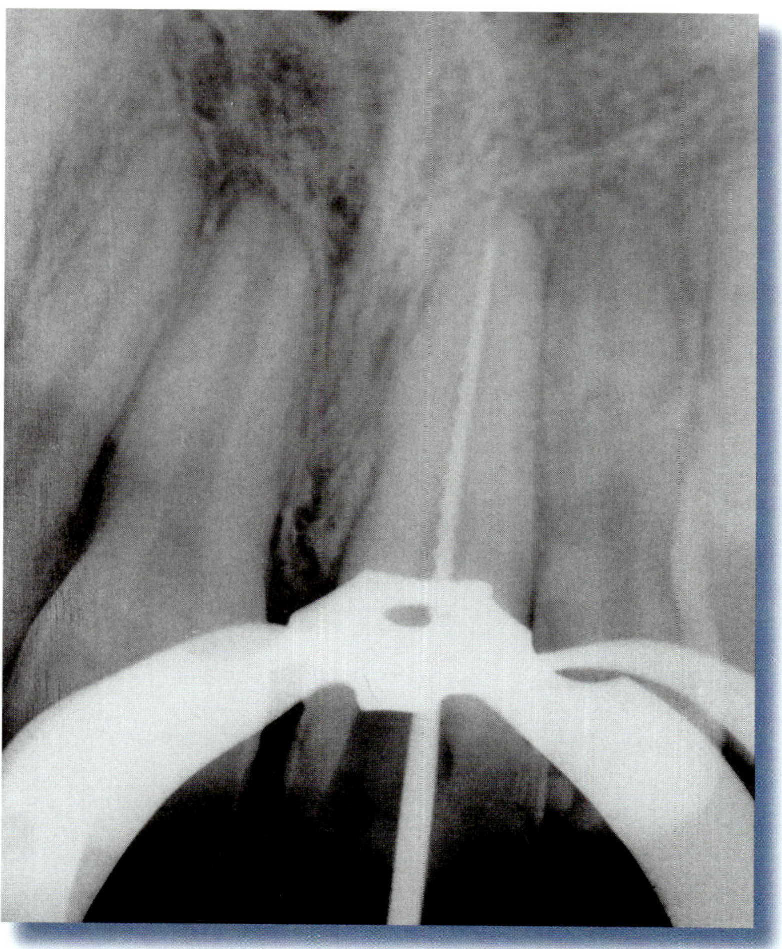

FIG. 2.V-18

To measure the difference between the instrument tip and the root apex in a working length radiograph. Later additional corrections will be made, in the event that the instrument does not reach the ideal point or if the instrument tip exits the apex. In this example, the difference between the instrument tip and the root apex was +1.5 mm.

Chart 2.V-3 – Mean, maximum and minimum length of the teeth, according to Pucci & Reig.

LENGTH OF TEETH IN MILLIMETERS (PUCCI & REIG)[64]			
MAXILLARY TEETH			
	Mean length	Maximum length	Minimum length
Central incisor	21.80	28.50	18.00
Lateral incisor	23.10	29.50	18.50
Canine	26.40	33.50	20.00
First premolar	21.50	25.50	17.00
Second premolar	21.60	26.00	17.00
First molar	21.30	25.50	18.00
Second molar	21.70	27.00	17.50
Third molar	17.10	22.00	14.00
MANDIBULAR TEETH			
Central incisor	20.80	27.50	16.50
Lateral incisor	22.60	29.00	17.00
Canine	25.00	32.00	19.50
First premolar	21.90	26.50	17.00
Second premolar	22.30	27.50	17.50
First molar	21.90	27.00	19.00
Second molar	22.40	26.00	19.00
Third molar	18.50	20.00	16.00

BREGMAN'S TECHNIQUE

The technique proposed by Bregman[6] consists of placing an instrument 10 mm long inside the root canal. After this, a radiograph is taken, and with the aid of a millimeter ruler, the length of the tooth is measured on the radiograph; having obtained these three values, a rule of three (Thales' theorem) is performed, which results in the real tooth length (RTL).

$$RTL = \frac{RLI \times ATL}{ALI}$$

RLI : *Real length of instrument*

ATL : *Apparent tooth length on the radiograph*

ALI : *Apparent length of instrument on the radiograph*

RTL : *Real tooth length*

ELECTRONIC WORKING LENGTH THIRD GENERATION DEVICES

Models of the Third Generation Devices

Some third generation devices are shown in Figs. 2.V-19 to 2.V-24.

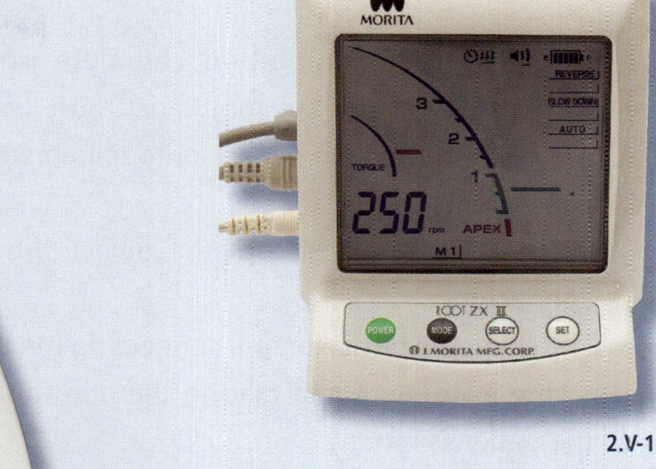

2.V-19

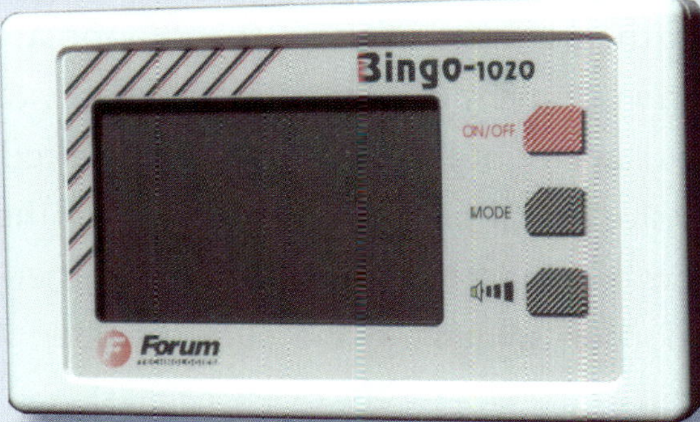

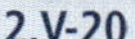

2.V-20

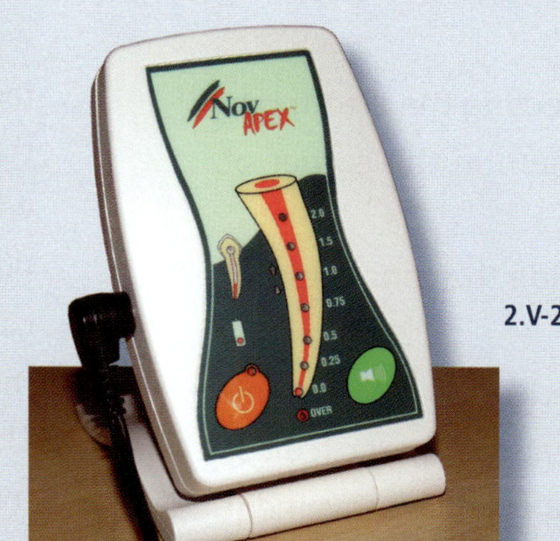

2.V-21

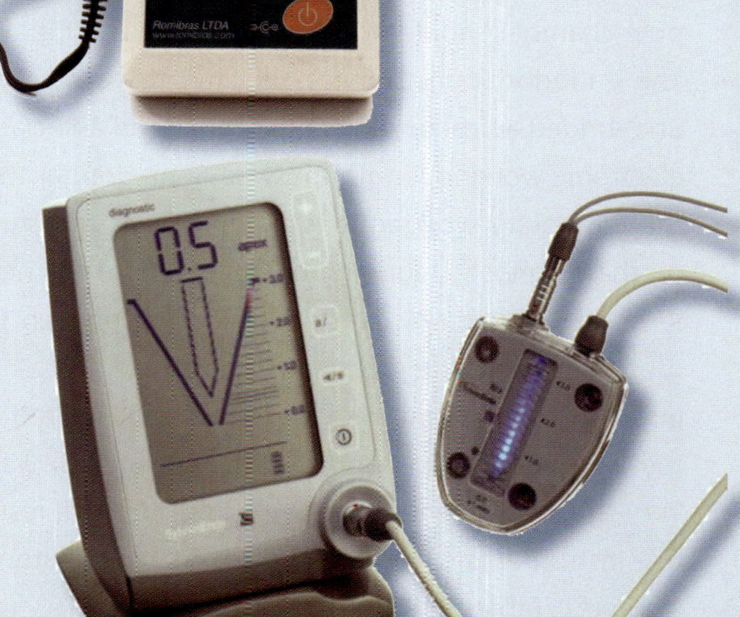

2.V-22

2.V-23

2.V-24

FIG. 2.V-19
Dentaport ZX (J Morita).

FIG. 2.V-20
Bingo 1020 (Forum).

FIG. 2.V-21
Novapex (Forum), Romiapex A-15 (Romidan).

FIG. 2.V-22
Romiapex D-30 (Romidan).

FIG. 2.V-23
Mini (SybronEndo).

FIG. 2.V-24
Components of Diagnostic Unit and Apex Locator (SybronEndo).

Operative Sequence

- After coronal opening and complete isolation of the operative field, the root canal must be carefully irrigated with sodium hypochlorite solution at different concentrations.
- Ensure that the cables to the device are properly connected.
- switch on the device before connecting the electrodes to the instrument and placing them in the corner of the patient's mouth.
- Before placing the instrument inside the canal, several precautions must be observed:
  - Contact between the electrodes (of the file and corner of the mouth). This will cause a short circuit of the signal. This procedure must result in movement of the signal on the equipment monitor, indicating a nearby point, in addition to the one with reference to the position of the apical foramen.
  - After access, verify whether the tooth is well isolated and that there are no metal restorations projecting into the canal entrances. Metal restorations divert the circuit, diminish impedance and give a false-positive result.

- The batteries must be fully charged. Precision equipment such as the electronic apex locators do not work correctly when the batteries are partially charged.
- In cases of biopulpectomy: A partial pulpectomy must be performed before electronic measurements can be performed. This must be limited to approximately 5 mm short of the tooth length on the radiograph, established by using the image of the preoperative radiograph. In case of hemorrhage it cannot exceed the limit of the root canal entrance(s). In extreme cases, a piece of cotton may be placed inside the pulp chamber, to prevent bleeding from interfering in the reading. The instrument can be inserted next to the piece of cotton.
- For cases of pulp necrosis: 1% hypochlorite sodium solution will cause initial cleaning of the necrotic remnants inside the pulp chamber. After the initial stage of progressive debridement, apically limited to a point 5 mm short of the radiographic apex (temporary working length) as measured on the diagnostic radiograph, an instrument of a size that matches with the anatomic diameter of the canal must be inserted, without excessive apical pressure. The file clip of the device will now be connected to the instrument. There can be no irrigation solution in the pulp chamber; it must be limited to the entrance(s) of the canal(s).
- The ground is placed in the corner of the patient's mouth.
- Opting for the debridement technique (crown-down), the largest size instruments can be used up to a limit of 5 mm before initial measurement (temporary working length), determined from the preoperative radiograph. At this time, the file clip is attached (Figs. 2.V-25 and 2.V-26) to the instrument in the operative sequence and a reading is taken. It is important that the canals contain an irrigation solution, while the pulp chamber should not contain an excess of it.
- The endodontic instrument selected to explore the undebrided apical portion of the canal, and associated electronic working length must be 5 mm longer than the temporary working length, which was measured on the diagnostic radiograph. This is due to the need for available space to place the file clip between the rubber stop and the instrument cable.
- Insert the instrument into the root canal. Ensure that the instrument is in contact with the internal walls. Very thin instruments may give a false-positive result. Use instruments of a diameter close to the anatomic diameter (Tables 2.V-1 and 2.V-2).

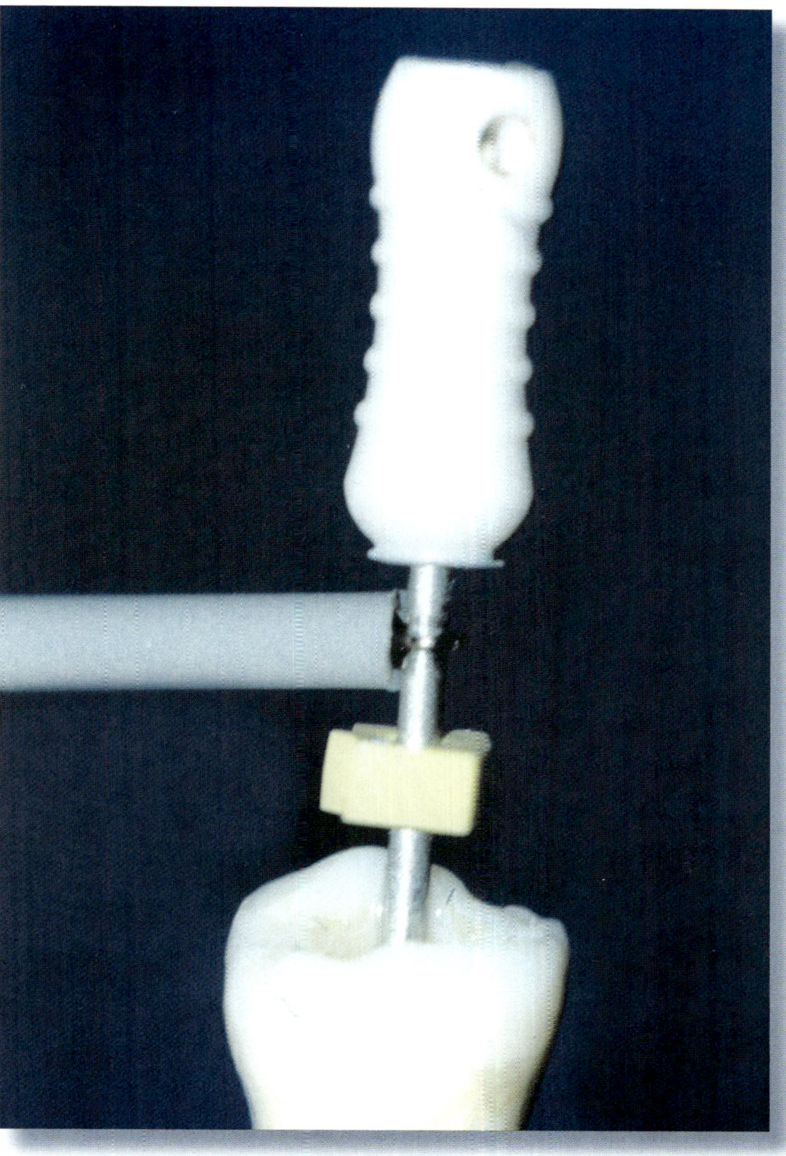

FIG. 2.V-25

Placement of the file clip in between the file handle and the rubber stop.

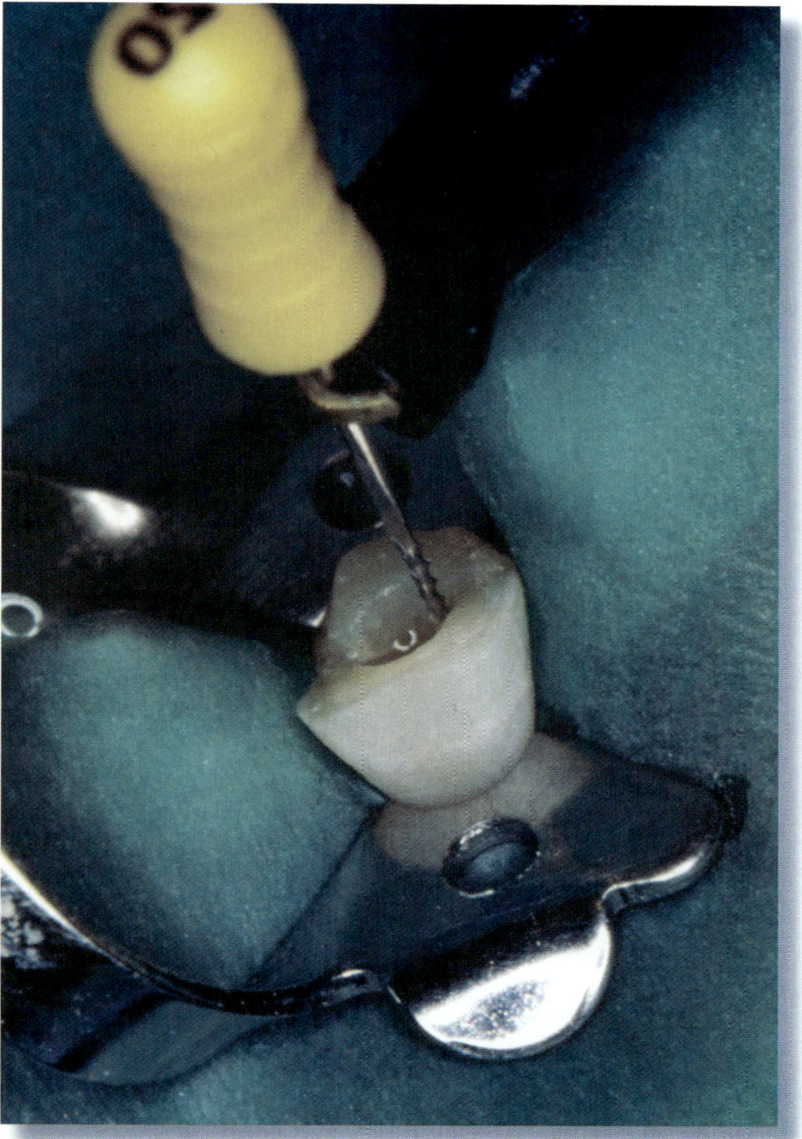

FIG. 2.V-26

Intra-oral view of the file placed in the root canal with the file clip attached during electronic measurements.

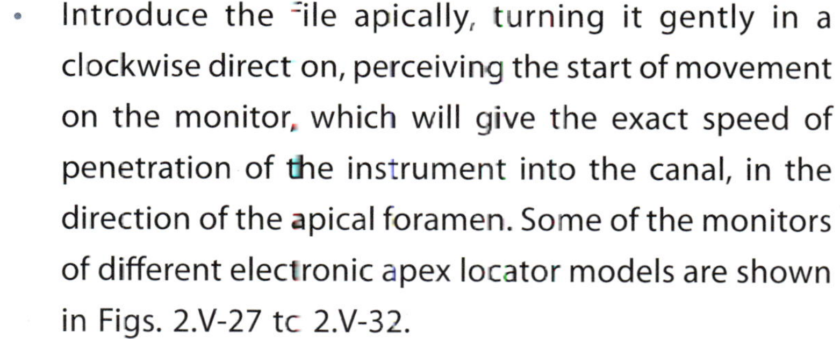

- Introduce the file apically, turning it gently in a clockwise direction, perceiving the start of movement on the monitor, which will give the exact speed of penetration of the instrument into the canal, in the direction of the apical foramen. Some of the monitors of different electronic apex locator models are shown in Figs. 2.V-27 to 2.V-32.
- When coming closer to the final reading, an intermittent alarm sounds. Continue with the instrument in an apical direction until the alarm sound is continuous, which will place the read-out in the position of the foramen exit. When reaching this mark, withdraw the instrument up to the point of the position of the apical constriction. The alarm will change from continuous to an intermittent sound. Note that each model identifies the read-out on the monitor in a different way.
- At this time, the operator must proceed to mark the real working length, sliding the rubber stop to the chosen occlusal or incisal reference point.

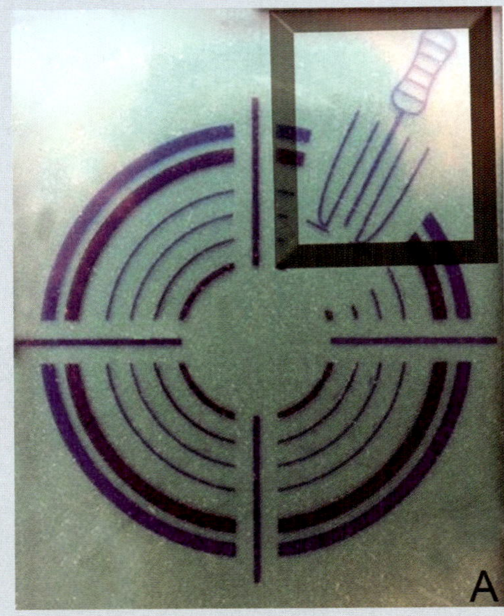

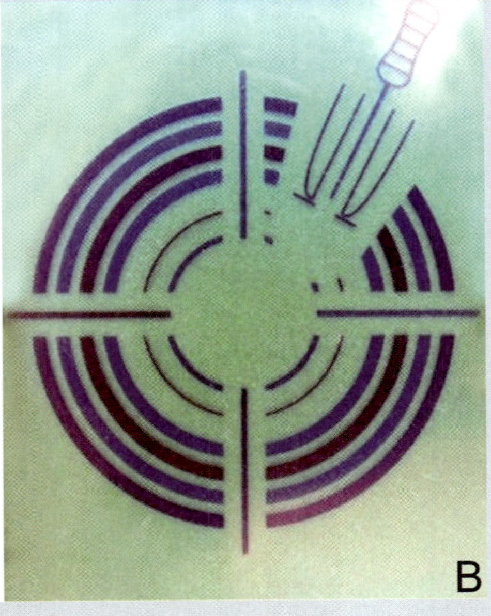

FIGS. 2.V-27A-B

A – Monitor of the model Romiapex D-30, showing the initial stages of measurement. From insertion of the instrument until it comes close to the last 3 millimeters of the root canal there will be no significant change in status of the bar.

B – When starting measurement, with the instrument at the apical third, the concentric circles surrounding the target are highlighted. In detail, the appearance on the panel indicating that measurement is being performed.

FIGS. 2.V-28A-B

Model Romiapex D-30 Screen, showing progression of measurement towards the last millimeters of the root canal.

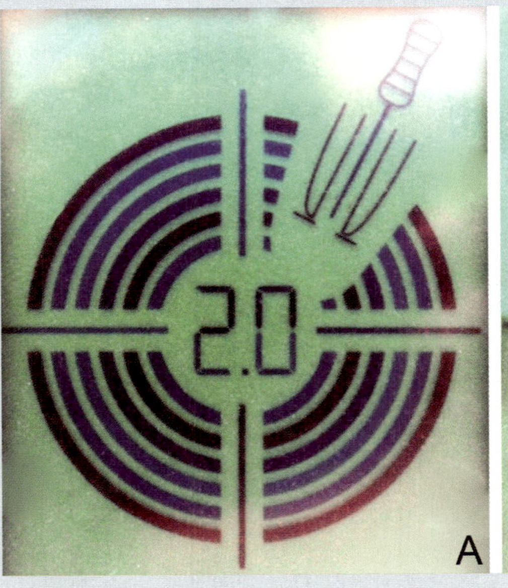

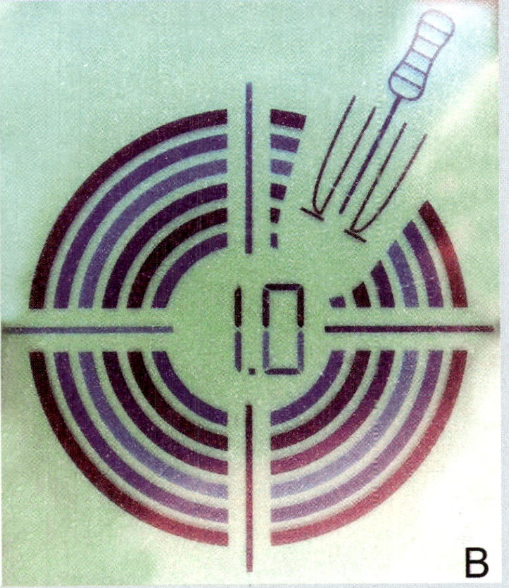

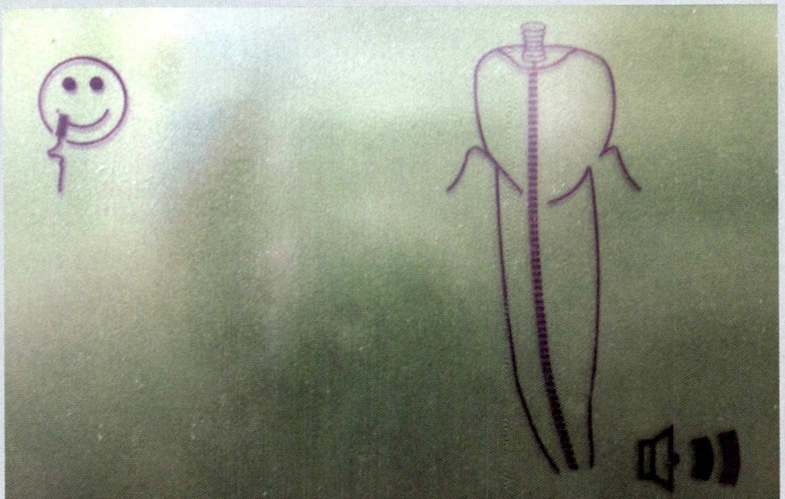

FIG. 2.V-29

Model Bingo 1020 monitor with on the right side a diagrammatic representation of a tooth and in a dotted line, which is used to measure the progress of the instrument when measuring the cervical, middle and apical thirds.

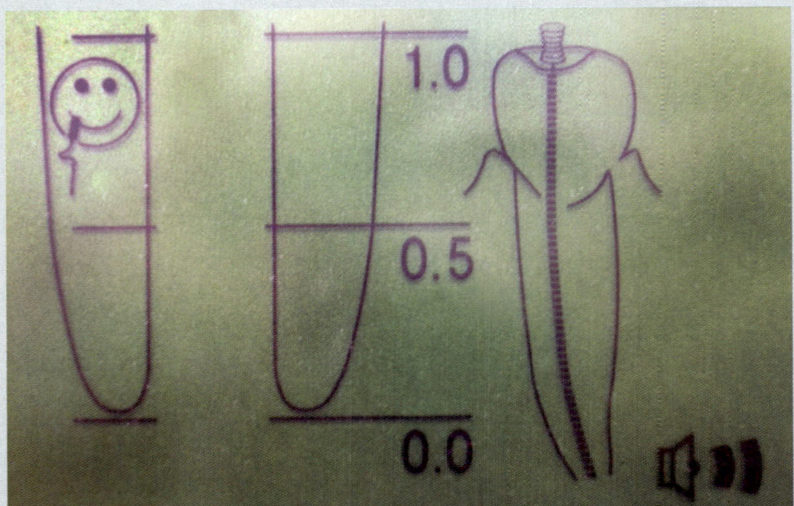

FIG. 2.V-30

Model Bingo 1020 Screen showing *Root Zoom.*

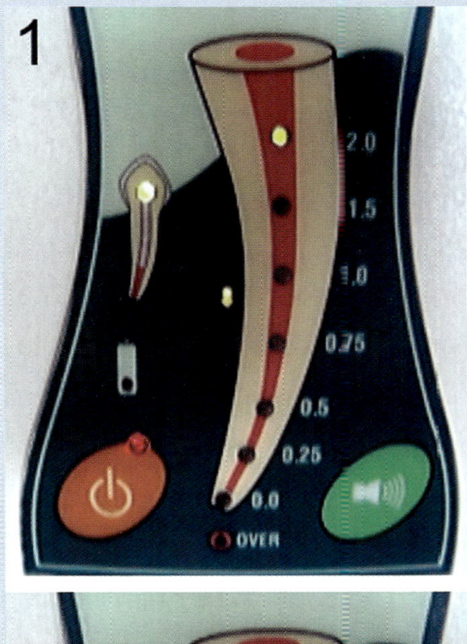

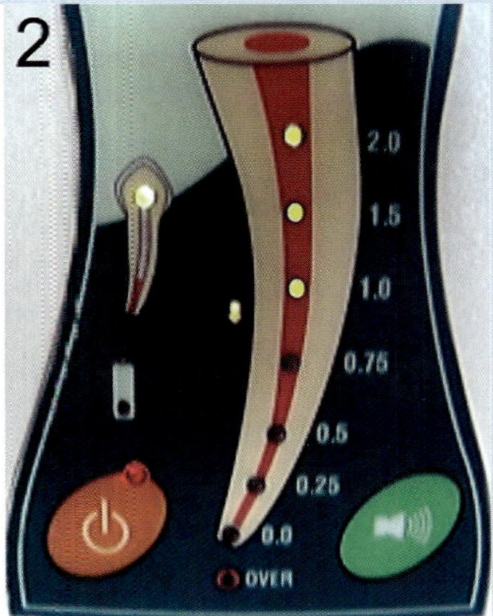

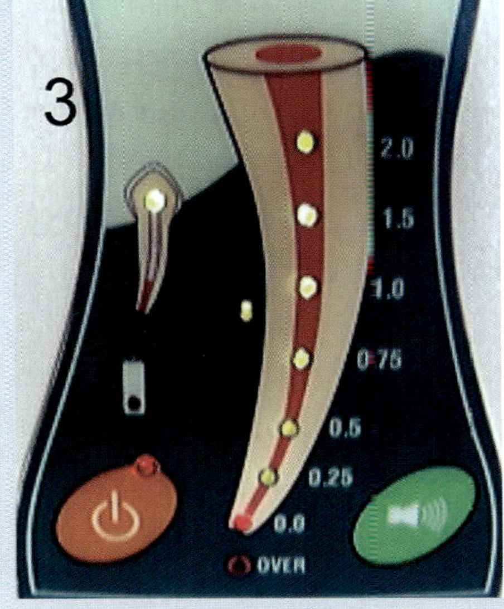

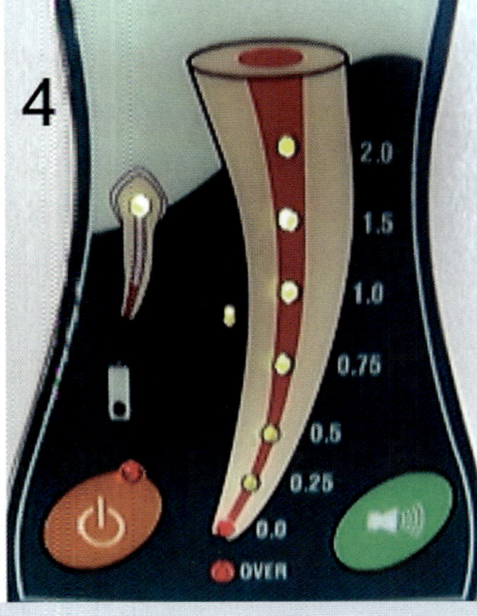

FIG. 2.V-31

View of the Novapex showing from left to right the sequence of electronic reading with the progression of the instrument in an apical direction, up to and beyond the foramen exit (over).

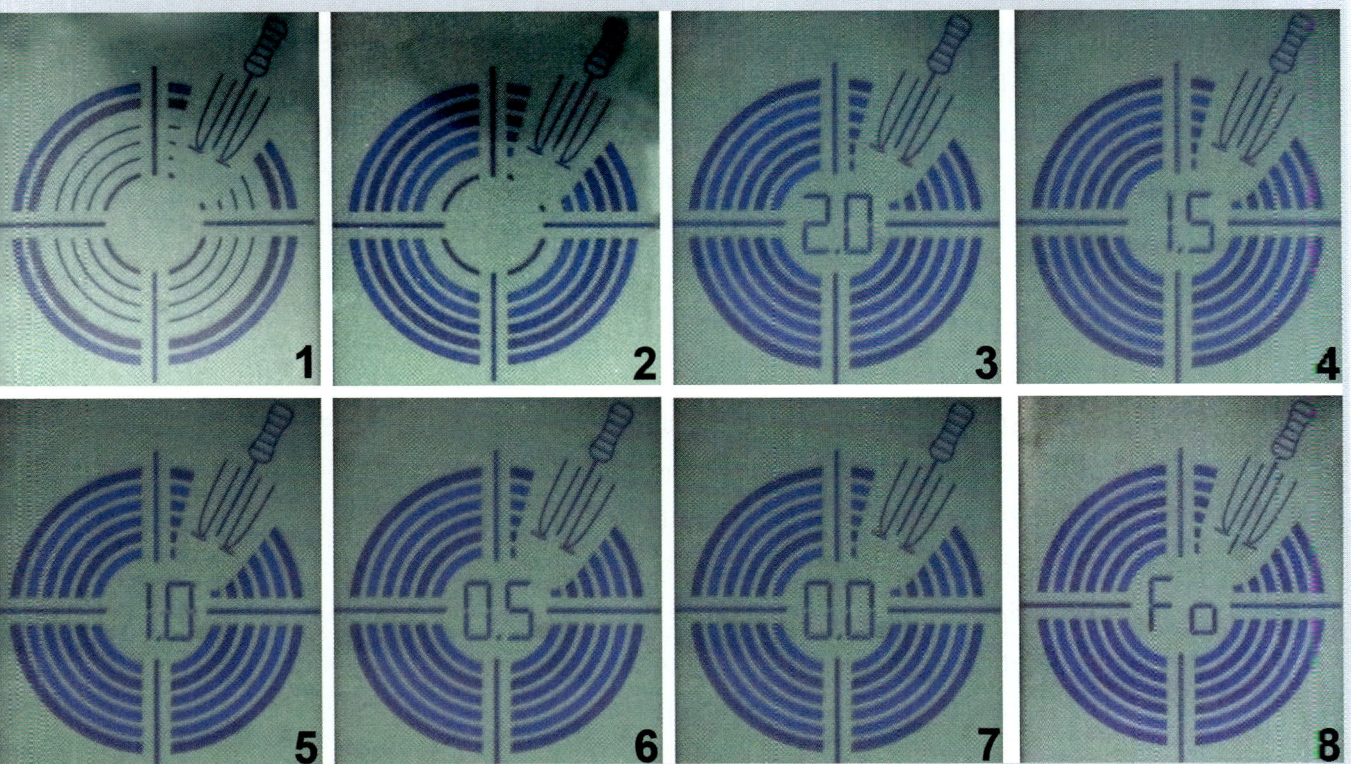

FIG. 2.V-32

View of the Romiapex D-30, from left to right, showing the progressive sequence of electronic readings of the instrument in an apical direction and beyond the foramen exit (Fo).

Precautions During Electronic Measurements

Some points must be observed during electronic measuring, irrespective of the model used:

- Before any attempt to use it in a patient, electronic measuring should be practiced *in vitro*. After familiarization with all the details of the method, in particular the way in which the equipment works, practice on a model with extracted teeth is highly recommended.
- Acquire a reliable diagnostic radiograph, preferably with the parallel technique, using locator cones (of the "indicator cone" type). Develop and process the radiograph carefully using standardized techniques and analyze it in a negatoscope without light bleeding from the borders, aided by a loupe and a flat metal millimeter ruler. The real temporary working length, measured from a proper initial radiograph normally differs from 0 to 15%[51] from the definitive working length measurement.
- In case the tooth is vital, perform a partial pulpectomy removing at least two thirds of pulp tissue volume. Clinically it has been noticed that in cases of irreversible pulpitis, placement of an instrument in the cervical third can result in a measurement that indicates a point close to the apical constriction. When partially removing tissues, abundant irrigation followed by aspirating excess fluid, the measurement tends to return to normal.
- The instrument used for measurement must match with the anatomic diameter of the canal (Tables 2.V-1 and 2.V-2). Larger size instruments will not reach the apical third. Thin instruments make apical placement and reading difficult, due to the lack of control over penetration. An important study of the anatomy of the last few millimeters of the root canal, in reference to the mean diameter, was performed by Wu et al.[80] The mean results are presented below in Tables 2.V-1 and 2.V-2.

Analysis of the data in the above tables indicates what would be the approximate anatomic diameter of the root canals to be measured, and consequently, what the instrument of choice to perform this procedure would be. It is of interest to note that in the majority of cases, the mesio-distal and bucco-lingual (or maxillary lingual) diameters do not coincide, indicating that we are dealing with an oval, rather than circular canal. The measuring instrument is not always capable of touching all the internal walls of the root canal. Several authors have shown that the measurement of the anatomic diameter, using the technique of the first instrument that fits to the apical limit, may lead to incorrect readings of the apical diameter. In the majority of cases, the instrument that is inserted fits to a point removed from the constriction, referring to a non-existent apical positioning, which is something the operator does not perceive because it is not possible to visualize the internal part of the canal. Frequently the tip of the instrument is free in the lumen of the canal, due to the taper of the instrument, whereas the thicker segment of this instrument would fit. The alternative for clinical detection of the anatomic diameter would be to perform the progressive debridement technique (crown-down). Thus, the interferences relative to the direction of the cervical and middle thirds and the beginning of the apical third of the root canal will be eliminated, facilitating the fit of the tip of the instrument in the anatomic lumen of the root canal. Based on the above-mentioned values, and after performing the crown-down technique, the operator will be able to perform this important operative step, aided by the electronic working length determination.

- The electrodes [file-holder and lip clips (contrary electrodes)] must be free from oxidation products, which may have developed as a result from contact with irrigation solutions.

TABLE 2. V-1 – Mean measurements of the bucco-lingual and mesio-distal diameter of the root canal of maxillary teeth at 1, 2 and 5 mm short of the apical foramen. The values are in millimeters (for example, 0.50 coincides with the D0 of the endodontic instrument 50, Wu et al.[80]).

POSITION SHORT OF THE APICAL FORAMEN	BUCCO-LINGUAL DIAMETER			MESIO-DISTAL DIAMETER		
	1 MM	2 MM	5 MM	1 MM	2 MM	5 MM
Maxillary teeth						
Central incisor	0.34	0.47	0.76	0.30	0.36	0.54
Lateral incisor	0.45	0.60	0.77	0.33	0.33	0.47
Canine	0.31	0.58	0.63	0.29	0.44	0.50
Buccal premolar	0.30	0.40	0.35	0.23	0.31	0.31
Lingual premolar	0.23	0.37	0.42	0.17	0.26	0.33
Mesio-buccal molar	0.19	0.37	0.46	0.13	0.27	0.32
Mesio-lingual molar	0.19	0.31	0.38	0.16	0.16	0.16
Disto-bucal molar	0.22	0.33	0.49	0.17	0.25	0.31
Lingual molar	0.29	0.40	0.55	0.33	0.40	0.74

TABLE 2. V-2 – Mean measurements of the bucco-lingual and mesio-distal diameter of the root canal of maxillary teeth at 1, 2 and 5 mm short of the apical foramen. The values are in millimeters (for example, 0.50 coincides with the D0 of the endodontic instrument 50, Wu et al.[80]).

POSITION SHORT OF THE APICAL FORAMEN	BUCCO-LINGUAL DIAMETER			MESIO-DISTAL DIAMETER		
	1 MM	2 MM	5 MM	1 MM	2 MM	5 MM
Mancibular teeth						
Incisors	0.37	0.52	0.81	0.25	0.25	0.29
Canine	0.47	0.45	0.74	0.36	0.36	0.57
Premolar	0.35	0.40	0.76	0.28	0.32	0.49
Mesio-buccal molar	0.40	0.42	0.64	0.21	0.26	0.32
Mesio-lingual molar	0.38	0.44	0.61	0.28	0.24	0.35
Distal molar	0.46	0.50	1.07	0.35	0.34	0.59

- The irrigation solution in the root canal can not be beyond the canal entrance(s). The canals must be moist when measurements are made, preferably using a 1% sodium hypochlorite solution.
- When the bar indicator on the display screen starts to oscillate up and down, remove the instrument from the canal. Irrigate, aspirate excess irrigation solution and start the procedure again. Verify the presence of contact between the file and metal restorations (if present). Do a preliminary test by touching the electrodes. Verify the presence of excess pulp tissue in case of an irreversible inflamed pulp. Verify that the battery is fully charged.
- It is recommended not to leave the batteries in the device for extended periods of time. When the measurements have been completed, switch off the device to prevent unnecessary drainage of the battery.
- Always keep the cable of the equipment straight, or rolled up on a large spool of the type used for fishing lines. Excessive bending of the cable may break the wires, damaging the equipment.
- Paiva and Antoniazzi[57] pointed out that the working length measurements do not remain constant during treatment, as the real working length is a dynamic measurement, which slowly undergoes changes during debridement. Electronic working length measurements may require confirmation of maintaining the real working length, and it may be made at any time of debridement, including when refining the apical stop, and before filling. This procedure we define as monitored debridement[64] (Figs. 2.V-33 to 2.V-35).

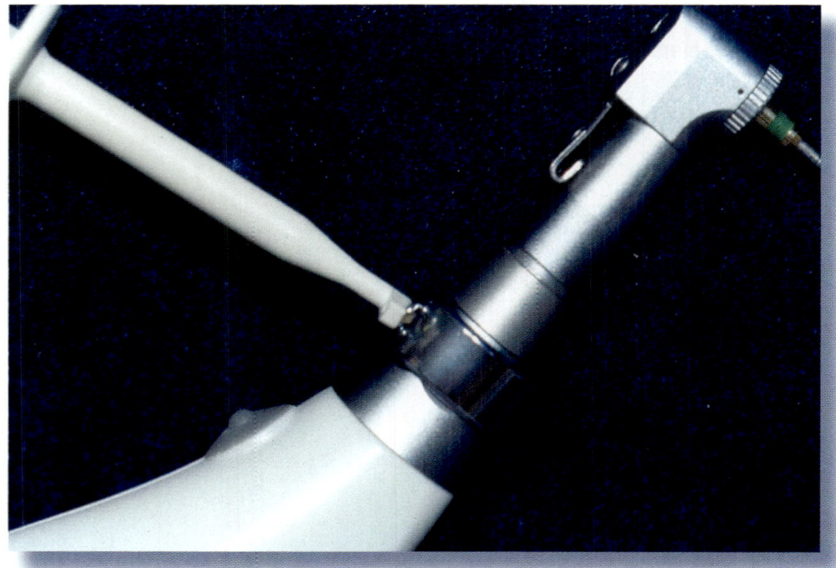

FIG. 2.V-33

Accessory attached to the wireless electric micromotor Endomate 2 (NSK, Japan). Rotary debridement can be performed, while the electronic apical locator file attached to the hand piece continuously monitors the real working length.

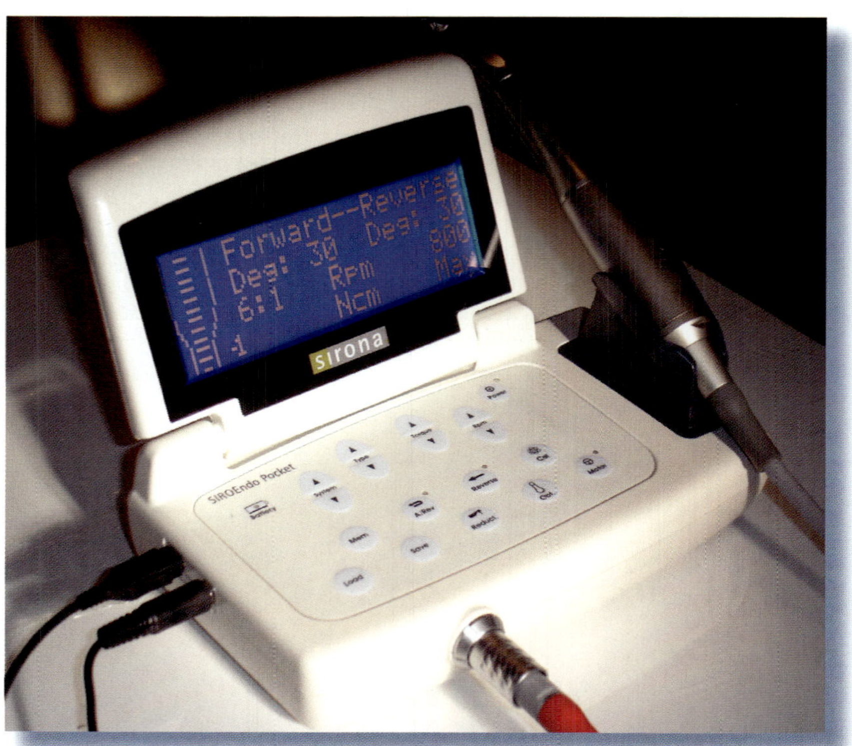

FIG. 2.V-34

Motor SiroEndo Pocket, Sirona, with attached foramin locator. Among the debridement options is one in which the operator can choose the monitored debridement.

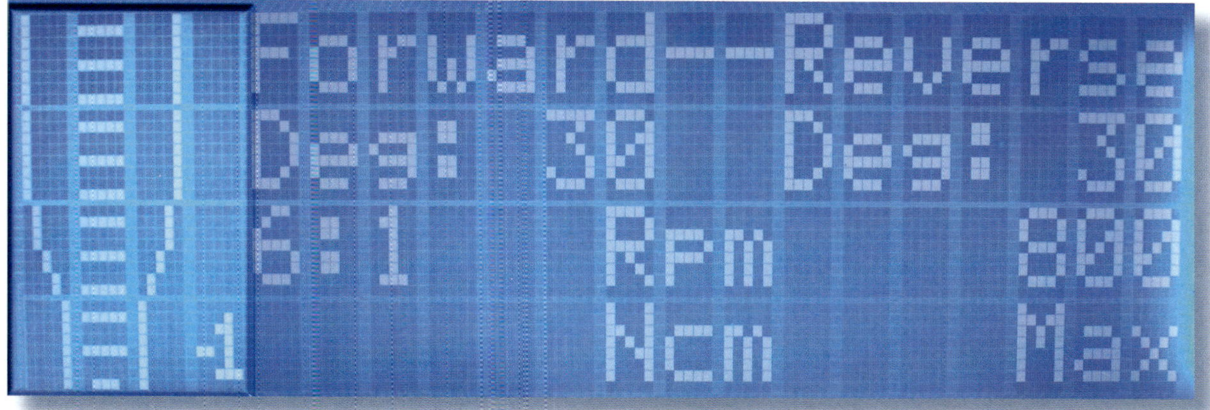

FIG. 2-V-35

The SiroEndo Pocket Motor monitor. Sirona, showing the information that is displayed during electronic measurement.

Taking a Radiograph for Measurement

One of the more important aspects when using electronic working length techniques is the need for taking a radiograph to verify the accuracy of the method. In this regard, we understand that there may be a conflict of objective, and not of procedure. The procedure of "making a radiograph after electronic working length measurement" must be performed even if the basic purpose of the procedure is not necessarily to confirm the accuracy of the apical limit established by the electronic reading. Many authors[4,8,13,19,20,22,26,38,44,46,52,58,65,61,62,76,78,80] have shown that the radiographic technique has minor and major limitations, depending on the root morphology of the tooth, the position in the arch, presence of anatomic structures that are superimposing the area of interest, presence of apical resorption. Furthermore there are the difficulties inherent to the making and processing of radiographs. Nevertheless, it should be pointed out that radiographs have to be made after electronic working length measurements in order to visualize the direction of the canal (or canals). The image of an instrument in a canal facilitates identification of details concerning the angle and radius of curvature, arch length, dilacerations, thickness of the dentin walls, as well as offering a representation of the relationship of the tip of the instrument and the radiographic apex.

In this case, the radiograph with an instrument in situ shows details, in addition to the ones of the diagnostic image, allowing identification of situations that may lead to different technical procedures. This step is valuable as it enables a novice operator to evaluate him or herself about the technical expertise that is required, which will improve confidence in the use of electronic working lengths measurements.

References

1. Arora RK, Gulabivala K. An in vivo evaluation of the Endex and RCM Mark II electronic apex locators in root canals with different contents. Oral Surg Oral Med Oral Pathol Oral Radiol Endod., v.79, n.4, p. 497-503, April 1995.
2. Berger CR. Obturação dos canais radiculares. In: ___. Endodontia. São Paulo, Pancast, 1998, p.420.
3. Best E. et al. A new method of tooth length determination for endodontic practice. Dent. Dig., v.66, p.450-454, 1960.
4. Blaskovic-Subat V, Maricic B, Sutalo J. Asymmetry of the root canal foramen. Int. Endod. J., v.25, n.3, p.42-47, May 1992.
5. Bramante CM, Berbert A. A critical evaluation of some methods of determining tooth length. Oral Surg Oral Med Oral Pathol Oral Radiol Endod., v.37, p.463-473, Mar. 1974.
6. Bregman RC. A mathematical method of determining the length of a tooth for root canal treatment and filling. J. Canad. Dent. Ass., v.16, p.305-306, 1950.
7. Brochado VHD, Silva Neto UX Da, Gonçalves Júnior JF, Ramos CAS. Avaliação da precisão de localizadores apicais eletrônicos na determinação do comprimento de trabalho. Pesqui Odontol Bras, v.15, Suplemento (Anais da 18ª Reunião Anual da SBPqO), p.79, 2001.
8. Burch JG, Hulen S. The relationship of the apical foramen to the anatomical apex of the tooth root. Oral Surg Oral Med Oral Pathol Oral Radiol Endod., v.34, n.2, p.262-268, Aug. 1972.
9. Busch LR. et al. Determination of the accuracy of the Sono-Explorer for establishing endodontic measurement control. J. Endod., v.2, n.10, p.295-297, Oct. 1976.
10. Chong BS, Pitt Ford TR. Apex locators in endodontics: which, when and how? Dent. Update, v.21, n.8, p.328-330, Oct. 1994.
11. Chunn CB, Zardiackas LD, Menke RA. In vivo root canal length determination using the Forameter. J. Endod., v.7, n.11, p.515-520, Nov. 1981.
12. Clouse HR. Electronic methods of root measurement. Gen. Dent., v.6, p.432-437, Nov./Dec. 1991.
13. Coolidge ED. Anatomy of root apex in relation to treatment problems. J. Amer. dent. Ass., v.16, p.1.456-1.465, 1929.
14. Crane AS. Discussion of nature methods of making perfect root fillings. Dent. Cosmos, v.63, p.1.039-1.040, 1921.
15. De Deus QD. Endodontia. 5.ª ed. Rio de Janeiro, Medsi, 1992.
16. Duinkerke ASH, Van Der Poel ACM. An analysis of apparently identical radiographs. Oral Surg Oral Med Oral Pathol Oral Radiol Endod., v.38, p.962-967, 1974.
17. Dummer PMH, McGinn JH, Rees DG. The position and topography of apical constriction and apical foramen. Int. Endod. J., v.17, p.192-196, 1984.
18. Dunlap CA. et al. An in vivo evaluation of an electronic apex locator that uses the ratio method in vital and necrotic canals. J. Endod., v.24, n.1, p.48-50, Jan. 1998.
19. Elayouti A. et al. Frequency of overinstrumentation with an acceptable radiographic working length. J. Endod., v.27, n.1, p.49-52, Jan. 2001.
20. Ferlini Filho J. Estudo radiográfico e microscópico das reabsorções radiculares na presença de periodontites apicais crônicas (microscopia ótica e de varredura). Bauru, 1999, 186 p. Tese (doutorado) – Faculdade de Odontologia de Bauru, Universidade de São Paulo.
21. Glickman GN, Mickel AK, Levin LG, Fouad AF, Johnson WT. Glossary of Endodontic Terms. American Association of Endodontists, 7.ª ed., 2003.
22. Goldman M, Pearson AH, Darzenta N. Endodontic success – Who's reading the radiographic? Oral Surg Oral Med Oral Pathol Oral Radiol Endod., v.33, p.432-434, 1972.
23. Gordon MPJ, Chandler NP. Electronic apex locators. Int Endod J, v.37, p.425-437, 2004.
24. Green D. A stereomicroscopic study of apices of 400 maxillary and mandibular anterior teeth. Oral Surg Oral Med Oral Pathol Oral Radiol Endod., v.9, p.1224-1235, 1956.
25. Grove CJ. An accurate new technique for filling root canals to the dentino-cemental junction with impermeable materials. J. Amer. dent. Ass., v.16, p.1594-1600, 1929.
26. Gutierrez JH, Aguayo P. Apical foraminal openings in human teeth – number and location. Oral Surg Oral Med Oral Pathol Oral Radiol Endod., v.79, n.6, p.769-777, June 1995.
27. Gutmann JL, Leonard JE. Problem solving in endodontic working-length determination. Comp. Continuing Educ. Dent., v.16, n.3, p.288-302, Mar. 1995.
28. Harrison JW, Baumgatner JC, Svec TA. Incidence of pain associated with clinical factors during and after root canal therapy. Part 2. Postobturation pain. J. Endod., v.9, n.10, p.434-438, Oct. 1983.
29. Huang L. The principle of electronic root canal measurement. Bull. 4th Milit. Med. Coll., v.8, p.32-34, 1959.
30. Ibarrola JL. et al. Effect of preflaring on Root ZX apex locators. J Endod., v.25, n.9, p. 625-626, Sep. 1999.
31. Iizuka H. et al. A study on electronic method for measuring root canal length. J. Nihon Univ. Sch. Dent., v.29, p.278-286, Nov. 1987.
32. Ingle JI. Endodontics instruments and instrumentation. Dent. Clin. N. Amer., v.1, p.805-822, Nov. 1957.
33. Kobayashi C. Electronic canal length measurement. Oral Surg Oral Med Oral Pathol Oral Radiol Endod., v.79, n.2, p.226-231, 1995.
34. Kobayashi C, Suda H. New electronic canal measuring device based on the ratio method. J. Endod., v.20, n.3, p.111-114, Mar. 1994.
35. Kobayashi C, Yoshioka T, Suda H. A new engine-driven canal preparation system with electronic canal measuring capability. J. Endod., v.23, n.12, p.751-754, Dec. 1997.
36. Kovačević M, Tamarut T. Influence of concentration of ions and foramen diameter on accuracy of electronic root canal length measurement. An experimental study. J. Endod., v.24, n.5, p.346-351, May 1998.
37. Kuttler Y. Microscopic investigation of root apexes. J. Amer. dent. Ass., v.50, p.544-52, May 1955.
38. Lambriandis T. Observer variations in radiographic evaluation of endodontic therapy. Endod. Dent. Traumat., v.1, p.235-241, 1985.
39. Langeland K. The histologic basis in endodontic treatment. Dent. Clin. N. Amer., p.491-520, 1967.
40. Leonardo MR. Contribuição para o estudo da reparação apical e periapical pós-tratamento de canais radiculares. Araraquara, 1973. 252 p. Tese (Livre-Docência). Faculdade de Odontologia de Araraquara, Universidade Estadual Paulista.
41. Leonardo MR, Leal JM. Endodontia: tratamento de canais radiculares. 3.ª ed., São Paulo, Editorial Médica Panamericana, 1998.
42. Levy AB, Glatt L. Deviation of the apical foramen from the radiographic apex. J. N. J. St. Dent. Soc., v.41, p.12-13, 1970.

43. Lucena CM, Robles GV, Ferrer LCM, Navajas RVJV. In vitro evaluation of the accuracy of three electronic apex locators. J. Endod., v.30, n.4, p.231-233, 2004.

44. Ludlow JB, Abreu M, Mol A. Performance of a new F-speed film for caries detection. Dentomaxilofacial Radiology, v.30, n.2, p.110-113, Mar 2001.

45. McQuillen JH. Fing Fillings. Dent. Cosmos, v.11, p.225-226, 1861.

46. Machado MEL, Pesce HF. Estudo da região apical de dentes tratados endodonticamente até o vértice radiográfico da raiz. Rev. Ass. Paul Cirurg. Dent., v.35, n.6, p. 534-537, nov-dez 1981.

47. Maculan N. Manual de eletrônica e eletrotécnica. Curitiba, Editec, 1974.

48. Masreliez CJ. Method and apparatus for apical detection with complex impedance measurement. United States Patent, n.5759 59, current U.S. class 600/547, 1998.

49. Mayeda DL. et al. In vivo measurement accuracy in vital and necrotic canals with Endex apex locator. J. Endod., v.19, n.11, p.545-548, Nov. 1993.

50. Meares WA, Steiman HR. The influence of sodium hypochlorite irrigation on the accuracy of the Root ZX electronic apex locator. J. Endod., v.28, n.8, p.595-598, 2002.

51. Milano NF, Silva CAG. Comprimentos e distorções na condutometria em pré-molares e molares superiores e inferiores. Rev. Gaúcha Odont., v.36, n.2, p.97-98, mar-abr. 1988.

52. Milano NF, Werner SM, Kapczinski M. Localização do forame apical; a real localização versus métodos usuais de condutometria. Rev. Gaúcha Odont., v.31, n.3, p.220-224, jul-set. 1983.

53. Morfis A, Sylaras SN, Georgopoulou M, Kernani M, Prountzoos F. Study of the apices of human permanent teeth with the use of a scanning electron microscope. Oral Surg Oral Med Oral Pathol, v.77, n.2, p. 172-176, Feb. 1994.

54. Oishi A, Yoshioka T, Kobayashi C, Suda H. Electronic detection of root canal constrictions. J. Endod., v.28, n.5, p.361-364, May 2002.

55. Olson AK, Goerig AC, Cavatio RE. The ability of the radiographic in determining the location of apical foramen. Int. Endod. J., v.24, p.28-31, 1991.

56. Ounsi HF, Haddad G. In vitro evaluation of reliability of the Endex electronic apex locator. J. Endod., v.24, n.2, p.120-121, Feb. 1998.

57. Paiva JG, Antoniazzi JH. Odontometria. In: ___. Endodontia. Bases para a prática clínica. 2.ª ed., São Paulo, Artes Médicas, 1988, p.488.

58. Palmer MJ, Weine FS, Healey HJ. Position of the apical foramen in relation to endodontic therapy. J. Canad. Dent. Ass., V.37, N.8, P.305-308, 1971.

59. Pratten DH, McDonald NJ. Comparison of radiographic and electronic working lengths. J. Endod., v.22, n.4, p.173-176, April 1996.

60. Ramos CAS. Avaliação in vivo da precisão de leitura de um modelo de localizador apical eletrônico. Bauru, 1998. 168p. Tese (doutorado). Faculdade de Odontologia de Bauru – Universidade de São Paulo.

61. Ramos CAS, Bernardineli N. Avaliação in vivo da precisão de leitura de um modelo de localizador apical eletrônico. Unopar Cient., Ciênc. Biol. Saúde, v.3, n.1, p.9-20, out. 2001.

62. Ramos CAS, Bernardineli N. Influência do diâmetro do forame apical na precisão de leitura de um modelo de localizador apical eletrônico. Rev. FOB, v.2, n.3, p.83-90, 1994.

63. Ramos CAS. Influência do diâmetro do forame apical na precisão de leitura de um modelo de localizador apical eletrônico. Bauru, 1993. 117p. Dissertação (mestrado). Faculdade de Odontologia de Bauru – Universidade de São Paulo.

64. Ramos CAS, Bramante CM. Instrumentação dos canais radiculares. In: ___. Endodontia. Fundamentos biológicos e clínicos. São Paulo, Santos Editora, 2001, Cap.8, p.159-206.

65. Reche MEA, Ramos CAS. Influência da determinação eletrônica do comprimento de trabalho, comprovada ou não radiograficamente, na qualidade do nível de obturação dos canais radiculares. Estudo in vivo. Londrina, 2001, 118 p. Monografia (especialização). Universidade Norte do Paraná.

66. Seltzer S, Soltanoff W, Smith J. Biologic aspects of endodontics. Oral Surg Oral Med Oral Pathol Oral Radiol Endod, v.36, p.725-737, 1973.

67. Shabahang S, Goon WWY, Gluskin AH. An in vivo evaluation of Root ZX electronic apex locator. J. Endod., v.22, n.11, p.616-618, Nov. 1996.

68. Simon JHS. The apex: how critical is it? Gen. Dent., v.42, n.4, p.330-334, Jul-Aug. 1994.

69. Sjögren, U. et al. Factors affecting the long-term results of endodontic treatment. J. Endod., v.16, p.498-504, Oct. 1990.

70. Suchde RV, Talim ST. Electronic ohmmeter. An electronic device for the determination of root canal length. Oral Surg Oral Med Oral Pathol Oral Radiol Endod., v.43, n.1, p.141-149, Jan. 1977.

71. Sunada I. New method for measuring the length of the root canal. J. Jap. Stomat. Soc., v.25, p.161-171, 1958.

72. Suzuki K. Experimental study in iontophoresis. J. Jap. Stomat. Soc., v.16, p.414-417, 1942.

73. Swartz DB, Skidmore AE, Griffin JR JA. Twenty years of endodontic success and failure. J Endod., v.9, n.5, p.198-202, May 1983.

74. Tidmarsh BG, Sherson W, Stalker NL. Establishing endodontic working length: a comparison of radiographic and electronic methods. N Z dent. J., v.81, p.93-96, 1985.

75. Ushiyama J. New principle and method for measuring the root canal length. J. Endod., v.9, n.3, p.97-104, Mar. 1983.

76. Vande Vorde HE, Bjorndahl AM. Estimating endodontic "working length" with paralleling radiographics. Oral Surg Oral Med Oral Pathol Oral Radiol Endod., v.27, p.106-109, 1969.

77. Yamaoka M, Yamashita Y, Saito T. Electrical root canal measuring instrument based on a new principle – makes measurements possible in a wet root canals. Osada Product Information, n.6, 12 p., June 1989.

78. Weine FS. Cálculo do comprimento de trabalho. In: ___. Tratamento Endodôntico. São Paulo, Santos, 5.ª ed., 1995, p.401.

79. Welk AR, Baumgartner JC, Marshall JG. An in vivo comparison of two frequency-based electronic apex locators. J. Endod., v.29, n.8, p.497-500, 2003.

80. Wu M. Wesselink PR, Walton RE. Apical terminus location of root canal treatment procedures. Oral Surg Oral Med Oral Pathol Oral Radiol Endod, v.89, n.1, p.99-103, Jan 2000.

2.VI

The Buchanan Concept

"Patency File"

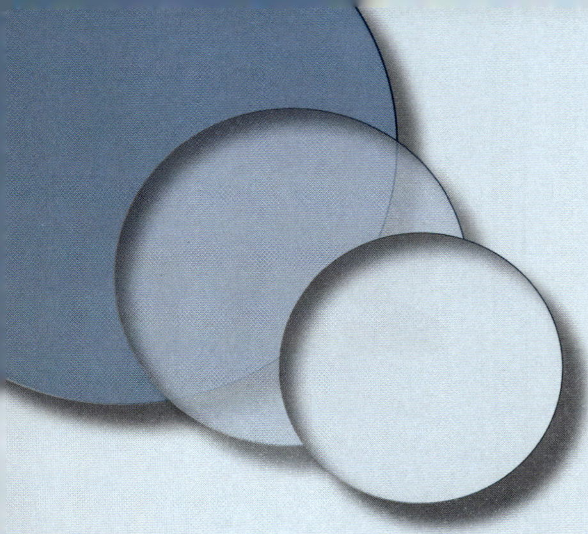

Mario Roberto Leonardo

Definitions

Patency[*]: unobstruction.

Apical patency: apical unobstruction (exploration/catheterization).

Patency file: file used to unobstruct, explore, open space, and feel the apical constriction of the root canal.

NOTE: The above-mentioned English terms do not have a translation in Portuguese. To use them, Dr. Quintiliano Diniz de Deus – ex-full Professor of the School of Dentistry of the Federal University of Minas Gerais – Brazil, used the term "patência", being influenced by the English word *patency*. The terms "patência", "lima patência" and "paténcia apical" were thus introduced in Brazilian endodontic terminology. In Spanish, the term used is "permeabilidad apical", which means apical permeability.

In 1989, Buchanan[1] defined the *patency file* as a small diameter instrument, such as the flexible type K file, numbers 10, 15 and/or 20, passively taken through the apical constriction of the root canal without enlarging it.

According to Buchanan[1] the objectives of apical patency are the following:

- Transmit the direction of the curvature of the root canal to the clinician in anticipation, through tactile sense, when the third dimension (bucco-lingual) is not observed radiographically.

This first objective of apical patency mentioned by Buchanan[1], to transmit the direction of the curvature of the root canal through tactile sense, is very important, particularly today with the

* Novo Michaelis – Dicionário ilustrado – Edições Melhoramentos: São Paulo, Brazil. 5.ª ed., 1964.

use of motor-driven nickel-titanium instruments, because in cases of a radius of curvature equal to 5 at the apex, we have a greater risk of fracture. For example, in 10% of cases the mesio-buccal root canal of the mandibular first molar has a buccal to lingual curvature at the apex, which is not observed radiographically, and terminates at the same foramen as the mesio-lingual canal[10]. In these cases, the fact is clinically confirmed when we perform apical patency using K files, numbers 10 and/or 15, and notice that these instruments, when withdrawn from the buccal canal of mandibular molars, are generally curved in the direction of the corresponding curvature.

- Use sodium hypochlorite solution over the total length of the entire root canal system, while activating it.
- False pathways (deviations) due to blockage are avoided when the patency is frequently confirmed during treatment.
- Possible formation of steps is minimized.
- Sodium hypochlorite solution, when activated by the action of a file, performs better and should be taken to the point of patency.
- Allows the clinician to by-pass pulp stones suspended in pulp tissue or adhering to the root canal walls, without the risk of carrying them beyond the instrument.

In 1997, a questionnaire by Cailleteau & Mullaney[3] and completed by 53 Faculties of Dental Schools in the USA, revealed that 50% taught the Buchanan concept to undergraduate and post-graduate students.

- 42% taught how to use the type K file No 10 to perform apical patency;
- 33% recommended the use of the type K file No 15;
- 25% recommended the use of the type K file No 25.

In an ex-vivo study, Goldberg & Massone[4] (2002) assessed transportation of apical foramen using (stainless steel) type K and nickel-titanium files numbers 10, 15, 20 and 25, as patency files.

In this study, the authors found that transportation of the apical foramen was detected in 18 of the 30 specimens analyzed, 9 being deviations observed in the group in which stainless steel K-type files were used, and 9 in the group in which the stainless steel type K file No 10, followed by nickel-titanium files No 15, 20 and 25, were used. They also observed that when the stainless steel type K file No 20 was used as a patency file, the possibility of transportation of the apical foramen increased to 56.6%. Furthermore, they showed that in 33.3% of the specimens, transportation of the apical foramen began with the use of the stainless steel type K file No 10. They drew attention to the fact that in the specimens the apical foramen usually emerged lateral to the apex, which means that the patency file frequently acted on one of the foramen walls but not completely on the entire foramen, irrespective of the diameter of the instrument or kinetics of use. Finally, they concluded that it is difficult to understand how the patency file can be safely used without modifying the shape and/or diameter of the apical foramen, particularly in curved root canals, as the Buchanan concept advocates.

Studies by Kuttler[7] (1961) contributed to justifying and confirming the conclusions of these authors, who reported that in 68% of young teeth and 80% of adult teeth, the cement canal – that is, the cement portion (end) of the root canal, does not continue in the same direction as the dentin canal, deviating towards the distal and/or lingual direction. Similarly, in 1972, Burch & Hulen[2] concluded that the foramen opens short of the anatomic apex in 92.4% of the cases.

Thus, with respect to the anatomic features, we fully agree with the conclusion of Goldberg & Massone[4], who found it difficult to understand how the patency file (Buchanan concept) can be safely used.

In our opinion, the use of the patency file, according to the definition itself, should be compatible with the anatomic conditions of the root canal, which are: use a stainless steel type K file No 10 for atresic and curved root canals; a stainless steel type K file No 15 for relatively atresic root canals and, finally, a type K file No 20 for wide and/or relatively wide root canals.

Furthermore, according in our opinion, the pathological conditions of the pulp and periapex, at the time of using the patency file, should also be considered and be an indication whether to use it or not.

With respect to the pathological conditions of the pulp and periapex, in cases of root canals of teeth with pulp necrosis (gangrene), without a radiographically visible periapical lesion, which root canal treatment we call **necropulpectomies I**, and particularly in the cases of pulp necrosis (gangrene) but with evident radiographic periapical lesion, denominated by us as **necropulpectomies II**, the use of a patency file may be an important operative procedure, providing the anatomic conditions and prior neutralization of the septic/toxic content of the root canal in a crown/apex direction has been performed.

However, in cases of root canals of teeth with a vital pulp, which we call **vital pulpectomies**, this procedure is completely contra-indicated by those who defend the application of a technique in which the biological principles are respected, preserving the vitality of the pulp stump (endoperiodontal stump) and the connective tissue located at the level of the cement canal. When its vitality is preserved during endodontic treatment, this tissue will allow the deposition of mineralized tissues, accomplishing a biological sealing of the apical foramen[5,6,8,9]. Therefore, according to these authors[5,6,8,9], the Buchanan concept is not indicated in cases of vital pulpectomies.

In 2005, Holland et al.[6] assessed the influence of the patency file and the type of filling material in apical and periapical post-treatment repair of root canal treatment in dog teeth with a vital pulp. Four groups were formed according to the following experimental conditions:

GROUP 1 – Without apical patency and filling of the root canals with Sealer Plus cement (Dentsply Ind. E Com. Ltda, Petrópolis-RJ – Brazil).

GROUP 2 – Without apical patency and filling of the root canals with zinc oxide and eugenol-based cement – Fill Canal (Ligas Odontológicas Ltda, Rio de Janeiro-RJ – Brazil).

GROUP 3 – With apical patency and filling of the root canals with Sealer Plus.

GROUP 4 – With apical patency and filling of the root canals with Fill Canal cement.

Seventy days after treatment, the animals were killed and biopsies obtained from the apical and periapical area of the treated teeth and prepared for histological analysis.

The data obtained, based on several histomorphologic parameters, were analyzed. The best results with regard to apical and periapical tissue repair were observed in the groups that were not subjected to apical patency ($p = 0.01$). The authors concluded that apical patency had an effect on the process of apical and periapical repair of teeth with a vital pulp, that undergo root canal treatment.

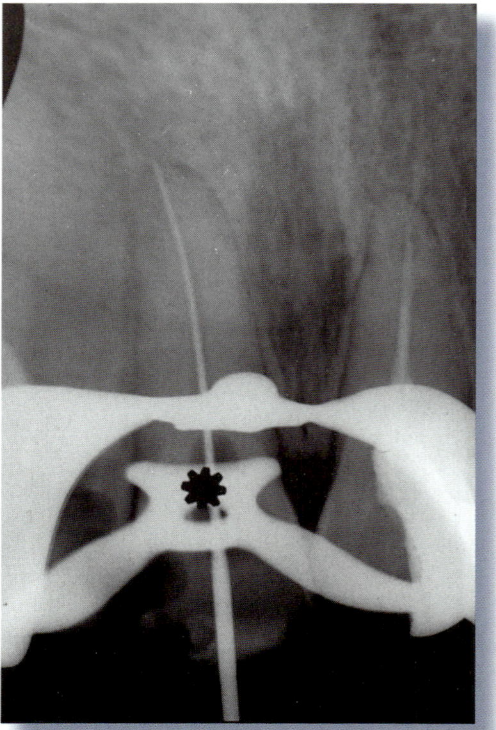

FIG. 2.VI-1

Periapical radiograph of a human maxillary right central incisor (1.1) with initial clinical diagnosis of acute irreversible pulpitis (4/14/1971). Note a stainless steel type K file No 20, passively taken through the apical constriction of the root canal, without enlarging it, inadvertently used as a patency file.

In 1973, while performing root canal treatment on a human maxillary right central incisor that was vital, (vital pulpectomy), Leonardo[8] explored the root canal with a stainless steel type K file No 20, passively taken it through the apical constriction, without enlarging it (Fig. 2.VI-1), in effect inadvertently using it as a patency file.

Forty days after this operative procedure, the tooth underwent an apiectomy and a biopsy of the apex and periapex was processed for histological analysis (Fig. 2.VI-2). It showed the following:

- An open space in the mesial portion of the foramen, at pulp stump level, approximating the shape of the tip of the type K file No 20.
- Presence of inflammatory infiltrate of moderate intensity, as a result of traumatic injury caused by the "patency file".

This histological analysis, in the case of vital pulpectomy, confirmed the ex vivo findings of Goldberg & Massone[4], who reported that in the vast majority of cases the foramen emerges lateral to the apex. In this case, the "patency file" acted on the mesial wall of the foramen, while the distal part histologically showed intact tissue, rich in Sharpey fibers, because this area was not reached by the "patency file" (Fig. 2.VI-2).

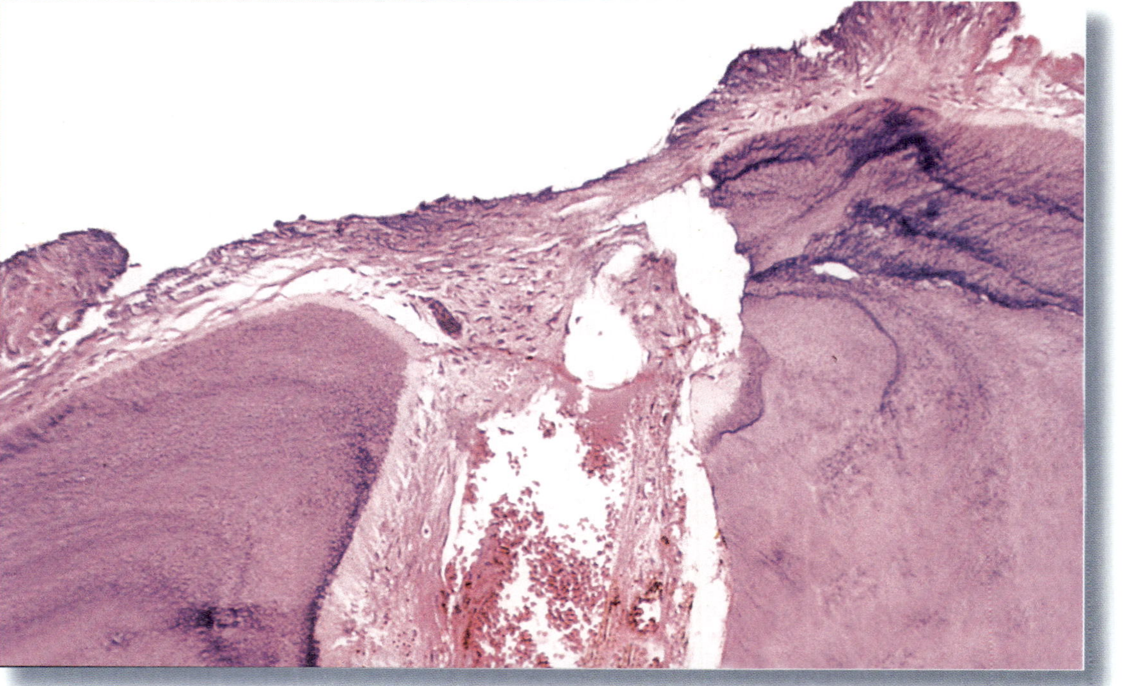

FIG. 2.VI-2

Histological section, obtained forty days after the operative procedure shown in the Figure 2.VI-1 (5/24/1971), showing the open space left by the action of the type K file tip No 20, inadvertently used as a patency file. Although a calcium hydroxide apical plug had been used, the pulp stump was dilacerated. Note the presence of inflammatory cells in the mesial portion of the foramen which, in reality, opened in a distal direction from the apical root. Note the presence of intact tissue, rich in Sharpey fibers, in the distal portion of the foramen, a region that was not reached by the patency file (H&E stain 40X).

Some practitioners suggest penetrating the patency file, slightly beyond the apical foramen.

The radiograph of Figure 2.VI-3 shows a stainless steel type K file No 20 used for exploring the root canal in a case of vital pulpectomy in a human maxillary right central incisor (1.1). Sixty days later, after the use of calcium hydroxide (Calen) as an apical plug, aiming at controlling post-treatment inflammation, the histological section of the apical and periapical region (Fig. 2.VI-4) showed partial destruction of the pulp stump, a basophilic area and a chronic inflammatory infiltrate. The cement in the proximities of the apical foramen showed small areas of resorption and mineralized tissue deposition.

However, if one respects the biological principles, then the cases of Leonardo[8] (1973) confirmed that the patency file must not be used in vital pulpectomies.

Fifteen days after the root canal treatment without apical patency and filling the root canal with Kerr Pulp Canal Sealer cement (Kerr Mg. Co. USA), with prior placement of calcium hydroxide (Calen) as an apical plug, histological sections of the apical and periapical regions (Fig. 2.VI-5) showed a live pulp stump, rich in fibroblasts.

Figure 2.VI-6 shows a periapical radiograph of the human maxillary right central incisor tooth (1.1) with pulp vitality (initial clinical diagnosis of acute irreversible pulpitis), showing a stainless steel type K file No 20, used to explore the root canal and to establish working length. Note that the file did not reach the pulp stump region. Figure 2.VII-7 shows a periapical post-operative radiograph fifty-seven days after treatment. It can be seen that the apical limit of filling is approximately 2 mm

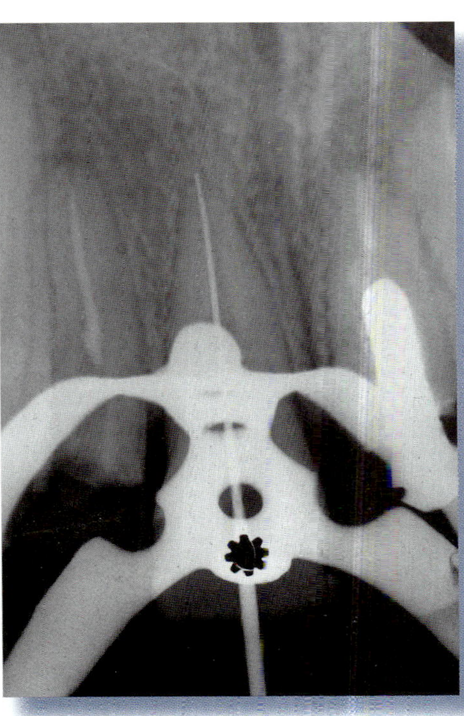

FIG. 2.VI-3

Periapical radiograph of a human maxillary right central incisor (1.1) with initial clinical diagnosis of acute irreversible pulpitis. Note a stainless steel type K file No 20, with slight radiographic penetration into the apical foramen (4/14/1971).

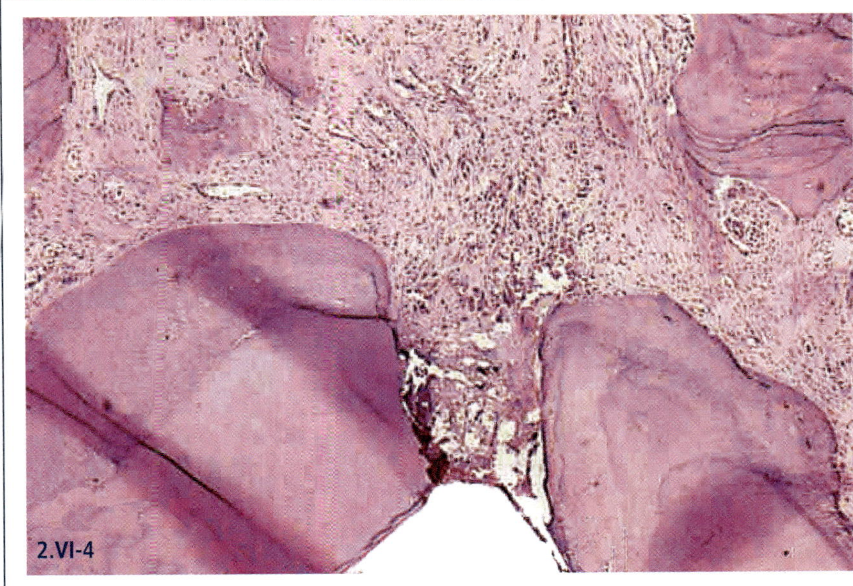

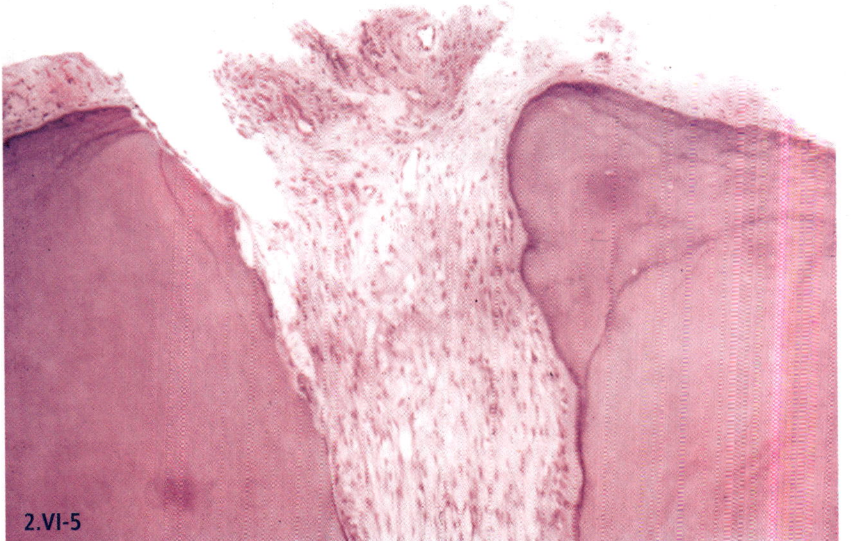

FIG. 2.VI-4

Histological section obtained sixty days after the operative procedure (vital pulpectomy) shown in the periapical radiograph of Figure 2.VI-3 (6/14/1971), showing partial destruction of pulp stump, which appeared dilacerated, with a minor chronic inflammatory infiltrate reaching the apical periodontal ligament. There are areas of apical cement resorption and new cement formation (H&E stain 40X).

FIG. 2.VI-5

Histological section of apical region, obtained fifteen days after the operative procedure (vital pulpectomy) without the use of the patency file and with the placement of calcium hydroxide (Calen) used as a temporary dressing. Note the intact pulp stump, absence of inflammatory cells and accentuated presence of fibers and/or fibroblasts (H&E stain 40X).

short of the radiographic apex. Filling material: Kerr Pulp Canal Sealer (Kerr Mg. Co. USA) and pulp stump protection with calcium hydroxide (Calen) apical *plug*. Fifty-seven days after filling the root canal of the tooth shown in Figure 2.VI-7, after an apiectomy and histological preparation of the biopsy involving the apex and periapical area, the sections showed the entire pulp stump, free of inflammatory cells and areas of resorption with mineralized tissue deposition (Fig. 2.VI-8).

Magnification of the previous figure shows a pulp stump free of inflammatory cells and areas of resorption and cement deposition (Fig. 2.VI-9).

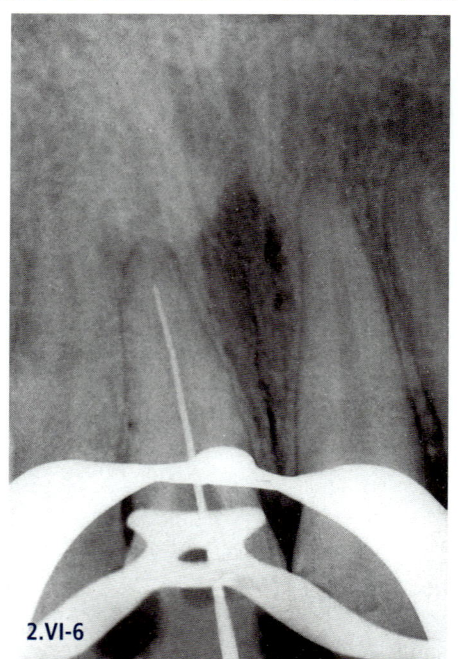

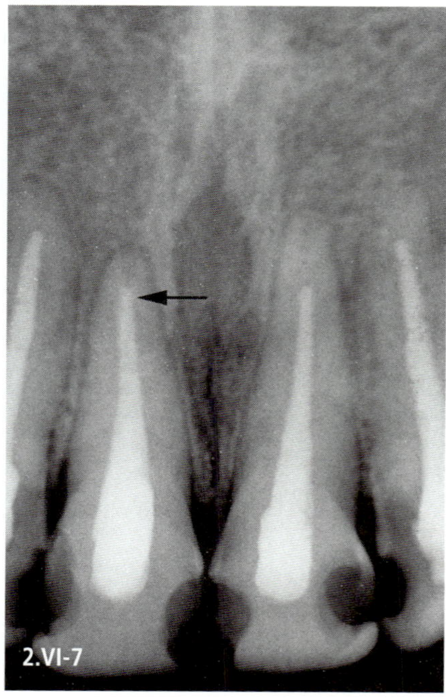

FIG. 2.VI-6

Periapical radiograph of a human maxillary right central incisor (1.1) with initial clinical diagnosis of acute irreversible pulpitis. Note a stainless steel type K file No 20, approximately 2 mm short of the radiographic apex (10/3/1970).

FIG. 2.VI-7

Postoperative periapical radiograph after treatment of the case shown in Figure 2.VI-6, obtained fifty days after vital pulpectomy without the use of the patency file. Note the root canal filled with gutta-percha cones and Kerr Pulp Canal Sealer cement, slightly short of the radiographic apex (arrow). Calcium hydroxide (Calen) was used as a temporary dressing to protect the pulp stump. Note the presence of lamina dura (11/29/1970).

FIG. 2.VI-8

Histological section of the apical region of the tooth shown in Figures 2.VI-6 and 7, obtained fifty-seven days after root canal filling and protection of the pulp stump with calcium hydroxide (Calen) plug. Note the intact pulp stump, with absence of inflammatory cells and also some areas of resorption and cement deposition (H&E stain 40X).

FIG. 2.VI-9

Magnification of previous figure, showing the intact pulp stump and absence of inflammatory cells (H&E stain 200X).

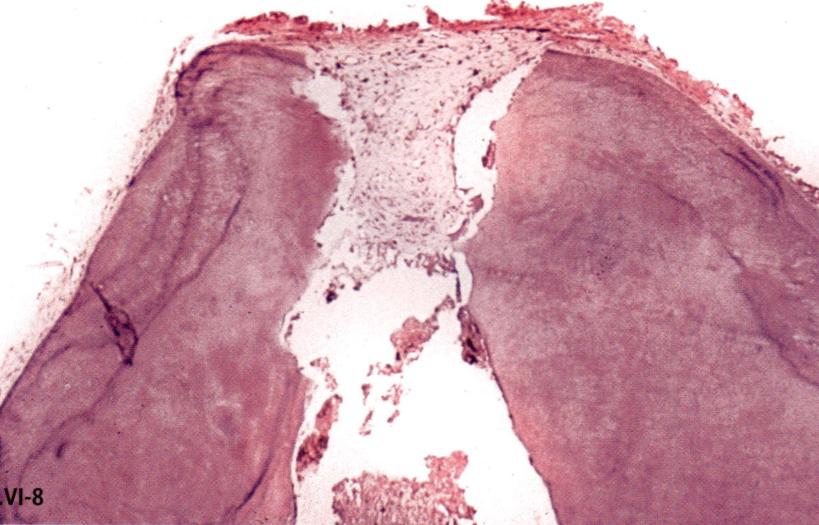

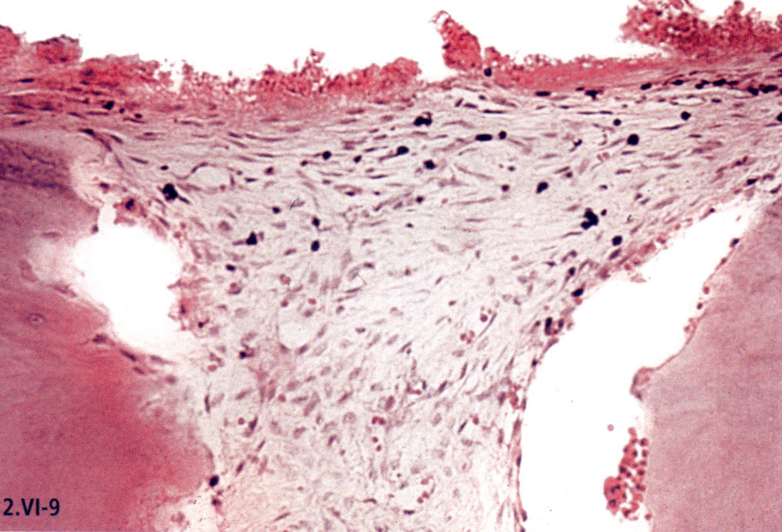

Figure 2.VI-10 shows a periapical radiograph for diagnostic purposes of a human maxillary right central incisor (1.1) and Fig. 2.VI-11 shows the filling of the root canal with Kerr Pulp Canal Sealer cement (Kerr Mg. Co. USA), and pulp stump protected by a calcium hydroxide (Calen) plug.

Figure 2.VI-12 shows a histological section of the apical and periapical region of the tooth in Figure 2.VI-11, one hundred and twenty days after the root canal filling, showing deposition of cement repairing resorption areas and isolating the entire pulp stump from the filling material.

Magnification of the previous figure Figure 2.VI-13 shows the pulp stump free of inflammatory infiltrate and extensive deposition of new cementum.

2.VI-10

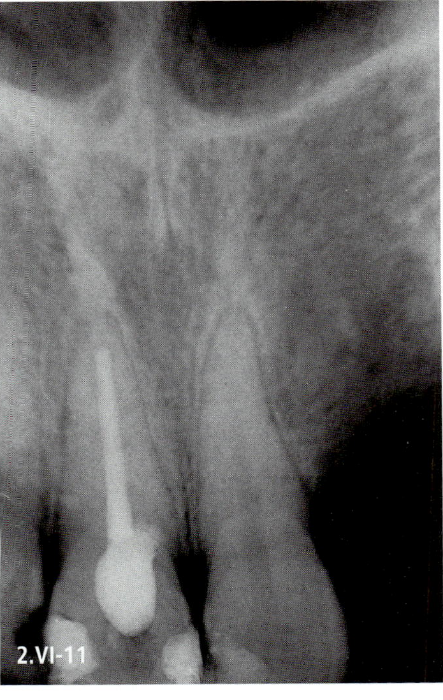

FIG. 2.VI-10

Periapical radiograph for clinical diagnosis of acute irreversible pulpitis in a human maxillary right central incisor (1.1) (11/17/1971). Note caries lesion in the distal area and normal apical periodontal ligament.

FIG. 2.VI-11

Post-treatment periapical radiograph of tooth shown in Figure 2.VI-10, obtained on the 3/17/1972, one hundred and seven days after the root canal filling by means of active lateral condensation of gutta-percha cones and Kerr Pulp Canal Sealer cement, protecting the pulp stump with calcium hydroxide (Calen). Five examiners considered the case a radiographic success: normal apical periodontal ligament, with evidence of intact lamina dura.

FIG. 2.VI-12

Histological section of apical and periapical regions, one hundred and twenty days after root canal filling of the human tooth (1.1), shown in Figures 2.VI-10 and 11, showing relatively extensive areas of apical cement resorption, repaired by the deposition of new cement formation, isolating the pulp stump that is vital and free of inflammatory cells. Normal apical periodontal ligament (H&E stain 40X).

FIG. 2.VI-13

Magnification of histological section presented in Figure 2.VI-12 showing pulp stump free of inflammatory cells and extensive new cement deposition (H&E stain 200X).

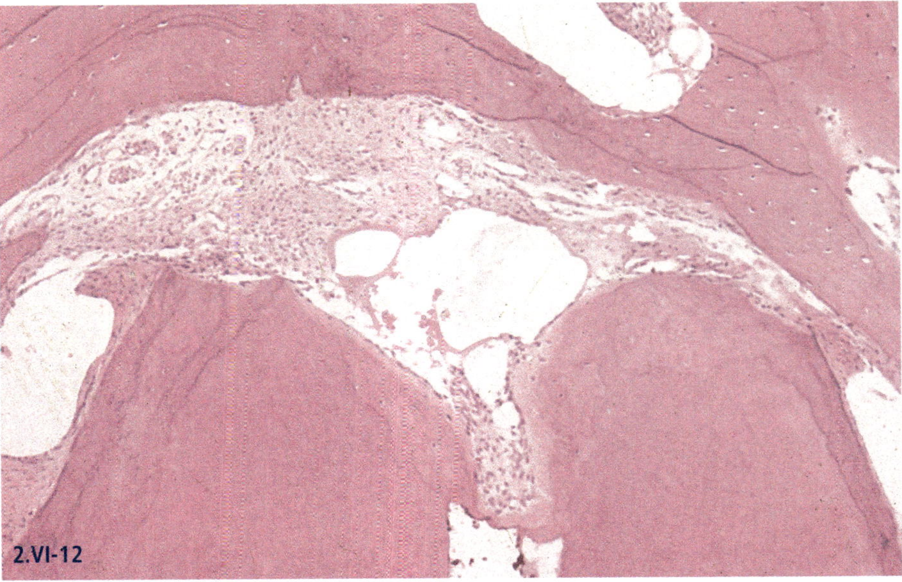

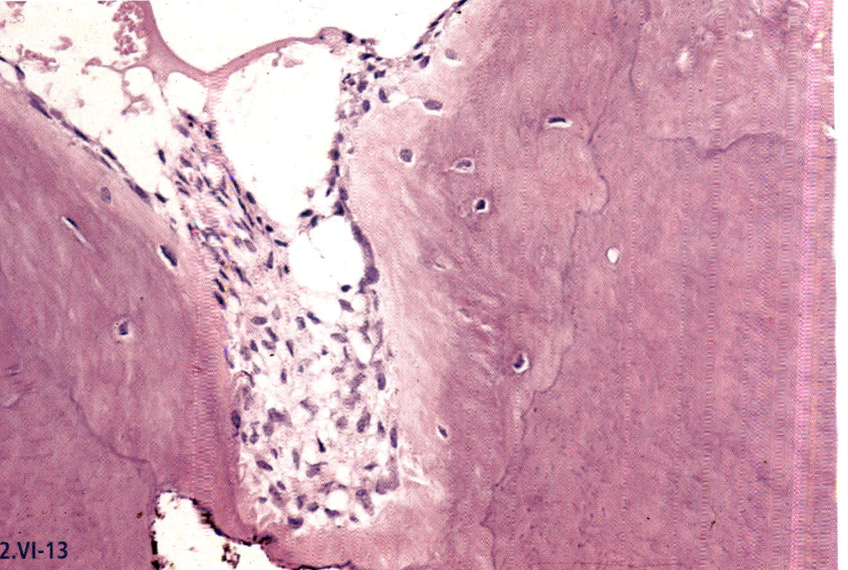

Furthermore, according to Leonardo[8] (1973), following biological principles, without apical patency, Figure 2.VI-14 shows radiographic confirmation of the clinical choice of the master gutta-percha cone at the time of root canal filling in a human maxillary left central incisor (2.1). Note the perfect adaptation of the gutta-percha cone at the apical stop, approximately 2 mm short of the radiographic apex, consequently respecting the pulp stump. During biomechanical preparation, a biologically compatible irrigation solution (1% sodium hypochlorite solution) and a calcium hydroxide plug (Calen) were used, isolating the pulp stump from the filling cement (Kerr Pulp Canal Sealer – Kerr Mg. Co. USA) (Fig. 2.VI-15).

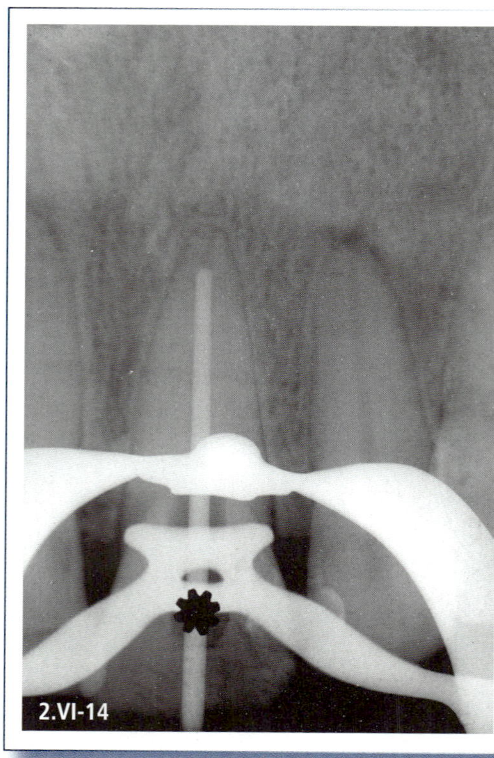

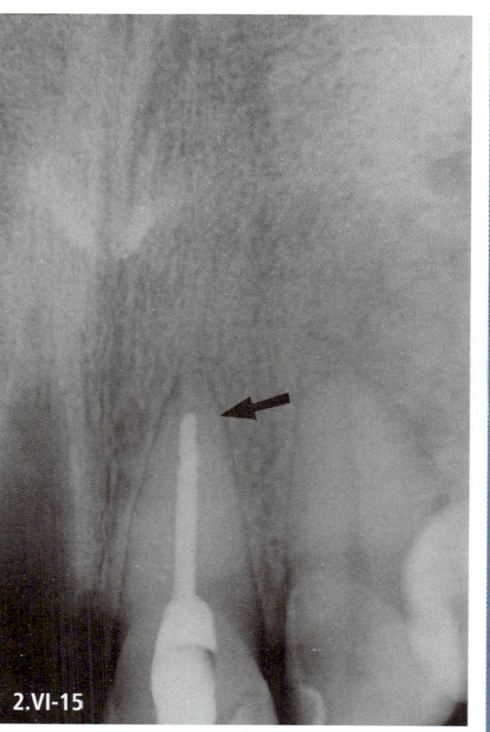

FIG. 2.VI-14

Periapical radiograph of a human maxillary left central incisor (2.1) with initial clinical diagnosis of acute irreversible pulpitis, submitted to vital pulpectomy without the use of a patency file. Note radiographic confirmation of clinical choice of master gutta-percha cone, approximately 2 mm short of the radiographic apex (8/31/1971).

FIG. 2.VI-15

Periapical radiograph of post-treatment follow up, obtained on 1/31/1972, one hundred and fifty days after the root canal filling with active lateral condensation of gutta-percha cones and Kerr Pulp Canal Sealer, protecting the pulp stump with calcium hydroxide (Calen).

After one hundred and fifty days had elapsed, an apiectomy of the tooth shown in Figures 2.VI-14 to 17 was performed, obtaining a biopsy (Fig. 2.VI-18). Sequential histological sections (Figs. 2.VI-19, 20, 21, 22 and 23) show a cement barrier isolating the filling material from the pulp stump that is vital and without inflammatory cells. These serial histological sections show continuity of the cement barrier formation.

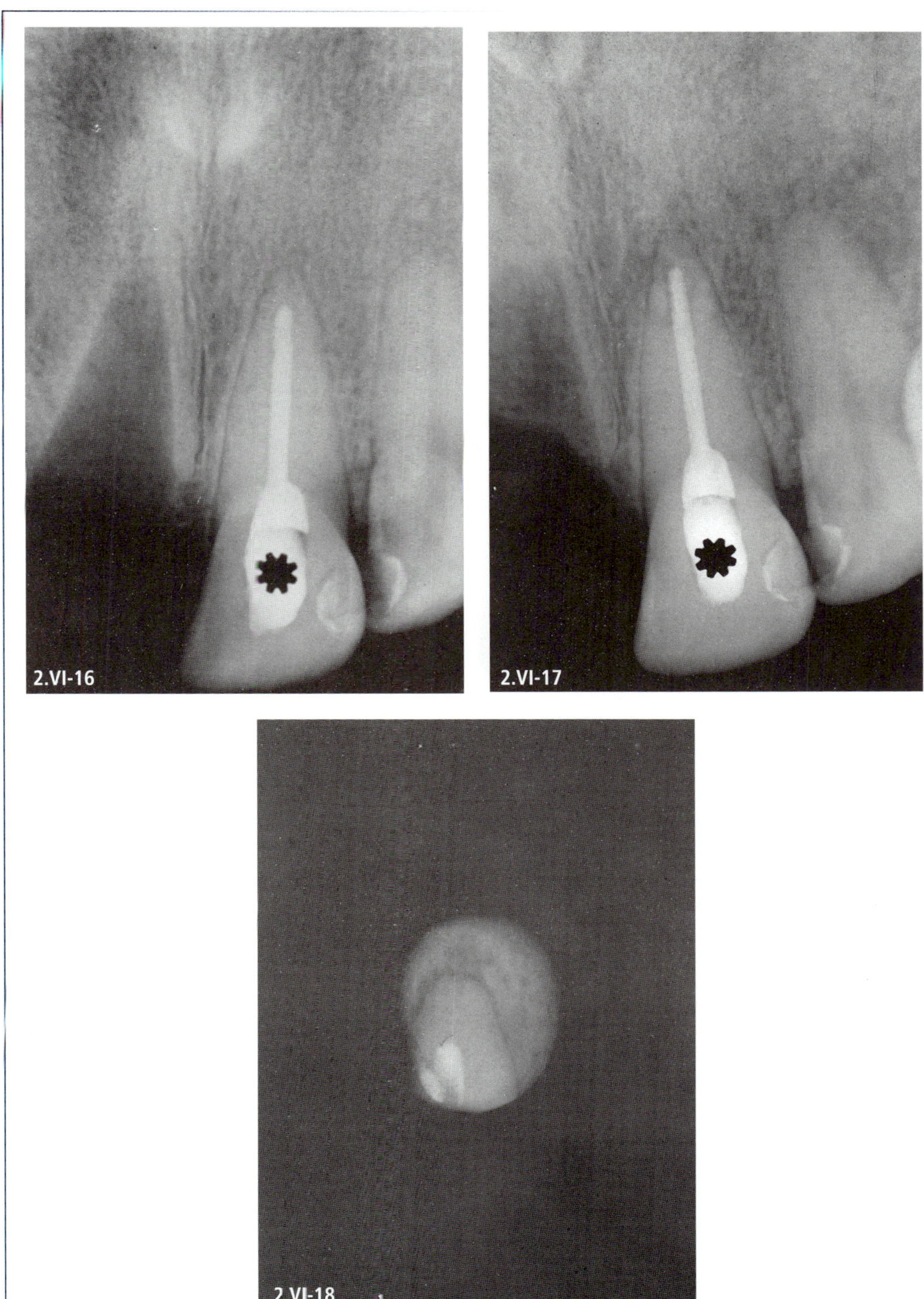

FIGS. 2-VI-16 and 17

Periapical radiographs of tooth shown in Figures 2.VI-14 and 15, at the time of periradicular surgery (apiectomy).

FIG. 2.VI-18

Radiograph of biopsy from apiectomy.

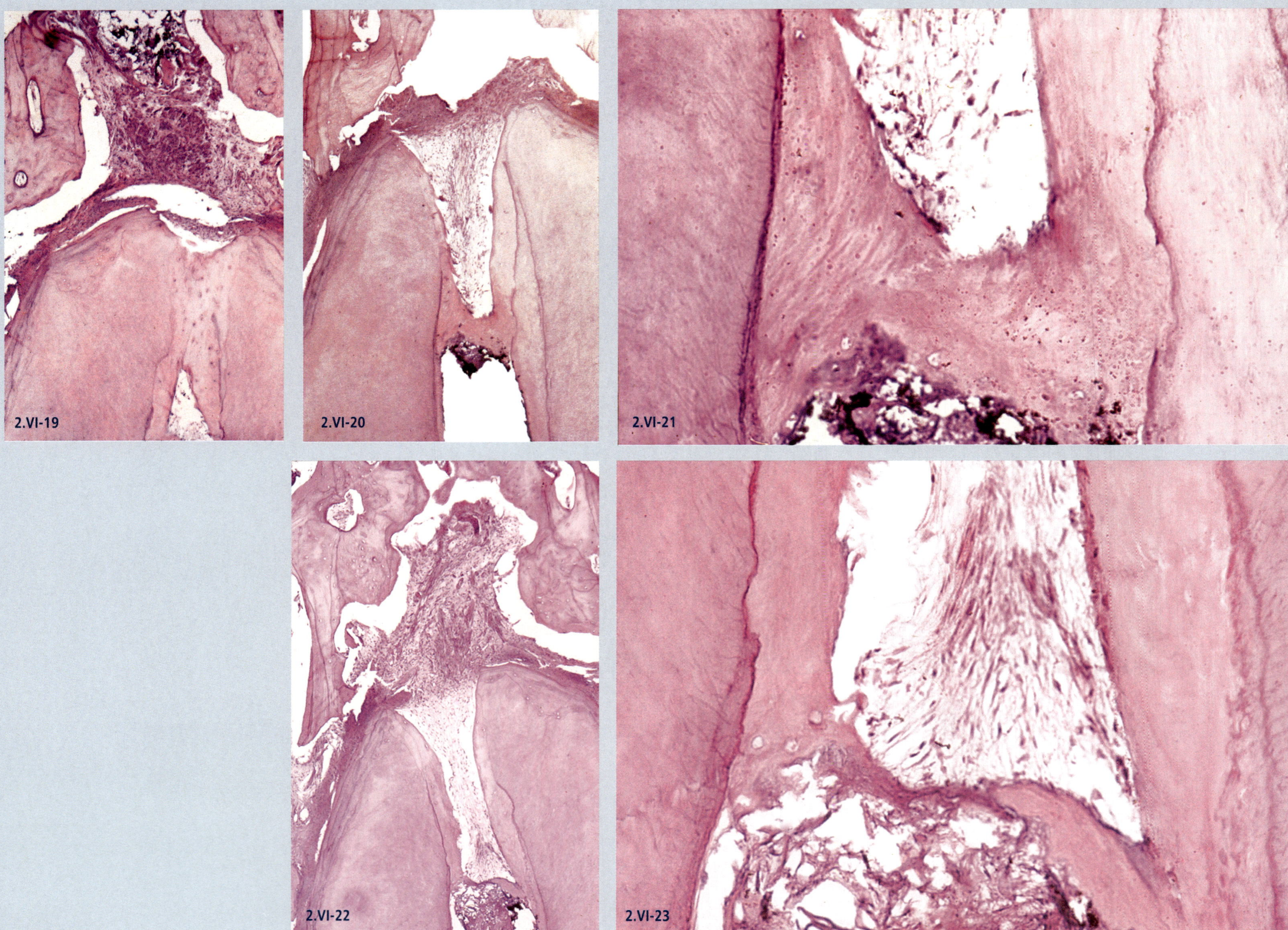

FIGS. 2.VI-19, 20, 21, 22 and 23

The majority of the serial histological; sections show a considerable barrier of new cement formation (Figs. 2.VI-19, 20 and 21), but a section in the center portion of the apical foramen, showed an very thick, but continuous barrier (Figs. 2.VI-22 and 23), isolating the intact pulp stump, which was free of inflammatory cells, from the filling material (H&E stain 40X).

Figure 2.VI-24 shows a periapical radiograph of a human maxillary right central incisor tooth (2.1) with a stainless steel type K file No 15 to explore the root canal without apical patency and to establish working length. Note that the instrument is approximately 2 mm short of the radiographic apex.

Figure 2.VI-25 shows a periapical post-operative radiograph, two years after performing a vital pulpectomy and root canal filling with Kerr Pulp Canal Sealer cement (Kerr Mg. Co. USA), gutta-percha cones and interim protection of the pulp stump with a calcium hydroxide (Calen) acting as an apical plug.

Figure 2.VI-26 shows the case of the previous figure at the time of the apiectomy and Figure 2.VI-27 shows the radiograph of the biopsy.

Figure 2.VI-28 is a transverse histological section at the level of the apex, showing sealing of the foramen by mineralized tissue. Figure 2.VI-29, is a higher magnification of the previous figure, showing sealing of the foramen by mineralized tissue deposition.

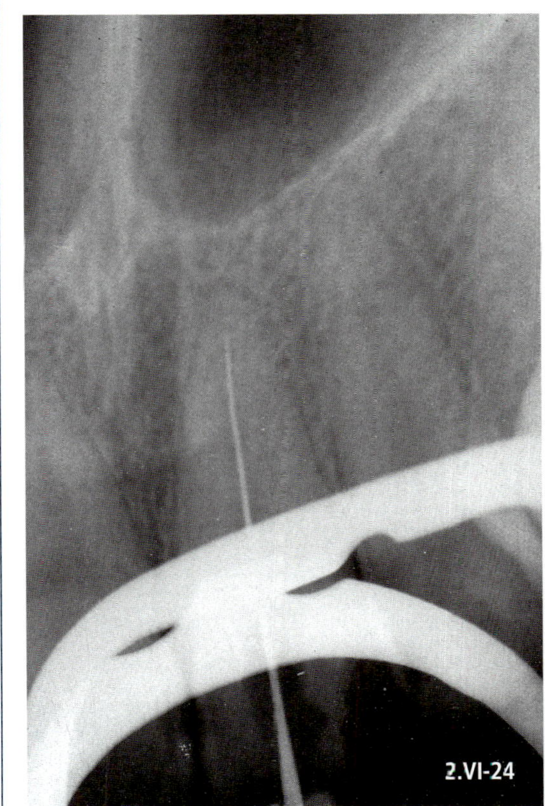

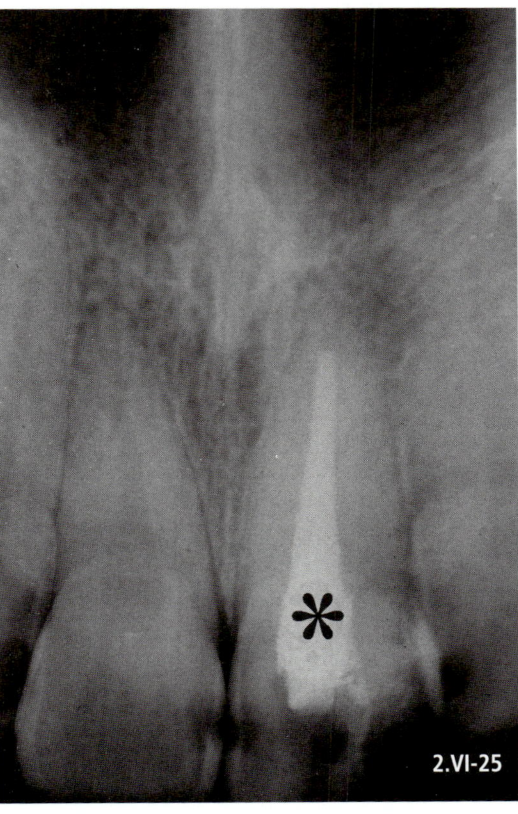

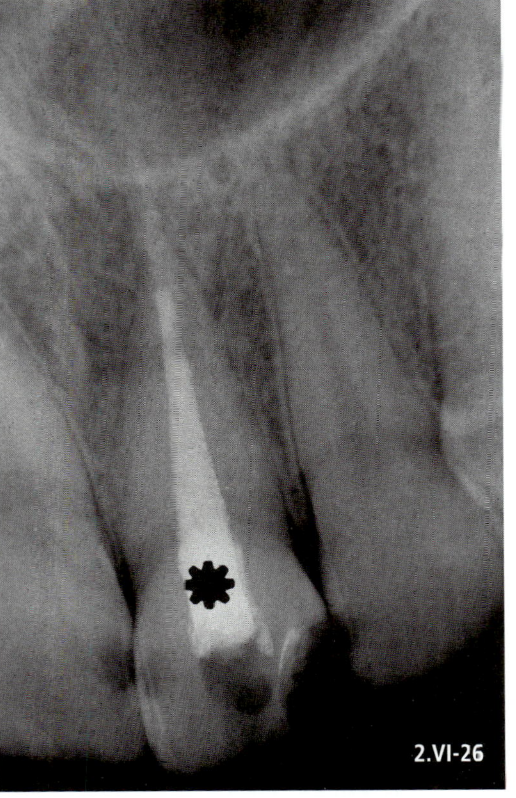

FIG. 2.VI-24

Periapical radiograph of a human maxillary left central incisor tooth (2.1) with initial clinical diagnosis of acute irreversible pulpitis, showing a stainless steel type K file No 15 at temporary working length, approximately 2 mm short of the radiographic apex, to establish working length (10/9/1980).

FIG. 2.VI-25

Post-treatment periapical radiograph (follow up) of the tooth shown in Figure 2.VI-24, two years after vital pulpectomy without the use of a patency file. Root canal filling by means of active lateral condensation of gutta-percha cones and Kerr Pulp Canal Sealer cement, with prior protection of the pulp stump with calcium hydroxide (Calen). Five examiners considered the case a radiographic success, highlighting the normal apical periodontal ligament and intact lamina dura (10/4/1982).

FIG. 2.VI-26

Periapical radiograph to confirm the direction of Sargenti's trephine (6 mm), used for surgical removal of apex and periapex of a human tooth (2.1) shown in Figures 2.VI-24 and 25.

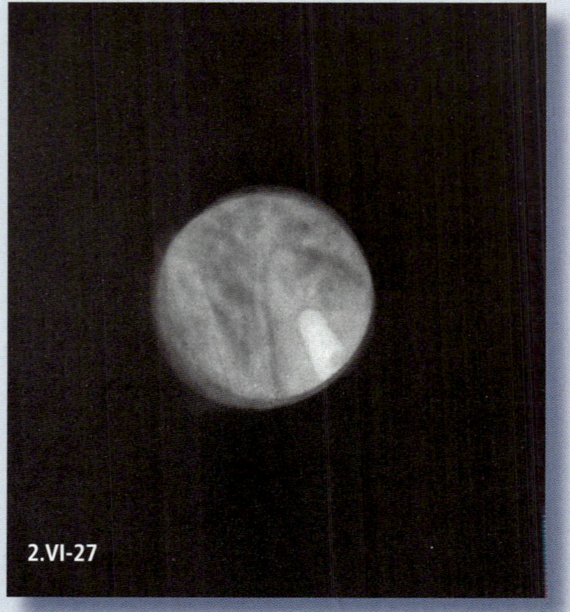

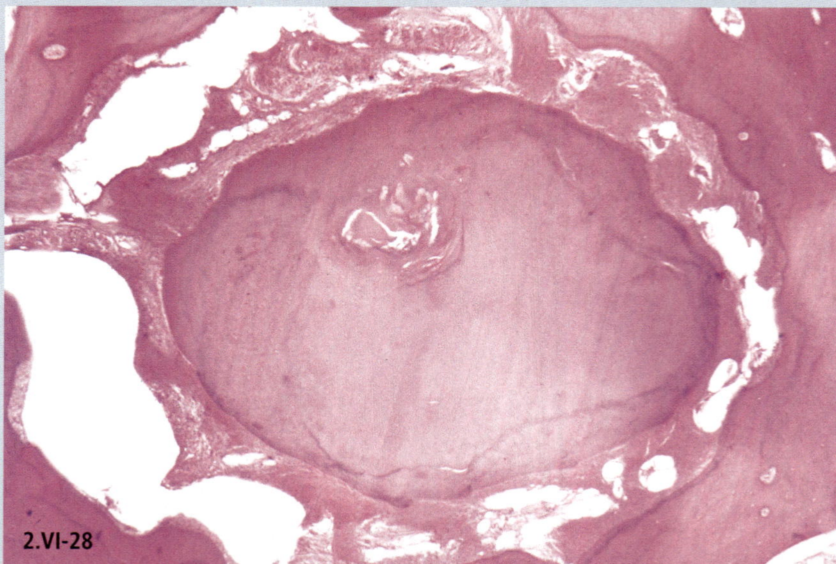

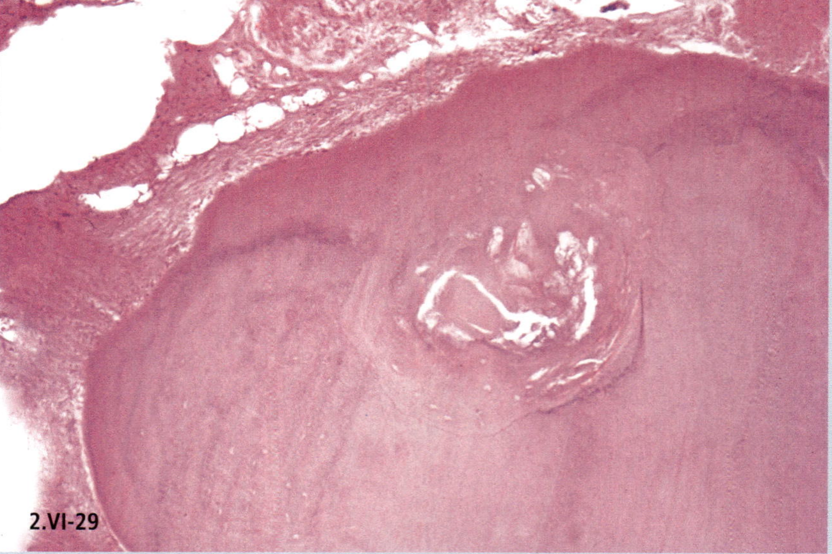

FIG. 2.VI-27

Radiograph of biopsy, involving the apex and periapex of a human tooth (2.1) shown in Figures 2.VI-24 and 25.

FIG. 2.VI-28

Transverse histological section of root apex of a human tooth (2.1) shown in Figures 2.VI-24 and 25, obtained two years after root canal filling with gutta- percha cones and Kerr Pulp Canal Sealer cement, previously covering the pulp stump with calcium hydroxide (Calen). This histological section was performed in a transverse direction, in relation to the long axis of the tooth. Note deposition of mineralized tissue of the cementoid type, in the space previously occupied by the pulp stump (H&E stain 40X).

FIG. 2.VI-29

Magnification of previous figure, showing clear mineralization of apical foramen, previously occupied by the pulp stump. The lines of new cement deposition clearly appear. The spaces seen inside the mineralized tissue refer to the artifacts of the technique (H&E stain 64X).

Note: All the human clinical/surgical cases mentioned where done during the 70`s, according to the Protocol of Helsinki (Finland) of 1964.

References

1. Buchanan LS. Management of the curved root canal. J Calif Dent Assoc, v.17, p.18-25, 1989.
2. Burch JG, Hulen S. The relationship of the apical forâmen (a palavra é acentuada, em inglês?) to the anatomic apex of the tooth root. Oral Surg, v.2, p.262-268, 1972.
3. Cailleteau JG, Mullaney TP. Prevalence of teaching apical patency and various instrumentation and obturation techniques in United States Dental Schools J Endod, v.6, p.394-396, 1997.
4. Goldberg F, Massone EJ. Patency file and apical transportation: an in vitro study. J Endod, v.7, p.510-511, 2002.
5. Holland R. et al. Reaction of human periapical tissue to pulp extirpation and immediate root canal filling with calcium hydroxide. J Endod, v.3, p.63-77, 1977.
6. Holland R. et al. Influence of apical patency and filling material on healing process of dog's teeth. Braz Dent J, v.1, p.9-16, 2005.
7. Kuttler Y. Endodoncia práctica. México: Alpha, 1961, p.23-25.
8. Leonardo MR. Contribuição para o estudo da reparação apical e periapical pós-tratamento de canais radiculares (tese de livre-docência) – Faculdade de Odontologia de Araraquara, SP, Brasil, 1973, p.87.
9. Leonardo MR, Leal JM, Simões Filho AP. Pulpectomy: immediate root canal filling with calcium hydroxide. Oral Surg. Oral Med. Oral Pathol, v.5, p.441-450, 1980.
10. Pucci FM, Reig R. Conductos radiculares. Montevideo: A Barreiro y Ramos, 1945, v.1-1960, p.216.

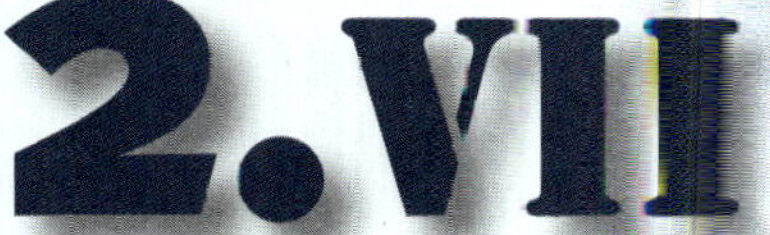

Foramen debridement

Concept and its clinical importance

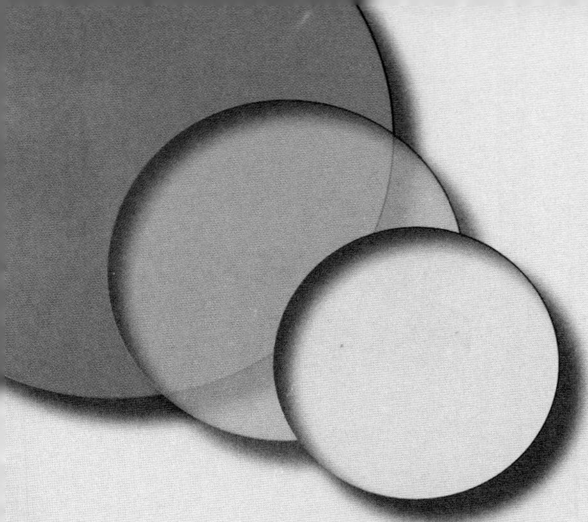

Mario Roberto Leonardo

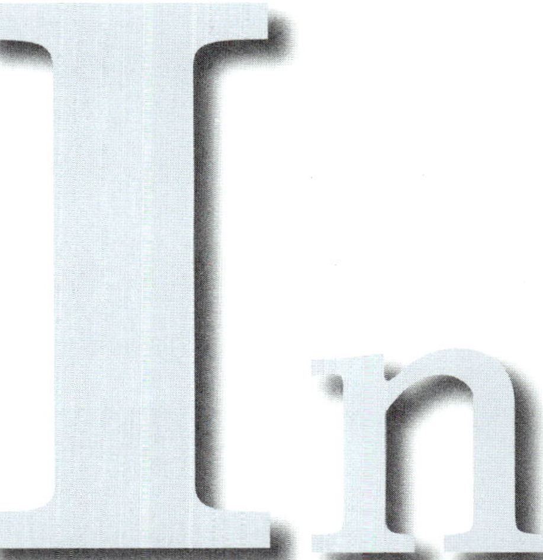

teeth with an **evident radiographically** chronic periapical lesion (apical periodontitis), as we have seen in Chapter 1 of this book, the apical cementum is shown to be resorbed (apical erosion), with veritable craters that promote **multiplication** and the proliferation of microorganisms, constituting a so-called **extra-radicular infection**. These microorganisms are kept isolated inside the apical bacterial biofilm[4] (Figs. 2.VII-1A-F) from the action of natural organic as well as immune defenses and the action of systemic antibiotic, when prescribed.

In these cases, the root canal is naturally wide or relatively wide at the apical five millimeters. Thus in order for **evident** chronic periapical lesion to exist, there needs to be sufficient space in the apical portion of the root canal to shelter bacteria (virulence), their products and by-products as well as bacterial LPS (endotoxins), responsible for the **evident periapical lesion**. Therefore, in these cases, because the root canal is wider at the apical five millimeters, it will naturally promote the operating procedure that we call **foramen debridement**.

According to the dictionary, *in medical terms, debridement means the act of dilating an orifice for therapeutic purposes.* **Debridement** can also be defined as the removal of dead, damaged, or infected tissue to improve the healing potential of the remaining healthy tissue. By correlating the medical terminology with the endodontic conditions of treatment in necropulpectomies II (apical periodontitis), we may consider that foramen debridement means the dilation, unobstruction and cleaning of the apical foramen for therapeutic purposes.

Studies we conducted in 1973[3], confirmed that in cases of teeth with evident periapical lesion, the apical foramen had an abundance of necrotic remnants, microorganisms and products resulting from tissue disintegration (carbonic anhydride and amines: cadaverine, putrescine and neuridine). These were all concentrated in the **apical five millimeters**, and were the main causes of chronic periapical reactions, which was exudative in nature (as in abscesses) and/or proliferative (as in cases of granulomas and apical cysts).

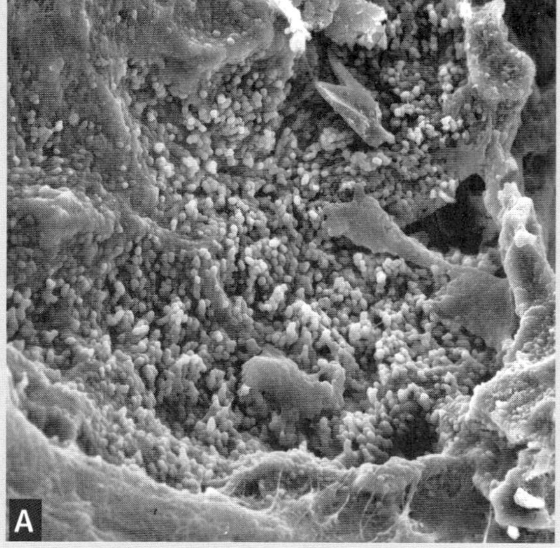

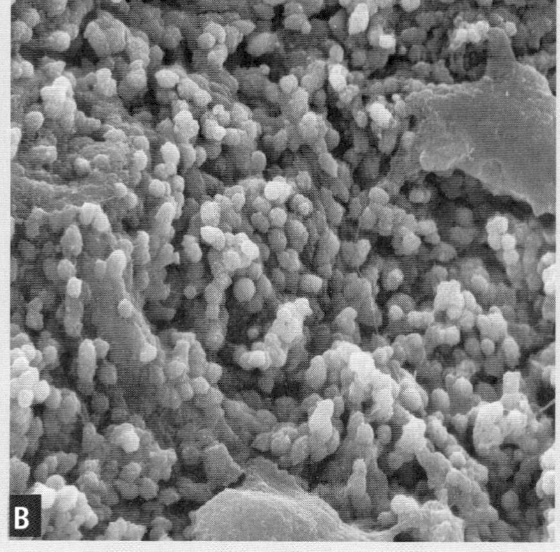

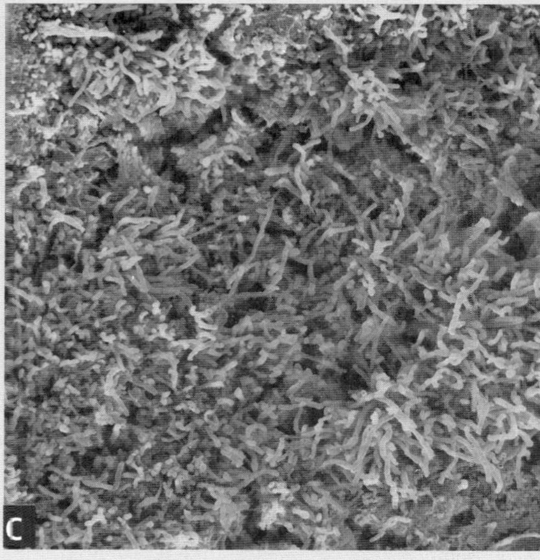

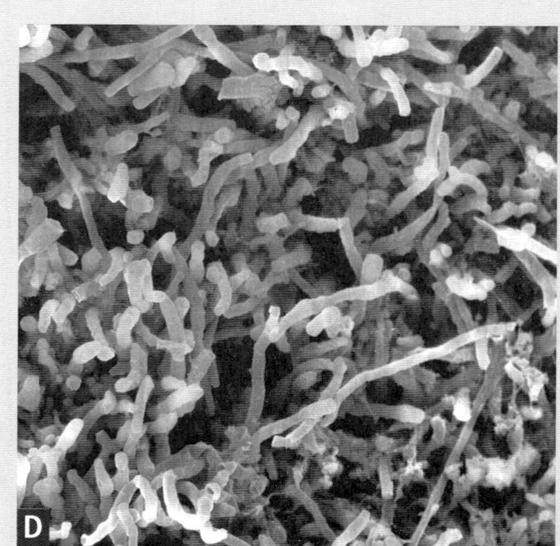

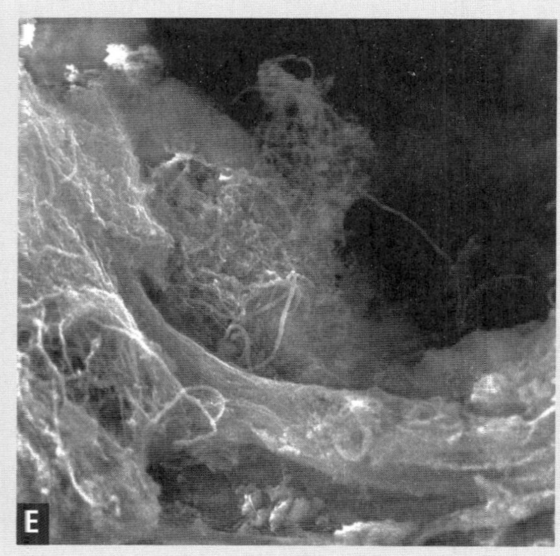

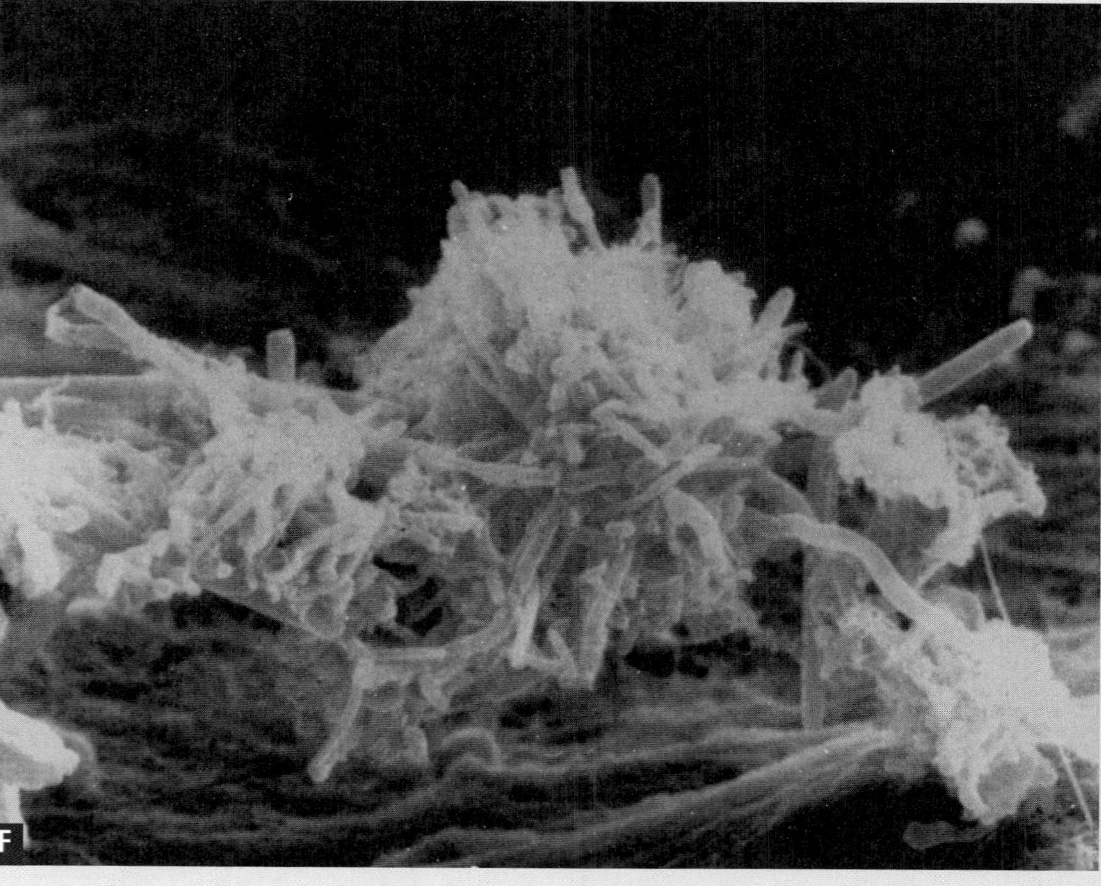

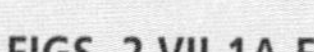

FIGS. 2.VII-1A-F

Scanning electron micrographs demonstrating the presence of different bacterial morphotypes on the surface of the root apex of a tooth with evident chronic periapical lesion. In A and B, the presence of coccus, C and D, bacillus and filamentous types, E and F bacillus and filamentous types. All figures show evidence of the presence of microorganisms inside the apical bacterial biofilm.

A – ZEISS – 1.850X - 16 µm.
B – ZEISS – 4.300X - 18 µm.
C – ZEISS – 1.850X - 16 µm.
D – ZEISS – 4.300X - 18 µm.
E – ZEISS – 3.600X - 9 µm.
F – ZEISS – 4.300X - 18 µm.

These periapical reactions are rich in blood vessels, phagocytary defense cells and cells constituting the adaptive immune response, which have the function of limiting the infectious process to the interior of the root canal system; that is, they prevent the infection microorganisms from reaching the surrounding anatomic structures and from disseminating systemically. On the other hand, the stimulus for the occurrence of apical cement and periapical alveolar bone resorption is determined both by the direct action of bacterial products (enzymes such as hyaluronidase and collagenase) and by toxic substances coming from the microorganisms themselves, such as bacterial lipopolysaccharide (the endotoxins), endol and various acids, such as sulfuric, butyric acid, etc., in addition to the indirect action of bacteria through the production of pre-inflammatory cytokines, such as the tumor necrosis factor, interleukin-1 and interleukin-6[5].

The perpetuation of these factors concentrated in the **apical five millimeters**, as well as their post-treatment continuation after a poorly performed root canal treatment, will be responsible for maintaining a chronic periapical reaction.

In the above-mentioned study, conducted by Leonardo[3] in 1973, root canal treatments were performed in anterior and posterior human teeth with evident chronic periapical lesion. When this work was carried out (in the 1970s), the predominant concept at the time recommended limiting root canal instrumentation and filling to approximately 1 mm short of the radiographic apex[2].

It is clear that if we followed this concept when we instrumented 1 mm short of the radiographic apex, necrotic remnants, microorganisms, and tissue remnants would naturally remain at the apical foramen, which was confirmed by post-treatment clinical/radiographic follow-up, and by means of histological analysis. For the purpose of histologically confirming the clinical importance of foramen debridement in cases of necropulpectomies II (apical periodontitis), we will show the following cases of the above-mentioned study[3] (Figs. 2.VII-2A-D and 2.VII-3A-C):

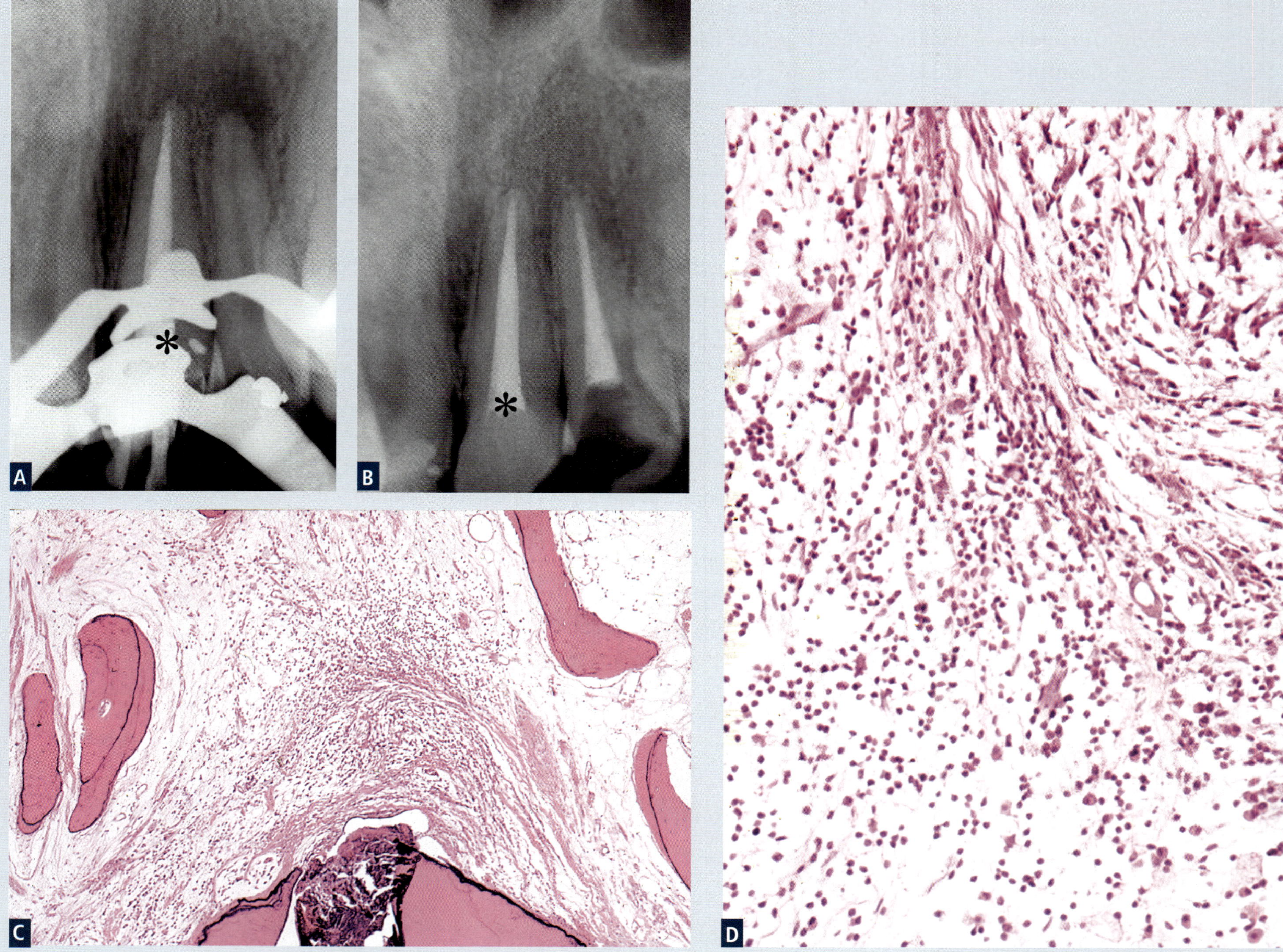

FIGS. 2.VII-2A-D – (CASE 4A)

A – Periapical radiograph obtained to prove the active lateral condensation of the root canal filling of a human maxillary left central incisor (2.1). Note the presence of chronic periapical lesion suggestive of apical granuloma – 2/28/1967.

B – Post-treatment follow-up periapical radiograph of the case in Figure 2.VII-2A, obtained five years and two months after root canal filling (10/9/1972) using active lateral condensation of gutta-percha cones and zinc oxide and eugenol cement. After radiographic assessment, six professors in endodontics considered the treatment a success. The clinical assessment made by the author also considered the treatment a success.

C – Histological section of the apical and periapical region of the tooth shown in Figure 2.VII-2-B, showing evidence that the apical foramen was obliterated by an amorphous, basophilic substance, with the presence of contaminated dentin debris, as a result of the instrumentation performed 1 millimeter short of the radiographic apex. The space corresponding to the apical periodontal ligament is very dilated (thickened), showing an intense chronic inflammatory infiltrate (H&E stain 40X).

D – Magnification of the previous figure, showing details of the chronic inflammatory infiltrate observed in the apical periodontal ligament (H&E stain 200X).

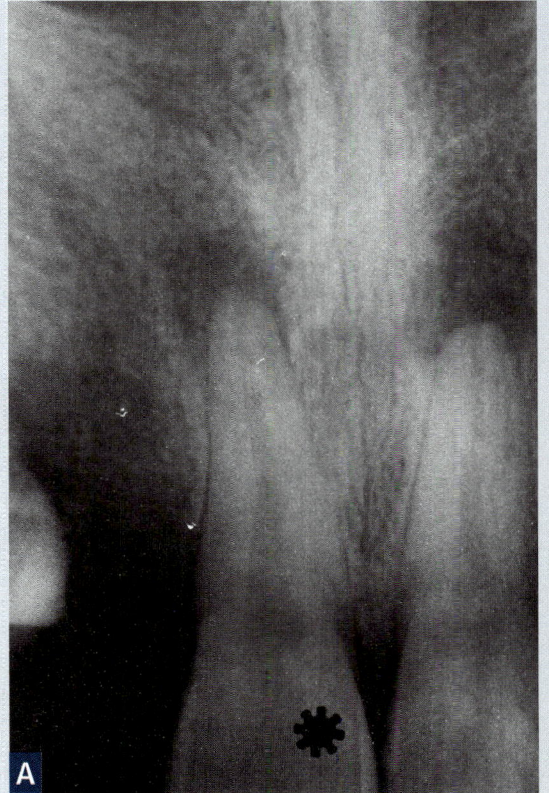

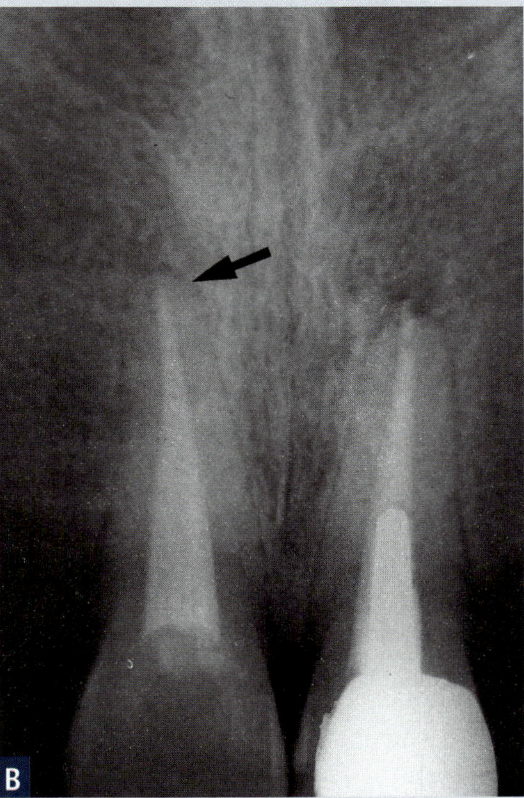

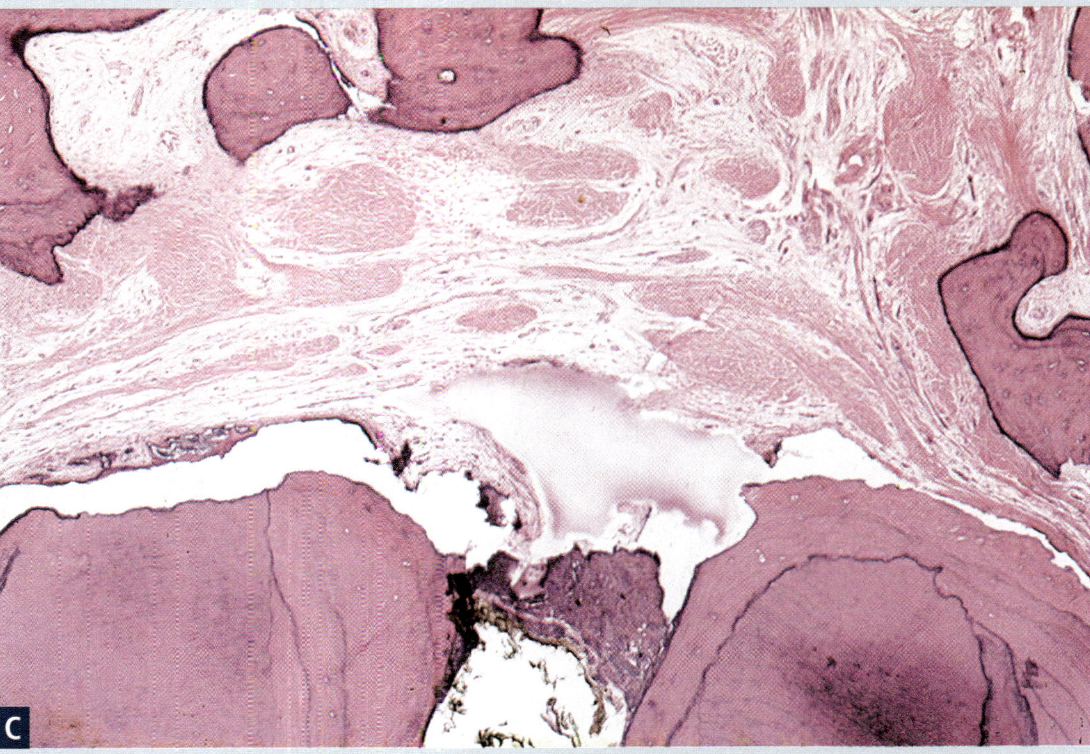

FIGS. 2.VII-3A-C – (CASE 12T)

A – A periapical radiograph for diagnostic purpose of a human maxillary right central incisor (1.1) (3/10/1964), showing evidence of an evident chronic periapical lesion, diagnosed as periapical diffuse rarefying osteitis, suggestive of chronic dento-alveolar abscess.

B – Post-treatment follow-up periapical radiograph of the case in Figure 2.VII-3A, obtained eight years and seven months after root canal filling (10/10/72) treated with active lateral condensation of gutta-percha cones and zinc oxide and eugenol cement. After radiographic assessment, six professors in endodontics considered the treatment a success. The clinical assessment made by the author also concluded that the treatment was a success.

C – Histological section of the apical and periapical region of the human tooth shown in Figure 2.VII-3-3, showing evidence that the apical foramen was filled by an amorphous substance, with the presence of dentin debris as a result of instrumentation, which was limited to 1 millimeter short of the radiographic apex, according to the concept at the time. Observe the thickened apical periodontal ligament, with an area close to the foramen, showing a chronic inflammatory infiltrate (H&E stain40X).

FINAL CONSIDERATIONS

Figures 2.VII-2A-D and 2.VII-3A-C confirm the need to remove the toxic septic contents located at the apical foramen in the cases of necropulpectomies II, by means of an operative procedure we call foramen debridement.

Initially, the author erroneously named this operative step apical patency, based on Buchanan[1] (*see* Chapter 2.VI). However, professor Dra. Liliana Glória Sierra, full professor of the School of Dentistry Chair of Endodontics at the National University of Buenos Aires – Argentina, in 1990, pointed out that she considered the operative procedure, which is today called **foramen debridement**, far broader and wider in scope, more comprehensive and particularly important in cases of necropulpectomies II (apical periodontitis), than merely overcoming the apical constriction of the canal with a small diameter instrument, without widening it, which is the function of patency file in the Buchanan[1] concept. **Foramen debridement** means cleaning, unobstructing and slightly enlarging the apical foramen, only applicable in cases of necropulpectomies II.

The foramen is explored with an apical foramen instrument (AFI), which is the first instrument, in the sequence of use from the largest to the smallest diameter, in the crown-apex direction without pressure, to reach and penetrate the apical foramen in a relatively forced manner, thus at the real tooth length (RTL), cleaning and unobstructing it.

After using the AFI, and consequently cleaning and unobstructing the apical foramen, we recommend withdrawing 1 millimeter from the real tooth length (RTL), and beginning to make the apical stop, with an instrument called the initial apical instrument (IAI).

We call the IAI the first instrument used in the clinical widening sequence, from the smallest to the largest diameter, to bind to the root canal walls at the real working length (RWI), which in cases of necropulpectomies II would be 1 millimeter short of the RTL. We use the IAI to start making the apical stop, which is the reason for the clinical, radiographic and histologic success of the treatment. The apical stop is concluded by using two or three instruments that have larger diameters than the IAI. Thus, for example, in the root canal of a maxillary central incisor with pulp necrosis and clear periapical lesion, the AFI could hypothetically be a stainless steel type K file No. 25. The IAI that will probably act on withdrawal of 1 millimeter, that is, at the RWL, must be a stainless steel type K file No. 30. Therefore, we conclude the apical stop with an instrument No. 40 and/or 45, which will be called the memory instrument (MI).

The above considerations technically constitute the critical time of biological endodontics in cases of necropulpectomies II, which if well applied, will be the reason for successful treatment.

Note: All the human clinical/surgical cases mentioned where done during the 70`s, according to the Protocol of Helsinki (Finland) of 1964.

References

1. Buchanan LS. Management of the curved root canal. J Calif Dent Assoc, v.17, p.18-25, 1989.
2. Kuttler Y. Endodoncia práctica. México: Alpha, 1961, p.217-219.
3. Leonardo MR. Contribuição para o estudo da reparação apical e periapical pós-tratamento de canais radiculares de dentes de humanos. Faculdade de Farmácia e Odontologia de Araraquara (tese de livre-docência), 1973, 103 p.
4. Leonardo MR, Rossi MA, Silva LAB, Ito IY, Bonifácio KC. EM (verificar EM: An?) evaluation of bacterial biofilm and microorganisms on the apical external root surface of human teeth. J Endod, v.28, p.815-818, 2002.
5. Siqueira JR JF, Dantas CJS. Mecanismos celulares e moleculares da inflamação. Medsi: Rio de Janeiro, 2000.

2.VIII

Periradicular surgery performed with the use of a microscope

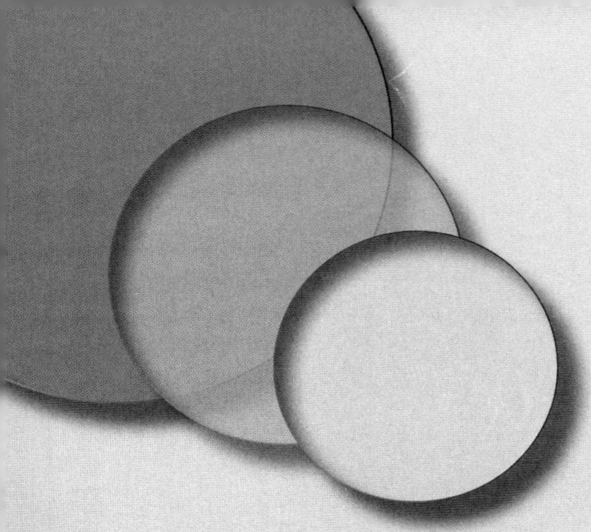

Gabriele Edoardo Pecora
Camilla Nicole Pecora
Jamil Awad Shibli

The development of concepts in the application of advanced technologies and the characteristics of material has provided notable improvement in the results and excellent predictability of the surgical technique in endodontics.

In particular, the use of operating microscopy in endodontic techniques has increased its indication in unsuccessful conventional treatments and diminished the need for radical surgical techniques (Fig. 2.VIII-1).

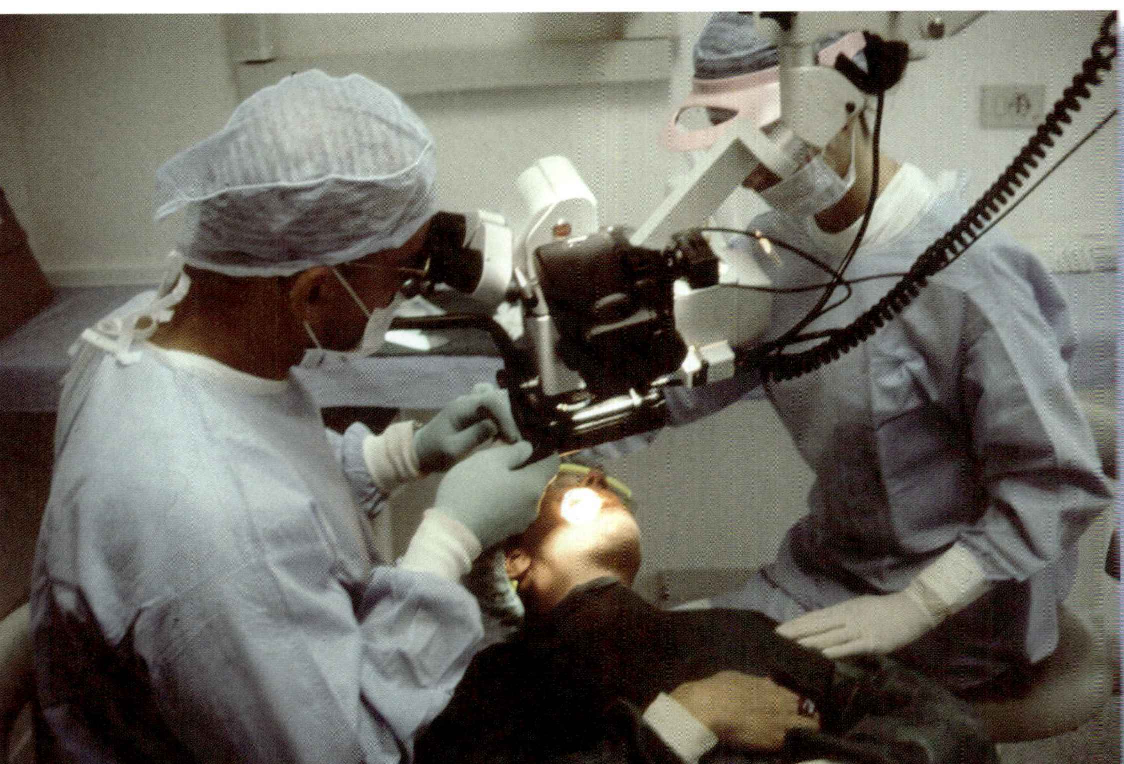

FIG. 2.VIII-1
Clinical aspect shows use of the surgical microscope.

The concept of surgery in endodontics is based on periradicular surgery, thus introducing the concept of endodontic microsurgery.

Indications of surgery in Endodontics are secondary when:

1. Treatment and re-treatment were not successful (Figs. 2.VIII-2 and 2.VIII-3);
2. In cases of operative errors that created situations that could only be solved with surgery (Figs. 2.VIII-4, 2.VIII-5, 2.VIII-6, 2.VIII-7, 2.VIII-8 and 2.VIII-9).

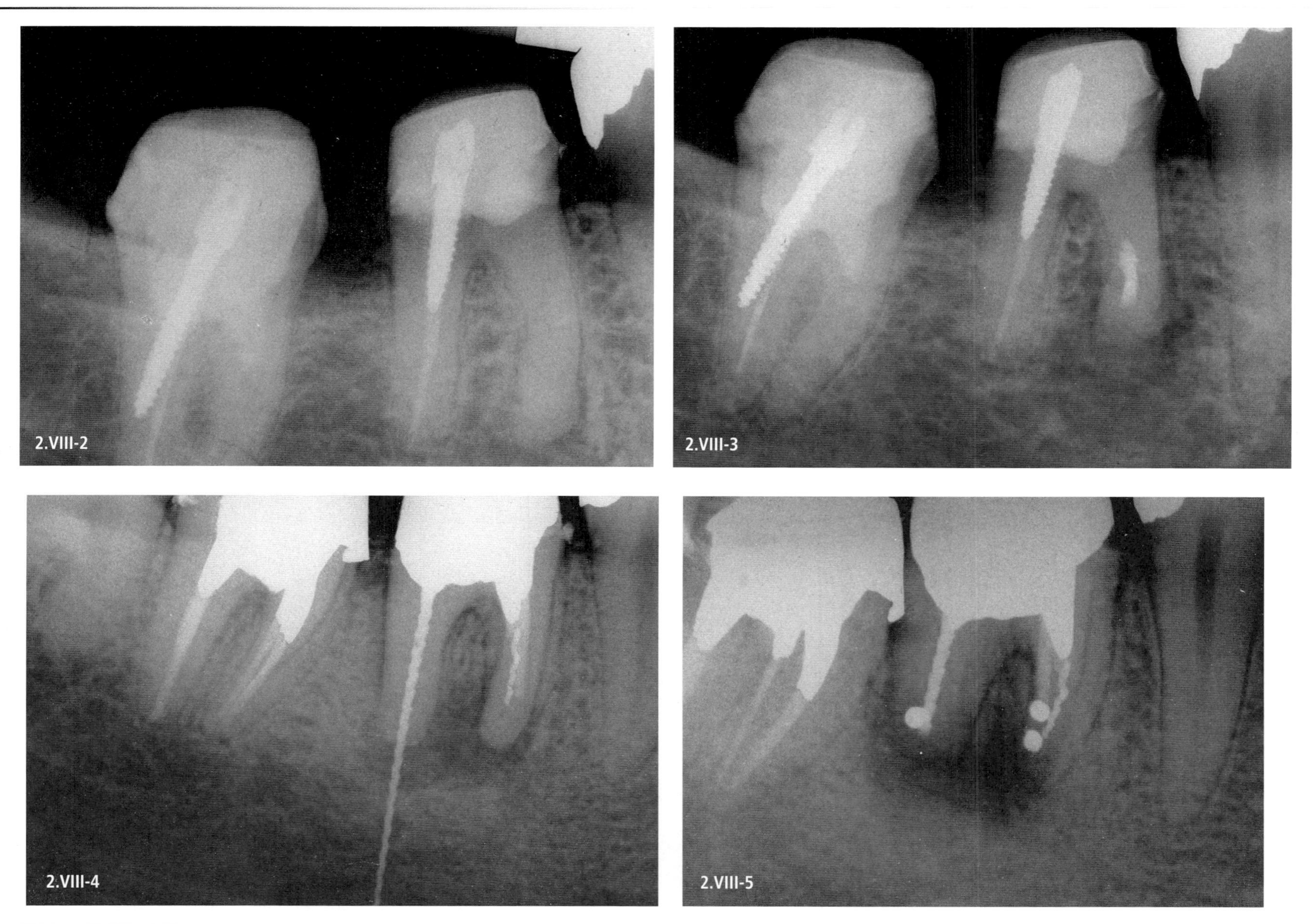
2.VIII-2
2.VIII-3
2.VIII-4
2.VIII-5

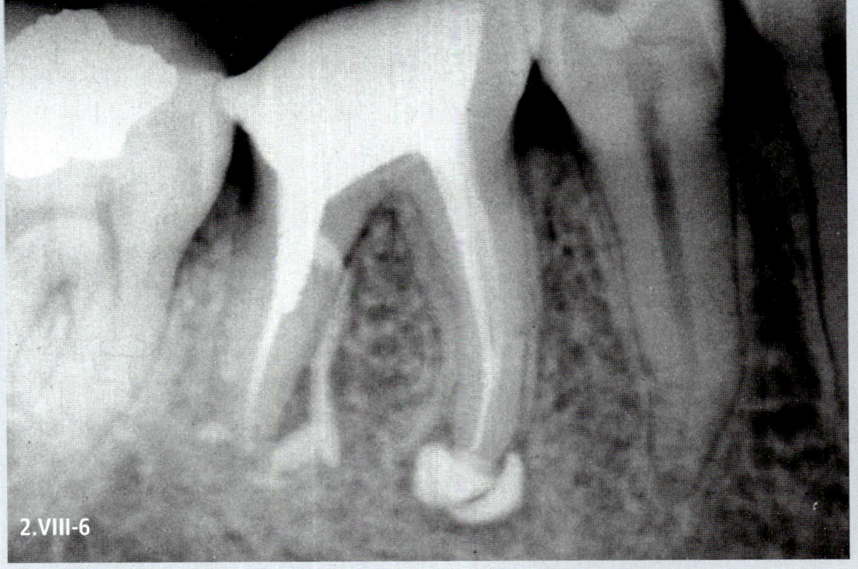

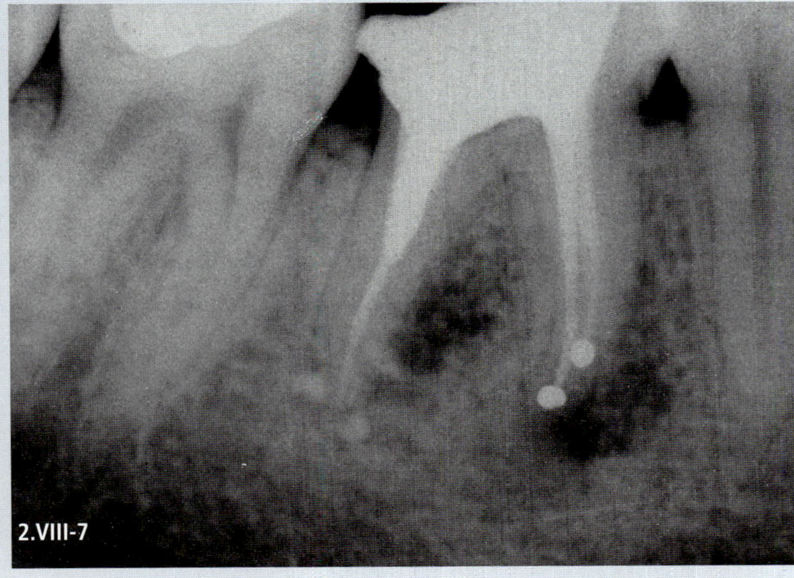

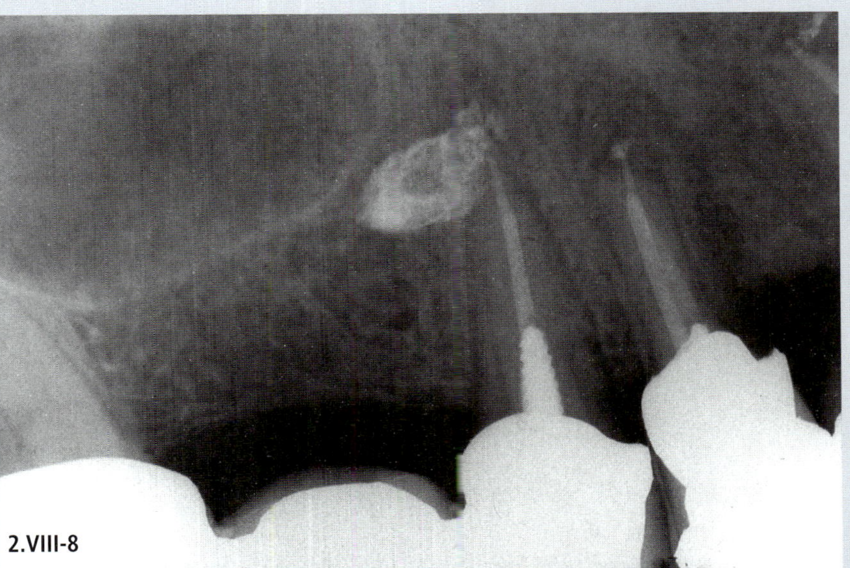

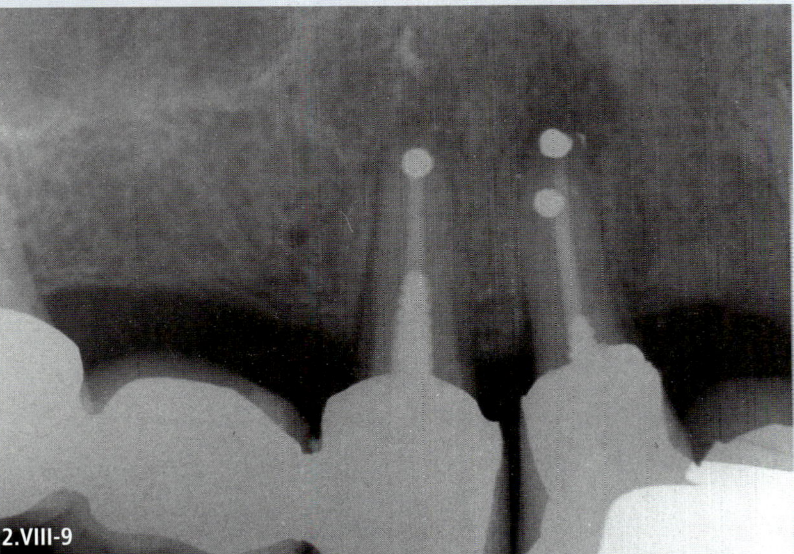

FIG. 2.VIII-2
Lesion of the mesial root of 4.6.

FIG. 2.VIII-3
Six months after surgery with retrograde filling.

FIG. 2.VIII-4
Iatrogenic lesion in 4.6.

FIG. 2.VIII-5
Two months after surgery.

FIG. 2.VIII-6
Extrusion of filled cement.

FIG. 2.VIII-7
Two months after surgery.

FIG. 2.VIII-8
Extrusion of filled cement in 1.5.

FIG. 2.VIII-9
Three months after surgery.

Primary indications, when the lesion cannot be treated via the root canal:

1. Large perforations;
2. Instrument fractures in the apical third;
3. Presence of crowns or restorations that are difficult to remove and prevent access to the root canal.

With the premise that success of endodontic treatment is related to the absence of bacteria in the endodontic system and that conventional treatment failure is due to the difficulty or impossibility of obliterating the complex ramification of the root canal system, we can easily understand why the use of the operating microscope has improved the results, increasing operative predictability and diminishing possible complications.

As far back as 1993, Pecora & Andreana[21] affirmed that the use of the operating microscope made visualization easier, by means of precise lighting, with significant improvement in operative precision and consequently in the quality of treatment.

In another study, Pecora et al.[24] (1993), in a multicenter study, established that the stages at which the surgical microscope brings benefits to the endodontic treatment are as follows:

- Isolation of the root apex;
- Evaluation of the prepared root surface and planning the cavity for retrograde filling;
- Cleaning and drying the cavity for retrograde filling;
- Filling the cavity with retro-filling material;
- Retrograde filling refinement;
- Cleansing of the bone crypt;
- Control of retrograde filling.

In two comparative studies between the conventional technique and the one that used the surgical microscope, Rubinstein & Kim[34,35] concluded that better longitudinal results were obtained with the technique that used the microscope.

The primary goal of surgical periradicular treatment is the same as that of conventional endodontics: to create conditions that promote healing of the periradicular tissues by regeneration or repair.

These conditions include:

- Necrotic tissue removal;
- Removal of products from degradation of the root canal system of the apical portion;
- Reduction in number of bacteria on the root surface;
- Reduction or elimination of the bacteria eventually present inside the root canal system;
- Removal of apical portion and accessory canals;
- Application of a biocompatible and hermetic sealing material in the apical portion.

Friedman et al.[10] and Pecora et al.[28] added that several factors may determine the result:

1. Pre-operative:

   - Presence of symptoms (Fig. 2.VIII-10);
   - Dimension of lesion (Fig. 2.VIII-11);
   - Level and quality of the root canal filling;
   - Patient's age;
   - Immunological conditions;
   - Concomitant presence of periodontal lesion (Fig. 2.VIII-12).

2. Operative:

   - Location of teeth: anterior or posterior;
   - Practitioner's ability;
   - Technical stage;
   - Level of the apicectomy;
   - Angle of cut;
   - Cutting surface assessment;
   - Correct cavity preparation;

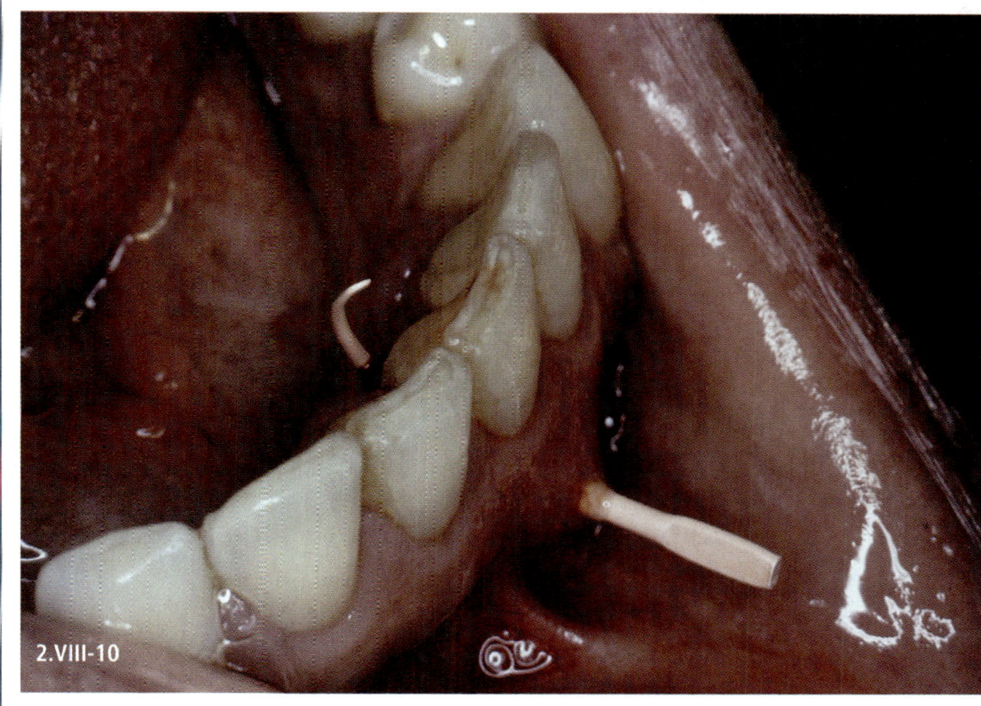

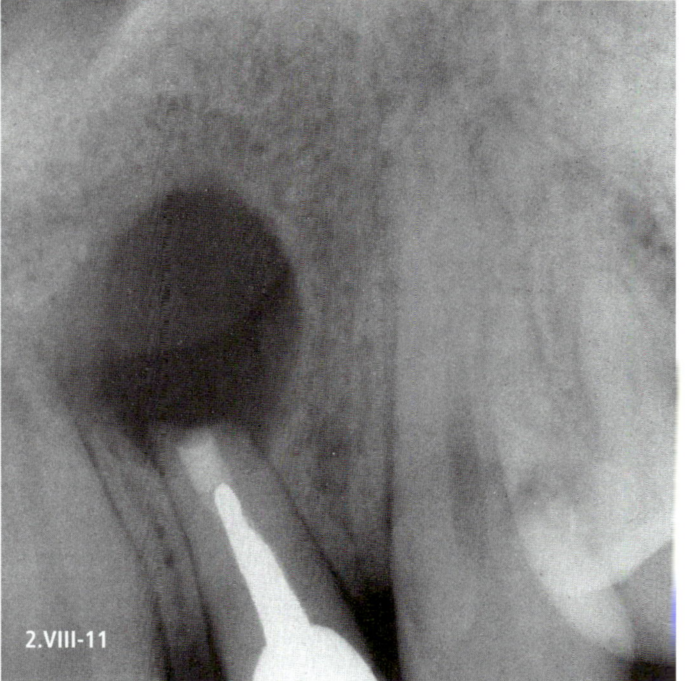

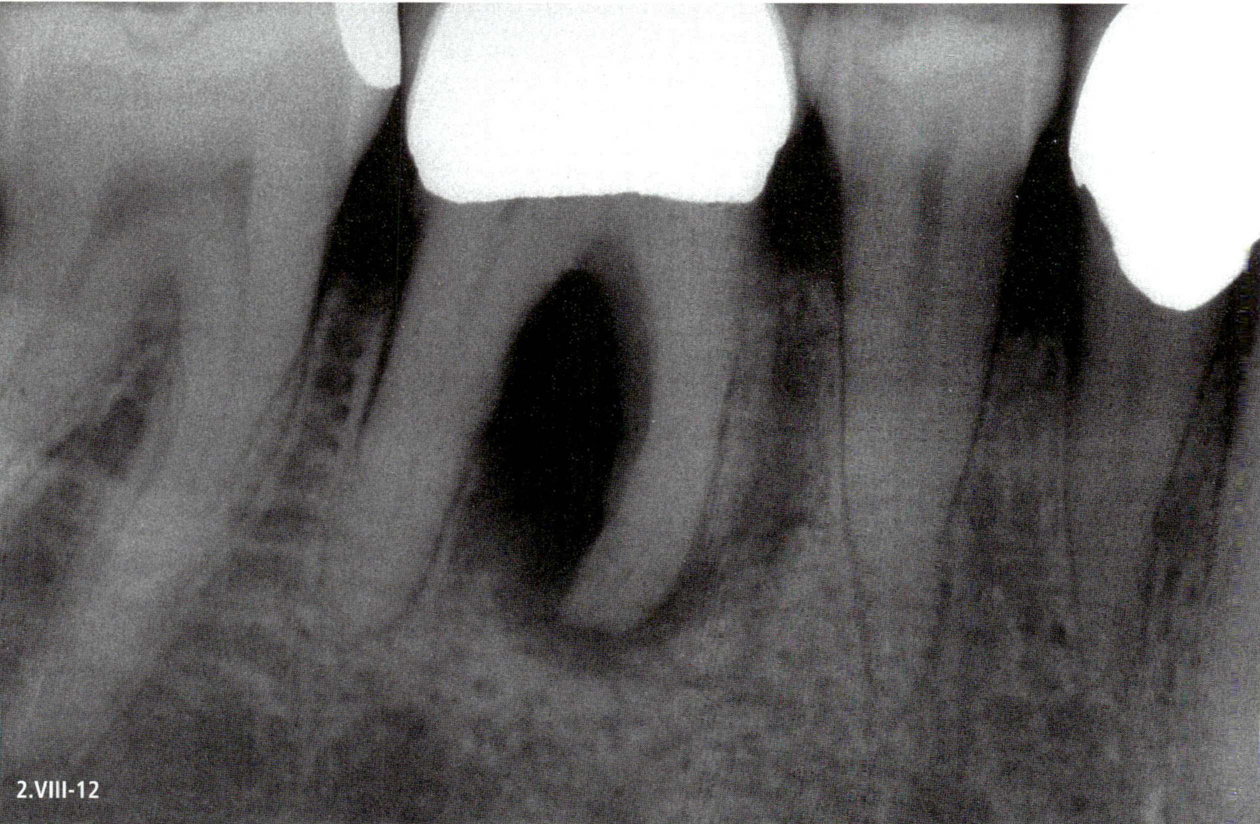

FIG. 2.VIII-10

Clinical aspect showing fistolography with gutta-percha cone on the fistula.

FIG. 2.VIII-11

Radiographic aspect after periradicular surgery on 2.2.

FIG. 2.VIII-12

Endo-perio lesion.

- Correct dose of preparation of retro-filling material;
- Lighting and ocular magnification system;
- Application of guided tissue regeneration technique (GRT).

3. Post-operative:

- Occlusion;
- Healing time;
- Restoration quality;
- Hygiene habits.

The evaluation of success or failure after periradicular surgery is based on several clinical and radiographical criteria.

In the literature, doubts have been expressed whether to consider the patient's periodontal condition as a conditioning factor. In a study performed by Leonardo[18], the authors affirmed that a persistent endodontic infection could be a risk factor for progression of loss of insertion after periradicular surgery. In the long term, healing of the periodontal tissue of a tooth with periodontal infection, shown by periradicular bone loss and loss of periodontal insertion, may result in slow and non homogeneous healing after periodontal therapy.

On the other hand, it is always opportune to treat periodontal infection before surgical endodontic treatment. Advanced periodontal lesions, with an increase in probing depth, associated with chronic periradicular infection, may lead to failure of surgical endodontic therapy (Rud et al.[36], 1972).

When the periradicular lesion advances, associated with loss of marginal bone tissue, there is less likelihood of a favorable result in the long term (Skoglund & Persson[40], 1985).

The high percentage of failure is attributed to the colonization of the root surface, exposed by a non-osteogenic tissue and to invasion of part of the epithelial tissue in the crown/apex direction along the root. In this anatomic situation, there is bacterial colonization from the gingival margin, in an apical direction, or from the apex, in a coronal direction.

Success in this situation depends on control of epithelial proliferation and bacterial decontamination of the root surface. The two situations may be summarized with the concept of "halting the progression of disease".

Therefore, the goals of surgical therapy are:

1. Elimination of symptoms;
2. Reduction in the area of radiographic rarefaction;
3. Reestablishment of function.

In addition:

4. Halting the progression of disease and controlling bacterial infection of the root.

Many periradicular surgery failures are attributed to insufficient apex sealing. Should the bacteria remain active in the root canal system (RCS), no conventional or surgical treatment will lead to solution of the problem.

Bacterial infiltration may occur:

- In lateral canals;
- In dentinal tubules;
- Between the dentinal wall and the retro-filling material.

Other factors may also influence the healing process:

- periodontal disease;
- microfractures (Fig. 2.VIII-13);
- occlusal trauma;
- the patient's immunological condition.

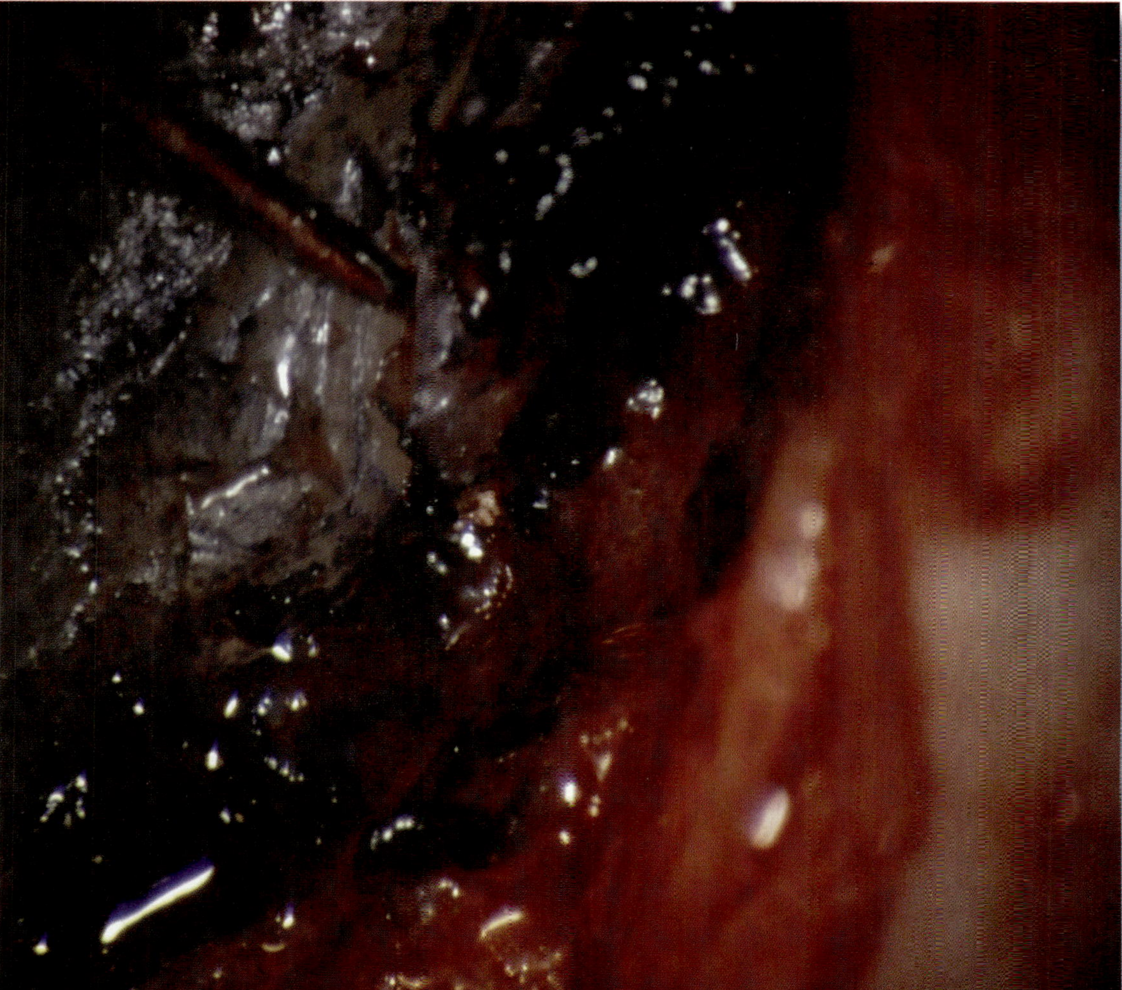

FIG. 2.VIII-13
Microfracture (16x) shown with methylene blue.

Endo-periodontal lesion therapy needs a correct diagnostic approach for a precise prognosis. In the majority of cases, the primary lesion is endodontic and if the time interval is brief and there is no deep bacterial colonization of the root surface, the treatment can accomplish complete regeneration of the destroyed tissue.

If the favorable time interval has elapsed and conventional endodontic therapy has not been successful, then one must evaluate the possibility of performing regenerative therapy, with the possibility of complete decontamination of the root surface and the use of regenerative materials.

In cases in which the periodontal lesion is primary, although sensitivity tests are suspect, the endodontic infection must first be treated and afterwards, the periodontal infection. It is very important to regenerate the root cementum, periodontal ligament and bone tissue at the level of the alveolar crest to prevent and impede bacterial infiltration via the gingival sulcus.

Essential conditions for guided tissue regeneration (GTR) are:

- hermetic sealing of the apex;
- etching the root surface with TTC;
- tooth stabilization;
- surgical wound stabilization;
- cellular migration (burying the root in bone, osteoconduction);
- maintaining the blood clot.

Previously, several techniques and materials were used, particularly resorbable and non-resorbable membranes.

In the last few years, calcium sulphate based materials (Surgiplaster, Ghimas, Italy) (Bonelli et al.[2], 2001; Piattelli et al.[32], 2002; Pecora et al.[31], 2001) have been used in cases of:

- hemostatic material in bone defects;
- perforation treatment of sinus membrane;
- osteoconductive material in extensive bone defects;
- in T and T lesions (Figs. 2.VIII-14, 2.VIII-15, 2.VIII-16, 2.VIII-17, and 2.VIII-18);
- in endoperiodontal lesions (Figs. 2.VIII-19, 2.VIII-20 and 2.VIII-21).

The fundamental question is: How important is the type of healing by regeneration or repair? As an answer, one could use the anatomical pathological classification into lesions of types I, II and III.

In **type I lesions**, the lesion extends above the apical region and the type of healing process is not so important. Only in particularly extensive lesions, for esthetic reasons, can one promote the formation of bone tissue by means of guided regeneration.

In **type II lesions**, the lesion extends to the root surface. Since the entire compromised root portion must not be removed, it is necessary to apply the GTR principle, for the purpose of obtaining the formation of cementum, periodontal ligament and alveolar bone.

In **type III lesions**, there is endo-perio marginal communication. To obtain regeneration, which completely seals this communication of fluids and bacteria, it is necessary to perform:

- an efficient root surface decontamination procedure
- clot and soft tissue stabilization
- intense osteoconduction
- inhibition of non-osteogenic cell competitiveness

It will be very difficult to answer what the healing potential of a limit case would be. The prognostic classification for evaluation may be the classes A, B, C, D and E (Pecora & Kim[29],1997):

- **Class A:** lesions limited to the apex;
- **Class B**: lesions limited to the apical third;
- **Class C:** class B lesions associated with periodontal lesion without communication with the gingival sulcus;

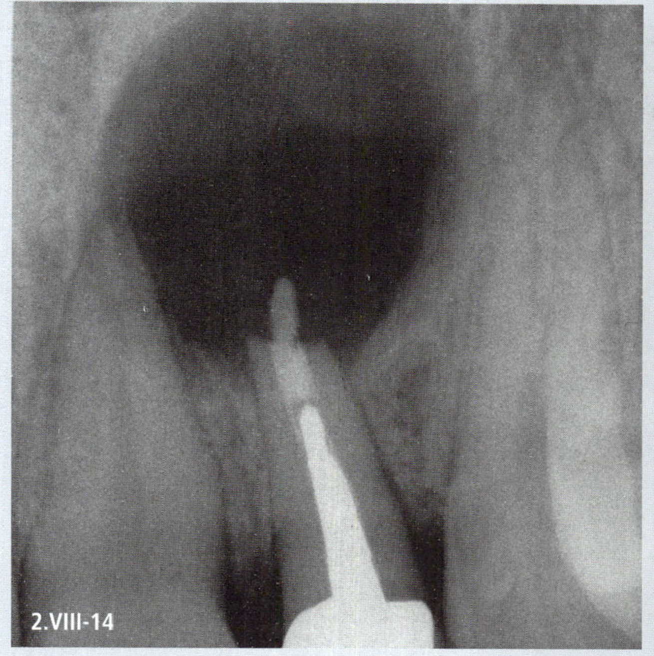
2.VIII-14

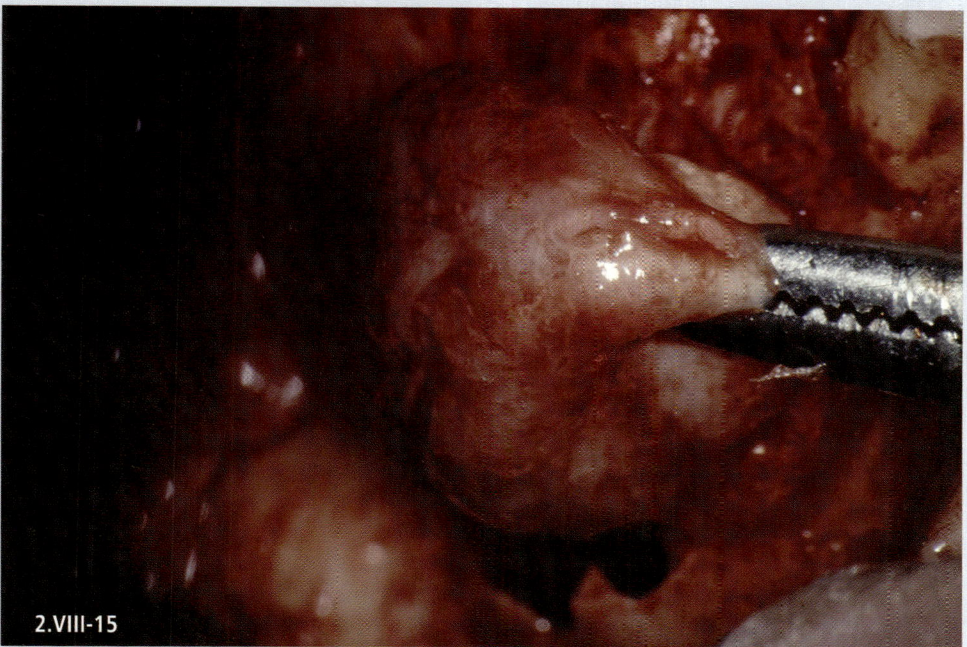
2.VIII-15

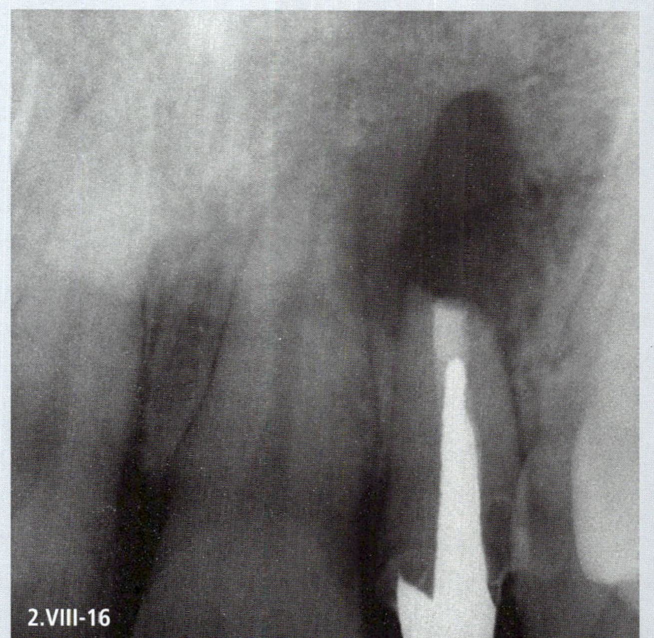
2.VIII-16

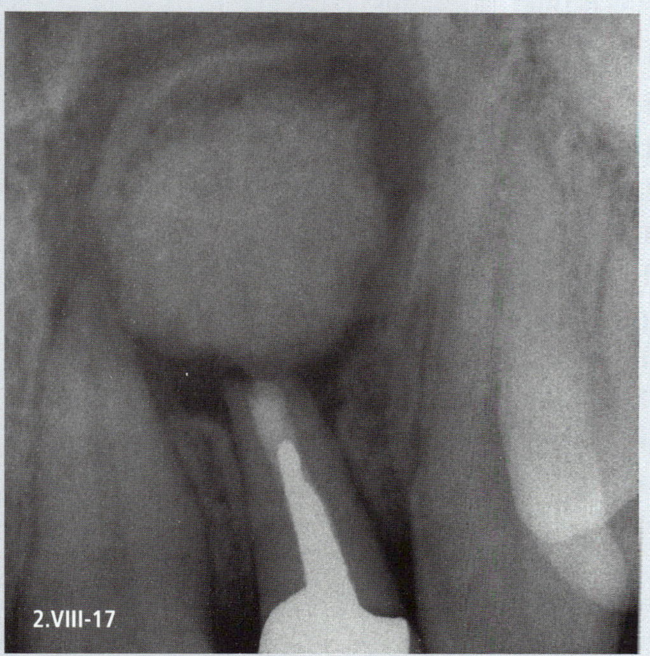
2.VIII-17

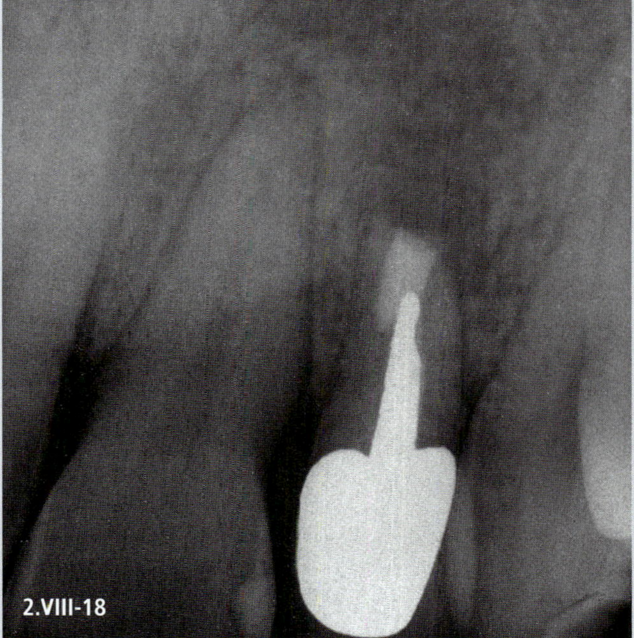
2.VIII-18

FIG. 2.VIII-14

Periapical radiograph showing pre-operative lesion in 2.2.

FIG. 2.VIII-15

Enucleation of the lesion.

FIG. 2.VIII-16

Periapical radiograph showing the progress of repair after 6 months.

FIG. 2.VIII-17

Re-opening due to symptoms; new retrograde filling and placement of Surgiplaster F30 (Ghimas, Casalecchio di Reno – Italy).

FIG. 2.VIII-18

Periapical radiograph showing repair after 6 months.

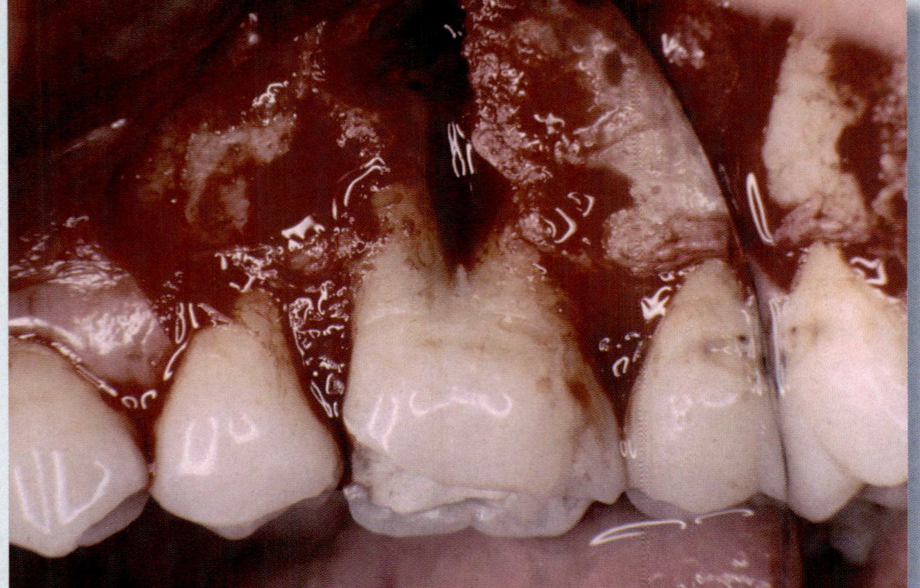

FIG. 2.VIII-19
Clinical aspect showing endo-perio lesion in 3.6.

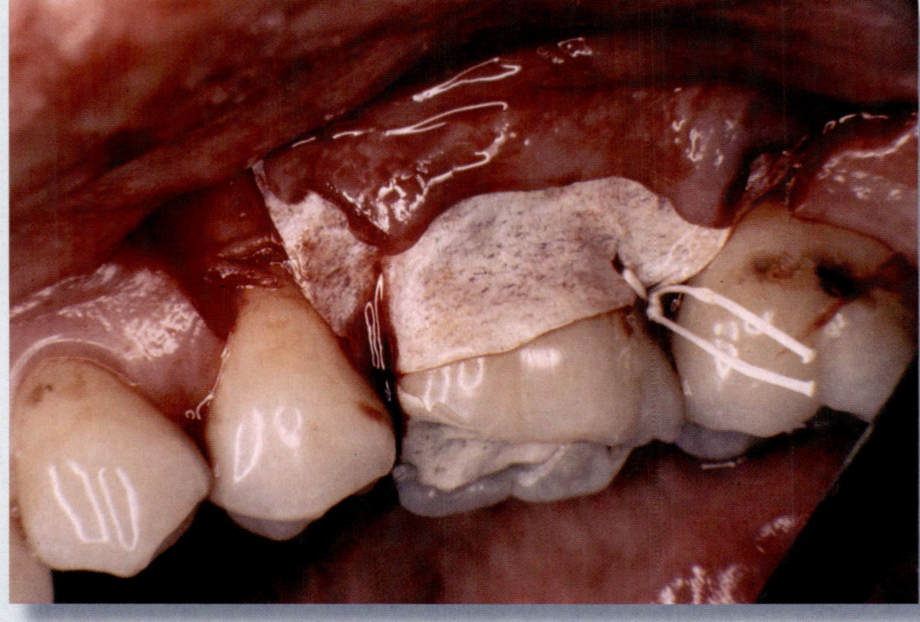

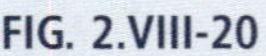

FIG. 2.VIII-20
Gore-tex membrane.

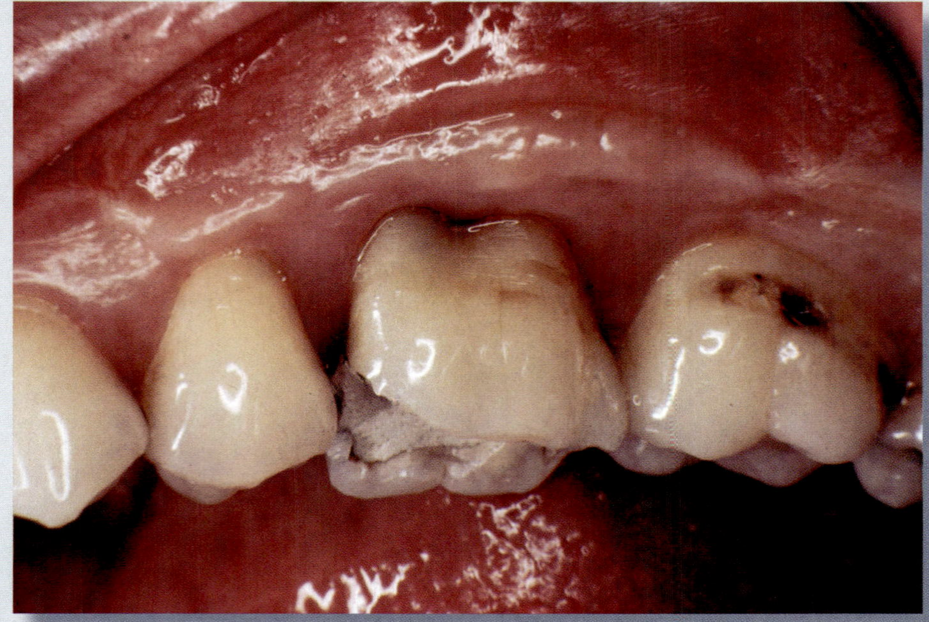

FIG. 2.VIII-21
Clinical view at 3 months.

- **Class D:** endodontic lesions with communication: Macro D1, micro D2 and microscopic D3;
- **Class E**: Absence of oral bone wall <E1; =E2; >E3; E4 with root at bone level; E5 with root in bone; E6 with root out of bone.

Classes A, B and C have a very favorable prognoses; classes D and E are the limit between conservative treatment and implant insertion.

Decisive criteria and evaluation are based on factors such as:

- bone tissue thickness;
- distance;
- root convexity;
- crown-root proportion.

After several years of experience with several membranes, many disadvantages were found:

- Difficult to use;
- frequent exposure and consequent infection (Figs. 2.VIII-22, 2.VIII-23 and 2.VIII-24);
- need for high predictability of the operator's technical ability;
- difficulty in maintaining space and the need to use filling materials (hydroxyapatite, DFDBA);
- high cost.

Due to these various disadvantages, the membrane fell into disuse in periradicular surgery and several researchers have investigated alternatives for the treatment of these lesions.

Another material that has been used on a large scale in clinical dentistry and in research is calcium sulphate-based Surgiplaster (Ghimas, Casalecchio di Reno, Italy). The application technique is stratified; the material is manipulated to a creamy consistency and applied in small quantities or compressed by sterilize gauze (TNT) until the defect is covered in excess. In large cavities Surgiplaster G170 may be used in grains; the material is extremely simple to use with highly predictable results. O Surgiplaster (Ghimas, Casalecchio di Reno, Italy) presents characteristics that make it indispensable to those who have used it in several clinical situations (Pecora et al.[22], 1997; Orsini et al.[20], 2004):

Properties:

- osteoconductor;
- completely resorbable;
- prevents bacterial growth;
- works as a space-maintainer for GTR and prevents non-osteogenic cell competitiveness;
- stimulates the growth and maturation of bone tissue;
- stimulates neo-angiogenesis.

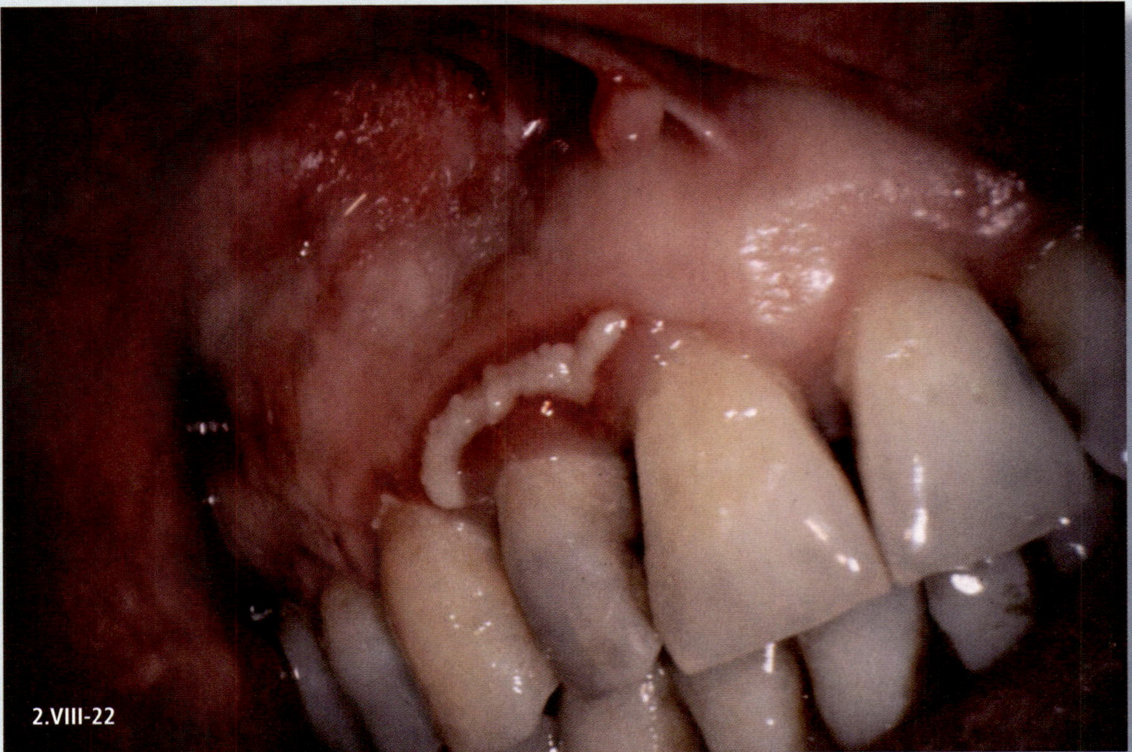

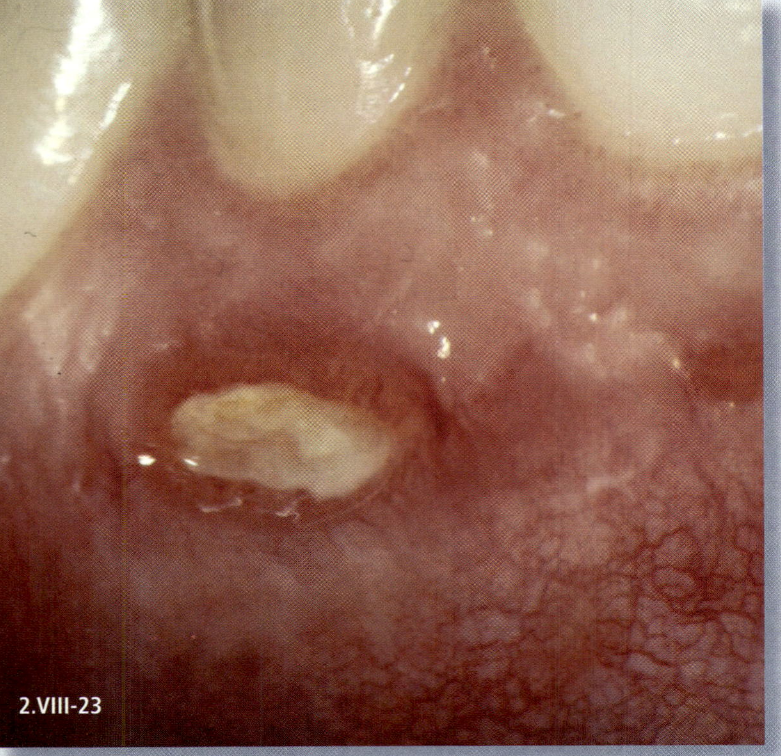

FIG. 2.VIII-22
Exposure of the Gore-tex membrane in 1.2.

FIG. 2.VIII-23
Exposure of the membrane at 12X magnification.

FIG. 2.VIII-24
Exposure of the membrane at 22X magnification.

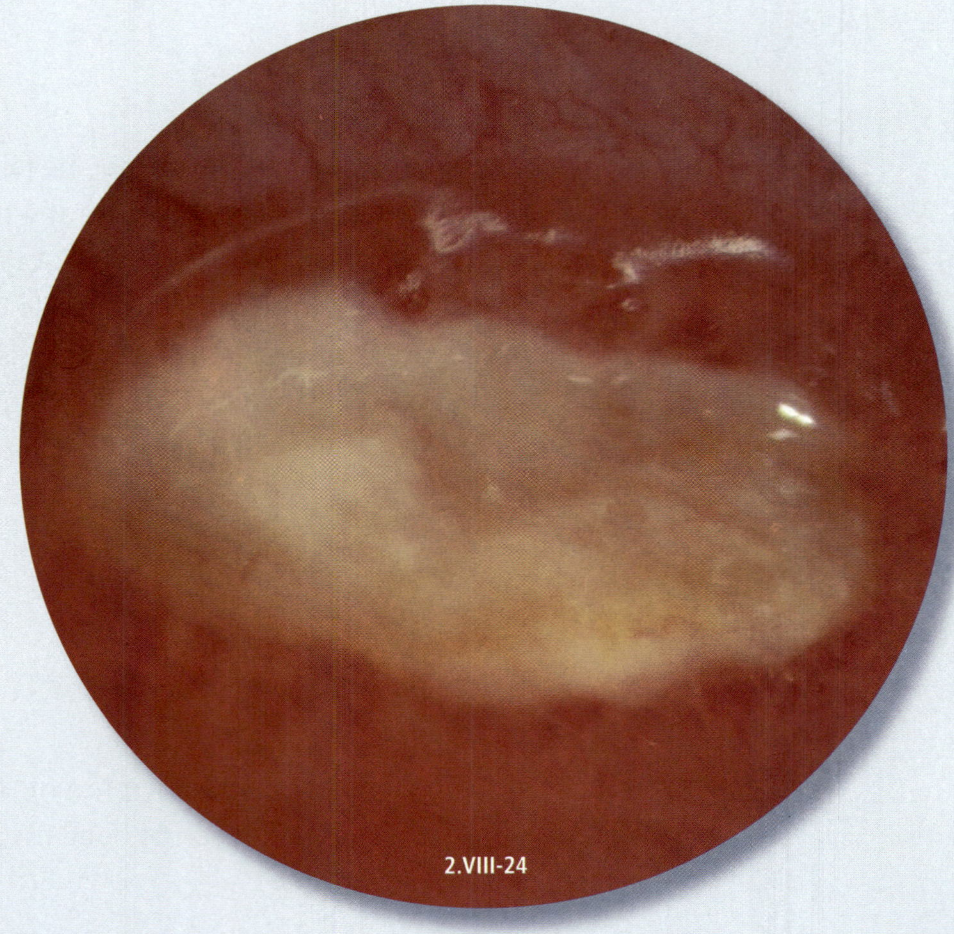

In 2001, in a clinical study, Pecora et al.[26] compared the use of Gore-Tex non-reabsorbable membrane and calcium sulphate (Surgiplaster P30) in the treatment of an endoperiodontal communication. The calcium sulphate presented the best result, due to the easy application and non-exposure to the oral environment, as usually occurs with the non-resorbable membranes. They concluded that in addition to the calcium sulphate working as an osteoconductive material, it prevents bacterial growth and enables healing of the regeneration type (Sottosanti[41], 1995; Coetzee[6], 1980; Bier & Sinensky[1], 1999).

Currently, the use of regenerative therapies optimizes the prognosis of many cases, limiting or improving eventual alternative implant therapy.

In some clinical situations, in which the type of healing is conditioned by the quality of therapy, the use of GTR is needed. Therefore, the use of calcium sulphate determines a series of favorable events, with high percentage of positive results in the regenerative technique.

The limit condition of the conservative therapy occurs when it is not possible to control root infection and tissue destruction compromises or makes it difficult to insert implants. At this critical stage, the decision to extract the tooth can be assessed by means of an exploratory flap, in order to evaluate the condition of the tooth. If the option is to remove the tooth, a series of therapeutic options may be applied:

a. guided bone regeneration soon after extraction;
b. immediate implant insertion;
c. immediate implant insertion followed by immediate restoration (Fig. 2.VIII-25).

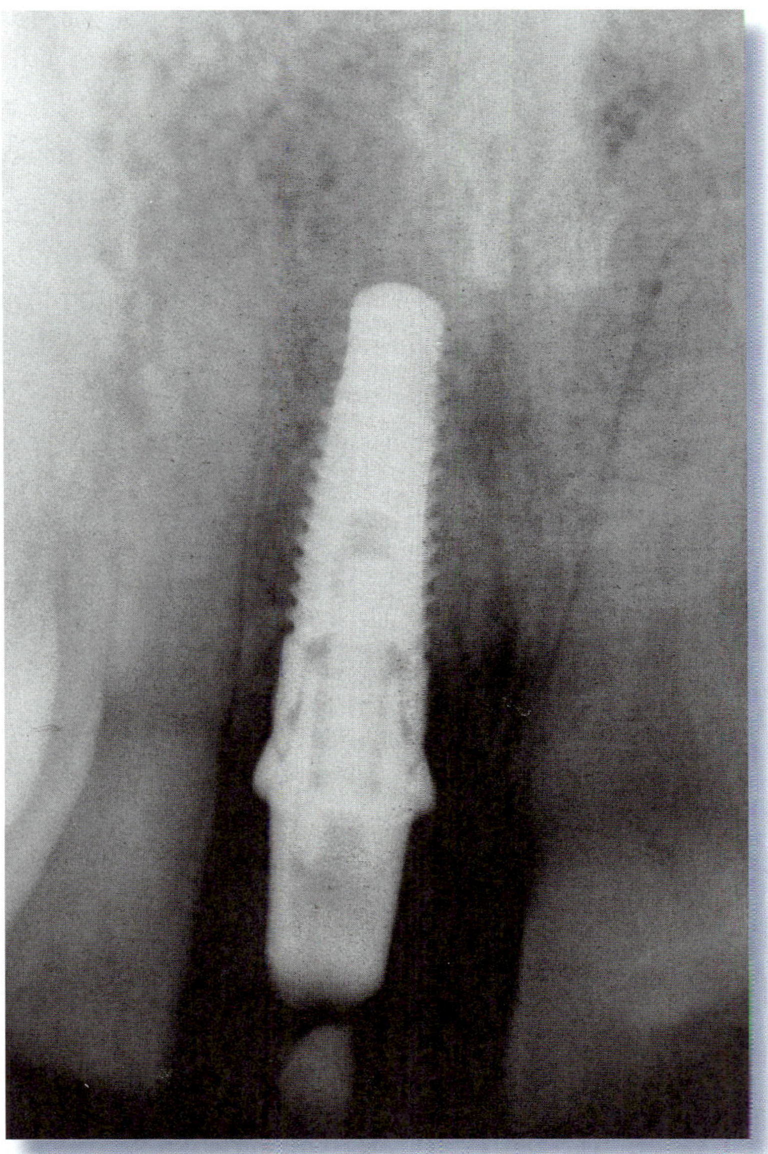

FIG. 2.VIII-25
Periapical radiograph showing FSI with immediate load.

Based on clinical experience, it can be affirmed that new clinical techniques, technologies and materials have been incorporated into the operating microsurgery protocol, creating a new dimension and providing new horizons for periradicular surgery (Kim et al.[16], 2001; Izawa et al.[12], 1994; Reuben & Apotherker[33], 1984; Scipioni & Bruschi[37], 1989; Scipioni & Bruschi[38], 1991; Carr[4], 1992; Carr[5], 1992).

OPERATIVE PROTOCOL OF PERIRADICULAR MICROSURGERY

1. Diagnosis
2. Flap
3. Osteotomy
4. Apiectomy
   - Periapical curettage
   - biopsy
   - root surface decontamination
   - hemostasis of surgical cavity (Fig. 2.VIII-26)
   - Evaluation of the cut surface (Figs. 2.VIII-27, 2.VIII-28, 2.VIII-29 and 2.VIII-30)
5. Cavity preparation for retrograde filling (Fig. 2.VIII-48)
   - Cavity drying
   - Cavity inspection with micro mirrors (Fig. 2.VIII-49)
6. Re-filling
7. Assessment of the need for GTR
8. Radiographic control
9. Suture

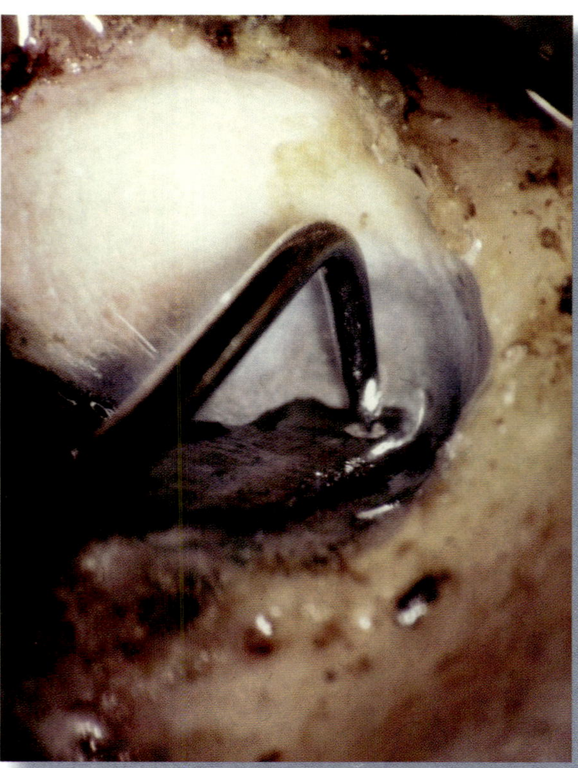

FIG. 2.VIII-26

Surgical aspect of the bone crest with Surgiplaster (Ghimas, Casalecchio di Reno – Italy) 16X magnification.

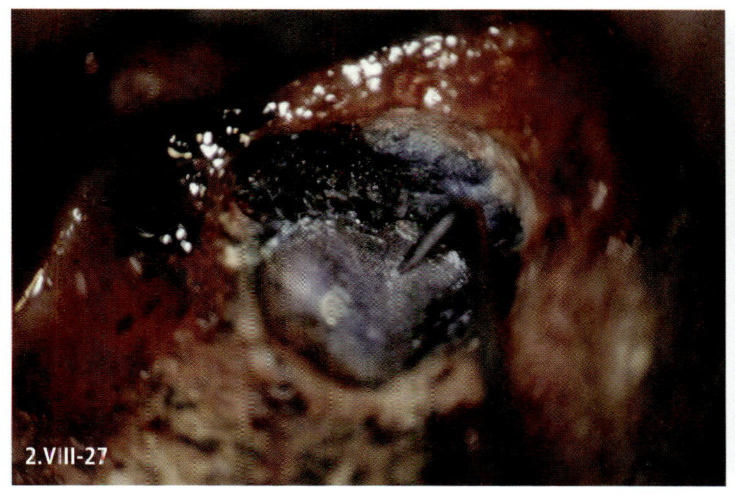

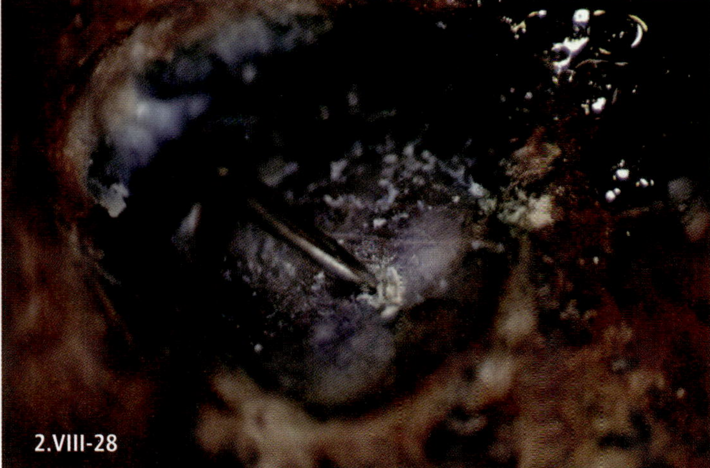

FIG. 2.VIII-27
Surgical aspect of the cut surface shown with methylene blue at 12X magnification.

FIG. 2.VIII-28
Seeking the foramen.

FIG. 2.VIII-29
Use of the micromirror at 14X magnification.

FIG. 2.VIII-30
Use of the microprobe at 32X magnification.

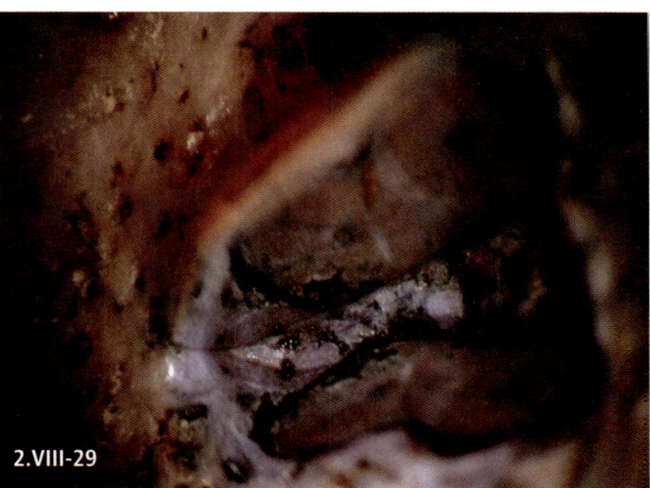

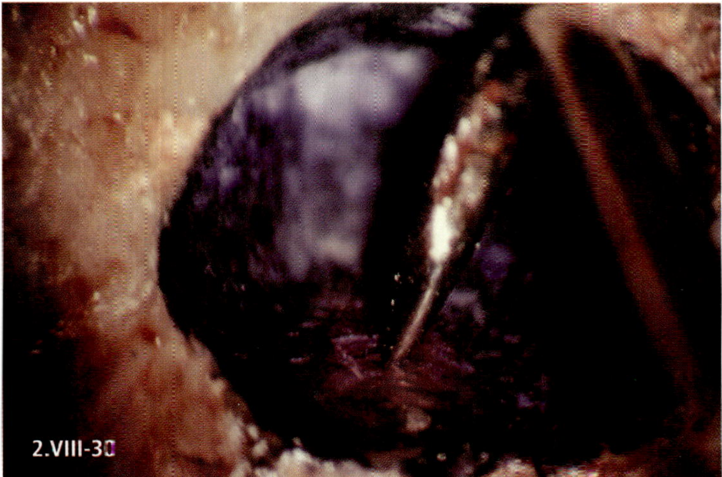

1. Diagnosis

Radiographic Assessment

Three periapical radiographs must be obtained with the use of a Rinn radiograph positioner (long cone technique). The radiographic exam allows careful evaluation of the root anatomy, as well as the extent of the lesion, paying special attention to:

a. root length and crown-root proportion;
b. root canal filling level;
c. posts and cores;
d. proximity of the root to the mandibular canal, maxillary sinus, mental nerve exit and nasal fossa;
e. location of lesion;
f. presence of fractures or microfractures (Figs. 2.VIII-31, 2.VIII-32 and 2.VIII-33);
g. presence of lateral and accessory canals;
h. periodontal lesions;
i. internal or external root resorption.

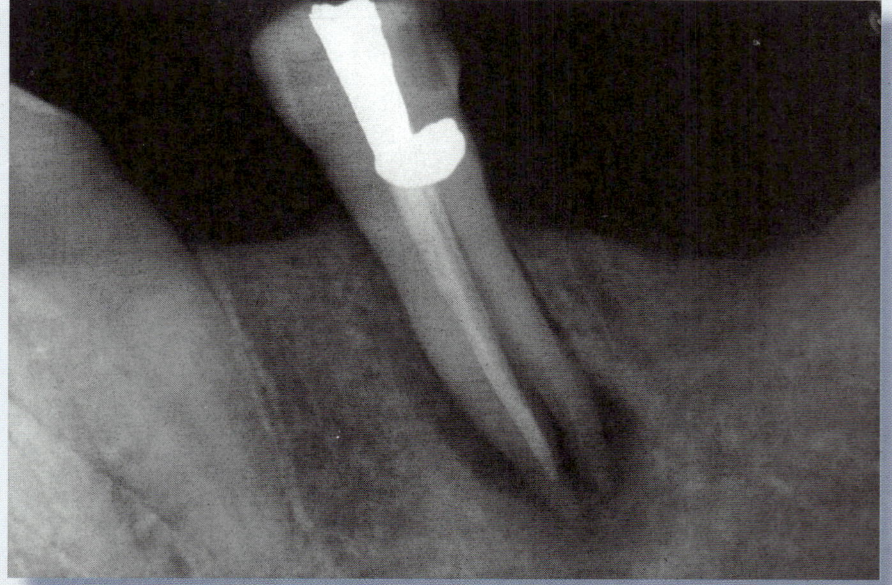

FIG. 2.VIII-31
Periapical radiograph showing a vertical fracture.

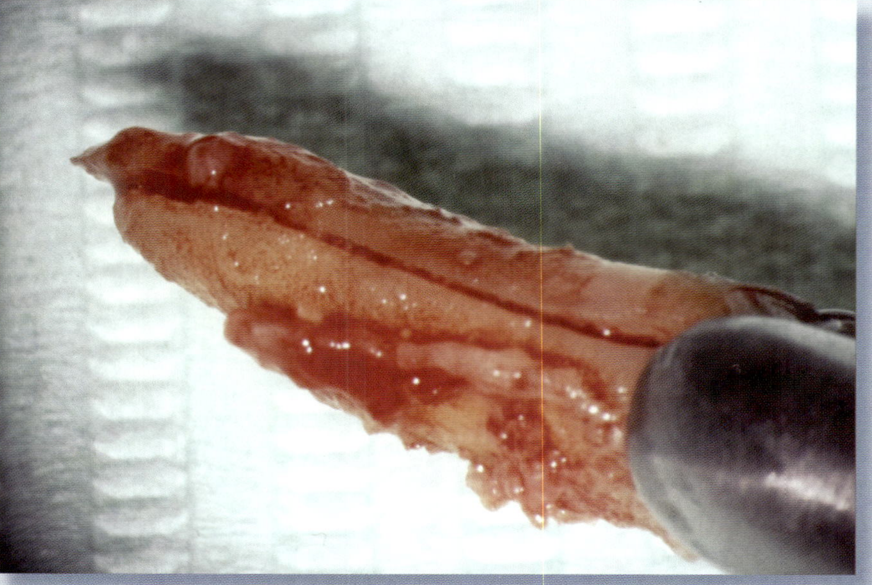

FIG. 2.VIII-32
Clinical view of the fracture after tooth extraction.

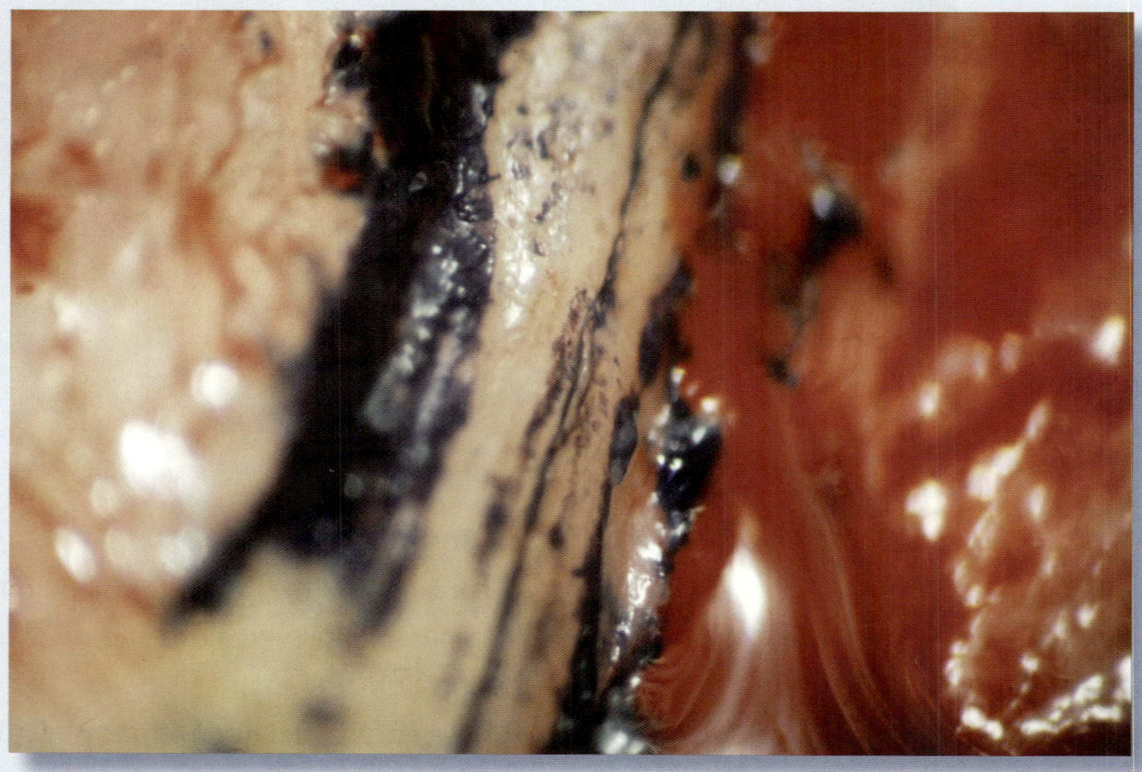

FIG. 2.VIII-33
Vertical fracture and methylene blue at 22X magnification.

Periodontal Assessment

Periodontal assessment is very important, with regard to pre-operative assessment or prognosis and particularly with respect to the type of flap to be performed and by the periodontal treatment itself to be instituted. Clinical assessment of probing depth and the clinical level of insertion must be performed before anesthesia, to avoid errors in measuring the bone level.

In the case of treating endoperiodontal lesions, clinical assessment of the following periodontal parameters must be made six months before surgery:

a. Silness & Loe plaque index[39];
b. LOE gingival index[19];
c. probing depth performed in six regions, per tooth (mesio-buccal, buccal, disto-buccal, disto-lingual, lingual and mesio-lingual);
d. clinical insertion level;
e. tooth mobility (Fleszar et al.[9], 1980);
f. palpation of root movement.

2. Flap

Anesthesia is important at this stage to control hemorrhage and because it promotes the procedure of performing the flap, allowing adequate access to the lesion and periapical area.

Hemorrhage control is based on three stages:

a. At the **pre-surgical** stage, it is important to use an anesthetic with an adequate percentage of vasoconstrictor (1:100.000). Mandibular block anesthesia must be followed by local infiltrations in the soft tissue adjacent to the area to be approached, thus reducing blood flow in the site. It must be administered 15-20 minutes before the intervention, in order to allow adequate vasoconstriction.
b. At the **surgical stage**, adequate planning of the flap is very important. The relaxing incision must be made vertically to place tension on the muscle fibers and prevent possible suture dehiscence. At this surgical stage, after apiectomy, curettage is performed to remove all the inflamed tissue. Cavity buffering can be performed by chemical means (for example, 17% ferric sulphate) or with resorbable material (collagen, calcium sulphate). Many researchers prefer to use calcium sulphate (Surgiplaster, Ghimas, Casalecchio di Reno, Italy) because of its characteristics, such as osteoconduction, biocompatibility and resorption (Whitherspoon & Gutmann[43], 1996; Jastak & Yagiela[13], 1983; Kim & Rethnam[17], 1997). The blood flow from the bone marrow tissue adjacent to the area to be operated can be controlled by aspiration.
c. **Post-surgical hemorrhage** is controlled with the use of an occlusive suture and eventually with sterile gauze compression.

The flap presents characteristics such as:

a. **Incision** (Figs. 2.VIII-34 and 2.VIII-35): comprised of the horizontal component, which may be sulcular or parasulcular, and one or two vertical components; mesial and distal. The shape of the flap must be triangular or rectangular. Vascularization is descendent; that is, a relaxing incision must be performed vertically. Special care must be taken with the muscular insertions. In the inferior region, precaution must be taken with the nerve exit, as well as the mental foramen itself. If the endodontic lesion is close to the mental foramen, computerized tomography of the region must be requested. As a precaution, a relaxing incision must be performed at the height of the mandibular incisor. The mental foramen is usually located close to the apex of the mandibular pre-molar.
b. **Divulsion**: Surgical spatulas with small and delicate tips must be used, because they facilitate access to

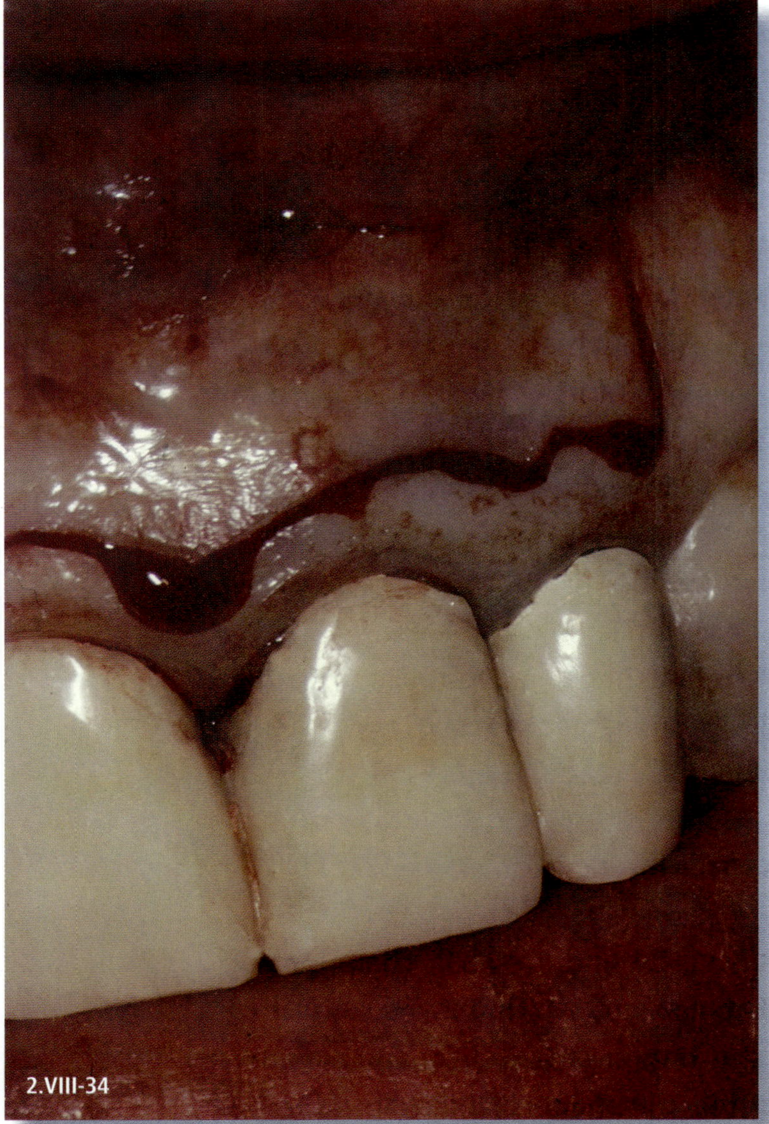

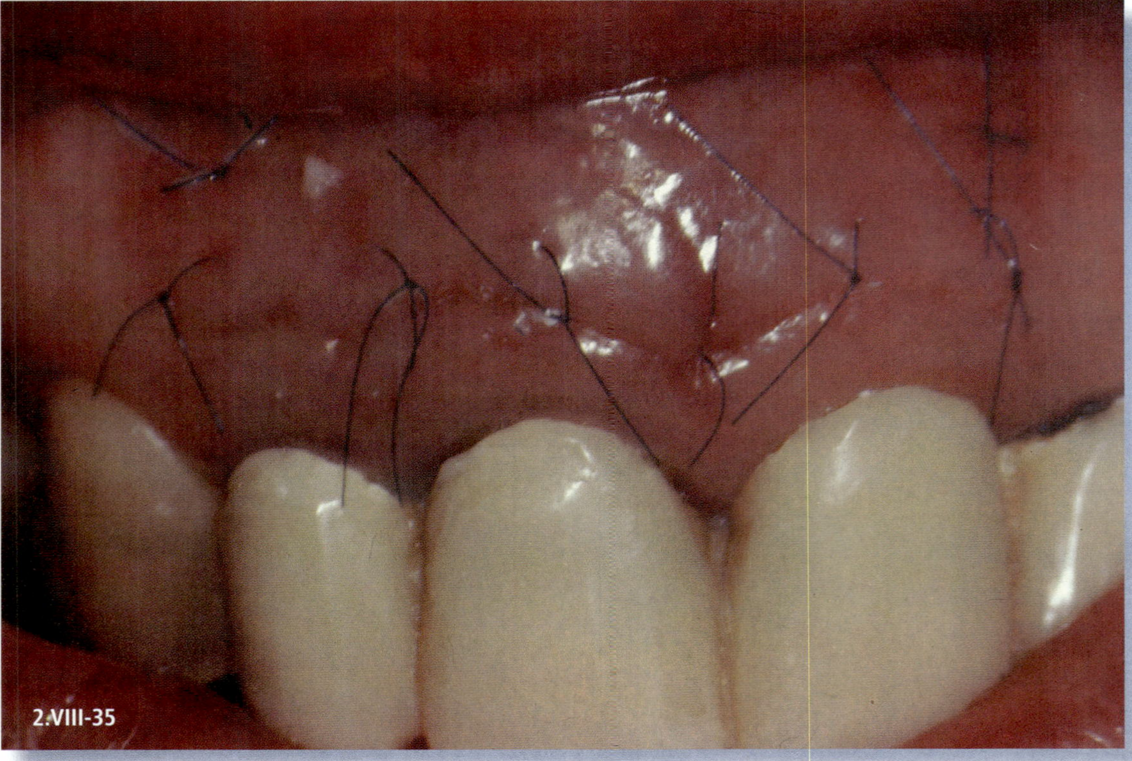

FIG. 2.VIII-34
Surgical view showing the rectangular shape of the flap.

FIG. 2.VIII-35
Repair (6 days).

the bone depressions and eminences and limit trauma during divulsion of the gingival sulcus. At this stage, as in the preceding one, low magnification of the microscope must be used to improve visualization of the operating field. It is worth emphasizing that a well-performed divulsion allows the flap to be easily manipulated and to heal more rapidly. Flaps of full thickness are obtained when the incision goes to the periosteum, which prevents them from suffering lacerations and ruptures. Incisions with acute angles must be avoided and rounded margins are recommended. The surgical spatula must be curved for curved surfaces and straight for flat surfaces, and have cutting edges of suitable dimensions. Divulsion begins at the most favorable point of the flap and continues, progressively, along the entire surface. Blood flow control of eventual ruptures of small vessels present in the flap must be obtained by obliterating these vessels by means of ligatures, compression and coagulation. Hemorrhage from the bone wall, although uncommon, can be controlled with aspiration. It must be possible to gain access to the operative area without placing stress or traction on the flap, by performing vertical relaxing incisions, whenever required.

c. **Flap separation**: the separator must rest on the bone tissue, however, without preventing the operating microscope from entering into the operating field. For this reason, separators must have a curved portion that is in stable contact with the bone, on which sulci or depressions may be made with greater firmness. Furthermore, the length of the separator must be appropriate for moving the lip away and keeping it in this position, creating adequate and stable access to the lower anatomical structures.

3. Osteotomy

Hjorting-Hansen & Andreasen[11], in a study on dogs, demonstrated that in endodontic lesions of up to 5 mm in size, with intact cortical bone, there was complete cicatrisation. Whereas, in lesions larger than 5 mm, with fibrous tissue formation, cicatrisation was incomplete.

In another study by Boyne *et at.*[3], who evaluated lesions from 5 to 8 mm in size in the maxilla of patients, by means of histological sections of biopsies performed in periods of between 4-5 and 8 months, observed complete formation of fibrous tissue. The study is important because it reinforces the idea that the bigger the defect, the less the possibility of obtaining a complete cicatrisation. Therefore, the aim of the osteotomy is to create an access of approximately 3 mm, in an apical direction to the lesion, by performing the smallest access osteotomy possible.

The osteotomy may be **guided** by the lesion, when a bone perforation is observed, or **non-guided**, when the cortical area is intact. In the latter case, one must assess the thickness of the bone tissue and the root anatomy to make it easier to locate the apex by means of two coordinates. One of them is horizontal and passes through the apexes of the neighboring teeth (mesial and distal areas); the length of the root will be verified in the radiograph and by means of a statistical arithmetic mean (for example: root length verified on the periapical radiograph – 20 mm/mean between 18 and 20 mm = 19 mm). The second coordinate is the extension of the longitudinal axis of the root. The apex of the tooth will be approximately where the two coordinates cross.

The osteotomy preparation technique is as follows: *by cutting* (using chisels) (Fig. 2.VIII-36), *by grinding* (drills) and *mixed* (by using both techniques). The aim of the cutting technique is to reduce the cortical-apical distance of the tooth and using the chip of bone tissue removed for a possible graft

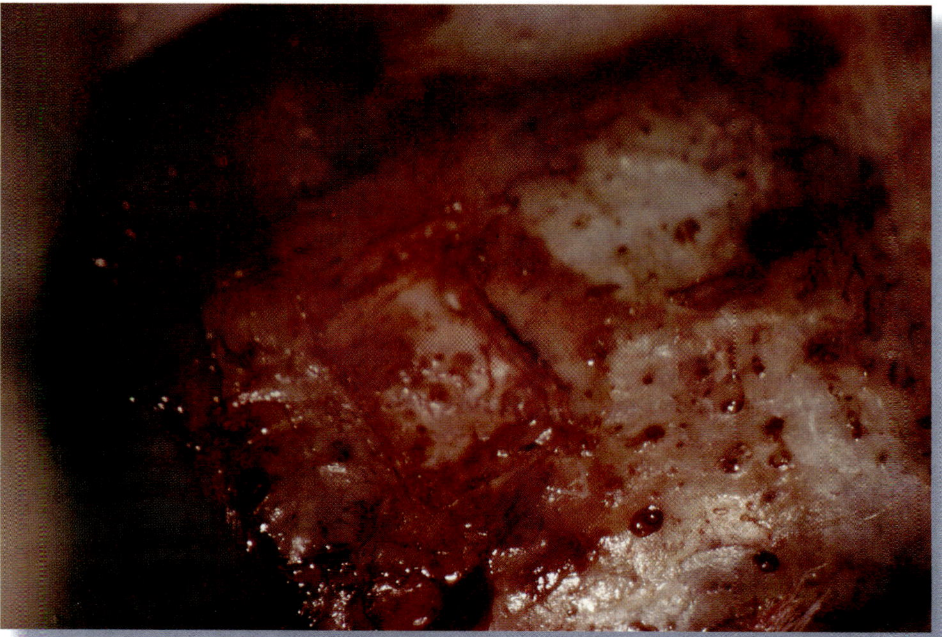

FIG. 2.VIII-36

Surgical view showing the osteotomy by cutting with a chisel.

in the region or in other areas (for example, in a small periodontal defect). Other authors have used the removed bone tissue to obliterate the surgical recess created during surgery.

In extreme cases, it may be easier to identify the root surface with the use of a microscope, because of the greater magnification and illumination, which show the following characteristics of the root: the absence of blood flow and a different bone tissue color, surrounded by periodontal space. With the surgical microscope, the mean ocular magnification ranges from 8 to 12x; magnifications of 16x are rarely used. Furthermore, it is necessary to have a wide visible field that allows good guidance and view of the operating field. Location of the apex and osteotomy are two closely connected stages and are frequently performed at the same time.

The osteotomy can be divided into:

1. access to the apical third;
2. showing evidence of the apical third (Fig. 2.VIII-37);
3. shape of the access;
4. adequate shape for better access;
5. guidance of the operating field (especially for posterior areas).

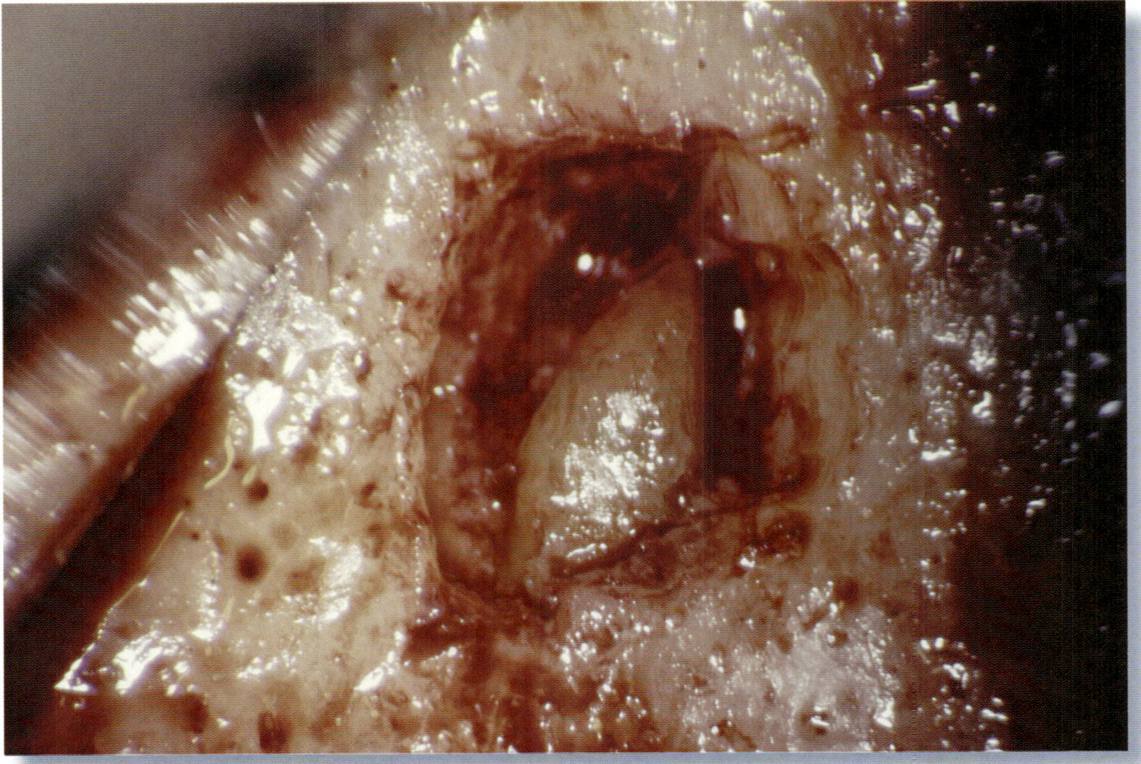

FIG. 2.VIII-37

Surgical view showing perforation and exposure of the apical third.

4. Apiectomy

After creating the access in the apical third, it is necessary to evaluate how much root tissue must be removed.

The anatomic premise is that the apical 5 mm constitute the critical zone of endodontic therapy, due to the presence of lateral canals, which are the main causes of endodontic treatment and re-treatment failures. The rule, however, cannot be considered absolute, because one cannot state that the apical 5 mm must always be resected.

There are many factors that can Influence an apiectomy:

a. **The root canal filling level:** retrograde filling must be performed in a canal that has already been prepared and filled. After cutting 3 mm and preparing a 3 mm-deep cavity it is possible to treat the apical 6 mm. If there is an untreated root canal portion remaining, one must evaluate the coronal-root proportion before the apiectomy.
b. **The level of cut of the root:** each level of cut corresponds to a different anatomy. This means that the apiectomy must be performed two times: first 1 to 2 mm of the apex must be removed; this is followed by a second cut to obtain a better anatomical shape of the apiectomy.
c. **The presence of pre-fabricated posts and cores:** cutting the posts is a purely theoretical idea. In the event the apical area is invaded, one must:
    - limit the cut to a minimum;
    - create a groove around the cores, which must be filled with Cavity-type material.

The aim of the strategy is to prevent micromovement of the core.

One concludes that for apiectomy, we must evaluate:

- the length of the cut between 2 and 3 mm;
- the slope of the cut ≤ 10 degrees;
- the total resection;
- the smoothness of the cut surface.

After apex resection, there is a series of important steps to be performed, preliminary to the following stage; that is, preparation and sealing of the new apex:

- *biopsy:* with the aim of providing the patient with a histological diagnosis as well as providing the dentist with a better prognosis in the process of cicatrisation.
- *curettage*: after the apicectomy, there is a better view for endodontic instrument control. It is necessary to make a radiographic evaluation in order to verify the anatomic structures that may have been injured during the procedure. Special attention should be paid to the mandibular canal and maxillary sinus.

Mandibular Canal

The possibility of damaging the mandibular canal and particularly the terminal portions of the canal, such as the mental foramen, arises in most cases from operative errors.

At this diagnostic stage, the coronal-root proportion should be evaluated; frequently done by using computerized tomography. In cases of close proximity to the mandibular canal, the osteotomy should be performed as far away from the nerve as possible, at all times when removing bone tissue using an operating microscope. Curettage is a very dangerous phase, especially when there is no sufficient opening (presence of a periapical cyst) or a subtle bone wall between the nerve and lesion. We have to locate the foramen through the exit opening of the mental foramen, and eventually protect it with the tip of a separator.

In reality, as the nerve could be injured with the separator when it is placed on the ramification of the nerve, a groove can be created over the mandibular canal or foramen, to help to support the tip of the separator (Kim & Kratchman[15], 2006).

Maxillary Sinus

Surgery on maxillary posterior tooth, frequently cause perforations of the maxillary sinus membrane. In these cases, it is very important to prevent foreign bodies and bacteria from entering the maxillary sinus. Irrespective of the size, the perforation should always be eliminated or closed before proceeding with the endodontic surgery stage. A very simple and safe technique is the one in which there is buffering with calcium sulphate (Surgiplaster P30, Ghimas, Casalecchio di Reno, Italy). The material can be introduced into the maxillary sinus without causing inflammation or obstructive problems in the ostium; furthermore, it stimulates the formation of bone tissue due to its osteoconductive capability. It is totally resorbable and, in particular, quickly induces a mechanical barrier, which prevents the foreign matter from penetrating into the maxillary sinus.

d. **Decontamination of the exposed root surface:** tetracycline in a saturated solution (250 mg in 5 cc of saline solution at 37°C) is the solution of choice, because it is technically easy, presents no side effects and has a prolonged action.

The characteristics of tetracycline are:

- it is powerful bactericidal (at high concentrations);
- is substantial (it has a prolonged effect on the root surface);
- has anti-collagenase properties;
- has anti-inflammatory properties;

- increases fibroblasts bonding;
- diminishes osteoclastic activity.

e. **Hemostasis:** it is easily performed with calcium sulphate (Surgiplaster P30, GHIMAS, Casalecchio di Reno, Italy), which should be placed on the bone ridge in the form of paste and kept in place with the aid of sterile gauze (TNT); it quickly produces efficient hemostasis and can remain in the cavity because it is totally resorbable and biocompatible.

f. **Evaluation of the cut surface** (Fig. 2.VIII-38): the use of biological markers, such as 2% methylene blue, is very useful. By combining the illumination of the microscope and a micromirror, evaluation with 12 to 16x magnification is a very accurate procedure. Our observation takes into consideration the following aspects:

    - root canal filling quality;
    - number of foramina in the endodontic system (Fig. 2.VIII-39);
    - non-treated root canals;
    - microfractures (Fig. 2.VIII-40);
    - vertical cracks;
    - lateral canals;
    - presence of an isthmus (Fig. 2.VIII-41);
    - presence of pre-fabricated posts and cores;
    - total to be sectioned.

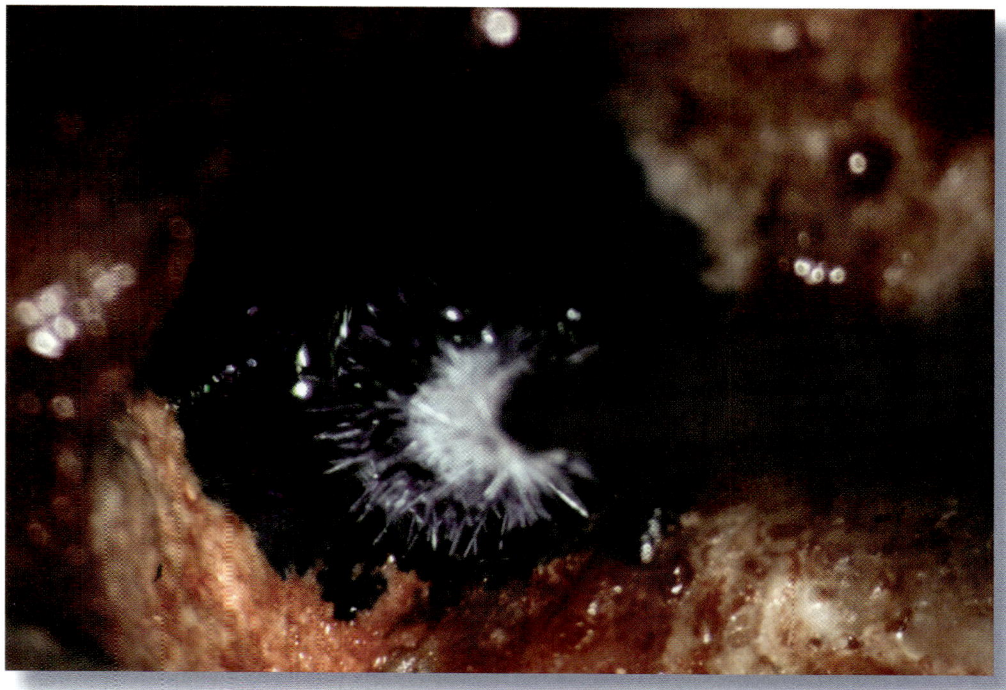

FIG. 2.VIII-38
Surgical view showing methylene blue applied to the root surface with a microbrush.

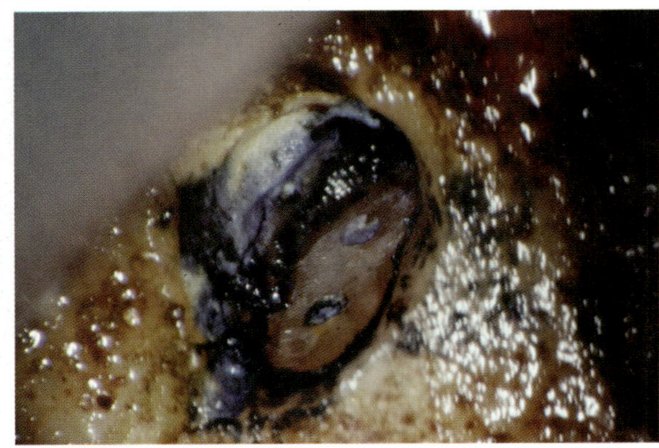

FIG. 2.VIII-39

Surgical view showing the presence of foraminas. Cut area at 12X magnification.

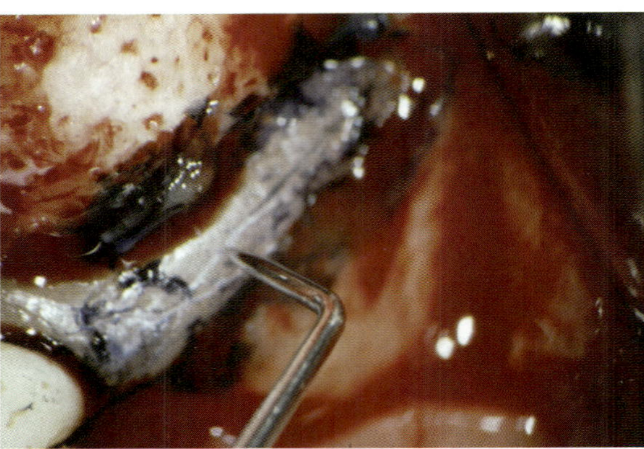

FIG. 2.VIII-40

Microfracture, methylene blue at 10X magnification.

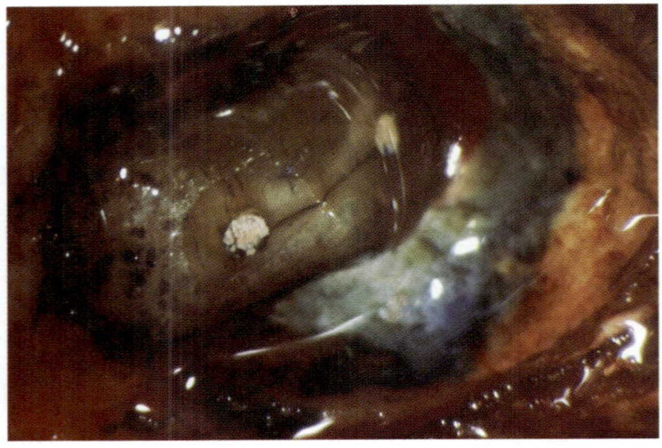

FIG. 2.VIII-41

Isthmus at 16X magnification.

Particularly when assessing fractures, it may be necessary to use an intraoral light source. Frequently the cut surface must be irrigated with a sterile saline solution and inspected with the aid of a micromirror.

Therefore, the ideal condition for evaluating the cut surface can be summarized as follows:

- correct cutting, with regard to both its totality and inclination;
- the possibility of performing another cut or grinding if necessary;
- shown with methylene blue or transillumination;
- adequate microinstruments for surface probing.

Two very important steps accompany preparation:

1. **Cavity drying:** this step frequently precedes cavity control, even before the filling material is applied. The surface must be dry to facilitate visualization and perfect adaptation of the filling material to the root surface. The Strokpo-method irrigation, a cannula that adapts to an irrigation syringe, is very useful for irrigation and air-drying the cavity, due to its good fit and precise dimensions.
   Many filling materials provide good sealing, even in the presence of moisture; however, the best adaptation takes place in dry cavities. In addition to this, it is not possible to dry the cavity in the presence of oozing. The surgical microscope and the micromirror enable correct visualization of a dry cavity (Fig. 2.VIII-42). However, after the last irrigation with sterile saline and tetracycline, at magnifications of 10 to 16x or 20 to 30x with Strokpo irrigation, one can achieve an optimum level of cavity drying. This method of irrigation consists of a syringe

with micro needles without cutting ends, with a 0.5 mm diameter. Although paper points are often used in this procedure, they are less efficient and practical, demanding a great deal of time and do not produce the same results as those obtained with aspiration.

2. **Cavity control with micromirrors:** one of the main causes of surgical therapy failure is the presence of filling material residue from the root canal, or materials that contaminate the buccal wall of the cavity. This should be very carefully noted when polishing the cut root section and during cavity preparation (Figs. 2.VIII-43 and 2.VIII-44).

   The use of points with proper curvature (Back Action Ultrasonic Tip) and the correct usage of condensers for gutta-percha, together with good illumination and correct magnification, provide more favorable conditions for sealing the retrograde filling.

We shall consider the following points:

- wall polishing;
- absence of blood;
- cavity depth;
- regularity of the margins and parallelism of the walls (Fig. 2.VIII-45);
- complete perforation;
- absence of microfractures.

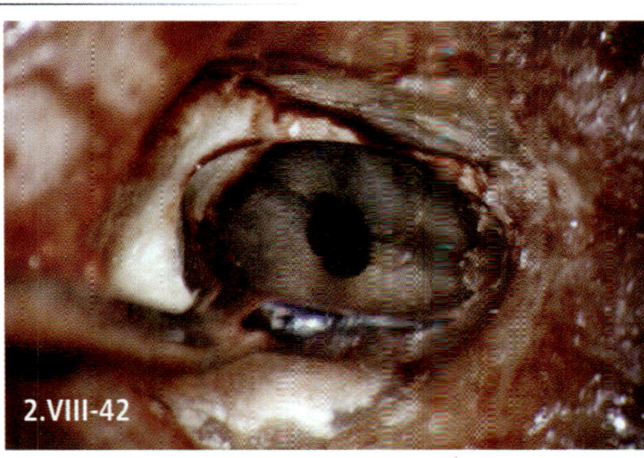

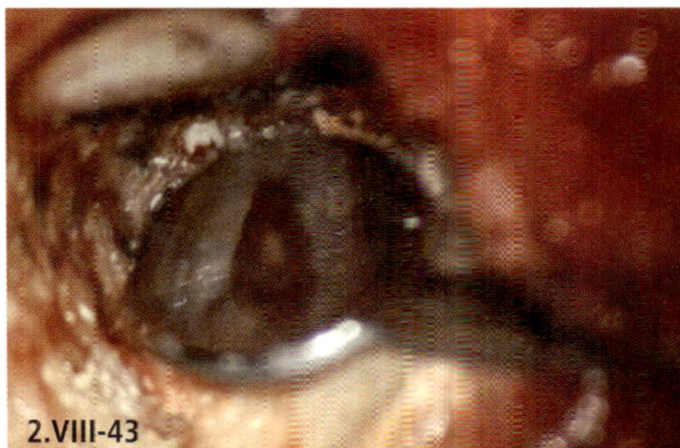

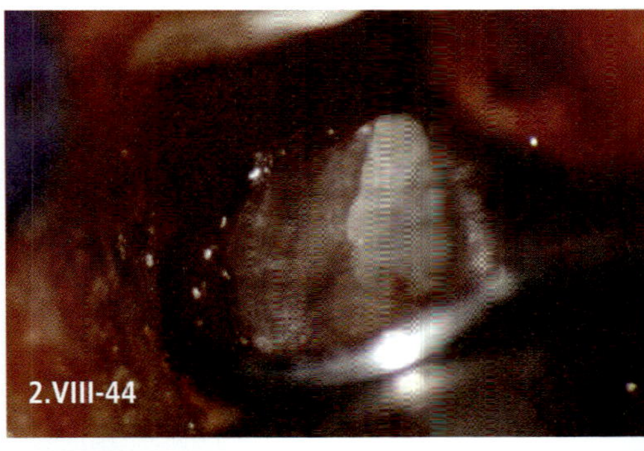

FIG. 2.VIII-42

Cavity visualization with micromirrors.

FIG. 2.VIII-43

Micromirror at 16X magnification.

FIG. 2.VIII-44

Retrograde filling at 22X magnification, and check-up with micromirror.

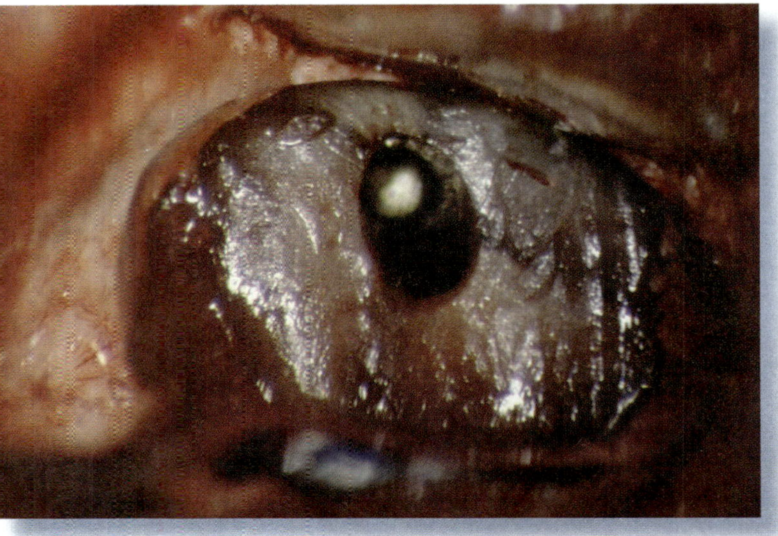

FIG. 2.VIII-45

Visualization of a post with a micromirror at 26X magnification.

Control of the above must be verified at higher magnifications – 20 to 30x – and with the aid of micro mirrors; without this equipment it is impossible to evaluate polishing of the cavity. These instuments are available in different shapes, sizes and qualities; they easily enter the bone crypt, allowing one to obtain a 45° inclination and optimum cavity visualization.

5. Cavity Preparation for Retrograde Filling

The following characteristics should be observed:

- inclusion of all apical foraminas and isthmus preparation, should they be present (Fig. 2.VIII-46);
- obtain a cross section, as small as possible (the smaller the filling surface, the lower the potential leakage);
- adequate root canal wall thickness;
- minimum depth of 3 mm;
- polished walls and as axial as possible (Pecora et al.[25], 1998) (Fig. 2.VIII-47).

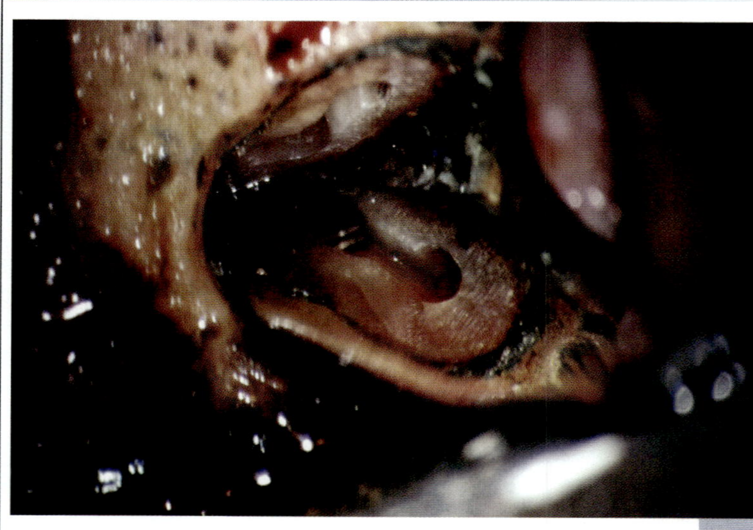

FIG. 2.VIII-46
Surgical view showing perforation of the isthmus.

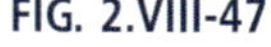

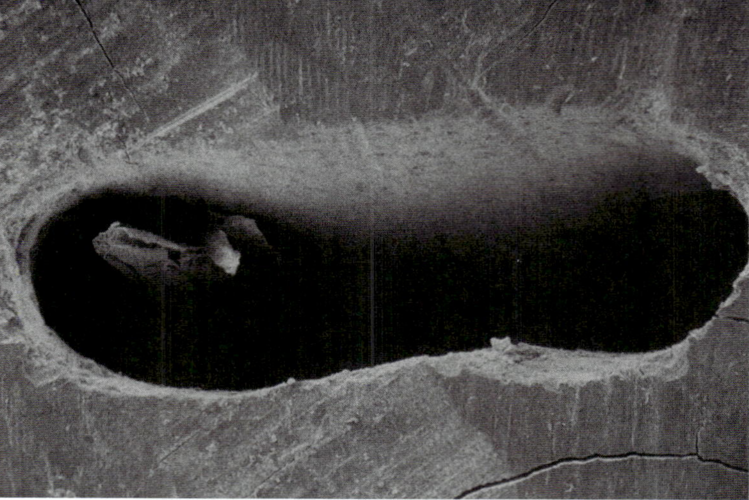

FIG. 2.VIII-47
Visualization of retropreparation as shown by scanning electron microscopy (preparation with ultrasound tips).

There is no doubt that the use of ultrasound activated instruments in cavity preparation for retrograde surgery in the apex represents a technical revolution that opens new horizons for endodontic surgery. The following observations cab be presented:

- the use of ultrasonic tips is extremely safe; the danger of perforating is minimal, whether due to the the type of axial preparation or due to the minimum pressure required for action of the points. The instrument tip is very easily inserted into the opening of the canal and into the filling when compacted into the dentin (Fig. 2.VIII-48);
- It is very easy to prepare the isthmus; all that is needed is to clearly identify the cut surface with a measuring device, possibly producing a small groove that serves to guide the tip;
- the irrigation tip should be ample and accurately directed onto the tip of the instrument; without proper irrigation, the instrument produces a smear layer and a heated zone, which can possibly burn the dentin. Therefore, copious irrigation is very important;
- the polished wall provides a better flow of the filling material at the bottom of the cavity, assuring its complete filling;

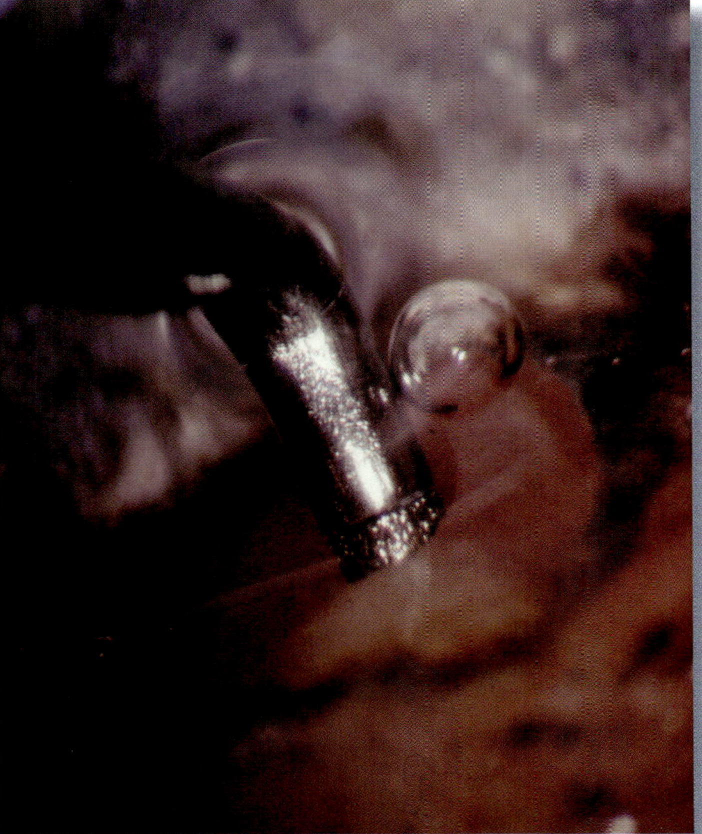

FIG. 2.VIII-48

Surgical view showing the perforation and cavity of the retropreparation at 26X magnification.

- when there is a preparation on the core, the points must make a groove around the post, which will then be cut with a spherical diamond tip at high speed, if possible.
- in some cases, in which soft tissue adhered to the root and prevented the precise limits of the lingual wall of the cavity, the tip is used to perform root curettage;
- in cases in which the presence of an unprepared canal was detected after the apex had been cut, very fine tips were used to assess the depth of the canal. Then a blunt tip was used to widen the preparation; This prevents possible complications or damage due to excessive pressure during the use of the tips;
- minor difficulties were found when polishing the buccal angle of preparations, due to the presence of gutta-percha; it was necessary to change the tip in order to find one that had an acute angulation.

The use of a surgical microscope and appropriate points allows the cavity to be prepared for retrograde filling in a very similar way to the cavity today considered ideal. In short, the advantages of using these instruments are:

1. preparation of small cavities, preserving apical dentin and preventing reduction or even wall fracture;
2. the use of ultrasound allows one to obtain a better polished wall;
3. The isthmus and foramens can be easily prepared, which would be virtually impossible with micro-contra-angles and tips that used to be available before the introduction of ultrasound;
4. access is easier than that possible with a micro contra-angle;
5. less operator effort and fatigue, due to greater safety during preparation;
6. unlike preparations made with burs, these tips allow an apical preparation to be parallel to the long axis of the root;
7. the less pressure, the more efficient the cutting action at the tip of the apex, thus allowing delicate refinement of the preparation.

6. Retrograde filling

According to studies on the anatomy of the endodontic system (very important in this connection are those conducted by Hess), the concept of "hermetic" filling in the surgical neo-apex is conditioned by a satisfactory root system filling, which is obtained conventionally. When one relies solely on the retrograde sealing of a canal that has not been debrided or filled, it is known that the long term result will not be satisfactory, because no material is capable of providing sealing that is really impermeable to bacterial fluids. The possibility of debriding and filling the canal by means of a neo-apex with a retrograde filling is part of what we call "acrobatic surgery", thus the quality of the result is very limited. Filling and hermetic sealing are conditioned to the type of the apex cut and to the type of the cavity preparation.

There is no broad consensus in the literature about what the best materials for retrograde filling are, which can be explained by the inadequate methodology used to evaluate these materials, usually carried out *in vitro*. Starting from the presupposition that although a retrograde filling is not completely hermetic, we have to accept the materials that have the best properties for this purpose. It is important to emphasize some anatomical and clinical data which are incontrovertible points of reference.

By reducing the apex cutting angle to 0 degree, we obtain a smaller cut surface, as well as less exposure of dentinal tubules and a smaller section of foramen or foramina. The less the leakage through the tubules, the smaller the circumference of the filling. The 3 mm depth allows better closing with all filling material used. Another interesting point of information is that in 1 mm deep cavities, sealing by filling material is significantly reduced. Therefore, in cavities 3 mm or more deep, the materials are equivalent, and the degree of sealing depends on the effectiveness of the filling material in the presence of moisture.

Suitable instruments are selected according to the cavity, while the assistant prepares the filling material. The various stages can be summed up as follows:

- material selection;
- mixing of material;
- insertion into the cavity;
- condensation (Fig. 2.VIII-49);
- shaping;
- filling refinement (Fig. 2.VIII-50);
- check-up.

The most frequently used materials are Super EBA and Mineral Trioxide Aggregate (MTA), which present different setting characteristics, but result in excellent sealing, even in a moist environment.

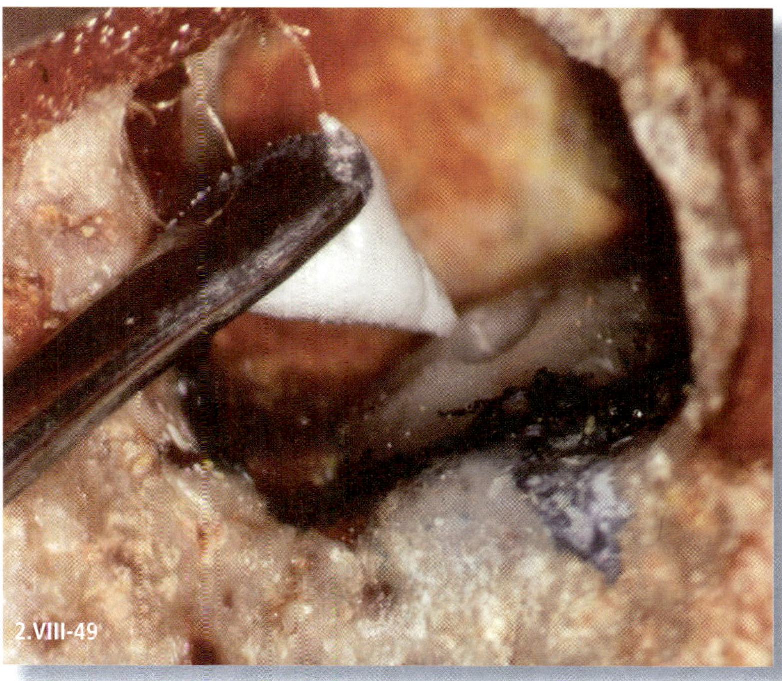
2.VIII-49

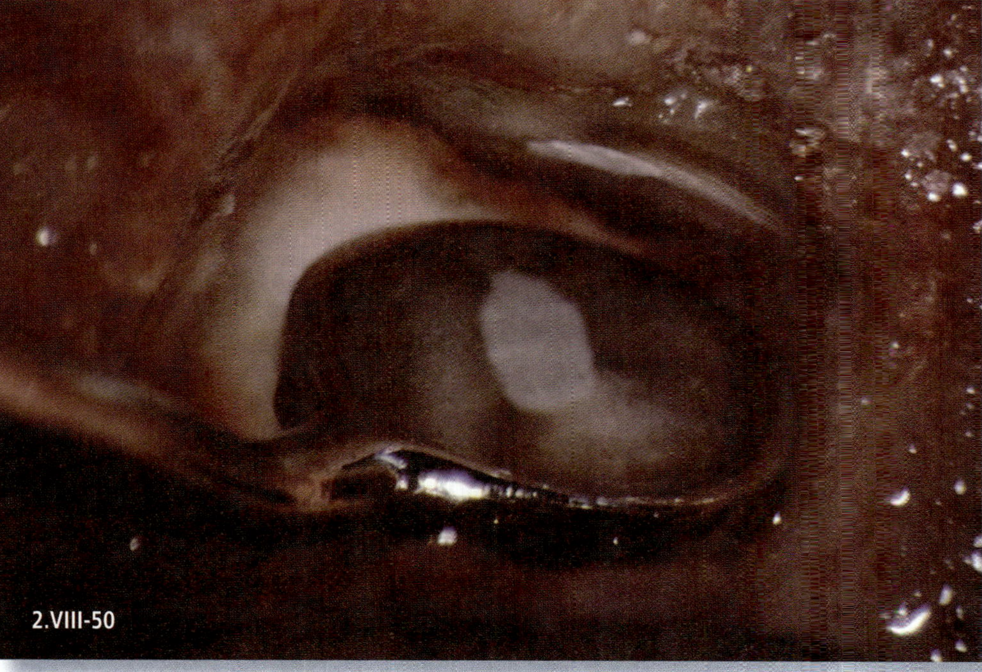
2.VIII-50

FIG. 2.VIII-49

Surgical view showing retrofilling with Superseal (OGNA, Milan – Italy).

FIG. 2.VIII-50

Retro-filling check with micromirror at 22X magnification.

7. Evaluation of Guided Tissue Regeneration (GTR)

The evaluation as to whether or not GTR is required should be simplified and planned. The indications are established according to clinical protocols found in the literature:

- large lesions that cover the entire root surface (Kellert et al.[14], 1994; Pecora et al.[30], 1995);
- bicortical lesions (Pecora et al.[26], 2001);
- endo-periodontal lesions (Duggings et al.[8], 1994; Pecora et al.[27], 2005).

With regard to suitable techniques and materials for GTR, there is no precise guide, because individual situations, different experiences and multidisciplinary aspects should be considered and each situation evaluated separately (Pecora et al.[23], 1997; De Leonardis et al.[7], 1999). According to our experience, we recommend the use of an osteoconductive, biocompatible and resorbable material that can be used in contaminated areas i.e. Surgiplaster (Ghimas, Casalecchio di Reno, Italy). The simplicity of use, predictability, low cost and suitability in a variety of clinical applications make it very useful in periradicular surgery.

8. Radiographic Postoperative Check-up

Under normal conditions, a radiographic postoperative check-up must be done at the following time intervals: initial (time 0), 1, 3, 6 and 12 months after surgery. In cases of cysts, a check-up should continue during the second and third consecutive years. Radiographs should always be taken with the aid of a radiographic long cone technique (Rinn), to allow for a better imaging and comparison of the images obtained.

9. Suture

Patients are almost always concerned about the esthetic aspect. Since microsurgical techniques allow microsutures to be performed, scars are almost imperceptible. The flap design and the use of 5.0 and 6.0 monofilament suture threads, allow the suture to be removed after 48 to 72 hours post-surgery, without leaving extensive scars (Figs. 2.VIII-51 and 2.VIII-52).

The papilla base incision technique (PBI – *papilla base incision*) (Velvart[42], 2002) prevents the loss of interdental papilla height due to flap recession.

The suture should be removed with the aid of the surgical microscope, to enable better visualization of the suture thread, thus preventing traumas to the flap.

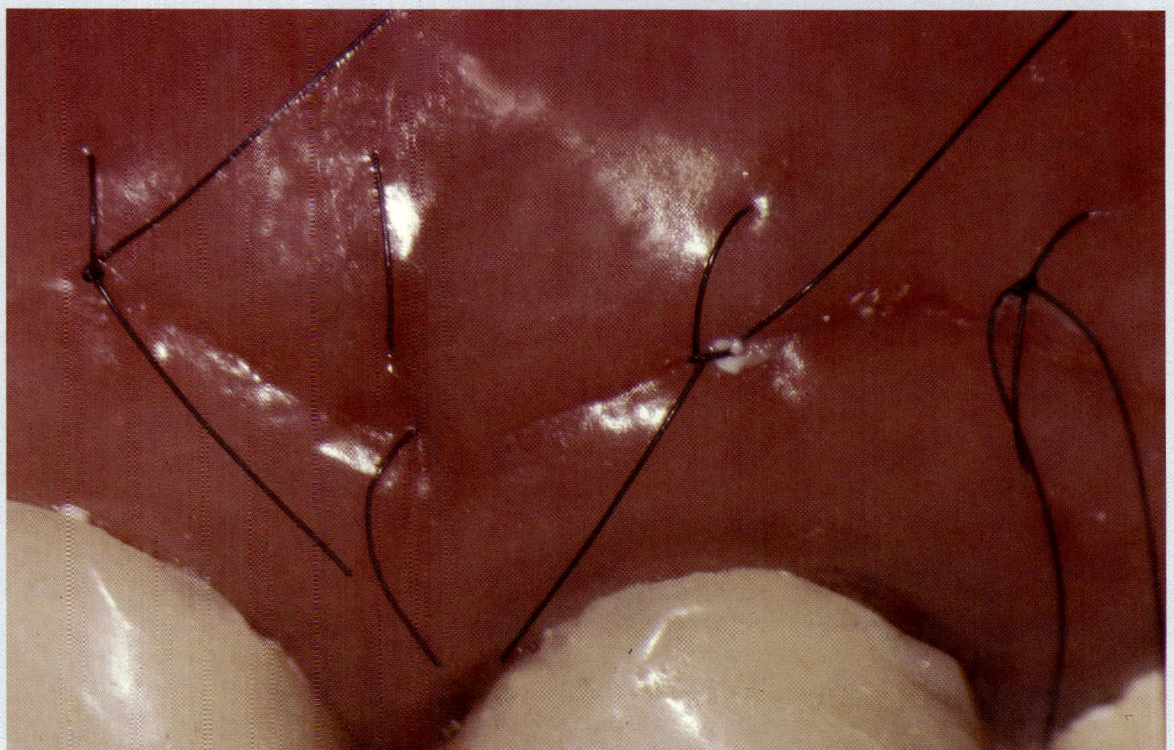

FIG. 2.VIII-51

Clinical view showing suture.

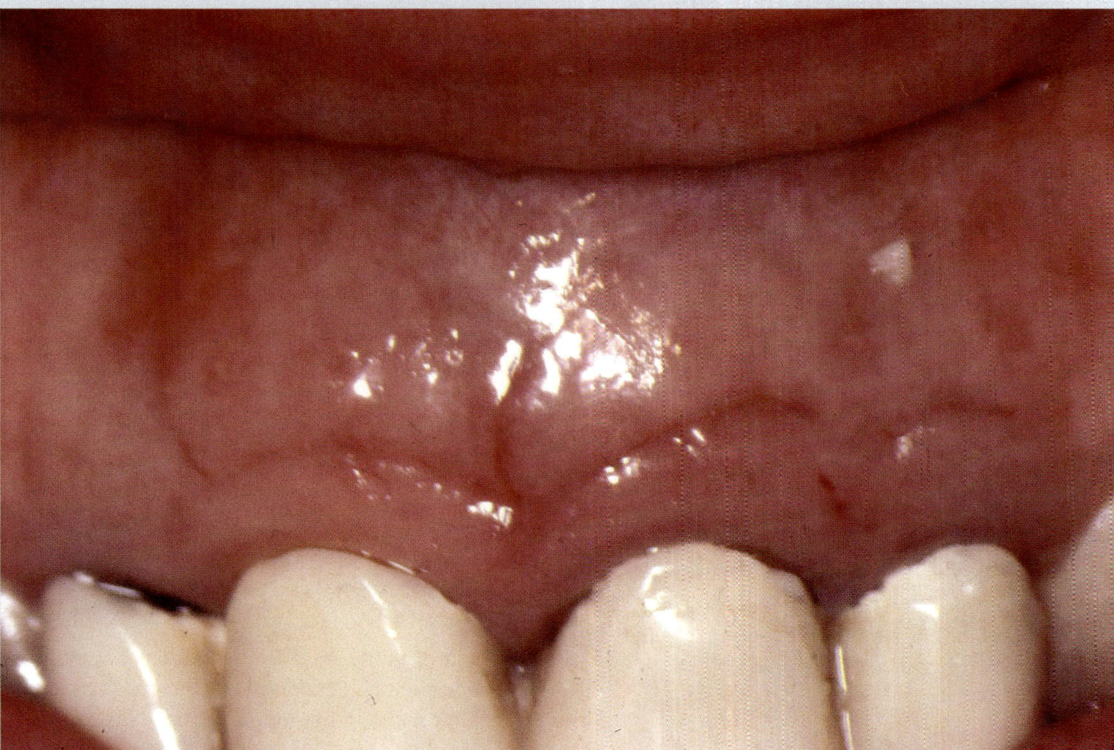

FIG. 2.VIII-52

Clinical view showing suture removal after 48 hours.

References

1. Bier SJ, Sinensky MC. The versatility of calcium sulfate: resolving periodontal challenges. Compend Contin Educ Dent, V.20, P.655-661, 1999.
2. Bonelli M, Bonetti I, de Leonardis D, Ricci J, Pecora G. L'uso del solfato di calcio in chirurgia endodontica. Trattamento delle larghe lesioni. Dental Cadmos, v.3, p.29-34, 2001.
3. Boyne P, Lyon H, Miller C. The effects of osseous implant materials on regeneration of alveolar cortex. Oral Surg Oral Med Oral Pathol, v.xx, p.369-378, 1961.
4. Carr GB. Advanced techniques and visual enhancement for endodontic surgery. Endodontic Report, p.48-51, 1992.
5. Carr GB. Microscope in endodontics. J. Californian Dental Association, p.20-55, 1992.
6. Coetzee AS. Regeneration of bone in the presence of calcium sulfate. Arch Otolaryngol, v.106, p.405-409, 1980.
7. De Leonardis D, Pecora G, Martuscelli G, Cornelini R, Andreana S. Impiego della GTR in chirurgia endodontica: studio clinico controllato. Dental Cadmos, v.1, p.31-38, 1999.
8. Duggins L, Clay J, Himel V, Dean J. A combined endodontic retrofill and periodontal guided tissue regeneration technique for repair of molar endodontic furcation perforation: a case report. Quintessence Int., v.25, p.109-114, 1994.
9. Fleszar TJ, Knowles JW, Morrison EC. et al. Tooth mobility and periodontal therapy. J Clin Periodontol, v.7, n.6, p.495-500, 1980.
10. Friedman S. et al. Treatment results of apical surgery in premolar and molar teeth Endod, v.17, p.30-33, 1991.
11. Hjroting-Hansen E, Andreasen JO. Incomplete bone healing of experimental cavities in dog mandibles. Br. J Oral Surg, v.9, p.33-40, 1971.
12. Izawa T, Kim S, Pecora G, Rubinstein R. Microscopic endodontic surgery. Quintessence, v.13, p.54-65, 1994.
13. Jastak JT, Yagiela JA. Vasoconstrictors and local anesthesia: a review and rationale for use. J Am Dent Assoc, v.107, p.623-630, 1983.
14. Kellert M, Chalfin H, Solomn C. Guided tissue regeneration: an adjunct to endodontic surgery. JADA, v.125, p.1.229-1.233, 1994.
15. Kim S, Kratchman S. Modern endodontic surgery concepts and practice: a review. JOE, v.7, n.32, p.601-623, 2006.
16. Kim S, Pecora G, Rubinstein R. Comparison of traditional and microsurgery on endodontics. In: Kim S, Pecora G, Rubinstein R, eds. Color atlas of microsurgery in endodontics. Philadelphia: W.B. Saunders, p.5-11, 2001.
17. Kim S, Rethnam S. Hemostasis in endodontic microsurgery. Dent. Clin. North America, v.41, p.499-511, 1997.
18. Leonardo MR. Endodontia: tratamento de canais radiculares – princípios técnicos e biológicos. 1.ª ed. São Paulo: Artes Médicas, 2006, 2v., 1.491 p.
19. Loe H. The gingival index, the plaque index, and the retention index systems. J Periodontol, v.38, p.610-616, 1967.
20. Orsini G, Ricci J, Scarano A, Pecora G, Petrone G, Lezzi G, Piattelli A. Bone defect healing with calcium sulfate particles and cement: an experimental study in rabbits. J. Biomed. Mat. Res. Post B: Appl Biomat, v.68B, p.199-208, 2004.
21. Pecora G, Andreana S. Use of dental operative microscope in endodontic surgery. Oral Surg Oral Med Oral Pathol, v.75 p.751-759, 1993.
22. Pecora G, Andreana S, Margarone JE. et al. Bone regeneration with a calcium sulfate barrier. Oral Surg Oral Med Oral Pathol Oral Radiol Endod, v.84, p.424-429, 1997.
23. Pecora G, Beek SH, Retnan S, Kim S. Barrier membrane techniques in endodontic microsurgery. Dental Clinics of North America, v.3, p.585-601, 1997.
24. Pecora G, Covani U, Giardino L, Rubinstein R. Valutazioni clinico-statistiche sull'uso dello stereo-microscopio in odontoiatria. RIS, v.8, p.425-431, 1993.
25. Pecora G, De Leonardis D, Fabi M, Meledandri R, Lattanzi U. Profondità della preparazione e sigillo del neoapice. Dental Cadmos, v.15, p.11-16, 1998.
26. Pecora G, De Leonardis D, Ibrahim N, Bovi M, Cornelini R. The use of calcium sulfate in the surgical treatment of a through and through lesion. Int Endod J, v.34, p.189-197, 2001.
27. Pecora G, De Leonardis D, Piattelli A. L'uso della microchirurgia endodontica da sola o associata all'innesto di solfato di calcio nel trattamento di lesioni endo-parodontali. Studio clinico controllato. Giornale Italiano di Endodonzia,(logo abaixo – 31 – a palavra aparece grafada com s) v.1, n.19, p.42-49, 2005.
28. Pecora G, De Leonardis D, Rubinstein R, Meledandri R, Lattanzi U. Preparazione apicale con utrasuoni. Dental Cadmos, v.16, p.49-56, 1998.
29. Pecora G, Kim S. Advanced endodontic microsurgery. Scientific Session IV American Association of Endodontis, 54th Annual Session; Seattle, May 7-10, 1997.
30. Pecora G, Kim S, Celletti R, Davarpanah M. The guided tissue regeneration principles in endodontic surgery: one year post-operative results of large periapical lesions. Int Endod J, v.28, p.41-46, 1995.
31. Pecora G, Rubinstein, R Giardino L, De Leonardis D. Il solfato di calcio nelle tecniche rigenerative in endodoncia.(ver 27) Rome: Elite Service, p.119-164, 2001.
32. Piattelli A, Orsini G, De Leonardis D, Scarano A, Lezzi G, Spoto G, Strocchi R, Pecora G. Il solfato di calcio nella rigenerazione ossea. Dental Cadmos, v.10, p.1-5, 2002.
33. Reuben HL, Apotherker H. Apical surgery with the dental microscope. Oral Surg Oral Med Oral Pathol, v.4, p.433-435, 1984.
34. Rubinstein R, Kim S. Short-term observation of the results of endodontic surgery and the use of a surgical operating microscope and Super EBA as root-end filling material. Endod, v.25, p.1, 1999.
35. Rubinstein R, Kim S. Long-term follow up of cases healed one year after apical microsurgery. J Endod, v.28, p.6, 2002.
36. Rud J, Andreasen JO, Moller Jensen JE. A multivariate analysis of various factors upon healing after endodontic surgery. Int J Oral Surg, v.1, p.258-271, 1972.
37. Scipioni A, Bruschi GB. Tecniche midificate (?) di apicectomia e otturazione retrograde. Riv. Amici di Brugg, v.2, p.59-66, 1989.
38. Scipioni A, Bruschi, GB. Uso dello stereomicroscopio in endodonzia (s ou z?) chirurgica. Gio It Endod, p.48-51, 1991.
39. Silness J, Loe H. Periodontal disease in pregnancy. Correlation between oral hygiene and periodontal conditions. Acta Odont Scand, v.22, p.121-135, 1964.
40. Skoglund A, Persson G. A follow up study of apicoectomized teeth with total loss of the buccal plate. Oral Surg Oral Med Oral Pathol, v.59, p.78-81, 1985.
41. Sottosanti JS. Calcium sulfate aided bone regeneration: a case report. Periodont. Clin Invest, v.17, p.10-15, 1995.
42. Velvart P. Papilla base incision: a new approach to recession-free healing of the interdental papilla after endodontic surgery. Int Endod J, v.35, p.453-480, 2002.
43. Witherspoon DE, Gutmann JL. Hemostasis in periradicular surgery. Int Endod J, v.29, p.135-149, 1996.

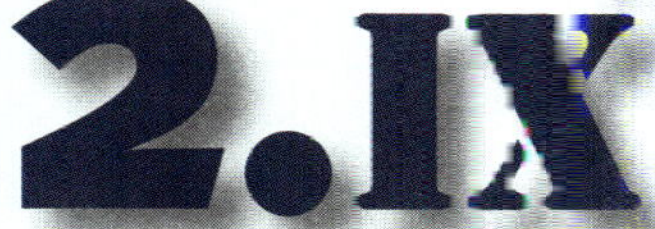

Use of calcium hydroxide (Calen paste) as a topical medication between sessions (temporary dressing)

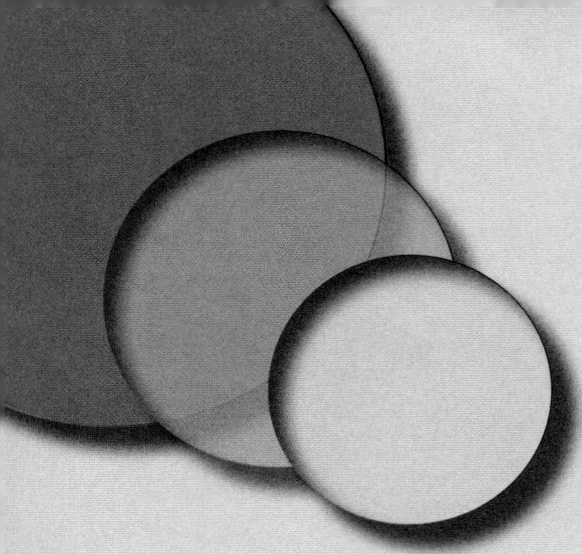

Raquel Assed Bezerra da Silva
Lea Assed Bezerra da Silva
Paulo Nelson-Filho

At present, Endodontics is going through a stage of one of the greatest technological-scientific advancements in all its history, justifying the specialty. The new methods of treating root canals, applying the crown/apex principle, the manufacturing of new endodontic instruments, particularly those made of nickel-titanium alloy of the motor-driven type, the use of electronic apex locators, new root canal filling materials and systems and the use of operative and surgical microscopes, coupled with the extensive clinical experience of outstanding professionals, have advanced Endodontics considerably.

Nevertheless, it is not admissible for a dentist to apply these up-to-date materials and techniques in daily practice unsupported by **scientific evidence**. Health professionals should not neglect the biological principles that are the basis of present-day endodontics and should not consider these principles outdated or banished.

At present two types of concepts of endodontics can be identified: *essentially technical endodontics (technologists) and endodontics based on biological concepts (bio-technologists).* Technical endodontics is based on materials and advanced treatment techniques. For example the use of instruments developed from knowledge in engineering, particularly in metallurgy. Biological endodontics is based on basic disciplines, such as histology, pathology, immunology, microbiology and molecular biology, among others, to support clinical practice.

Obviously, as health professionals, we must use all the recourses that can be transformed into benefits for the patients. Thus, the two types of concepts of endodontics, with the same objectives, are useful in clinical practice and must be used simultaneously: technical endodontics, because it provides the patient with a comfortable, painless, fast and anatomically better performed treatment; biological endodontics, because it considers the patient's health, reduces apical periodontitis, as well as the intensity of acuteness and retreatments, and raises the status of the specialty.

Therefore, at the conclusion of endodontic treatment, the dentist must be aware that the absence of post-operative pain alone is not the determining factor of the success of the therapy, as the lack of clinical symptoms is not the only indicator of success. It cannot be disputed that continuation of the lesion, or even post-treatment partial radiographic repair means a persistence of the infection in the root canal system or at the surface of the external apical root. This will prevent repair and is associated with a persistent chronic periapical inflammatory infiltrate and areas of cement and bone resorption.

In view of the above discussion, during the endodontic treatment of primary and permanent teeth with pulp necrosis and radiographically evident chronic periapical lesion (apical periodontitis), the practitioner should bear in mind that regardless whether the therapy is technological, biological or mixed, it will only be effective when it is successful from a clinical, radiographical but above all, a histological point of view. The treatment techniques that result in success based on the three above mentioned parameters should be used in clinical practice.

TEETH WITH PULP NECROSIS AND CHRONIC PERIAPICAL LESION (APICAL PERIODONTITIS): ENDODONTIC TREATMENT IN A SINGLE SESSION OR IN TWO SESSIONS?

A chronic periapical lesion or apical periodontitis is a chronic inflammatory condition of the periapical tissues, caused by etiologic agents of endodontic origin (Fig. 2.IX-1). This process can persist when root canal treatment does not adequately eliminate the microbial infection.

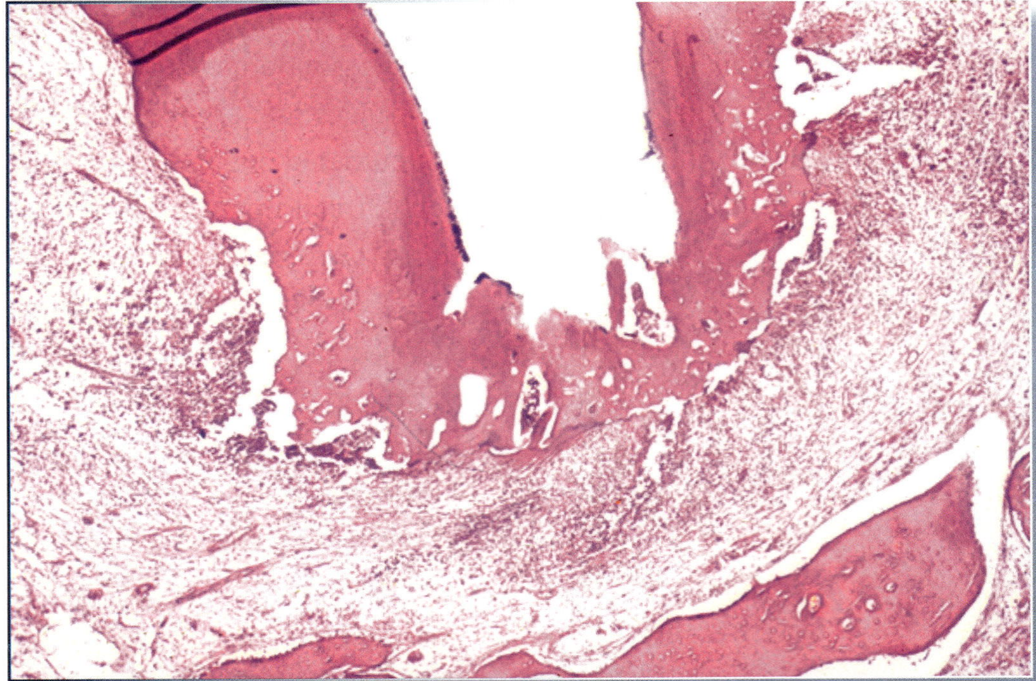

FIG. 2.IX-1

Histological section of the apical region of a dog's tooth with pulp necrosis and chronic periapical lesion, showing evidence of intense inflammatory infiltrate, areas of cement resorption and extensive bone resorption.

Among the problems that cause the persistence of apical periodontitis are the following: Inadequate control of asepsis, unsatisfactory coronal opening, inadequate instrumentation, coronal leakage via the restoration and persistence of infection in the root canal system, and extraradicular infection[106].

In the pertinent literature, different opinions are expressed with respect to the number of sessions required for endodontic treatment of teeth with pulp necrosis and chronic periapical lesion as well as the need to use *a temporary dressing between sessions*.

Based on studies limited to clinical and radiographic evaluations, some authors believe that the success rate is similar for a single session treatment (without the use of a temporary dressing) and two session treatment (using calcium hydroxide as the temporary dressing)[86,98,121]. Other authors have reported that clinical and radiographic success is significantly greater when a temporary dressing is used between sessions[71,74,153].

It should be pointed out that more studies observed no difference between treatments in a single or in two sessions in which the dressing remained in place for a period of only 7 days. According to Nerwich *et al.*[109] (1993) this time is considered insufficient for calcium hydroxide to diffuse through dentinal tubules, apical cementum and accessory/collateral canals. The temporary dressing should be kept in place for a minimum of 14 days, in order to have an effect[57,76].

The literature also reports conflicting results with respect to postoperative pain and *flare-ups* (chronic periapical pathological processes that developed into an acute flare-up). For some, the use of the temporary dressing is not significant[6,86], while for others it reduces post-operative pain and the occurrence of *flare-ups to an insignificant extent* [184].

In a systematic review of the literature published in 2008, Sathorn et al.[133] concluded that there is lack of evidence indicating significant differences in postoperative pain and *flare-ups* between root canal treatment performed in a single or in multiple sessions. According to Lin et al.[87] (2007), further randomized clinical studies are necessary.

As previously pointed out, treatment cannot be considered successful if it is evaluated only from a clinical and radiographic point of view. It is necessary to prove efficacy of treatment by means of histological techniques.

Katebzadeh et al.[68] (1999) induced periapical lesions in dog's teeth and made a histological comparison between treatment in a single session and treatment using a temporary dressing with calcium hydroxide. After 6 months the results demonstrated that the use of the antimicrobial temporary dressing resulted in significantly less periapical inflammation.

Holland et al.[57] (2003) evaluated histologically the repair process after endodontic treatment in a single session, or in two sessions, using a calcium hydroxide based dressing for 7 or 14 days. They concluded that the use of a temporary dressing for 14 days between sessions offered the best results.

In 2006, Leonardo et al.[76] conducted a histological study of periapical repair in dogs comparing endodontically treated teeth with periapical lesions in a single session or in two sessions. They used Calen paste as temporary dressing for 15 days and the results of this study demonstrated that it is indispensable (Figs. 2.IX-2A-D and 2.IX-3A-D), and that the repair in the periapical region was significantly better when the temporary dressing was used between sessions. The histological results of the single session treatment were unsatisfactory.

In a recent study, Silveira et al.[149] (2007) did a histological evaluation of the response of apical and periapical tissues of dog's teeth with pulp necrosis and periapical lesion induced by *Enterococcus faecalis*, after root canal treatment in a single or in two sessions (using a calcium hydroxide-based temporary dressing). After 6 months of follow-up, they showed 46% success in teeth treated in a single session, and 74% success with the use of the temporary dressing. The

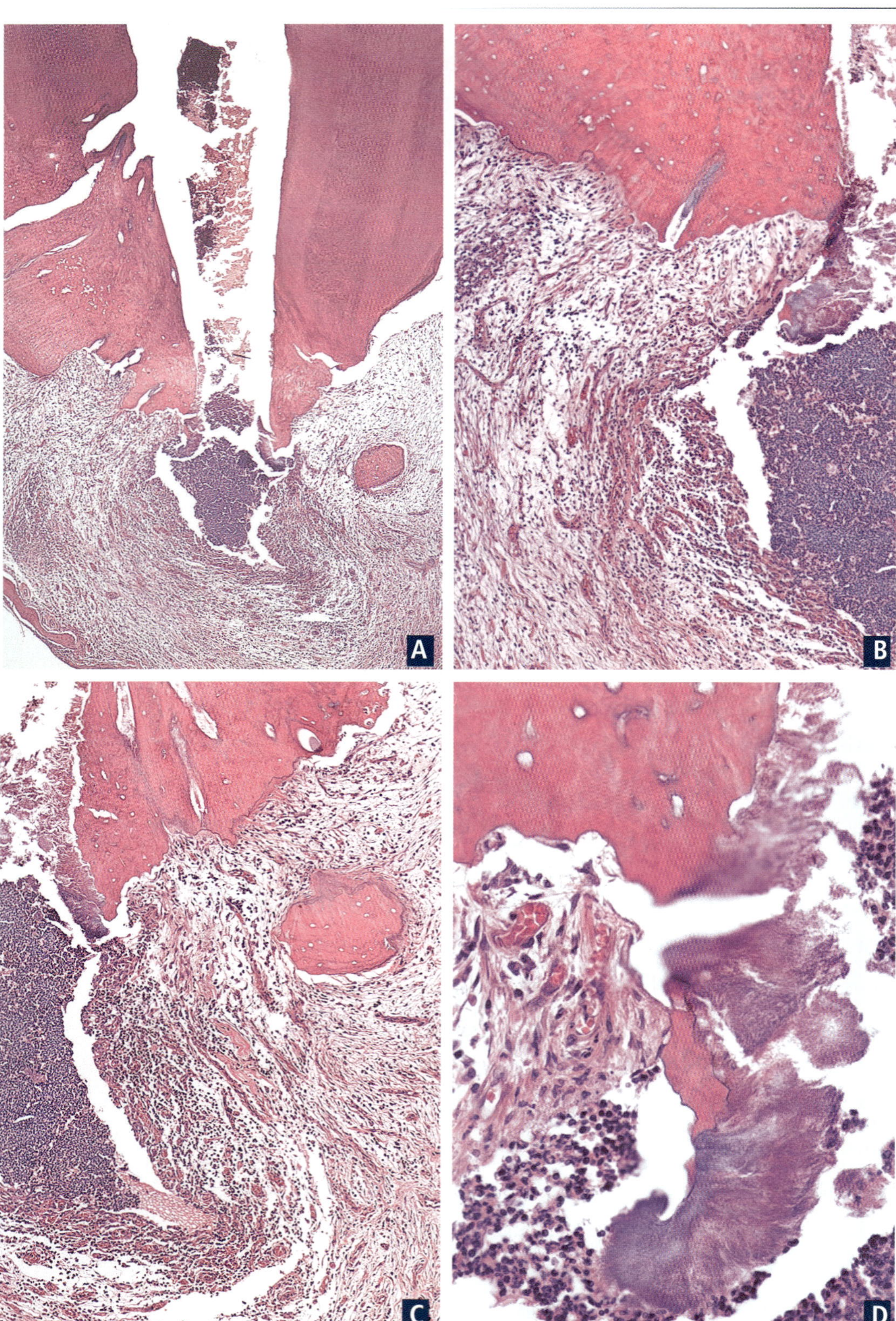

FIGS. 2.IX-2A-D

A – Histological panoramic view of the root apex and periodontal ligament of a dog's tooth with pulp necrosis and chronic periapical lesion, showing evidence of severe inflammatory infiltrate, absence of fibers in the periodontal ligament and extensive area of bone resorption. (H&E – 24X). B and C – Detail of the previous figure, showing an abscess next to the foraminal opening and areas of cement resorption. (H&E – 40X). D – Necrotic remnants and microorganisms at the root apex. (H&E.100X).

results of this study demonstrated that, using histology as a parameter, the use of a temporary dressing offered significantly higher success rates.

TEETH WITH PULP NECROSIS AND CHRONIC PERIAPICAL LESION (APICAL PERIODONTITIS): WHY IS THE TEMPORARY DRESSING NECESSARY?

Irrespective of the number of sessions, specific bacteriological control of the root canal system is critical for the success of endodontic therapy. Although the treatment may fail due to multiple factors, including perforations, transportation through the foramen, failures in instrumentation and/or filling (incorrect working length, use of unsuitable irrigation solutions, use of irritating sealer cements or sealers that allow considerable leakage, etc.), coronal leakage via the restorative material, vertical root fractures, presence of foreign bodies and low resistance of the host, among others, the primary etiology of failure after endodontic treatment is the refractory bacterial infection present in the root canal system[66,86,99,105].

Currently it is acknowledged that even after biomechanical preparation of teeth with pulp necrosis (gangrene) and chronic periapical lesion, bacteria may persist in the ramifications of the canal, in the exposed dentinal tubules, in the gaps of the cellular cement and in the apical foramen; that is, removed from the open space of the root canal. Therefore, there is the possibility that the techniques that are routinely used during endodontic treatment do not totally eliminate bacteria; in particular, the oxygen-sensitive bacteria may survive and consequently maintain the infectious process, with repercussions on the periapical tissues[47,169,173]. The low percentage of success observed in the evaluation of cases of pulp necrosis and chronic periapical lesions [29,71,94,154,170] to some extent confirms this.

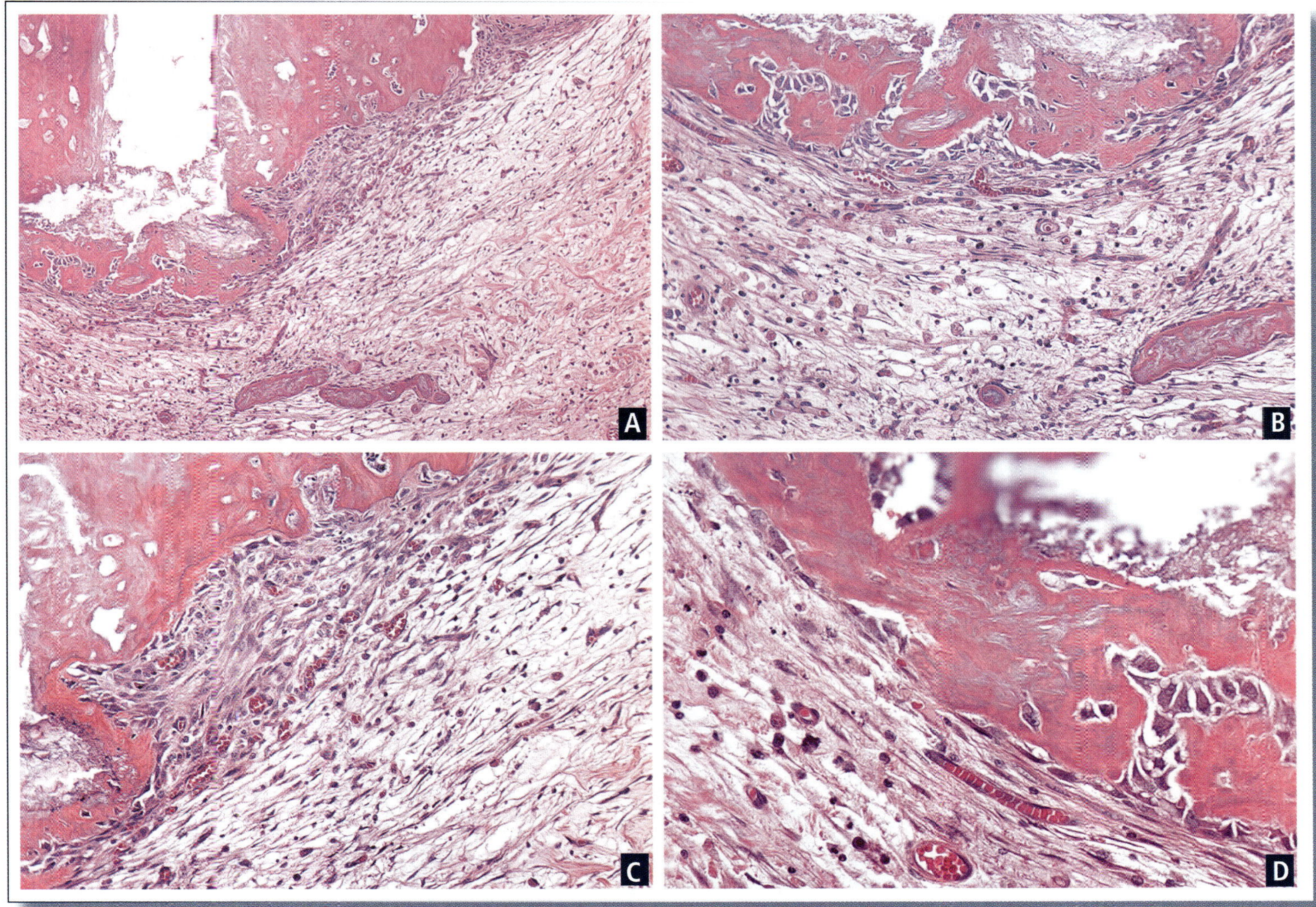

FIGS. 2.IX-3A-D

Histological section of the apical region of dog's tooth with pulp necrosis and chronic periapical lesion, after biomechanical preparation and temporary dressing with Calen paste. A – Apical and periapical region show mild presence of inflammatory cells in the periodontal ligament and newly formed mineralized tissue deposition at the foraminal opening (H&E – 40X). B – Periodontal ligament in a developmental stage of repair (H&E – 64X). C and D – Newly formed fibrous barrier, with high concentration of cells. External to it, note the matrix, collagenous fibers and blood vessels (H&E –100 and 200X).

In order for repair to occur in teeth with periapical lesions, it is important to control/eliminate the microorganisms present in the root canal system, before the are filled[153]. It is the opinion of the authors of this chapter that this objective is not reached when treatment is performed in a single session, since it is not possible to control the infection located beyond the main root canal (the endodontist's field of action) without the use of an antimicrobial temporary dressing between sessions.

As a result of the advances that have taken place, particularly in the microbial culture and molecular biology techniques, numerous studies have demonstrated that the infection in primary and permanent teeth with pulp necrosis and periapical lesion is polymicrobial, with a predominance of anaerobic microorganisms[1,71,115,120,129,138,148,151,152,157,161], particularly the Gram-negative types[7,163].

The polymicrobial infection is located not only in the open space of the root canal and dentinal tubules, but also in the gaps in the cement, apical craters and throughout the entire root canal system[71,139,165]. Moreover, it is present in the external areas of the root surface (apical biofilm) and in the periapical lesion, areas also inaccessible to biomechanical preparation[77,78,127] (Figs. 2.IX-4A-D).

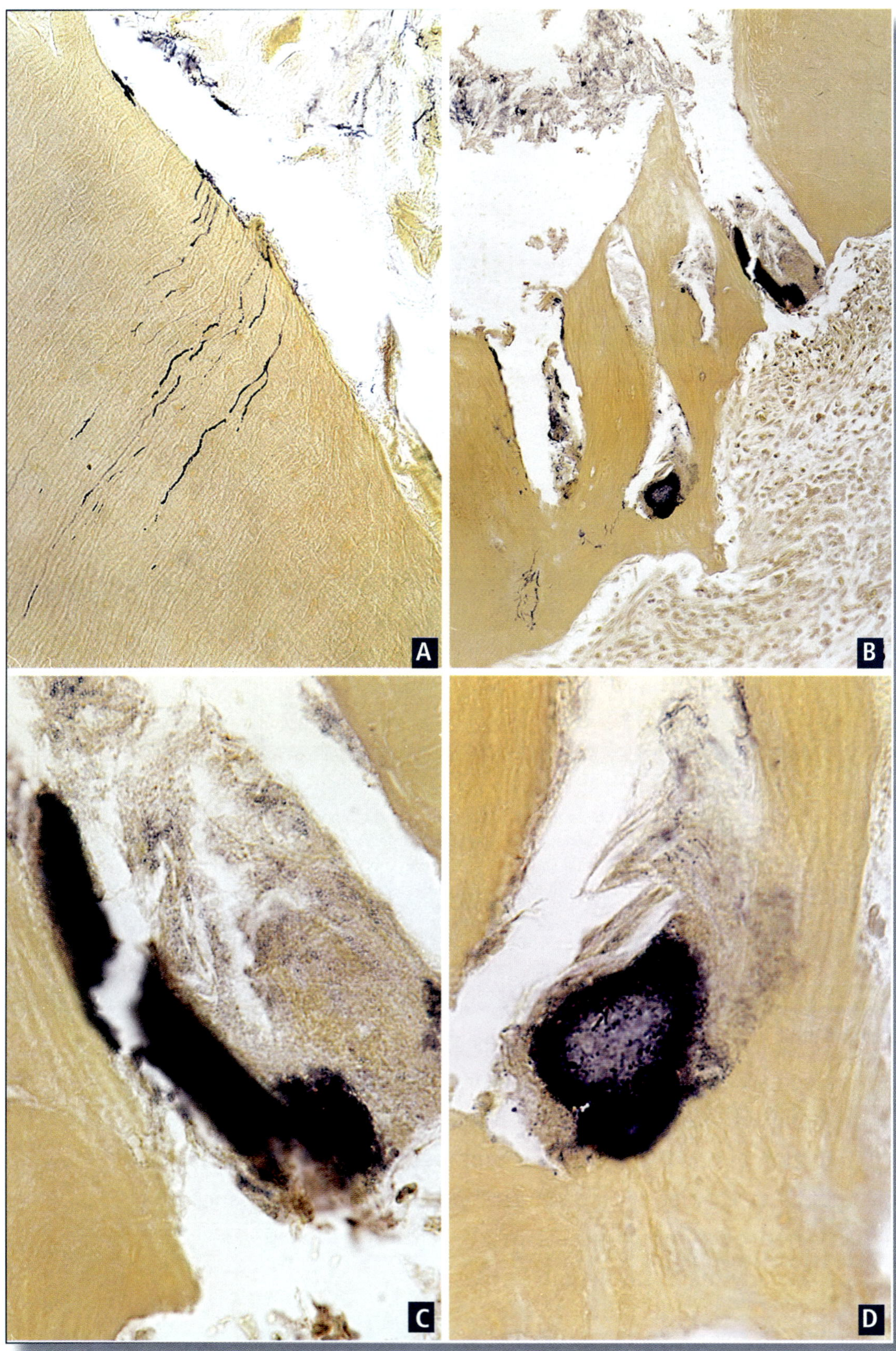

FIGS. 2.IX-4A-D

Dog's teeth with pulp necrosis and chronic periapical lesion. A – Dentinal tubules with large number of microorganisms (Brown & Brenn 40X). B – Apical region with innumerable aggregates of microorganisms in the lumen of the main root canal and in the ramification of the apical delta (Brown & Brenn 100X). B and C – Detail of the previous figure, showing evidence of large number of microorganisms (Brown & Brenn 400X). D – Large number of microorganisms in the ramifications of the apical delta (Brown & Brenn 400X).

The predominance of Gram-negative anaerobic bacteria, the high concentration of bacterial endotoxins and their implications in the apical and periapical regions that determine the appearance of cement erosions that constitute veritable craters in which microorganisms are lodged that are protected by bacterial biofilm[78,127](Figs. 2.IX-5A-F), are the main causes of endodontic therapy failure.

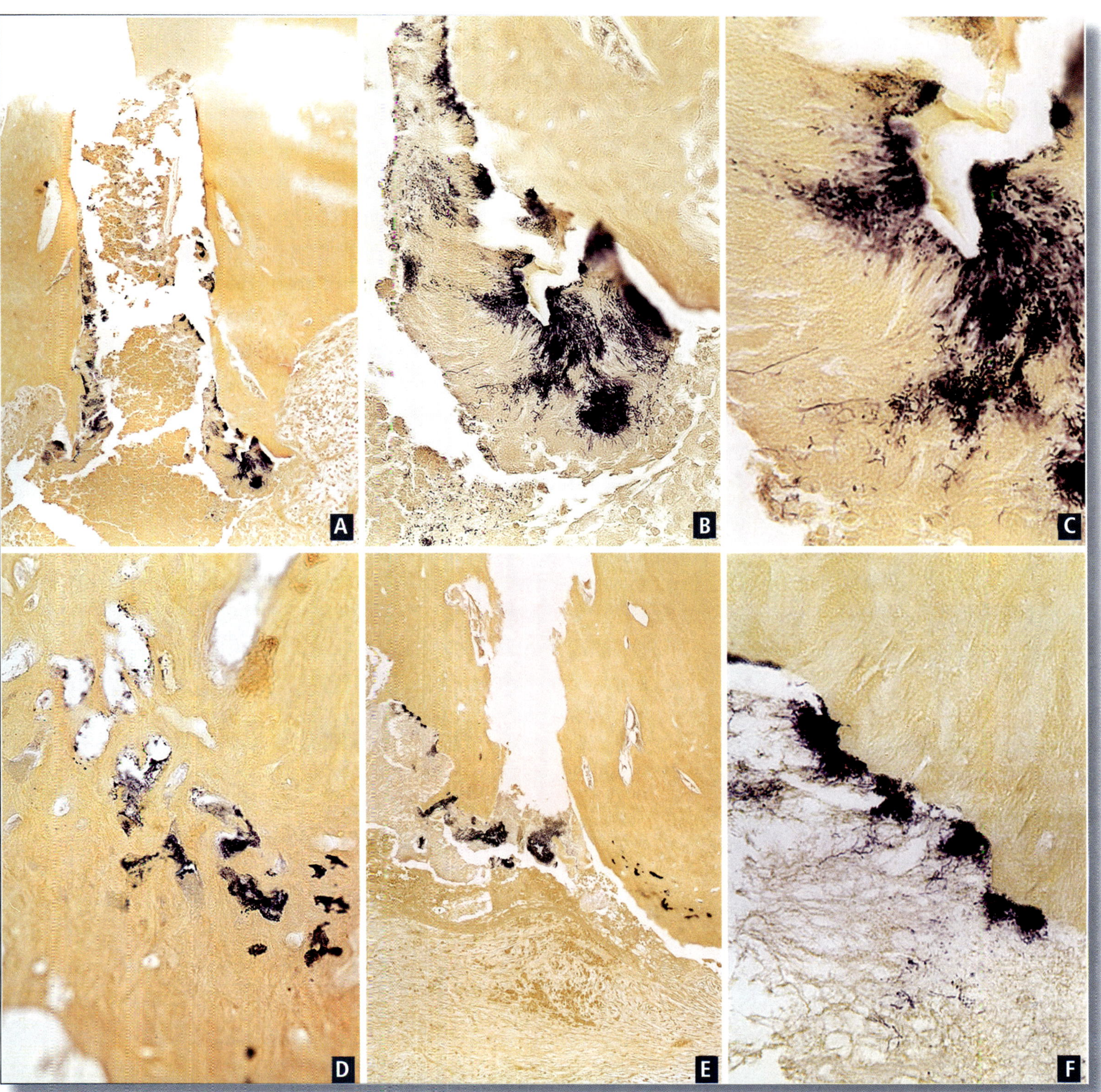

FIGS. 2.IX-5A-F

Dog's tooth with pulp necrosis and chronic periapical lesion. A – Histological section of apical and periapical region with aggregates of microorganisms in the lumen and on the walls of the root canal, extending into the periapical region (Brown & Brenn 60X). B – Bacterial biofilm formed on the apical cementum (Brown & Brenn 100X). C – Higher magnification of the previous figure, showing evidence of innumerable microbial morphotypes (cocci, bacillus and filamentous types) (Brown & Brenn 400X). D – Presence of cocci and bacillus in gaps in the cementum (Brown & Brenn 100X). E – Microorganisms in the form of biofilm in the apical region (Brown & Brenn 60X). Higher magnification of the Apical Biofilm observed in the previous figure (Brown & Brenn 200X).

In addition to having different virulence factors and generating products and by-products that are toxic to the apical and periapical tissues, the cell walls of these Gram-negative microorganisms contain endotoxin[126]. This knowledge is particularly important, as endotoxin, also known as lipopolysaccharide or LPS, is released during multiplication or after death of the bacteria, causing a series of significant biological events[10,97]. These events lead to an inflammatory reaction[126,146], followed by cement and bone resorption[64,108,160,180], contributing to the genesis, development or persistence of a chronic periapical lesion (Figs. 2.IX-6A-B).

Furthermore, LPS acts as a powerful stimulator of nitric oxide production (NO)[14,16], which is involved in the periapical bone resorption process[162] and plays a fundamental role in the regulation of periapical inflammatory reactions, associated with other cytokines[49].

The LPS of live or dead bacteria, whole or in fragments, acting on macrophages[126], neutrophils[101] and fibroblasts[24], sets off the release of a large number of chemical, bioactive inflammatory mediators or cytokines[97], such as interleukins and TNF[9,15,27,96,97,122], involved in the development, maintenance and repair of periapical lesions[159].

LPS also activates the Hageman factor (factor XII of the coagulation cascade), has a lethal effect on animals[97], induces fever[59], activates the complement system[21,59,100] acting in events of the inflammatory response such as the increase in vascular permeability. It also activates neutrophil and macrophage chemotaxis, lysozyme and lymphokine release[100], activates the cycle of arachidonic acid metabolism [21,97], is mytogenic for lymphocytes B[97] and causes degranulation of mastocytes[58]. In infected root canals, according to Seltzer & Farber[138] (1994), endotoxin can contribute to a rise in the release of vasoactive and neurotransmitter substances in the region of the periapical tissue nerve endings, leading to the occurrence of pain.

In addition to causing an inflammatory reaction, LPS adheres to the mineralized tissues, acting as a powerful stimulant of bone resorption[135,180], promoting the synthesis and release of osteoclast activating cytokines[64,67,130,175], causing osteoclastogenesis[64]. According to Torabinejad et al.[168] (1985), the products of arachidonic acid metabolism and activation of the complement system play an important role in bone resorption that presents itself in human teeth with periapical lesions.

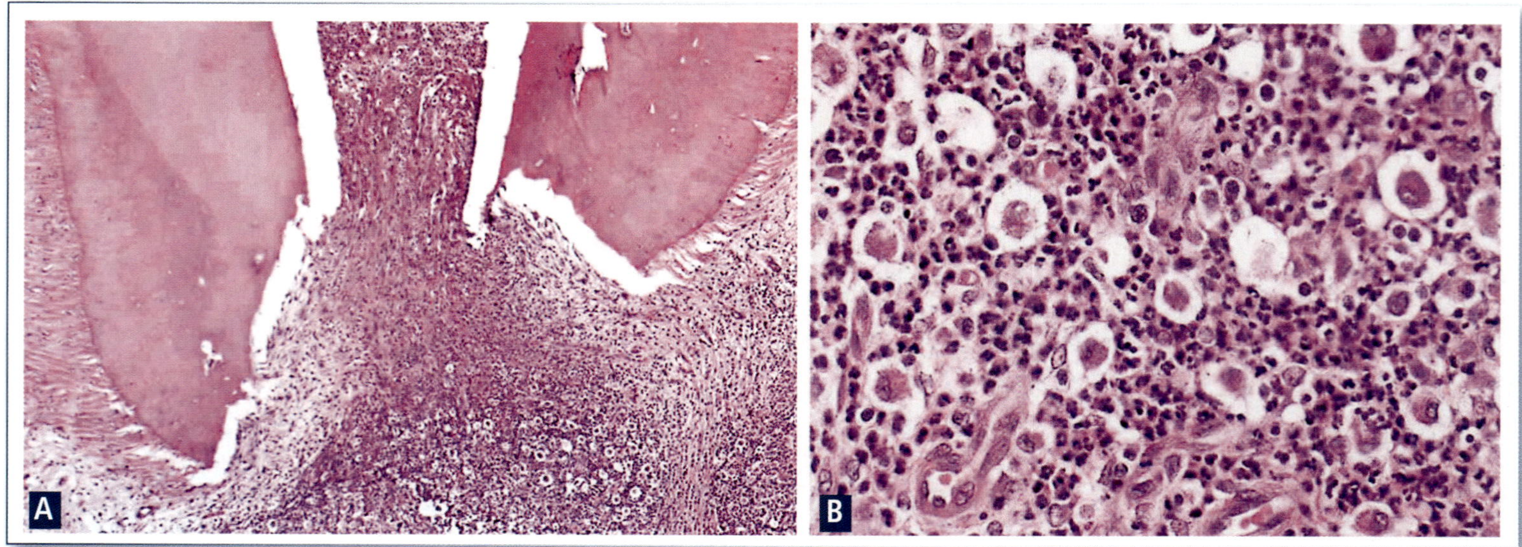

FIGS. 2.IX-6A-B

Histological section of apex of dog's tooth 30 days after biopulpectomy and root canal filling with bacterial endotoxin (LPS) solution. A – Bone resorption and intense inflammatory infiltrate in the interstitial tissue and periapical region. Cement resorption with absence of cementoblasts (H&E.20X). B – Detail of previous figure. Concentration of mixed inflammatory infiltrate with predominance of macrophages. Considerable dissociation of collagenous fibers (H&E –128X).

TEMPORARY DRESSING BETWEEN SESSIONS: IS IT IMPORTANT TO INACTIVATE BACTERIAL ENDOTOXIN (LPS) DURING ENDODONTIC TREATMENT OF TEETH WITH PULP NECROSIS AND PERIAPICAL LESION (APICAL PERIODONTITIS)?

From the above discussion, the important role LPS plays in the pathogenesis of periapical lesions is unquestionable. Therefore, currently, in root canal treatment of teeth with pulp necrosis and chronic periapical lesions called by us as necropulpectomy II, the professional's major goal must not only be to kill bacteria, but to inactivate endotoxins as well [71,141]. Martinho and Gomes[95] (2008) observed in a clinical study the presence of microorganisms and LPS in 100% of the root canals of teeth with pulp necrosis and periapical lesion, with elevated levels in symptomatic teeth.

The literature has reported studies that have been conducting investigations of medications or substances that inactivate the bacterial endotoxins present in teeth that present pathological changes to eliminate their biologically toxic potential. Using different experimental models, the following products were tested for this purpose: caustic soda[30,110], polymixin B[114], neutrophilic enzymes[101], formocresol[132], chlorhexidine[113] and sodium hypochlorite solutions in concentrations ranging from 0.58 to 5.25%[19,95,113,164], without significant results.

Nevertheless, *in vitro* and *in vivo* studies have revealed that calcium hydroxide as a temporary dressing between sessions is capable of inactivating bacterial LPS [10,64,108,113,114,130,146,164] (Figs. 2.IX-7A-B and 2.IX-8A-B), which even further reinforces and justifies the indication of this material. This knowledge has revolutionized the concepts with regard to temporary dressings between sessions, pointing towards calcium hydroxide as the most ideal medication up to now, capable of promoting LPS inactivation[71,81,141], without causing complications in tissue repair.

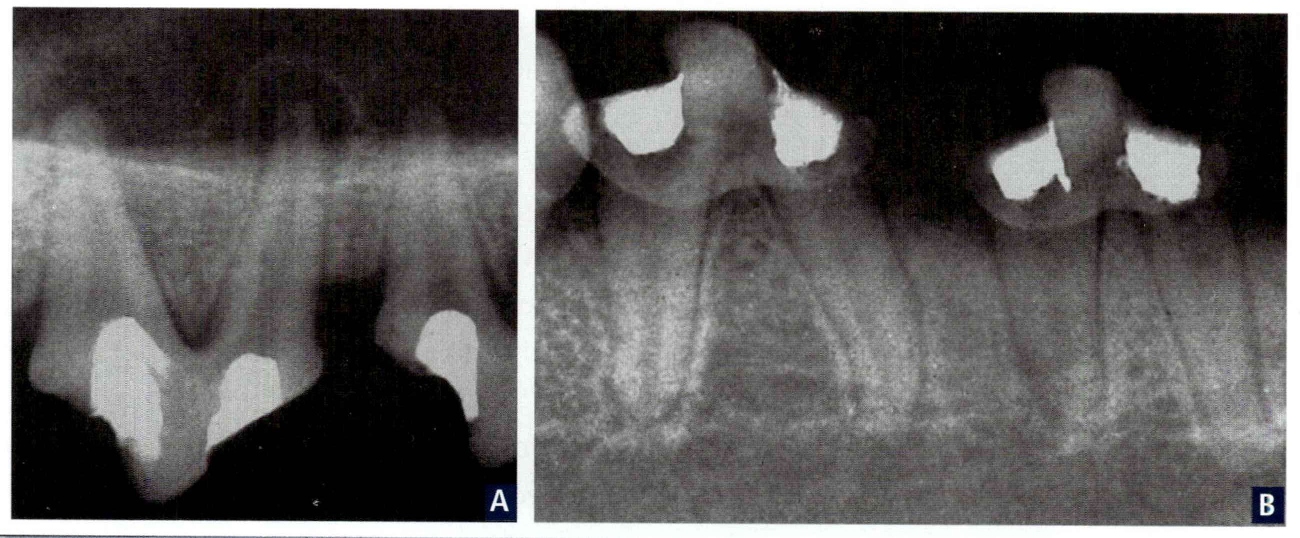

FIGS. 2.IX-7A-B

A – Periapical radiograph, 30 days after biopulpectomy and root canal filling of a dog's tooth with bacterial endotoxin (LPS). Radiolucent image suggestive of chronic periapical lesion. B – Periapical radiograph, 30 days after biopulpectomy and root canal filling with (LPS) associated with calcium hydroxide. Aspect of normal appearance in the apical and periapical regions.

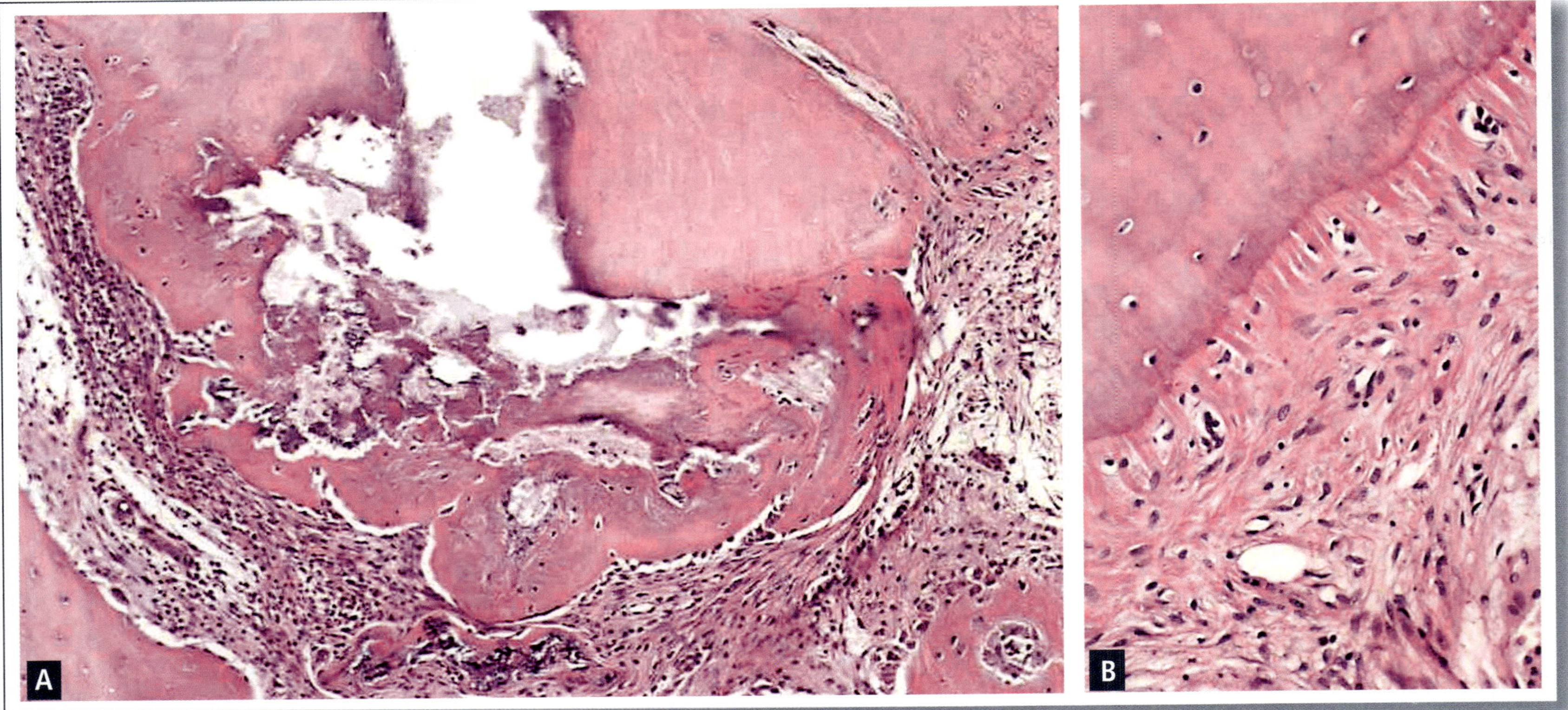

FIGS. 2.IX-8A-B

A – Histological section of dog's tooth 30 days after pulpectomy and root canal filling with (LPS) associated with calcium hydroxide. Panoramic view of root apex showing evidence of mineralized tissue formation surrounding the foraminal opening. Normal periodontal ligament (H&E – 25X). B – Dog's tooth 30 days after pulpectomy and root canal filling with (LPS) associated with calcium hydroxide. Apical cement region with absence of resorption. Normal periodontal ligament (H&E – 80X).

JUSTIFICATIONS FOR THE CHOICE OF CALCIUM HYDROXIDE AS TOPICAL MEDICATION BETWEEN SESSIONS (TEMPORARY DRESSING)

At present, the emphasis in endodontics is to seek medicaments that combine antibacterial and anti-inflammatory properties as well as inducing mineralization of tissues, so that the interaction of these properties provides the medication with a beneficial effect on live tissue in the periapical region, whose integrity depends on tissue repair. Among these substances, calcium hydroxide is outstanding. It is the most studied, used and discussed as a temporary dressing material, due to properties such as, antibacterial [41,71,92,140], and anti-exudative actions[3,51], action of inducing mineralized tissue formation[4,80,76,137], biocompatibility[90,103,107], dissolving necrotic tissues[50] and of promoting bacterial endotoxin (LPS) hydrolysis *in vitro*[10,64,113,130,131] and *in vivo*[108,114,146,164].

Murakami et al.[102] (1997) reported that calcium hydroxide promoted an increase in the synthesis of collagen and proteins after it was incorporated into PMMA (polymethylmethacrylate) spheres during osteogenesis. Similarly, Jaunberzins et al.[61] (2000) and Silva et al.[143] (2008) described that primary cultures of rat calvaria exposed to calcium hydroxide presented an increase in the expression of collagenous and non-collagenous proteins of the extracellular matrix, which could favor the repair process. The results of studies using different experimental animal models showed that the exposure of periapical tissues to this material promotes different aspects of the tissue repair process, including the neoformation of cement and alveolar bone[31,72,79,146].

THE USE OF CALEN PASTE AS TOPICAL MEDICATION BETWEEN SESSIONS (TEMPORARY DRESSING)

Calen paste (Fig. 2.IX-9) has been marketed by S. S. White Artigos Dentários Ltda. since 1993, and has the following composition:

Calcium hydroxide .... 2.5 g
Zinc oxide .... 0.5 g
Colophonia (staybelite resin) .... 0.05 g
Polyethylenoglycol 400 .... 1.75 mL

FIG. 2.IX-9

Commercial presentation of Calen paste (S. S. White Artigos Dentários Ltda., Rio de Janeiro, RJ, Brazil).

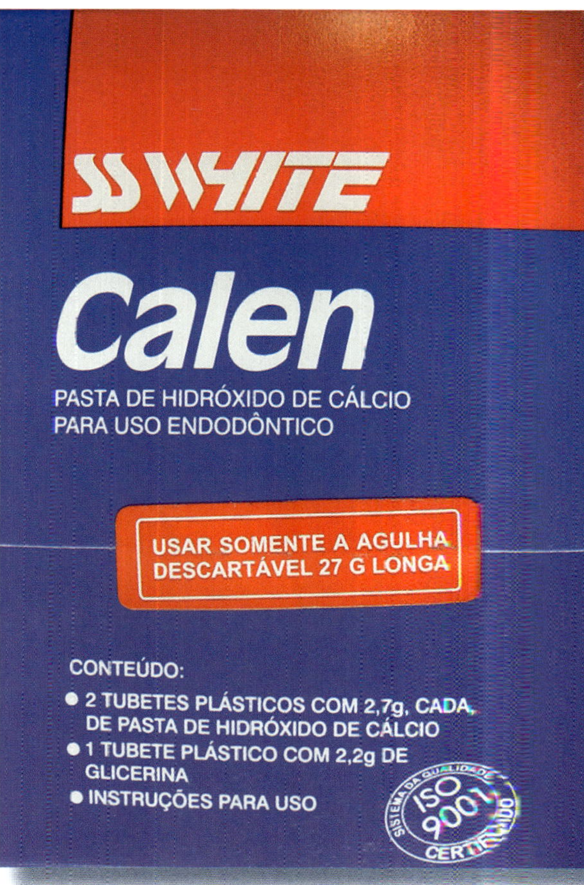

The paste is a calcium hydroxide-based product associated with a viscous vehicle, polyethylenoglycol "400", which keeps the calcium hydroxide in the desired area for a longer time, prolonging its action, diminishing solubilization and increasing its penetration into root dentin. In addition, the paste has a pH of around 12.4, therefore, offering high antibacterial activity [71]. Its biocompatibility[73,107] (Figs. 2.IX-10 and 2.IX-11) has been proven by means voluminous clinical evaluations in human teeth (Figs. 2.IX-12A-C, 2.IX-13A-C, 2.IX-14A-B, 2.IX-15A-C, 2.IX-16A-B and 2.IX-17A-B).

The difficulty of the dispersion of polyethylenoglycol "400" theoretically makes Calen paste less prone to be diluted (solubilized), allowing a reduced speed of releasing Ca^{++} and OH^- ions, when compared with an aqueous vehicle (distilled water, physiological solution, or anesthetic solutions, amongst others), which are very rapidly diluted. This is very important, bearing in mind that calcium hydroxide undergoes changes when it is in an aqueous vehicle, while there is a need to maintain the pH during the release of calcium and hydroxyl ions. This disadvantage does not occur with Calen paste, which ionic dissociation speed is lower, allowing a slow and progressive release of calcium and hydroxyl ions of up to 60 days.

Dozens of studies have analyzed Calen paste, particularly its biological properties, and it is now recommended by many authors and widely used in Brazil and other countries, also because of its low cost.

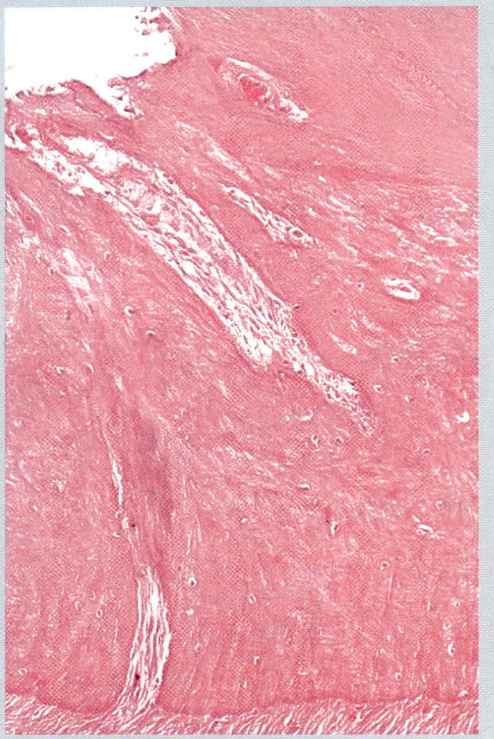

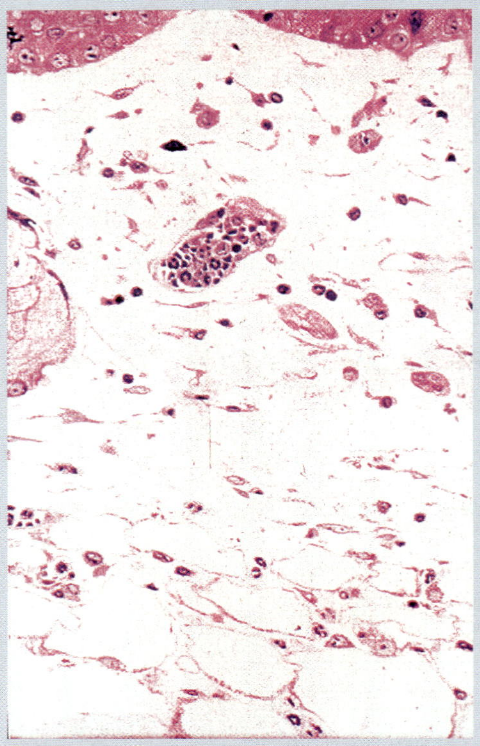

FIG. 2.IX-10

Histological section of root apex of dog's tooth after use of temporary dressing using Calen paste. Connective tissue of all ramifications of the delta and periapex (H&E – 64X).

FIG. 2.IX-11

Histological section of complete tissue repair, 15 days after Calen paste injection into the subcutaneous connective tissue of isogenic Balb/c mice.

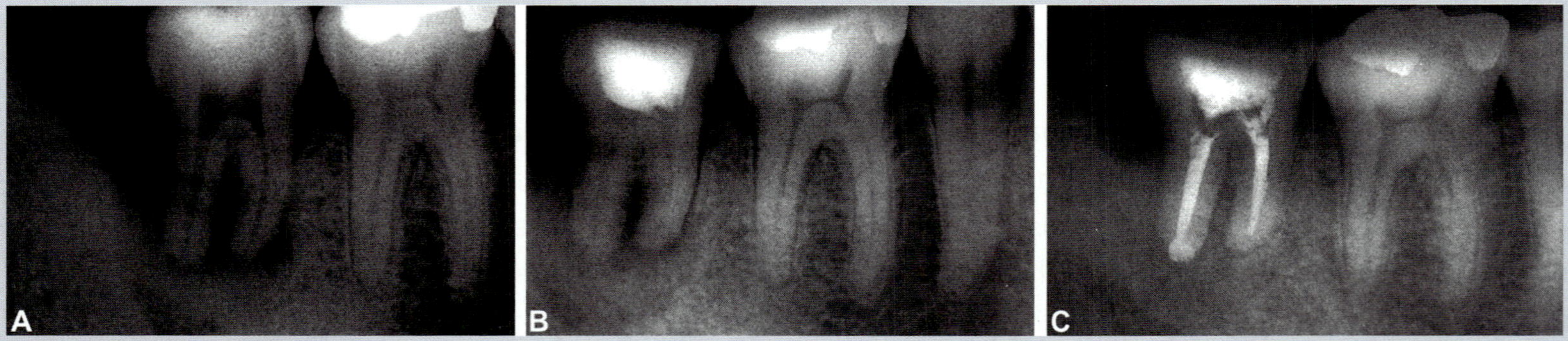

FIGS. 2.IX-12A-C

A- Periapical radiograph for diagnosis of mandibular right 2nd molar, with pulp necrosis and extensive endo-perio lesion. B – Periapical radiograph 3 months after dressing with Calen paste, with considerable extrusion into the periapical region. C – Follow-up radiograph one year and two months after endodontic treatment. Note the complete repair of the endo-periodontal lesion. (Courtesy of Dr. Guilherme Rothier Washsolz – Endodontist in Rio de Janeiro – Brazil.)

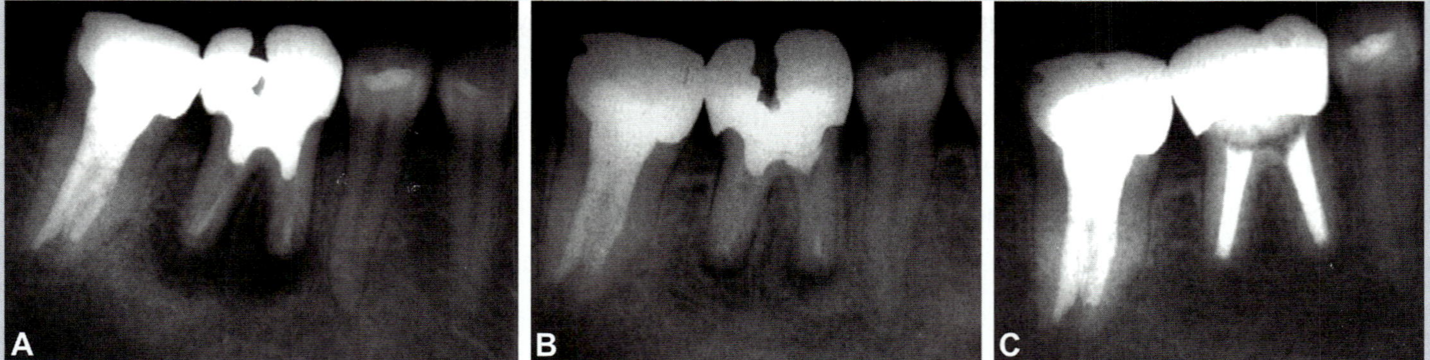

FIGS. 2.IX-13A-C

A – Periapical radiograph for diagnosis, showing evidence of a mandibular right first molar with partially filled root canals, with extensive periapical lesion and clinical presence of fistula. According to the clinical history, the case had been submitted for apical surgery. B – Radiograph after removal of the filling material, biomechanical preparation and temporary dressing with Calen paste. C – Radiograph showing periapical repair, two years after 3 bi-monthly changes of Calen paste and filling of root canals. (Courtesy of Dr. Vicente G. N. Rocha, endodontist in Goiânia – Goias – Brazil.)

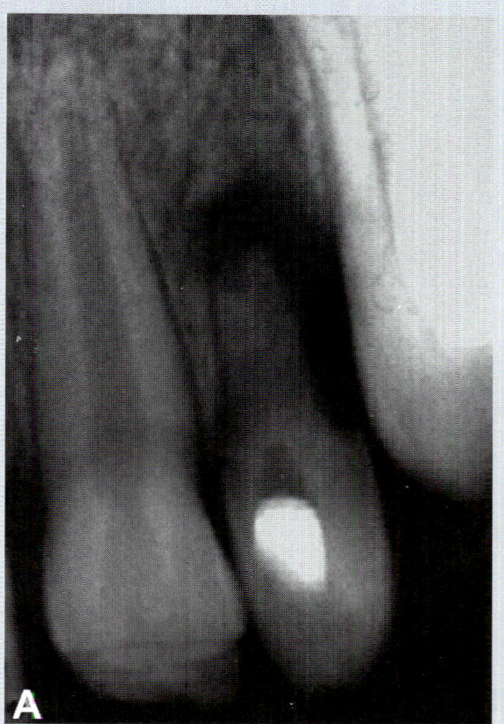
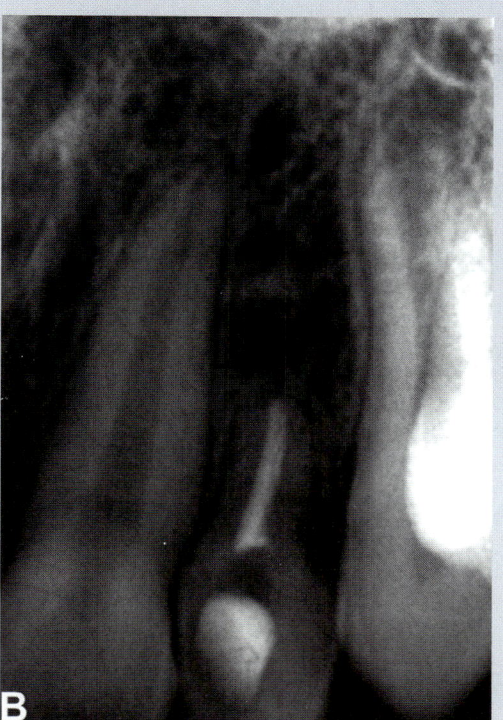

FIGS. 2.IX-14A-B

A – Periapical radiograph for diagnosis of maxillary lateral incisor showing evidence of extensive endo-perio lesion. B – Radiograph showing evidence of endo-perio lesion repair, 2 years after 3 bi-monthly changes of Calen paste, used as temporary dressing and after filling the root canal. (Courtesy of Dr. Paulo Tadeu da Silva, endodontist in São Carlos – São Paulo – Brazil.)
Note: In cases considered special, 2 or 3 changes of temporary dressing (Calen) every 2 weeks may be necessary. In cases considered routine, only one application of Calen paste for a minimum period of 14 days is indicated.

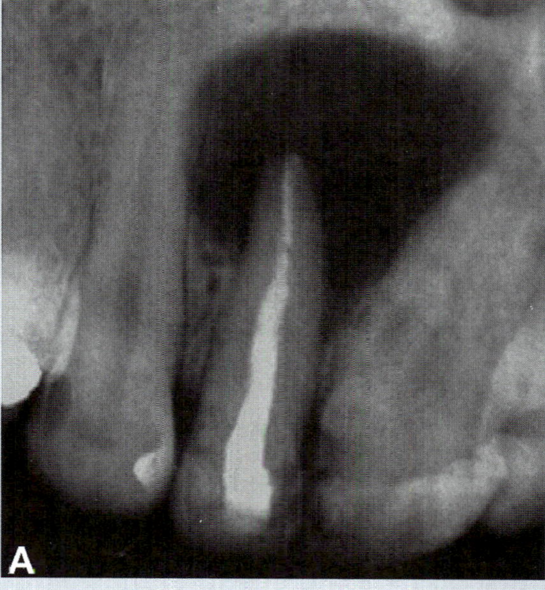
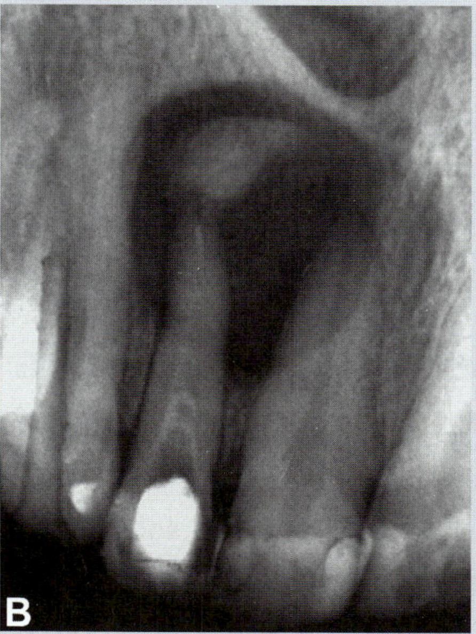
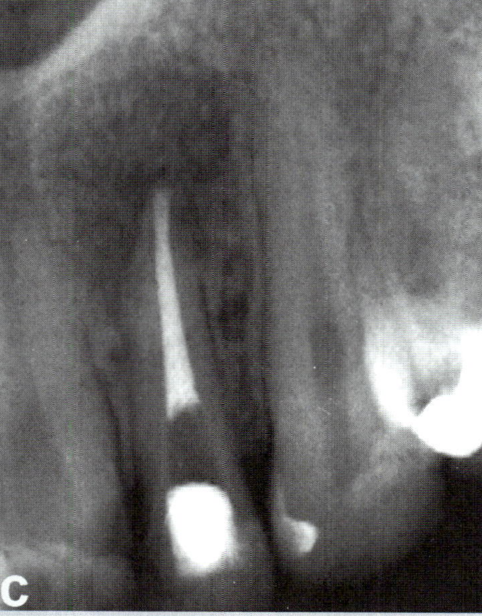

FIGS. 2.IX-15A-C

A – Periapical radiograph for diagnosis of a filled maxillary lateral incisor, but with an extensive periapical lesion. B – Radiograph after temporary dressing with Calen paste and slight extrusion into the periapical region. C – Radiograph one and a half years after root canal filling, showing evidence of lesion repair. (Courtesy of Dr Sebastião Azevedo, endodontist in Ribeirão Preto – São Paulo – Brazil.)

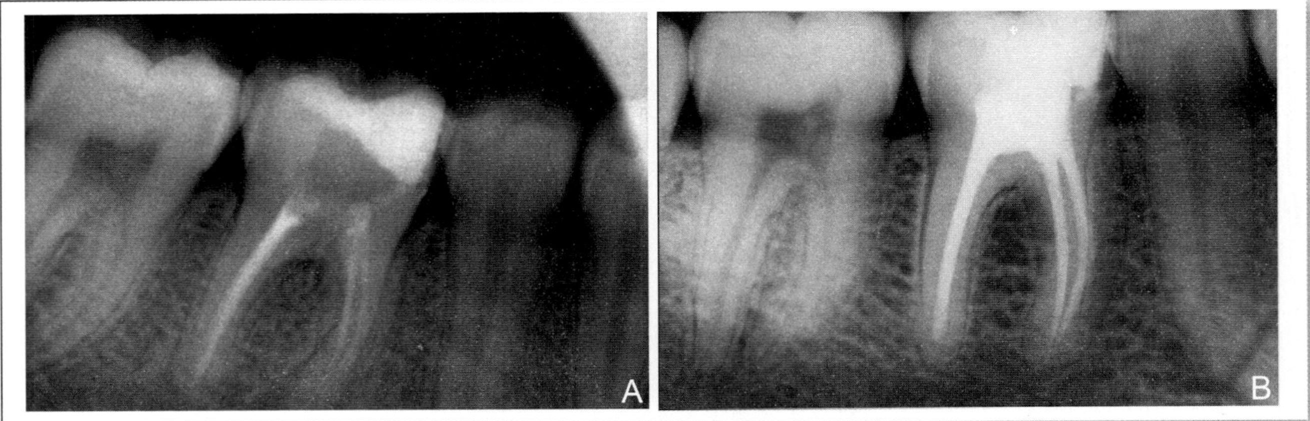

FIGS. 2.IX-16A-B

A – Periapical radiograph for diagnosis of mandibular right first molar showing a chronic periapical lesion on the mesial root, with indication of retreatment. B – Follow-up radiograph taken 15 months after endodontic retreatment, with the use of Calen paste as temporary dressing between sessions. (Courtesy of Prof. Dr. Maria de Los Angeles Bulacio – Tucuman – Argentina.)

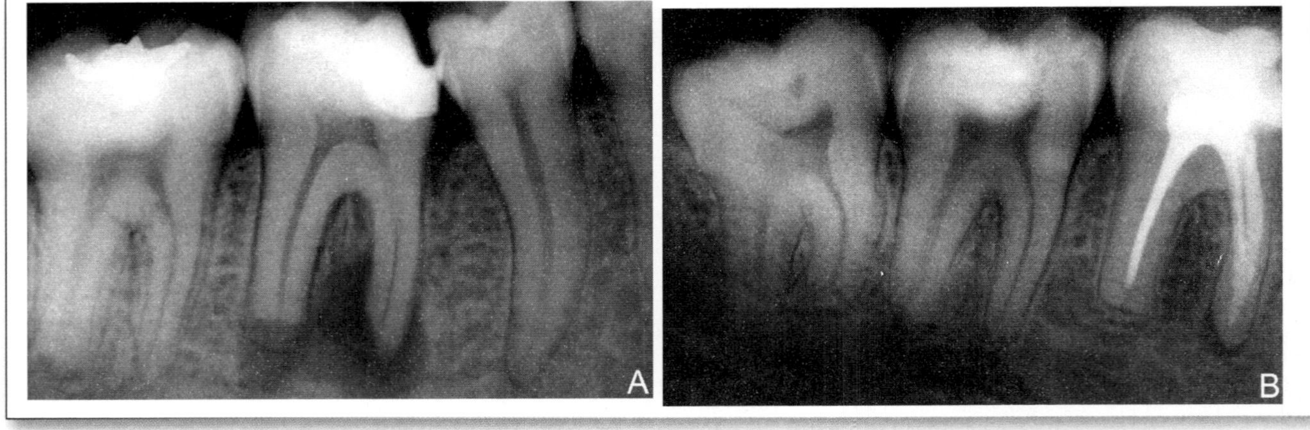

FIGS. 2.IX-17A-B

A – Periapical radiograph for diagnosis of the mandibular right first molar, showing clear evidence of chronic periapical lesion and apical resorption in the mesial and distal roots. B – Follow-up radiograph taken 3 years after endodontic treatment, with the use of Calen paste as temporary dressing between sessions. (Courtesy of Prof. Dr. Maria de Los Angeles Bulacio – Tucuman – Argentina.)

THE RESULTS OF PERTINENT STUDIES USING CALEN PASTE AS TOPICAL MEDICATION BETWEEN SESSIONS (TEMPORARY DRESSING)

Leonardo et al.[74] (1993), in a histopathological study, evaluated two calcium hydroxide-based pastes (Calasept and Calen), which was replaced every month for a period of 90 days, in dog`s teeth with immature apex and periapical lesions. They observed that both helped in sealing the apical and in the repair of the periapical region, however, better results were obtained with Calen paste.

In a further study in 1993, Leonardo et al.[73] evaluated the effect of Calen paste as a temporary dressing in dog`s teeth with incomplete rhizogenesis and periapical lesions. After 3 months of use, they observed apexification with considerable mineralized tissue at the foramen, repair of the periapical lesion, absence of inflammatory infiltrate, a significant quantity of collagen fibers, and a normal apical periodontal ligament (Figs. 2.IX-18 and 2.IX-19).

In 1999, Nelson-Filho et al.[107] evaluated the inflammatory response induced by Calen and Calasept pastes in subcutaneous tissues of isogenic BALB/c mice. They observed that Calen paste caused an inflammatory response of short duration, while Calasept generated a more extensive response. At the end of the experiment, both pastes allowed the repair process to occur, but they differed with respect to the speed of the repair process.

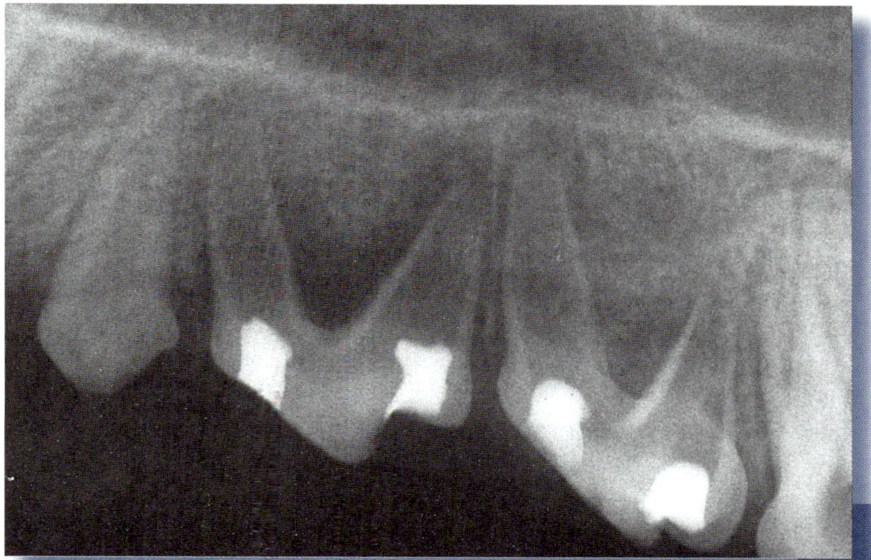

FIG. 2.IX-18

Periapical radiograph of dog's teeth showing evidence of the presence of extensive chronic periapical lesion.

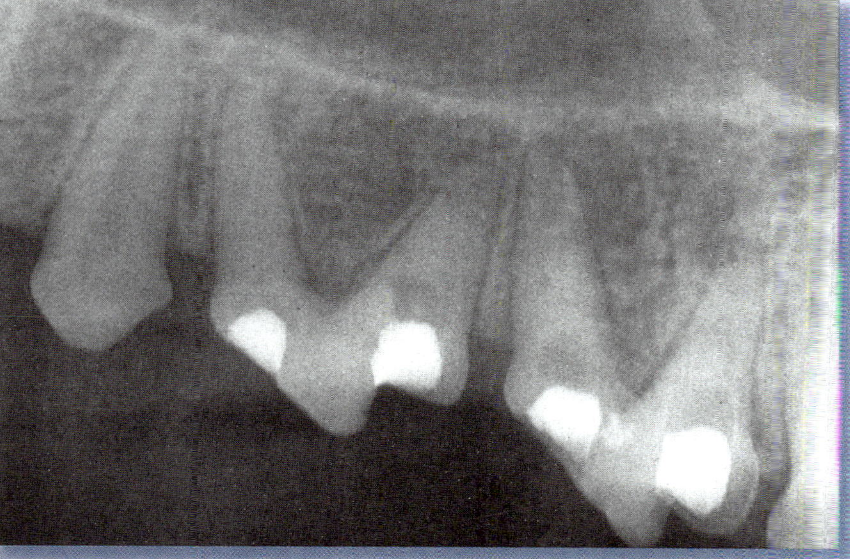

FIG. 2.IX-19

Radiograph of the case in the previous figure, showing evidence of repair process in the periapical region, 90 days after biomechanical preparation and temporary dressing with Calen paste.

Leonardo et al.[75] (2000) evaluated *in vitro* antimicrobial activity of Calen and Calasept pastes against 7 microbial strains (*Micrococcus luteus, Staphylococcus aureus, Pseudomonas aeruginosa, Streptococcus mutans, Staphylococcus epidermidis, Escherichia coli and Enterococcus faecalis*), inoculated into a culture medium directly or by means of paper points. Both materials exhibited antimicrobial activity against all microorganisms that were evaluated.

In 2003, Camões et al.[20] evaluated the Ca^{++} diffusion of Calen paste and observed that it showed a slow and steady Ca^{++} ion release.

Ferreira et al.[39] (2004) conducted an *in vitro* study to evaluate the release of calcium ions and the pH of calcium hydroxide-based pastes, including Calen paste (viscous vehicle), LC paste (oily vehicle), and calcium hydroxide paste in a saline solution (aqueous vehicle). They concluded that Calen paste and the aqueous paste were shown to have higher calcium release and pH levels.

In 2005, Faria et al.[36] verified, *in vivo*, that biomechanical preparation was effective in eliminating the microorganisms from the root canals of primary teeth with pulp necrosis and periapical lesion in 20% of the cases, and the temporary dressing with Calen paste in 62.5%, whereas the cumulative action of biomechanical preparation and the temporary dressing eliminated the microorganisms in 70.0% of the cases. They concluded that biomechanical preparation alone presented microbiological results inferior to those obtained when it was associated with the temporary dressing.

In 2007, Herrera et al.[55] reported a case of complete repair of the periapical region after the use of Calen paste as temporary dressing in a permanent molar submitted to autogenous transplant.

Gurgel-Filho et al.[46] (2007), by means of an *in vitro* study, observed that Calen paste used as a temporary dressing was effective controlling infection by *Enterococcus faecalis*.

Tanomaru et al.[166] (2007) evaluated the *in vitro* antimicrobial activity of Calen paste against 5 species of microorganisms (*Escherichia coli, Staphylococcus epidermidis, Staphylococcus aureus, Pseudomonas aeruginosa and Micrococcus luteus*). They observed that the paste presented activity against all the evaluated microorganisms.

Furthermore, in 2007, Soares et al.[156] observed that Calen paste presented residual antibacterial activity after remaining in place for 21 days in root canals of dog`s teeth with pulp necrosis and periapical lesion.

TEMPORARY DRESSING WITH CALEN PASTE: HOW IS IT PERFORMED?

After instrumentation and drying with sterile paper points, the root canal has to be flooded with solution of ethylenediaminetetracetic acid (EDTA) for 3 minutes, using constant agitation with for instance a type K file, to remove the *smear layer*[11,181]. After 3 minutes the EDTA solution has to be removed and neutralized by irrigation/aspiration with a 1% sodium hypochlorite solution, followed by drying with sterile paper points. This method will promote diffusion of the temporary dressing throughout the root canal system, allowing it to reach left behind microorganisms.

After this the root canals must be filled with Calen Paste by means of a special threaded plunger syringe (ML – SS. White – Artigos Dentários Ltda., RJ, Brazil) and a long 27G needle (Septoject XL – Septodont), with a rubber or silicone stop set to the working length (Fig. 2.IX-20). The description of the use of Calen paste together with the ML threaded plunger syringe, as well as its advantages, was published by Leonardo et al.[83] in 1993 in the Journal of Endodontics (v. 19, p. 319-20), in an article entitled *Safe and easy way to use calcium hydroxide as a temporary dressing*.

First, the small carpule of glycerin supplied with the Calen paste kit should be inserted in the syringe. The rubber plunger must be compressed and flow of glycerin should be verified by checking the tip of the needle, indicating that there are no obstructions. After removal of the glycerin carpule from the

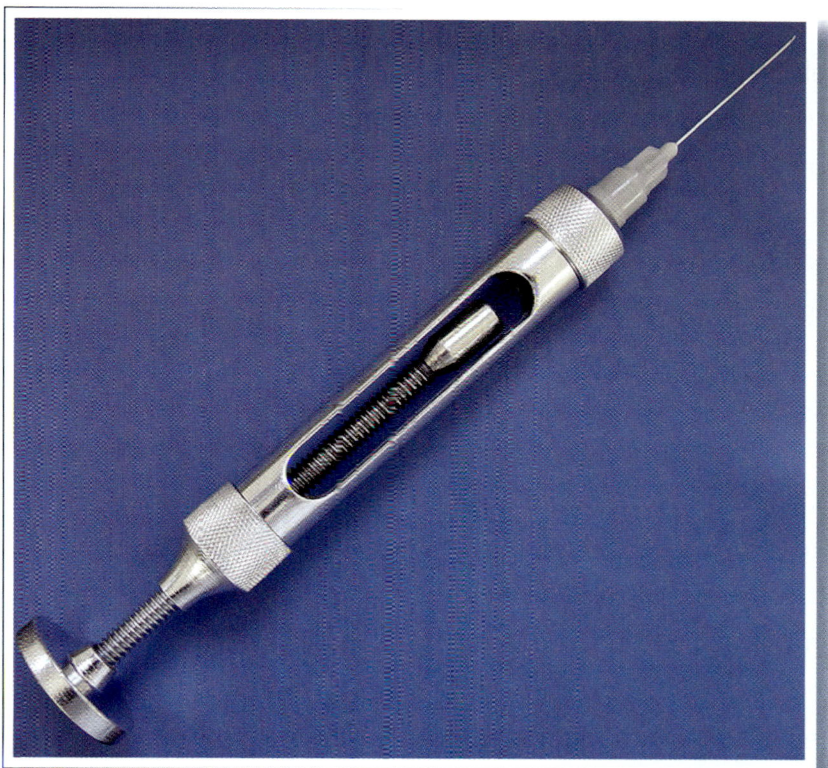

FIG. 2.IX-20
ML Syringe fitted with needle.

syringe the carpule with paste can be inserted. The plunger of the syringe must be turned clockwise until the paste begins to flow through the needle, discarding the first drop that contains glycerin. The needle must then be introduced into the canal, turning the syringe to extrude the paste. The root canal must be progressively filled to the real working length (RWL), observing the appearance of excess paste at the level of the pulp chamber.

While the root canal is being filled with paste, the needle must initially remain at the real tooth length (RTL) for a few seconds in the case of treating teeth with a periapical lesion, in order to cause a little extrusion of the paste. The objective here is to reach the apical biofilm.

After this, a radiographic examination must be performed to confirm that the root canal has been correctly filled. Remember that the paste has a radiopacity similar to that of dentin, and thus, in order for the dressing to be considered adequate (the image of the root canal space is not visible), there must be no voids along the entire RTL. In other words, the radiograph should show that the entire lumen of the root has been filled. If filling is inadequate, the needle has to be re-introduced into the canal to address the shortcomings that were observed.

After using the temporary dressing between sessions, a piece of sterile cotton must be placed at the orifice of the canals and the pulp chamber must be sealed with a zinc oxide and eugenol-based cement (IRM – Dentsply Indústria e Comércio Ltda.), or glass ionomer-based restorative cement. In anterior teeth, preference is given to a glass ionomer. Temporary coronal sealing is of fundamental importance to avoid microleakage, which will certainly lead to treatment failure.

The temporary dressing must remain in place until the following session, when it will be removed by hydrodynamic action, through successive irrigation with sodium hypochlorite solution and mechanical agitation with a file. This can be done successfully as this paste does not set.

This method will promote diffusion of the temporary dressing throughout the root canal system allowing it to reach left behind microorganisms.

HOW LONG MUST THE TEMPORARY DRESSING BE KEPT IN PLACE IN TEETH WITH PULP NECROSIS AND CHRONIC PERIAPICAL LESION (APICAL PERIODONTITIS)?

The antibacterial activity of calcium hydroxide results from its alkalizing action, which in turn results from the concentration of hydroxyl ions. Therefore, calcium hydroxide applied in the root canal should diffuse, by means of its hydroxyl ions, through the apical foramen[25], secondary and accessory canals, as well as the dentinal tubules[2,109], with the goal of reaching the areas of apical cement resorption and extra-radicular microbial infection.

The temporary dressing must remain in place inside the root canal for a period of time that allows the hydroxyl ions from the paste to diffuse through the dentin. Knowing that this diffusion is primarily determined by the molecular weight, it is to be expected that the diffusion would be faster in aqueous pastes. Nevertheless, *in vivo* studies have suggested that this rapid diffusion does not occur, since the hydroxyl ions can interact with the components of dentin, such as hydroxyapatite, which can buffer the OH^- ions[176].

Nerwich et al.[109] (1993) demonstrated that the diffusion capacity of the paste in dentin varied according to the root canal third being evaluated, as there is a difference in permeability between the cervical, middle and apical thirds. According to Paslhey[118] (1990), dentinal permeability depends on the diameter of the tubules, size and load. The diffusion of these OH^- ions is therefore affected by the buffering capacity of dentin, absorption and load. Thus, in vitro studies cannot always be correlated to *in vivo* studies.

Although satisfactory microbiological results were obtained when using the calcium hydroxide-based temporary dressing for 7 days[7,85,117], more recent studies have shown that when the dressing remains in place for longer periods, the reduction in microbiota is greater.

Nerwich et al.[109] (1993) also verified that in the apical third, a minimum period of 21 days was necessary to allow the OH^- ions to reach the external surface of the cement. This was further supported by Tronstad et al.[169] (1981) *in vitro*, who reported that calcium hydroxide takes 28 days to reach the external surface of dentin. For calcium hydroxide to diffuse, it must remain in the root canal for a minimum period, in order to perform its bactericide action. This minimum time required for calcium hydroxide to raise the pH in external apical root dentin is around 14 to 21 days[109].

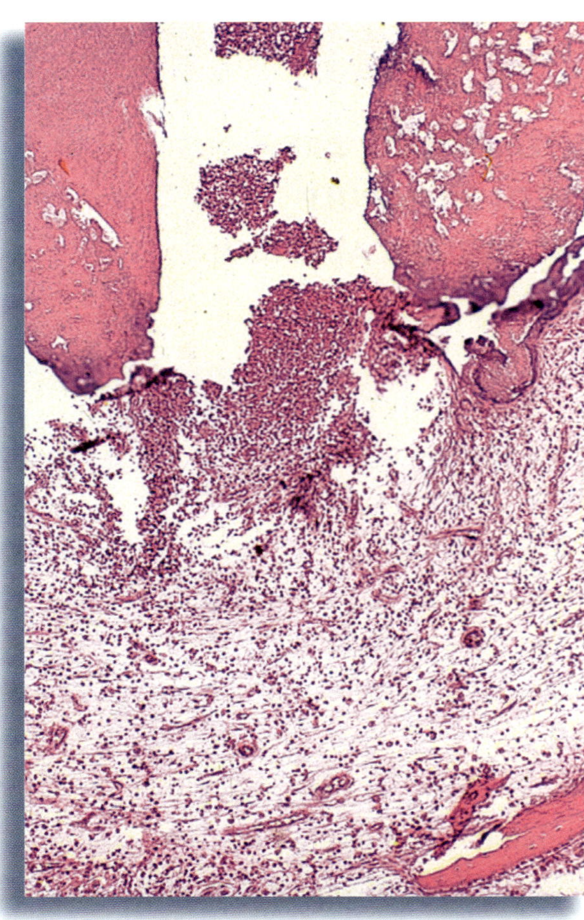

The periods of 15 and 30 days of temporary dressing were the ones that presented the best histopathological results[78], whereas the results after 7 days were undesirable.

Recently, Soares et al.[156] (1999), using Calen paste, verified greater reduction in anaerobic and aerobic microbiota in a period of 15 days, as well as a better histopathological condition (Figs. 2.IX-21 and 2.IX-22A-F). In this study, the authors confirmed that the physical presence of the dressing, blocking the exudate and reducing the transport of nutrients to the bacteria originating from the periapical region also helped the apical and periapical repair.

The literature therefore shows that the ideal time of use of the temporary dressing material in primary and permanent teeth with pulp necrosis and chronic periapical reaction, should be a minimum of 14 days[71,141]. This may explain the unsatisfactory results that have been reported when a period of 7 days was used.

FIG. 2.IX-21

Panoramic view of root apex of a dog's tooth with pulp necrosis and chronic periapical lesion, after biomechanical preparation and calcium hydroxide-based temporary dressing for 7 days. Note the widened periodontal ligament, containing abscessed foci, inflammatory infiltrate, and areas of necrosis and resorption (H&E – 40X).

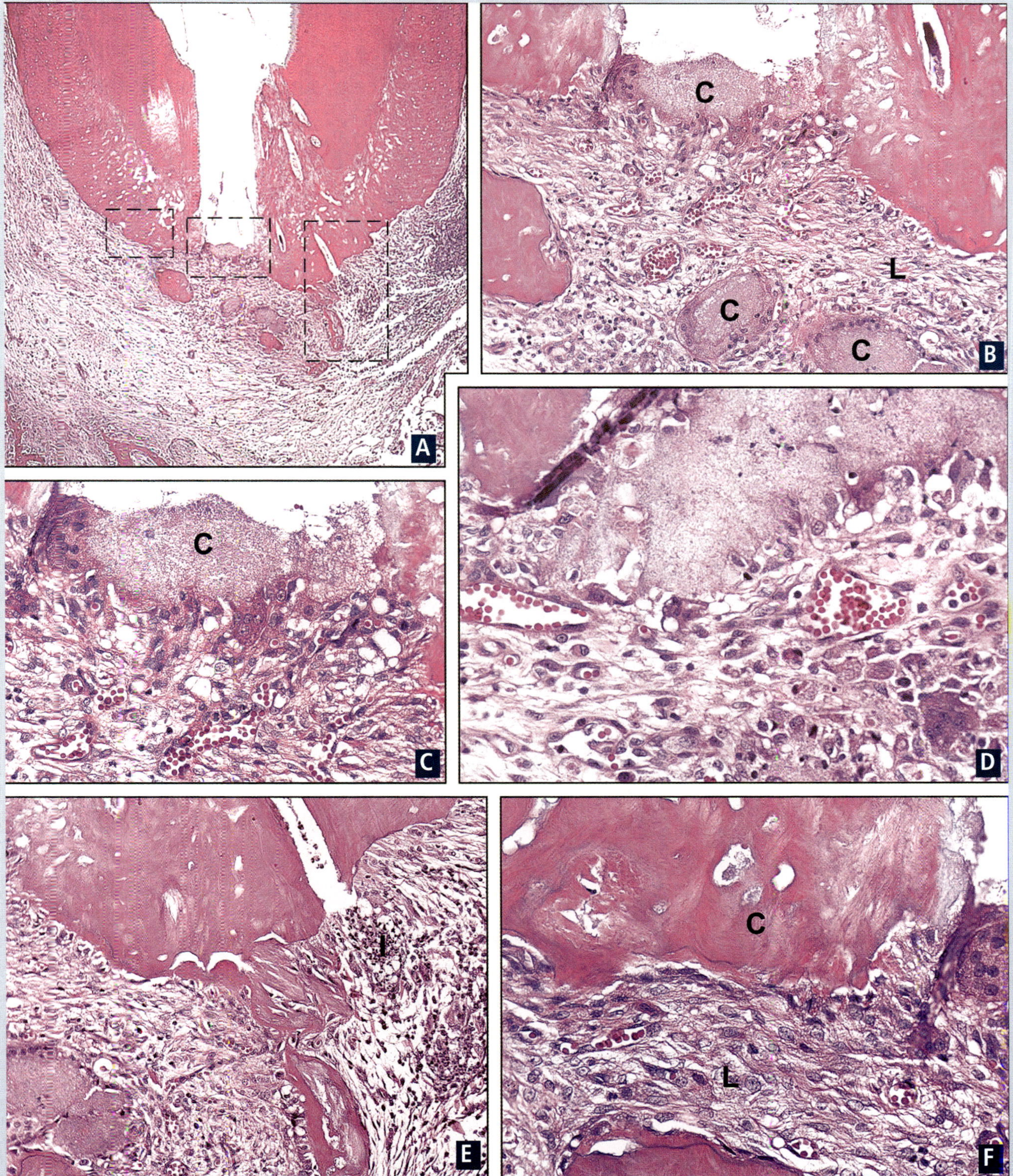

FIGS. 22.IX-22A-F

Histological section of dog's tooth with pulp necrosis and chronic periapical lesion, after biomechanical preparation and temporary dressing with Calen paste for 14 days. A – Apical and periapical region in the developmental stage of repair (H&E – 24X). B – Detail of the previous figure, showing evidence of Calen paste (c) extruded into the foraminal opening and periodontal ligament (L) (H&E – 60X). C and D – Large number of fibers, vessels and cells adjacent to the material (c) (H&E – 200X. E – Region of the root apex and periodontal ligament with presence of inflammatory cells (I) (H&E – 100X). F – Apical cement (c). Periodontal ligament (L) containing collagenous fibers, cells and vascular neoformation (H&E – 200X).

COMBINATION OF CALCIUM HYDROXIDE WITH CHLORHEXIDINE: CURRENT STATUS

Different materials have been added to calcium hydroxide in an effort to improve some of its properties, such as radiopacity, viscosity, flow, antimicrobial action spectrum, ionic dissociation speed and other physical-chemical properties, that promote the clinical conditions[12].

Among these substances, chlorhexidine digluconate has outstanding properties. It is an active antimicrobial agent of the group consisting of biguanides, which has been investigated as a new alternative in combination with calcium hydroxide as a temporary dressing[26,128,187], with the aim of increasing its antibacterial action against resistant microorganisms[5,12,13,54,123,150, 174,178]. Although it is incapable of inactivating bacterial LPS[18,25,147] and dissolving tissues[104,112,186] on its own, chlorhexidine presents substantiality [60,63,70,84,128,178], biocompatibility[22,158,167], low toxicity[45,62,89,182] and a broad spectrum of action against Gram-positive, Gram-negative, aerobic, anaerobic bacteria, yeasts and fungi[54,62,134,171,172].

Moreover, chlorhexidine has been shown to be effective, even in low concentrations, against the microorganisms most frequently found in endodontic infections[23,28,38,111]. The association of calcium hydroxide with chlorhexidine results in a greater synergistic antimicrobial effect than the sole use of calcium hydroxide[123,174,187]. *In vitro* studies have demonstrated that this combination has no adverse effects on the solubility or activity of the two substances[12,37,42,123].

From the above discussion, one can derive that the combination of calcium hydroxide with chlorhexidine can be of benefit to the endodontic treatment of teeth with pulp necrosis and radiographically visible chronic periapical lesions. This combination has been evaluated *in vitro*, *ex vivo* and *in vivo*[12,26,31,156,183,185,187].

However, the literature presents conflicting evidence with respect to the toxicity of chlorhexidine when used alone. Some authors have shown evidence that chlorhexidine has a beneficial effect[17,40,52,57], while others have reported that depending on concentration, it has a toxic effect on various types of cells, such as human erythrocytes[53], HeLa cells[177], rat peritoneal macrophages[69], human gingival fibroblasts [8,93] and osteoblasts[119].

It has also been reported that the use of chlorhexidine alone may affect the synthesis of proteins[43,124] and cell proliferation[91] to different degrees. Faria et al.[35] (2007) evaluated the effect of chlorhexidine digluconate in various concentrations on fibroblasts L929 after exposure for 24 hours, with the objective of observing cell death by apoptosis/necrosis. The authors observed that chlorhexidine caused stress of the endoplasmatic reticulum (ER) as a result of the accumulation of proteins in the cisterns. In addition, it induced apoptosis and/or necrosis, via stress in the ER, and an increase in protein expression as an indicator of cellular stress. Nevertheless, these effects are dose-dependent and among the concentrations evaluated, the intermediate concentration of 0.4% did not promote an increase in cell death.

As a result of the scarcity of studies evaluating the biocompatibility and antimicrobial activity of the combination of calcium hydroxide and chlorhexidine in low concentrations, Silva et al.[142] (2008) carried out a series of experiments, with the objective to evaluate a calcium hydroxide-based paste (Calen) combined with chlorhexidine digluconate in a low concentration (0.4%). Cell viability, immunostimulating properties, (dosage of nitric oxide – NO) and anti-inflammatory properties (dosage of NO, TNF-α and IL-1α) were studied in cultures of RAW 264.7 macrophages. The results demonstrated that the Calen and Calen+0,4% chlorhexidine pastes, in general, did not cause immunostimulation. They did not raise the production of NO in comparison with the control, and were therefore non-cytotoxic. On the other hand, LPS (control) behaved as a powerful inflammatory agent and stimulator of NO production.

These authors also performed an anti-inflammatory activity test, by means of pre-treating cells with different materials, including Calen and Calen+0.4% of chlohexidine pastes, and exposed the cells afterwards to an inflammatory stimulus (LPS) and dosage of NO, IL-1α and TNF-α. According to their results, Calen+0.4% chlohexidine paste presented anti-inflammatory activity at the higher concentration used; that is 25μg/ml, inhibiting the production of NO, IL-1α and TNF-α.

Although the literature has published studies related to the effect of chlorhexidine by itself on various types of cells and with conflicting reports, there have been few studies describing the effect of the combination of chlorhexidine and calcium hydroxide, especially on osteogenic cultures. Silva et al.[143] (2008) evaluated the effect of Calen paste with and without 0.4% chlorhexidine digluconate, with respect to cell viability, total protein content, alkaline phosphatase activity, non-collagenous matrix proteins and mineralized nodule formations in the matrix, in primary cultures of cells of the osteoblastic lineage. As osteoblastic differentiation markers, they used the alkaline phosphatase molecules, bone sialoprotein and osteopontin. No statistically significant differences were observed between the Groups Calen, Calen+ chlohexidine and control as regards to the predetermined parameters (cell viability, alkaline phosphatase activity, total protein content and proportion of nodule areas in the mineralized matrix). In the three groups the primary cultures exhibited an osteogenic phenotype at 14 days (Figs. 2.IX-23A-O). These results indicated that exposure to the culture medium containing Calen paste at the concentration used did not alter the osteogenic potential of the primary cultures. However, the non statistically significant increase in mineralization areas in the Calen+0.4% chlohexidine group, in the order of 35% (interpreted only as a tendency), indicated the need to evaluate this parameter in more studies, or under different conditions or using different experimental models, both *in vitro* and *in vivo*.

The antimicrobial activity of Calen paste associated with 0.4% chlorhexidine digluconate was evaluated by Silva et al.[144] (2008) by means of the agar diffusion test, against 2 indicator microorganisms (*Enterococcus faecalis* and *Kocuria rhizophila*). Chlorhexidine digluconate alone (control) presented the highest antimicrobial activity (microbial growth inhibition halo ranging from 16 to 17 mm) for *E. faecalis*, although without statistically significant difference. The antimicrobial activity of chlorhexidine was reduced when it was combined with calcium hydroxide (halo of 11 to 12 mm).

Furthermore, the antimicrobial activity of calcium hydroxide was elevated by this combination (halo of 9 to 10 mm when used alone and a halo of 11 to 12 mm when combined with chlorhexidine). The numerical results showed only a tendency towards higher antimicrobial activity of the Calen-chlorhexidine paste in comparison with Calen paste alone, although without a statistically significant difference. The authors also observed no statistically significant differences between the antimicrobial activity of Calen and Calen-chlohexidine pastes against *E. faecalis* and *K. rizophila*.

As Haenni et al.[48] (2003) have pointed out, the addition of chlorhexidine to calcium hydroxide did not elevate the antimicrobial efficacy against *E. faecalis*, by the agar diffusion test, bearing in mind that they observed a larger inhibition halo with the use of 0.5% chlorhexidine alone (15.2±0.3 mm) compared to the combination with calcium hydroxide (13.8±0.3 mm).

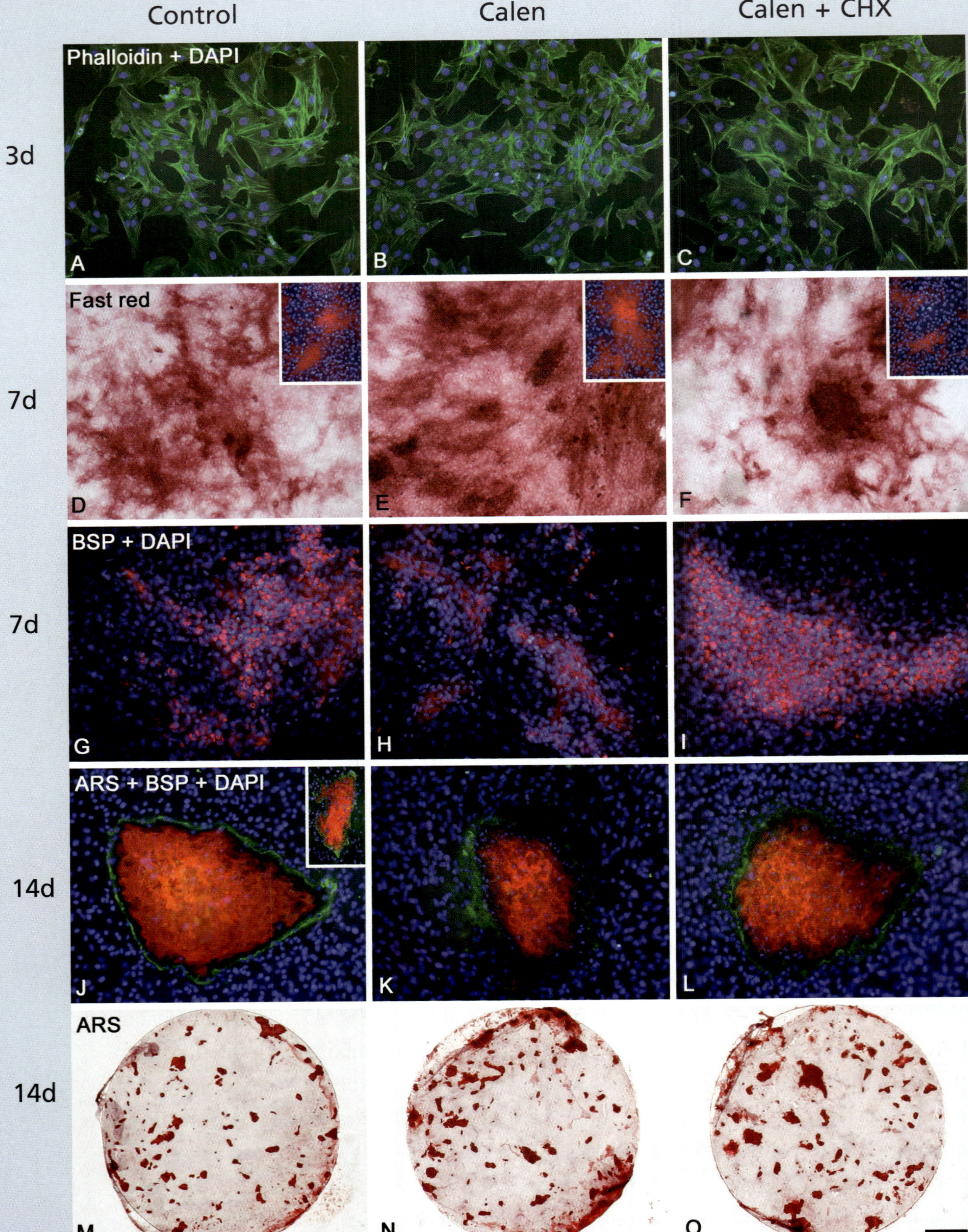

FIGS. 2.IX-23A-O

Aspects of osteogenic cultures grown on Thermanox in the presence of a control culture medium (A, D, G, J and M) and containing Calen (B, E, H, K and N) and Calen + Chlorhexidine (C, F, I, L and O) pastes, over time periods of 3 (A-C), 7 (D-I) and 14 (J-O) days. In 3 days, epifluorescence of cultures marked with phalloidine (green) and DAPI (blue), showed that the cells were adhered and spread out on the substrate in the three groups (A-C), with predominantly polygonal morphology. In 7 days, the cultures presented in confluence, and areas with the beginning of multiple layer formation exhibited alkaline phosphatase activity (areas colored in red by the Fast red method, observed by light transmitted in D-F and by epifluorescence, in the details in D-F) and expression of bone sialoprotein (areas of red fluorescence in G-I). At 14 days, areas with calcified matrix formations, stained with Alizarin red (observed by epifluorescence in J-L and macroscopically in M-O), occurred in all the groups, together with bone sialoprotein and osteopontin markings (green fluorescence in J-L and detail in J, respectively) were observed. The scale bar represents 100 µm for A-C and G-L, 200 µm for D-F and detail in J, 300 µm for details in D-F and 2.3 mm for M-O. BSP= bone sialoprotein and ARS= Alizarin red.

In 2001, Estrela et al.[34] also showed no additional antimicrobial effect when they combined calcium hydroxide with chlorhexidine. They did demonstrate that calcium hydroxide did not lose its antibacterial activity when combined with chlorhexidine. In 2006, Ercan et al.[32] compared the antimicrobial activity of calcium hydroxide p.a., without or in combination with 2% chlorhexidine, against *E. faecalis in vitro*. They concluded that chlorhexidine alone was significantly more effective then when combined with calcium hydroxide.

This would logically lead to the question: "*Why is the antimicrobial activity of calcium hydroxide maintained and that of chlorhexidine diminished when these two materials are combined?*" A possibly explanation is that the antimicrobial properties of calcium hydroxide are directly related to the pH[33]; that is, its capacity to release hydroxyl ions. However, according to Haenni et al.[48] (2003), the pH is not altered by the addition of chlorhexidine, as calcium hydroxide is a highly alkaline substance. Therefore, the combination of these two materials does not reflect changes in ionic release, maintaining the alkaline pH, and consequently, the antimicrobial activity of calcium hydroxide. On the other hand, according to Gomes et al.[44] (2006), the reduction of the antimicrobial effect of chlorhexidine occurs when it is combined with calcium hydroxide, and is probably the result of the precipitation of chlorhexidine that occurs at a high pH.

In 2003, Haenni et al.[48] reported that the combination of chlorhexidine with calcium hydroxide resulted in an inhibition of the antimicrobial activity of chlorhexidine, probably as a result of the high pH, which causes deprotonation of the biguanide at a pH of over 10, and therefore, reduction in the solubility and changes in the interaction with the bacterial surfaces, due to alterations in the molecular load[65].

Additional studies from a physical-chemical and antimicrobial point of view are necessary in order to explain the mechanism of possible loss of effectiveness of chlorhexidine when it is combined with calcium hydroxide.

It is known that the initial aggressiveness, characteristic of alkalinity (area of superficial necrosis) of Calen paste is reduced when it is in contact with live tissues, due to the vehicle used (polyethylenoglycol 400), which releases H^+, which unites with the hydroxyl group (OH^-) of calcium hydroxide, thus neutralizing the reaction, which partly justifies its biocompatibility[107]. On the other hand, several authors have emphasized the irritating properties of chlorhexidine when used alone, and when in contact with connective tissue[35,115,182].

Silva et al.[145] (2008) evaluated the tissue biocompatibility after implantation of polyethylene tubes containing Calen paste combined with 0.4% chlorhexidine digluconate and an experimental UltraCal™ paste (calcium hydroxide and 2% chlorhexidine digluconate – Ultradent Product Inc. USA) on subcutaneous connective tissue of isogenic mice. They observed that based on the parameters, (fibrosation, tissue thickness and inflammatory infiltrate), the 0.4% Calen+ chlohexidine paste presented microscopic results similar to those of the control group, over periods of 7 and 21 days, with a return to normal appearance after 63 days (Figs. 2-IX-24A-F). Therefore, the results obtained with the combination of Calen paste with 0.4% chlorhexidine were similar to those described in the literature with the use of

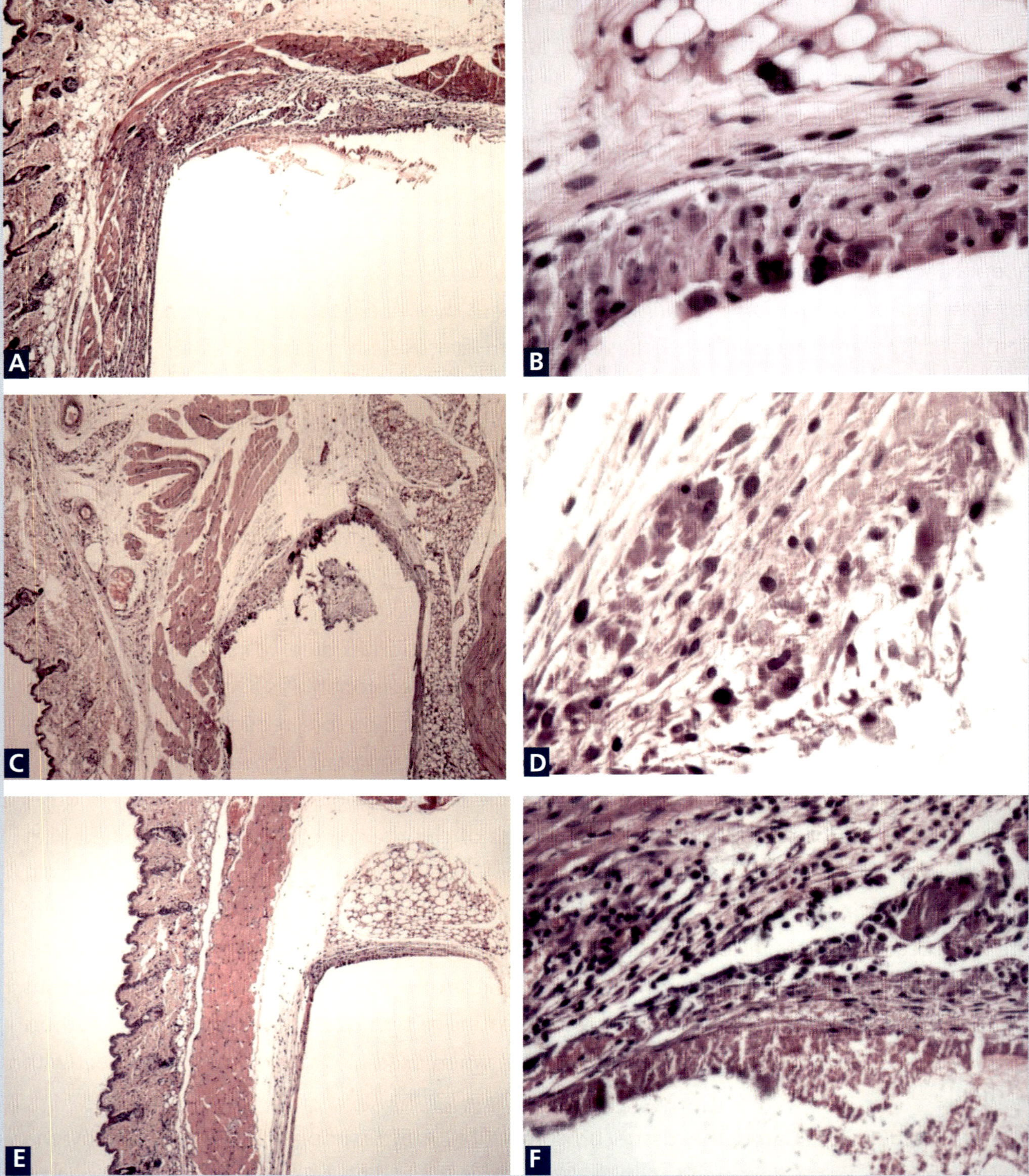

FIGS. 2.IX-24A-F

Microscopic aspects of the subcutaneous connective tissue reaction of rats against Calen® + Chlorhexidine paste in polyethylene tubes in the different experimental periods. A and B – At 7 days, the reaction tissue was not very thick, poor in exudate and rich in young macrophages and fibroblasts with discrete fibrosation. Neutrophils were observed among the macrophages and fibroblasts. (H&E.; A=4X and B=40X). C and D – At 21 days, reaction tissue thickness was discrete, with few neutrophils, with discrete degree of fibrosation. Macrophages predominated, interlaced by fibroblasts and at the interface with the material there were inflammatory multinucleated giant cells. (H&E.; C=4X and D=40X). E and F – At 63 days, in the reaction tissue, the collagen fiber bundles were distributed in the same way as they were at the interface of the lateral wall of the tube with normal connective tissue. It was not very thick, without negative spaces, and eventually a few neutrophils were present. At the interface with the material, small inflammatory multinucleated giant cells were noted. (H&E.; E=4X and F=40X).

pure Calen paste, when in contact with live tissues[71,107]. The reaction was initially characterized (7 days) by the presence of a mild neutrophilic infiltrate, sparse macrophages phagocyting the material and organized reaction tissue. At 21 and 63 days the reaction tissue was practically normal, demonstrating that the paste allowed tissue repair.

The tissue response of chlorhexidine combined with calcium hydroxide seems to be dose-dependent, bearing in mind that in the study of Silva et al.[145] (2008), the results obtained with the use of an experimental Ultracal paste were unsatisfactory. In the periods of 7, 21 and 63 days, Ultracal (experimental) paste, in general, presented worse results than the Calen+ 0.4% chlorhexidine paste, with respect to the parameters fibrosation, tissue thickness and inflammatory infiltrate. These results are in agreement with Schilder and Amsterdam[136] (1959), who confirmed that the use of a drug does not depend only on its biocompatibility, but also on its correct use, and at a suitable concentration.

With regard to biocompatibility, Soares *et al.*[155] (2003), observed that in dog`s teeth with pulp necrosis and periapical lesion, the temporary dressings Calen, Calen/CMCP (Camphorated mono paraclorofenol), calcium hydroxide P.A.+ anesthetic solution (Citanest) and calcium hydroxide P.A.+ 2% chlorhexidine digluconate solution maintained in place in the root canals for 21 days, provided a significant improvement in apical and periapical repair, demonstrated by an increase in reduction in the periapical inflammatory process, together with intense collagenous fiber deposition and new bone formation.

In 2005, De Rossi et al.[26] evaluated the effect of the temporary dressing with calcium hydroxide-based paste combined with 1% chlorhexidine on the repair of chronic periapical lesions, by means of a histopathological study in dog`s teeth. They verified that the application of the calcium hydroxide-based/1% chlorhexidine paste resulted in a significant reduction in the radiographic images and better histopathological repair of periapical lesions in comparison with the teeth filled in a single session. Although the results with the use of this paste were significantly better in comparison with those of the single session, some undesirable effects were observed, which could be attributed to the concentration of chlorhexidine (1%).

However, by and large the addition of chlorhexidine has not been shown to add benefits to the calcium hydroxide-based paste. Further studies are necessary combining calcium hydroxide-based pastes with different concentrations of chlorhexidine, before it can be recommended for clinical use.

FINAL CONSIDERATIONS

Considering the scientific and biological trends on which Endodontics at present is based, the goal of endodontic treatment in teeth with pulp necrosis and periapical lesions must be repair, not only from a clinical and radiographic, but also from the histological point of view.

Considering this goal, research has shown that the use of a calcium hydroxide-based temporary dressing materials between sessions (14 days minimum), helps to raise the percentage of endodontic post-treatment success.

References

1. Abou-Rass M, Bogen G. Microorganisms in closed periapical lesions. Int Endod J, v.31, p.39-47, 1998.
2. Alaçam TH, Yoldas O, Gulen O. Dentin penetration of 2 calcium hydroxide combinations. Oral Surg Oral Med Oral Pathol Oral Radiol Endod, v.86, p.469-472, 1998.
3. Allard U, Stromberg U, Stromberg T. Endodontic treatment of experimentally induced apical periodontitis in dogs. Endod Dent Traumatol, v.3, p.240-244, 1987.
4. Almushayt A, Narayanan K, Zaki AE, George A. Dentin matrix protein 1 induces cytodifferentiation of dental pulp stem cells into odontoblasts. Gene Ther, v.13, p.611-620, 2006.
5. Almyroudi A, Mackenzie D, McHugh S, Saunders WP. The effectiveness of various disinfectants used as endodontic intracanal medications: an in vitro study. J Endod, v.28, p.163-167, 2002.
6. Al-Negrish AR, Habahbeh R. Flare up rate related to root canal treatment of asymptomatic pulpally necrotic central incisor teeth in patients attending a military hospital. J Dent, v.34, p.635-640, 2006.
7. Assed S, Ito IY, Leonardo MR, Silva LAB, Lopatin D. Anaerobic microorganisms in root canals of human teeth with chronic apical periodontitis detected by immunofluorescence. Endod Dent Traumatol, v.12, p.66-69, 1996.
8. Babich H, Wurzburger BJ, Rubin YL, Sinensky MC, Blau L. An in vitro study on the cytotoxicity of chlorhexidine digluconate to human gingival cells. Cell Biol Toxicol, v.11, p.79-88, 1995.
9. Barkhordar RA, Hayashi C, Hussain MZ. Detection of interleukin-6 in human dental pulp and periapical lesions. Endod. Dent. Traumatol., v.15, p.26-27, 1999.
10. Barthel CR, Levin LG, Reisner HM, Trope M. TNF-alpha in monocytes after exposure to calcium hydroxide treated Escherichia coli LPS. Int End J, v.30, p.155-159, 1997.
11. Baumgartner JC, Mader CL. A scanning electron microscopic evaluation of four root canal irrigation regimens. J Endod, v.13, p.147-157, 1987.
12. Basrani B, Ghanem A, Tjäderhane L. Physical and chemical properties of chlorhexidine and calcium hydroxide-containing medications. J Endod, v.30, p.413-417, 2004.
13. Basrani B, Santos JM, Tjäderhane L, Grad H, Gorduysus O, Huang J, Lawrence HP, Friedman S. Substantive antimicrobial activity in chlorhexidine-treated human root dentin. Oral Surg. Oral Med. Oral Pathol. Oral Radiol Endod, v.94, p.240-245, 2002.
14. Bellows CF, Alder A, Wludyka P, Jaffe BM. Modulation of macrophage nitric oxide production by prostaglandin D2. J Surg Res, v.132, p.92-97, 2006.
15. Bertolini DR, Nedwin GE, Bringman TS, Smith DD, Mundy GR. Stimulation of bone resorption and inhibition of bone formation in vitro by human tumour necrosis factors. Nature, v.319, p.516-518, 1986.
16. Blix IJS, Helgeland K. LPS from Actinobacillus actinomytcetemcomitans and prodution of nitric oxide in murine macrofages J774. Eur. J Oral Sci, v.106, p.576-581, 1998.
17. Brennan SS, Foster ME, Leaper DJ. Antiseptic toxicity in wounds healing by secondary intention. J Hosp Infect, v.8, p.263-267, 1986.
18. Buck RA, Cai J, Eleazer PD, Staat RH, Hurst HE. Detoxification of endotoxin by endodontic irrigants and calcium hydroxide. J Endod, v.27 p.325-327, 2001.
19. Buttler TK, Crawford JJ. The detoxifying effect of varying concentrations of sodium hypochloride on endotoxins. J Endod, v.8, p.59-66, 1982.
20. Camões IC, Salles MR, Chevitarese, O. Ca2+ diffusion through dentin of Ca(OH)2 associated with seven different vehicles. J Endod, v.29, p.822-825, 2003.
21. Cotran RS, Kumar V, Robbins SL. Patologia estrutural e functional. 4.ª ed. Rio de Janeiro: Guanabara Koogan, 1991.
22. Dammaschke T, Schneider U, Stratmann U, Yoo JM, Schäfer E. Effect of root canal dressings on the regeneration of inflamed periapical tissue. Acta Odontol Scand, v.63, p.143-152, 2005.
23. D'Arcangelo C, Varvara G, De Fazio P. An evaluation of the action of different root canal irrigants on facultative aerobic-anaerobic, obligate anaerobic, and microaerophilic bacteria. J Endod, v.25, p.351-353, 1999.
24. Day AE, Langkamp HH, Bowen LL, Ascencio F, Agarwal S, Piesco NP. Signal transduction during LPS-mediated activation of pulp fibroblasts. J Dent Res, v.77, p.673, 1998.
25. De Oliveira LD, Jorge AO, Carvalho CA, Koga-Ito CY, Valera MC. In vitro effects of endodontic irrigants on endotoxins in root canals. Oral Surg Oral Med Oral Pathol Oral Radiol Endod, v.104, p.135-142, 2007.
26. De Rossi A, Silva LA, Leonardo MR, Rocha LB, Rossi MA. Effect of rotary or manual instrumentation, with or without a calcium hydroxide/1% chlorhexidine intracanal dressing, on the healing of experimentally induced chronic periapical lesions. Oral Surg Oral Med Oral Pathol Oral Radiol Endod, v.99, p.628-636, 2005.
27. Dewhirst FE, Stashenko PP, Mole JE, Tsurumachi T. Purification and partial sequence of human osteoclast-activating factor: identity with interleukin 1 beta. J Immunol, v.135, p.2562-2568, 1985.
28. Do Amorim CV, Aun CE, Mayer MP. Susceptibility of some oral microorganisms to chlorhexidine and paramonochlorophenol. Braz. Oral Res, v.18, p.242-246, 2004.
29. Doyle SL, Hodges JS, Pesun IJ, Baisden MK, Bowles WR. Factors affecting outcomes for single-tooth implants and endodontic restorations. J Endod, v.33, p.399-402, 2007.
30. Dwyer TG, Torabinejad M. Radiographic and histologic evaluation of the effect of endotoxin on the periapical tissues of the cat. J Endod, v.7, p.31-35, 1981.
31. Ercan E, Dalli M, Duulgergil CT, Yaman F. Effect of intracanal medication with calcium hydroxide and 1% chlorhexidine in endodontic retreatment cases with periapical lesions: an in vivo study. J Formos Méd Assoc, v.106, p.217-224, 2007.
32. Ercan E, Dalli M, Dülgergil CT. In vitro assessment of the effectiveness of chlorhexidine gel and calcium hydroxide paste with chlorhexidine against Enterococcus faecalis and Candida albicans. Oral Surg Oral Med Oral Pathol Oral Radiol Endod, v.102, p.e27-e31, 2006.
33. Evans MD, Baumgartner JC, Khemaleelakul SU, Xia T. Efficacy of calcium hydroxide: chlorhexidine paste as an intracanal medication in bovine dentin. J Endod, v.29, p.338-339, 2003.
34. Estrela C, Estrela CRA, Bammann JC, Pecora JD. Two methods to evaluate the antimicrobial action of calcium hydroxide paste. J Endod 2001; 27:720-3.
35. Faria G, Celes MR, De Rossi A, Silva LA, Silva JS, Rossi MA. Evaluation of chlorhexidine toxicity injected in the paw of mice and added to cultured l929 fibroblasts. J Endod, v.33, p.715-722, 2007.
36. Faria G, Nelson-Filho P, Freitas AC, Assed S, Ito IY. Antibacterial effect of root canal preparation and calcium hydroxide paste (Calen) intracanal dressing in primary teeth with apical periodontitis. J Appl Oral Sci, v.13, p.351-355, 2005.

37. Fava LR, Saunders WP. Calcium hydroxide pastes: classification and clinical indications. Int Endod J, v.32, p.257-282, 1999.

38. Ferreira CM, Da Silva Rosa OP, Torres SA, Ferreira FB, Bernardineli N. Activity of endodontic antibacterial agents against selected anaerobic bacteria. Braz Dent J, v.13, p.118-122, 2002.

39. Ferreira FBA, Souza PARS, Vale MS, Moraes IG, Granjeiro JM. Evaluation of pH levels and calcium íon release in various calcium hydroxide endodontic dressings. Oral Surg Oral Med Oral Pathol Oral Radiol Endod, v.97, p.388-392, 2004.

40. Gendron R, Grenier D, Sorsa T, Mayrand D. Inhibition of the activities of matrix metalloproteinases 2, 8, and 9 by chlorhexidine. Clin Diagn Lab Immunol, v.6, p.437-439, 1999.

41. Georgopoulou M, Kontakiotis E, Nakou M. In vitro evaluation of the effectiveness of calcium hydroxide and paramonochlorophenol on anaerobic bacteria from the root canal. Endod Dent Traumatol, v.9, p.249-253, 1993.

42. Geurtsen W, Leyhausen G. Biological aspects of root canal filling materials-histocompatibility, cytotoxicity, and mutagenicity. Clin Oral Investig, v.1, p.5-11, 1997.

43. Goldschmidt P, Cogen R, Taubman S. Cytopathologic effects of chlorhexidine on human cells. J Periodontol, v.48, p.212-215, 1977.

44. Gomes BPFA, Vianna ME, Sena NT, Zaia AA, Ferraz CCR, Souza-Filho FJ. In vitro evaluation of the antimicrobial activity of calcium hydroxide combined with chlorhexidine gel used as intracanal medicament. Oral Surg Oral Med Oral Pathol Oral Radiol Endod, v.102, p.544-550, 2006.

45. Greenstein G, Berman C, Jaffin R. Chlorhexidine. An adjunct to periodontal therapy. J Periodontol, v.57, p.370-377, 1986.

46. Gurgel-Filho ED, Vivacqua-Gomes N, Gomes BPFA, Ferraz CCR, Zaia AA, Souza-Filho FJS. In vitro evaluation of the effectiveness of the chemomechanical preparation against Enterococcus faecalis after single or multiple-visit root canal treatment. Braz Oral Res, v.21, p.308-313, 2007.

47. Haapasalo M, Udnaes T, Endal U. Persistent recurrent and acquired infection of the root canal system post-treatment. Endod Top, v.6, p.29-56, 2003.

48. Haenni S, Schmidlin PR, Mueller B, Sener B, Zehnder M. Chemical and antimicrobial properties of calcium hydroxide mixed with irrigating solutions. Int Endod J, v.36, p.100-105, 2003.

49. Hama S, Takeichi O, Hayashi M, Komiyama K, Ito K. Co-production of vascular endothelial cadherin and inducible nitric oxide synthase by endothelial cells in periapical granuloma. Int Endod J, v.39, p.179-184, 2006.

50. Hasselgren G, Olsson B, Cvek M. Effects of calcium hydroxide and sodium hypochlorite on the dissolution of necrotic porcine muscle tissue. J Endod, v.14, p.125-127, 1988.

51. Heithersay GS. Periapical repair following conservative endodontic therapy. Aust Dent J, v.15, p.511-518, 1970.

52. Heitz F, Heitz-Mayfield LJ, Lang NP. Effects of post-surgical cleansing protocols on early plaque control in periodontal and/or periimplant wound healing. J Clin Periodontol, v.31, p.1012-1018, 2004.

53. Helgeland K, Heyden G, Rölla G. Effect of chlorhexidine on animals cells in vitro. Scand. J Dent Res, v.79, p.209-215, 1971.

54. Heling I, Steinberg D, Kenig S, Gavrilovich I, Sela MN, Friedman M. Efficacy of a sustained-release device containing chlorhexidine and Ca(OH)2 in preventing secondary infection of dentinal tubules. Int Endod J, v.25, p.20-24, 1992.

55. Herrera H, Herrera H, Leonardo MR, de Paula e Silva FW, da Silva LA. Treatment of external inflammatory root resorption after autogenous tooth transplantation: case report. Oral Surg Oral Med Oral Pathol Oral Radiol Endod, v.102, p.e51-e54, 2006.

56. Hirst RC, Egelberg J, Hornbuckle GC, Oliver RC, Rathbun WE. Microscopic evaluation of topically applied chlorhexidine gluconate on gingival wound healing in dogs. J South Calif Dent Assoc, v.41, p.311-317, 1973.

57. Holland R, Otoboni Filho JA, de Souza V, Nery MJ, Bernabé PF, Dezan Jr E. A comparison of one versus two appointment endodontic therapy in dogs' teeth with apical periodontitis. J Endod, v.29, p.121-124, 2003.

58. Hook WA, Snyderman R, Mergenhagem SE. Histamine releasing factor generated by the interation of endotoxin with hamster serum. Infect Immun, v.2, p.462-467, 1970.

59. Horiba N, Maekawa Y, Yamauchi Y, Ito M, Matsumoto T, Nakamura H. Complement activation by lipopolysaccharides purified from gram-negative bacteria isolated from infected root canals. Oral Surg Oral Med Oral Pathol, v.74, p.648-651, 1992.

60. Huang J, Wong HL, Zhou Y, Wu XY, Grad H, Komorowski, R, Friedman S. In vitro studies and modeling of a controlled-release device for root canal therapy. J Control Release, v.67, p.293-307, 2000.

61. Jaunberzins A, Gutmann JL, Witherspoon DE, Harper RP. Effects of calcium hydroxide and tumor growth factor-ß on collagen synthesis in subcultures I and V of osteoblasts. J Endod, v.26, p.494-499, 2000.

62. Jeansonne MJ, White RR. A comparison of 2.0% chlorhexidine gluconate and 5.25% sodium hypochlorite as antimicrobial endodontic irrigants. J Endod, v.20, p.276-278, 1994.

63. Jenkins S, Addy M, Wade W. The mechanism of action of chlorhexidine. A study of plaque growth on enamel inserts in vivo. J Clin Periodontol, v.15, p.415-424, 1988.

64. Jiang J, Zuo J, Chen SH, Holiday LS. Calcium hydroxide reduces lipopolysaccharide-stimulated osteoclast formation. Oral Surg Oral Med Oral Pathol Oral Radiol Endod, v.95, p.348-354, 2003.

65. Jones DS, Brown AF, Woolfson AD, Dennis AC, Matchett LJ, Bell SE. Examination of the physical state of chlorhexidine within viscoelastic, bioadhesive semisolids using raman spectroscopy. J Pharm Sci, v.89, p.563-571, 2000.

66. Kakehashi S, Stanley HR, Fitzgerald RJ. The effects of surgical exposures of dental pulps in germ-free and conventional laboratory rats. Oral Surg Oral Med Oral Pathol, v.20, p.340-349, 1965.

67. Katagiri T, Takahashi N. Regulatory mechanisms of osteoblast and osteoclast differentiation. Oral Dis, v.8, p.147-159, 2002.

68. Katebzadeh N, Hupp J, Trope M. Histological periapical repair after obturation of infected root canals in dogs. J Endod, v.25, p.364-368, 1999.

69. Knuuttila M, Söderling E. Effect of chlorhexidine on the release of lysosomal enzymes from cultured macrophages. Acta Odontol Scand, v.39, p.285–289, 1981.

70. Lenet BJ, Komorowski R, Wu XY, Huang J, Grad H, Lawrence HP, Friedman S. Antimicrobial substantivity of bovine root dentin exposed to different chlorhexidine delivery vehicles. J Endod, v.26, p.652-655, 2000.

71. Leonardo MR. Endodoncia: tratamiento de conductos radiculares. Princípios técnicos y biológicos. 1.ª ed. São Paulo: Artes Médicas, 2005.

72. Leonardo MR, Almeida WA, Ito IY, da Silva LA. Radiographic and microbiologic evaluation of posttreatment apical and periapical repair of root canals of dogs' teeth with experimentally induced chronic lesion. Oral Surg Oral Med Oral Pathol, v.78, p.232-238, 1994.

73. Leonardo MR, Bezerra da Silva LA, Utrilla LS, Leonardo RT, Consolaro A. Effect of intracanal dressings on repair and apical bridging of teeth with incomplete root formation. Endod Dent Traumatol, v.9, p.25-30, 1993.

74. Leonardo MR, da Silva LA, Leonardo RT, Utrilla LS, Assed S. Histological evaluation of therapy using a calcium hydroxide dressing for teeth with incompletely formed apices and periapical lesions. J Endod, v.19, p.348-352, 1993.

75. Leonardo MR, da Silva LA, Tanomaru Filho M, Bonifácio KC, Ito IY. In vitro evaluation of anti-

microbial activity of sealers and pastes used in endodontics. J Endod, v.26, p.391-394, 2000.

76. Leonardo MR, Hernandez ME, Silva LA, Tanomaru-Filho M. Effect of a calcium hydroxide-based root canal dressing on periapical repair in dogs: a histological study. Oral Surg Oral Med Oral Pathol Oral Radiol Endod, v.102, p.680-685, 2006.
77. Leonardo MR, Rossi MA, Bonifácio KC, da Silva, L.A.; Assed, S. Scanning electron microscopy of the apical structure of human teeth. Ultrastruct Pathol, v.31, p.321-325, 2007.
78. Leonardo, M.R.; Rossi, M.A.; Silva, L.A.; Ito, I.Y.; Bonifácio, K.C. EM evaluation of bacterial biofilm and microorganisms on the apical external root surface of human teeth. J Endod, v.28, p.815-818, 2002.
79. Leonardo MR, Salgado AA, da Silva LA, Tanomaru Filho M. Apical and periapical repair of dogs' teeth with periapical lesions after endodontic treatment with different root canal sealers. Pesqui Odontol Bras, v.17, p.69-74, 2003.
80. Leonardo MR, Silva LA, Utrilla LS, Assed S, Ether SS. Calcium hydroxide root canal sealers – histopathologic evaluation of apical and periapical repair after endodontic treatment. J Endod, v.23, p.428-432, 1997.
81. Leonardo MR, Silva RAB, Assed S, Nelson-Filho. P. Importance of bacterial endotoxin (LPS) in endodontics. J Appl Oral Sci, v.12, p.93-98, 2004.
82. Leonardo MR, Silveira FF, Silva LA, Tanomaru Filho, M, Utrilla LS. Calcium hydroxide root canal dressing. Histopathological evaluation of periapical repair at different time periods. Braz Dent J, v.13, p.17-22, 2002.
83. Leonardo MR, Simões Filho AP, Esberard RM, Bonetti Filho I, Leonardo RT. Safe and easy way to use calcium hydroxide as a temporary dressing. J Endod, v.19, p.319-320, 1993.
84. Leonardo MR, Tanomaru Filho M, Silva LA, Nelson Filho P, Bonifácio KC, Ito IY. In vivo antimicrobial activity of 2% chlorhexidine used as a root canal irrigating solution. J Endod, v.25, p.167-171, 1999.
85. Leonardo MR, Almeida WA, da Silva LA, Utrilla LS. Histopathological observations of periapical repair in teeth with radiolucent áreas submitted to two different methods of root canal treatment. J Endod, v.21, p.137-141, 1995.
86. Lin NY, Gao XJ. A short-term clinical study of one-visit endodontic treatment for infected root canals. Zhonghua Kou Qiang Yi Xue Za Zhi, v.41, p.525-528, 2006.
87. Lin LM, Lin J, Rosenberg PA. One-appointment endodontic therapy: biological considerations. J Am Dent Assoc, v.138, p.1.456-1.462, 2007.
88. Lin LM, Di Fiore PM, Lin J, Rosenberg PA. Histological study of periradicular tissue responses to uninfected and infected devitalized pulps in dogs. J Endod, v.32, p.34-38, 2006.
89. Löe H. Discussion of methods and criteria in evaluation of gingival and periodontal response. Int Dent J, v.20, p.502-504, 1997.
90. Lu Y, Liu T, Li X, Li H, Pi G. Histologic evaluation of direct pulp capping with a self-etching adhesive and calcium hydroxide in beagles. Oral Surg Oral Med Oral Pathol Oral Radiol Endod, v.102, p.e78-e-84, 2006.
91. Lucarotti ME, White H, Deas J, Silver IA, Leaper DJ. Antiseptic toxicity to breast carcinoma in tissue culture: an adjuvant to conservation therapy? Ann R. Coll Surg Engl, v.72, p.388-392, 1990.
92. Manzur A, González AM, Pozos A, Silva-Herzog D, Friedman S. Bacterial quantification in teeth with apical periodontitis related to instrumentation and different intracanal medications: a randomized clinical trial. J Endod, v.33, p.114-118, 2007.
93. Mariotti AJ, Rumpf DA. Chlorhexidine-induced changes to human gingival fibroblast collagen and non-collagen protein production. J Periodontol v.70, p.1443-1448, 1999.
94. Marquis VL, Dao T, Farzaneh M, Abitbol S, Friedman S. Treatment outcome in endodontics: the Toronto Study. Phase III: initial treatment. J Endod, v.32, p.299-306, 2006.
95. Martinho FC, Gomes BP. Quantification of endotoxins and cultivable bacteria in root canal infection before and after chemomechanical preparation with 2.5% sodium hypochlorite. J Endod, v.34, p.268-272, 2008.
96. Matsushita K, Tajima T, Tomita K, Takada H, Nagaoka S, Torii M. Inflammatory cytokine production and specific antibody responses to lipopolysaccharide from endodontopathic black-pigmented bacteria in patients with multilesional periapical periodontitis. J Endod, v.25, p.795-799, 1999.
97. Mc Gee JOD, Isaacson PG, Wright NA. Oxford textbook of pathology. Principles of pathology. Oxford: University Press; 1992.
98. Molander A, Warfvinge J, Reit C, Kvist T. Clinical and radiographic evaluation of one- and two-visit endodontic treatment of asymptomatic necrotic teeth with apical periodontitis: a randomized clinical trial. J Endod, v.33, p.1145-1148, 2007.
99. Möller AJ, Fabricius L, Dahlén G, Ohman AE, Heyden G. Influence on periapical tissues of indigenous oral bacteria and necrotic pulp tissue in monkeys. Scand J Dent Res, v.89, p.475-484, 1981.
100. Morrison B, Kline L. Activation of the classical and properdin pathways of complement by bacterial lipopolysaccharides (LPS). J Immunol, v.118, p.362-368, 1977.
101. Munford RS, Hall CL. Detoxification of bacterial lipopolysaccharides (endotoxins) by a human neutrophil enzyme. Science, v.234, p.203-205, 1986.
102. Murakami T, Murakami H, Ramp WK, Hudson MC, Nousiainen MT. Calcium hydroxide ameliorates tobramycin toxicity in cultured chick tibiae. Bone, v.21, p.411-418, 1997.
103. Murray PE, García Godoy C, García Godoy F. How is the biocompatibilty of dental biomaterials evaluated? Med Oral Patol Oral Cir Bucal, v.12, p.E258-E266, 2007.
104. Naenni N, Thoma K, Zehnder M. Soft tissue dissolution capacity of currently used and potential endodontic irrigants. J Endod, v.30, p.785-787, 2004.
105. Nair PN, Sjögren U, Krey G, Kahnberg KE, Sundqvist G. Intraradicular bacteria and fungi in root-filled, asymptomatic human teeth with therapy-resistant periapical lesions: a long-term light and electron microscopic follow-up study. J Endod, v.16, p.580-588, 1990.
106. Nair PN. On the causes of persistent apical periodontitis: a review. Int Endod J, v.39, p.249-281, 2006.
107. Nelson Filho P, Silva LAB, Leonardo MR, Utrilla LS, Figueiredo F. Conective tissue responses to calcium hydroxide based root canal medicaments. Int Endod J, v.32, p.303-311, 1999.
108. Nelson-Filho P, Leonardo MR, Silva LAB, Assed S. Radiografic evaluation of the effect of endotoxin (LPS) plus calcium hydroxide on apical and periapical tissues of dogs. J Endod, v.28, p.694-696, 2002.
109. Nerwich A, Figdor D, Messer HH. pH changes in root dentin over a 4-week period following root canal dressing with calcium hydroxide. J Endod, v.19, p.302-306, 1993.
110. Niwa M, Milner KC, Ribi E, Rudbach JA. Alteration of physical, chemical, and biological properties of endotoxin by treatment with mild alkali. J Bacteriol, v.97, p.1069-1077, 1969.
111. Ohara P, Torabinejad M, Kettering JD. Antibacterial effects of various endodontic irrigants on selected anaerobic bacteria. Endod Dent Traumatol, v.9, p.95-100, 1993.
112. Okino LA, Siqueira EL, Santos M, Bombana AC, Figueiredo JA. Dissolution of pulp tissue by aqueous solution of chlorhexidine digluconate and chlorhexidine digluconate gel. Int Endod J, v.37, p.38-41, 2004.
113. Oliveira LD, Jorge AO, Carvalho CA, Koga-Ito CY, Valera MC. In vitro effects of endodontic irrigants on endotoxins in root canals. Oral Surg Oral Med Oral Pathol Oral Radiol Endod, v.104, p.135-142, 2007.

114. Oliveira LD, Leão MVP, Carvalho CAT, Camargo CHR, Valera MC, Jorge AOC, Unterkircher CS. In vitro effects of calcium hydroxide and polymyxin B on endotoxins in root canals. J Dent, v.33, p.107-114, 2005.

115. Onçag O, Hosgor M, Hilmioglu S, Zekioglu O, Eronat C, Burhanoglu D. Comparison of antibacterial and toxic effects of various root canals irrigants. Int Endod J, v.36, p.423-432, 2003.

116. Oppenhein JJ, Perry S. Effects of endotoxins on cultured leukocytes. Proc Soc Exp Biol Med, v.118, p.1.014-1.019, 1965.

117. Orstavik D, Kerekes K, Molven O. Effects of extensive apical reaming and calcium hydroxide dressing on bacterial infection during treatment of apical periodontitis: a pilot study. Int Endod J, v.24, p.1-7, 1991.

118. Pashley DH. Dentine permeability: theory and practice. In: Spangberg LSW. Experimental Endodontics. Boca Raton: CRC Press, 1990. p.19-49.

119. Patel P, Ide M, Coward P, Di Silvio L. The effect of a commercially available chlorhexidine mouthwash product on human osteoblast cells. Eur J Prosthodont Restor Dent, v.14, p.67-72, 2006.

120. Pazelli LC, Freitas AC, Ito IY, Souza-Gugelmim MCM, Medeiros AS, Nelson-Filho P. Prevalence of microorganisms in root canals of human deciduos teeth with necrotic pulp and chronic periapical lesions. Pesqui Odontol Bras, v.17, p.367-371, 2003.

121. Penesis VA, Fitzgerald PI, Fayad MI, Wenckus CS, BeGole EA, Johnson BR. Outcome of one-visit and two-visit endodontic treatment of necrotic teeth with apical periodontitis: a randomized controlled trial with one-year evaluation. J Endod, v.34, p.251-257, 2008.

122. Perrier S, Kherratia B, Deschaumes C, Ughetto S, Kemeny JL, Baudet-Pommel M, Sauvezie B. IL-1ra and IL-1 production in human oral mucosal epithelial cells in culture: differential modulation by TGF-beta1 and IL-4. Clin. Exp. Immunol., v.127, p.53-59, 2002.

123. Podbielski A, Spahr A, Haller B. Additive antimicrobial activity of calcium hydroxide and chlorhexidine on common endodontic bacterial pathogens. J Endod, v.29, p.340-345. 2003.

124. Pucher JJ, Daniel JC. The effects of chlorhexidine digluconate on human fibroblasts in vitro. J Periodontol, v.63, p.526-532, 1992.

125. Rehman K, Saunders WP, Foye RH, Sharkey SW. Calcium ion diffusion from calcium hydroxide – containing materials in endodontically-treated teeth: an in vitro study. Int Endod J, v.29, p.271-279, 1996.

126. Rietschel ET, Brade H. Bacterial endotoxins. Sci Am, v.267, p.26-33, 1992.

127. Rocha CT, Rossi MA, Leonardo MR, Rocha LB, Nelson-Filho P, Silva LA. Biofilm on the apical region of roots in primary teeth with vital and necrotic pulps with or without radiographically evident apical pathosis. Int Endod J, 2008.

128. Rosenthal S, Spångberg L, Safavi K. Chlorhexidine substantivity in root canal dentin. Oral Surg Oral Med Oral Pathol Oral Radiol Endod, v.98, p.488-492, 2004.

129. Ruviére DB, Leonardo MR, da Silva LA, Ito IY, Nelson-Filho P. Assessment of the microbiota in root canals of human primary teeth by checkerboard DNA-DNA hybridization. J Dent Child, v.74, p.118-123, 2007.

130. Safavi K, Nichols FC. Effect of calcium hydroxide on bacterial lipopolyssaccharide. J Endod, v.19, p.76-78, 1993.

131. Safavi KE, Nichols FC. Alteration of biological properties of bacterial lipopolysaccharide by calcium hydroxide treatment. J Endod, v.20, p.127-129, 1994.

132. Sant'anna AT, Spolidório LC, Ramalho LT. Histological analysis of the association between formocresol and endotoxin in the subcutaneous tissue of mice. Braz Dent J, v.19, p.40-45, 2008.

133. Sathorn C, Parashos P, Messer H. The prevalence of postoperative pain and flare-up in single- and multiple-visit endodontic treatment: a systematic review. Int Endod J, v.41, p.91-99, 2008.

134. Schäfer E, Bossmann K. Antimicrobial efficacy of chloroxylenol and chlorhexidine in the treatment of infected root canals. Am J Dent, v.14, p.233-237, 2001.

135. Schein B, Schilder H. Endotoxin content in endodontically involved teeth. J Endod, v.1, p.19-21, 1975.

136. Schilder H, Amsterdam M. Inflamatory potencial of root canal medicaments. Oral Surg Oral Med Oral Pathol, v.12, p.211-221, 1959.

137. Schroder U. Effects of calcium hydroxide-containing pulp-capping agents on pulp cell migration, proliferation, and differentiation. J Dent Res, v.64, p.541-548, 1985.

138. Seltzer S, Farber PA. Microbiologic factors in endodontologt. Oral Surg, v.78, p.634-645, 1994.

139. Shovelton DS. The presence and distribution of microorganisms within non-vital teeth. Br Dent J, v.117, p.101-107, 1964.

140. Shuping GB, Orstavik D, Sigurdsson A, Trope M. Reduction of intracanal bacteria using nickel-titanium rotary instrumentation and various medications. J Endod, v.26, p.751-755, 2000.

141. Silva LAB. Tratado de Odontopeediatría. Caracas: AMOLCA, 2008.

142. Silva RAB, Leonardo MR, Silva LAB, Faccioli LH, Medeiros AI. Effect of a calcium hydroxide-based paste associated to chlorhexidine on raw 264.7 macrophage cell line culture. Oral Surg Oral Pathol Oral Méd Oral Radiol Endod, 2008a (Aceito).

143. Silva RAB, Leonardo MR, Silva LAB, Castro LMS, Rosa AL, De Oliveira PT. Effects of the association between a calcium hydroxide paste and 0.4% chlorhexidine on the development of the osteogenic phenotype in vitro. J Endod, 2008b (Enviado).

144. Silva RAB, Nelson-Filho P, Silva LAB, Leonardo MR, Ito IY. In Vitro Antimicrobial Activity Of A Calcium Hydroxide-Based Paste Associated To Chlorhexidine. Braz Oral Res, 2008c (Enviado).

145. Silva RAB, Assed S, Nelson Filho P, Silva LB, Consolaro A. Subcutaneous tissue response of isogenic mice to calcium hydroxide-based pastes in association with chlorhexidine. Oral Surg Oral Pathol Oral Méd Oral Radiol Endod, 2008d (Enviado).

146. Silva L, Nelson-Filho P, Leonardo MR, Rossi MA, Pansani CA. Effect of calcium hydroxide on bacterial endotoxin in vivo. J Endod, v.28, p.94-98, 2002.

147. Silva LA, Leonardo MR, Assed S, Tanomaru Filho M. Histological study of the effect of some irrigating solutions on bacterial endotoxin in dogs. Braz Dent J, v.15, p.109-114, 2004.

148. Silva LA, Nelson-Filho P, Faria G, de Souza-Gugelmin MC, Ito IY. Bacterial profile in primary teeth with necrotic pulp and periapical lesions. Braz Dent J, v.17, p.144-148, 2006.

149. Silveira AM, Lopes HP, Siqueira JR JF, Macedo SB, Consolaro A. Periradicular repair after two-visit endodontic treatment using two different intracanal medications compared to single-visit endodontic treatment. Braz Dent J, v.18, p.299-304, 2007.

150. Siqueira JR JF, Batista MM, Fraga RC, de Uzeda M. Antibacterial effects of endodontic irrigants on black-pigmented gram-negative anaerobes and facultative bacteria. J Endod, v.24, p.414-416. 1998.

151. Siqueira Jr JF, Rôças IN, Alves FR, Santos KR. Selected endodontic pathogens in the apical third of infected root canals: a molecular investigation. J Endod, v.30, p.638-643, 2004.

152. Siqueira Jr JF, Rôças IN, Favieri A, Oliveira JCM, Santos KRN. Polymerase chain reaction detection of Treponema denticola in endodontic infections within root canals. Int Endod J, v.34, p.280-284, 2001.

153. Sjögren U, Figdor D, Persson S, Sundqvist G. Influence of infection at the time of root filling on the outcome of endodontic treatment of teeth with apical periodontitis. Int Endod J, v.30, p.297-306, 1997.

154. Sjogren U, Hagglund B, Sundqvist G, Wing K. Factors affecting the long-term results of endodontic treatment. J Endod, v.16, p.498-504, 1990.

155. Soares JA, Leonardo MR, Silva LAB, Tanomaru Filho M, Ito IY. Effect of biomechanical preparation and calcium hydroxide pastes on the antisepsis of root canal systems in dogs. J Appl Oral Sci, v.13, p.93-100, 2005.

156. Soares JA, Leonardo MR, Tanomaru Filho M, Silva LA, Ito iY. Residual antibacterial activity of chlorhexidine digluconate and camphorated p-monochlorophenol in calcium hydroxide-based root canal dressings. Braz Dent J, v.18, p.8-15, 2007.

157. Socransky SS, Haffajee AD, Smith C, Martin L, Haffajee JA, Uzel NG, Goodson JM. Use of checkerboard DNA-DNA hybridization to study complex microbial ecosystems. Oral Microbiol Immunol, v.19, p.352-362, 2004.

158. Southard SR, Drisko CL, Killoy WJ, Cobb CM, Tira DE. The effect of 2% chlorhexidine digluconate irrigation on clinical parameters and the level of Bacteroides gingivalis in periodontal pockets. J Periodontol, v.60, p.302-309, 1989.

159. Stashenko P, Teles R, D'Souza R. Periapical inflammatory responses and their modulation. Crit Rev Oral Biol Med, v.9, p.498-521, 1998.

160. Stashenko P. The role of immune cytokines in the pathogenesis of periapical lesions. Endod Dent Traumatol, v.6, p.89-96, 1990.

161. Sundqvist G. Ecology of the root canal flora. J Endod, v.18, p.427-430, 1992.

162. Takeichi O, Hayashi M, Tsurumachi T, Tomita T, Ogihara H, Ogiso B, Saito T. Inducible nitric oxide synthase activity by interferon-gamma-producing cells in human radicular cysts. Int Endod J, v.32, p.124-130, 1999.

163. Tani-Ishii N, Wang CY, Tanner A, Stashenko P. Changes in root canal microbiota during the development of rat periapical lesions. Oral Microbiol Immunol, v.9, p.129-135, 1994.

164. Tanomaru JM, Leonardo MR, Tanomaru Filho M, Bonetti Filho I, Silva LA. Effect of different irrigation solutions and calcium hydroxide on bacterial LPS. Int Endod J, v.36, p.733-739, 2003.

165. Tanomaru JM, Leonardo MR, Tanomaru-Filho M, Silva LA, Ito IY. Microbial distribution in the root canal system after periapical lesion induction using different methods. Braz Dent J, v.19, p.124-129, 2008.

166. Tanomaru JMG, Pappen FG, Tanomaru-Filho M, Spolidorio DMP, Ito IY. In vitro antimicrobial activity of different gutta-percha points and calcium hydroxide pastes. Braz Oral Res, v.21, p.35-39, 2007.

167. Tanomaru-Filho M, Leonardo MR, Silva LA, Aníbal FF, Faccioli LH. Inflammatory response to different endodontic irrigating solutions. Int Endod J, v.35, p.735-739, 2002.

168. Torabinejad M, Eby WC, Naidorf IJ. Inflammatory and immunological aspects of the pathogenesis of human periapical lesions. J Endod, v.11, p.479-488, 1985.

169. Tronstad L, Barnett F, Riso K, Slots J. Extraradicular endodontic infections. Endod Dent Traumatol, v.3, p.86-90, 1987.

170. Trope M, Delano EO, Orstavik D. Endodontic treatment of teeth with apical periodontitis: single vs. multivisit treatment. J Endod, v.25, p.345-350, 1999.

171. Vahdaty A, Pitt Ford TR, Wilson RF. Efficacy of chlorhexidine in disinfecting dentinal tubules in vitro. Endod Dent Traumatol, v.9, p.243-248, 1993.

172. Vianna ME, Gomes BP, Berber VB, Zaia AA, Ferraz CC, de Souza-Filho FJ. In vitro evaluation of the antimicrobial activity of chlorhexidine and sodium hypochlorite. Oral Surg Oral Med Oral Pathol Oral Radiol Endod, v.97, p.79-84, 2004.

173. Waltimo TM, Sen BH, Meurman JH, Ørstavik D, Haapasalo MP. Yeasts in apical periodontitis. Crit Rev Oral Biol Med, v.14, p.128-137, 2003.

174. Waltimo TM, Sirén EK, Orstavik D, Haapasalo MP. Susceptibility of oral Candida species to calcium hydroxide in vitro. Int Endod J, v.32, p.94-98, 1999.

175. Wang CY, Stashenko P. Characterization of bone-resorbing activity in human periapical lesions. J Endod, v.19, p.107-111, 1993.

176. Wang JD, Hume WR. Diffusion of hydrogen ion and hydroxyl ion from various sources through dentine. Int Endod J, v.21, p.17-26, 1988.

177. Wennberg A. Biological evaluation of root canal antiseptics using in vitro and in vivo methods. Scand. J Dent Res, v.88, p.46-52, 1980.

178. White RR, Hays GL, Janer LR. Residual antimicrobial activity after canal irrigation with chlorhexidine. J Endod, v.23, p.229-231, 1997.

179. Wolff S. Biological effects of bacterial endotoxins in man. J Infect Dis, v.128, p.S259-S269, 1973.

180. Yamasaki M, Nakane A, Kumazawa M, Hashioka K, Horiba N, Nakamura H. Endotoxin and gram-negative bacteria in the rat periapical lesions. J Endod, v.18, p.501-504, 1992.

181. Yamashita JC, Tanomaru Filho M, Leonardo MR, Rossi MA, Silva LA. Scanning electron microscopic study of the cleaning ability of chlorhexidine as a root-canal irrigant. Int Endod J, v.36, p.391-394, 2003.

182. Yesilsoy C, Whitaker E, Cleveland D, Phillips E, Trope M. Antimicrobial and toxic effects of established and potential root canal irrigants. J Endod, v.21, p.513-515, 1995.

183. Yeung SY, Huang CS, Chan CP, Lin CP, Lin HN, Lee PH, Jia HW, Huang SK, Jeng JH, Chang MC. Antioxidant and pro-oxidant properties of chlorhexidine and its interaction with calcium hydroxide solutions. Int Endod J, v.40, p.837-844, 2007.

184. Yoldas O, Topuz A, Isçi AS, Oztunc H. Postoperative pain after endodontic retreatment: single- versus two-visit treatment. Oral Surg Oral Med Oral Pathol Oral Radiol Endod, v.98, p.483-487, 2004.

185. Yucel AC, Aksoy A, Ertas E, Guvenc D. The pH changes of calcium hydroxide mixed with six different vehicles. Oral Surg Oral Med Oral Pathol Oral Radiol Endod, v.103, p.712-717, 2007.

186. Zehnder M, Grawehr M, Hasselgren G, Waltimo T. Tissue-dissolution capacity and dentin-disinfecting potential of calcium hydroxide mixed with irrigating solutions. Oral Surg Oral Med Oral Pathol Oral Radiol Endod, v.96, p.608-613, 2003.

187. Zerella JA, Fouad AF, Spångberg LS. Effectiveness of a calcium hydroxide and chlorhexidine digluconate mixture as disinfectant during retreatment of failed endodontic cases. Oral Surg Oral Med Oral Pathol Oral Radiol Endod, v.100, p.756-761, 2005.

2.X

Rotary Systems in Endodontics

Renato de Toledo Leonardo
Maria Guiomar Azevedo Bahia
Carlos Garcia Puente
Alejandro Jaime

When

the success rates after endodontic treatment are clinically and radiographically evaluated using longitudinal statistical criteria, it is verified that after following up treatments for two years, an average of 30% need to be redone. There are many factors that contribute to the high level of failure – for example, many professionals do not even perform endodontic treatment under absolute isolation. In 2005, only 4% of Danish dentists routinely used the rubber dam[11]. Taking into consideration the importance of bacterial infiltration in the crown-apex direction, we begin to understand and explain the reasons for endodontic failures. On the other hand, when analyzing the materials and substances used in endodontic treatments, we find the large-scale use of type K and Hedströen files, calcium hydroxide, sodium hypochlorite solution, zinc oxide and eugenol-based cements, materials that have been used in endodontic treatments for over 80 years. In the view of these facts, it is rather surprising that the failure levels are not higher.

The operating microscope, third generation electronic apex locators, reappearance of ultrasound, and adhesive root canal adhesive filling techniques are new technologies that endeavor to modify the *status quo* of present day endodontics.

There are new technologies to be considered in root canal preparations, such as rotary instruments made of nickel-titanium alloy. The search for a metal alloy that is more flexible than stainless steel, which could turn inside the root canal, cleaning and modeling more efficiently, has been in progress for a long time.

In an endeavor to overcome the limitations of stainless steel instruments when they are used in curved root canals, nickel-titanium alloy (NiTi) instruments were introduced into endodontics by Walia *et al.* (1988)[65], as an alternative. By means of mechanical tests, the authors observed that these instruments presented two or three times more flexibility than those made of stainless steel, as well as a higher resistance to torsion fracture, attributed to the low modulus of elasticity of the alloy.

Nickel-titanium alloys with antimagnetic properties and resistance to corrosion, were developed by Buehler *et al.*[15], in the early 1960s, for application in parts and instruments for the space program. The alloys were generically called Nitinol, because they had been developed at the *Naval Ordnance Laboratory* – NOL, a North American marine research center (Thompson, 2000)[83].

NiTi alloys are widely used because of two special properties: superelasticity (SE) and the form memory effect (FME), in addition to having high resistance to corrosion and biocompatibility (Serene *et al.*[58], 1995; Thompson[63], 2000). Their mechanical properties and behavior vary according to their chemical composition, production characteristics and the thermo-mechanical treatment applied during manufacturing (Thompson[63], 2000; Kuhn *et al.*, 2001).

Among the multiple commercial applications of NiTi alloys in medical and dentistry areas, the catheters and stents for arterial unobstruction, used in cardiovascular surgeries, deserve to be mentioned, as well as the wires used in orthodontic appliances and in the manufacture of manual and rotary endodontic instruments.

MARTENSITIC TRANSFORMATION (MT), SHAPE-MEMORY EFFECT (SME) AND SUPERELASTICITY (SE).

Both the FME and SE are associated with a change of phase of the solid state of the alloy: martensitic transformation (MT), which may be induced by **stress application** or by a **reduction in temperature** (Otsuka & Wayman[45], 1998; Thompson[63], 2000). Martensitic transformation is a transformation between a high symmetry crystalline structure phase, called austenite or parent phase, and a low symmetry phase, called martensite. During this transformation, the atoms move cooperatively by a shear-like mechanism, without altering the chemical composition of the matrix, and are rearranged into a more stable new crystalline structure (Otsuka & Wayman[45], 1998; Thompson[63], 2000). Typically, austenite is stable when exposed to high temperatures and low stress values, while martensite is stable at low temperatures and high stress values. The phase transformation between the austenite and martensite states is the key to explaining the FME and SE (Otsuka & Wayman[45], 1998).

The shape-memory effect is the ability to recover large non-linear deformations by means of moderate heating, although the material has apparently undergone permanent deformation. In other words, deformations that occur in "conventional" metals or alloys by the plastic flow regime, that is, which would be permanent, can be annulled in shape-memory alloys by simply increasing the temperature of the material by a few degrees. NiTi alloys can be "programmed" by selecting their chemical composition and using the appropriate thermomechanical treatments, so that their shape is recovered by stress withdrawal only, without the need for heating. This effect allows the instantaneous recovery of large non-linear deformations, providing the material with a feature conventionally called "superelasticity", which is a particular case of SMF. While the SMF involves thermal and mechanical processes, in SE the driving force for the transformation is mechanical (Otsuka & Wayman[45], 1998; Thompson[63], 2000).

The superelastic behavior of NiTi alloy is illustrated in the tension-deformation curve obtained in a uniaxial tensile test (Fig. 2.X-1) in comparison with austenitic stainless steel, previously deformed. When testing is interrupted after 8% of deformation, the stainless steel recovers approximately 0.3% from this deformation, while the NiTi superelastic alloy recovers to its original shape from an 8% deformation (Otsuka & Wayman[45], 1998).

When a material that undergoes MT is cooled below certain temperature, the transformation starts by a shear mechanism, as illustrated in Figure 2.X-2. The martensitic regions in A and B have the same crystalline structure, but the spatial orientations of the crystals are different. These regions are called variants of martensite. As the martensite shows low symmetry, many variants may be formed from the same parent phase (Kennon & Dunne[30], 1981; Otsuka & Wayman[45], 1998).

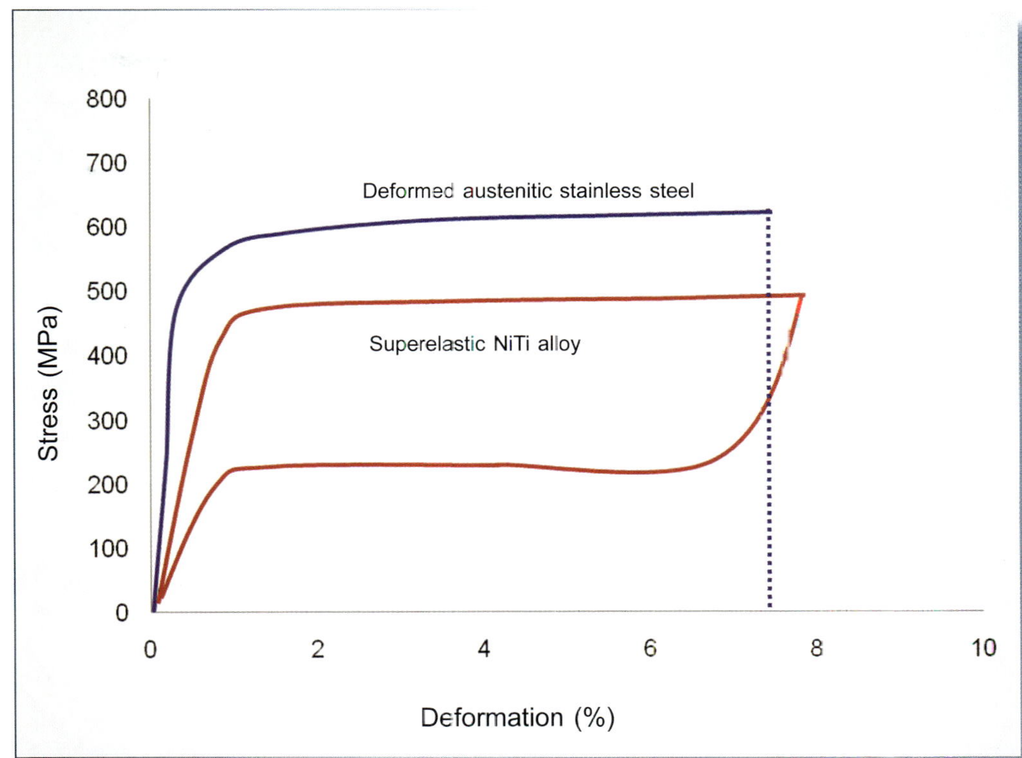

FIG. 2.X-1
Schematic tension-deformation curves in traction for deformed austenitic stainless steel and a superelastic NiTi alloy.

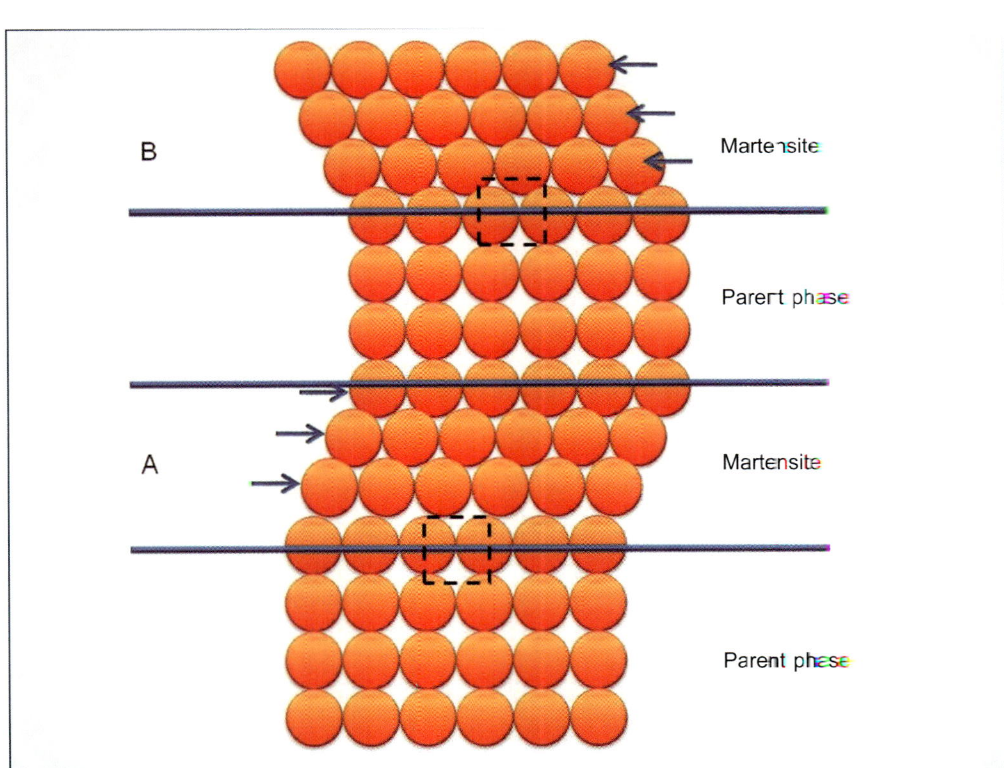

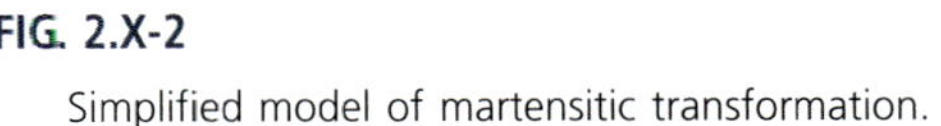

FIG. 2.X-2
Simplified model of martensitic transformation.

When the material in martensitic state is heated, the martensite becomes unstable, and reverse transformation occurs; that is, the martensite returns to its parent phase. Due to the low symmetry of martensite, return to the high temperature phase occurs by the inverse pathway to that of MT, and the parent phase is formed in its original orientation (Kennon & Dunne[30], 1981; Otsuka & Wayman[45], 1998).

It is possible to vary the NiTi alloy composition in order to obtain wires with FME or SE characteristics. The differences between the alloys will lie in their nickel content and in the temperature range of the martensitic transformation. The NiTi alloy used in endodontics contains approximately 51% of nickel and 49% of titanium, which results in an equiatomic combination of its main components (Serene *et al.*[58], 1995; Thompson[63], 2000, Bahia *et al.*[9], 2005).

When the martensitic transformation takes place during cooling, it begins at a temperature designated as M_s and finishes at a lower temperature, M_f. If cooling is interrupted between the two temperatures, transformation stops. This is another characteristic that differentiates martensitic transformation from other phase changes in the solid state: it is athermal (non-isothermal); that is, it does not occur if the temperature is kept constant. Another important characteristic of martensitic transformation is its high speed, to the order of the speed of sound in the material.

During heating, reverse transformation from martensite into the parent phase occurs, generally referred to as austenite, analogous to the high temperature phase of steels. Reverse transformation has the same characteristics as those of martensitic transformation and starts at a temperature designated A_a, ending at A_t, as illustrated in Figure 2.X-3.

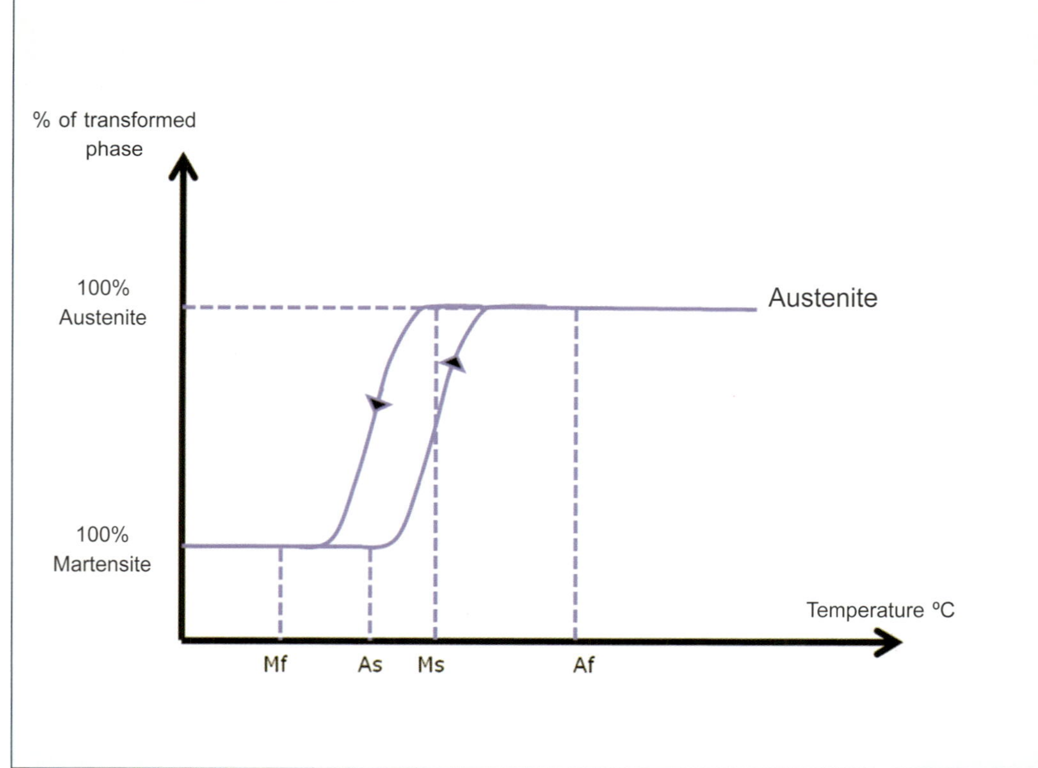

FIG. 2.X-3
Characteristic temperatures of martensitic and reverse transformations.

The theoretical thermogram of martensitic transformation temperatures, in which Ms is the initial temperature of the transformation from austenite into martensite; Mf is the final temperature of transformation, in which all the alloy is martensitic; As is the initial temperature of the reverse transformation and Af the final temperature of the reverse transformation, in which the alloy is completely austenitic.

The mean martensitic and reverse transformation temperatures, determined in samples of NiTi endodontic instruments, are as follows: 18.2°C for Ms; -2.3°C for Mf; 3.4°C for As and 22.9°C for Af. It is found that the alloy is completely austenitic at room temperature, thus showing superelasticity characteristics (Bahia *et al.*[9], 2005).

At temperatures sufficiently above Af, the NiTi alloys in the austenitic phase, behave like a conventional metal, with plastic flow and deformation beginning normally at a low stress level. At temperatures below Ms, the austenite is unstable and is transformed into self-accommodated variants of martensite. At a low stress level, the variants of martensite most favorably oriented grow at the expense of the others, resulting in great deformation. A large amount of this deformation remains after discharge, being capable of recovery by heating and consequent reverse transformation into the austenitic phase. At temperatures slightly above Af, the austenite is transformed into martensite by the application of stress, and undergoes great deformations under constant stress (A-B). During discharge, the stress-induced martensite is reverted into austenite at a lower stress level, with complete recovery from deformation, which characterizes superelasticity (Fig. 2.X-4) (Bahia *et al.*[9], 2005).

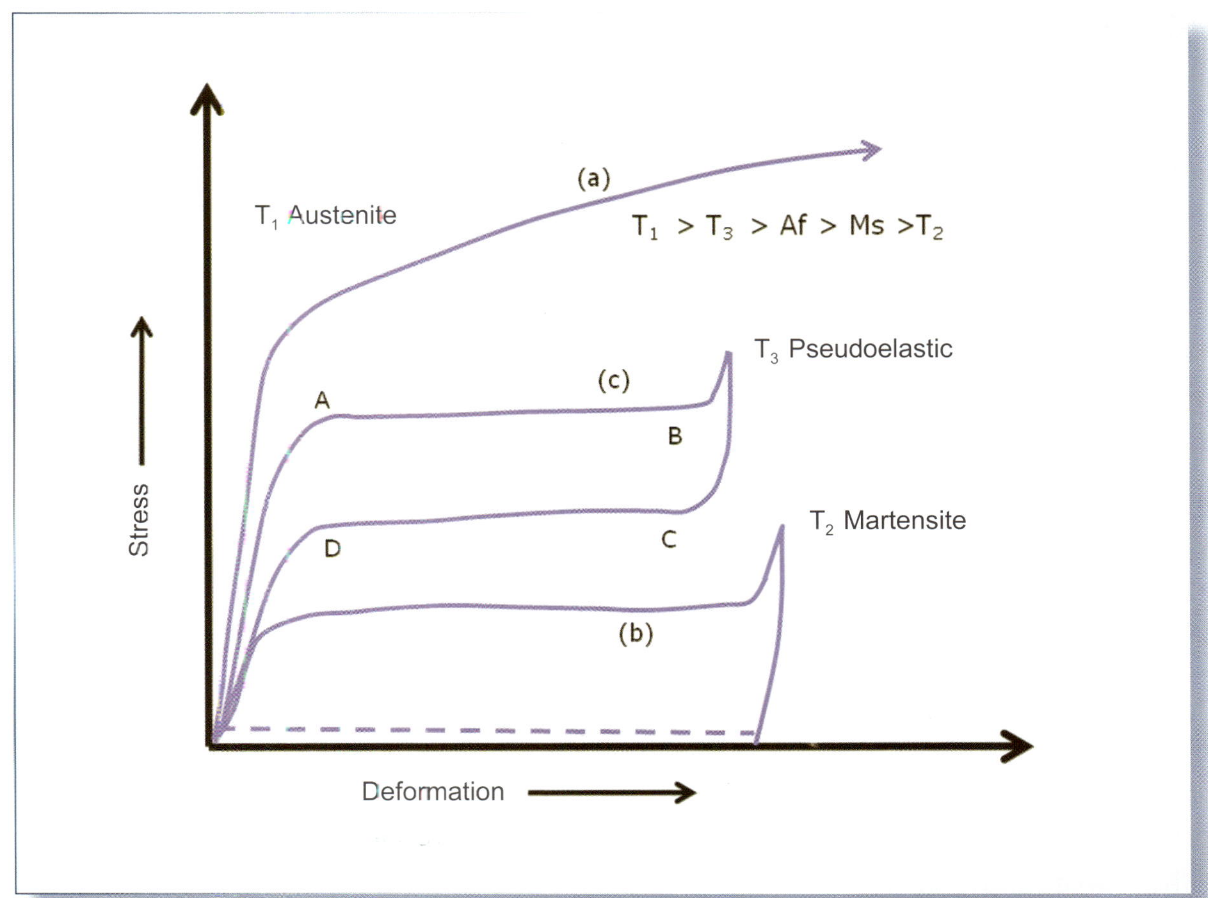

FIG. 2.X-4

Tension-deformation curves for (**a**) stable austenite, (**b**) temperature-induced martensite, and (**c**) tension-induced martensite, where A-B is the deformation undergone by the material during phase transformation and C-D is the recovery of the original form by reverse transformation.

In cases of endodontic instruments, the MT occurs due to the stress imposed by the curvature inside the root canal. Rotary NiTi endodontic instruments are completely austenitic at room temperature. These instruments show superelastic behavior during clinical use, in which the imposition of stress induced by the root curvature, results in cycles of martensitic and reverse transformation, due to the rotary movement. When stress is finally removed by withdrawing the instrument from the interior of the root canal, consequent reverse transformation into the original austenitic structure occurs (Brantley *et al.*[14], 2002). The martensite is capable of absorbing up to 8% of recoverable deformation. In the presence of minimal additional deformation, the self-accommodated martensite undergoes an elastic deformation. Any deformation in addition to this will result in plastic deformation, and later fracture (Gambarini[21], 2000).

NiTi instruments show a superelastic behavior, and remain within this regime in situations that would cause permanent deformations in stainless steel instruments (Bahia *et al.*[9], 2005). Due to the increased flexibility, NiTi instruments have the advantage of causing less canal transportation during instrumentation (Glosson *et al.*[26], 1995). Owing to their high flexibility, NiTi instruments are produced by the machining process because the superelasticity of the alloy makes it impossible to twist the shaft in order to produce the spiral (Thompson[63], 2000). Generally, machining of the instruments results in surfaces with a high concentration of defects, such as barbs, cavities, machining scratches, as well as pits and thick cutting edges, which may compromise their cutting ability, favor instrument corrosion, and potentially cause the nucleation of microcracks (Serene *et al.*[58], 1995; Melo *et al.*[43], 2002; Martins *et al.*[40], 2002. Bahia *et al.*[9], 2005).

Moreover, the flexibility of the alloy has provided the advantage of manufacturing rotary instruments capable of performing 360-degree movements in curved canals, making it possible to prepare them quickly and efficiently. Instrumentation thus performed creates favorable conditions: effective cleaning and shaping, due to a good cutting ability, and deeper penetration of the irrigation syringe into the root canal, allowing adequate, abundant and easy flow of auxiliary chemical substances. In addition to these actions, there is also the possibility of dense and tridimensional gutta-percha compaction during filling of the root canal system.

MORPHOLOGICAL CHARACTERISTICS OF ROTARY INSTRUMENTS MADE OF NITI

It is imperative to know the design features of the rotary instruments. This knowledge will enable professionals to obtain and use all the advantages and benefits this type of instrumentation offers. The introduction of new instruments, with new designs, could lead to significant improvements in clinical performance, bearing in mind that when the professional keeps instruments that lead to inefficient preparation, and is unaware of this fact, it allows industry to re-introduce low quality instruments on the market under the guise of innovations. Any improvement or advancement in endodontic treatment is preceded by full knowledge of the instrument the professional owns. Thus, it is imperative to present and describe the features of the rotary instrument (Fig. 2.X-5).

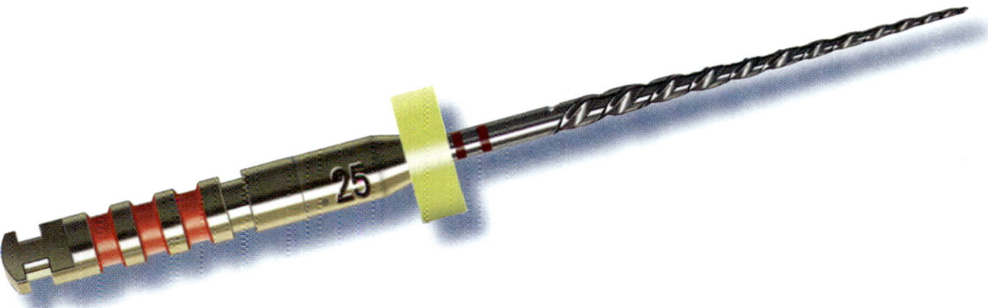

FIG. 2.X-5
Rotary instrument.

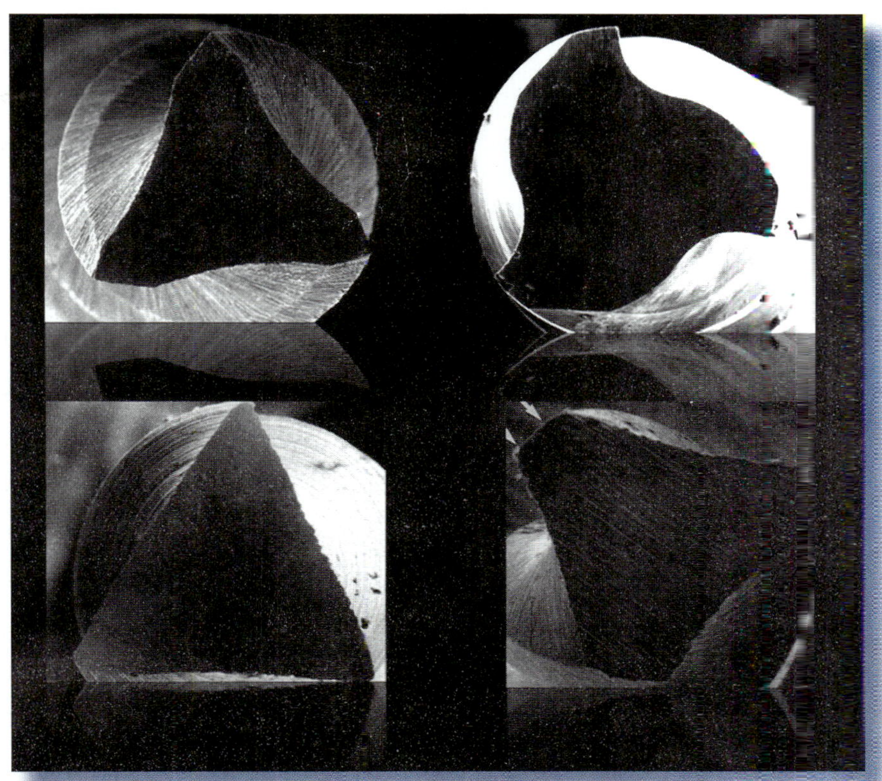

FIG. 2.X-6
Cross section of the active part of different rotary instruments.

Cross Section

When the active part of an instrument is cut in a perpendicular direction, one can see a characteristic geometric figure of each rotary system.

In Figure 2.X-6, note the different cross sections, differing for each instrument, and also in different areas of its active part.

Active Part

This represents the area of the instrument that has the cutting edge, and is effective in root canal preparations (Fig. 2.X-7).

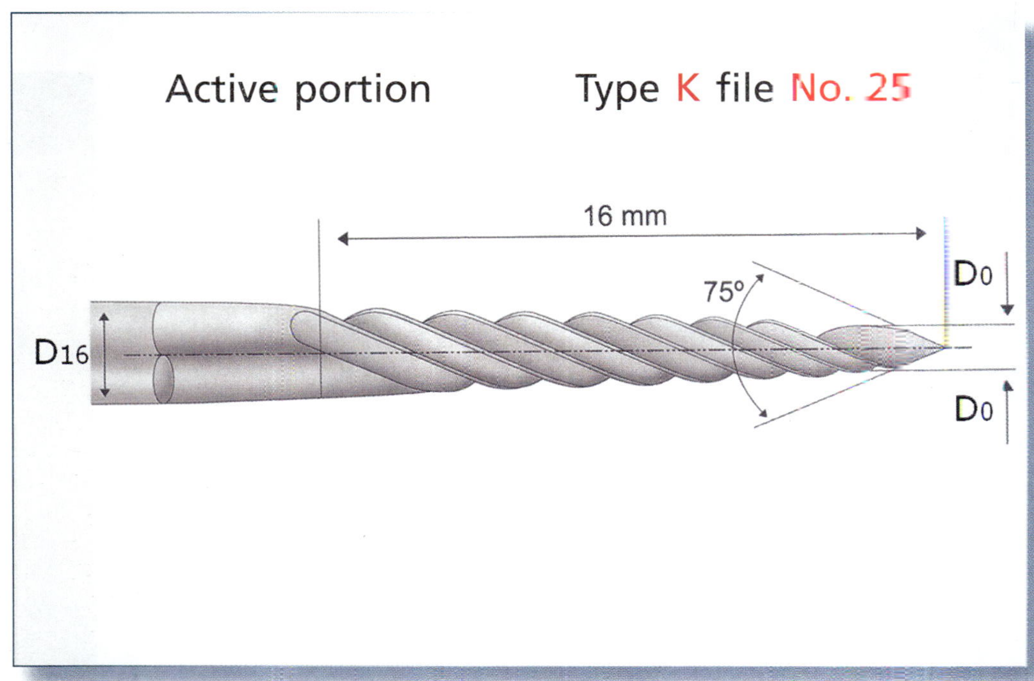

FIG. 2.X-7
Characteristics of the active portion.

Taper

The taper of rotary NiTi instruments is the increase in diameter that exists from D_0, in the direction towards D_{16}, expressed as mm/mm (Fig. 2.X-8). For example, a standardized type K file No. 25 has a diameter equal to 0.25 mm at the beginning of the active part (D_0). These standardized instruments have 0.02 mm/mm taper; that is, for each millimeter in the direction of (D_{16}) there is an increase of 0.02 mm in diameter. Thus, if we cut off 1 mm from the tip of the active part, we will obtain an instrument No. 27. If we cut off 2 mm, we shall have an instrument No. 29, and so on successively.

Some manufacturers express taper in percentage, for example, an instrument with 0.02 mm/mm taper (the case of all standardized K type and Hedströen instruments) is referred to as having a 2% taper.

When the root canal is instrumented with standardized manual instruments, only files with a 0.02 mm/mm taper are used. To compensate this deficiency, one varies the diameter D_0 of the instrument to be used, either in the apex-crown or crown-apex sequence.

For instrumentation with rotary files, we have instruments with a variety of tapers (0.02 - 0.04 - 0.06 - 0.08 - 0.10... mm/mm) at our disposal.

Radial Land

The area of the instrument in direct contact with the root canal wall is called the radial land (Fig. 2.X-9). The direct result of contact between the radial land area and the root canal walls is called frictional resistance. Thus, the smaller this area, the easier it is for the instrument to overlap on the dentinal walls when pressed in the apical direction. The larger the area, the lower the tendency to overlap.

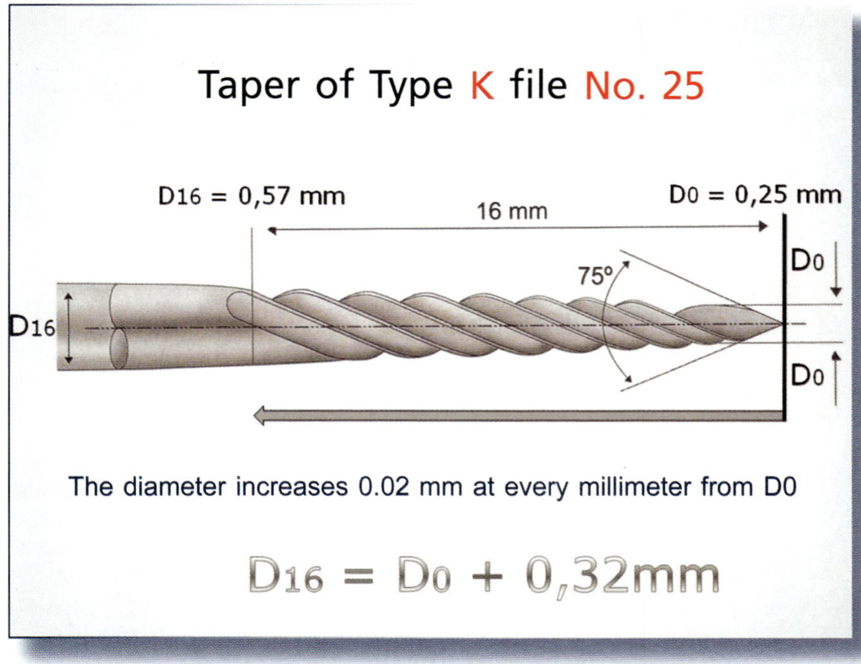

FIG. 2.X-8
Taper of standardized endodontic instruments.

FIG. 2.X-9
Radial land of the rotary instruments (arrow).

Moreover, the wider and larger the radial lands, the higher the frictional resistance, and therefore, the greater the torque demanded for the instrument to rotate inside the root canal. In the same way, instruments with small diameter radial lands and tapers are better able to "negotiate" the curved portions of the root canal, preventing the occurrence of deviations and formation of steps. Therefore, the radial land reduces the screwing effect of the instrument inside the root canal and the propagation of microfractures in it. With the purpose of relieving and diminishing the frictional resistance or the abrasion resulting from the radial land. some instruments present a "relief" of this surface (Fig. 2.X-10).

Stria

The wavy groove of the active part of the NiTi instrument, called stria (Fig. 2.X-11), is the receptacle in which dentin scrapings and tissues removed from root canal walls accumulate. The efficiency of the stria depends on its depth, width, configuration and surface finish. The most external edge of the groove forms the cutting flute (Fig. 2.X-12), which may be sharper or not as sharp, depending on the angulation (Fig. 2.X-13).

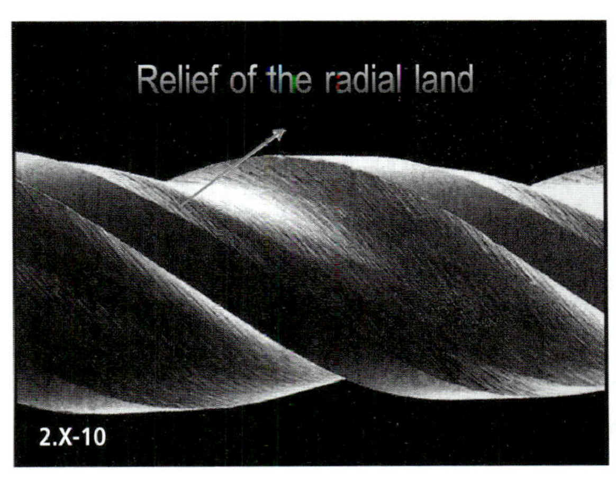

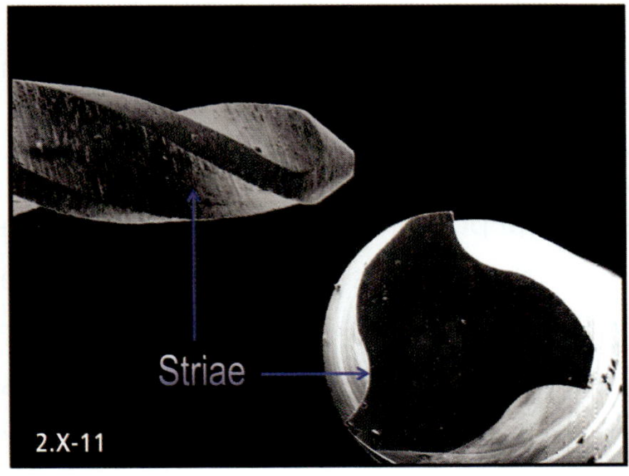

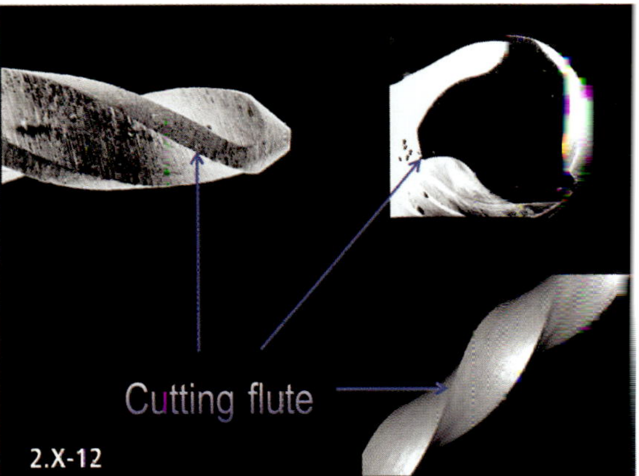

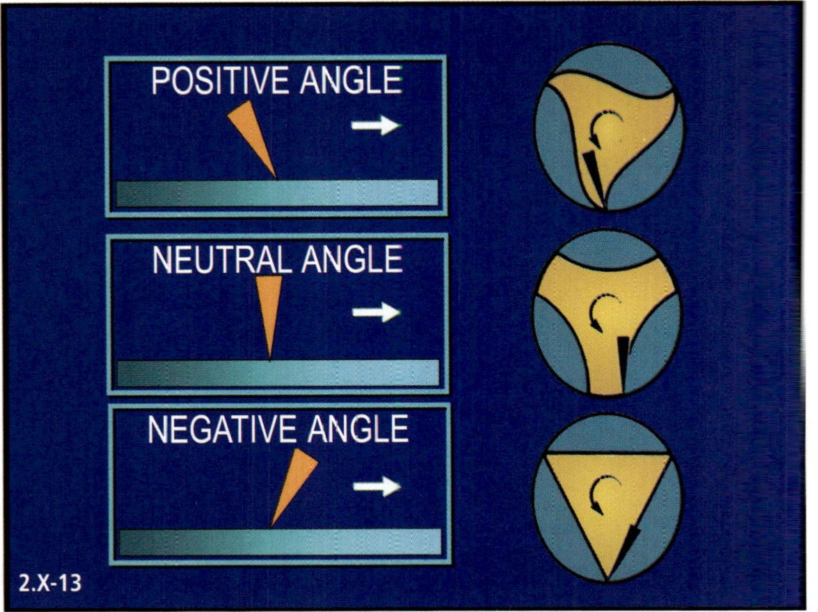

FIG. 2.X-10
Relief of the radial land (arrow).

FIG. 2.X-11
Arrow shows wavy groove (striae) (arrows).

FIG. 2.X-12
Cutting flute (arrows)

FIG. 2.X-13
Different cross-sectional cuts of instruments with different angles of cut.

- Negociation – American endodontists expression that means instrument capacity, through operator's action, of contouring root canal curvatures or even other anatomical accidents.

Spiral Angle

The angle formed between the cutting edge and the long axis of the instrument is called spiral angle. The bigger this angle (maximum of 89º), the higher the number of striae there will be per unit of area, which increases the flexibility of the instrument, number of areas or contact points, cutting efficiency and probability of fracture. On the contrary, the smaller the spiral angle (minimum of 1%), the lower the number of striae will be, which decreases flexibility, contact points and cutting efficiency.

Tip Design

The tips (the thinnest end of the active portion) (Fig. 2.X-14) are classified as active, inactive and partially active and depend on the proximity to the end of the cutting flute and stria, in relation to the effective end of the instrument (D_0).

Rigidity, flexibility and ability to remain along the root canal axis depend on the activity or inactivity of the tip and its proximity to the radial land. These are the features that make the tip of the instrument more or less effective and enable it to continue without deviations.

Internal Mass (Core)

The cylindrical central portion of the instrument is called the core (Fig. 2.X-15).

The ratio between the distance that goes from the core up to the most external portion of the instrument, generally the most external portion of the stria, in the cutting flute, determines the variation in the flexibility of the instrument and its resistance to torsion. This ratio may vary, depending on the area of the active portion, allowing optimization of the instrument working inside the root canal.

The Distance Between the Cutting Flutes (Pitch)

Depending on the instrument, the distance may constant or variable (Fig. 2.X-16). One of the major problems associated with instrument locking inside the root canal is its ability to move in a rotating motion inside it. By changing the pitch on the active portion, there is less risk.

Surface Finish

The surface finish is as important as the alloy and the instrument design as far as its efficiency and fracture risk are concerned (Fig. 2.X-17).

According to the technology used for manufacturing the instrument: torqued or machined, with or without chemical or electrolytic polishing; it may have microfissures (Fig. 2.X-18) that concentrate and propagate the stress, leading to fracture.

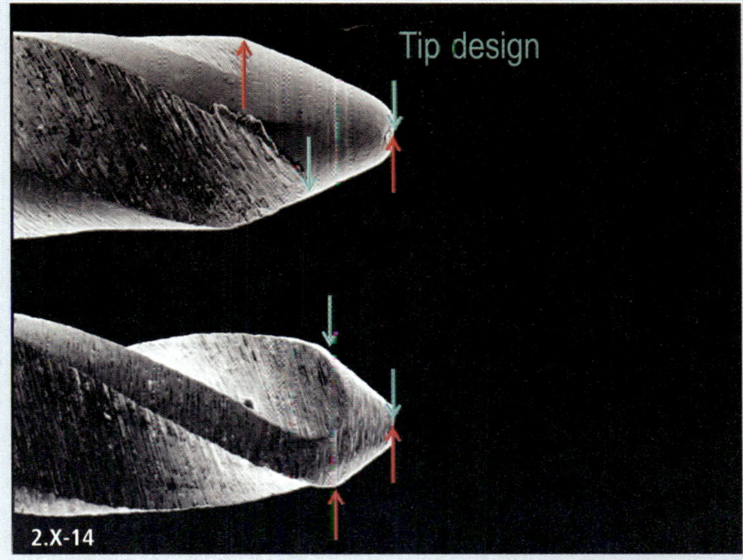

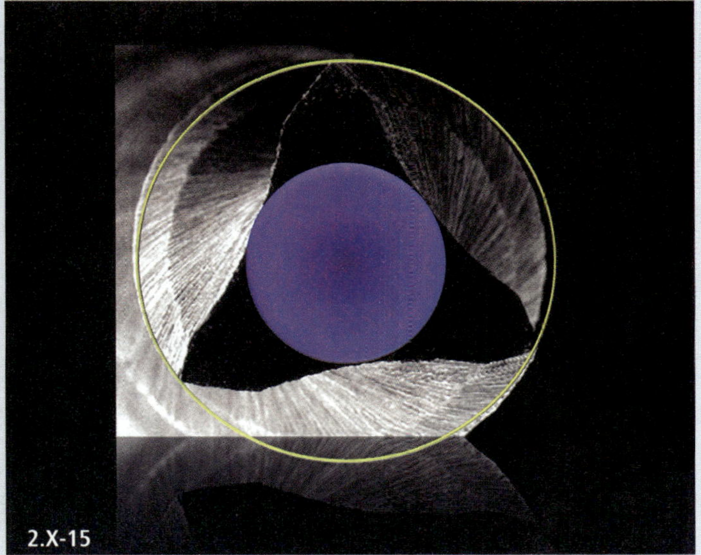

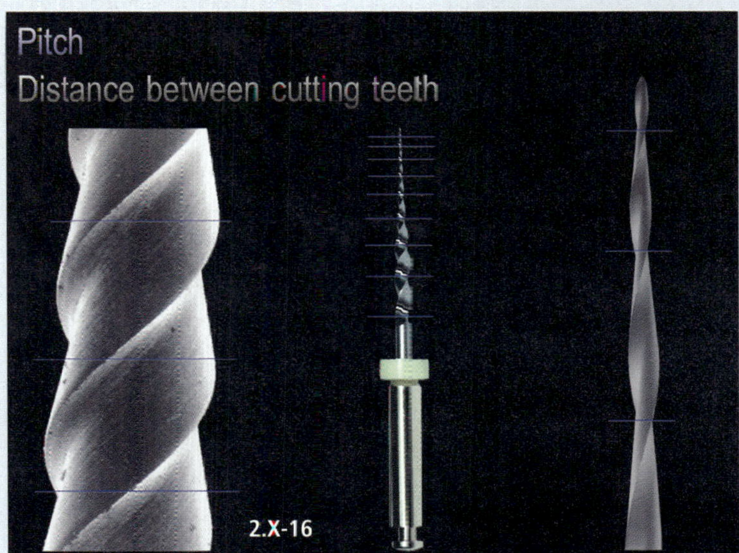

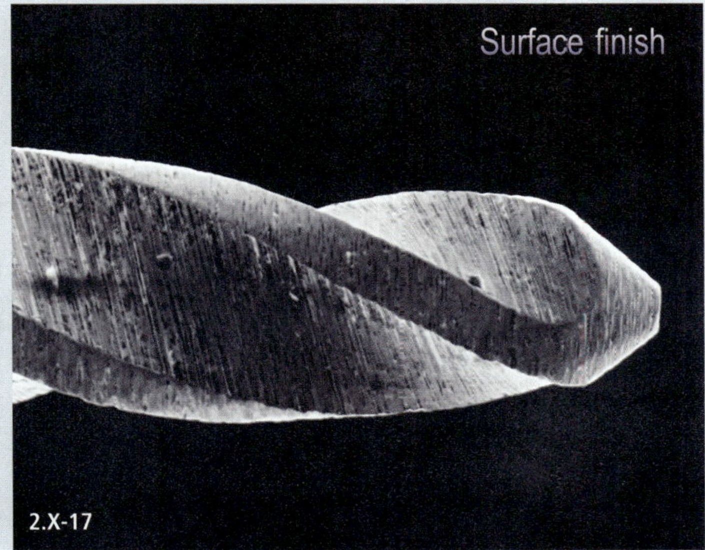

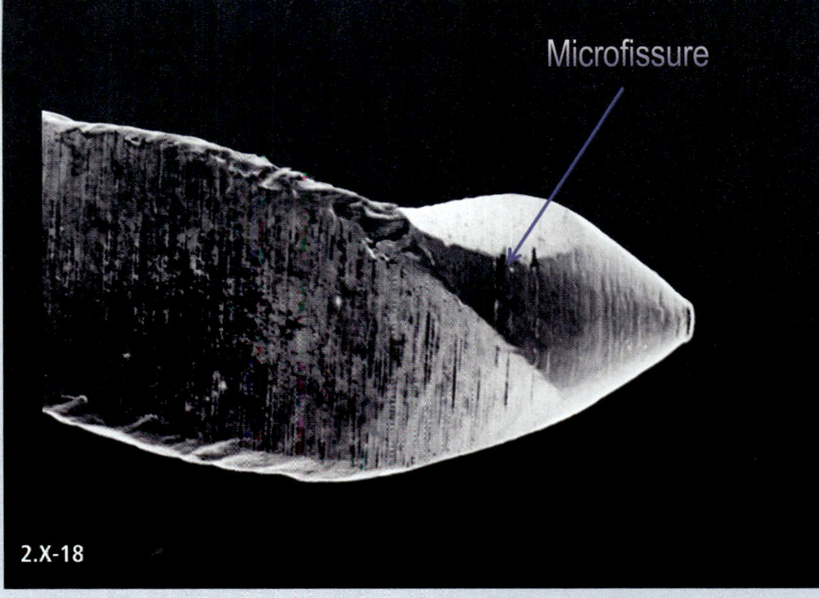

FIG. 2.X-14
Different tip designs.

FIG. 2.X-15
Core of the rotary instrument.

FIG. 2.X-16
Pitch of the instrument.

FIG. 2.X-17
Surface finish.

FIG. 2.X-18
Microfissure showing evidence of inadequate surface finish.

THE RELATIONSHIP BETWEEN THE IMPORTANCE OF KNOWLEDGE OF THE MORPHOLOGICAL CHARACTERISTICS OF THE INSTRUMENT, ITS PHYSICAL PROPERTIES, AND THE ANATOMY OF THE ROOT CANAL (John T. McSpadden)[42]

- An instrument with a better design and a greater cutting capacity requires less torque (force that makes the instrument rotate) to provide the same degree of root canal widening. 2.X-19).
- In straight root canals, the capacity of an instrument to resist to torque varies directly according to the instrument diameter (Fig. 2.X-20). In curved canals, the opposite occurs; that is, thinner instruments show better resistance in curvatures.
- The torque required to rotate an instrument varies directly according to the surface area of the instrument in contact with the root canal walls and the design of the cutting flute (Fig. 2.X-21).
- Instrument fatigue increases with the number of rotations it undergoes inside the root canal, and according to its anatomy. The greater the curvature, the greater the fatigue (Fig. 2.X-22).

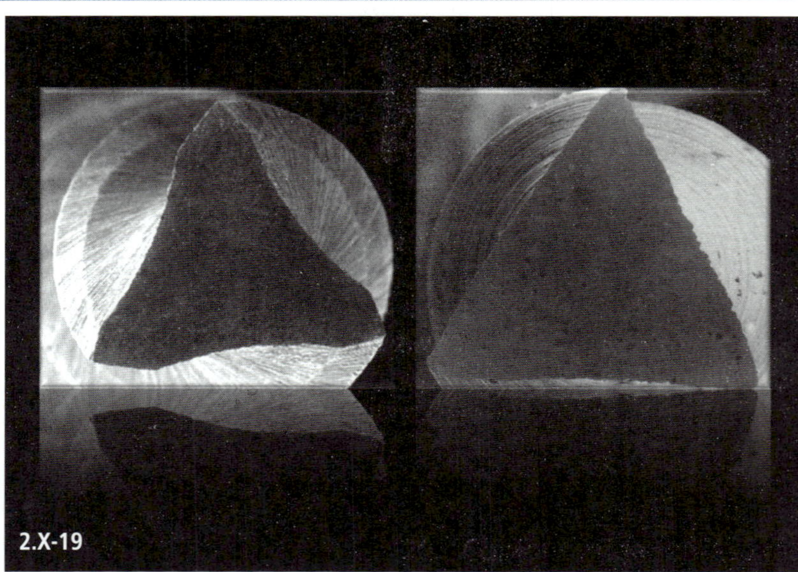

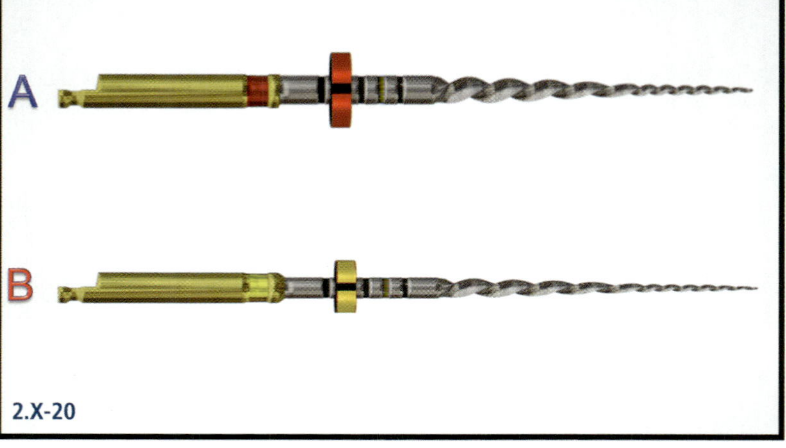

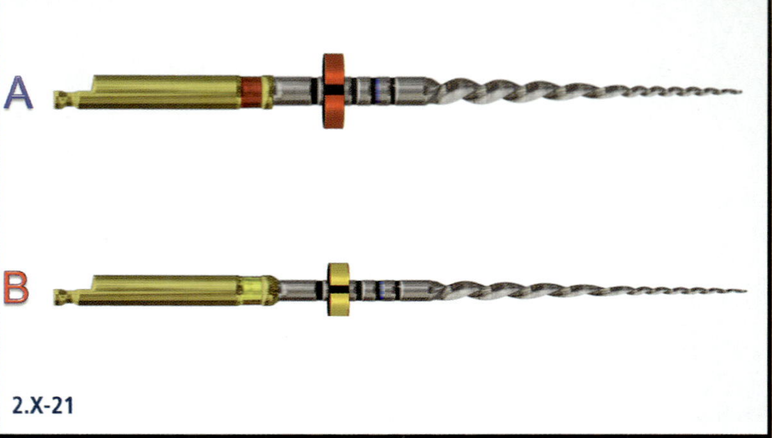

FIG. 2.X-19

Different drawing of the cross sectional cut of the active part of the instrument.

FIG. 2.X-20

The instrument A resists torque better in straight canals. In curved portions, the instrument B is more resistant.

FIG. 2.X-21

The larger the contact area, the greater the torque.

- To improve instrument efficiency, the smaller the surface area of the instrument in contact with the root canal walls, the higher the rotation speed that can be used (Fig. 2.X-23).
- The higher the number of striae per unit of area around the active part of the instrument, the higher the torque required to rotate it, and the more points of stress concentration there are, which potentiates fracture, but with a gain in flexibility. 2.X-24).
- The fewer the striae per unit of area on the active cutting surface, the greater the resistance to deformation the instrument undergoes, thus making it more rigid and less flexible (Fig. 2.X-25).

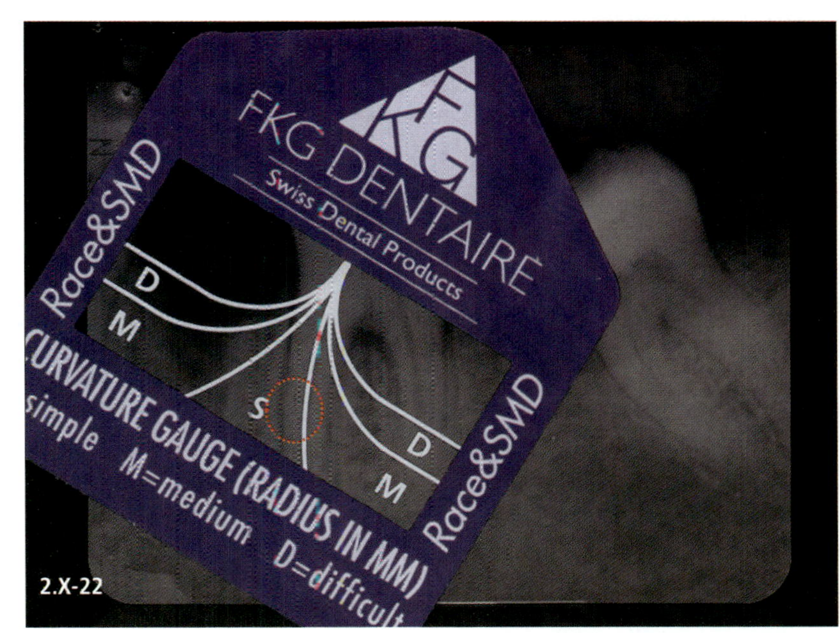

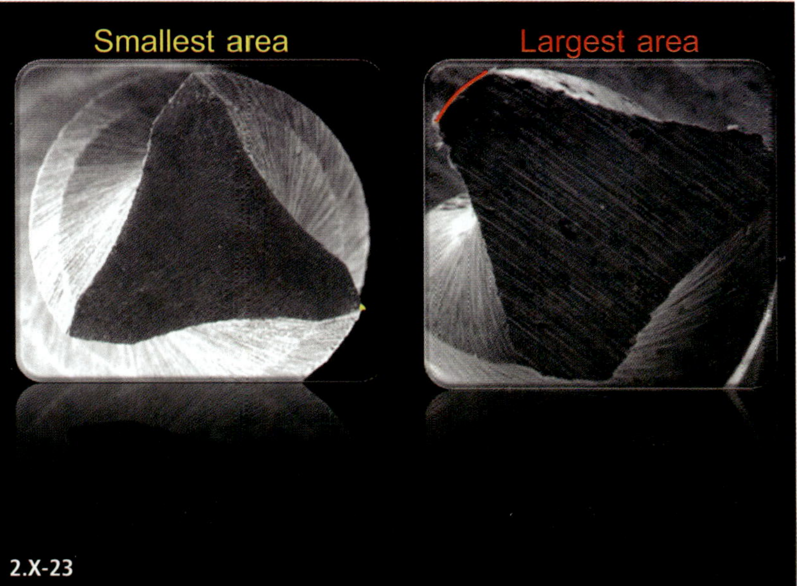

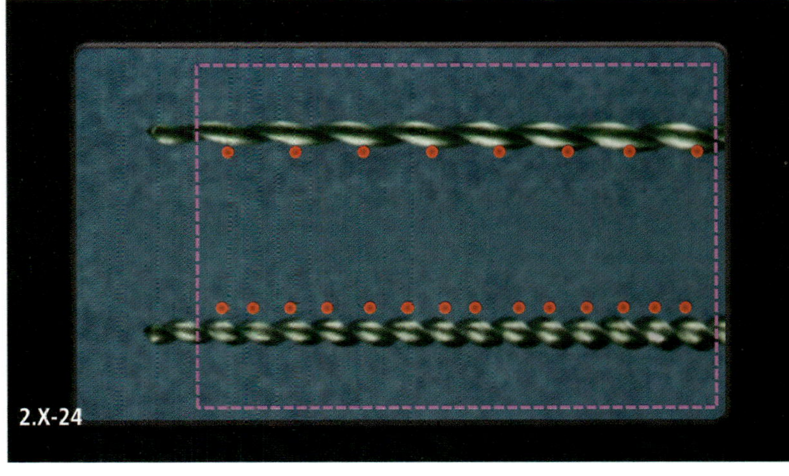

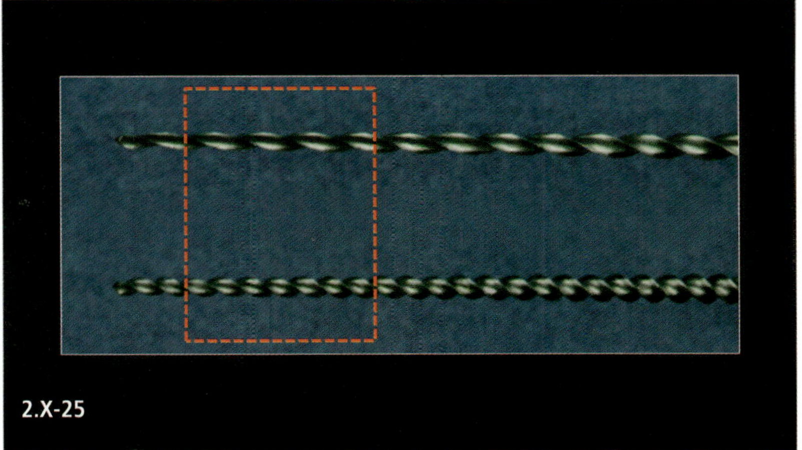

FIG. 2.X-22

Devices to qualify different canal curvatures, provided by FKG Dentaire, Switzerland.

FIG. 2.X-23

The smaller the contact area, the higher the rotary speed.

FIG. 2.X-24

The higher the number of points, the more flexible, the greater the stress, the greater the torque required.

FIG. 2.X-25

The fewer the striae, the lower the flexibility, the less the torque.

- The sharper the cutting surface of an instrument, the smaller the number of striae required (Fig. 2.X-26).
- The higher the number of striae with the same cutting angle, the greater the tendency of an instrument to cling to root canal walls, become stuck and enable fractures (Fig. 2.X-27).
- Greater area of contact of an instrument with the root canal walls occurs when it is introduced more deeply into the canal, in a proportion equal to that of the pressure in the direction of the apex. 2.X-28).
- Less transportation of the root canal occurs when one uses instruments with great flexibility, asymmetric cross section and radial land (Fig. 2.X-29).

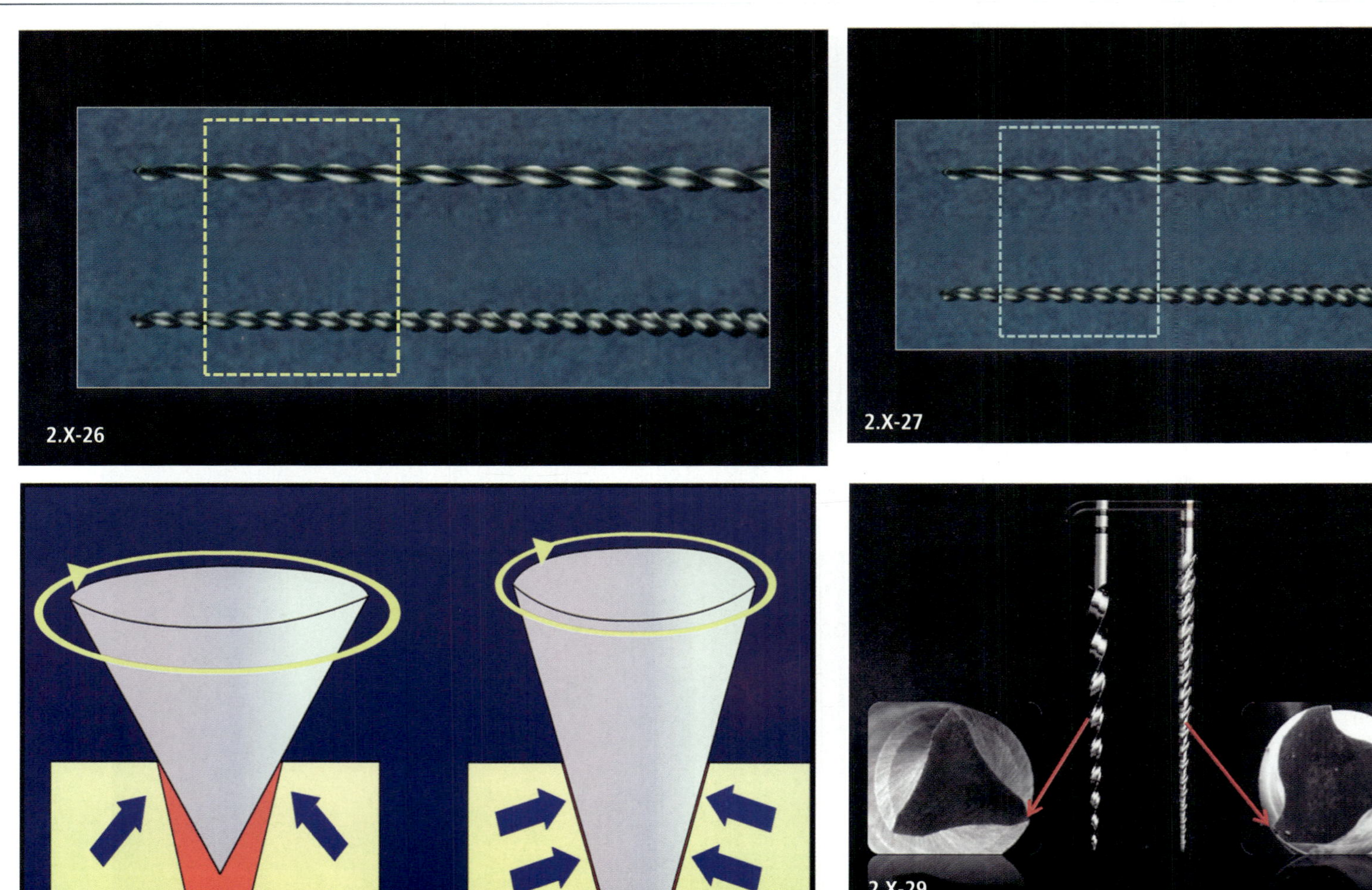

FIG. 2.X-26
The more striae, the greater the rotating effect.

FIG. 2.X-27
The higher the number of striae, the greater the probability of becoming stuck.

FIG. 2.X-28
The greater the depth, the greater the contact.

FIG. 2.X-29
The higher the number of striae, the greater the flexibility, the radial land, the less transport of the canal.

CLINICAL CRITERIA IN ROTARY INSTRUMENTATION

"Technological development requires increased knowledge"
John McSpadden

In this part of the chapter, there will be a review of the knowledge available at present, with regard to rotary instrument engineering, applied to the surgical anatomy of root canals, as well as the development of techniques and sequences for the efficient and safe use of the instruments.

In 1974, Herbert Schilder[56] established, that the conformation to be attributed to the root canal during biomechanical preparation should not only be done based on the unique and individual anatomy of each canal, but also on the technique and filling material. He also recommended that when using filling techniques with thermoplasticized gutta-percha, the basic shape of the root canal should be that of a funnel with a continuous taper, following the original shape of the root canal, thus attributing an appropriate conformation for the filling.

According to the author, there are five mechanical objectives to determine the conformation of a fillable endodontic cavity. Although published in 1974, they remain in absolute force and it is the goal of mechanical instrumentation to attain these objectives.

1. To establish a continuously narrowing tapered shape. To create a continuously tapered funnel (infundibuliform preparation) from the access cavity to the canal up to the apex.
2. To make the root canal diameter become smaller and smaller in the direction of the canal apex.
3. To make a tapered root canal preparation; that is, performed in multiple planes, so that it is continuous, like the original and tridimensional anatomic shape of the root canal.
4. The apical foramen should remain in its original spatial position, without external and internal transportation.
5. The apical foramen should remain as small as possible.

When endeavoring to reach these mechanical objectives, especially in the curved root canals of molars, there may be errors in the operating procedure, such as the transportation of foramens, "zips", steps, perforations, largely due to the rigidity of stainless steel alloys.

In 1988, Walia *et al.*[65] researched nickel-titanium (NiTi) endodontic instruments for the first time, and stated that they had three times more elastic flexibility, as well as higher resistance to fracture by torsion, in comparison with stainless steel files of similar designs and sizes.

Because of the characteristics of the metal, NiTi alloy seems to be the solution to problems of canal shaping. The torsional and bending properties of NiTi, in addition to an appropriate design, made it possible for these instruments to be used for preparing the curved root canals of molars, with little or no deviation from their original trajectories[19,26,32,62].

Despite the efforts of industry to offer a wide range of NiTi instruments of different sequences and designs, it has been unable to prevent them from fracturing to a considerable extent[31, 47, 55, 60].

In reality, the operator has no faithful, concrete and universally disseminated parameters to use as a guide to foresee and prevent these accidents, differing from what happens with manual stainless steel instruments. NiTi instruments can fracture without previous visible deformation[35,66]. Therefore, visual inspection is not a safe method to evaluate their functional conditions[51,60,64].

Since the beginning, rotary instrumentation has been associated with an increase in the speed of using it, which goes to show that speed will increase risks, with the resultant loss of its objectives.

The main commitment with the use of rotary instrumentation is not the reduction in the operating time, but the safety.

Clinicians know that the speed of rotary instrumentation does not depend on the speed of intracanal procedures, but on correct planning and ergonomic involvement of the entire endodontic procedure.

One can safely obtain a reduction in root canal preparation time with an optimum strategy in each clinical situation, by replacing the risky and unnecessary components of technique with effective and controlled actions. This would allow one to change the commercial slogan *"easy, simple and fast endodontics"* to *"conscious, responsible and predictable endodontics".*

The information available at present is provided by two points of view. On the one hand, there are few recommendations from manufacturers and opinion leaders, who try to convince professionals to use only one kit, with a few instruments, generally manufactured by them and indicated for use in all clinical situations. On the other hand, there is information from researches, frequently of a highly technical nature, making it difficult to understand and apply to clinical conditions. Moreover, due to methodological problems, it is difficult or impossible to compare the different evaluations. In addition, the regulations related to the standards in force do not reflect the clinical and dynamic situations as far as rotary instruments are concerned[42].

As a result, clinicians perform root canal instrumentation based on uncertainties, because they do not understand the physics of rotary instrumentation technology, which would allow them to arrive at the ideal model, according to disclosed standards.

Frequently, when following such suggestions, the stress level of the instrument is so high that a fracture is most likely to occur. One can hardly indicate that the instrument is disposable, because it could fracture the first time it is used[1].

As the clinician's knowledge increases, he/she will slowly set aside the guidance of the "recipe book" type, which served as an introduction to the world of rotary instrumentation.

The passage of time, added to the experience and knowledge accumulated, allows one to establish that today, rotary instrumentation is understandable and accessible, and favors full use of the potential this technology has to offer. Thus, one is able to use the knowledge that indicates the appropriate technique for each anatomy.

The art of endodontics is transformed into endodontic science, harmonizing the instruments with the root canal anatomy.

Causes and Prevention of Instrument Fractures

The most frequent and feared accident when using NiTi instruments is the occurrence of fracture. The situation generally surprises the clinician, who is endeavoring to improve the quality of the preparation, and is suddenly faced with the difficult and sometimes impossible task of removing the fractured instrument from inside the root canal[24].

Instrumentation is subject to and adversely influenced by the huge variability in the anatomy of root canals[4,5,28,44,50,54]:There are canals that unite, have simple and double curvatures, dilacerations or divisions[54].

The causes of instrument fracture, for didactic purposes, can be grouped into **clinical** and **metallographic fractures**. In most situations, however, there are multiple causes that add up, since one leads to the other[16].

Ultimately, fracture is produced because the stress to which the instrument is submitted during its action inside the root canal generates fracture forces that overcome the traction force of the atoms of the metal[39,46,71].

CLINICAL CAUSES

1. **Inadequate coronal opening (access surgery).** It has been widely demonstrated that the elimination of cervical and coronal interferences is a previous and indispensable requisite of canal preparation, for both stainless steel and NiTi instruments 53, 57. The previous dilation of the cervical third of the root canal (anti-curvature wear) allows the instruments used afterwards in the apical preparation to have access in a straight line, and to be submitted to minimal stress, so that it diminishes their cutting effort and possibility of rotating[34,61].
2. **Absence of previous exploration (catheterization).** As a basic principle, manual stainless steel type K files must be used for exploration, catheterization and previous dilation of the root canal segment that will be soon submitted to the action of rotary instruments[10,48,53]. This will equal or diminish the difference between the diameter of the instrument tip and root canal. The axiom "*mechanized instruments are always preceded by manual instruments*" is a dogma in endodontics.
3. **Adequate kinematics.** The details of the kinematics of use of NiTi instruments will be presented as follows.

Metallographic Causes

When turning inside the root canal, the instrument undergoes two types of stress: **torsional stress** (responsible for torsion fractures) and **bending stress** (responsible for cyclical fatigue fracture).

Torsional Stress

Torsional stress occurs when a segment of the instrument, generally the tip, is stuck and immobilized by the root canal walls, unable to overcome dentin resistance in order to cut; at the other extreme, the instrument is submitted to the axial torsional force generated by the motor when turning. Stress is then generated, exceeding the elastic limit of the metal, which presents a plastic deformation, followed by fracture (Fig. 2.X-30B).

The torque required to make the instrument turn and cut dentin is directly proportional to its contact surface with the canal walls and its cutting capacity.

Therefore, an instrument with highly efficient cutting ability will require less torque, lower pressure and rotation, and thus, a shorter working time. That is why the present trend in the production of new instruments is that designs emphasize the cutting efficiency, so that they can do the same work with fewer risks.

If the instruments were cylindrical, the torque requirements would be the same, since the radius does not vary. But as the instruments are tapered, they have different radii at different levels, the torque required for cutting will vary according to the segment of the instrument acting against the walls (r1, r2, r3) (Fig. 2.X-31).

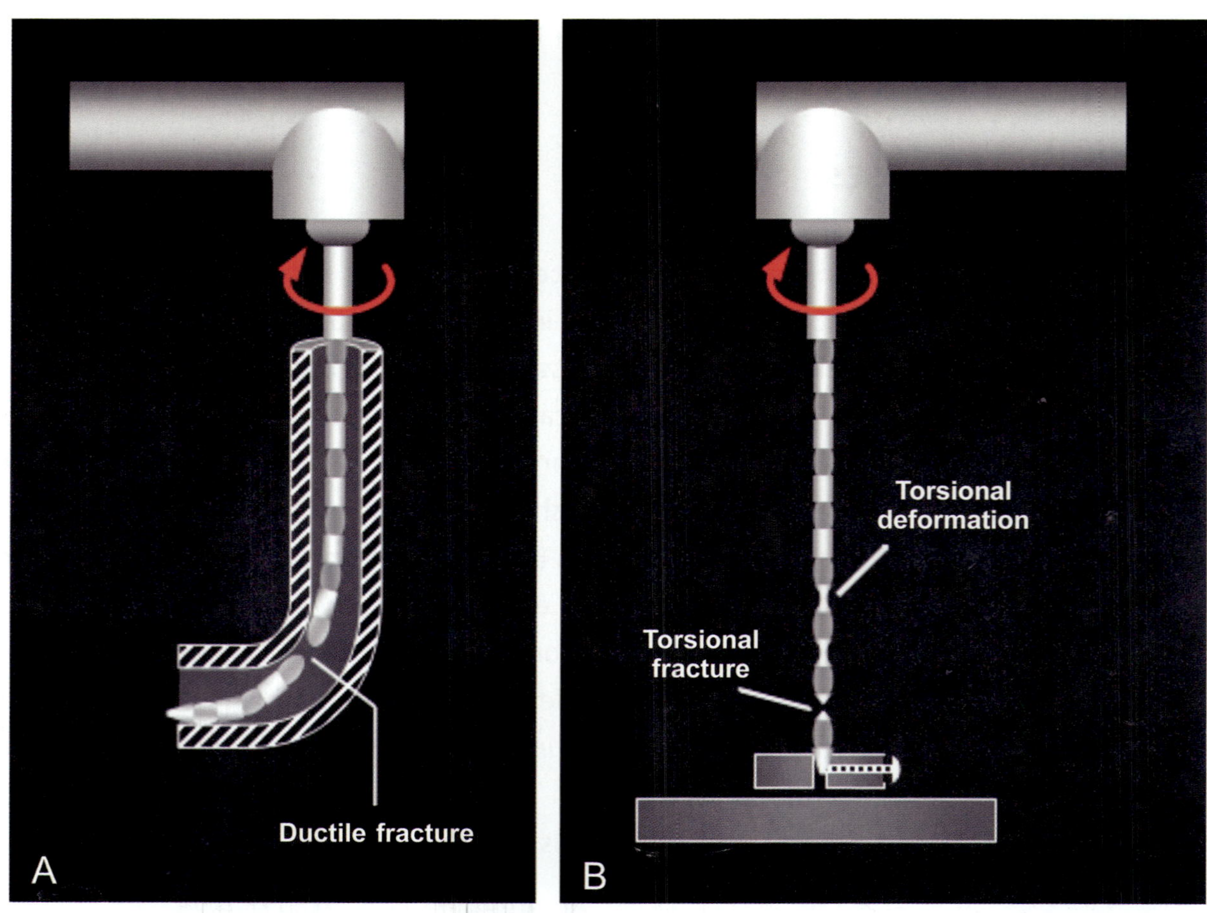

FIGS. 2.X-30A-B

A – Bending stress – it is the repetition of alternate cycles of tension-compression on one point of the instrument when turning inside a curved root canal.
B – Torsional stress – when the tip of the instrument is stuck and the other part is submitted to axial torsion force, generated by the motor when it turns. Torsional fracture or deformation.

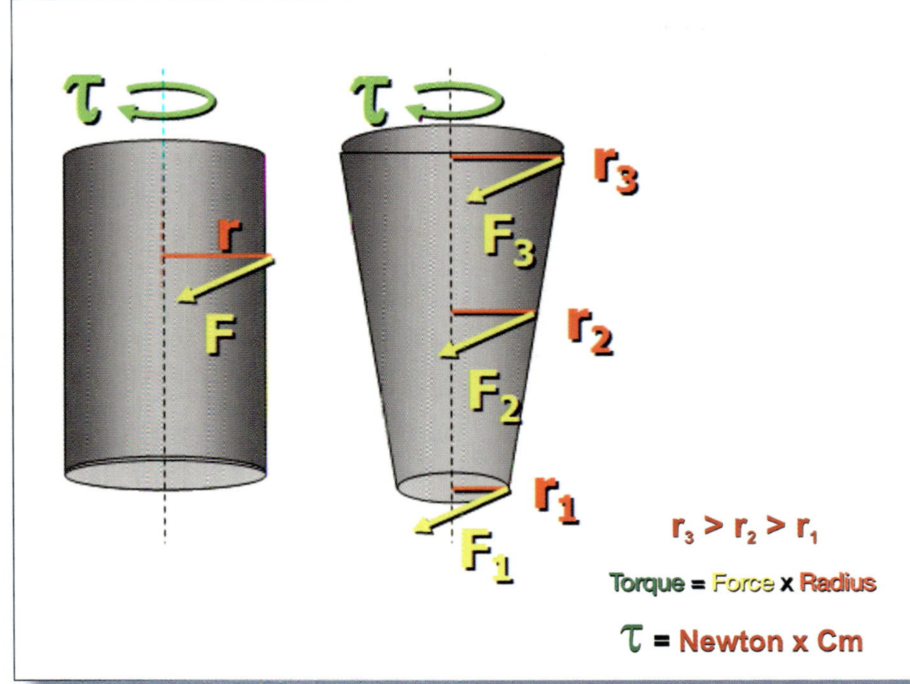

FIG. 2.X-31
The taper of the active part of rotary instruments provides different radii at different levels; thus, the torque required to cut dentin will differ according to the segment of the instrument.

In clinical situations, it is really impossible to establish an adequate torque for each segment of the instrument in relation to the anatomy of the canals, considering the risk that would be involved in working with a high torque in a sequence that does not protect the tip of the instrument.

The maximum torque required for instrument fracture to occur also varies with the diameter and cross section[41].

Considerations about motors with torque control available for the use of NiTi instruments:

The motors proposed for use with NiTi rotary instruments offer speeds ranging between 150 and 700 rpm, and torques between 0.1 and 10 N.cm. The ideal torque to program the motor should be lower than the limit of resistance to fracture by torsion of the instrument. To this one must add the difficulty of choosing a torque suited to the continual changes in the instrument resistance to dentin due to the anatomic variability of the cross sections and root canal tapers[23].

Therefore, one cannot suggest torque values for instruments without considering root canal anatomy, as manufacturers do. In addition to not informing the necessary determination of these values, they do not take the irrigation and the lubrication processes into consideration.

From the foregoing explanation, one infers that the priority in fracture prevention is not controlling the torque loading on the motors.

What does the torsional stress depend on?

1. ***Instrument cross section***: The larger section will tend to have a greater torsional resistance. Therefore, between two instruments that have the same tip diameter, the one with the greater taper will bear torsional stress better than the one with smaller taper.

2. **Torque**: The higher the torque demanded to make the instrument turn and cut the canal dentin, the greater will be the torsional stress generated.
3. **Adjustment surface:** A greater surface of instrument adjustment to the root canal walls will determine a greater contact area, causing a greater friction, what will demand more torque and cause a greater torsional stress.
4. **Cutting efficiency:** An instrument with a greater cutting power will require less torque to cut the dentin and will have a lower torsional stress.
5. **Irrigation and lubrication**: Both factors are important at the instrument level of contact with the root canal walls, reducing torsional stress. With lubrication, the instrument surface will demand less torque, without diminishing its cutting ability. The use of lubricants reduces torsional stress by approximately 20%[6,12,13,25,49,59,69] (Fig. 2.X-32).
6. **Kinetics of use:** Greater pressure in the apical direction will cause the instrument to tend to "stick" to the canal walls, and undergo a greater torsional stress. For the use of kinetics with less risk, it is recommendable to use slight apical pressure, not forcing the instrument into the canal and previously control the degree of adjustment and depth of insertion.
7. **Exploration:** As previously explained, maintaining accessibility to the canal system reduces torsional stress.

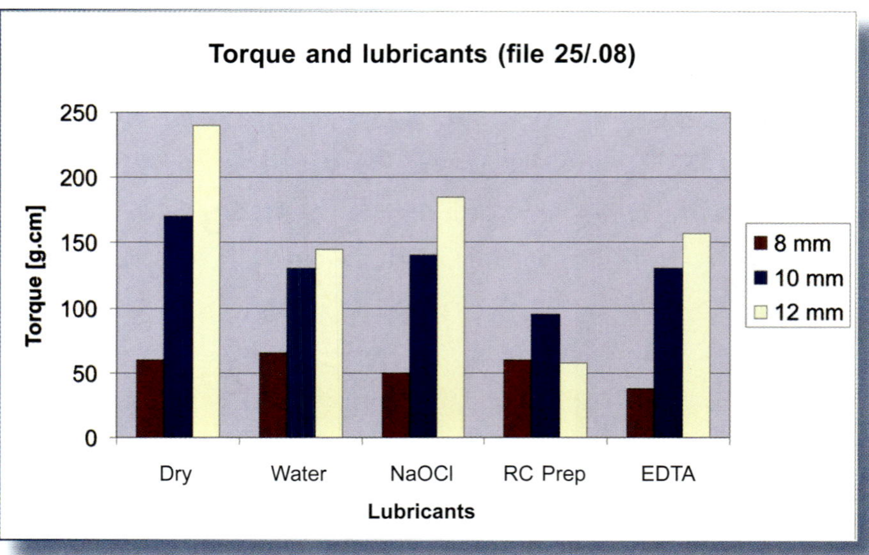

FIG. 2.X-32
Relationship between torque and lubricants. Adapted from McSpadden[42].

Bending Stress

Bending stress is the repetition of alternate cycles of tension-compression on one point of the instrument when it is turning inside a curved root canal[37,68] (Fig. 2.X-30A), which is closely related to the inversion of the square of the radius of the instrument at the bending point. Thus, an instrument with smaller taper will bear bending better than an instrument with a larger taper[51] (Fig. 2.X-33).

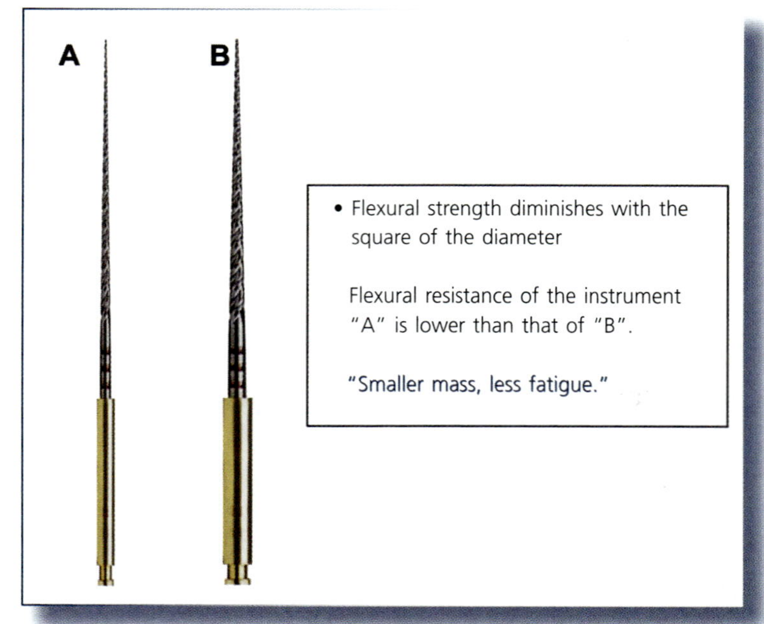

FIG. 2.X-33
Flexural Strength.

Bending stress is directly related to the curvature of canals, instrument diameter and to the rotation speed, which are variables that determine the useful life of the instrument.

Fatigue begins to manifest itself by small fissures on the instrument surface, which soon propagate to its interior, producing fracture. Thus it is necessary to examine the surface of instruments with a magnifying glass after use, to prevent them from being discarded too soon.

What does the bending stress depend on?

1. **Radius of curvature:** It is the factor of greatest incidence, since the smallest radius of curvature determines the greatest cyclical fatigue[22,51]. Therefore, it is important to make a previous clinical selection of an instrument that can safely turn in this curvature (Figs. 2.X-34 and 2.X-35).

2. **Speed and time:** Greater speed and longer time increase the cyclical fatigue because of the larger number of repetitions of cycles[17,20,67,70].

3. **Kinetics of use:** Rotation in a fixed point of a root canal curvature increases fatigue. For this reason it is always suggested to use back and forth movements, and to prevent the instrument from turning in the same point (length).

FIG. 2.X-34
Radius of curvature.

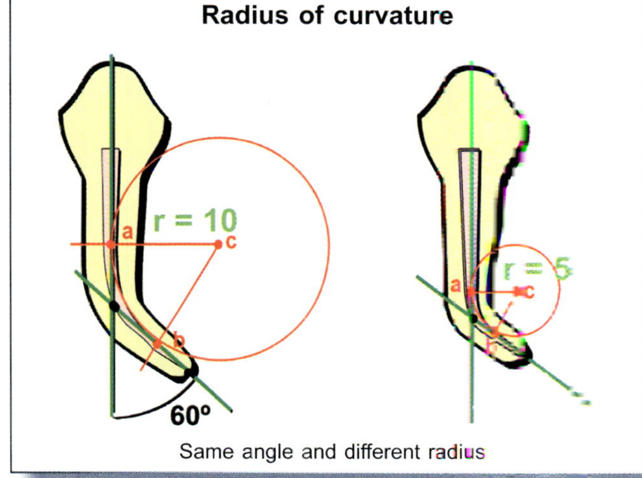

FIG. 2.X-35
Maximum diameter recommended for 45° and 8 mm radius curvatures (in red).

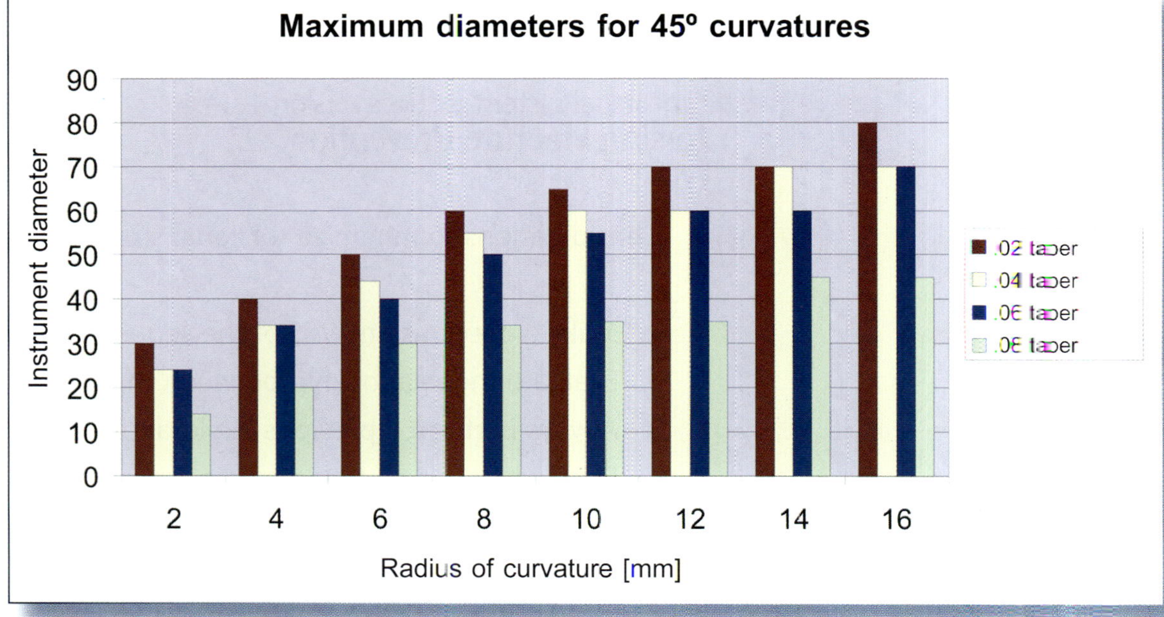

4. **Section:** The larger diameter of the instrument at the point of inflection of the root canal curve will bear greater fatigue. 2.X-36).

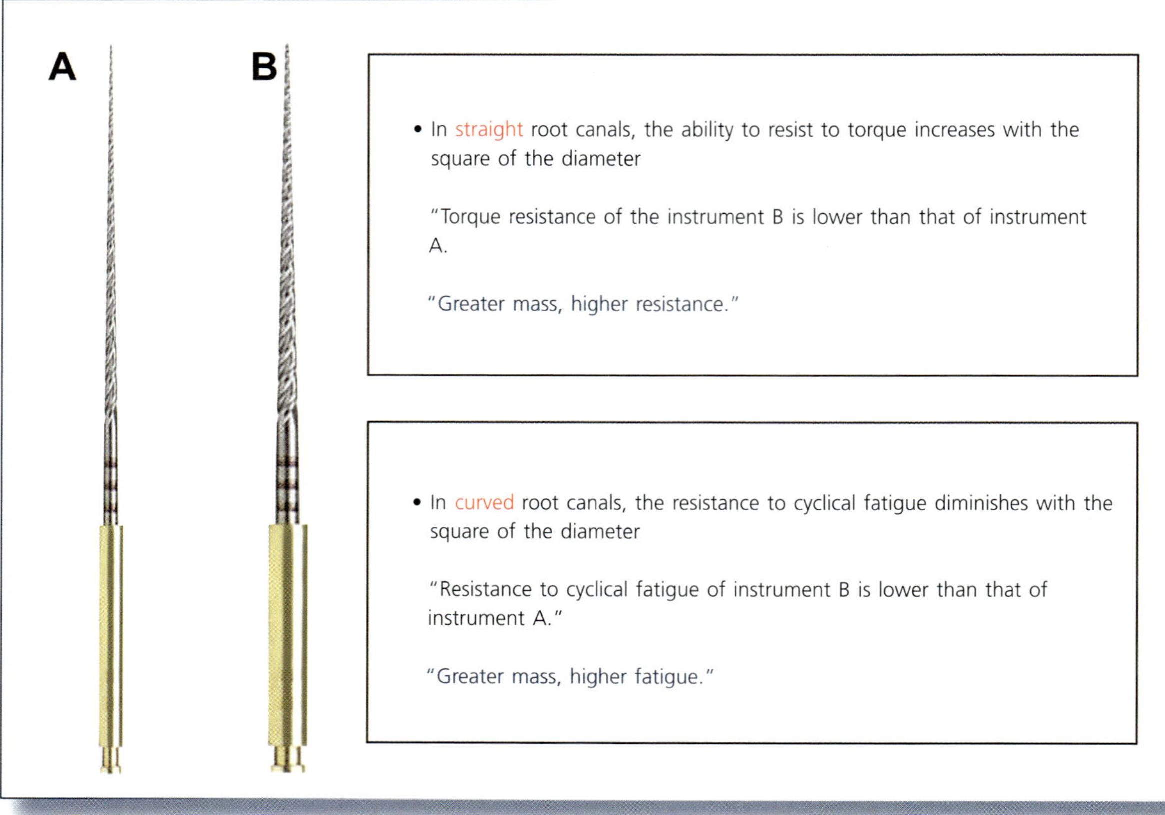

FIG. 2.X-36

Greater mass, higher resistance. In straight root canals, torque resistance of the instrument A is higher than that of instrument B. **Greater metal mass, greater fatigue.** In curved root canals, the cyclical fatigue resistance of instrument A is lower than that of instrument B.

INSTRUMENT FRACTURE PREVENTION

Torsion Fracture Prevention

Considerations to minimize torsional stress:

1. Make a previous analysis of the sequence of instruments for the technique to be used.
2. Evaluate the relationship between the instrument dimension and the root canal anatomy.
3. Always perform a previous exploration (*glide path*).
4. Ensure that the cutting stress is supported by the body of the instrument, leaving the point free, as it is the part most vulnerable to torsional stress[36].
5. Reduce the segment of the instrument in contact with the root canal walls.
6. Try to irrigate and lubricate continuously.

7. Keep the surface of the instruments free of debris accumulated in their striae[2,3]. The accumulation of dentinal scrapings will cause rotation and an increase in friction.

Prevention of Bending Fracture

To minimize bending stress:

1. Do not increase the speed recommended by manufacturers.
2. Do not leave the instrument turning in the same length of the curved portion. It is important to emphasize that the instrument also undergoes bending stress simply by turning In a curvature, even without cutting.
3. Always use smaller diameters and tapers in curvatures with small radii.

A sudden curvature with a small radius in the apical third of the canal may be less dangerous than a moderate curvature in the cervical middle third, since the instrument, due to its taper, will turn in the middle and cervical thirds with large diameter and large mass of metal. The situation requires the operator to take all the necessary precautions[18,22,27,31,37].

4. Do not exceed the critical diameters suggested for 45°, 8 mm radius and smaller curvatures (Figs. 2.X-37 to 2.X-39).

When increasing the instrument taper, one diminishes the segment of the file that can go beyond the curvature. It is important to have a visual representation of the diameter and the taper of the instrument that can be taken beyond a 45° and 8 mm radius curvature.

In the diagram of Figure 2.X-38 one can graphically note the depth of the instrument penetration into the curvature: as its taper increases, the segment of the instrument that can pass through the curvature diminishes. This enables one to calculate the risks and anticipate accidents. The red color indicates the segments of the instruments that should not pass through a curvature of 45° and 8 mm radius.

The Table in Figure 2.X-39 shows that starting from this diameter, the passage of the instrument through the curvature will involve high bending stress. The graph was made to serve as a quick reference clinical guide for selecting the suitable instrument, used in the learning and training process by students of the specialization course in Endodontics at FOUM (Buenos Aires – Argentina).

When applying these concepts to the clinical case in Figure 2.X-40, one notes that the real working length in the radiograph of the mesial root is 23 mm; the distance from the reference point to the main curve is 17 mm, which is equivalent to saying that the main curve is approximately 6 mm from the real work length (RWL).

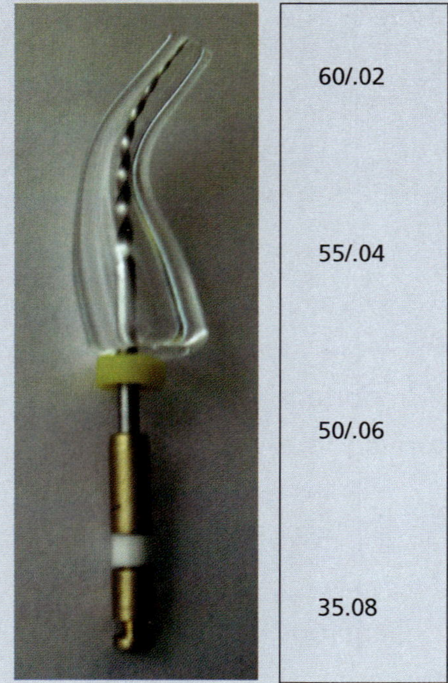

FIG. 2.X-37

Critical diameters for 45° curvatures and 8 mm and/or smaller radius.

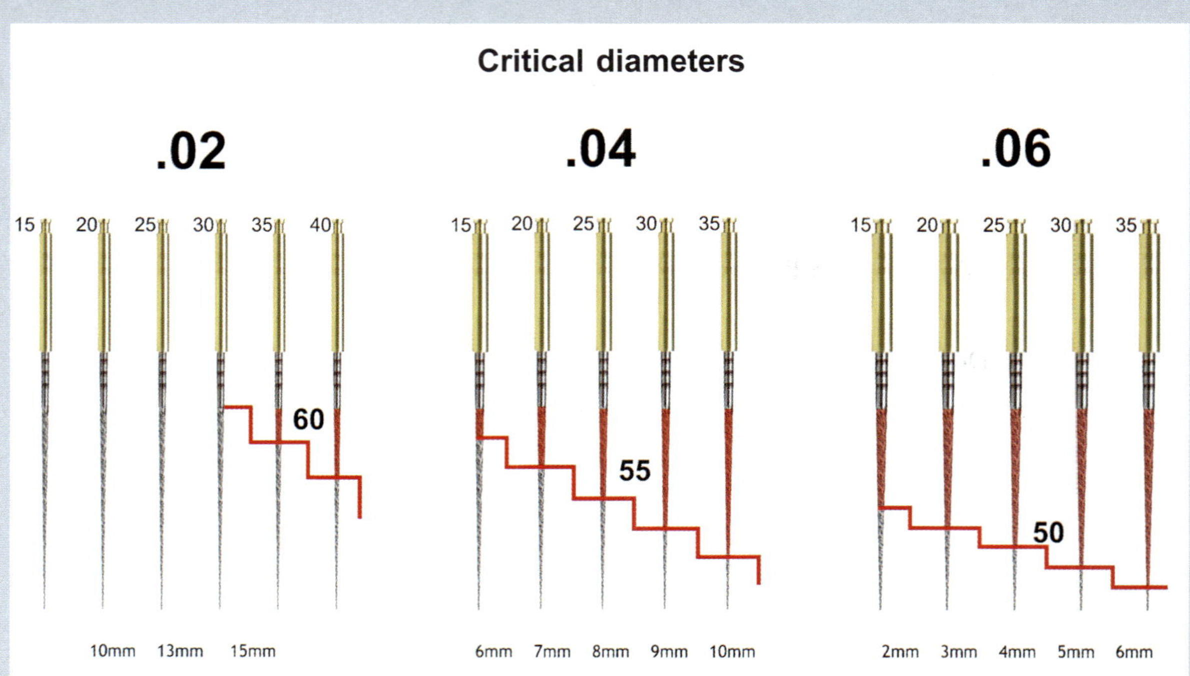

FIG. 2.X-38

Critical diameters. Adapted from McSpadden[42].

Table of safe diameters to turn the instrument in a 45° angle and 8 mm radius curvature

Once the canal curvature is detected in the diagnostic radiograph and clinically confirmed, select the instrument and the sequence of instrumentation following the safe radii of the table.

	16	15	14	13	12	11	10	9	8	7	6	5	4	3	2	1
15/04	79	75	71	67	63	59	**55**	51	47	43	39	35	31	27	23	19
15/06	111	105	99	93	87	81	75	69	63	57	**51**	45	39	33	27	21
20/02	48	46	44	42	40	38	36	34	32	30	28	26	24	22	20	18
20/04	84	80	76	72	68	64	60	**56**	52	48	44	40	36	32	28	24
20/06	116	110	104	98	92	86	80	74	68	62	56	**50**	44	38	32	26
25/02	57	55	53	51	49	47	45	43	41	39	37	35	33	31	29	27
25/04	89	85	81	77	73	69	65	61	**57**	53	49	45	41	37	33	29
25/06	121	115	109	103	97	91	85	79	73	67	61	55	**49**	43	37	31
30/02	62	**60**	58	56	54	52	50	48	46	44	42	40	38	36	34	32
30/04	94	90	86	82	78	74	70	66	62	58	**54**	50	46	42	38	34
30/06	126	120	114	108	102	96	90	84	78	72	66	60	54	**48**	42	36
35/02	67	65	63	**61**	59	57	55	53	51	49	47	45	43	41	39	37

Diameters that must not be exceeded
Taper .02 = 60 mm
Taper .04 = 55 mm
Taper .06 = 50 mm

FIG. 2.X-39

This figure represents the diameters from which the passage through the curvature will implicate high bending stress.

Figure 2.X-41 presents the different diameters that the instruments have at the point of inflection of the main curvature, when using a .02 mm/mm taper.

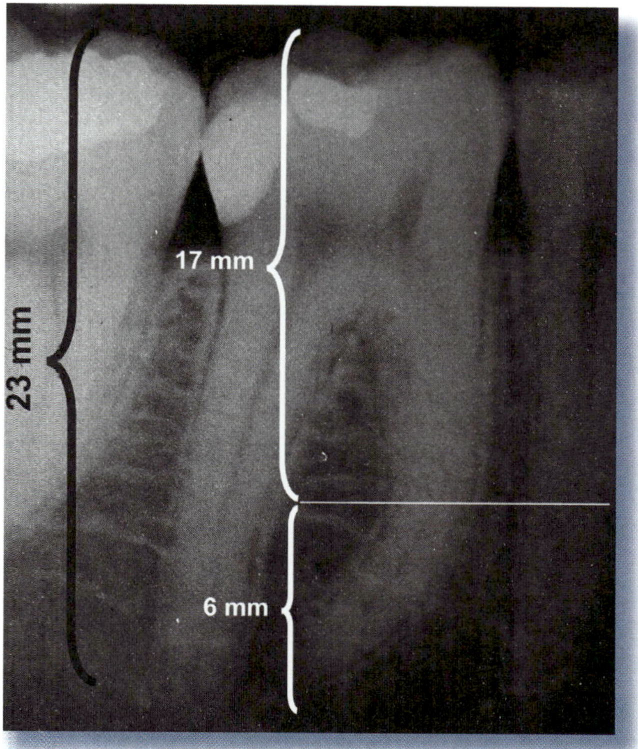

FIG. 2.X-40
According to the text.

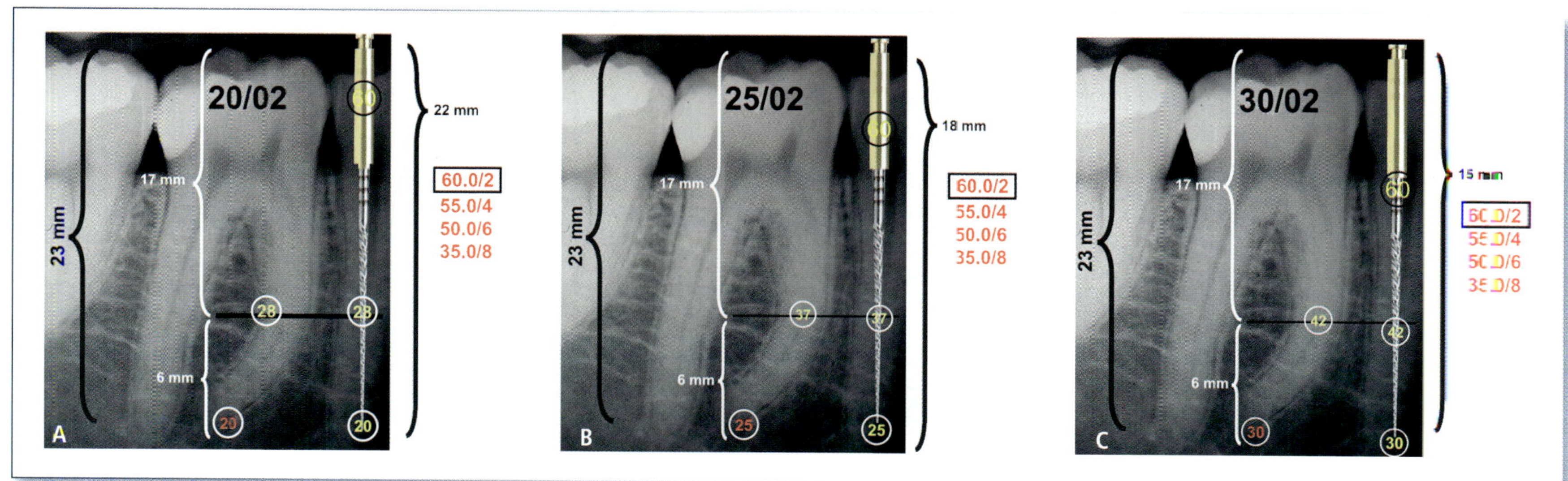

FIGS. 2.X-41A-C
Different diameters the instruments have at the point of inflection of the main curvature, according to the 02 mm/mm taper.

Critical Diameters for .02 Tapered Instruments

When one takes a 20/.02 instrument (Fig. 2.X-42A), 25/.02 (Fig. 2.X-42B), 30/.02 (Fig. 2.X-42C) to the RWL, the diameter these instruments will reach at the point of inflection of the main curvature will be 0.28 mm for No. 20, 0.37 mm for No. 25 and 0.42 mm for No.30.

In these three situations, the diameter of the instruments with .02 mm/mm tapers at the point of inflection of the curvature is far from being unsafe. Therefore, all the instruments could reach the RWL with a *low* bending stress.

Manufacturers generally tend not to include instruments of .02 mm/mm taper in their kits, but these are absolutely necessary for debriding the root canal at the real working length in the presence of middle or cervical third curvatures.

Critical Diameters for .04 mm/mm Tapered Instruments

When one takes 20/.04, 25/.04, 30/.04 instruments to the RWL, the diameter at which they reach the point of inflection of the curvature is 0.44 mm for No. 20, 0.49 mm for No. 25 and 0.54 mm for No. 30 (Figs. 2.X-43A-C).

In the three situations, the critical diameter for .04 mm/mm tapered instruments has not been exceeded. Therefore, all the instruments could be used at the RWL with moderate bending stress.

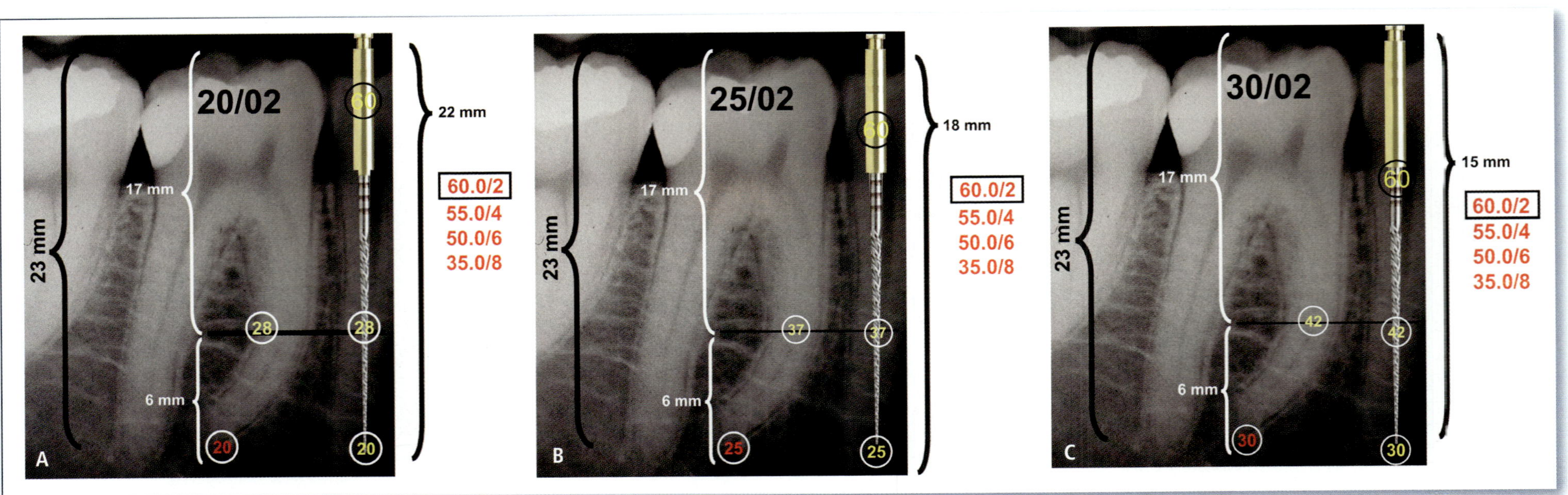

FIGS. 2.X-42A-C

A – Instrument No. 20, with .02 mm/mm taper. The point of inflection of the main curvature is 28.
A – Instrument No. 25, with .02 mm/mm taper. The point of inflection in the main curvature is 37.
C – Instrument No. 30, with .02 mm/mm taper. The point of inflection in the curvature is 42.

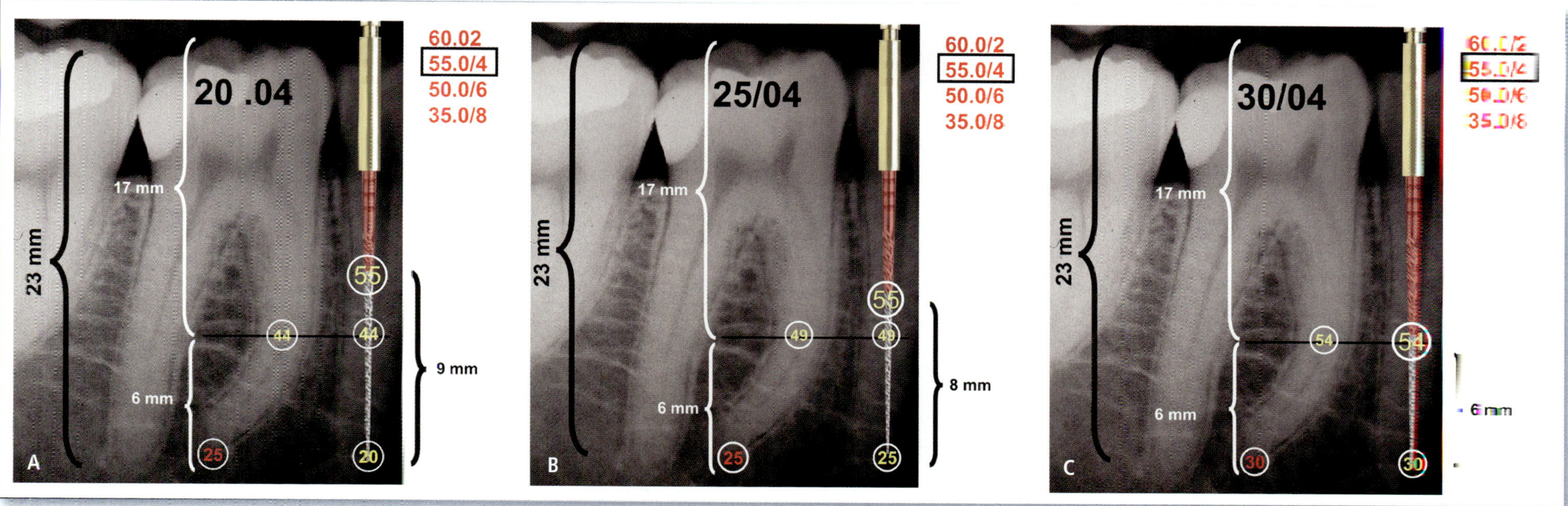

FIGS. 2.X-43A-C

Different diameters the instruments have at the point of inflection in the curvature, with .04 mm/mm taper.
A – Instrument No. 20, with .02 mm/mm taper. The point of inflection in the curvature is 44.
B – Instrument No. 25, with .04 mm/mm taper. The point of inflection in the curvature is 49.
C – Instrument No. 30, with .04 mm/mm taper. The point of inflection in the curvature is 54.

Critical Diameters for .06 mm/mm Tapered Instruments (Fig. 2.X-44)

When one takes 20/.06, 25/.06, 30/.06 instruments to the RWL, the diameter at which they reach the point of inflection of the curvature is 0.56 mm for No. 20, 0.62 mm for No. 25 and 0.66 mm for No. 30 (Figs. 2.X-44A-C).

In the three situations mentioned above, the critical diameter of 50 for .06 tapers is exceeded, from which the bending stress is high and the risk of fracture increases.

Therefore, in this case, these instruments should not reach the RWL.

Figure 2.X-45 shows a clinical case in which one notes the fracture of the Protaper F2 in the mesial root canal of a maxillary left first molar. Figure 2.X-46 shows a similar situation. Those fractures could probably have been avoided if the instruments had remained a few millimeters short of the RWL[7].

This other clinical case (Fig. 2.X-47), with a double curvature, shows a real working length of 22 mm of the mesial root. The distance up to the first curve is 13 mm, and up to the second curvature, 17 mm. As one may note, the first curvature is very far from the RWL, therefore special care must be taken when reaching the RWL with instruments that have large tapers. Remember that the diameter of these instruments should not exceed the critical values at the first curvature.

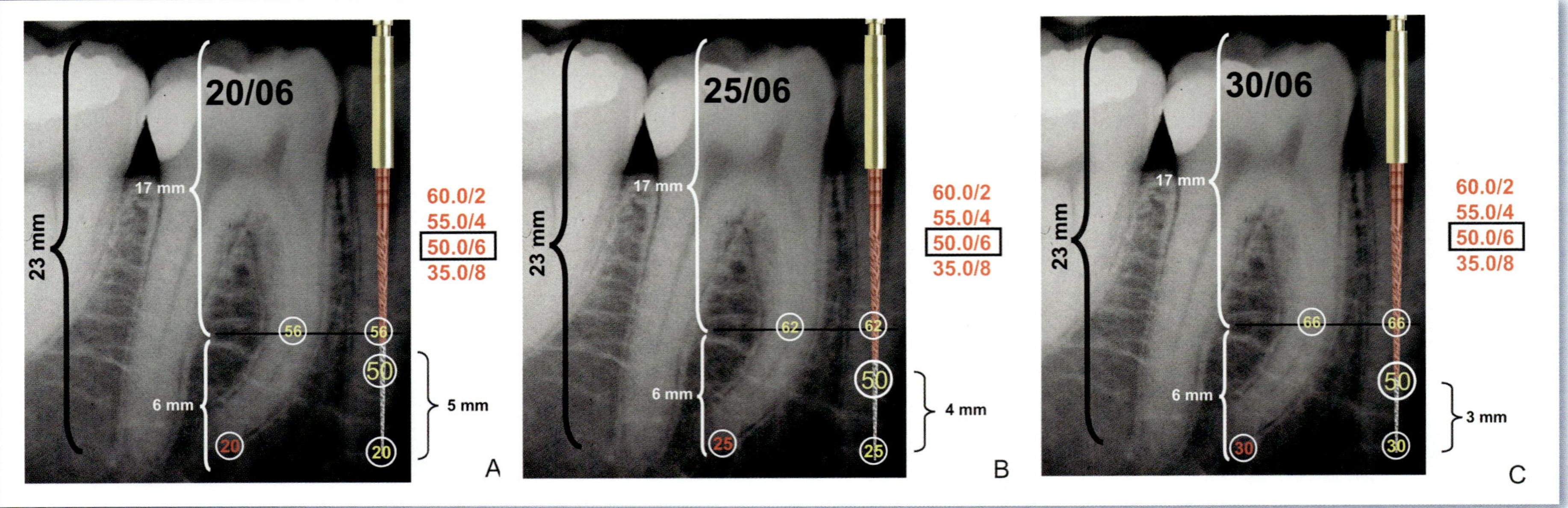

FIGS. 2-X-44A-C

Different points of inflection of the instruments with .06 mm/mm tapers, at the point of inflection in the curvature.
A – Instrument No. 20, with .06 mm/mm taper. The point of inflection of the curvature is 56.
B – Instrument No. 25, with .06 mm/mm taper. The point of inflection in the curvature is 62.
C – Instrument No. 30, with .06 mm/mm taper. The point of inflection in the curvature is 66.

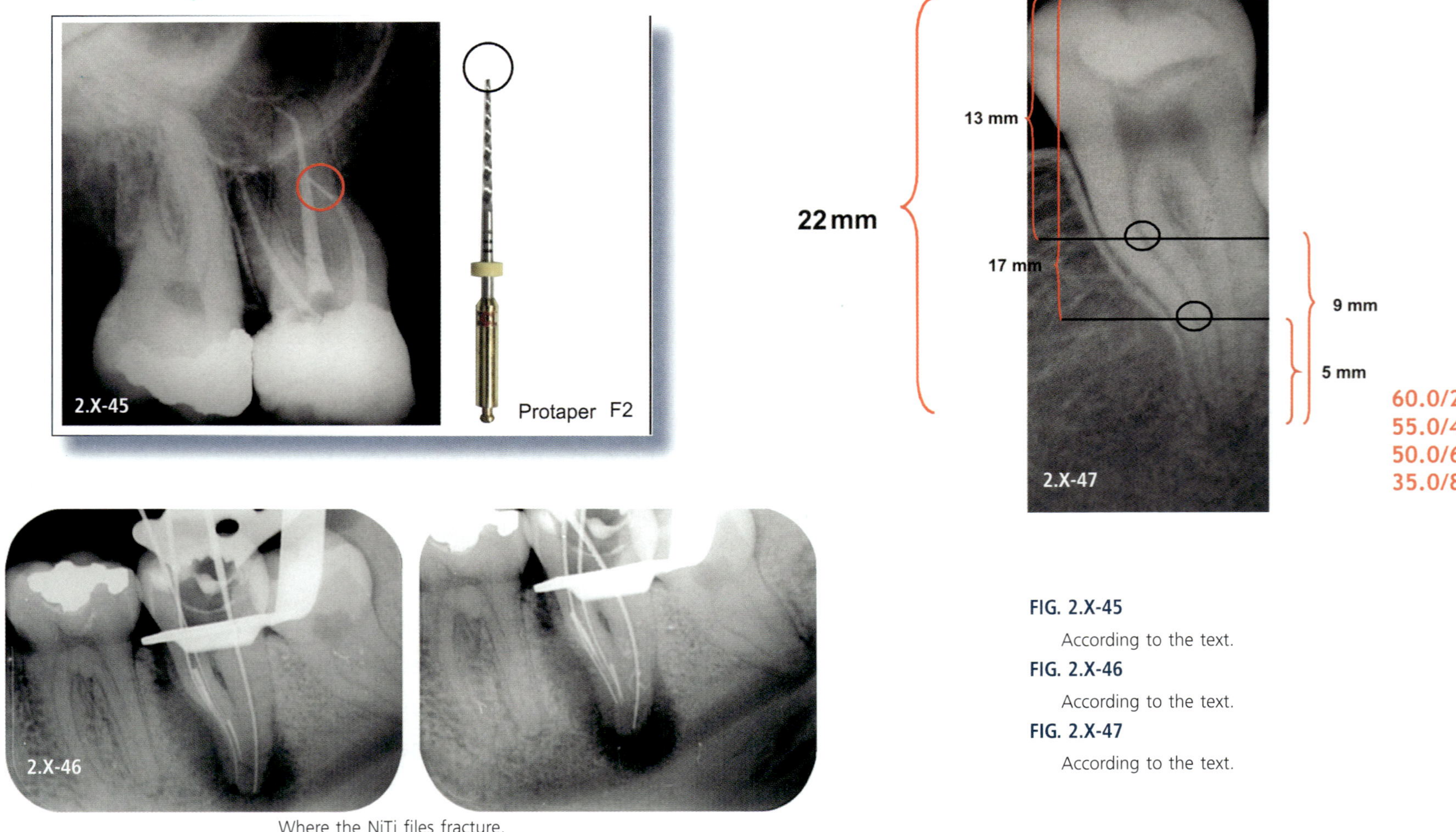

Where the NiTi files fracture.

FIG. 2.X-45

According to the text.

FIG. 2.X-46

According to the text.

FIG. 2.X-47

According to the text.

GENERAL CONSIDERATIONS ABOUT MECHANIZED ROOT CANAL SHAPING TECHNIQUES

Irrespective of the techniques to be used and with the understanding of the causes of fracture and how to prevent them, as detailed before, there are important aspects to be taken into consideration, when one decides to debride root canals in a mechanized rotary manner.

1. **Give priority to the root canal anatomy, not the technique**
   The anatomy will always dictate the shaping strategy and the most convenient sequence of instruments.
2. **Know the design of instruments and their clinical implications** (Fig. 2.X-48).
   As important as knowing the terrain in which one will intervene (the root canal), is the type of instruments one will use to modify it. The behavior of the instrument inside the canal according to its cutting power, helicoidal angle and taper (design), are important details that the operator must not overlook.

There is a wide offer of instruments with different designs and brands on the market. One of the most frequent errors professionals make is to confuse the characteristics of instrument with the techniques recommended by the companies. One must bear in mind that the final forms of shape can be obtained with the use of any brand of instrument, provided that they present the diameters and tapers required for an ideal clinical sequence.

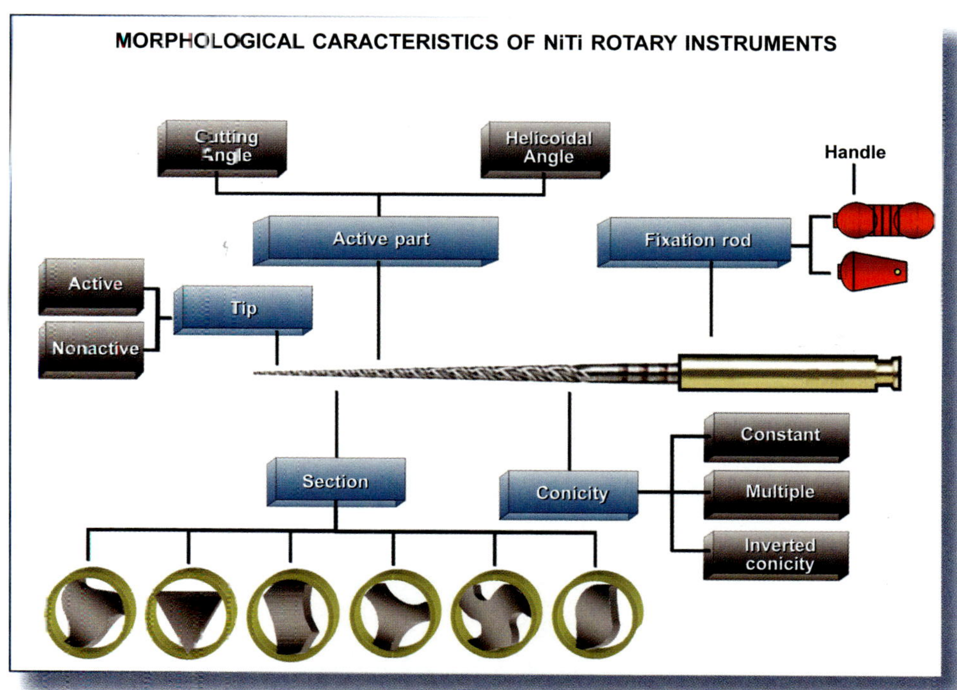

FIG. 2.X-48
According to the text.

3. **Correctly apply the kinematics of the use of instruments** (Fig. 2.X-49).
   Application of the correct kinematics in the use of instruments is an aspect of the utmost importance in the safety of rotary instrumentation. Kinematics of use is directly related to the instrument design and root canal anatomy. However, it is not sufficient to understand only the kinematics of use, since it also demands a great deal of training.

The kinematics of rotary instrumentation comprises six variables: movement, speed, pressure and time.

Movement

- Test the instrument inside de root canal, without activating it, up to the point where it fits. Instruments must be "introduced to" the root canal before being used. Consider the distance to run in instrumentation, which should not be more than 2 mm starting from the point where it fits.
- After testing, penetrate into the root canal, always with the instrument turning, in a small-amplitude advance and withdrawal (back and forth) movement.
- The withdrawal movement may be done against the canal walls, and by traction (as with the use of a Hedströen type file). In cases of oval root canals, this procedure will allow a better cleaning of the poles of the oval shape.

Pressure

- Always apply slight pressure, never forcing the instrument in the apical direction.
- If the necessary pressure to advance needs to be greater, or if the instrument tends to "rotate" inside the canal, it should be replaced by another with a different taper.

When using a stainless steel instrument, the difference is that one intends to "feel the tip of the instrument" (tactile sensitivity), whereas with NiTi instruments, one only feels the degree of fit (the instrument engaging or locking inside the root canal).

Speed

- Generally one uses a speed ranging from 250 to 350 rpm, but some instruments demand 500 and/or 600 rpm.
- Speed may vary according to the portion of the canal: in the straight segments of the root canal, instruments can turn at greater speed.
  - Speed may vary according to the contact surface.
  - In cases of smaller contact surfaces between the instrument and the wall, as for example, with the RaCe, Race S. Apex and Light Speed systems[17], the speed is greater.

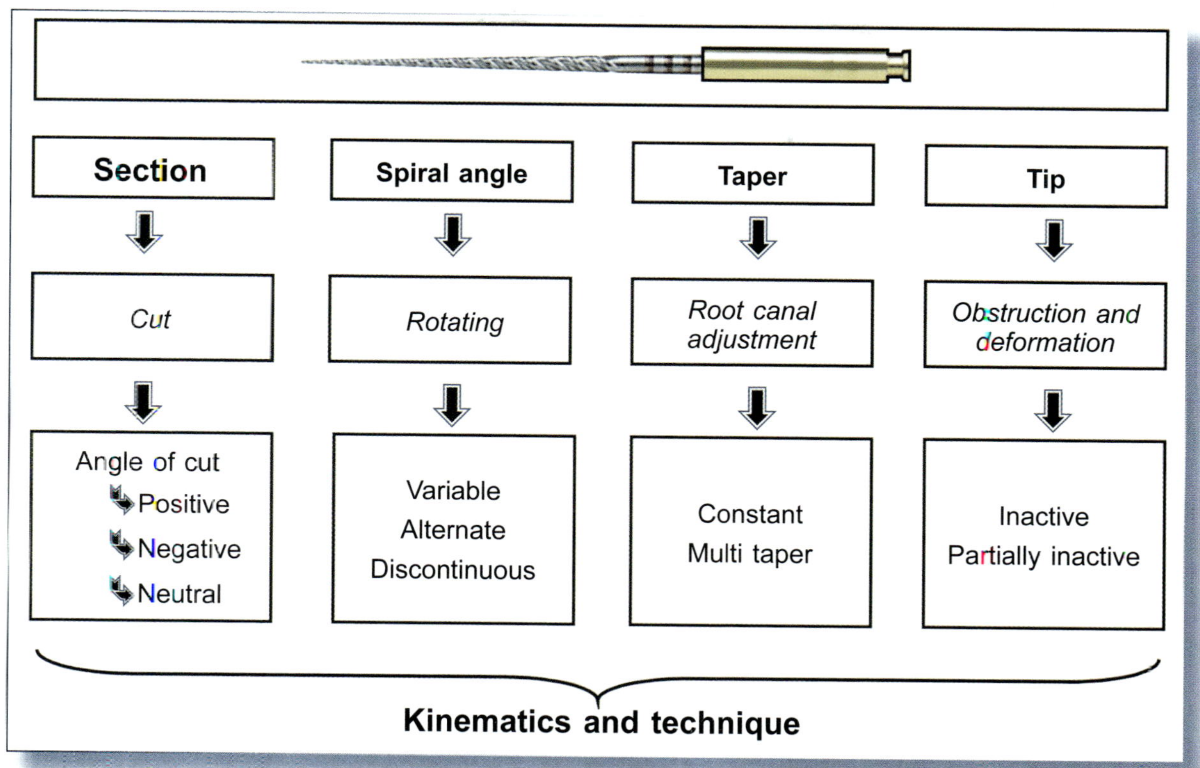

FIG. 2.X-49

The kinematics of use is directly related to the design of the instrument.

Time

- Once the cut has been produced, remove the instrument, because a greater accumulation of dentin scrapings occurs and the canal becomes obstructed, making a higher demand for torque necessary, with a greater risk of fracture by torsion.
- Do not leave the instrument turning in curves in the same length, because it increases cyclical fatigue.

4. Use sequences of instruments that demand low stress.

- A technique will be safer when instrument stress is smaller, according to the proposed sequence. Although there is a wide range of sequences nowadays, it is opportune to make it clear that the two basic shaping techniques, when one uses stainless steel or nickel-titanium instruments, present different variables.
- Stainless steel instruments with a standard .02 mm/mm taper, are used by increasing or decreasing their diameters and the depth of insertion in the crown-apex (crown-down) or apex-crown (step-back) sequences.
- In the case of NiTi instruments, a very important variable is added: taper, which will allow the conventional techniques to be performed in the following manner:

IN CROWN-DOWN PREPARATION (FIG. 2.X-50)

This sequence is convenient for the stage of anti-curvature wear, and for root canals with a low degree of difficulty (wide canals and those with a high radius of curvature).

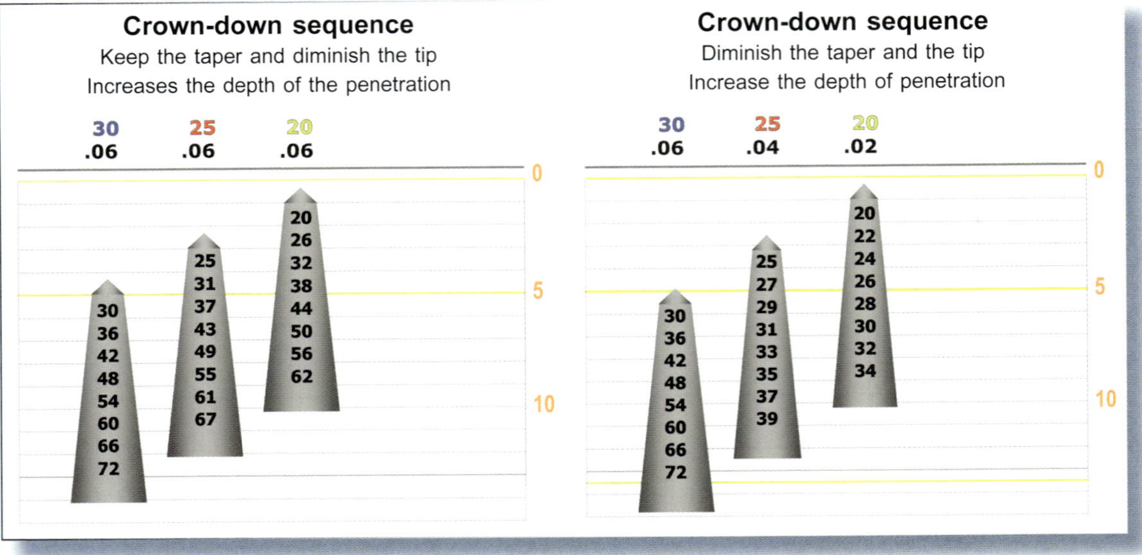

FIG. 2.X-50
Crown-down sequence, indicated for anticurvature wear and wide root canals.

IN STEP BACK PREPARATION (FIG. 2.X-51)

The sequence is convenient for apical dilation and for root canals with a medium and high degree of difficulty (atresic canals and those with a low radius of curvature or double curvatures).

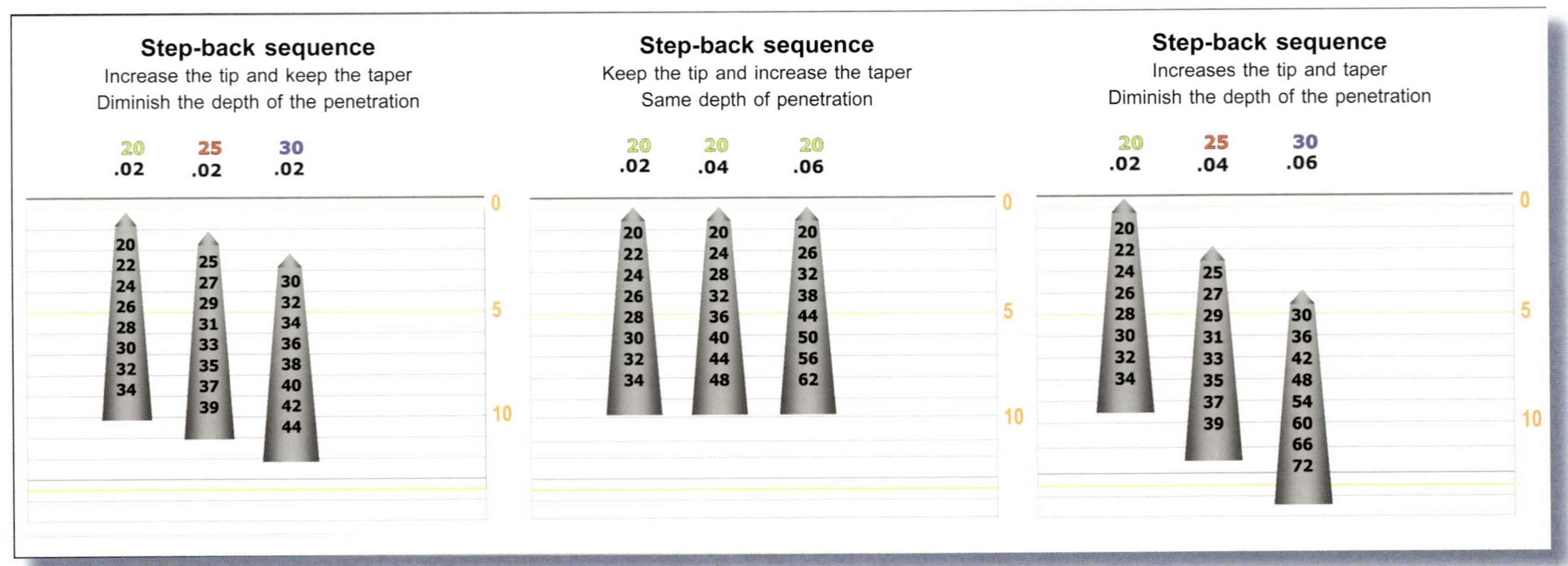

FIG. 2.X-51
Staged sequence (step-back), indicated for atresic and curved root canals.

Irrespective of the technique used, the suggestion is to:

1. Calibrate the root canal with .02 mm/mm taper (Fig. 2.X-52A).
2. Increase taper with .04 and .06 tapered instruments, without involving the tip (Fig. 2.X-52B).
3. Avoid performing instrumentation by working with the entire active part, which will adjust itself along the root canal (Fig. 2.X-52C).

In a comparative study of four root canal preparation techniques, no differences were detected between step-back and crown-down root canal preparations in terms of rectification, but the crown-down preparation produced more steps[38].

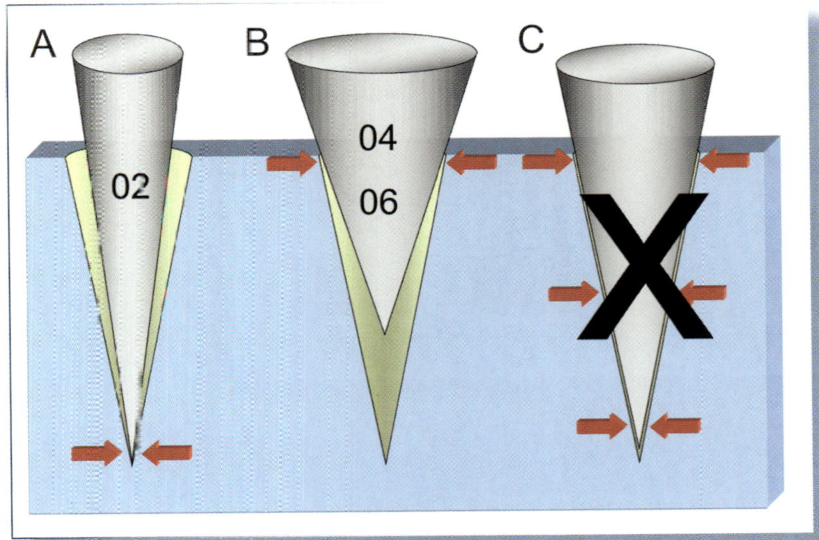

FIGS. 2.X-52A-C

A – According to the text.
B – According to the text.
C – According to the text.

STRESS CALCULATION

This calculation is a graphic representation (arbitrary) which endeavors to make a theoretical demonstration of the stress that each instrument could undergo and the technique in general, for later analysis, as follows:

1. This is a graphic representation of the instrument with its diameter at each millimeter of its active part.
2. Therefore, by comparing it with the next instrument in the sequence, one can calculate the increase and decrease in volume of each millimeter.
3. This calculation also gives us an idea of which segment of the instrument is most exposed to cutting.

In the cases of Figures 2.X-53A-B, the sequence is 15/02 and 15/04: the partial stress is high and the contact surface is wide, in comparison with the case of Figures 2.X-53A-B, with the sequence 15/06 and 20/02, in which the stress is low and the contact surface is reduced.

Partial stress is the sum of the changes of diameter in each segment of the instrument.

Total stress is the sum of the changes of diameter in the entire active part of the instrument.

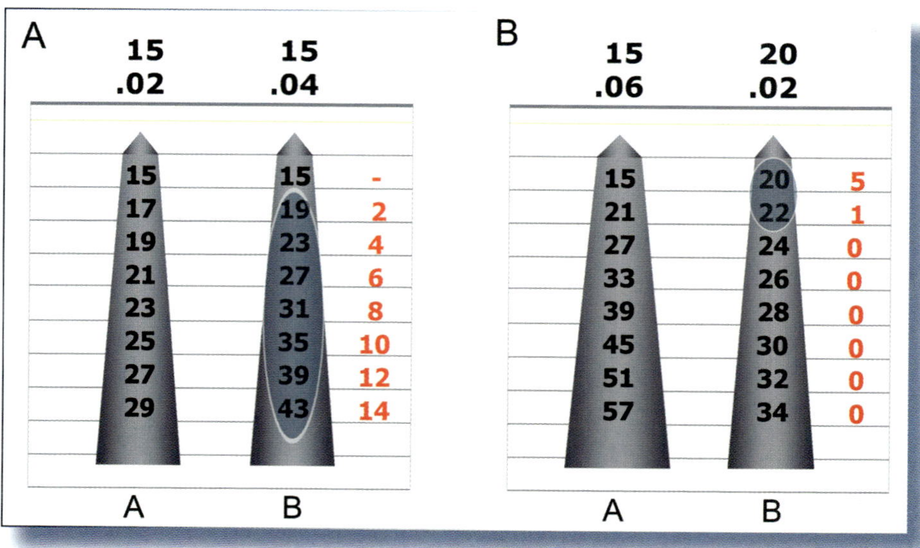

FIGS. 2.X-53A-B

A – In the sequence 15/.02 and 15/.04, the partial stress is high and the contact surface is wide.
B – In the sequence 15/0.06 and 20/0.02, the stress is low and the contact surface is reduced.

THE MINIMUM STRESS TECHNIQUE

This sequence was developed by, and is used in the Specialization Course in Endodontics at the Faculty of Dentistry of the University of Maimónides (FOUM), Buenos Aires, Argentina.

The minimum stress technique has a sequence of nine-instruments, as is noted in Figure 2.X-54, and can be performed with any commercial brand of instruments that have the diameters and tapers demanded by this technique.

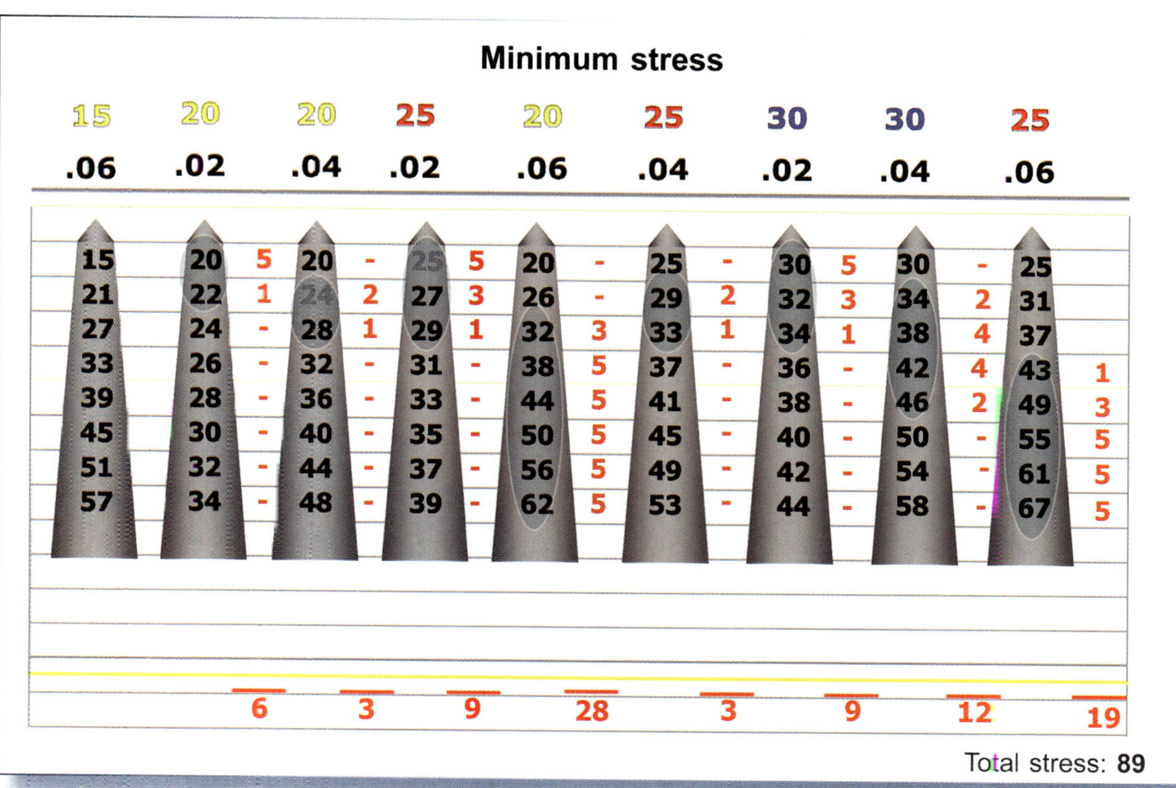

FIG. 2.X-54
According to the text.

Considerations about the minimum stress technique:

The values of increase in stress are minimum.

The contact surfaces are small.

The instruments with greater tapers work with tips that remain free.

The instruments with smaller tapers determine the diameter of the apical stop.

It covers the majority of clinical situations with a high margin of safety.

The technique, therefore, allows stress to be minimized, increases the cutting efficiency of instruments, diminishes their contact surfaces and increases in their useful life.

It is not imperative to use motors with torque control, since the “fit” or the “rotation” of the instrument in the root canal is minimum.

DEVELOPMENT OF THE MINIMUM STRESS TECHNIQUE SEQUENCE

Radiographic Analysis and Operative Strategy

Irrespective of the technique to be used, the clinician must make a detailed study of the information provided by the radiographic exam, taking into consideration its limitations (a two dimensional image of a three dimensional structure). He/she will then be able to prepare an endodontic "map" as closely as possible to reality. The operative strategy should adapt the technique to the canal, not the canal to the technical sequence.

Undoubtedly, one of the major limitations Endodontics still has is diagnosis from images. Not only does the clinician operate without seeing the surgical area, but he/she also does not have complete prior information about the area in which he/she will intervene.

To optimize the radiographic resource, a radiographic positioner (Multiplanex) has been developed and is at present being used at FOUM. This device allows angulations to be obtained in the vertical and horizontal planes simultaneously, and it is considered an accurate, quantifiable and reproducible procedure.

The time invested, and the resources used in the previous analysis of the case to be treated, bring great benefits, because they enable one to anticipate difficulties, thus optimizing the resources for preventing accidents.

Planning and Strategies

Dentists usually have a very limited view to evaluate the difficulty of the case under treatment, first observing the apical thirds of the root canals, focusing on the curvatures and apical endings, without paying sufficient attention to the first important obstacle, which is the angulation of the cervical third of the canal in relation to the pulp chamber[52].

As observed in Figure 2.X-55A, the first inconvenience to be overcome would be to change in the angulation of the canal cervical third with the pulp chamber, modifying the angle of incidence or attack of the instruments. All known advantages of access to the root (anti-curvature wear) are beneficial and necessary for shaping both with steel or with NiTi instruments.

In the mesial root canals of mandibular molars, the case shown in Figure 2.X-56A, one can note a medium-high curve. It is a situation that should be complemented with the high probability of a more accentuated curve in the vestibulolingual plane, which cannot be seen in the radiograph, but can be imagined due to the loss of radiolucence of the root canal in this zone.

As previously explained, the cases of curvatures that are distant from the RWL are the ones that require special care, particularly when one reaches the RWL with instruments with large tapers.

In the distal root canal one notes a medium-low curvature and a counter curvature in the apical third, as well as the loss of radiolucence of the canal, which could indicate an accentuated dilaceration and/or apical delta. When exploring the distal root shortly after coronal opening is performed, one must be extremely careful to maintain accessibility to the apical third with stainless steel instruments, before using rotary instruments. The real challenge will then be not to obstruct this surgically inaccessible zone[52].

As observed in the post-operative Figure 2.X-55B, the radius of curvature of the cervical third was modified, to allow more direct access to the main curve of the canals of both roots.

The mesial canals could be instrumented without inconvenience up to the RWL, with special care not to reach the RWL with files with large tapers, because one would be passing through the main curve with critical diameters, in which cyclical fatigue is important, as previously explained in detail, when dealing with the causes of bending fractures.

In the distal root canal one notes dilation up to the apical delta zone, preventing the tips of the rotary instruments from being blocked and fractured in the attempt to shape a surgically inaccessible zone with instruments with large tapers through the apical radius of curvature[52].

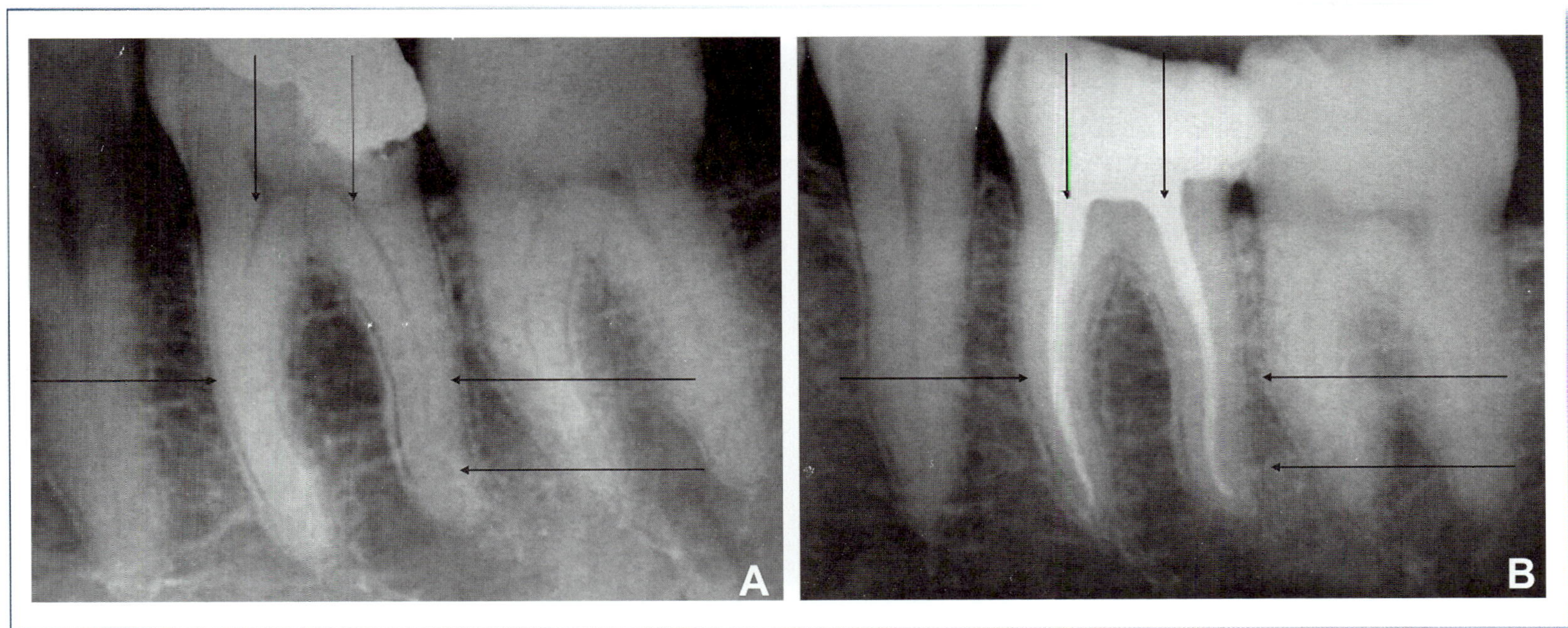

FIGS. 2.X-55A-B

According to the text.

Establish an Estimated Length at the Level of the Main Curvature

- Locate the main curvature and establish whether it is cervical, middle or apical, because it will be subject to the surgical strategy to be used[29] (Figs. 2.X-56A-D).

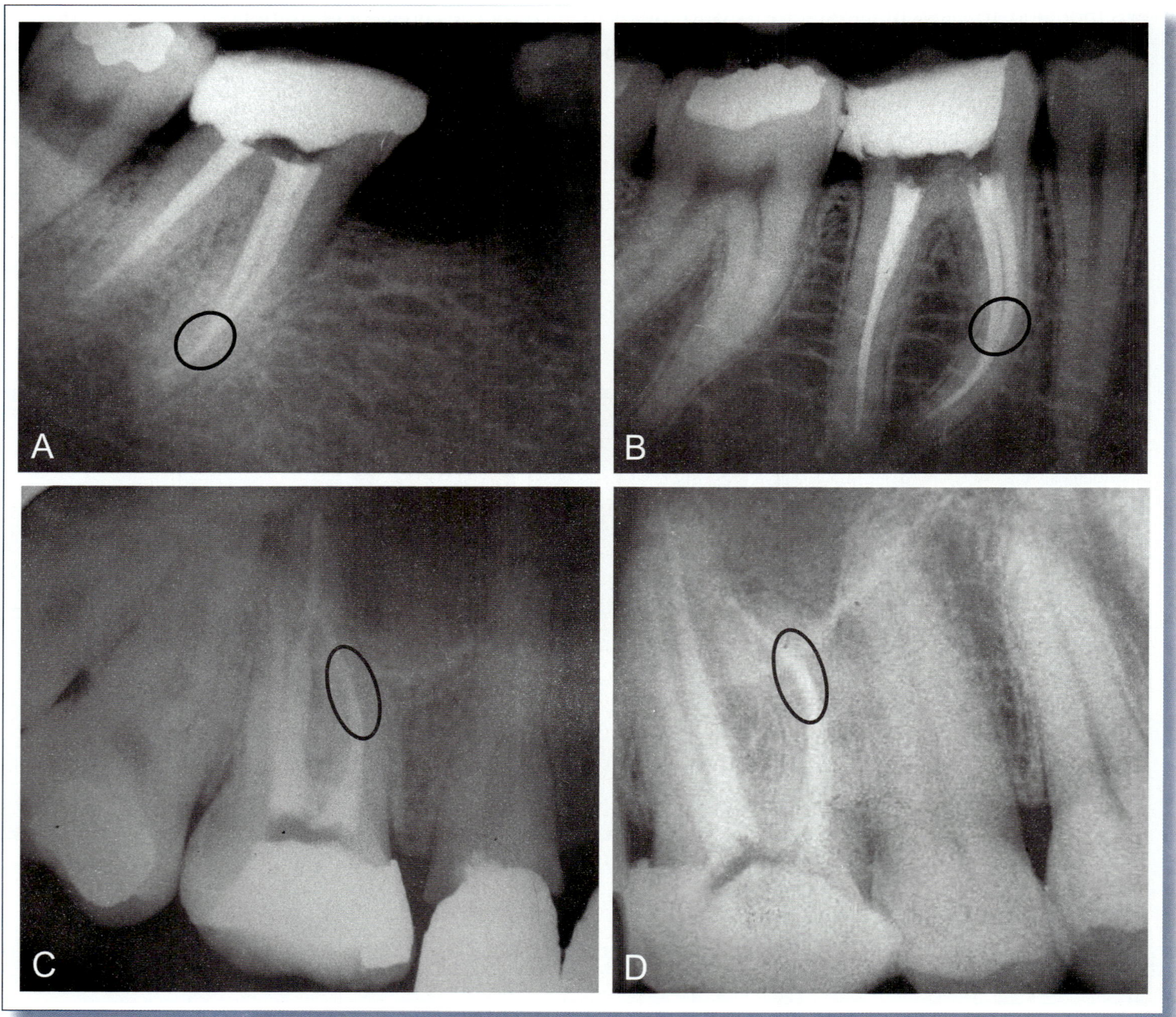

FIGS. 2.X-56A-D

Radiographs of clinical cases with different levels of main curvatures.

Once the case has been clinically and radiographically analyzed, one prepares a strategy. Its main steps are:

1. **Root access (anti-curvature wear):** Once the canal is located, it should be explored at the level of its cervical (and middle) thirds, using manual type K files, with the purpose of familiarizing oneself with the field of action, noting the changes of angulation and opening the pathway for achieving the corresponding root access (anti-curvature wear). In this maneuver, one can use a wide range of steel rotary instruments: Gates Glidden cutters (drills) 1,2,3 and/or Peeso burs 1,2 and/or NiTi instruments. During exploration, one must detect the following clinical situations: canals that unite, curvatures, double curvatures, divisions, which are risk factors for instrument fractures.
2. **Apical access:** After performing anti-curvature wear, the entire canal should be explored with stainless steel manual type K files. Determine the real work length (RWL), with a radiograph and/or and electronic foramen locator. Take the first instrument in the sequence, a 15/.06, into the canal and evaluate its depth of insertion and fit.
   - If this instrument (15/.06) is over 3 mm short of the RWL, one should manually improve the shape of the canal with type K file No. 15 and the step-back technique (by retroceding approximately 1 mm), followed by the instruments Nos. 20, 25 and 30, dilating the canal and thus improving access to the apical third.
   - If the instrument (15/.06) is 3 mm or less short of the RWL, activate it up to the RWL (always advancing 1 or 2 mm). The body of the instrument will cut, without involving the tip, which is of the same diameter as the one obtained by exploration with the manual stainless steel file. Shaping performed by this instrument is fundamental for the later development of the sequence, since it allows the following instruments to cut with a level of low stress. If this step is successfully finished, a great part of the optimization of the final geometry of the canal is assured.
3. **Apical dilation:** With instruments of smaller taper, one starts to increase the section and the taper of the apical third, working with the step-back technique in the following sequence, without involving the tips of instruments with larger tapers:

   20/02 Cuts by the tip
   20/04 Cuts by the body (free tip)
   25/02 Cuts by the tip

4. **Final taper and apical calibration:** Using instruments with larger tapers, and without involving the tip, one continues modeling the rest of the canal. Depending on the root canal anatomy and its relationship with the depth of insertion of the instrument, the .06 tapered instruments should not necessarily reach the RWL.

   20/06
   25/04 to the RWL
   30/02 to the RWL
   25/06
   30/04 to the RWL

If the clinical case allows, and its clinical criterion demands it, one may continue with apical dilation (apical stop) with 35/.02 and 40/.02 optional instruments.

Note: it is necessary to remember that the instruments should be "introduced to" the root canal before being used, to consider their level of fit, since the distance to be covered during instrumentation must not exceed 2 mm, from the point of fit up to the apical limit.

This sequence is adaptable to the majority of clinical situations. However, in cases of difficult surgical accessibility the sequence can be adapted to each clinical case, by reducing the number of instruments in some cases, and in others, by varying the depth of the apical insertion.

References

1. Alapati SB, Brantley WA, Svec TA, Powers JM, Mitchell JC. Scanning electron microscope observations of new and used nickel-titanium rotary files. J Endod, v.29, p.667-669, 2003.
2. Alapati SB, Brantley WA, Svec TA, Powers JM, Nusstein JM, Daehn GS. Proposed role of embedded dentin chips for the clinical failure of nickel-titanium rotary instruments. J Endod, v.30, p.339-341, 2004.
3. Alapati SB, Brantley WA, Svec TA, Powers JM, Nusstein JM, Daehn GS. SEM observations of nickel-titanium rotary endodontic instruments that fractured during clinical Use. J Endod, v.30, p.40-43, 2005.
4. Al-Omari MAO, Dummer PMH, Newcombe RG. Comparison of six files to prepare simulated root canal. Part 1. J Endod, v.25, p.57, 1992.
5. Al-Omari MAO, Dummer PMH, Newcombe RG, Doller R, Hartles F. Comparison of six files to prepare simulated root canal. Part 2. Int Endod J, v.25, p.67, 1992.
6. Anderson D, Joyce A, Roberts S, Runner R. A comparative photoelastic stress analysis of internal root stresses between RCprep and saline when applied to the Profile/GT rotary instrumentation system. J Endod, v.32, p.222-224, 2006.
7. Ankrum MT, Hartwell GR, Truit JE. K3 Endo, ProTaper, and ProFile systems: breakage and distortion in severely curved roots of molars. J Endod, v.30, p.234-237, 2004.
8. Root canal files and reamers, type K for hand use Am. Dent. Assoc. Specification nº`28. 1988
9. Bahia MGA, Martins RC, Gonzalez BM, Buono VTL. Physical and mechanical characterization and the influence of cyclic loading on the behavior of nickel-titanium wires employed in the manufacture of rotary endodontic instruments. Int Endod J, v.38, p.795-801, 2005.
10. Berutti E, Negro A, Lendini M, Pasqualinl D. Influence of Manual Preflaring and Torque on the Failure Rate of ProTaper Rotary. J Endod, v.30, p.228-239, 2004.
11. BjORndal L, Reit C. The adoption of new endodontic technology amongst Danish general dental practioners. Int Endod J, v.38, n.1, p.52-58, 2005.
12. Boessler C, Peters OA, Zehnde, M. Impact of Lubricant Parameters on Rotary Instrument Torque and Force. J Endod., v.33, 2007.
13. Bramante C. Betti L. Comparative analysis of curved root canal preparation using nickel-titanium instruments with or without EDTA. J Endod, v.26, p.278-280, 2000.
14. Brantley WA, Svec TA. Iijima M. Powers JM. Grentzer TH. Differential scanning calorimetric studies of nickel-titanium rotary endodontic instruments after simulated clinical use. J Endod, v.28, n.11, p.774-778, 2002.
15. Buehler WJ, Gilfrich JV, Wiley RC. Effect of low temperature phase changes on the mechanical properties of alloys near composition TiNi. J Appl Phys, v.34, p.1475-1477, 1963.
16. DI Fiore PM, Genov E, Komaroff Y, LI L. Nickel–titanium rotary instrument fracture: a clinical practice assessment. Int Endod J, v.39, p.700-708, 2006.
17. Dietz D, Di Fiore PM, Bahcall JK, Lautenschager E. Effect of rotational speed on breakage of nickel–titanium rotary files. J. Endod., v.26, p.68-71, 2000.
18. Fife D, Gambarini G, Britto LR. Cyclic fatigue testing of ProTaper NiTi rotary instruments after clinical use. Oral Surg Oral Med, Oral Path, Oral Radiol Endod, v.97, p.251-256, 2004.
19. Frick K, Deguzman J, Walia HD, Austin BP. Comparison of Quantec Series 2000 and Profile Series 29 to handfiling. J Dent Res, p.76-304, 1997.
20. Gabel WP, Hoen M, Steiman HR, Pink FE, Dietz R. Effect of rotational speed on nickel-titanium file distortion. J Endod, v.25, p.752-754, 1999.
21. Gambarini G. Rationale for the use of low-torque endodontic motors in root canal instrumentation. End Dent Traumat, v.16, p.95-100, 2000.
22. Gambarini G. Cyclic fatigue of profile rotary instruments after prolonged clinical use. Int Endod J, v.34, p.386-389, 2001.
23. Gambarini G, Dell'Agnola A. Prevenzione della fractura di strumenti rotanti al nichel-titanio valutazioni ed accorgimenti patrici. G It Endo, v.1, p.17-28, 1988.
24. García Jerónimo FJ. Doble fractura de limas rotatorias NITI en un molar inferior. ENDODONCIA.
25. Girard S, Paque F, Badertscher M, Sener B, Zehnder M. Assessment of a gel-type chelating preparation containing 1-hydroxyethylidene-1, 1-bisphosphonate. I. J Endod, v.38, p.810-816, 2005.
26. Glosson CR, Haller RH, Dove SB, Del Río CE. A comparison of root canal preparation using Ni-Ti hand, Ni-Ti engine-driven, and K-Flex endodontic instruments. J Endod, v.21, p.146-151, 1995.
27. Haıkel Y, Serfaty R, Bateman G, Senger B, Allemann C. Dynamic and cyclic fatigue of engine-driven rotary nickel–titanium endodontic instruments. J Endod, v.25, p.434-440, 1999.
28. Hübscher W, Barbakow F, Peters OA. Root canal preparation with FLEXMASTER: canal shapes analysed by micro-computted tomography. International Endod J, v.36, p.740, 2003.
29. Jerome CE, Hanlon RJ. Identifying Multiplanar Root Canal Curvatures Using Stainless-Steel Instrument. J Endod, v.29, 2003.
30. Kennon NF, Dunne DP. Shape memory behaviour. Metals Forum, v.4, n.3, p.130-134, 1981.
31. Kerlins V, Phillips A. Modes of fracture. In: Mill K, Davis J, Destejani J, Dieterich D, Frissell H, Crankovic G. et al. eds. Fractography, ASM Handbook, v.12, 3rd edn. Materials Park, OH, USA. ASM International, p.12-71, 1987.
32. Knowles KI, Ibarrola JL, Christiansen RK. Assessing apical deformation and transportation following the use of LightSpeed™ root canal instruments. Int. Endod. J., v.29, p.113-117, 1996.
33. Kuhn G, Tavernier B, Jordan L. Influence of structure on nickel-titanium endodontic instruments failure. J. Endod., v.27, n.8, p.516-520, 2001.
34. Laguna Contreras MA. Comparison of the first file that fits at the apex, before and after earl flarng. J Endod, v.27, p.113-116, 2001.
35. Laustren L, Luebke N, Brantley W. Bending properties of nickel-titanium rotary endodontic instruments. J. Dent. Res., p.75-384, 1996.
36. Leonardo MR. Endodoncia, 1.ª ed., Artes Medicas, São Paulo, 2008, p.814.

37. Li UM, Lee BS, Shih CT, Lan WH, Liu CP. Cyclic fatigue on endodontic nickel-titanium rotary instruments: static and dynamic tests. J Endod, v.28, p.448-451, 2002.

38. Luiten DJ, Morgan LA, Baumgartner JC, Marshall JG. A comparison of four instrumentation techniques on apical canal transportation. J. Endod., v.21, p.26-32, 1995.

39. Martın B, Zelada G, Varela P. Factors influencing the fracture of nickel-titanium rotary instruments. I J Endod, v.36, p.262-266, 2003.

40. Martins RC, Bahia MGA, Buono VTL. Surface analysis of ProFile instruments by scannig electron microscopy and X-ray energy-dispersive spectroscopy: a preliminary study. Int Endod J, v.35, n.10, p.848-853, 2002.

41. Matheus, T.C.U. Fractura por torcão de instrumentos de niquel-titânio, K3 endo e ProFile. RBO, v.60.p.202-204, 2003.

42. McSpadden JT. Mastering Endodontic Instrumentation, 1.ed, Cloudland Institute, Chattanooga, p.105-123, 2007.

43. Melo MCC, Bahia MGA, Buono VTL. Fatigue resistance of engine-driven rotary nickel-titanium endodontic instruments. J Endod, v.28, n.11, p.765-769, 2002.

44. Nagy CD, Bartha K, Bernath M, Verdes E, Szabo J. A comparative study of seven instruments in shaping the root canal in vitro. Int Endod J, v.30, p.124, 1997.

45. Otsuka K, Wayman CM. Shape Memory Materials. 1ed. United Kingdom: Cambridge University Press, p.284, 1998

46. Parashos P, Gordon I, Messer HH. Factors influencing defects of rotary nickel–titanium endodontic instruments after clinical use. J Endod, v.30, p.722-725, 2004.

47. Parashos P, Messer HH. Questionnaire survey on the use of rotary nickel-titanium endodontic instruments by Australian dentists. Int Endod J, v.37, p.249-259, 2004.

48. Patiño PV, Biedma BM, Rodríguez Liébana C, Cantatore G, González Bahillo J. The Influence of a Manual Glide Path on the Separation Rate of NiTi Rotary Instruments. JOE, v.31, 2002.

49. Peters OA, Boessler C, Zehnder M. Effect of liquid and paste-type lubricants on torque values during simulated rotary root canal instrumentation.. IEJ, v.38, p.223-229, 2005.

50. Peters OA, Peters CI, Schönenberger K, Barbakow F. ProTaper rotary root canal preparation: effects of canal anatomy on final shape analysed by micro CT. Int Endod J, v.36, p.86, 2003.

51. Pruett JP, Clement DJ, Carnes DL. Cyclic fatigue testing of nickeltitanium endodontic instruments. J Endod, v.23, p.77-85, 1997.

52. Pucci F. Conductos Radiculares, Ed. Medico Quirúrgica, Montevideo, 1945, p.301.

53. Roland DD, Andelin WE, Browning DF, Hsu GH, Torabinejad M. The effect of preflaring on the rates of separation for 0.04 taper nickel titanium rotary instruments. J Endod, v.28, p.543-545, 2002.

54. Ruddle C. Cleaning and shaping the root canal system. In: Choen, S.; Burns, R.C. Pathways of the Pulp. 2002.

55. Satapan B, Nervo G, Palamara J, Messer H. Defects in Rotary NiTi Files After Clinical Use. J Endod, v.26, p.161-165, 2000.

56. Schilder H. Cleaning and shaping the root canal. Dent Clin North Am, v.18, p.269-296, 1974.

57. Schroeder KP, Walton RE, Rivera EM. Straight Line Access and Coronal Flaring: Effect on Canal Length. J Endod, v.28, 2002.

58. Serene TP, Adams JD, Saxena A. Nickel-Titanium instruments: Applications in Endodontics. St. Louis, MO, USA:Ishiaku EuroAmerica, Inc., 1995.

59. Stewart G, Kapsimalas P, Rappaport H. Hedta and urea peroxide for root canal preparation. J Am Dent Assoc, v.78, p.335-338, 1969.

60. Svec TA, Powers JM. The deterioration of rotary nickel-titanium files under controlled conditions. J Endod, v.28, p.105-107, 2002.

61. Tan BT, Messer HH. The effect of instrument tipe and preflaring on apical file size determantion. Int Endod J, v.35, p.752-758, 2002.

62. Tharuni SL, Parameswaran A, Sukumaran VG. A comparison of canal preparation using the K-file and LightSpeed in resin blocks. J Endod, v.22, p.474-476, 1996.

63. Thompson SA. An overview of nickel-titanium alloys used in dentistry. Int Endod J, v.33, p.297-310, 2000.

64. Tripi TR, Bonaccorso A, Tripi V, Condorelli GG, Rapisarda E. Defects in GT Rotary instruments after use: an SEM study. J Endod, v.27, p.782-785, 2001.

65. Walia H, Brantley WA, Gerstein HN. A initial investigation of the bending and torsional properties of nitinol root canal files. J Endod, v.14, n.7, p.346-351, 1988.

66. West JD, Roane JB, Goerig AC. Cleaning and shaping the root canal system. In: Cohen, S.; Burns, R.C. St. Louis: Mosby. Pathways of the pulp, 6th ed. p.206-207, 1994.

67. Yared GM, Bou Dagher FE, Machtou P, Kulkarni GK. Influence of rotational speed, torque, and operator proficiency on failure of greater taper files. Int Endod J, v.35, p.7-12, 2002.

68. Yared GM, Dagher FEB, Machtou P. Cyclic fatigue of profile rotary instruments after simulated clinical use. International Endod J, v.32, p.115-119, 1999.

69. Zehnder M, Schmidlin P, Sener B, Waltimo T. Chelation in root canal therapy reconsidered. J Endod, v.31, p.817-820, 2005.

70. Zelada G, Varela P, Martin PB, Bahillo JG, Magan F, Ahn S. The effect of rotational speed on the breakage of rotary endodontic instruments. J Endod, v.28, p.540-542, 2002.

71. Zinelis S, Margelos J. Failure mechanism of endodontic files in vivo. J Endod, v.28, p.471-473, 2002.

EndoSequence System and ACTIV GP

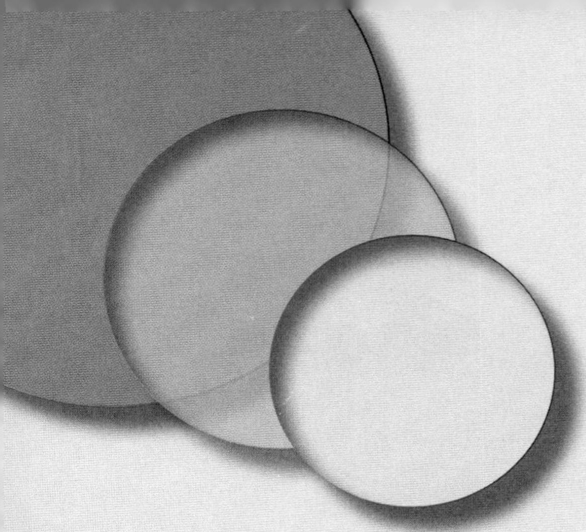

Daniel Silva Herzog Flores
Tatiana Ramirez Mora

During

the last few years, considerable changes have occurred in Endodontics, which will undoubtedly continue in the future. The introduction of new technologies has made this specialty clinically easier, faster and more reliable with more predictable results[2]. One of the most important changes was the introduction of nickel-titanium (NiTi) instruments, which enabled a more consistent, predictable and reproducible instrumentation of the root canal. This predictability did not only affect debridement, but also the final result of the filling[11].

Many dentists and researchers have become aware of the significant changes that have occurred in this area of Dentistry, such as the use of disposable endodontic products and the concept of hermetic sealing when filling the root canal systems, facilitating endodontics and making it more simpler and better.

The introduction of rotary systems with nickel-titanium-based metal alloy files with different tapers, replacing those that had been used for many years, led to a considerable number of endodontists beginning to use the new systems. However, since these rotary systems produce a larger canal diameter, they may cause greater risks that could multiply during the course of the procedure. However, as time passed, practitioners perceived that this did not occur and that these systems indeed simplified endodontic procedures.

As a result of the search for a simpler and easier technique, a new system was realized by Real World Endo, in conjunction with Brasseler-USA, called EndoSequence. It is expected that this new rotary system will satisfy the current demands of modern root canal therapy, since the design of the instruments achieve the goal to obtain an ideal shaping of the root canal[3].

Preparation using nickel-titanium instruments with 0.06 mm/mm or 0.04 mm/mm tapers, when performed in an adequate manner, has surprised dentists by being fast, simple and predictable.

Real World Endo idealizing a completely tapered root canal preparation, offers 0.06 mm/mm and 0.04 mm/mm files (the latter used in cases of calcified root canals or with curvatures greater than 30º), which use in all cases makes filling easier.

REAL WORLD ENDO ENDOSEQUENCE SYSTEM[5,8]

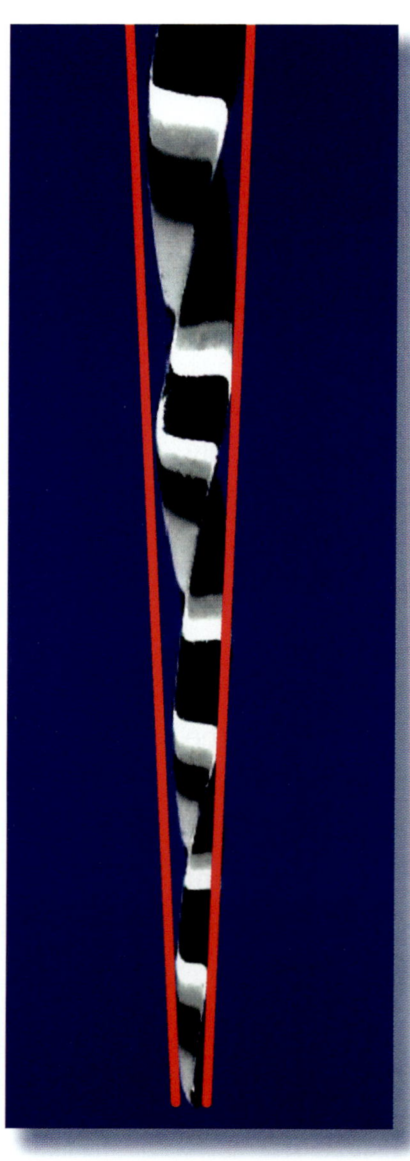

FIG. 2.X-1-1

Graphic representation of alternate contact points (ACPs) between the file and the root canal.

Blank Design

The design of the EndoSequence file is considered revolutionary because it has alternate contact points (ACPs) along the body of the instrument. This innovative design does not only keep the file centered in the root canal, but the ACPs significantly reduce the torque requirements for the file, resulting in a reduction of the resistance of the file when turned (Fig. 2.X-1-1).

There are other significant features in the design of the ACPs in combination with a precision point (inactive), which keeps the file centered in the root canal, and therefore there is no need for radial lands. This change in design, represented by the lack of radial lands, allows the instrument to be sharper and subsequently more efficient. Furthermore, the lack of radial lands also enables a decrease in metal thickness, which results in increased flexibility.

Metal Treatment

Another characteristic of this system is the electropolishing process to which the instruments are subjected, which removes many imperfections of NiTi. The presence of these imperfections can hook onto dentin and predispose the instruments to fracture. For example, electropolishing is very effective in inhibiting crack propagation in NiTi blades (Fig. 2.X-1-2). On several occasions, it has been shown that these cracks are one of the major causes of nickel-titanium instrument fractures. Moreover, superior finishing gives the sharp edge of the instrument greater cutting capacity, a lower degree of impurities and more durability. This system offers a file with more cutting efficiency, less lateral resistance and increased resistance to wear. Although electropolishing can extend the useful life of the rotary file, the EndoSequence system recommends that the instruments should be used only once.

It is worth mentioning, that up to now, the EndoSequence system is the only constant taper rotary system that is submitted to a process of improvement by electropolishing.

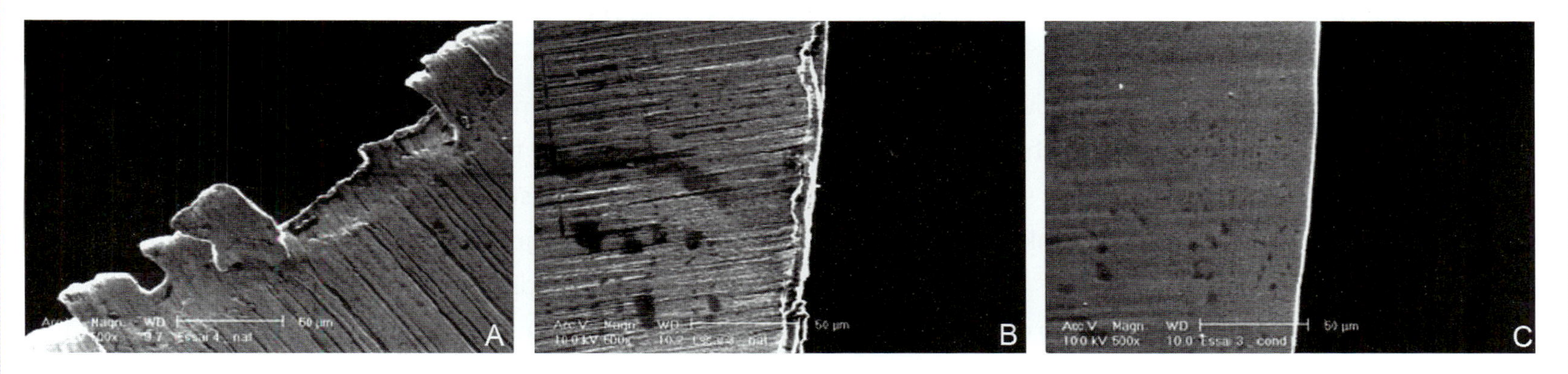

FIGS. 2.X-1-2A-C

A – Scanning electronic micrograph (SEM) of a file.
B – After conventional polishing.
C – After finishing with electro polishing[6].

Taper

The instruments of the EndoSequence system are available in both 0.04 and 0.06 mm/mm tapers. It should be emphasized that these files maintain their taper throughout the entire extent of the active part; that is, the working shank is 16 mm. This is important, because it allows the clinician to perform a precise tapered shaping in a crown/apex direction. The technique for the application of these instruments does not only contribute to a more biological treatment, it also makes filling easier, since the master cone will fit precisely in the root canal.

Point Design

This system uses a precision point, which is defined as inactive, and which becomes active precisely at the level of D-1 (Fig. 2.X-1-3). This makes the file safer (non perforating) and efficient, with the added benefit of keeping the file centered in the root canal. The precision point combined with the blank design of the ACPs is considered to be a new and revolutionary concept.

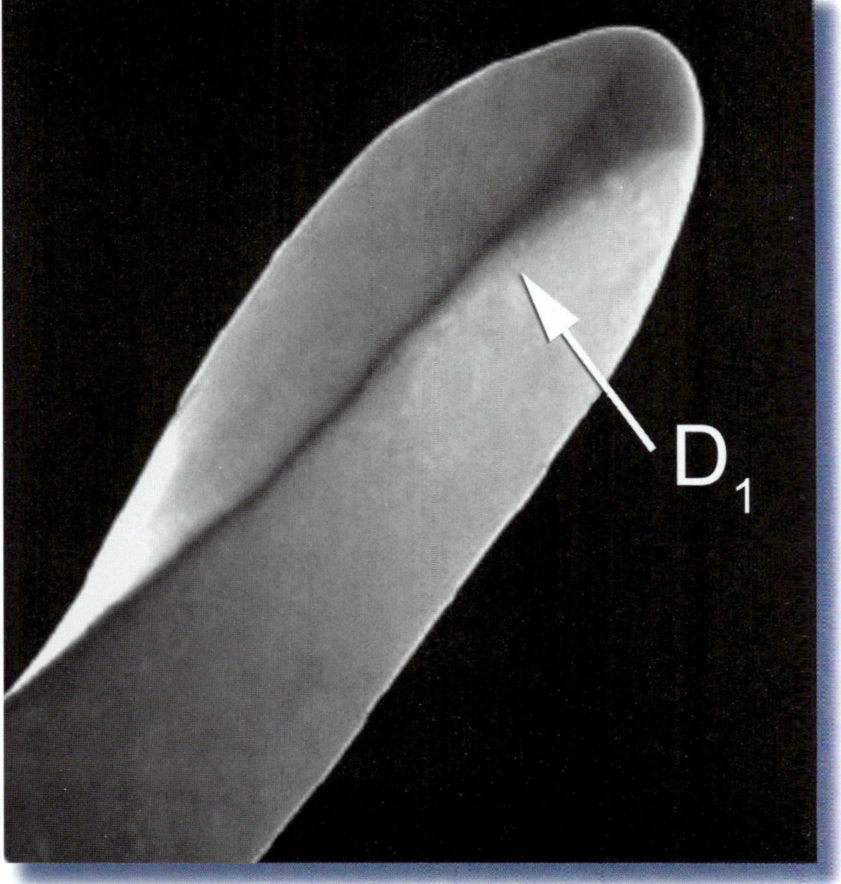

FIG. 2.X-1-3

Blank tip (SEM)[6], with cutting activity at level D_1.

Cutting Efficiency

The files of this system have been shown to have great cutting efficiency, and are comparable with the instruments of the ProTaper system only, which have similar efficiency. The ProTaper system uses a triangular blank design, while in this system it has been modified.

What gives the EndoSequence file extra cutting efficiency is the electropolishing process, which results in extremely sharp blades. Furthermore, the ACP design also allows the portion of the instrument in contact with dentin to work efficiently, because the entire shank is not totally engaged with the entire dentin surface.

Since these files cut very efficiently, the practitioner has to clean them, or change them after three pecks of the file (in and out). After a brief period (3 to 5 seconds), one can see debris between the spirals, due to the high cutting capacity of the file. Consequently, the clinician and his/her assistant need to be aware of the need to clean the files, which can only be inserted into the root canal again after being cleaned.

Another important aspect of the high cutting efficiency of these files is how fast root canal preparation is performed.

Resistance

The instruments of this system generate one of the lowest resistances to the lateral walls of the root canal when compared with instruments of other systems. This is due to its triangular design, extremely sharp edges, electropolishing and absence of radial lands. At present, this rotary file system is the one that requires the lowest torque.

Flexibility

The creation of a file that remains centered in the root canal, without radial lands, has given it greater flexibility; a very important characteristic during rotary debridement, particularly in difficult cases. Flexibility of the file is of the utmost importance in performing quality endodontic treatment.

Pitch/Helical Angles

The EndoSequence system has both variable pitch and variable helical angles (Fig. 2.X-1-4). The result is that this file has less tendency to being pulled into the direction of the foramen, which is also attributable to the design of the ACPs

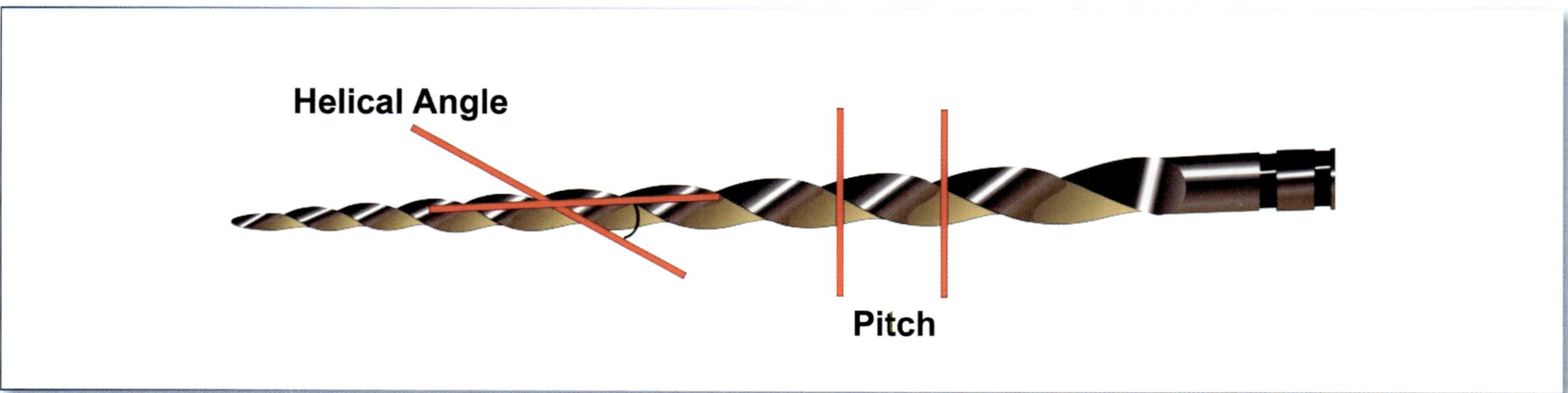

FIG. 2.X-1-4
Helical angles and variable pitches.

and absence of radial lands. The sum of all these qualities provides greater control over the file, resulting in greater operating control and debris removal.

Speed

After laboratory and clinical tests, it was determined that the best working speed for the instruments of this system is in the range of 450 to 600 rpm. It should be emphasized that the ideal speed may vary according to the operator's personal preferences and the motor that is used.

Experience has shown that portable motors constitute a challenge when using 0.06 mm/mm tapered rotary files, since the majority of them have radial lands that generate excessive lateral resistance, and as previously explained, this does not occur with the EndoSequence system.

It must also be pointed out that the files of this system have a tendency to click when they are rotating inside the root canal, which initially was a cause of alarm among users. However, this is normal for files with a triangular design. When there is a strong click; that is, when there is excessive noise, this indicates that excessive force is being exerted on the file. In this situation, it is not necessary to reduce speed, rather pressure.

Clinical experience has shown that when rotary files are used at very low speed (150-175 rpm), there is a higher percentage of fracture, because when the file is working very slowly, the clinician tends to compensate by exerting undesirable pressure on the file.

TECHNICAL SEQUENCE

The EndoSequence system files are available in both 0.04 mm/mm (15-40) and 0.06 mm/mm (15-40) tapers, and total lengths of 21, 25 and 31 mm. These files are offered as individual instruments or in procedure packages (small, medium or large) (Fig. 2.X-1-5). The system has an initial file called Expeditor (Fig. 2.X-1-6), for the purpose of determining the initial diameter of the root canal[6].

OPERATING PROCEDURE

The preparations begin after access to the coronal third has been done. For this a K file No 10 is used and introduced half way down the root canal with small amplitude up and down movements. Exploration of the coronal third is important,

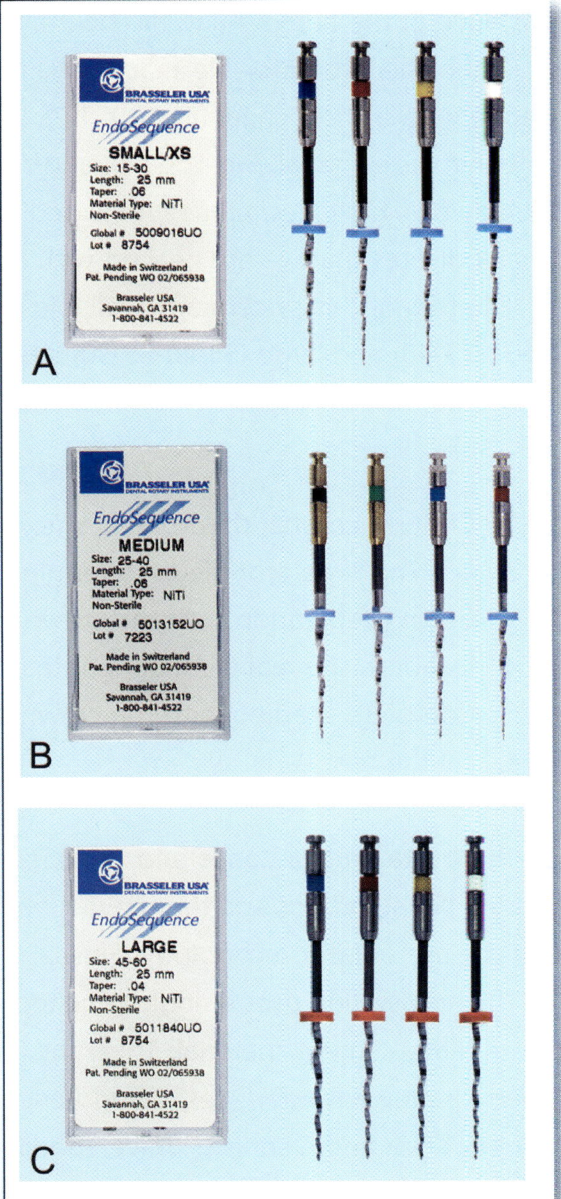

FIGS. 2.X-1-5A-C
Presentation of different sizes of the EndoSequence system.

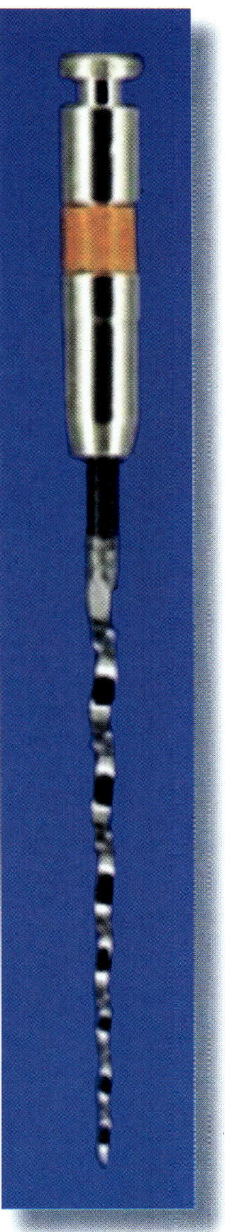

FIG. 2.X-1-6
Expeditor file.

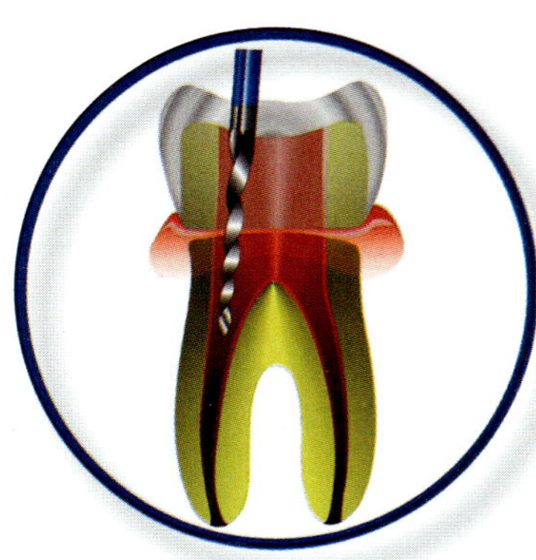

FIG. 2.X-1-7

Hand file – Expeditor file – canal length – short.

because when it is accessible, the remaining two thirds to the apex will also be accessible. When the root canal is extremely atresic, the use a type K file No 15 is recommended.

When coronal third patency has been confirmed, an Expeditor rotary file, which is different from the others as it is 27/.04 and has a 16 mm working shank and overall length of 21 mm, is introduced. The purpose of the Expeditor is to determine the approximate length of the canal and guide the length of the files to be used next.

Once inside the root canal, the Expeditor rotary file must be taken down in the canal, and as soon as it encounters resistance must be removed. At this point it has to be decided what file length will be used next. This decision is based on the information provided by the initial radiograph, resistance of the type K hand file No 10, and the depth of penetration of the Expeditor file.

When the Expeditor file reaches halfway down the root canal it is an indication that we are dealing with a short canal (Fig. 2.X-1-7). When it penetrates more than halfway into the canal it is a medium sized canal (Fig. 2.X-1-8) and the medium package should be selected starting with file No 40 (*crown-down technique*). An Expeditor file that penetrates freely to the full extent of the root canal indicates that we are dealing with a long canal (Fig. 2.X-1-9).

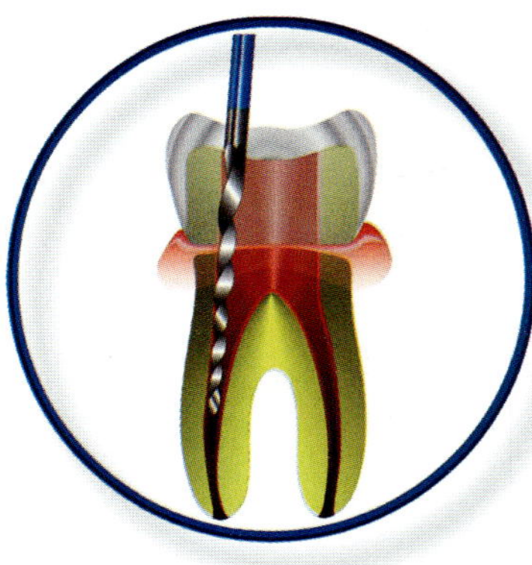

FIG. 2.X-1-8

Expeditor file. Root canal of medium length.

The files of this system are available in packages of individual or small (15-20-25-30), medium (25-30-35-40) and large (35-40-45-50) sizes.

The following sequence summarizes the basic technique of the EndoSequence system (Fig. 2.X-1-10):

1. Confirm coronal third patency (exploration);
2. Use the Expeditor file to determine the root canal length;
3. Begin preparation with the crown down debridement technique;
4. Establish the real working length after the second rotary file;
5. Complete shaping with the crown down technique;
6. Fill the root canal system.

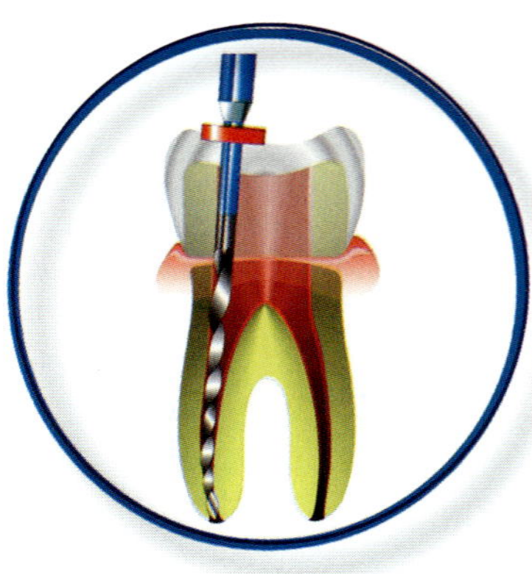

FIG. 2.X-1-9

Expeditor file. Wide root canal.

The gutta-percha cones and EndoSequence absorbent paper points are made in accordance with the ISO standards and they have high and consistent precision, because they are manufactured with the use of laser technology (Figs. 2.X-1-11A-B).

The new system uses a single cone technique with gutta-percha cones lined with glass ionomer, also a filling cement material. Thus, the manufacturer affirms to have created a true monoblock system that avoids interfaces, called Activ GP (Brasseler). Its manufacturer, in cooperation with Drs. Kenneth Koch and Dennis G Brave, modified the glass ionomer particles to prolong working time and increase bonding properties[4].

As regards working time, the Activ GP sealer is presented in the form of powder or liquid that allows the operator to manipulate it to the desired consistency, and modify the working time. This takes 12 minutes when manipulated on paper, and 20 minutes when it is done on a cold glass slide.

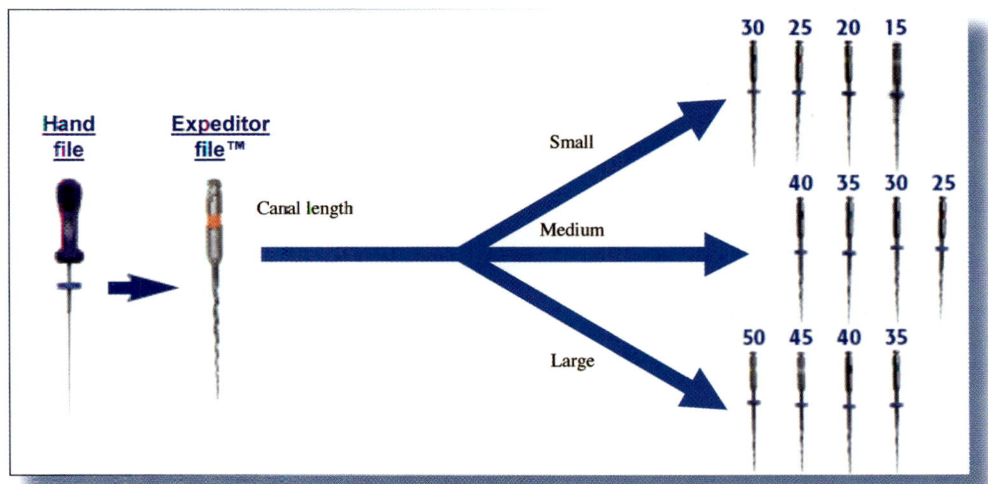

FIG. 2.X-1-10
According to the text.

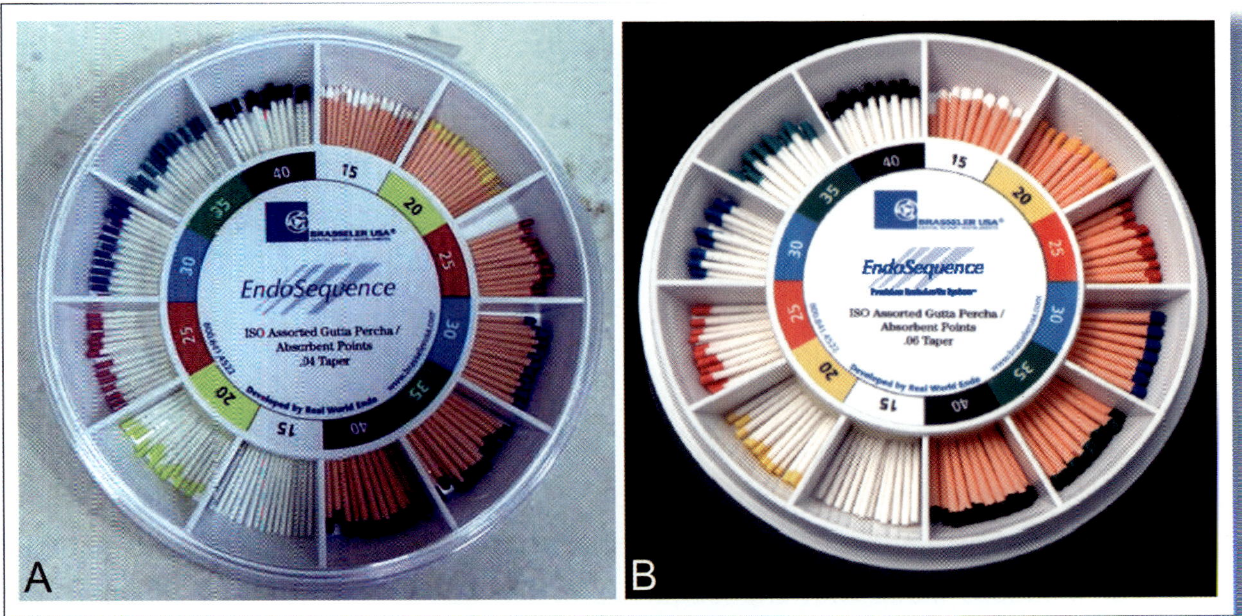

FIGS. 2.X-1-11A-B
According to the text.

With regard to bonding, to avoid interfaces, the Activ GP sealer was idealized with the purpose of bonding the glass ionomer to the cone, and uniting them with the cement. The fact that the filling cones are enveloped in glass ionomer does not affect the properties of the gutta-percha. The new cones have been lined with a 2 micrometer thick layer of ionomer. By means of scanning electronic microscopy, it has been shown that there is perfect bonding between the Activ GP cone and the sealer, and between the sealer and dentin, creating a truly impermeable monoblock system[7], as shown in Figure 2.X-1-12.

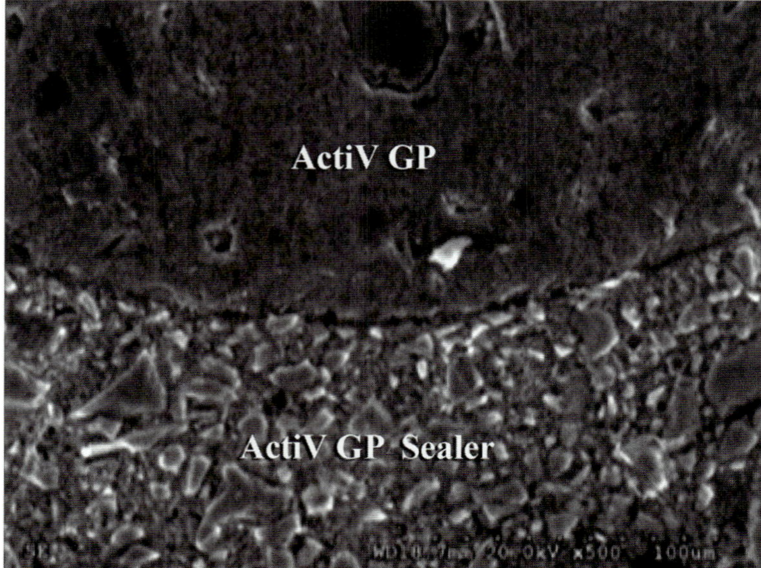

FIG. 2.X-1-12
SEM showing bond between the Activ GP cone and cement.

TECHNIQUE FOR USE OF ACTIV GP

Activ GP points are standardized and colored in accordance with the ISO standards, and are available in the traditional design and a new improved version (Activ GP Plus). The improved version has two marks to facilitate measuring the barrel-shaped end which, when used with a transportation instrument (included in the introductory package), facilitates cone placement in the root canal. (Figs. 2.X-1-13A-B).

It is important to mention that during root canal system preparation with this system, a sodium hypochlorite solution or any other irrigation solution can be used.

The Activ GP system allows a monoblock filling with the single cone technique, but it requires synchronization between the file and the master cone that is selected. The measurements of the Activ GP points are calibrated, constant and precise and they have laser quality control, being indicated for preparations made with EndoSequence rotary system files with 0.04 mm/mm and 0.6 mm/mm tapers. Because the master cone corresponds to the preparation, it minimizes the quantity of sealer that is required and therefore diminishes polymerization shrinkage to which it is subjected[12].

The technique associated with the Activ GP system is very simple. Once root canal preparation has been completed, the Activ GP cone adjustment is radiographically determined. The cone is then removed and a hand file, which matches with the final apical size, is chosen and used to insert the sealer into the root canal.

The cement is mixed in a powder/liquid ratio of a half measure of powder to three drops of liquid and mixed on a cold glass slab. After mixing the cement with a spatula and when a thinner consistency is needed, another drop of liquid may be added. The mixing technique is very similar to that of zinc phosphate cement (Figs. 2.X-1-14A-C).

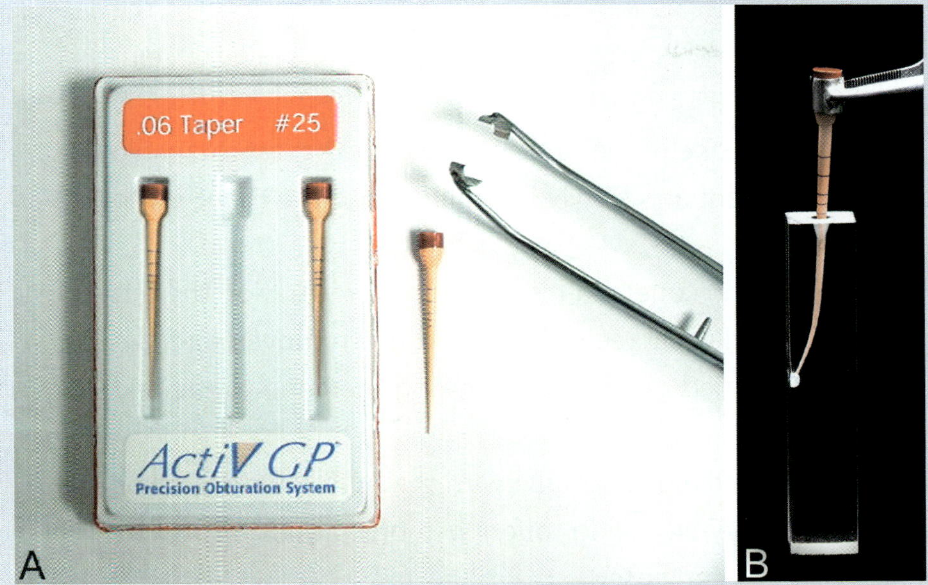

FIGS. 2.X-1-13A-B
According to the text.

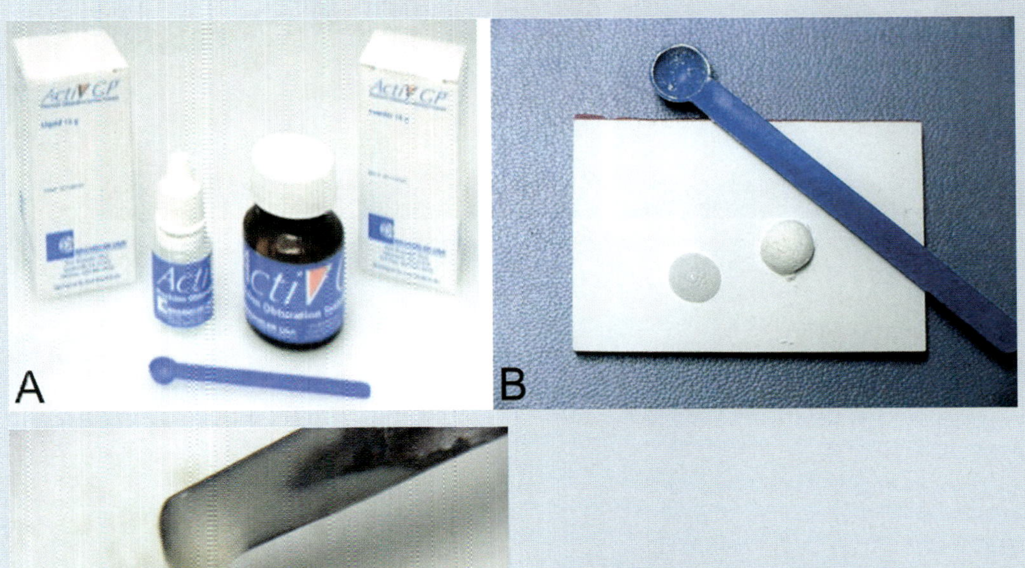

FIGS. 2.X-1-14A-C
According to the text.

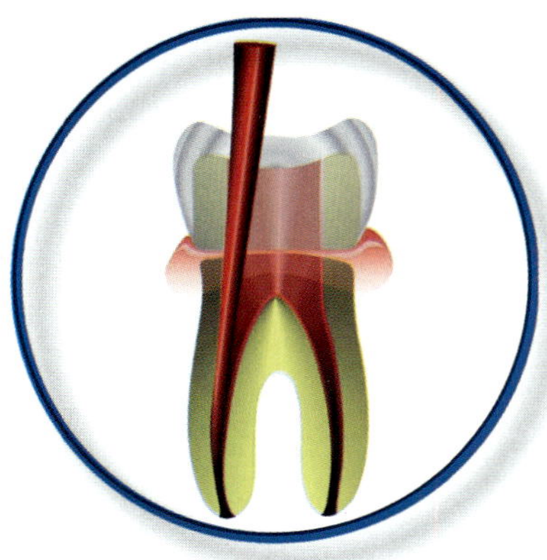

FIG. 2.X-1-15
According to the text.

Once the cement has been mixed it must be introduced into the root canal with the selected hand file with rotary movements. As in all filling techniques, the sealer cement must be placed short of the apical foramen (Fig. 2.X-1-15).

After placing the cement, the Activ GP cone of the same diameter as the last rotary file that was used has to be covered with cement and slowly introduced into the canal, up to the real working length.

Due to the tight adjustment between the cone and the root canal preparation there is the potential for extravasation into the periapical region if up and down movements are made during filling. Filling must be performed gently, slowly taking the cone to the real working length (Figs. 2.X-1-16A-C)

In conclusion, it can be stated that the filling technique with the Activ GP system has the advantage of establishing an impermeable filling, offering more promising results when compared to techniques that are currently used.

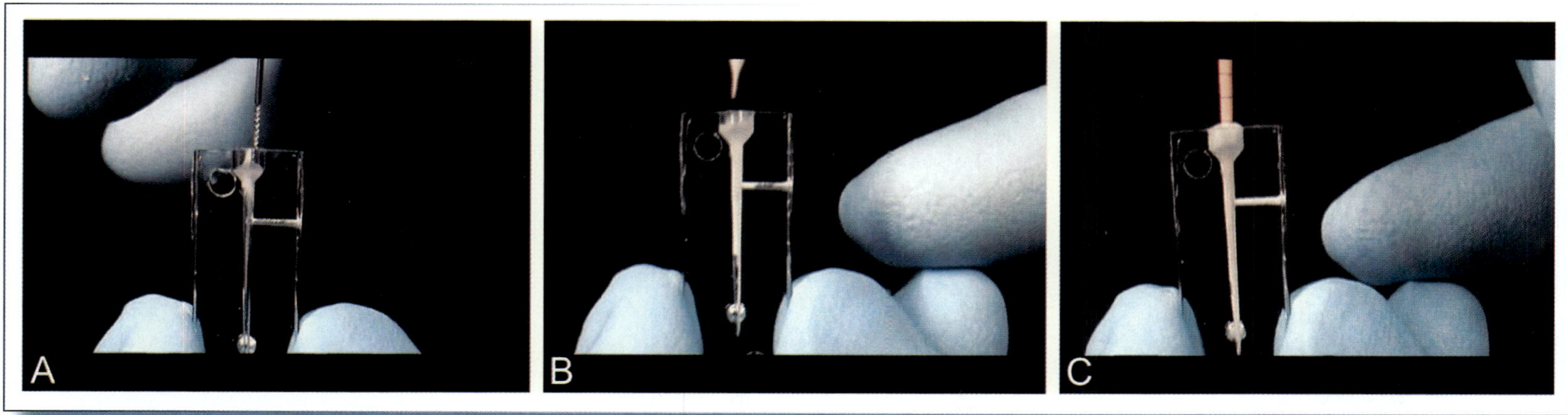

FIGS. 2.X-1-16A-C
According to the text.

CLINICAL CASES USING THE ENDOSEQUENCE SYSTEM AND ROOT CANAL FILLING WITH THE ACTIV GP SYSTEM

Courtesy of Dr. Carlos Tinajero M. (Figs. 2.X-1-17A-B).

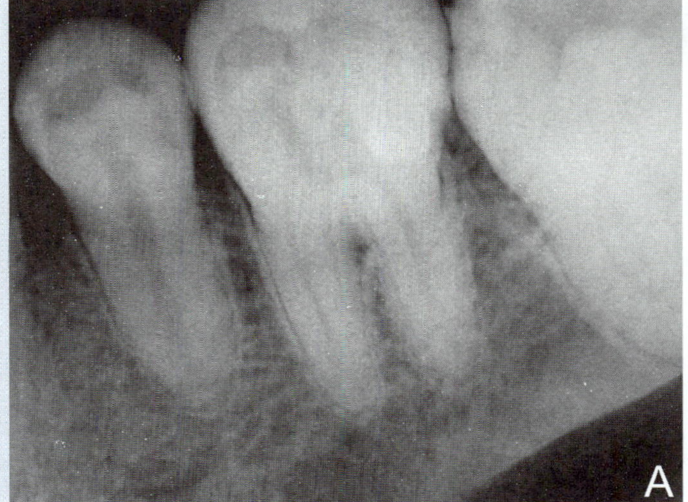

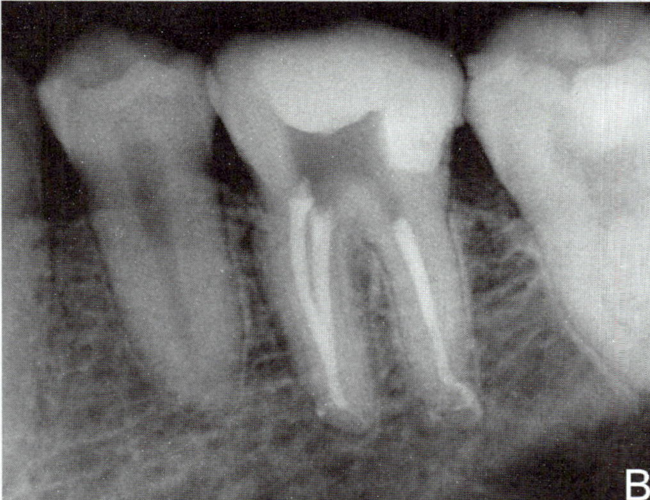

FIGS. 2.X-1-17A-B

Courtesy of Dr. Ali Nasseh (Figs. 2.X-1-18A-B).

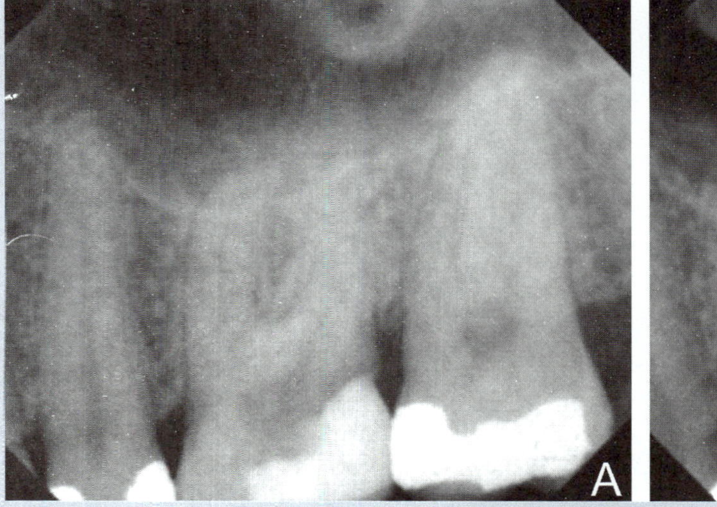

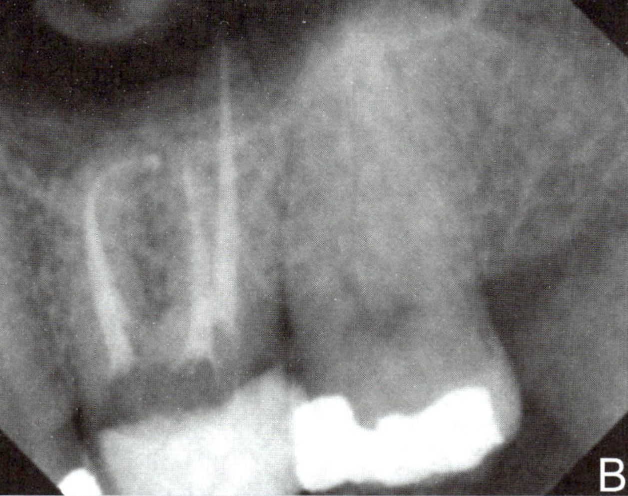

FIGS. 2.X-1-18A-B

Courtesy of Dr. Arianna Gomez (Figs. 2.X-1-19A-C

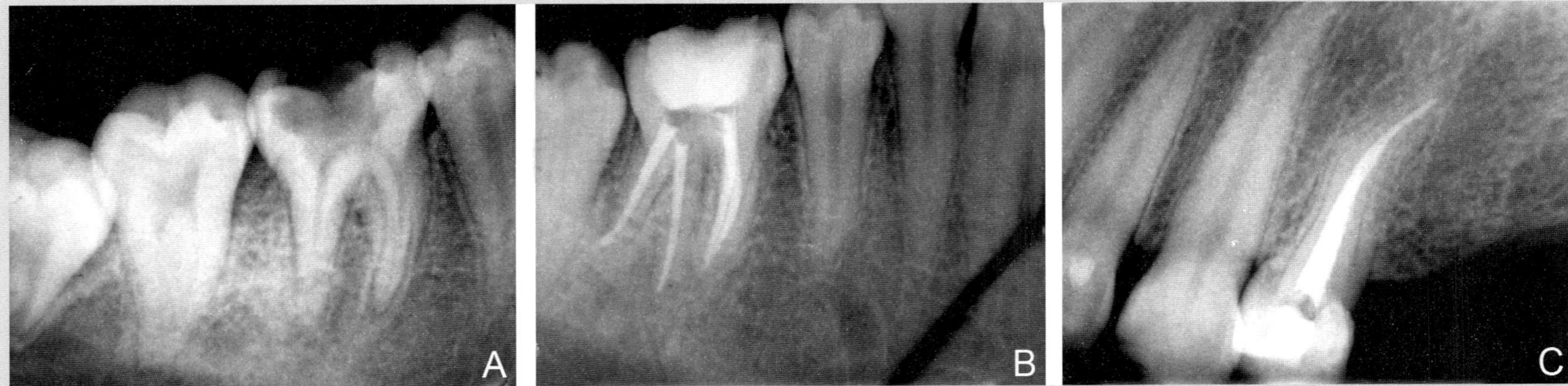

FIGS. 2.X-1-19A-C

References

1. Diemer F, Caldas P. Effect of pitch length on the behavior of rotary triple helix root canal instruments. J Endod, v.30, n.10, 2004.
2. Kim S. Modern endodontic practice instruments and techniques. Dent Clin N Am, v.48, p.1-9, 2004.
3. Koch AK. Real World Endo Sequence File. Dent Clin N Am, v.48, p.159-182, 2004
4. Koch K, Brave D. Activ GP Precision Obturation System. (Por publicarse)
5. Koch K, Brave D. Endodontic synchronicity. Comped Contin Educ Dent, v.26, n.3, p.220-224, 2005.
6. Koch K, Brave D. The EndoSequence file: a guide to clinical use. Compend. Contin. Educ. Dent., v.25. n.10A, p.811-813, Oct. 2004.
7. Koch K, Brave D. The future of endodontics. Dent Today, v.27, n.4, p.80-84, 2008.
8. Kurtzman MG. Simplifying endodontics with EndoSequence rotary instrumentation. CDA Journal, v.35, n.9, 2007.
9. Leonardo MR, Leonardo RT. Sistemas Rotatorios en Endodoncia. São Paulo: Ed. Artes Médicas, 2002.
10. Leonardo MR, Leonardo RT. Tratamiento de Conductos Radiculares. v.2, São Paulo: Ed. Artes Médicas, 2005.
11. Walsch H. The hybrid concept of nickel-titanium rotary instrumentation. Dent Clin N Am, v.48, p.183-202, 2004.
12. www.brasselerusa.com
13. Yang GB, Zhou XD, Zhang H, Wu HK. Shaping ability of progressive versus constant taper instruments in simulated root canals. Int Endod J, v.39, n.10, p.791-799, 2006.

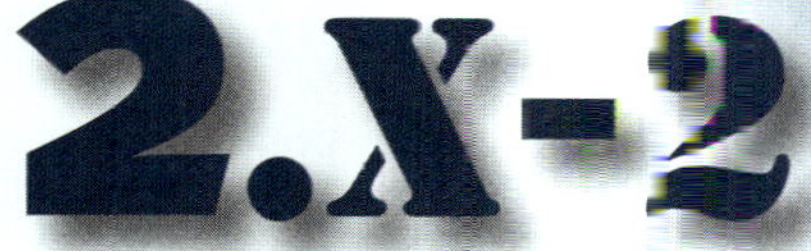

ProTaper Universal System

Combining rotary and manual instrumentation
in root canal preparation.
Filling with gutta-percha cones with different tapers –
simplicity, speed and safety

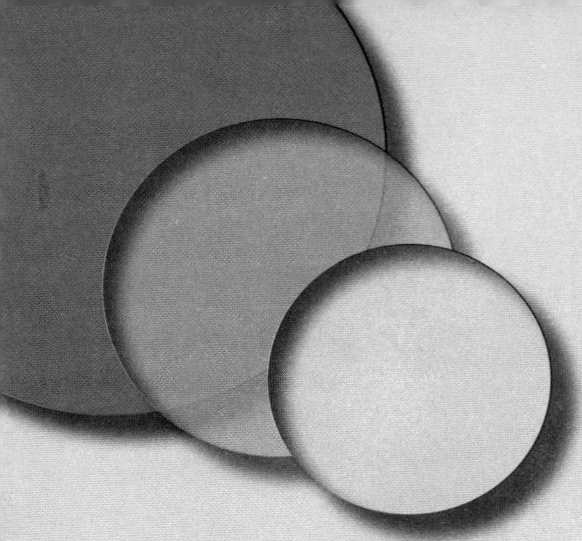

Idomeo Bonetti Filho

Protaper

Universal (Dentsply/Maillefer – Ballaigues – Switzerland) is a new rotary endodontic system and is offered in three versions: Protaper Treatment, Protaper Filling and Protaper Retreatment[3].

Protaper treatment is composed of 8 nickel titanium instruments with variable tapers (Fig. 2.X-2-1), offered for rotary (requiring an electric or computerized motor), or manual instrumentation (Figs. 2.X-2-2 and 2.X-2-3).

Three rotary and/or manual instruments are offered, designated *shaping files,* indicated for modeling the root canal, denominated **SX, S1 and S2** (Fig. 2.X-2-4). These instruments are characterized by having an active part with variable tapering (Eiffel Tower-shaped); the final portion of the active part having a smaller, and the base a larger diameter, and are indicated for widening the cervical and middle parts of root canals[2] (Fig. 2.X-2-5).

The instrument **SX**, which the manufacturer considers an accessory, has a total length of 19 mm, with an active part of 14 mm, an initial taper of 0.035 mm/mm, tip diameter (D0) of 0.19 mm and final diameter at the base of the active part (D14) of 1.10 mm. It does not have a colored identification ring on its metal shaft (handle). It is used after exploring (patency) the root canal with a manual K type file, to widen the canal entrance, rectifying it and allowing better direct access. It must be used with brush-stroke movements, applying light force against the root canal walls[2] (Fig. 2.X-2-4).

Instruments **S1** have a total length of 21, 25 and 31 mm, with an active part of 14 mm and active part tip diameter (D0) of 0.18 mm, with an initial taper of 0.02 mm/mm, reaching D14 with a diameter of approximately 1.10 mm. It has a purple identification ring on its metal shank (rotary instruments) and purple handle (manual instruments)[2] (Fig. 2.X-2-4).

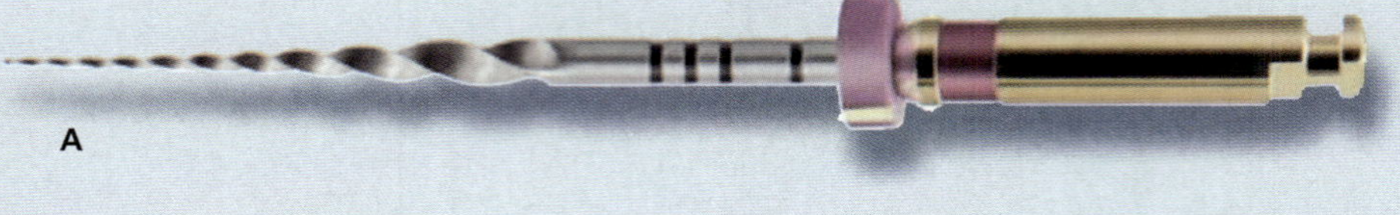

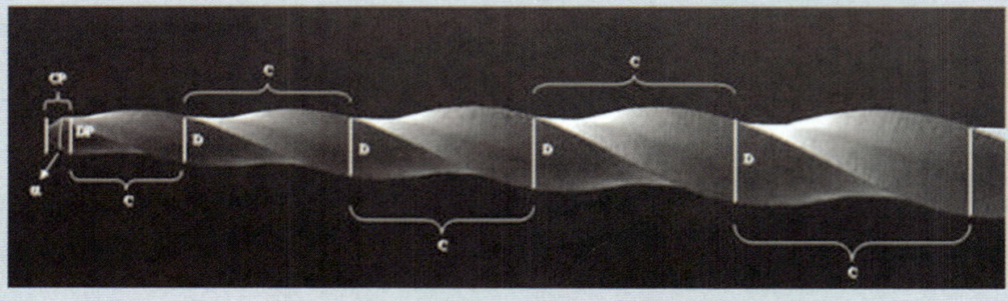

2.X-2-1 B

FIGS. 2.X-2-1A-B

A – Active part of instrument S1, with different tapers.

B – Scanning electron micrograph showing the tip angle (α); tip length (CP); tip diameter (DP); length of each pitch along the cutting shaft (C) and diameters of the instrument at every millimeter of the active part (D). (Photo provided by Dr. Alexandre Câmara.)

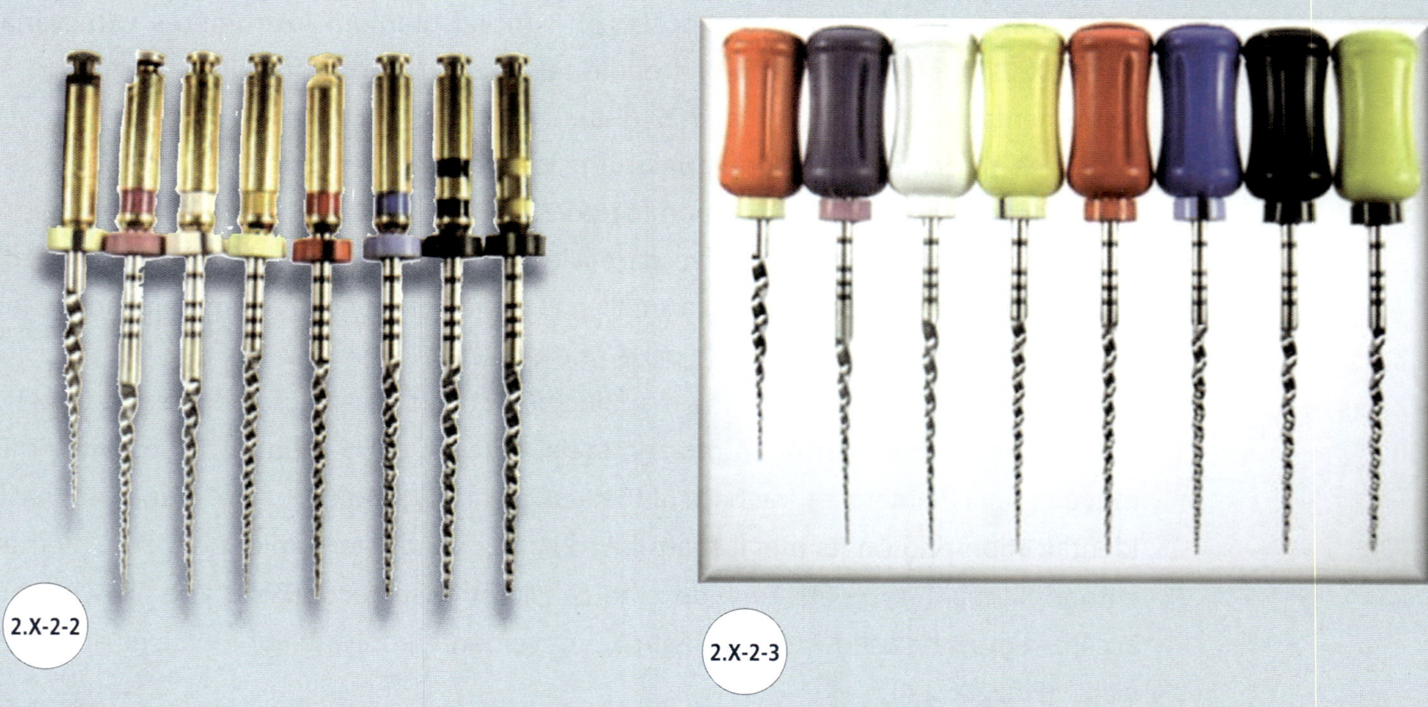

2.X-2-2

2.X-2-3

FIGS. 2.X-2-2 AND 2.X-2-3

Sequence of rotary and manual instruments – SX, S1, S2, F1, F2, F3, F4 and F5.

Instruments **S2** have a total length of 21, 25 and 31 mm, with an active part of 14 mm and active part tip diameter (D0) of 0.20 mm, with an initial taper of 0.04 mm/mm, reaching D14 with a diameter of approximately 1.10 mm. It has a white identification ring on its metal shank (rotary instruments) and white handle (manual instruments) [2] (Fig. 2.X-2-4).

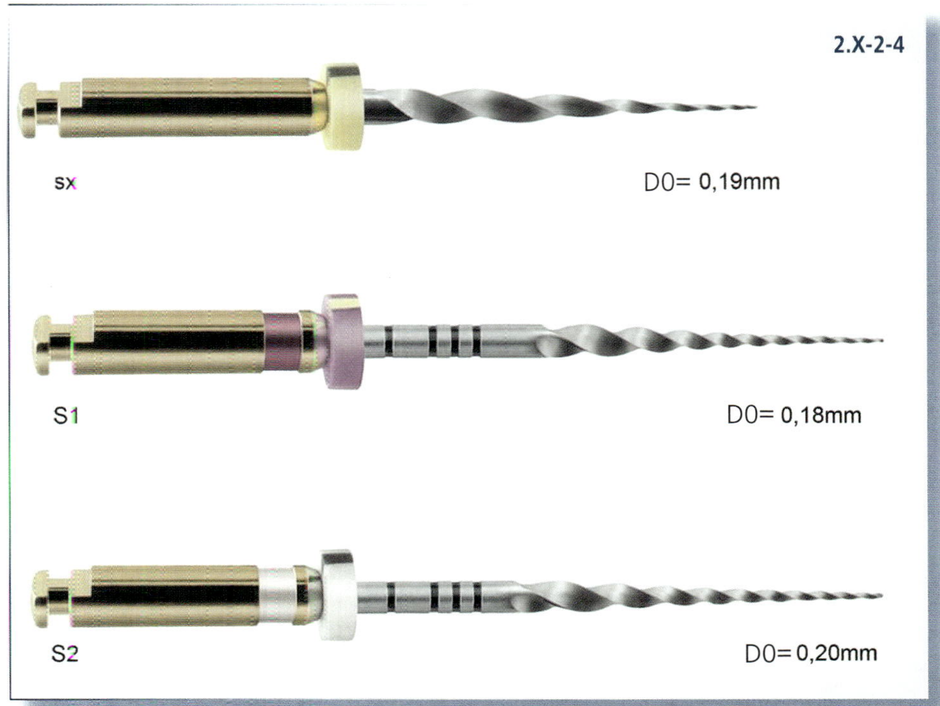

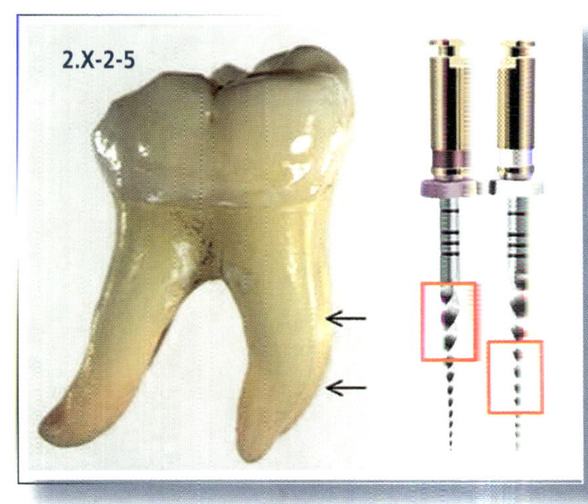

FIG. 2.X-2-4

Rotary instruments – shaping files SX, S1 and S2 with D0 of 0.19 mm, 0.18 mm and 0.20 mm respectively. (Courtesy of Dentsply/Maillefer, Baillagues, Switzerland.)

FIG. 2.X-2-5

Instruments S1 and S2, with their active areas demarcated, inside the root canal (arrows).

Rotary or manual finishing files comprise five instruments, denominated **F1, F2, F3, F4 and F5** (Fig. 2.X-2-6) and are characterized by having an active part with variable tapering that decreases, specifically to allow them to cut more in the apical part of the root canal[2].

Finishing instrument **F1**, with a yellow identification ring on its metal shank (rotary instruments) and yellow handle (manual instruments), has a tip diameter (D0) of 0.20 mm, with a 0.07 mm/mm taper in the apical 3 mm (Fig. 2.X-2-6).

Finishing instrument **F2**, with a red identification ring on its metal shank (rotary instruments) and red handle (manual instruments), has a tip diameter (D0) of 0.25 mm, with a 0.08 mm/mm taper in the apical 3 mm (Fig. 2.X-2-6).

Finishing instrument **F3**, with a blue identification ring on its metal shank (rotary instruments) and blue handle (manual instruments), has a tip diameter (D0) of 0.30 mm, with a 0.09 mm/mm taper in the apical 3 mm (Fig. 2.X-2-6).

Finishing instrument **F4**, with a metal fixation shaft that has two black identification rings (rotary instruments) and black handle (manual instruments), has a tip diameter (D0) of 0.40 mm, with a 0.06 mm/mm taper in the apical 3 mm (Fig. 2.X-2-6).

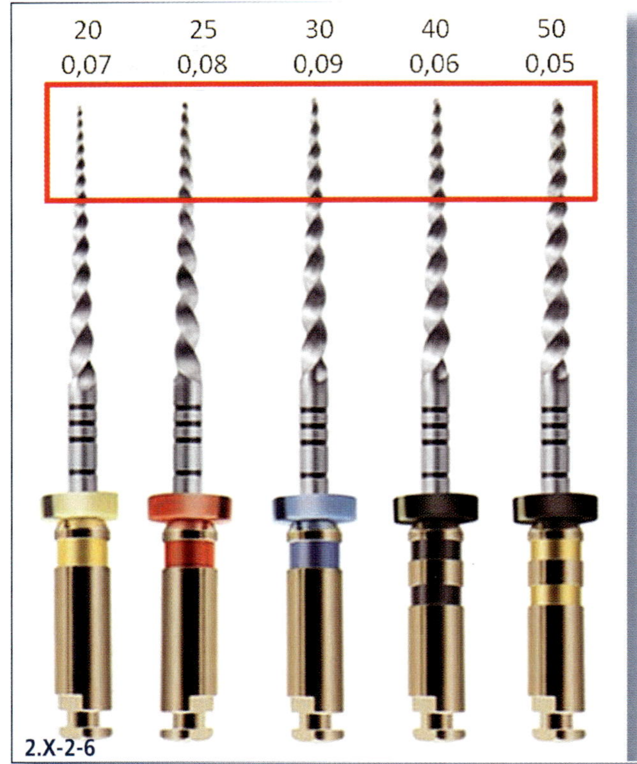

Finishing instrument **F5**, with a metal fixation shaft that has two yellow identification rings (rotary instruments) and yellow handle (manual instruments), has a tip diameter (D0) of 0.50 mm, with a 0.05 mm/mm taper in the apical 3 mm (Fig. 2.X-2-6).

The shaping files (S) have an active part (Eiffel Tower-shaped), enabling good widening of the cervical and middle parts of the root canal with a flexible apical extremity. After this has been used, the finishing file (F) (obelisk-shaped), will act more in the apical part, thus diminishing the effect on the surface that each instrument of this group will have on the coronal walls of the root canal, as well as diminishing the locking action (variable taper instrumentation)[2] (Fig. 2.X-2-7).

All the instruments of this system have cutting blades, increasing the cutting efficiency without *radial lands, as occurs with Profile instruments* (Fig. 2.X-2-8).

Instruments **S1, S2, F1 and F2** have a convex triangular cross section, with the purpose of increasing fracture resistance, and instruments **F3, F4 and F5**

FIG. 2.X-2-6

Finishing files (F) F1, F2, and F3 with colored identification rings, yellow, red and blue, respectively, tip diameters of 0.20 mm, 0.25 mm and 0.30 mm and 0.07 mm/mm, 0.08 mm/mm and 0.09 mm/mm tapers in the apical 3 mm, respectively, and F4 and F5, with two colored identification rings, black and yellow, with tip diameter of 0.40 mm and 0.50 mm and with 0.06 mm/mm and 0.05 mm/mm taper in the apical 3 mm, respectively. (Courtesy of Dentsply/Maillefer, Baillagues, Switzerland.)

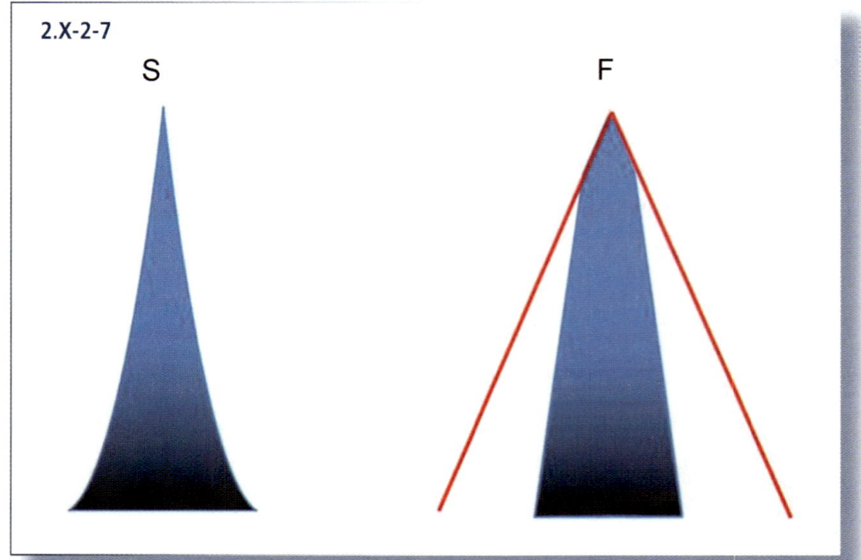

FIG. 2.X-2-7

Image representative of Eiffel Tower-shaped instruments (S), and obelisk-shaped finishing instruments (F). (Courtesy of Dentsply/Maillefer, Baillagues, Switzerland.)

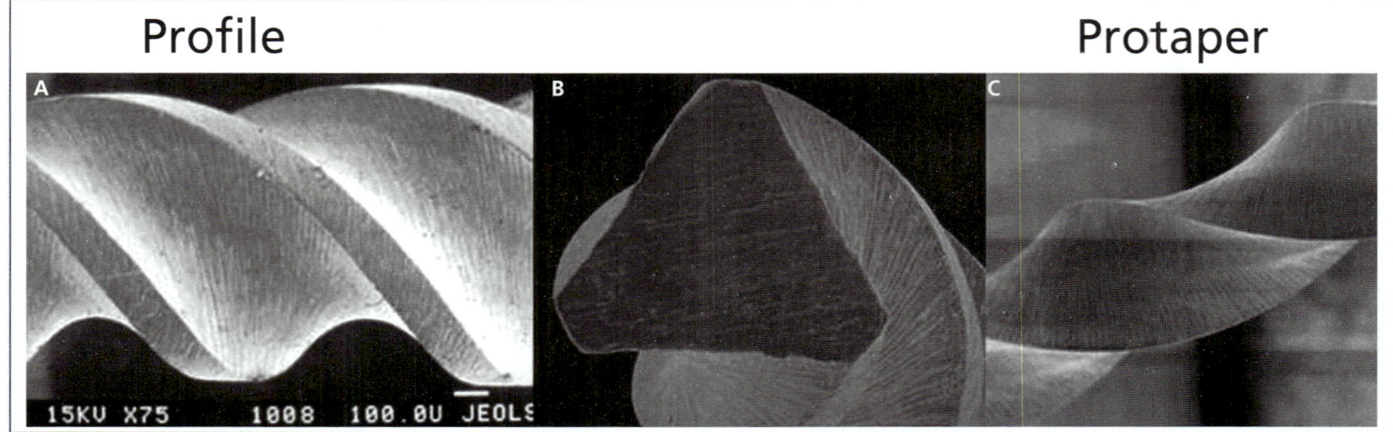

FIG. 2.X-2-8

Scanning electron micrographs:
A – Profile Instrument with cutting area presenting radial lands.
B – Cross-section of the same instrument.
C – Protaper Instrument with cutting blades without radial lands. (Courtesy of Dentsply/Maillefer, Baillagues, Switzerland.)

have a concavity in the triangular cross section, to increase flexibility[2] (Fig. 2.X-2-9)

The Protaper instruments have a non-cutting tip, which serves as a guide inside the root canal, diminishing zip or step formation[2] (Fig. 2.X-2-10).

Protaper Filling consists of gutta-percha cones with variable taper similar to the finishing files F1, F2, F3, F4 and F5 (Fig. 2.X-2-11). These gutta-percha cones are used to fill the root canal, with the single or heated technique, according to the system chosen, or by the Thermafil[2] system, in a one-step operation (Fig. 2.X-2-12).

There are sterile absorbing paper points for drying the root canal, with the same diameters and tapers as the instruments (Fig. 2.X-2-13).

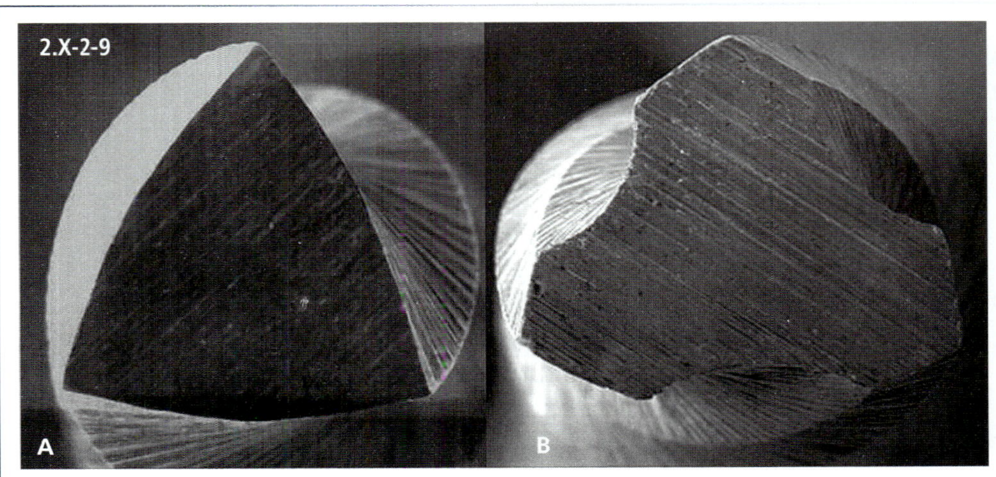

2.X-2-10

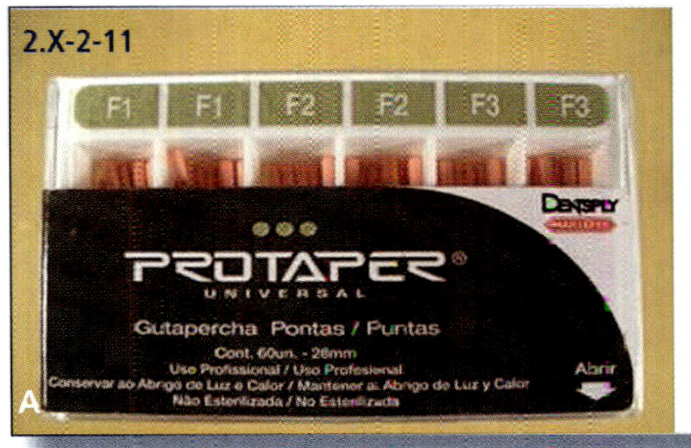

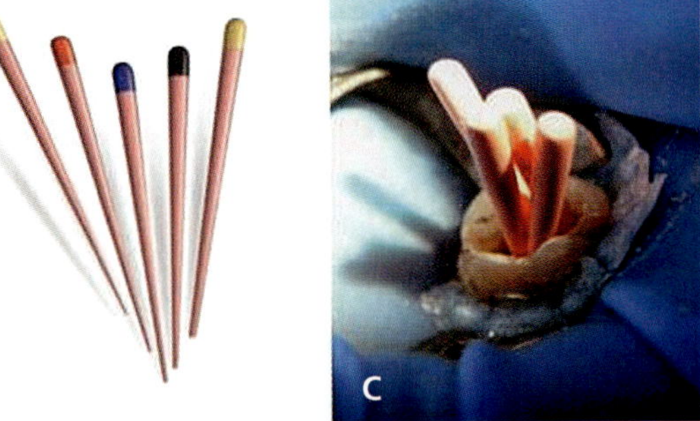

C

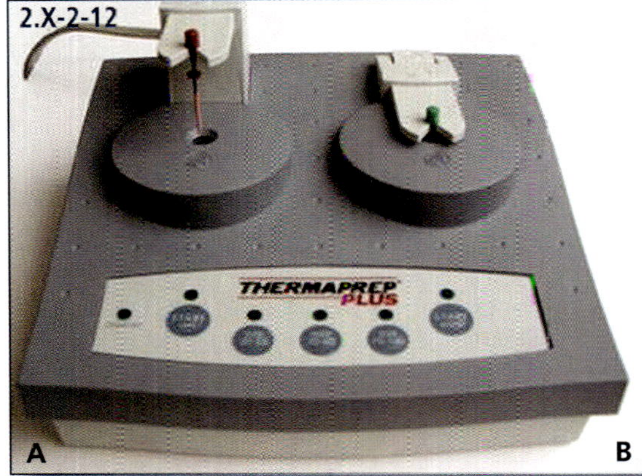

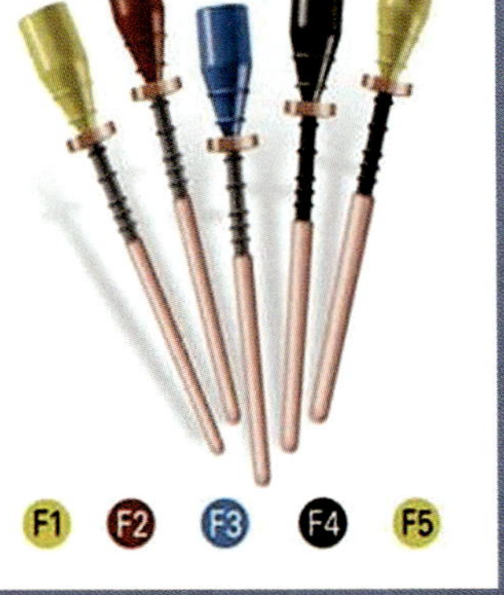

FIG. 2.X-2-9

Scanning electron micrograph of Universal Protaper instrument:
A – Instruments S1, S2, F1 and F2 with triangular convex cross-section.
B – Instruments F3, F4 and F5 with triangular conical cross-section. (Courtesy of Dentsply/Maillefer, Baillagues, Switzerland.)

FIG. 2.X-2-10

Scanning electron micrograph of non-cutting tip of Protaper instrument. (Courtesy of Dentsply/Maillefer, Baillagues, Switzerland.)

FIGS. 2.X-2-11A-C

A – Box with gutta-percha cones F1, F2 and F3.
B – Tapered gutta-percha cones; shown with colors according to the ISO.
C – Tapered gutta-percha cones placed inside a root canal.

FIGS. 2.X-2-12A-B

A – Thermaprep Plus appliance for heating and plasticizing the carriers.
B – Carriers with colors corresponding to instruments F1, F2, F3, F4 and F5. (Courtesy of Dentsply/Maillefer, Baillagues, Switzerland.)

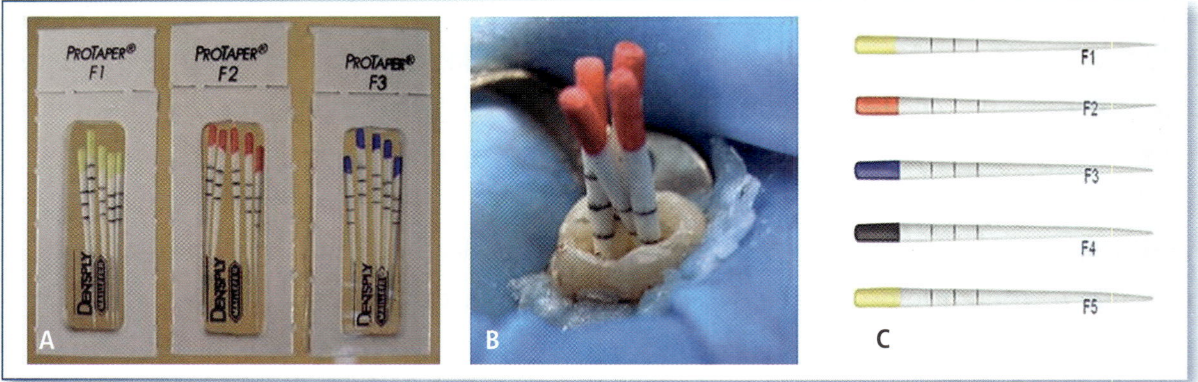

FIGS. 2.X-2-13A-C

A – Sterile paper points with the same diameters and tapers as the instruments.
B – Clinical aspect of paper points drying the root canal.
C – Paper points with colors corresponding to the standardized color code of the instruments (ISO).

Protaper Retreatment comprises three instruments denominated **D1, D2 and D3**[2] (Fig. 2.X-2-14).

Instrument **D1** has an 11 mm metal fixation shank, with a white identification ring (rotary Instruments) and white handle (manual instruments) and an active part measuring 16 mm, with a tip diameter of 0.30 mm and 0.09 mm/mm continuous taper, and is indicated for opening the cervical portion of the root canal and removing the filling material from it. This instrument is the only one that has an active cutting tip to facilitate its initial penetration into the filling material (Fig. 2.X-2-15).

Instrument **D2** has an 11 mm metal fixation shank, with two white identification rings (rotary Instruments) and white handle (manual instruments), and an active part measuring 18 mm, with a tip diameter of 0.25 mm and a 0.08 mm/mm continuous taper. It is used to remove the deeper situated filling material in the middle portion of the root canal, and does not have an active tip (Fig. 2.X-2-14).

Instrument **D3** has an 11 mm metal fixation shank, with three white identification rings (rotary Instruments) and white handle (manual instruments), and an active part measuring 22 mm, with a tip diameter of 0.20 mm and a 0.07 mm/mm continuous taper. It is used to remove the deeper situated filling material, beyond the point to which instrument D2 penetrated, in the most apical portion of the root canal, and does not have an active tip (Fig. 2.X-2-14).

The (D) instruments have decreasing tip diameters and tapers, D1=30/09, D2=25/08 and D3=20/07 (Fig. 2.X-2-14). This makes the D1 instrument more resistant and more tapered, as it begins to remove the filling material, opening space for the following instruments (D2 and D3) to penetrate more easily into the root canal, acting more in apical portions, safely and efficiently[2] diminishing the area of action, as shown in Fig. 2.X-2-16.

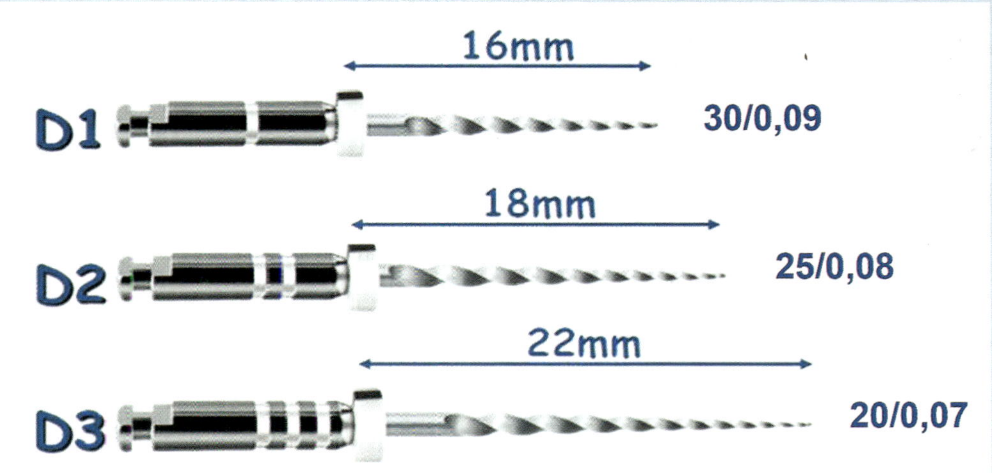

FIG. 2.X-2-14

Protaper instruments for re-treatment, with measurements, different active tip diameters and tapers. (Courtesy of Dentsply/Maillefer, Baillagues, Switzerland.)

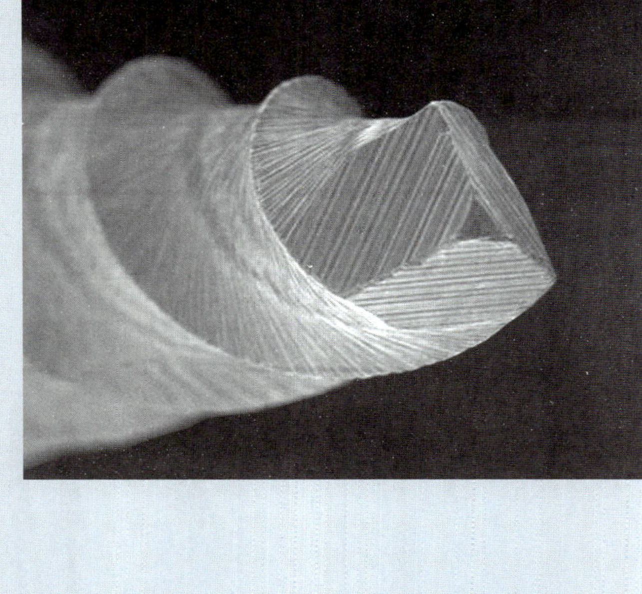

FIG. 2.X-2-15

Scanning electron micrograph of active tip of instrument D1. (Courtesy of Dentsply/Maillefer, Baillagues, Switzerland.)

FIGS. 2.X-2-16A-B

A – Diagrammatic drawing representing action of instruments D1 with larger diameter and taper.

B – Diagrammatic drawing representing action of instruments D2 and D3 with smaller diameters, and being longer, penetrating deeper into the root canal and acting on small areas inside the root canal. (Courtesy of Dentsply/Maillefer, Baillagues, Switzerland.)

INITIAL CONSIDERATIONS FOR ROOT CANAL INSTRUMENTATION WITH THE PROTAPER UNIVERSAL SYSTEM

All root canals must always be explored (patency), initially with manual Type K files, up to Nº 20, in order to establish a pathway that transmits the real conditions of the root canal (wide, atresic, etc) to the practitioner, avoiding very aggressive locking with the use of rotary instruments. Manual files must initially penetrate into the cervical and middle portions of the root canal, without apical pressure, respecting their anatomic shape, without ever exceeding the temporary working length (TWL). Once a pathway has been established, one must use instrument S1 (rotary instruments), but without exceeding the depth reached by the type K file No.20, thus guaranteeing cervical widening without the tip becoming locked in the root canal (Fig. 2.X-2-17). Knowing that the tip diameter of the active part (D0) of instrument S1 is approximately 0.18 mm and that the canal has been instrumented up to type K file No. 20, we must remember that this instrument (S1) will act only in the cervical region, widening it, because of its tapered shape.

To use the rotary instruments, it is necessary to choose equipment to drive them. One can use a counter-angle reducer with torque control coupled directly to the micromotor of the dental equipment (Fig. 2.X-2-18) or preferably a special endodontic electric motor with speed and torque control, as well as programming (Fig. 2.X-2-19).

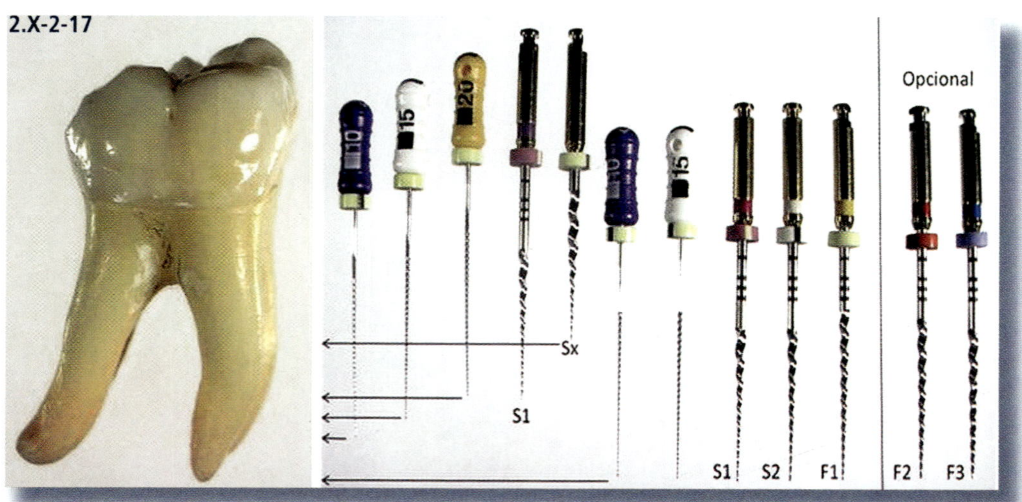

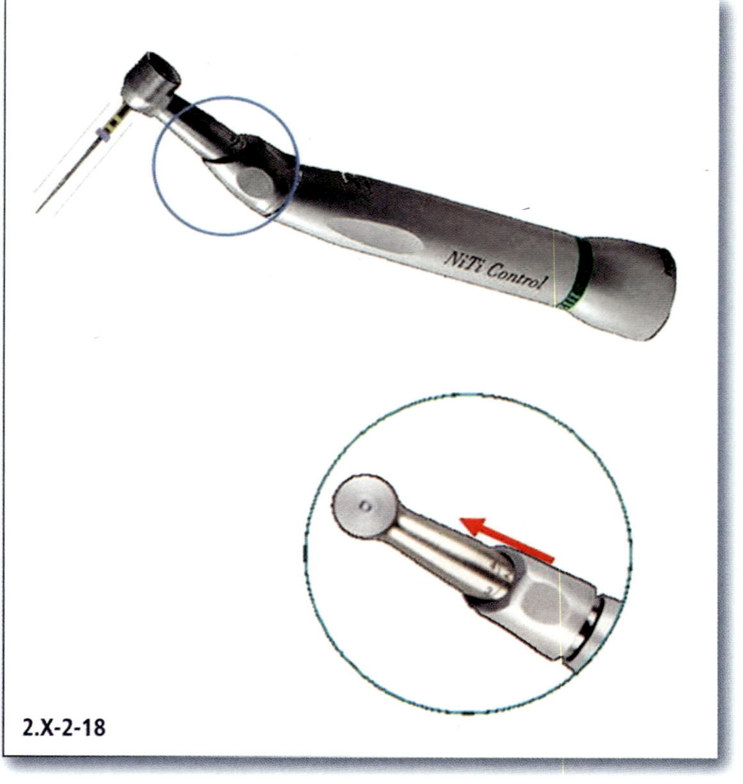

FIG. 2.X-2-17

Diagrammatic rotary instrumentation sequence with the penetration limits of both the manual files and rotary instruments.

FIG. 2.X-2-18

Contra angle reducer with torque control. (Courtesy of Dentsply/Maillefer, Baillagues, Switzerland.)

When beginning to use rotary instrumentation, doubts arise about the speed and torque to use for the different instruments and root canal regions.

One of the greatest concerns with the use of rotary systems is instrument fracture inside the root canal. To avoid or reduce the possibility of this occurrence, one can use higher speed and torque for the instruments that will be used in the cervical and middle thirds, and a lower speed and torque for instruments that will work in the apical thirds. Generally speaking, one can work with a speed of 250 to 300 rpm and a torque of 2-3 N.cm in the cervical and middle thirds, and 1 N.cm in the apical third of the root canal. The X-Smart appliance comes with a card indicating torques with constant speed, and different torques for the different instruments (Fig. 2.X-2-19).

It is very important for the practitioner to pay careful attention – if the instrument is locking frequently, he/she should take the actions indicated **in the following order**:

Pass the initial K type files again, to make sure that the initial pathway was well made.

Use the manual rotary instruments to increase the sense of touch of the root canal.

Increase the torque and speed of the electric motor, to avoid accidents.

The practitioner could use a sequence of rotary instrumentation or manual instrumentation, as shown in Figs. 2.X-2-17 and 2.X-2-20.

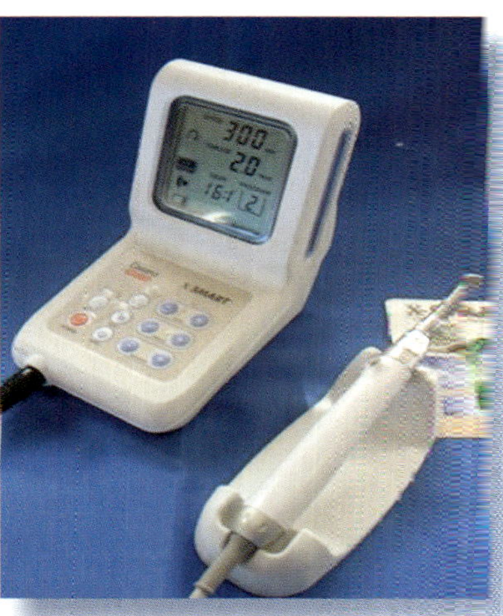

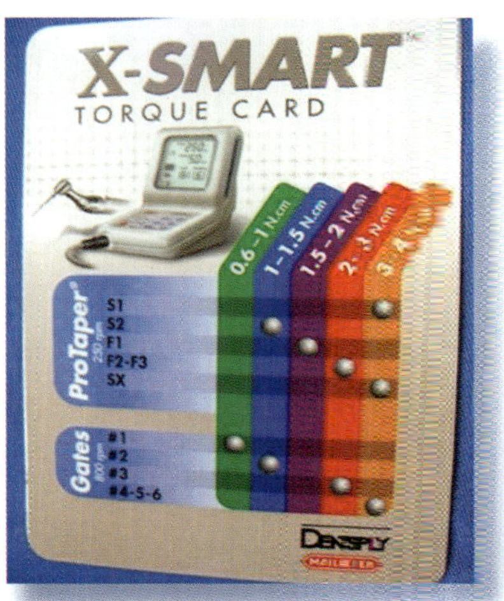

FIG. 2.X-2-19

S-Smart (Dentsply/Maillefer, Baillagues, Switzerland) and torque card.

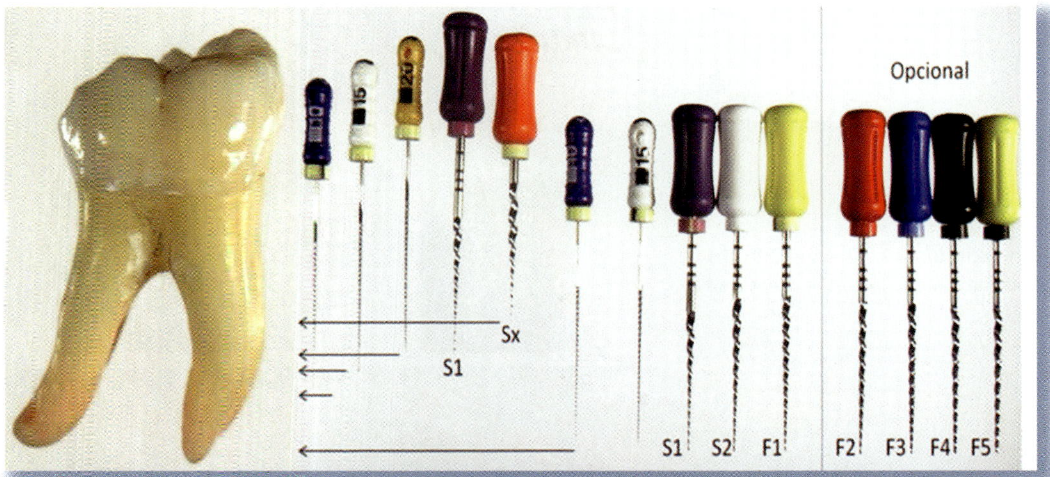

FIG. 2.X-2-20

Diagrammatic sequence of rotary instruments combined with manual instrumentation, indicating the penetration limit of the stainless steel files and Protaper treatment instruments.

Hybridization of the manual and rotary instrumentation sequences will give the practitioner more confidence and assurance to perform perfect instrumentation of the root canal (Fig.2.X-2-26).

A microscopic evaluation was done of the apical preparation of curved root canals with rotary, manual, and oscillatory instrumentation, by the action of the Protaper Universal system. This demonstrated the efficiency and safety of manual rotary instrumentation, followed by rotary when compared to oscillatory instrumentation, with regard to the area instrumented and the displacement of the center of the root canal (Figs. 2.X-2-21, 2.X-2-22 and 2.X-2-23).[1]

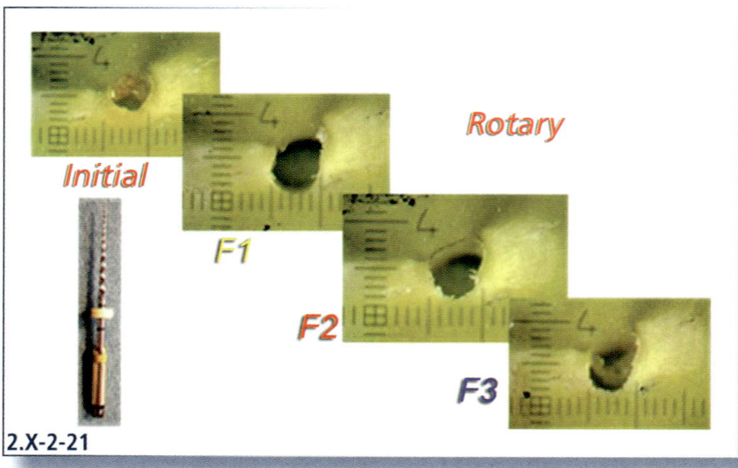

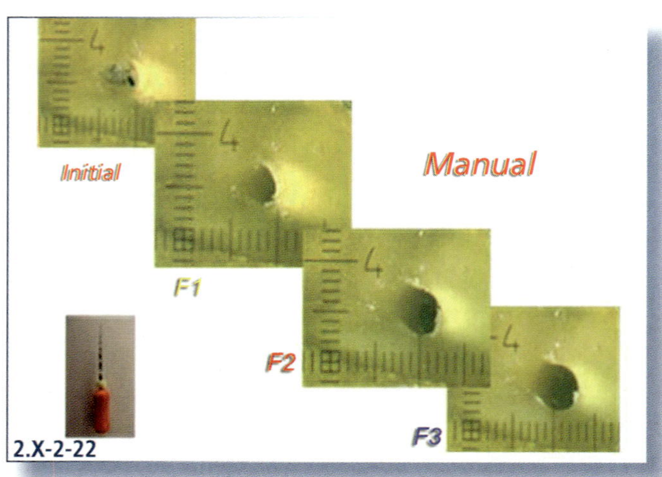

FIG. 2.X-2-21

Action sequence of rotary instruments F1, F2 and F3 in the apical third of mesial root canals of mandibular molars. Note the areas and the displacement caused by the instruments.

FIG. 2.X-2-22

Action sequence of manual rotary instruments F1, F2 and F3 in the apical third of mesial root canals of mandibular molars. Note the areas and the displacement caused by the instruments.

FIG. 2.X-2-23

Action sequence of rotary instruments with oscillatory F1, F2 and F3 in the apical third of mesial root canals of mandibular molars. Note the areas and the displacement caused by the instruments.

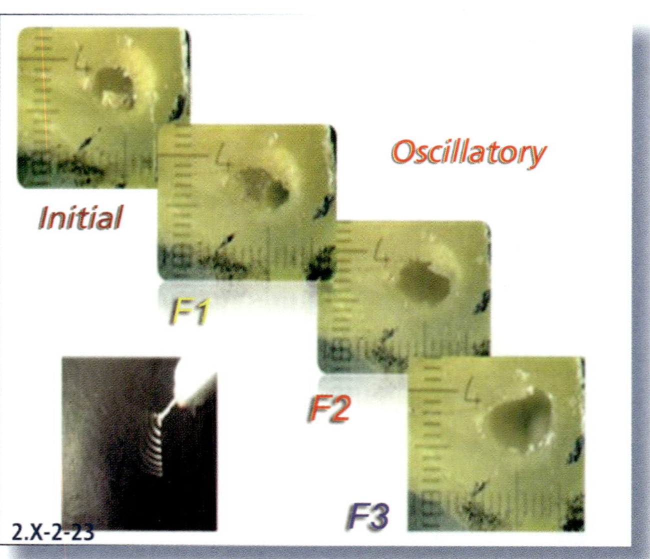

When observing Figure 2.X-2-24, one notes that manual instrumentation removed an area statistically equal to that removed by rotary instrumentation. In Figure 2.X-2-25 one can see that the displacement of the root canal center (deviation from the natural canal, degree) with the rotary instrument used manually was lower, being statistically superior to that of oscillatory instrumentation in F3. In view of the results offered by these and other studies, in addition to clinical experience, one can suggest that root canal instrumentation should be performed combining rotary with manual instrumentation.

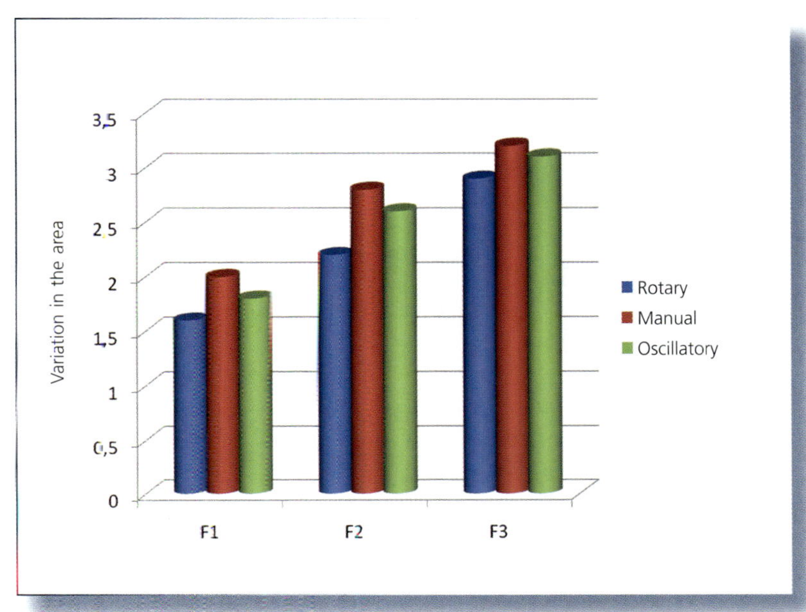

FIG. 2.X-2-24

Chart showing sample means and subsequent intervals of confidence of variation in the area after the use of instruments F1, F2 and F3.

FIG. 2.X-2-25

Chart showing sample means and subsequent intervals of confidence of variation in displacement of the center of the root canal after the use of instruments F1, F2 and F3.

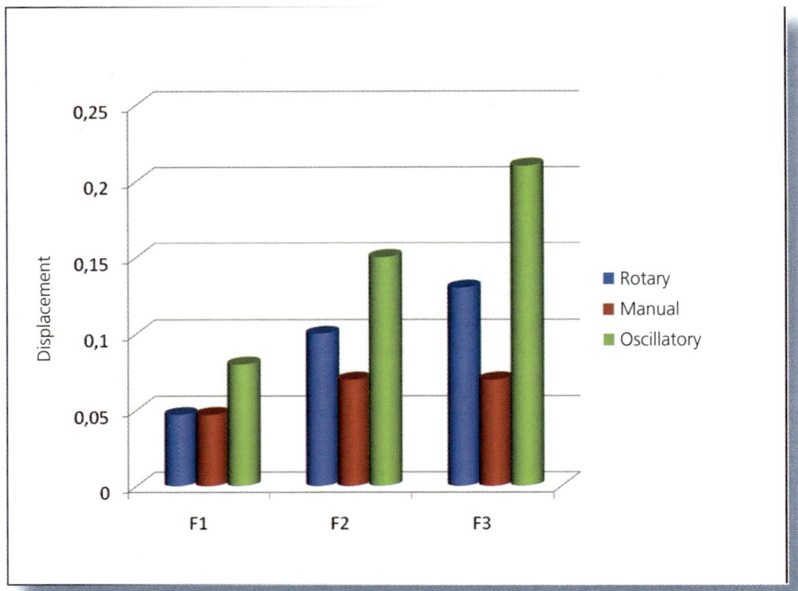

Hybrid instrumentation sequence, combining the Universal Protaper, rotary and manual instruments, and filling with a single gutta-percha cone method

In this sequence (Fig. 2.X-2-26), the mechanically driven instrument will receive a letter **m** (for mechanical) below the instrument, for example, S1-**m**. The manual instruments will receive a letter **d** (for digital) above the instrument, for example, S1-**d**.

By means of radiography for diagnosis (Fig. 2.X-2-27), the TWL (temporary working length) should be determined and the measurements transferred to type K files, 10, 15 and 20, or C$^+$ to start exploration (patency), widening and familiarization with the anatomic shape of the root canal (Figs. 2.X-2-28 and 2.X-2-29).

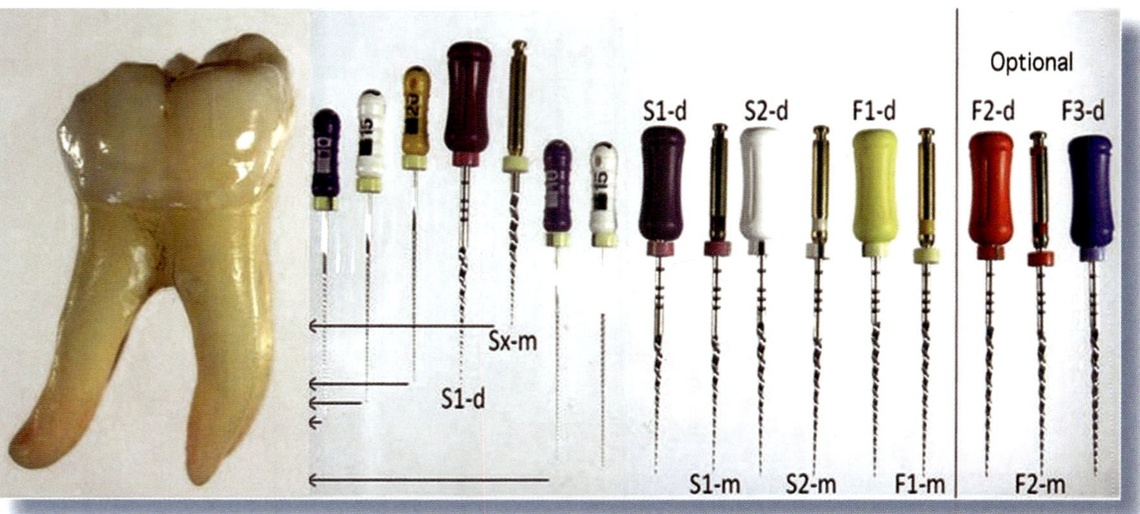

FIG. 2.X-2-26
Illustration of sequence of hybrid rotary and manual instrumentation. The penetration limits of the stainless steel files and Protaper treatment instruments are indicated with arrows.

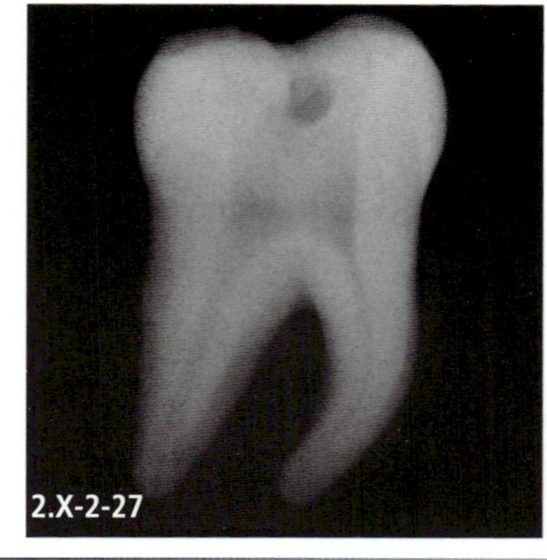

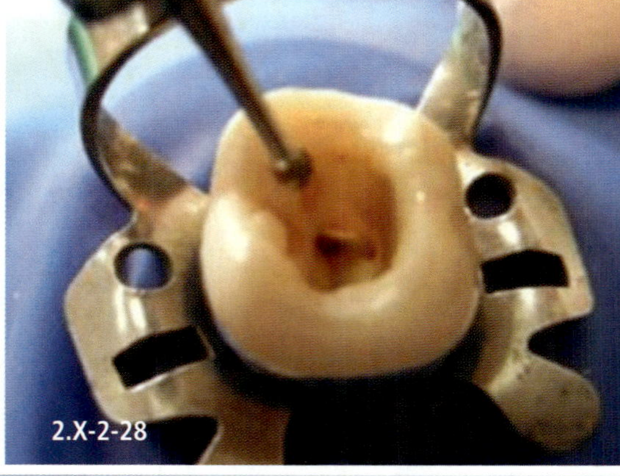

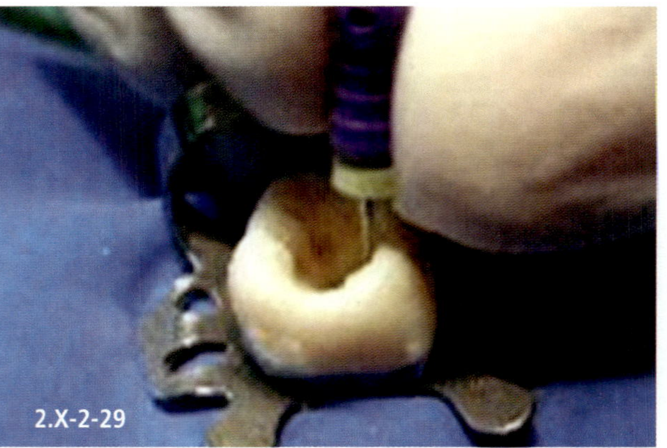

FIG. 2.X-2-27
Radiograph for diagnosis of mandibular molar.

FIG. 2.X-2-28
Laboratory aspect, showing coronal opening of mandibular molar.

FIG. 2.X-2-29
Laboratory aspect of exploration with C+ (10) files at the entrance of root canals.

All procedures performed in the root canal must be preceded by irrigation, aspiration and flooding with a sodium hypochlorite solution.

The manual files must penetrate inside the anatomical root canal, without apical pressure, with oscillatory movements, widening and filing, applying greater pressure on the wall opposing the furcation region, for example, the mesial wall of the maxillary molar. The depth of file penetration must be measured. This is an easy step to perform. The silicone stops of all the files used previously were set at the TWL when exploration (patency) was concluded. This stop lined up to an occlusal reference point, thus determining the temporary working length of the rotary instrument (Figs. 2.X-2-30 and 2.X.32).

The instrument S1-d must be introduced into the root canal with rotary movements in a clockwise direction, applying apical pressure. The process should be repeated until the pre-determined length (TWL) has been reached (Figs. 2.X-2-30 and 2.X-2-31). Should lock-in occur, it should be turned in a counter-clockwise direction, which will free it from the root canal.

With instrument Sx-m in a contra-angle hand piece operated at a speed of 300 rpm and torque of 2 N.cm, a temporary working length somewhat shorter than that reached with instrument S1-d (Fig. 2.X-2-26) is established. Instrumentation begins with in-and-out movements and pressure on the lateral walls opposite the furcation. These brush strokes must be applied only during the withdrawal of the instrument, until the pre-establish length is attained.

Instrument SX must never be used beyond the penetration level of instrument S1 or the manual stainless steel K type files. The root canal must be frequently irrigated, aspirated and flooded to eliminate dentin debris. With the help of a *clean stand,* dentin debris must be removed from the instrument.

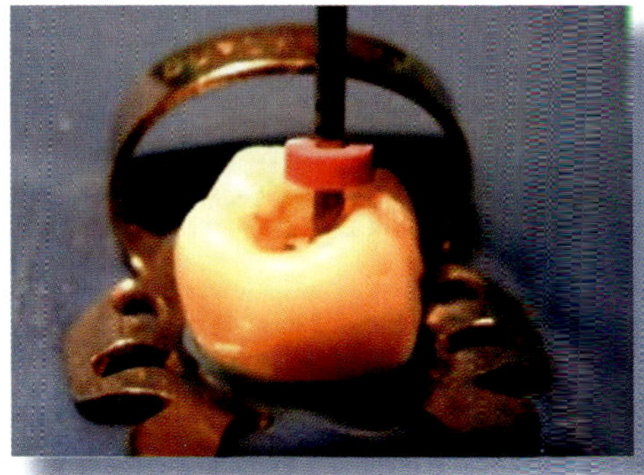

FIG. 2.X-2-30

Laboratory aspect showing the S1-d instrument at the temporary working length (pre-determined length), reached with K-file N° 20.

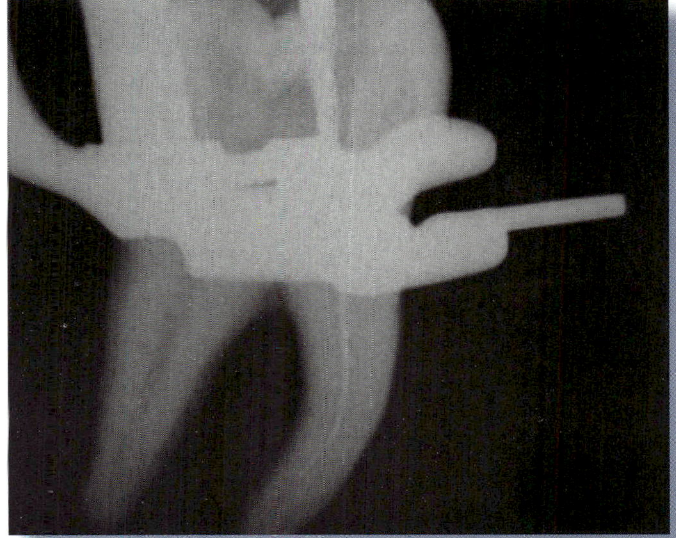

FIG. 2.X-2-31

Radiograph showing penetration depth of instrument S1-d.

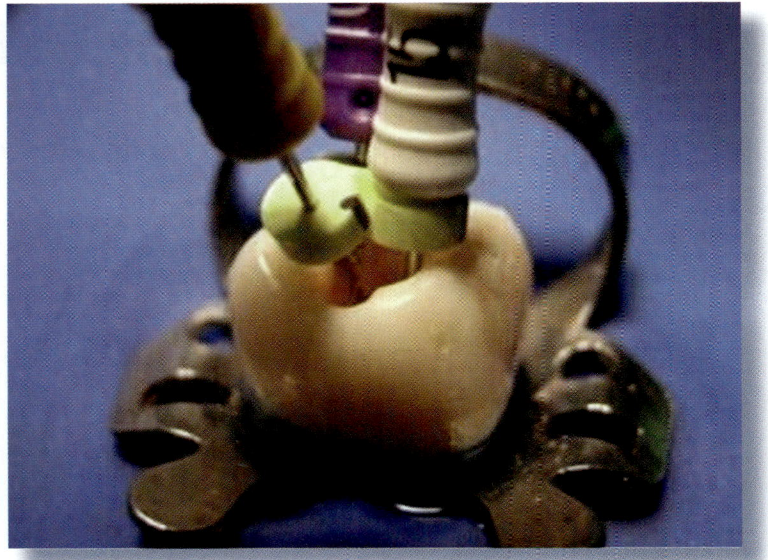

FIG. 2.X-2-32

Laboratory aspect showing penetration depth of instruments used for exploration.

WORKING LENGTH DETERMINATION

After widening the cervical and middle thirds of the root canal, working length is established with pre-curved K type files using an electronic apex locator, in order to obtain the real working lengths for each root canal (Figs. 2.X-2-33, 2.X-2-34 and 2.X-2-35).

At the real working length, instrumentation is performed with stainless steel type K files until No.15 experiences no resistance (Fig. 2.X-2-36).

After the canal has been instrumented with type K file No. 15, the manual instrument S1-d should be inserted in the root canal using short turning movements, with minimal apical pressure, until the real working length is reached. After this, instrument S1-m is used at a speed of 250 rpm and torque of 1 N.cm, with in-and-out movements (pecking) and pressure on the lateral walls only when withdrawing the instrument (brush strokes), until the real working length is reached (Figs. 2.X-2-37 and 2.X-2-38).

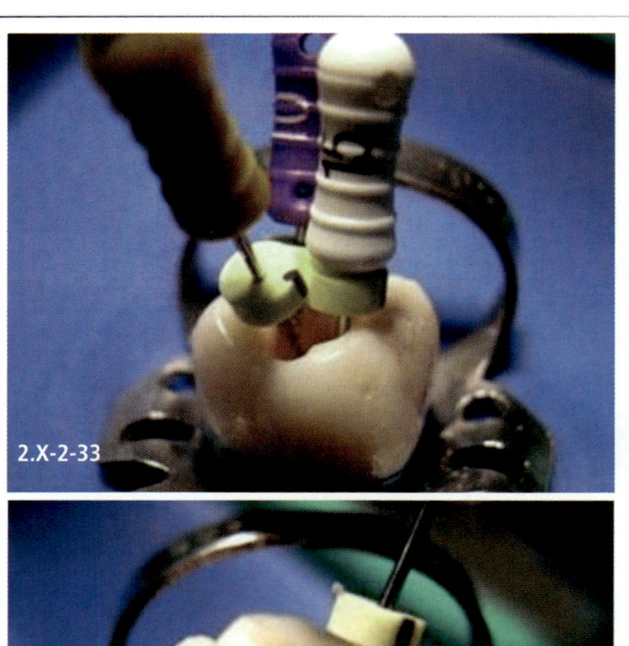

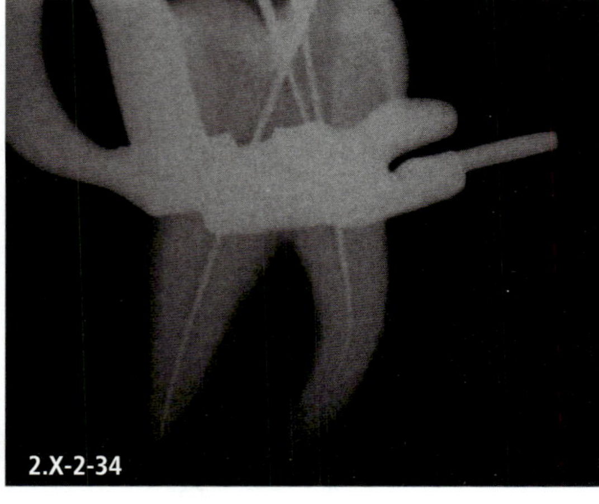

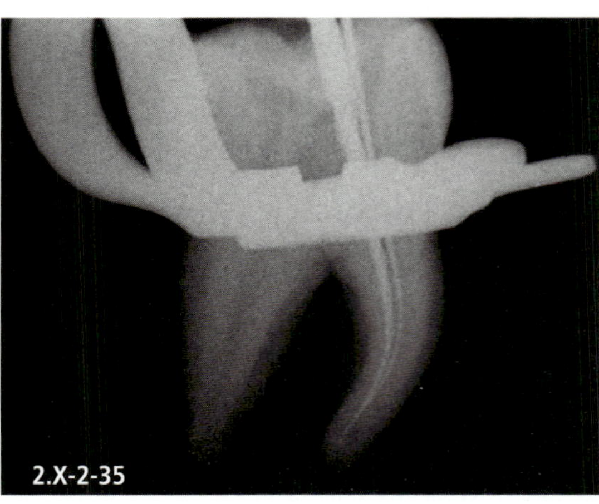

FIG. 2.X-2-33
Laboratory aspect showing establishing working length with stainless steel type K files.

FIG. 2.X-2-34
Radiograph with type K files in root canals, to determine the real working length.

FIG. 2.X-2-35
Radiograph with type K files inside the root canals, to confirm the real working length.

FIG. 2.X-2-36
Laboratory aspect of root canal instrumentation up to type K file No.15.

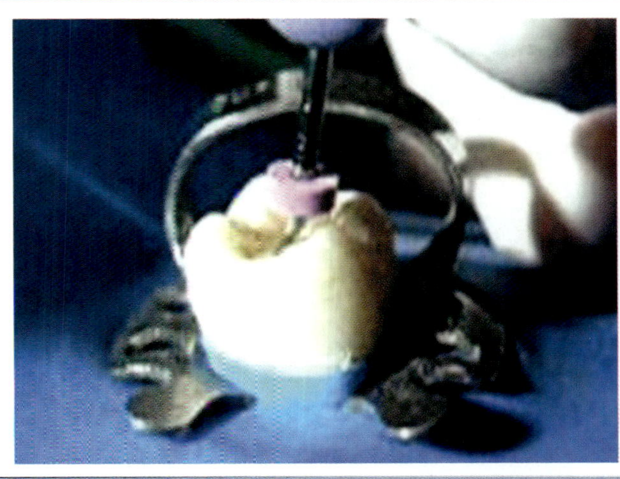

FIG. 2.X-2-37

Laboratory aspect of instrument S1-d being turned to the real working length.

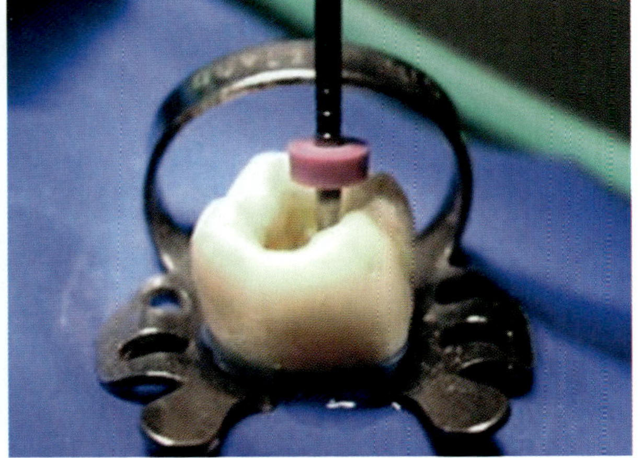

FIG. 2.X-2-38

Laboratory aspect of instrument S1-m activated to the real working length, with in-and-out movements with light pressure on the lateral walls of the root canal.

Next, instruments S2-d and S2-m are used, exercising the same care as with S1-d and S1-m, to widen the apical and middle parts of the root canal (Fig. 2.X-2-39). Should there be any undue resistance, the previous instrument should be used again when necessary, re-working the stainless steel K type files, without losing the real working length.

After completion, instruments S1 and S2 determine the tapered shape in the two coronal thirds of the root canal, with apical enlargement of 0.20 mm, leaving them prepared to receive the finishing files (F).

Caution: Never use brush stroke movements with the *finishing files*. They must enter and leave the root canal following its long axis.

The finishing files (F) series of rotary instruments must be immediately removed when they reach the real working length. The instrument must be inserted and removed (pecking) a maximum of three times, make sure that the silicone stop is touching the occlusal reference point previously established for each root canal..

To continue the hybrid instrumentation, use instrument F1-d, yellow handle, with the same movements as instrument S1-d (turning in a clockwise direction and when locked-in turning in a counter-clockwise direction), until the real working length is reached (Fig. 2.X-2-40). This is followed by instrument F1-m, exercising the same care as mentioned above (Fig. 2.X-2-41,) thus widening the apical region of the canal with a 0.07 mm/mm taper.

Note: Note that in Figure 2.X-2-42 dentin debris can be seen in the middle portion of the active part of instrument F1-m and not on the coronal and apical portions. This shows that the apical region of the root canal has been instrumented with instrument S2, which has an apical diameter of 0.20 mm, equal to the apical diameter of instrument F1, and that the cervical region was widened with instruments SX and S1, demonstrating cutting efficiency in a small area of the root canal, without locking in and causing accidents.

The Universal Protaper System manufacturer indicates measuring the apical diameter of the root canal with a stainless steel type K file, No.20. If the file is adjusted at this length, this means that the diameter of the apical stop is 0.20 mm, and the root canal is prepared for filling. If the type K file, No. 20 has a loose fit, preparation should continue with the other instruments, F2 and F3, and in wider canals, instruments F4 and F5 should be used.

It is important to decide up to which number the root canal should be widened. With the initial apical instrument (IAI), one can determine which stainless steel type K file is the first to reach the real working length and become stuck in this region. For example: If a type K file No.10 or 15 is not loose at the real working length and has the function of filing and widening, instrumentation up to F1 is appropriate. If this does not occur, one can continue with instrumentation up to F2 and/or F3.

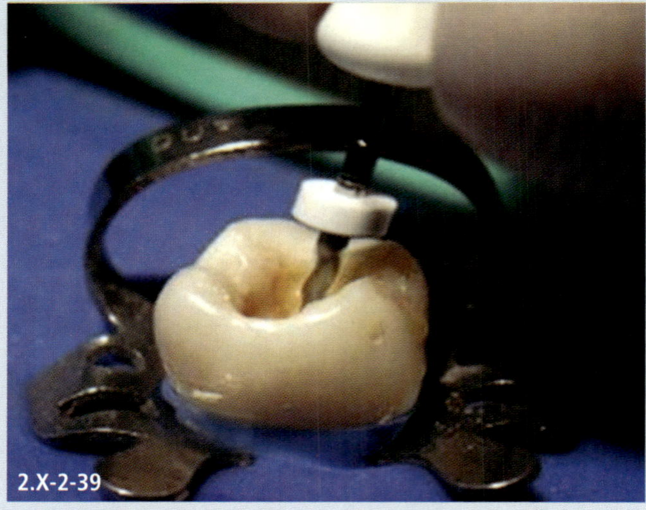
2.X-2-39

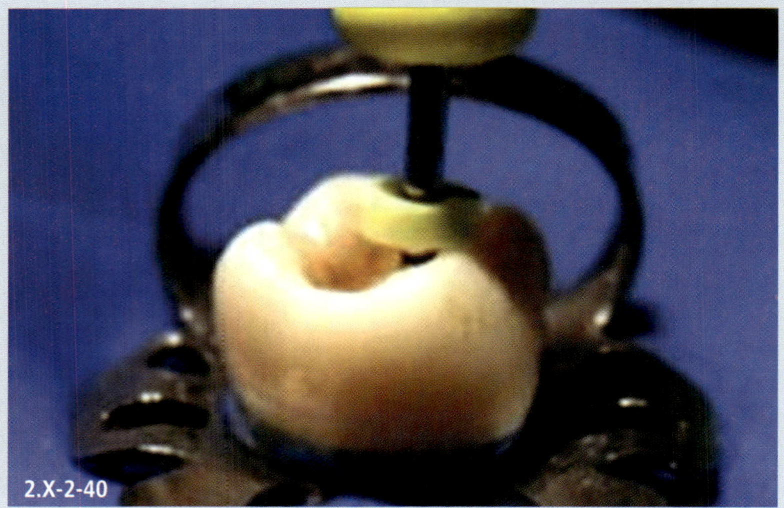
2.X-2-40

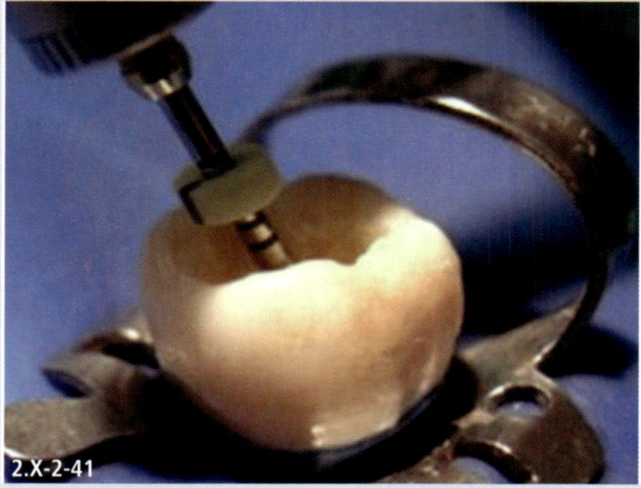
2.X-2-41

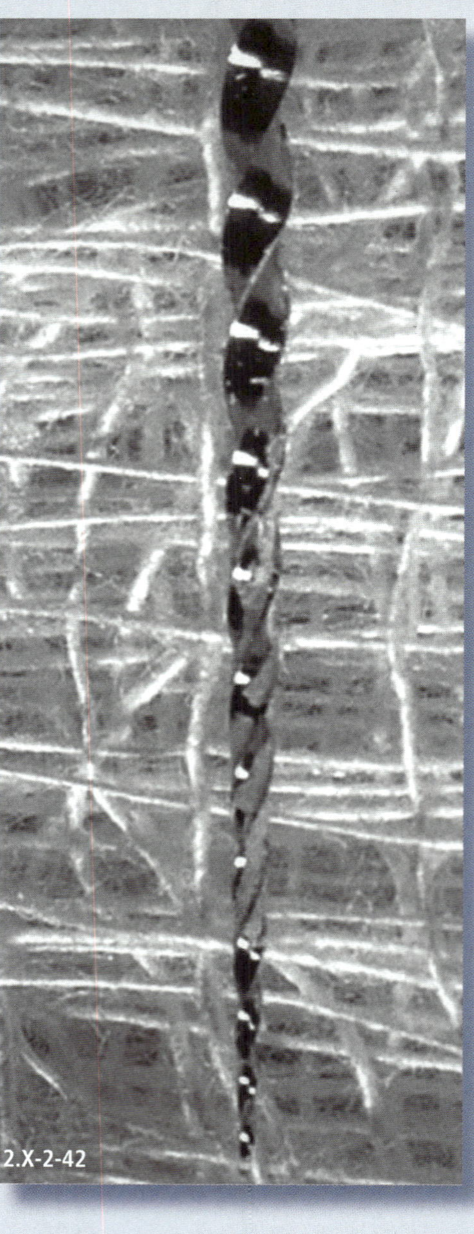
2.X-2-42

FIG. 2.X-2-39

Laboratory aspect of instrument S2-d being turned to the real working length.

FIG. 2.X-2-40

Laboratory aspect of instrument F1-d being turned at the real working length.

FIG. 2.X-2-41

Laboratory aspect of instrument F1-m, activated to the real working length, with in-and-out movements (pecking).

FIG. 2.X-2-42

Instrument F1-m with dentin debris on the central portion of the active part.

Another important factor is the root canal curvature radius. If the root canal presents a very pronounced curvature and a small radius, there will frequently be a risk of fracture with the use of mechanical rotary instruments. Thus, a good evaluation and the previous use of conventional instrumentation or the combination of rotary/manual instrumentation will be necessary.

In the case presented in Figures 2.X-2-43, 2.X-2-44 and 2.X-2-45, the mesial root canals were instrumented up to instruments F2-d and F2-m (Fig. 2.X-2-43) and the distal canal, up to instrument F3, both digital and rotary (Figs. 2.X-2-44 and 2.X-2-45).

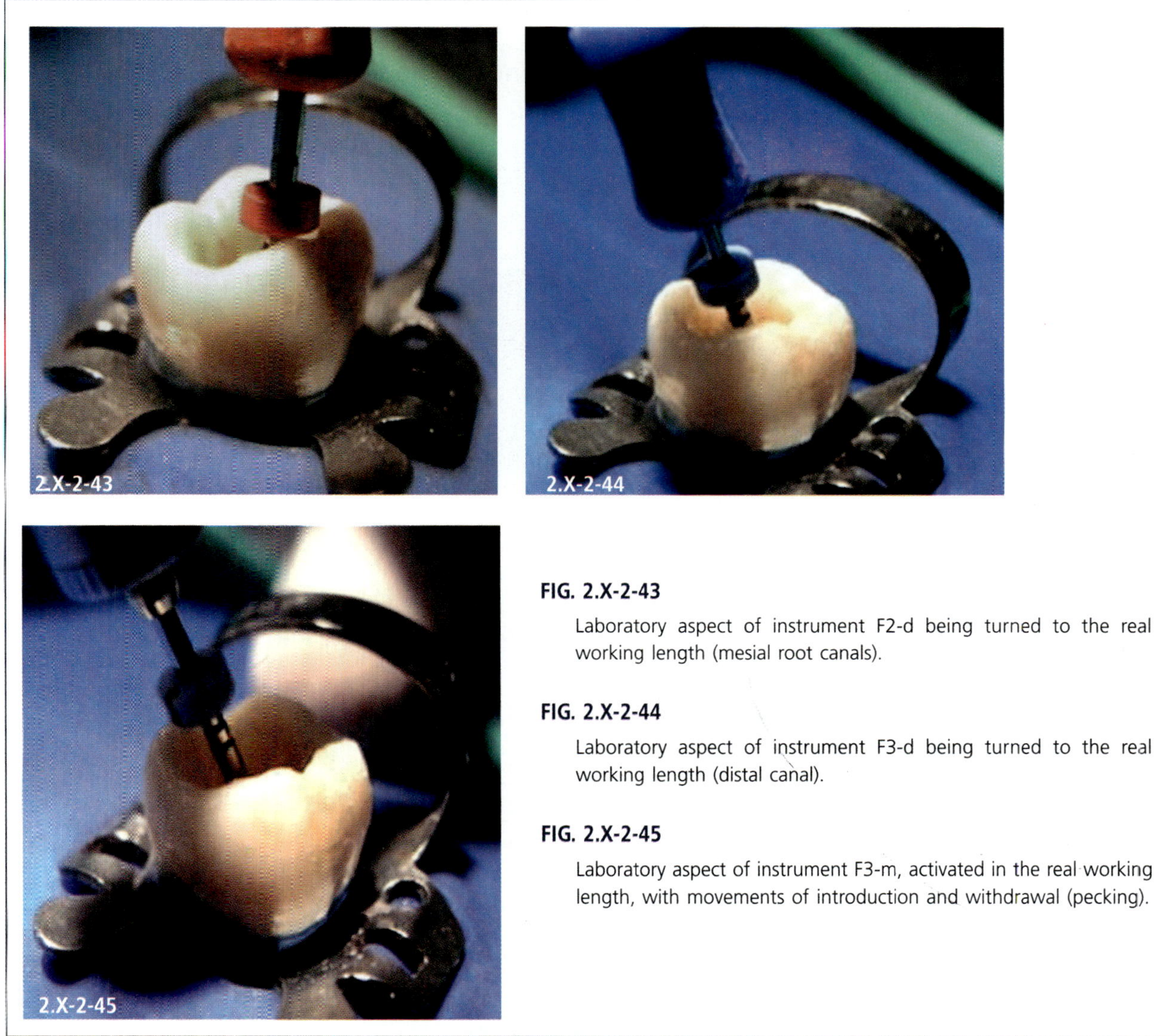

FIG. 2.X-2-43
Laboratory aspect of instrument F2-d being turned to the real working length (mesial root canals).

FIG. 2.X-2-44
Laboratory aspect of instrument F3-d being turned to the real working length (distal canal).

FIG. 2.X-2-45
Laboratory aspect of instrument F3-m, activated in the real working length, with movements of introduction and withdrawal (pecking).

FILLING

After instrumentation, irrigation and flooding with EDTA solution to remove the *smear layer*, the root canals had to be dried with sterile paper points, matching the last instrument used. For the two mesial root canals, paper points F2 were selected, and for the distal canals, F3 (Figs. 2.X-2-13a and 2.X-2-13c). Paper points with tapers that are similar to the instruments that were used, provide excellent fit and dry the entire root canal.

The next step was to test the gutta-percha cones to determine their adaptation to the root canal, both clinically and radiographically, as shown in Figures 2.X-2-46, 2.X-2-47 and 2.X-2-48.

Depending on the instrumentation performed and experience with the technique, the gutta-percha cone may not reach the real working length. Note that in one of the mesial canals shown in Figure 2.X-2-48, the cone could have extended a bit further. Thus, with the aid of cotton pliers, the gutta-percha cone is held to its occlusal reference point, withdrawn and lined-up on a millimeter ruler to measure the length attained (Fig. 2.X-2-49). When the new measurement has been corrected, the root canal is re-instrumented with the manual Protaper instruments, or with stainless steel (pre-curved) K type files, and another radiograph is made.

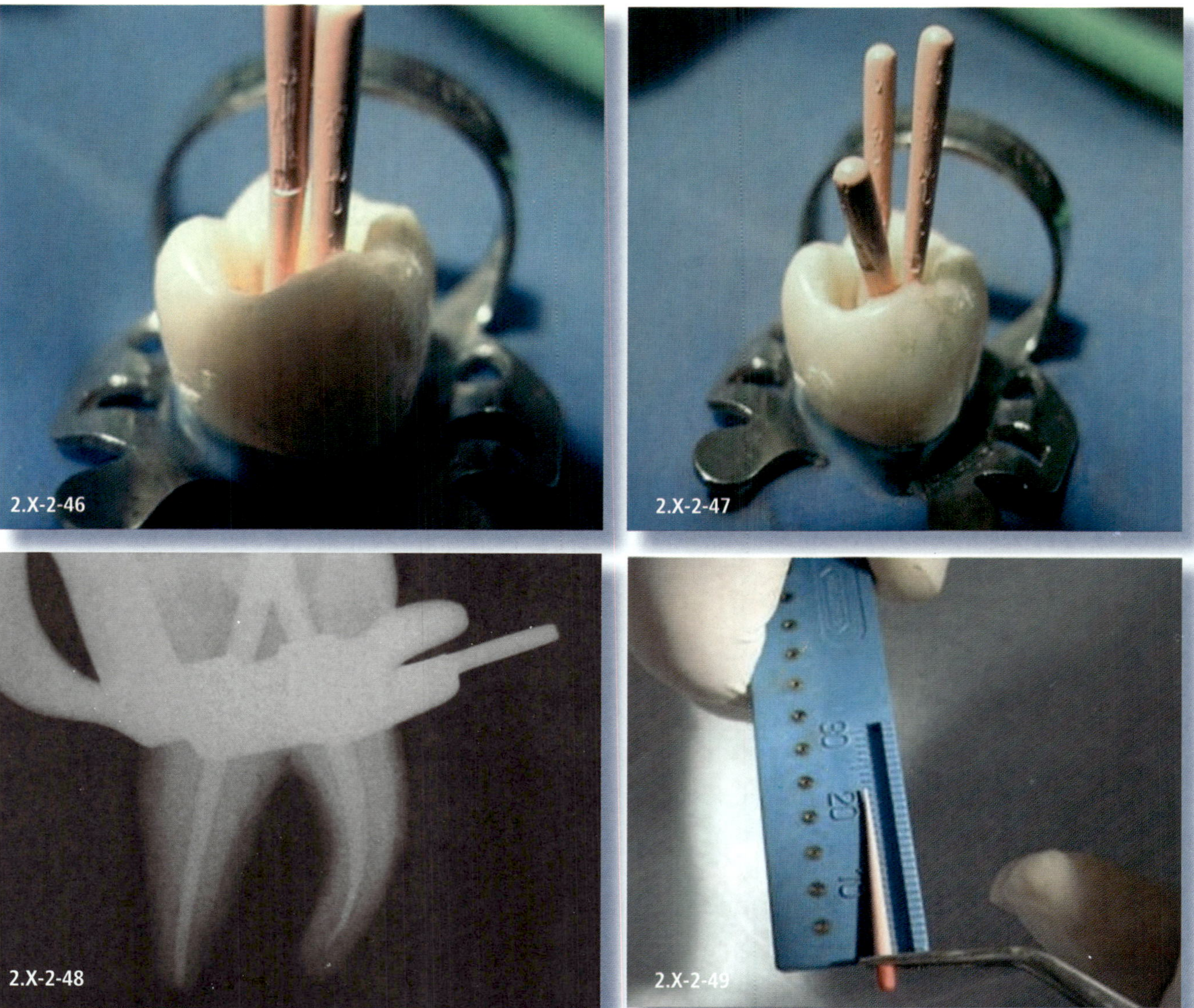

FIG. 2.X-2-46
Laboratory test of tapered gutta-percha cones in mesial root canals.

FIG. 2.X-2-47
Laboratory test of tapered gutta-percha cones in all root canals.

FIG. 2.X-2-48
Radiographic proof of clinical fit of gutta-percha cones.

FIG. 2.X-2-49
Measurement with a millimeter ruler to confirm whether the gutta-percha coned reached the real working length.

Doubts and Questions

Should filling be done with a single gutta-percha cone or with the active lateral condensation technique? Is a root canal filling with a single cone better, equal to or worse than the active lateral condensation technique?

When filling a root canal with the lateral condensation technique, in reality one only fills the apical region with the main cone (Fig. 2.X-2-50). In curved root canals, the auxiliary cones remain more distant from the lock-in length (adjustment) of the main gutta-percha cone. Figure 2.X-2-51 shows evidence that the silicone stop of the finger spreader is not in contact with the occlusal reference point, indicating a real working length that is too short.

When instrumenting and filling root canals with tapered gutta-percha cones, the apical regions will have a quantity of gutta-percha equal to or larger than with conventional instrumentation and filling (Fig. 2.X-2-52).

In oval-shaped root canals (distal of mandibular molars, lingual of the maxillary molars, etc.), we can perform a smooth lateral condensation, complementing it with the placement of auxiliary cones, which fuse well with the main gutta-percha point (Fig. 2.X-2-53).

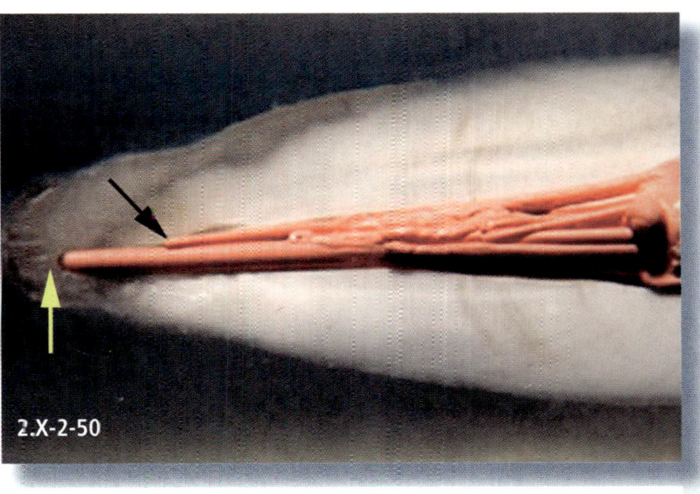

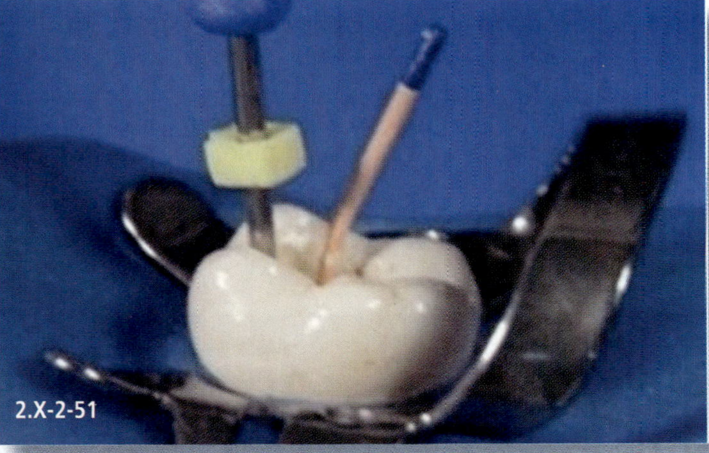

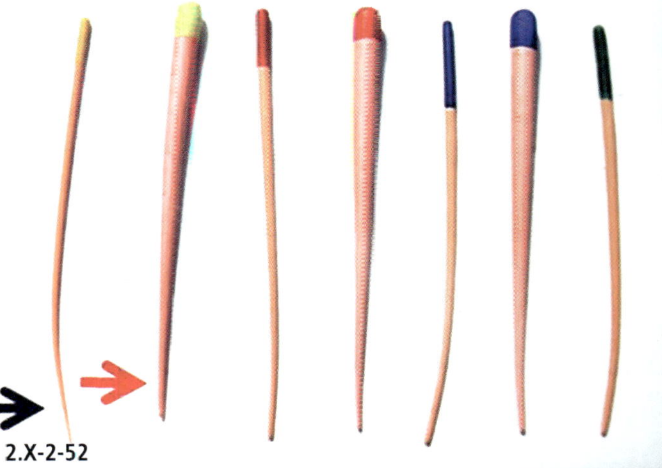

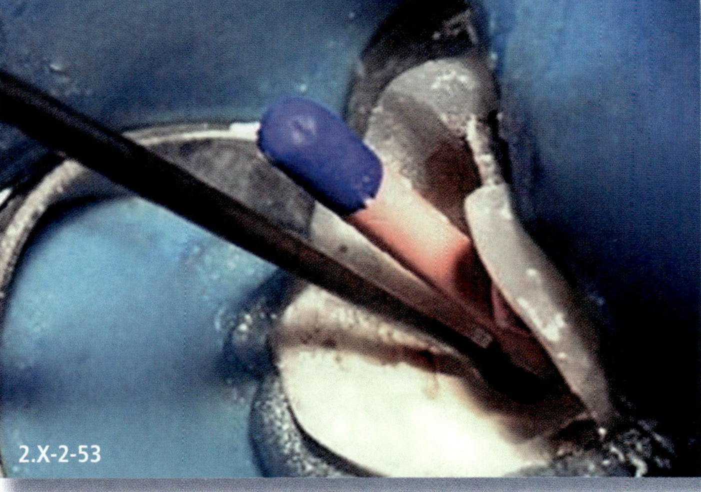

FIG. 2.X-2-50

Example of ex-vivo laboratory study, showing the difference in penetration of the master gutta-percha cone (yellow arrow) in relation to the auxiliary cones (black arrow), inside the root canal.

FIG. 2.X-2-51

Finger spreader with silicone stop, showing the distance at which the auxiliary cones will be positioned inside the root canal in relation to the master gutta- percha cone.

FIG. 2.X-2-52

Difference in diameter between conventional gutta-percha cones in comparison to tapered cones.

FIG. 2.X-2-53

Laboratory view showing the opening of space with a finger spreader to place auxiliary gutta-percha cones.

Choice of Filling Cement (Sealer)

AHPlus resin cement, marketed by Dentsply/DeTrey, Switzerland, has shown to be an excellent filling cement, with respect to both its physical-chemical and biological properties. Early data of a study currently being conducted* shows that the material has the capacity to penetrate into the dentinal tubules, as can be seen in Figures 2.X-2-54 and 2.X-2-55.

An endodontic cement in the development stage, derived from caster oil polymer, a trifunctional polyester for filling with a single point technique appears to be very promising. It presents good biocompatibility[7], cytotoxicity[9], sealing capacity[10] and expansion during hardening, as well as a short working time, around 15 to 25 minutes (Figs. 2.X-2-56A and 2.X-2-56B). This promotes filling with a single cone technique, because at the time of cutting excess coronal material with a heated spatula (Fig. 2.X-2-60) the cement has already started expanding, lightly locking-in the cone and preventing it from being displaced.

How to take the Sealer into the Root Canal

It is important to first take the endodontic cement to the root canal with the last instrument used in root canal preparation; next, the gutta-percha cone is coated with cement, which is then inserted in the root canal. Thus the cement will be pressed against the root canal walls without causing voids in the sealer (Figs. 2.X-2-57, 2.X-2-58 and 2.X-2-59).

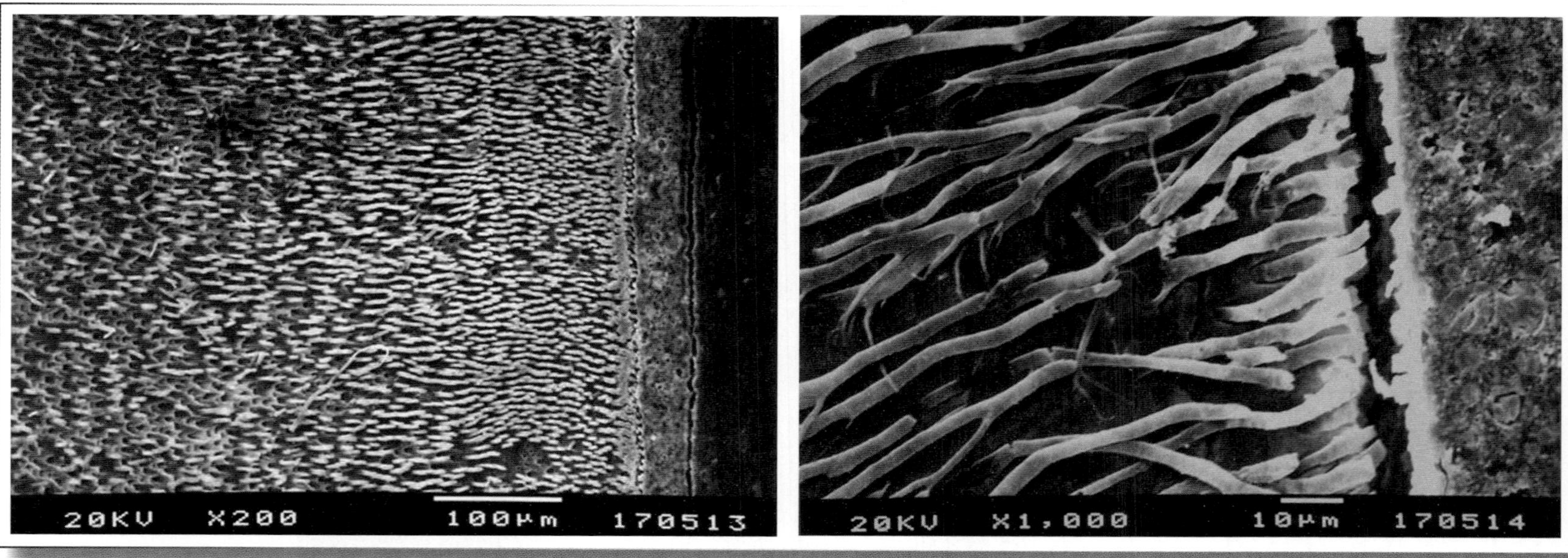

FIG. 2.X-2-54

Image obtained by scanning electronic microscopy (SEM), showing evidence of AHPlus cement penetration into the dentinal tubules.

FIG. 2.X-2-55

Image obtained by scanning electronic microscopy (SEM), showing evidence of AHPlus cement penetrating into the dentinal tubules.

* Bonetti Filho I, Farac RV, Gutierrez JCR, Góes MF. Avaliação microscópica da adaptação e penetração de diferentes cimentos endodônticos nas paredes e túbulos dentinários de dentes bovinos. SBPqO (2008).

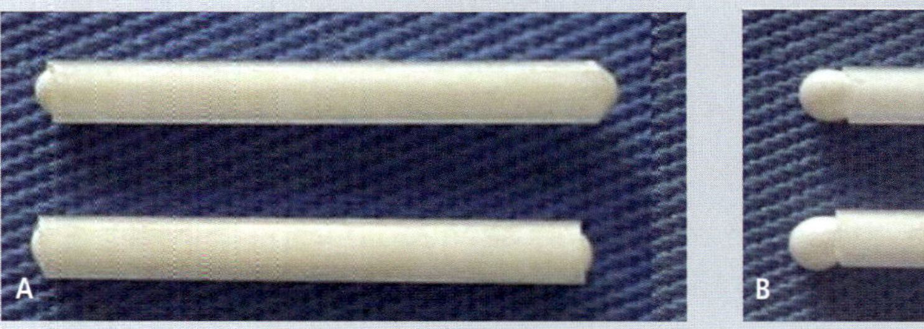

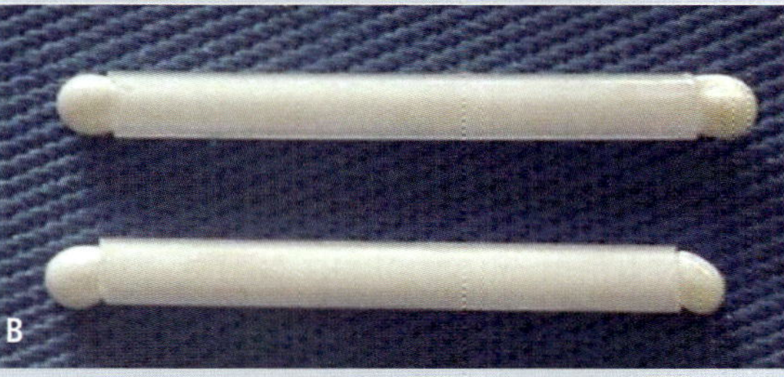

FIGS. 2.X-2-56A-B

A – Experimental endodontic cement (trifunctional polyester), immediately after manipulation, completely filling the interior of polyethylene tubes.

B – Experimental endodontic cement (trifunctional polyester), twenty minutes after manipulation, completely filling the interior of the polyethylene tubes. Note ballooning at the ends of the tubes indicative of the expansion during setting.

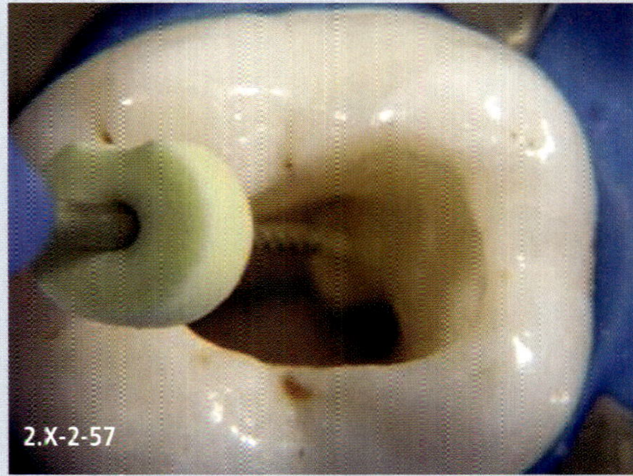

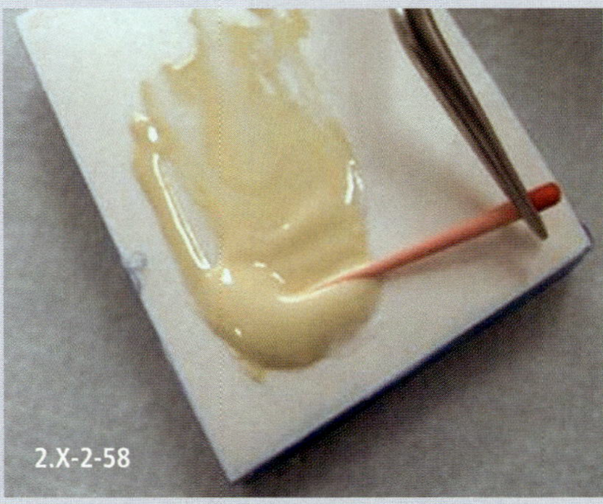

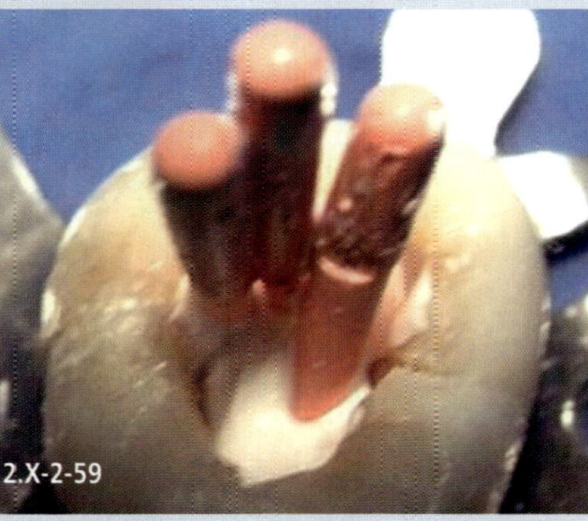

FIG. 2.X-2-57

Laboratory view, showing placement of the cement in the root canal.

FIG. 2.X-2-58

Coating of a gutta-percha cone F2 with experimental cement (trifunctional polyester).

FIG. 2.X-2-59

Laboratory view showing gutta-percha cones cemented with experimental sealer inside the root canals.

The gutta-percha cone is then cut with a heated plastic instrument, followed by using vertical condensers, condensing the gutta-percha vertically inside the root canal.

Warning: The excess gutta-percha cones must be cut with a heated plastic instrument, without causing displacement inside the root canal (Fig. 2.X-2-60).

Note: Hybrid instrumentation with the Universal Protaper system maintained the tapered shape of the root canal curvature; the single cone filling, seen radiographically, filled the entire root canal in a simple, fast and safe manner.

Final radiograph with the filled root canals (Fig. 2.X-2-61).

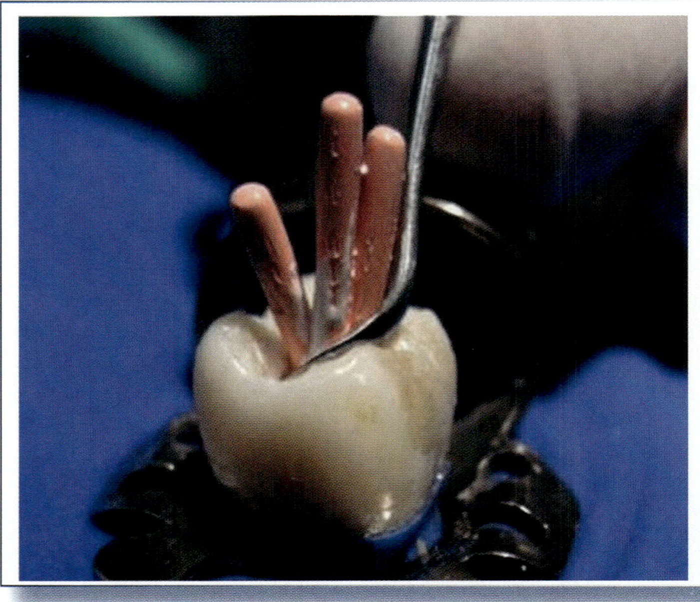

FIG. 2.X-2-60

Laboratory view showing the gutta-percha cones being cut with a heated plastic instrument.

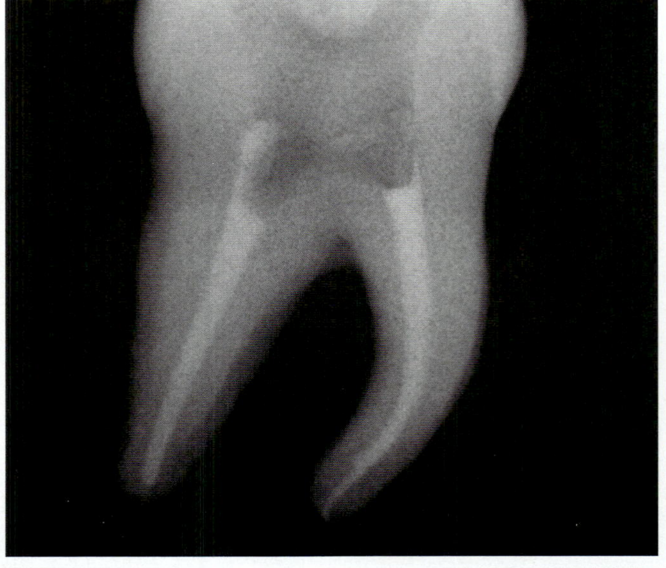

FIG. 2.X-2-61

Radiograph of mandibular molar root canal filling.

CLINICAL CASES INSTRUMENTED AND FILLED USING THE UNIVERSAL PROTAPER SYSTEM

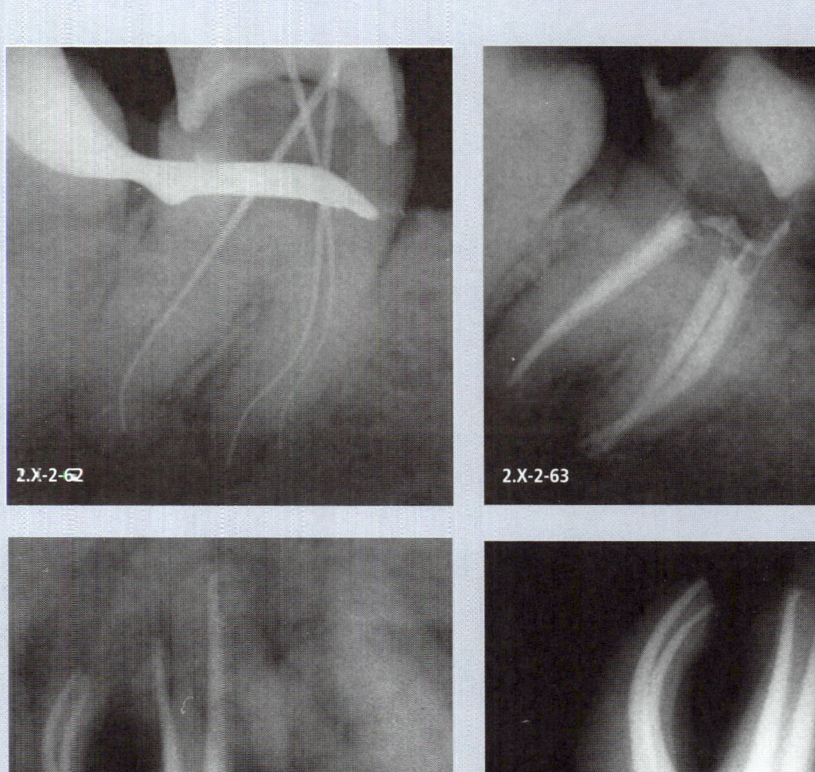

FIG. 2.X-2-62

Radiograph for determining working length in a mandibular molar.

FIG. 2.X-2-63

Post operative radiograph of mandibular molar filling. Note that the mesial root canal curvatures have been maintained.

FIG. 2.X-2-64

Radiograph of testing the fit of the tapered gutta-percha cones in the four root canals of a maxillary molar.

FIG. 2.X-2-65

Post operative radiograph of the filling of the four root canals of the maxillary molar in Figure 2.X-2-64. Note that the curvatures have been maintained.

FIG. 2.X-2-66

Radiograph of testing the fit of the tapered gutta-percha cones in the three root canals of a maxillary molar.

FIG. 2.X-2-67

Post operative radiograph of the filling of the three root canals of a maxillary molar. Note that the curvatures have been maintained.

FIG. 2.X-2-68

Post operative radiograph of a maxillary molar with a considerable curvature of the mesio buccal canal. The filling was done by an undergraduate student during a laboratory exercise.

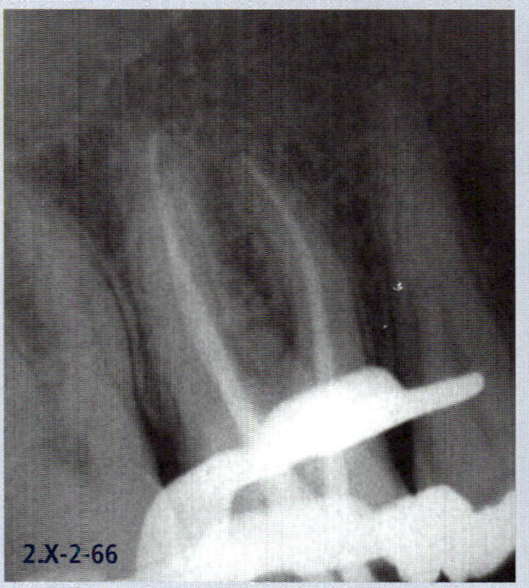

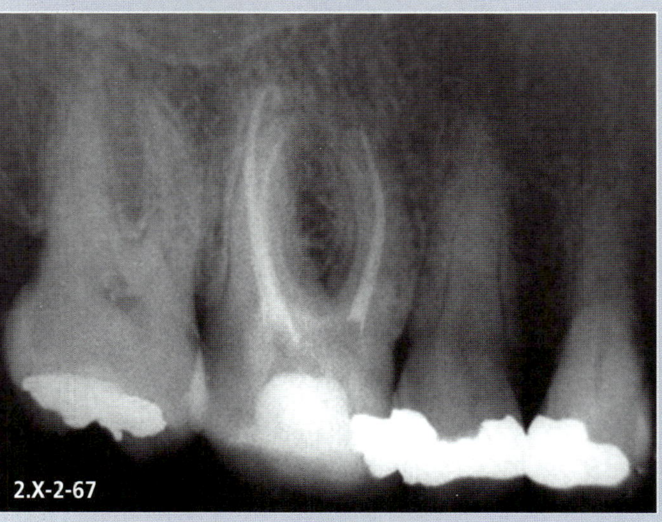

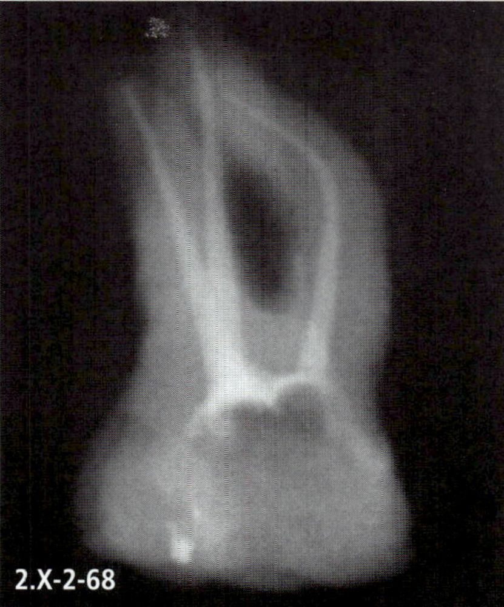

Undergraduate Students at Araraquara Dental School-UNESP, SP, Brazil, are using the conventional techniques and the Universal Protaper System for root canal instrumentation and filling, with optimum results with respect to quality, in both the laboratory and clinic.

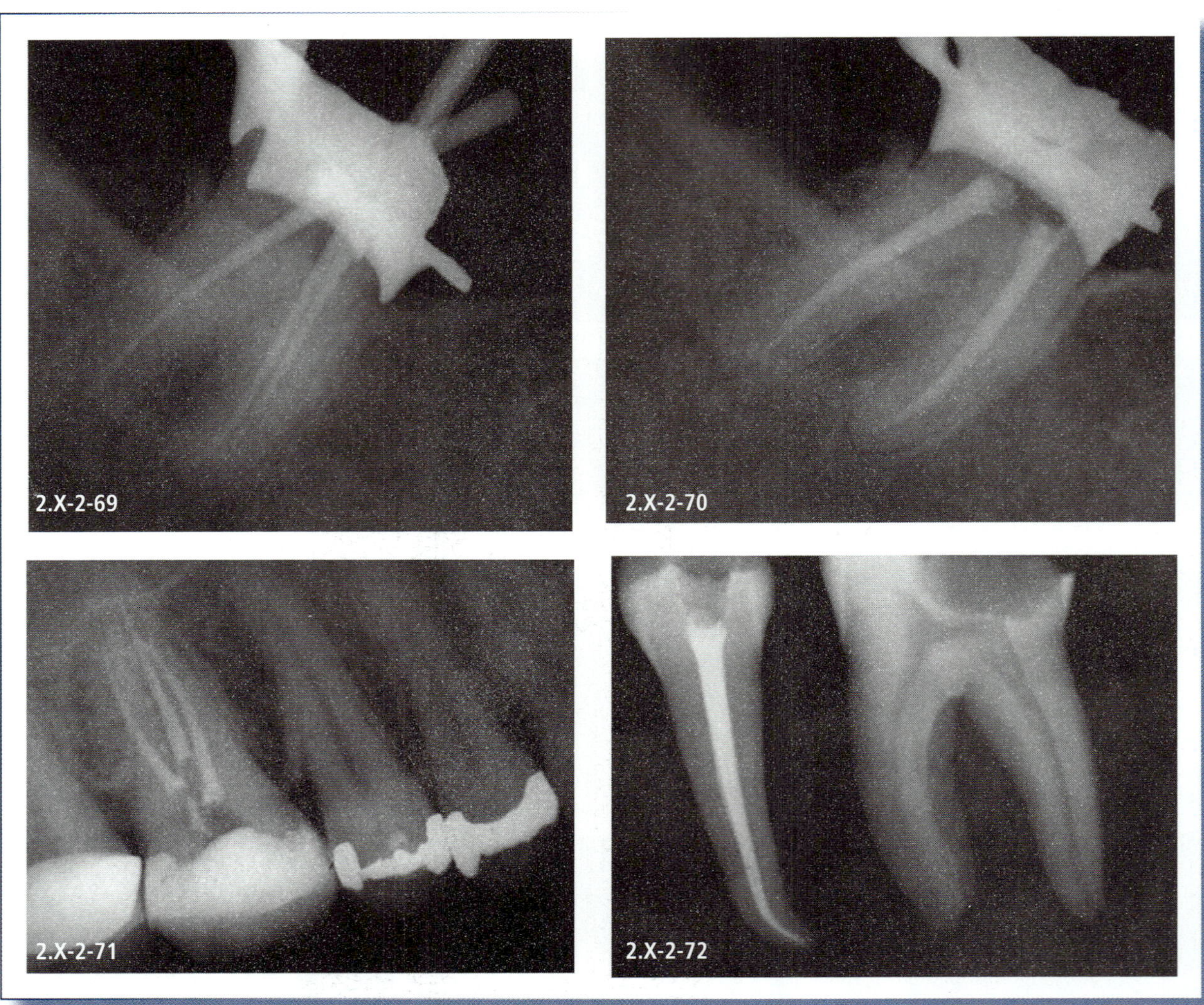

FIG. 2.X-2-69

Radiograph confirming the fit of tapered gutta-percha cones in the three root canals of a mandibular molar.

FIG. 2.X-2-70

Post operative radiograph of the filling of the three root canals of a mandibular molar. Note that the root curvatures have been maintained.

FIG. 2.X-2-71

Post operative radiograph of maxillary molar root canal fillings.

FIG. 2.X-2-72

Post operative radiograph of a mandibular premolar root canal filling maintaining the root curvature (laboratory exercise).

Problems and Solutions

P: *Fracture of Instruments*

S: a. The following steps are indicated for each type of instrumentation.

b. Always work with Protaper instruments after determining a pathway with stainless steel type K files.

c. Use motors or contra angles with torque and speed control.

d. After and during the use of instruments, if possible, examine them with a loupe to verify whether there are deformations.

e. Preferably use the hybrid sequence; that is, combining manual rotary with mechanical instrumentation.

P: *After instrumentation, the gutta-percha cones with F1, F2 or F3 tapers do not reach the real working length*

S: a. Normally, when this occurs, the tapered cones become locked in the root canal body, due to the taper.

b. Verify whether the finishing files are penetrating into the real predetermined working length, and compare this measurement with the penetration measurement of the gutta-percha cones. If this has not occurred, re-instrument the root canal, and attempt to reach the real working length.

c. Rotary mechanical instruments for modeling must be used with a brush stroke movement (on withdrawal they must be pressed against the root canal walls, widening the cervical and middle regions even further).

d. When only manual rotary instrumentation is used (without the possibility of using brush stroke movements), instrument **Sx** should be used again at the end of the sequence, in order to better widen the cervical region of the root canal.

P: *Failures in Filling*

S: In the clinical gutta-percha cone test, when it is removed from the root canal, one may observe that the tip is bent into the shape of the letter "s".

This means that the root canal was wider than the cone diameter, or a smaller gutta-percha cone was used. Try a larger diameter cone, and verify whether it returns to the real working length.

P: *Radiographical observation of lack of filling cement in the middle third of the root canal*

S: Some root canals present a larger diameter in the middle region than in the cervical region. In the filling technique with a tapered single cone, it is important to place cement into the root canal before inserting the gutta-percha cone, so that it fills the entire canal. Perform a smooth lateral condensation with auxiliary gutta-percha cones. Alternatively, gutta-condenser compactors can be used to plasticize the cones to correct the problem.

Note: The material capable of sealing the root canal is the filling cement. The gutta-percha fills the bulk of the root canal space, enabling future re-treatment, or making it easy to create a space for an intra-radicular post.

In all canals, an attempt should be made to perform smooth lateral condensation with the auxiliary gutta- percha cones, locking the master gutta-percha cone preferably in the distal and lingual canals of molars and in very wide canals.

Questions and Answers

Q: *What is the difference between the Protaper and Universal Protaper Systems?*

A: 1. The Universal Protaper System is presented with two additional finishing files (F4 and F5,) for wider apexes (ISO sizes: 0.40 and 0.50 mm tip diameters D0).

2. Instruments F3, F4 and F5 were reduced of metal mass and have concavities in the active part, which gives them greater flexibility (Fig. 2.X-2-9). Kim et al.[4], in 2008, compared the forces generated during root canal preparation as well as the residual stress, and determined that this was higher in the instruments of the Protaper system, followed by the Universal Protaper and Profile systems.
3. The Manual Universal Protaper instruments are manufactured with silicone handles, offering the practitioner greater comfort.
4. They have a new, non-cutting guide tip (Fig. 2.X-2-10).
5. They are also manufactured with a total length of 31 mm.

Q: *Are the manual Protaper instruments as efficient as the mechanical Universal Protaper instruments?*

A: 1. In simulated root canals, Pasqualini et al.[6] (2008) made a comparison between mechanical rotary and manual instrumentation, with respect to the required working time to effectively complete instrumentation of the root canal, and the number of rotations necessary. They concluded that the manual Protaper demanded a significantly lower number of rotations than the rotary Protaper, however, the effective working time to completely instrument the root canal was significantly longer with the manual Protaper.

2. Note that the manual instrumentation demands a longer time, but is efficient, provided that one follows the steps in Figure 2.X-2-20, [1] (Figs. 2.X-2-21 and 2.X-2-25).
3. From clinical and laboratory experience, it can be concluded that the sum of the two instrumentations, as shown in Figure 2.X-2-26, reduces the instrumentation time and improves the safety with regard to fracture of the instrument and root canal transport (step).

Q: *Is prior training necessary when using the mechanical or manual Universal Protaper instrument?*

A: Before attempting a new technique, it is important to first get training in order to master and understand the technique, thus diminishing failures and/or accidents. This should be done on simulated root canals, preferably on extracted teeth, to become familiar with the motor (torque and speed) and the insertion and withdrawing technique of the instrument from the root canal without getting it locked-in. With manual instrumentation, one has to develop a feel for and master the force (pressure) that is being used, to know when to turn or not to turn the instrument inside the root canal, going from left to right and returning from the right to left, until achieving a 360 degree turn, without getting the instrument locked-in, until the real working length is attained.

Q: *How many times can the Universal Protaper instruments be used?*

A: The ideal would be to use them only once, but with training and knowledge of the sequence of instruments and root canal anatomy, on average, one can use them for 5 to 8 molars. Vieira et al.[12], in 2007, in a study on Protaper instrument resistance to fatigue, conducted in patients whose root canals had been instrumented by an experienced endodontist and by undergraduate students without any experience, concluded that with experience, resistance to fatigue was reduced, but no significant change was observed between the instruments used for root canal preparation of 5 and 8 molars.

Q: *Can Gates-Glidden burs and stainless steel type K files be used together with Universal Protaper instruments?*

A: Mechanical and manual nickel and titanium rotary instruments should be used only after the root canal has been initially prepared with stainless steel type K files (10 and 15). Gates-Glidden burs can help widening the cervical and middle root canal, when necessary.

Q: *Is filling with a tapered single cone better than the lateral condensation technique?*

A: There are few studies in the literature comparing the efficacy of the sealing capacity of root canals filled with a single tapered gutta-percha cone and active lateral condensation. Some studies have demonstrated statistically that there is no significant difference (Wu et al.[13], 2003; Zmener et al.[14], 2005; Sagsem et al.[8], 2006; Monticelli et al.[5], 2007). In a recent study, Souza et al.[11], 2008, demonstrated that the lateral condensation procedures are not standardized, reaching a gutta-percha density of 71 to 87% in the apical region, in addition to the possibility of the spacers leaving defects in the gutta-percha material. The technique can easily be used for filling with a single tapered cone, using smooth lateral condensation, when this is dictated by the (wide and oval) root canal.

References

1. Aguirre Balseca GM. Avaliação microscópica do preparo apical de canais radiculares curvos pela instrumentação manual rotatória e mecanizada rotatória e oscilatória utilizando o sistema ProTaper Universal. 2008. 135f. Tese (Doutorado em Endodontia) – Faculdade de Odontologia de Araraquara, Universidade Estadual Paulista, Araraquara, 2008.
2. Dentsply Maillefer. ProTaper Universal. Ballaigues – Switzerland, 2007. Folder.
3. Dentsply Maillefer. ProTaper Universal: a melhor performance em qualquer circunstância. Petrópolis, 2007. Folder.
4. Kim HC. et al. Comparison of forces generated during root canal shaping and residual stresses of three nickel-titanium rotary files by using a three-dimensional finite-element analysis. J Endod, Chicago, v.34, p.743-747, Jun. 2008.
5. Monticelli F. et al. Sealing properties of two contemporary single-cone obturation systems. Int Endod J, Oxford, v. 40, p. 374-85, May 2007.
6. Pasqualini D. et al. Hand-operated and rotary ProTaper instruments: a comparison of working time and number of rotations in simulated root canals. J Endod, Chicago, v.34, p.314-317, Mar. 2008.
7. Perassi FT. et al. Estudo morfológico da resposta tecidual a quatro cimentos endodônticos. Rev Odont Unesp, v.37, n.º 2, abr./jun. 2008. No prelo.
8. Sagsen B, Ozgür E, Kahraman Y, Rucoblu H. Evaluation of microleakage of roots filled with different techniques with a computerized fluid filtration technique. J Endod, Chicago, v.32, p.1168-1170, Dec. 2006.
9. Silva PT. et al. Evaluation of cell culture cytotoxicity of new root canal ealers. Braz Dent J, Ribeirão Preto, 2008. No prelo.
10. Souza EM. et al. Comparability of results from two leakage models. Oral Surg. Oral Med. Oral Pathol. Oral Radiol. Endod, St. Louis, v.106, p.309-313, Aug. 2008.
11. Souza EM. et al. Effects of different techniques and area on the quality of laterally compacted root fillings. Int Endod J, Oxford, 2008. In press.
12. Vieira EP. et al. Influence of multiple clinical use on fatigue resistance of ProTaper rotary nickel-titanium instruments. Int Endod J, Oxford, v.41, p.163-172, Aug. 2008.
13. Wu MK. et al. Fluid movement along the coronal two-thirds of root fillings placed by three different gutta-percha techniques. Int Endod J, Oxford, v.36, p.533-540, Aug. 2003.
14. Zmener O, Pameijer CH, Macri E. Evaluation of the apical in root canals prepared with a new rotary system and obturated with a methacrylate based endodontic sealer: an in vitro study. J Endod, Chicago, v.31, p.392-395, May 2005.

2.X-3

Rotary System Twisted File

Richard Mounce
Renato de Toledo Leonardo

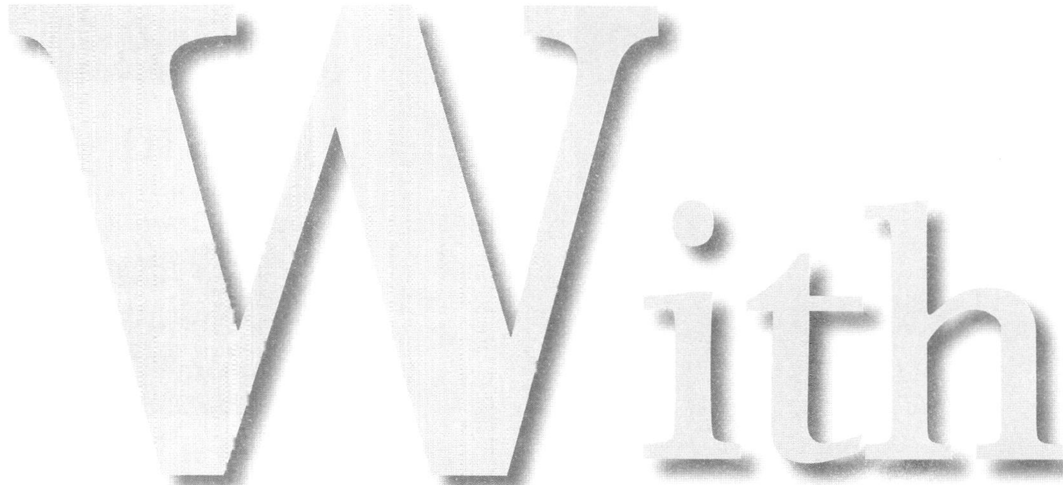

the exception of the Light Speed LSX* instruments, which are manufactured by stamping nickel titanium (NT)[3], the other nickel-titanium rotary instrument systems available on the market are manufactured by lathe, which grinds and machines cross and longitudinal sections of NT[4] wires. This machining process has two primary limitations. The first is that it impedes the making of possible forms and designs that could be made from NT[5] wires. The second limitation is that the procedure results in microfractures in the active portion, which act as a point of stress concentration, creating a scenario of instrument fracture when it is submitted to excessive torsion or cyclic fatigue[6].

The Twisted** rotary system is composed of five files manufactured from torqued NT alloy (Figs. 2.X-3-1, 2.X-3-2 and 2.X-3-3), which is capable of being twisted, provided that an intermediate crystal phase, called Rhombohedra (R) is obtained by heat treatment. The R phase is an intermediate crystalline structural phase of the austenite and martensite phases[1,2]. At room temperature, the NT alloy cannot be twisted if it is in the austenite or martensite phase. With the alloy in the R phase, reached by heating and cooling, it is possible to twist the instrument and create grooves and cutting teeth. It is important to emphasize that with this manufacturing procedure no microfractures are created (Fig. 2.X-3-4). Moreover, the Twisted instruments are submitted to deoxidation process, which maintains the hardness and sharpness of the cutting blade.

* Discus Dental Products, Culver City, CA-USA.
** SybronEndo, Orange CA, USA.

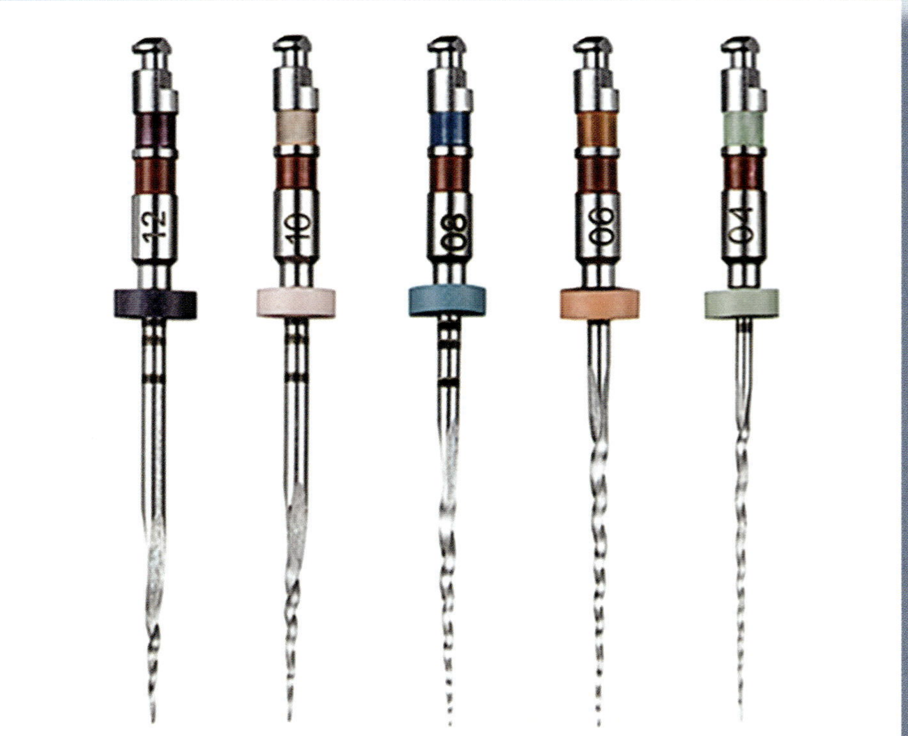

FIG. 2.X-3-1

Twisted files (TF) (SybronEndo Orange Ca-USA).

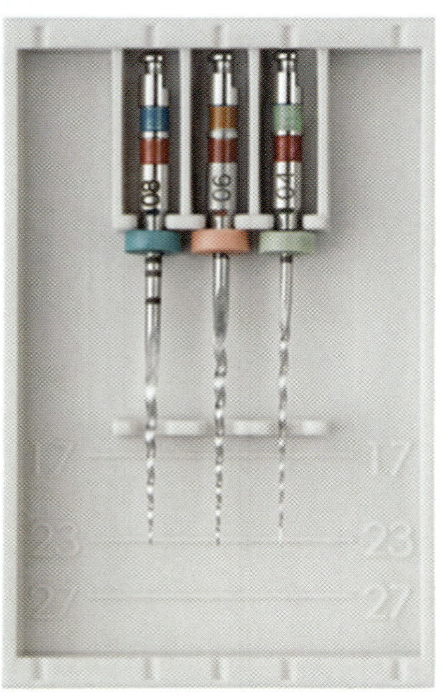

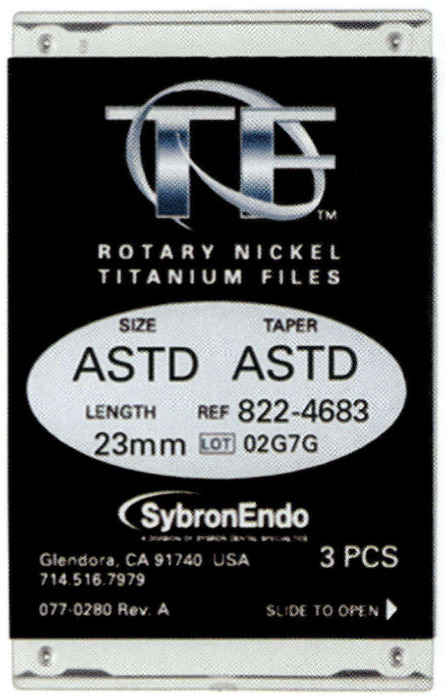

FIG. 2.X-3-2

Small box with files TF .04, .06, .08 mm/mm.

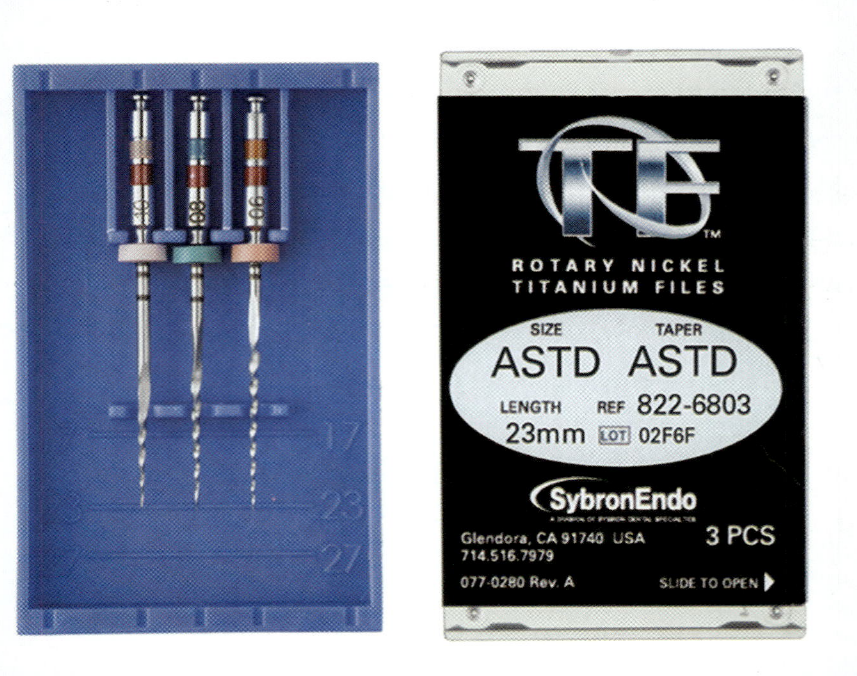

FIG. 2.X-3-3

Large box with files TF .06, .08, .10 mm/mm.

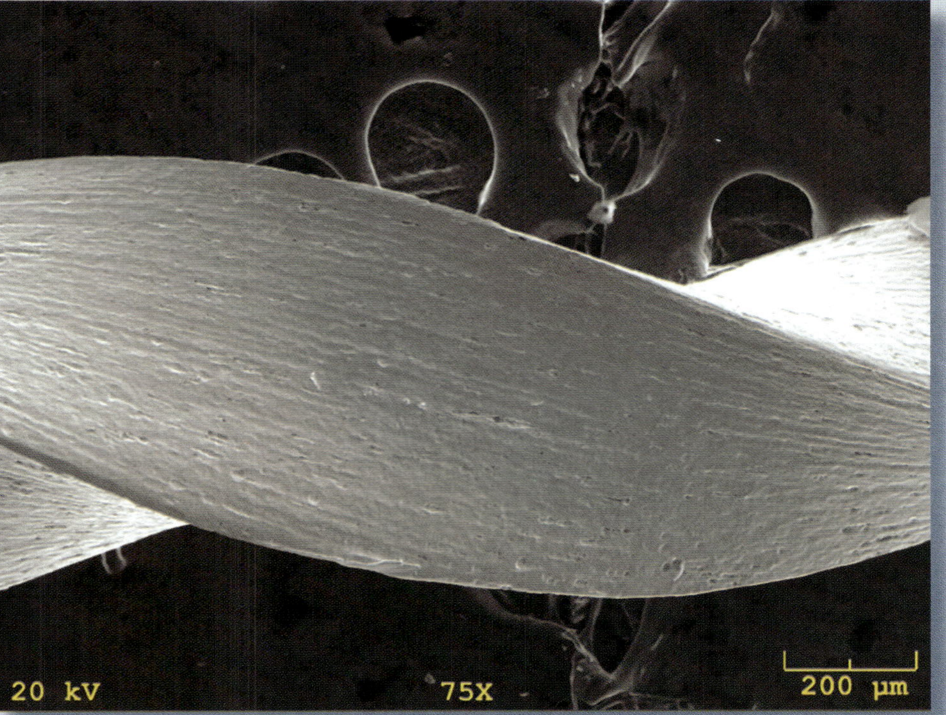

FIG. 2.X-3-4

Scanning Electronic Microscopy image of TF file.

The manufacturing process that creates the Twisted instrument results in one with several exceptional functional abilities, which differentiates it from other rotary instruments, such as:

1. During routine clinical work, in 1/3 of cases in which endodontic treatment is indicated, only one Twisted instrument is used, provided that the apical preparation does not exceed 0.25 mm in diameter. In these cases, the instrument of choice is frequently No. 25, with a 0.08 mm/mm or 25-.08 taper.
2. Another third of the clinical routine can be performed with only 2 instruments, frequently the 25-.08 and/or the 25-.10.
3. The last third, representing atresic root canals, requires 3 instruments: 25-.10, 25-.08 and 25-.06, while only in exception, in cases of very complex anatomy, more than 3 instruments are required, and the apical widening limit is always up to 0.25 mm.
4. Root canal preparation can be completed with a minimum number of insertions. With straight, wide root canals, only one instrument and 3 or 4 insertions are sufficient.
5. While many practitioners would like a more apical widening than the classical norm recommended by the endodontic literature, others differ on this point. It must be emphasized that with the Twisted instruments, the limit and real working length are more easily, quickly, safely and efficiently reached with an instrument that has an active point of 0.25 mm and tapers of 0.10 and 0.08 mm/mm, than with other systems.
6. Further to the explanation in topic 5, as the Twisted instruments are extremely flexible and fracture resistant, it is not only possible to achieve the real working length with instrument No. 25, but it is possible to widen the apical preparation with Instruments that have large tapers. Normally, with the use of machined instruments in root canals of moderate anatomic complexity, the apical preparation is performed with instruments that have tapers of up to 0.06 mm/mm. Whereas, when using machined instruments in cases of great anatomic complexity, tapers exceeding 0.04 mm/mm must not be used in apical preparation. When using Twisted instruments, however, even in cases of considerable anatomic complexity, apical preparation can be performed with instruments that have tapers greater than 0.06 mm/mm.

FACTORS THAT OPTIMIZE THE USE OF TWISTED INSTRUMENTS

1. The instrumentation sequence should preferably be crown-apex; that is, first the cervical third is enlarged, followed by the middle and finally, the apical third. In the cervical portion straight access preparation is important. In short, one should remove the dentinal triangle, which impedes the free and direct entry of instruments into the cervical third. The better and more efficiently this task is performed, the easier it will be to reach the middle thirds and apical thirds, without iatrogenic

risks. Irrespective of the anatomic portion to be worked on, the root canal must have been instrumented with a manual instrument No.15 at a minimum; either manually or by oscillatory instrumentation. Obviously, it the root canal diameter is wider than 0.15 mm in the apical third, this stage is unnecessary. When using the instrument No. 15 it is possible to create a glide pathway, which is imperative for the subsequent use of rotary instruments; with the same instrument, it is necessary to perform apical patency.

3. Although it is not a sine qua non condition, root canal visualization can be optimized with an operating microscope, which will greatly facilitate endodontic treatment.
4. After each insertion of the Twisted instrument, copious irrigation and a review with a small diameter manual instrument (Numbers 06, 08 or 10) are required. The purpose of the review is only to remove the residues and to make sure that there has been no deviation.
5. The tactile insertion of Twisted instruments must be delicate, passive and relatively slow (from 2 to 3 seconds), always with pecking movements.

GENERAL INFORMATION ON USE

1. Generally, the instrumentation must follow the crown-apex direction, from an instrument with larger taper to one with smaller taper. In wide root canals, one must start with instruments that have a 0.10 mm/mm taper; in canals with little anatomic complexity, with instruments that have a 0.08 mm/mm taper, and in those that are complex, with instruments that have 0.06 mm/mm taper.
2. After making the glide pathway manually or by oscillatory means, the Twisted instrument must be inserted with movements of small amplitude and penetration depth, every 2 mm, in the direction of the apex. In case one does not feel that it is necessary to increase pressure significantly, one can continue to use the same instrument until the apex is reached; otherwise an instrument with a smaller taper must be used afterwards.
3. In cases of curvature in more than two planes, after preparing the glide pathway, one must reach the real working length in the crown apex direction with Twisted instrument .04, and afterwards increase the taper in the crown-apex direction, with apical widening using instruments with a .06 and .08 mm/mm tapers.
4. The rotation speed indicated for the system is 500 rpm.
5. The use of electric motors with torque control is not recommended. The use of a hand piece itself, and the fact that the instruments are very flexible, cause loss of tactile sensitivity. In addition to this, a wide range of different torques and the anatomic complexity, make it difficult to obtain proprioception of the system. Therefore, it is advisable to use only one torque, preferably higher than 6 N.cm, in order to become accustomed to the system.
6. Twisted instruments may be used with any electric motor, or with a hand piece with a reduction gear in a micromotor.
7. Twisted instruments are manufactured to be used in one tooth only, whether it has 1 or 5 root canals. The use of these instruments in more than one tooth is contrary to manufacturer's recommendations.
8. For lubrication during instrumentation, a 5.25% sodium hypochlorite (USP) or a 2% chlorhexidine solution is recommended. EDTA gel or other similar substances are not necessary.
9. In order to widen the apical preparation with instruments larger than a number 25, the use of K3 or Lightspeed numbers 30, 35 or larger instruments is recommended. It is always important to widen the apical third with 5 instruments above the initial apical instrument (IAI) or anatomic (IA) (whichever instrument first fits the anatomic diameter at the real working length of the tooth).

10. The Twisted instruments may be used in conjunction with any other system. However, this defeats the purpose of using an instrument with different standards with regard to manufacture (machined or twisted).
11. Since instruments with large tapers are used, it is not necessary to use Gates-Glidden, Largo or Peeso drills.
12. When filling root canals prepared with Twisted instruments, it is recommended to use cones with the same taper as the largest diameter instrument last used to the real working length. For example, if the last instrument used to the real working length was a 25/.10, the cone must be a 25-.10 (Figs. 2.X-3-5A-F).

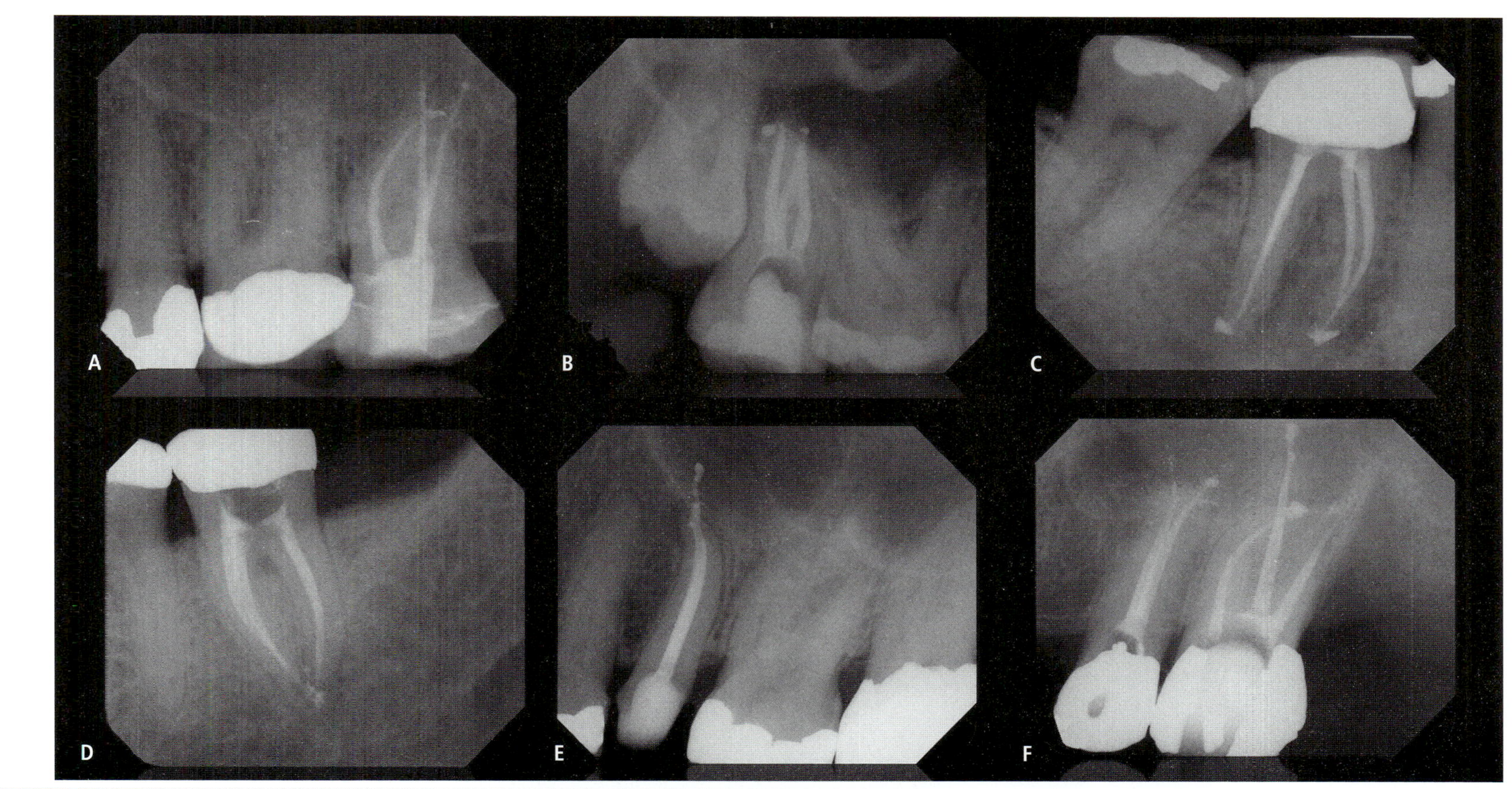

FIGS. 2.X-3-5A-F

Clinical cases in which instrumentation was performed with TF.

References

1. Gambarini G, Gerosa R, De Luca M, Garala M, Testarelli L. Mechanical properties of a new and improved nickel-titanium alloy for endodontic use: an evaluation of file flexibility. Oral Surg, Oral Med, Oral Pathol, Oral Radiol, Endod, v.105, n.6, p.798-800, 2008.
2. Gambarini G, Grande NM, Plotino G, Somma F, Garala M, De Luca M, Testarelli L. Fatigue resistance of engine-driven rotary nickel-titanium instruments produced by new manufacturing methods. J Endod, v.34, n.8, p.1003-1005, 2008.
3. Iqbal MK, Banfield B, Lavorini A, Bachstein B. A comparison of lightspeed LS1 and lightspeed LSX NiTi rotary instruments in apical transportation and length. J Endod, v.33, n.3, p.268-271, 2007.
4. Leonardo MR, Leonardo RT. Sistemas rotatórios em endodontia. Instrumentos de níquel-titânio. Artes Médicas: São Paulo, 2002. 323 p.
5. Melo MC, Pereira ES, Viana AC, Fonseca AM, Buono VT, Bahia MG. Dimensional characterization and mechanical behaviour of K3 rotary instruments. Int Endod J, v.41, n.4, p.329-338, 2008.
6. Ounsi HF, Al-Shalan T, Salameh Z, Grandini S, Ferrari M. Quantitative and qualitative elemental analysis of different nickel-titanium rotary instruments by using scanning electron microscopy and energy dispersive spectroscopy. J. Endod., v.34, n.1, p.53-55, 2008.

2.XI

Use of mineral trioxide aggregate (MTA) in Endodontics

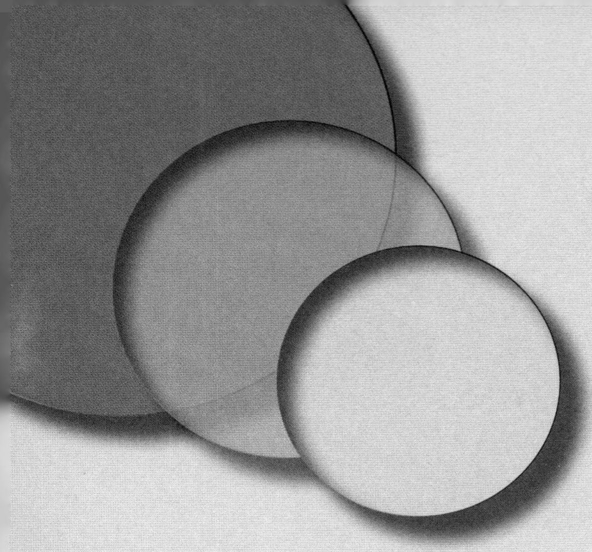

Clóvis Monteiro Bramante
Ivaldo Gomes de Moraes
Alexandre Silva Bramante

In the early 1990s, an experimental material for use in endodontics was developed at the University of Loma Linda, California, USA, by Mohamoud Torabinejad, and named mineral trioxide aggregate (MTA). In 1993, Lee, Monsef, Torabinejad[99], for the first time reported the use of MTA in root perforations. After numerous publications by the author, either as a single authors or in participation with others [1,11,15,91,93,94,99,103,110,123,134, 135,136,137,138,139,140] MTA was finally evaluated and approved in 1998 by the a FDA (*US Food and Drugs Administration*), and in 1999, a gray-colored material, under the trade name Pro Root MTA®, was commercially launched by Dentsply/Tulsa Dental (Oklahoma, USA). Subsequently in 2004 white MTA was launched by Dentsply/Tulsa Dental (Oklahoma, USA).

In Brazil, in 2001, the industry Angelus Soluções Odontológicas (Londrina, PR), was the first to offer MTA, labeled MTA-Angelus®, originally gray-colored, and later in 2004, white-colored MTA-Angelus®. In 2004 also, in Argentina, EGEO launched commercial MTA under the label CPM. This was also the first company to launch an MTA-based cement for root canal filling, called Endo CPM sealer[27]. At present, MTA is offered in white and gray, and the fundamental difference is the presence of iron oxide in the first[16,25,26,45,55]. Basically all these products have the same composition as the MTA Pro-Root (Dentsply/Tulsa), with small variations of some of the components.

MTA is a powder composed of fine hydrophilic particles, mainly of tricalcium silicate, dicalcium silicate, tricalcium aluminate, tricalcium ferroaluminate, tetracalcium, tricalcium oxide, di-hydrated calcium sulphate, as well as bismuth oxide, which is added to make the aggregate radiopaque[45,46,55,65,68,95,126,131,136,145].

MTA has been extensively evaluated and has shown to be an excellent endodontic sealer, capable of providing a seal of communications between the pulp cavity and the external surface of the tooth, both of the crown and root. Initially used for sealing dental perforations, it subsequently was introduced for different clinical situations, such as indirect or direct pulp protection, internal or external resorptions, apexification, root canal filling, and in apiectomy surgery, as a retrograde filling material.

Mainly composed of mineral oxides, when mixed with water MTA is converted into a colloidal gel, which crystallizes, and later expands, promotion excellent sealing action[40,59,111,131].

According to Torabinejad et al.[136], the initial pH of MTA is 10.2, and after 3 hours, it increases to 12.5, and remains constant. Because of this high pH, close to that of calcium hydroxide, it stimulates mineralization when used as reparative material. The calcium and phosphorous ions, constituents of mineralized dental tissues, are the main components of MTA and an influential factor in the repair process. Also the material has excellent biocompatibility, being well tolerated when placed in contact, with organic cells and tissues[56,78,90,91,93,110,115].

The action mechanism of MTA is similar to that of calcium hydroxide. MTA contains calcium oxide, and when mixed with water, forms calcium hydroxide. This dissociates into Ca- ions and OH-ions. When the Ca- ions come into contact with connective tissue, they cause an area of necrosis and form carbon dioxide. This and calcium hydroxide form calcite crystals (calcium carbonate) that serve as the core for calcification. The alkalinity of the medium stimulates the connective tissue secretion of glycoprotein, called fibronectin; this together with the calcite crystals stimulate the formation of Type 1 collagen, which together with calcium, induces mineralization[81,148].

Figure 2.XI-1 shows a diagram of the action mechanism of MTA.

ACTION MECHANISM OF MTA

MTA (calcium oxide) + Water ⇨ Calcium hydroxide

Calcium Hydroxide ⇨ dissociation of Ca+ and OH- ions

Ca+ Ions ⇨ Tissue necrosis ⇨ Carbon dioxide

Carbon dioxide + Calcium Hydroxide ⇨ Calcite crystals (Calcium carbonate) ⇨ Serve as calcification core

Alkalinity of the medium ⇨ Connnective tissue secretes Glycoprotein (Fibronectin)

Fibronectin + Calcite crystals ⇨ Deposit collagen type I

Collagen type I + Calcium ⇨ Mineralization

FIG. 2.XI-1
Action mechanism of MTA.

With regard to its clinical use, MTA has the advantage of not requiring a completely dry field, and can be used in locations with moisture, while excess MTA can easily be removed with moist gauze.

The difficulties practitioners commonly find are related to the setting time, which is very long. Furthermore, its sandy consistency makes clinical handling and placement and condesing in the desired location very difficult.

These problems have generated numerous research projects, particularly in Brazil, with the aim to resolve or diminish the problems. Thus, the goal of diminishing the quantity of calcium sulphate, or completely removing it, was to accelerate the setting time. The objective of adding calcium chloride to accelerate the setting time and make it more workable, and the use of different vehicles to facilitate handing, was to transform the material into a more user-friendly product that was easier to work with[29,30,31,66,83,88,92,100,113,133,143].

Based on a stucy by Wucherpfenning & Green[147], in 1999, who reported that MTA basically possessed the same composition as Portland cement, various studies have been conducted with the objective to compare the two products, while aiming at diminishing the cost of MTA and making it more accessible to the general practitioner[25,26,30,31,40,41,43,45,49,53,54,59,66,68,76,80,83,95,107,113,145].

The ideal material for use in endodontics should present the following requisites:

- Be biocompatible;
- Offer an adequate setting time;
- Induce repair by mineralized tissue formation;
- Have antimicrobial properties;
- Have dimens onal stability;
- Offer slight expansion during the setting period;
- Offer good sealing;
- Have low solubility in tissue fluids;
- Be easy to handle;
- Be radiopaque.

Among the mineral trioxide aggregate-based products available, the following are outstanding: ProRoot MTA from Dentsply/Tulsa Dental (Fig. 2.XI-2), the MTA, from Angelus, in the original (Fig. 2.XI-3) and in the new packaging (Fig. 2.XI-4), CPM (Fig. 2.XI-5) and Endo CPM Sealer, from EGEO (Fig. 2.XI-6). The latter, since it is indicated for filling root canals, has a special liquid in its package, which differs from the others that use distilled water for preparing the cement.

Recently, new mineral trioxide aggregate-based products have been developed, such as Dental Crete, light polymerizable MTA, MTA Obtura (Fig. 2.XI-7) and MTA Bio (Fig. 2.XI-8), the former two in the United States and the latter two in Brazil. The studies conducted with these material have shown promising results[50,51,54,61,67].

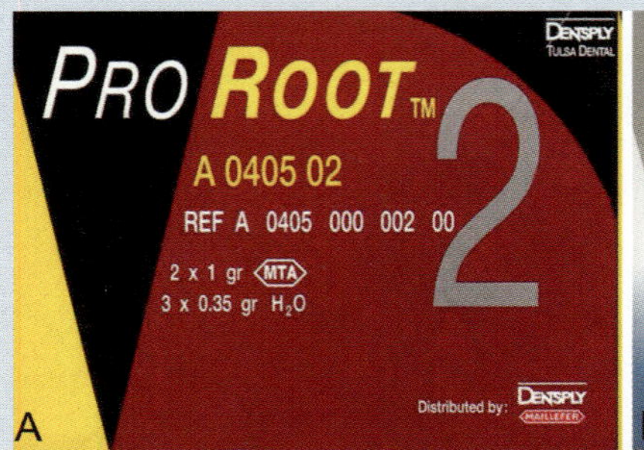

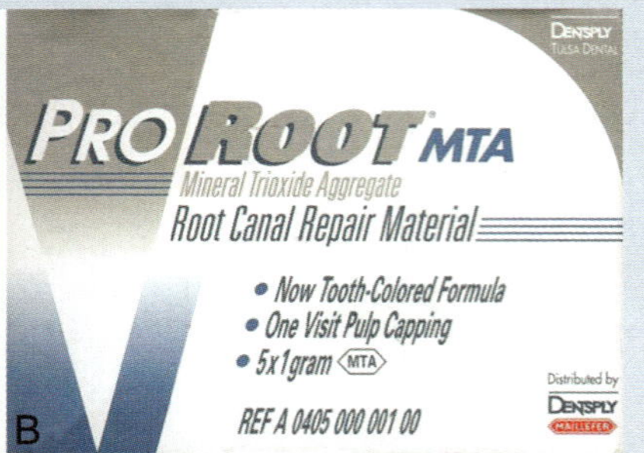

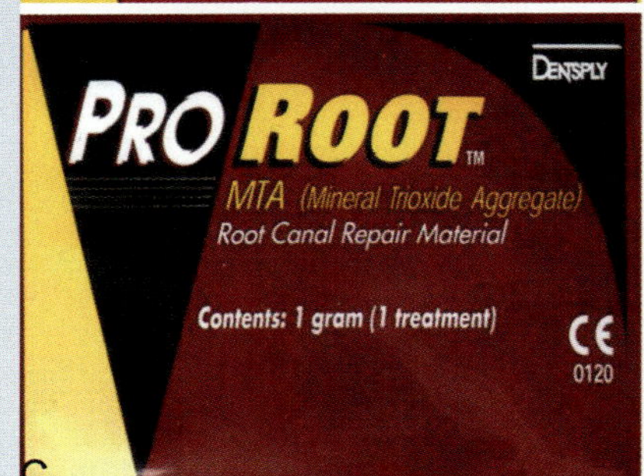

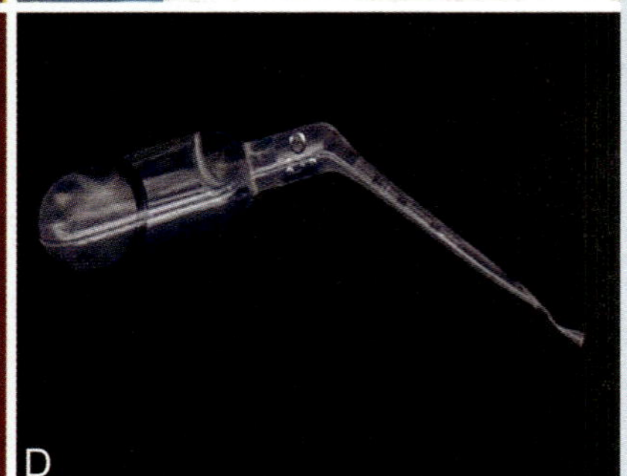

FIG. 2.XI-2

ProRoot MTA (gray and white), from Dentsply/Tulsa Dental, USA.

Composition of ProRoot MTA (Dentsply/Tulsa Dental, USA)	
Powder	
Portland Cement	
Tricalcium silicate	
Dicalcium Silicate	75%
Tricalcium Aluminate	
Tetracalcium Ferroaluminate	
Bismuth oxide	20%
Di-hydrated calcium sulphate	5%
Liquid – Distilled Water	

FIG. 2.XI-3

MTA (gray and white), from Angelus.

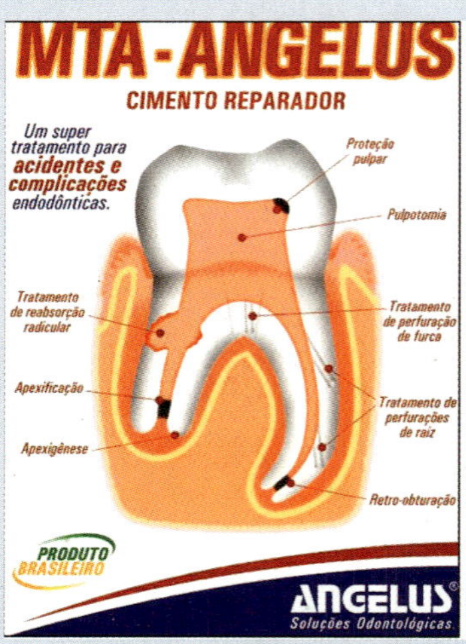

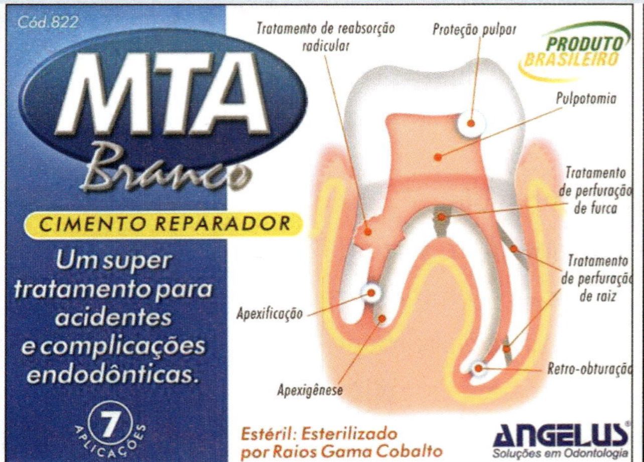

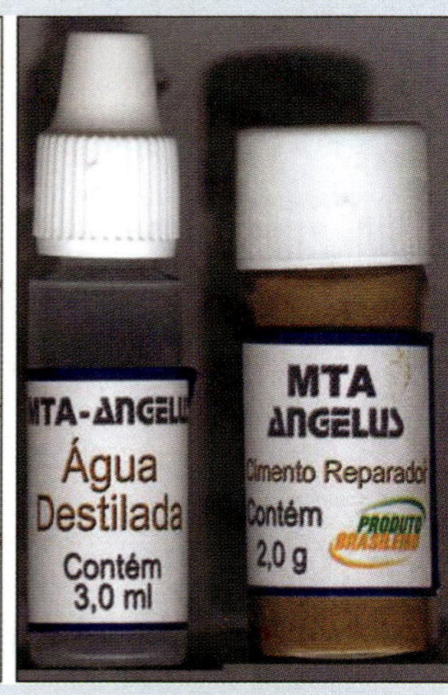

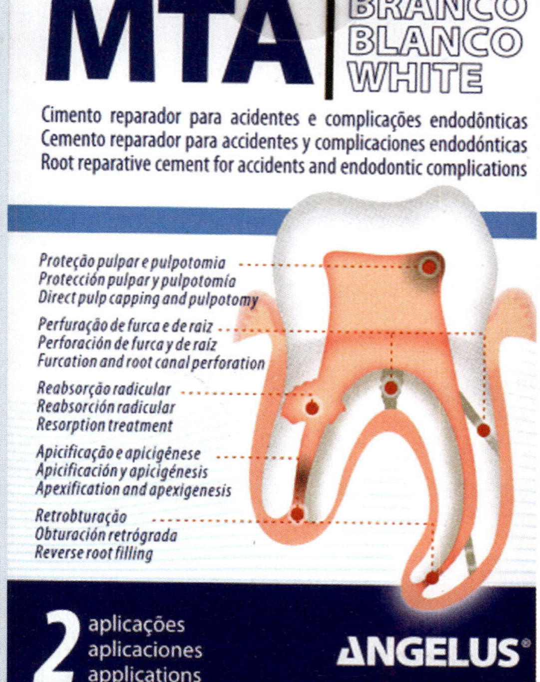

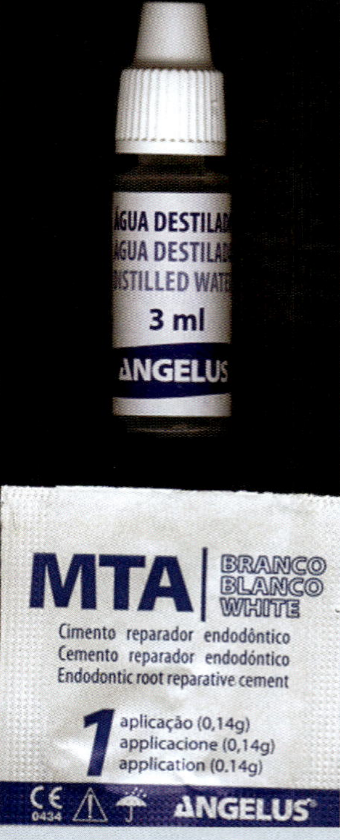

FIG. 2.XI-4

New packaging of MTA Angelus.

Composition of MTA (Angelus, Brazil)	
Powder	
Portland cement	
Tricalcium silicate	
Dicalcium silicate	80%
Tricalcium aluminate	
Tetracalcium ferroaluminate	
Bismuth oxide	20%
Note: This cement contains no calcium sulphate	
Liquid – Distilled water	

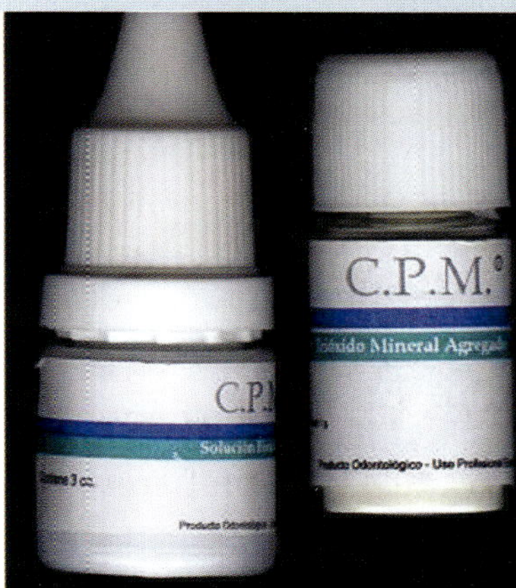

FIG. 2.XI-5

CPM from EGEO, Argentina.

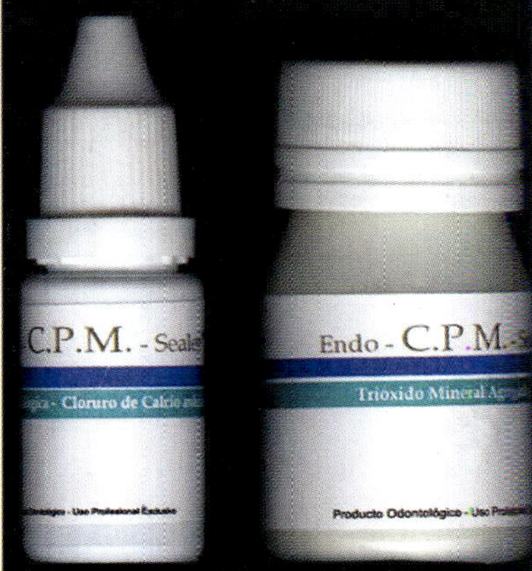

FIG. 2.XI-6

Endo CPM Sealer from EGEO, Argentina.

Composition of CPM (EGEO S, Argentina)

Powder
- Silica dioxide
- Potassium oxide
- Aluminum trioxide
- Magnesium oxide
- Calcium oxide
- Calcium carbonate
- Barium sulphate
- Bismuth trioxide
- Note: The latter two components are radiopacifiers

Liquid – Distilled water

Composition of Endo CPM Sealer (EGEO, Argentina)

Powder
- Mineral trioxide aggregate.......... 50%
- Silica dioxide
- Calcium carbonate
- Bismuth trioxide
- Barium sulphate

Liquid
- Propylene Glycol Alginate
- Propylene Glycol
- Sodium citrate
- Calcium chloride

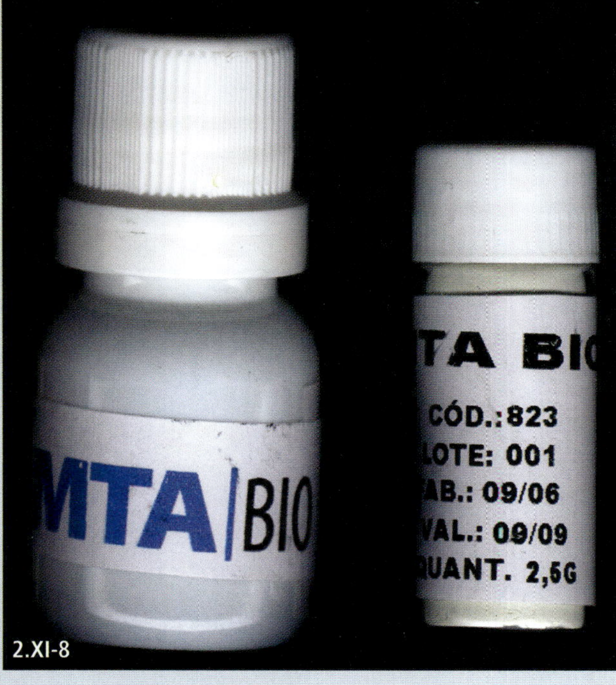

FIG. 2.XI-7

MTA Obtura from Angelus, Brazil.

FIG. 2.XI-8

MTA Bio from Angelus, Brazil.

METHOD FOR USE OF MTA

Manipulation

MTA is mixed with distilled water that comes with the product, in a ratio of 3:1 powder/liquid; a proportion that can be altered according to the location in which the material will be used [65,122]. If it is to be inserted into the pulp chamber, where access is easier, MTA can have less liquid, whereas inside the root canal, where access is more difficult, a bit more water is required to make it flow more readily (Fig. 2.XI-9).

Insertion

MTA must immediately be inserted into the location after it is prepared, to prevent it from dehydrating. Should this occur, a little liquid can be added, which has to be spatulated into the mixture. Depending on the location, MTA can be inserted with a plastic instrument (Hollenback), Dycal applicator, excavator, chisel, small amalgam delivery tip), or with a Lentulo spiral or type K file (Fig. 2.XI-10).

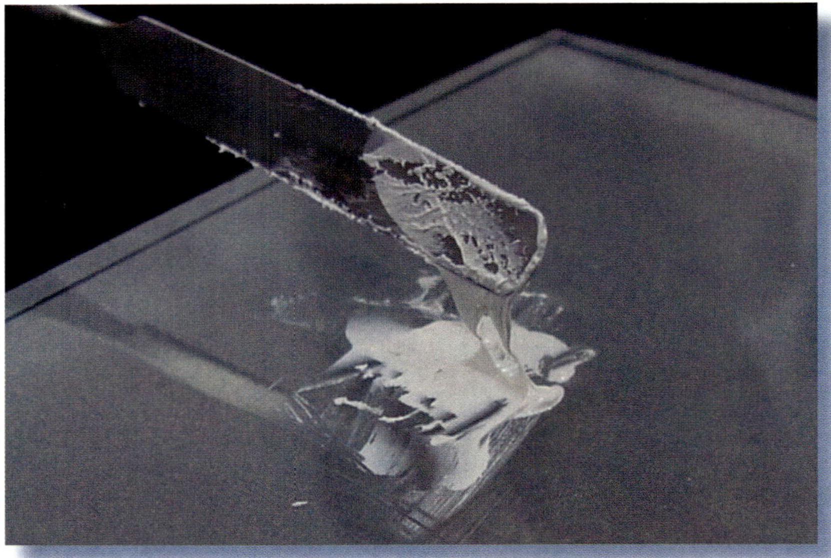

FIG. 2.XI-9
Mixture of MTA (note the consistency of the paste).

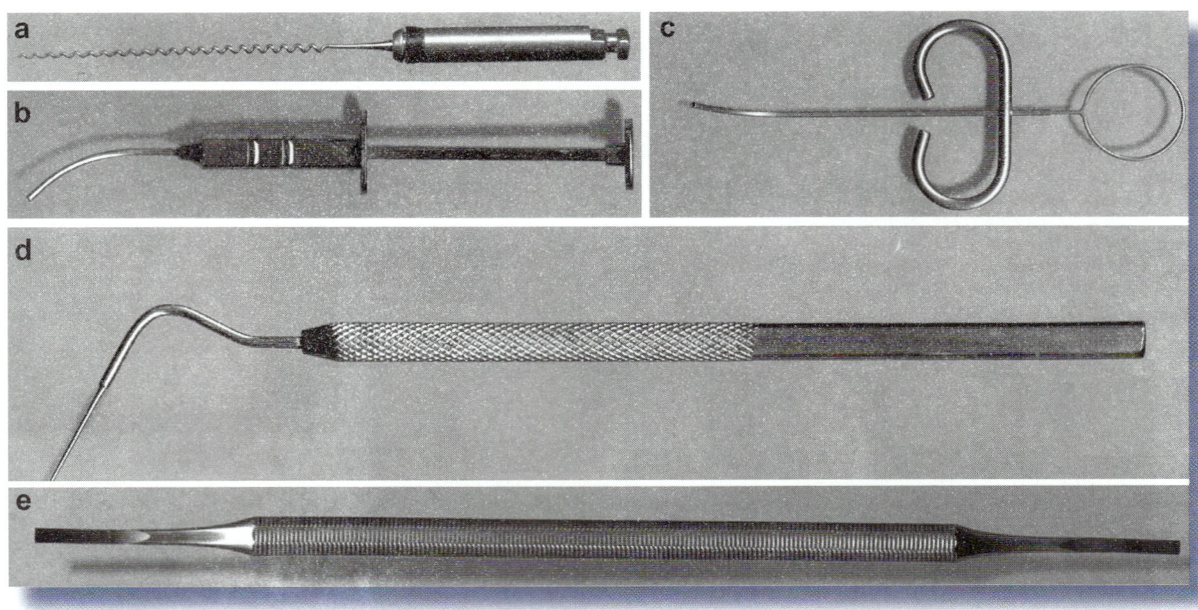

FIGS. 2.XI-10
Devices for inserting MTA:
A – Lentulo Spiral
B – Micro amalgam carrier.
C – MTA Holder.
D – Paiva Pluggers.
E – Chisel.

In the pulp chamber, a plastic instrument or excavator is used. Inside a canal a type K file or Lentulo spiral is preferred, while for a retrograde filling, a chisel or small amalgam delivery tip is used. It has also been reported that ultrasound can be used in placement[10].

CLINICAL USE OF MTA

Among the indications for MTA, the following are outstanding[21,33,34,35,81,134]:

a. Direct pulp capping;
b. Pulpotomy;
c. Incompletely formed apices;
d. Perforation;
e. Root canal filling;
f. Apiectomy surgery.
g. Root resorption;
h. Root fracture.

The different clinical applications of MTA are presented below:

a. Direct Pulp Protection (Capping)

Direct pulp protection is indicated when the pulp is accidentally exposed. After irrigating the cavity with a physiologic saline solution and hemostasis has been established, MTA is carefully applied taking care not to compress the material into pulpal tissues. Excess material that is on the surrounding dentin must be removed with a curette, and the cavity closed with IRM, a light polymerizable resin or a glass ionomer (Fig. 2.XI-11).

In direct pulp protection, MTA has been shown to be an excellent material, providing the formation of a mineralized barrier (dentin bridge)[1,2,4,44,60,76,82,86,121,124,141].

b. Pulpotomy

This is the procedure by which the coronal pulp is removed, while the root pulp is retained, and is indicated when irreversible inflammation of the coronal pulp occurs, making is possible to maintain the vitality of the root pulp, particularly in teeth with incompletely formed apices, allowing for root formation to continue.

After removing the roof of the pulp chamber, the coronal pulp is curetted, followed by irrigation with physiological saline to stop hemorrhage. A corticosteroid medication (Otosporin or Maxitrol) can be placed on the pulp stump for 5 minutes to minimize inflammation that will result from cutting pulp tissue.

MTA is mixed with distilled water in the recommended proportion and placed on the injured pulp, without pressure, in a thickness of approximately 3 mm. This is covered with a calcium hydroxide paste of firm consistency (Dycal) and the cavity is closed with IRM (Fig. 2.XI-12). The purpose of the layer of calcium hydroxide is to prevent direct contact of the sealing material with MTA, particularly when the restoration is performed in the same session.

Soares[130], in 1996, observed similar dentin bridges in pulpotomies performed with calcium hydroxide and MTA. Whereas Holland et al.[82] (2001), who performed pulpotomies in dog teeth, found when MTA was used, better formation of a complete tubular dentin bridge was observed than in teeth with calcium hydroxide. Other authors also found MTA efficient in pulpotomies[19,29,51].

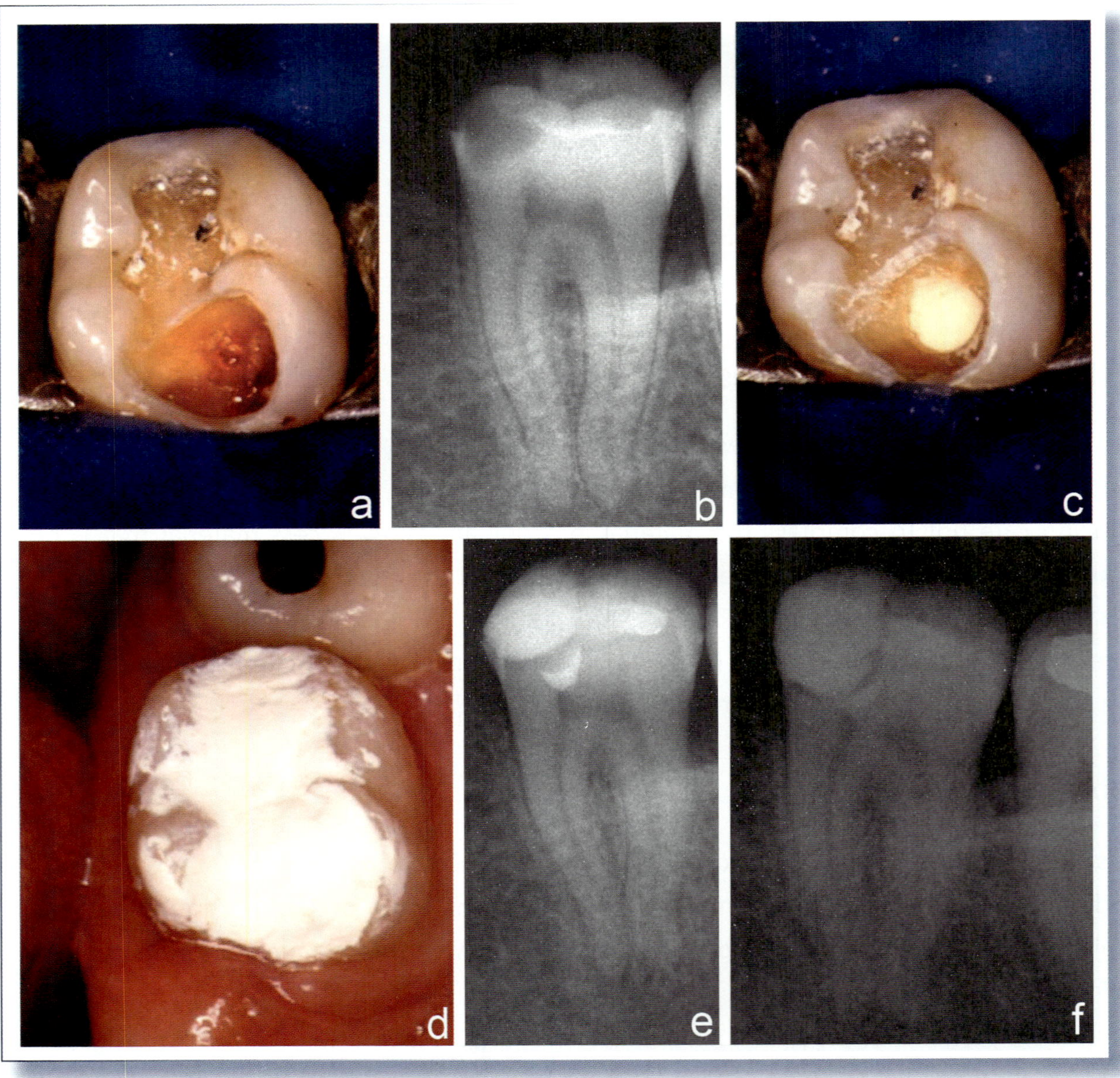

FIGS. 2.XI-11A-F

Direct pulp protection with MTA.

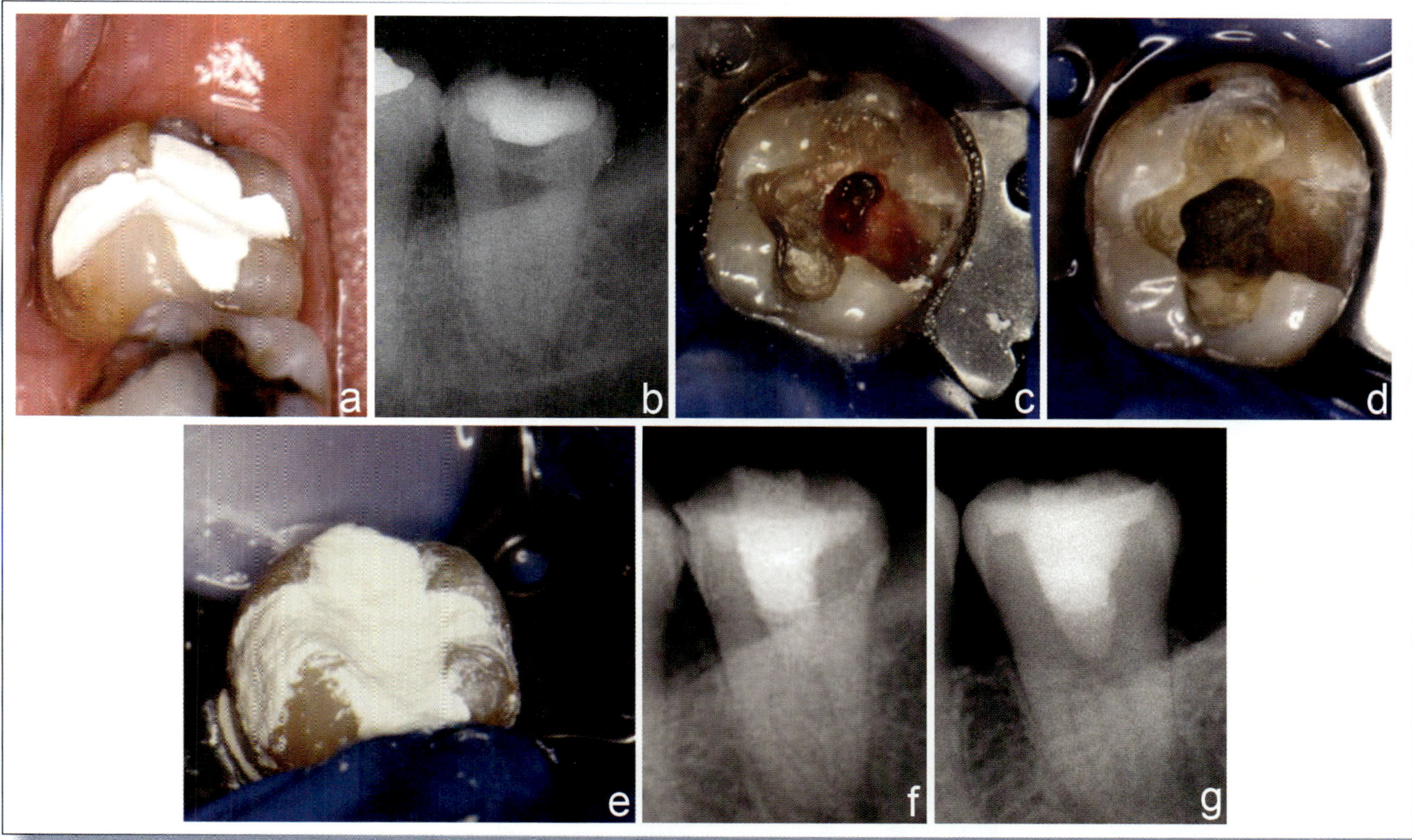

FIGS. 2.XI-12A-G
Pulpotomy with MTA.

The repair process takes place by a mineralized tissue being deposited on the root pulp remainder, isolating and protecting it (Fig. 2.XI-13).

c. Incompletely Formed Apices

The tooth with incompletely formed apices poses a serious problem for root canal treatment, as the apical region of the root is not completely formed, which makes it difficult to perform instrumentation and subsequent filling using gutta-percha cones. For these cases, MTA can be used as an apical *plug*[105]. When the canal is completely prepared (Fig. 2.XI-14A), the material is placed in the apical region with a Lentulo spiral, in a quantity that establishes a 5 mm apical plug (Figs. 2.XI-14B-C). After placement of the MTA an endodontic file wrapped in cotton is used for vertical compaction (Fig. 2.XI-14D). After this the root canal is filled with gutta-percha cones and a sealer cement. If the filling is not done during the same session, the canal can be filled with calcium hydroxide paste (Calen), which will serve as a temporary dressing (Figs. 2.XI-14A-F).

An alternative technique for making the plug is to completely fill the canal with MTA, and then remove part of it, leaving only enough for an apical plug. The technique is as follows. When the canal has been instrumented (Fig. 2-XI-15A), it is completely filled with MTA using a Lentulo spiral (Figs. 2.XI-15B-C). This is followed with a type K file (Fig. 2.XI-15D), to remove part of the material. When the desired amount of material has been removed, the MTA is compacted with a type K file wrapped in cotton, thus making the plug (Fig. 2.XI-15E). With the same type K file, now with the cotton slightly moist, all canal walls are cleaned (Fig. 2.XI-15F). This removal must be done in the same session, because if the MTA is left

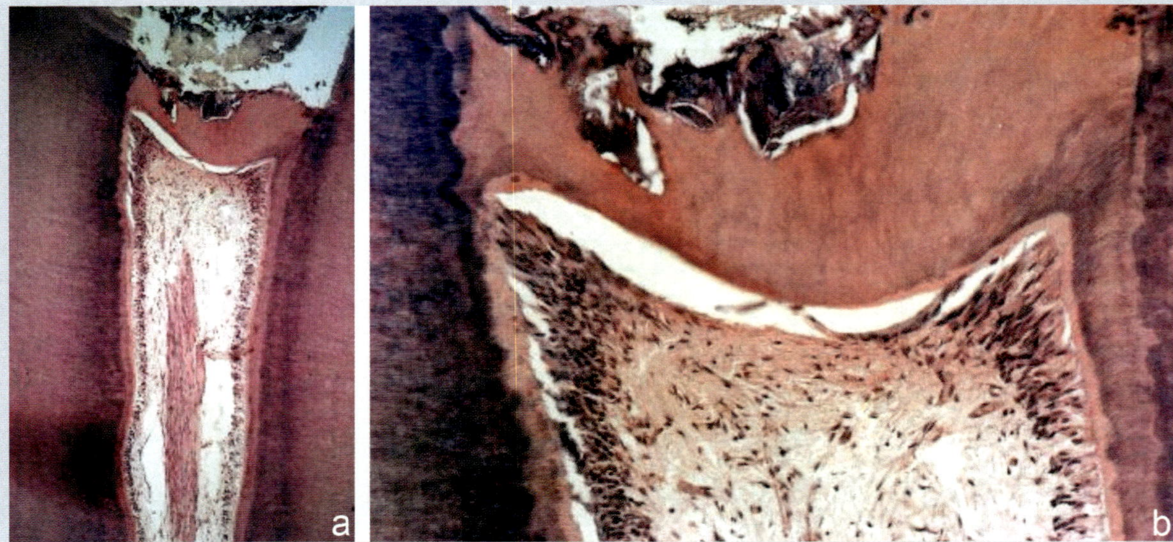

FIGS. 2.XI-13A-B

Mineralized tissue bridge after pulpotomy with MTA.

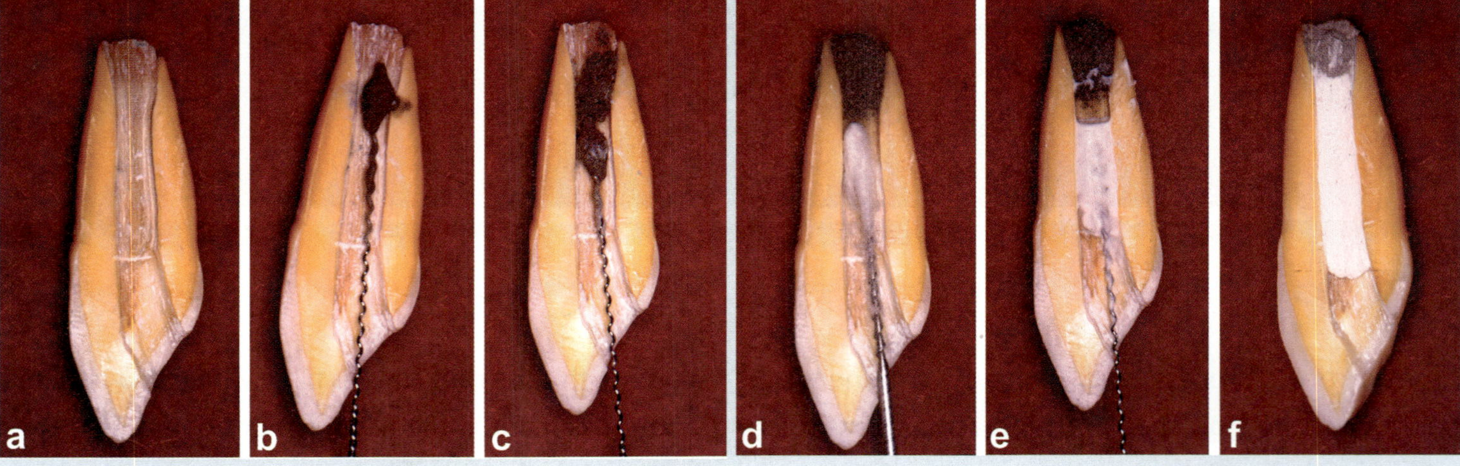

FIGS. 2.XI-14A-F

Making apical plug with the aid of Lentulo spiral and endodontic file.

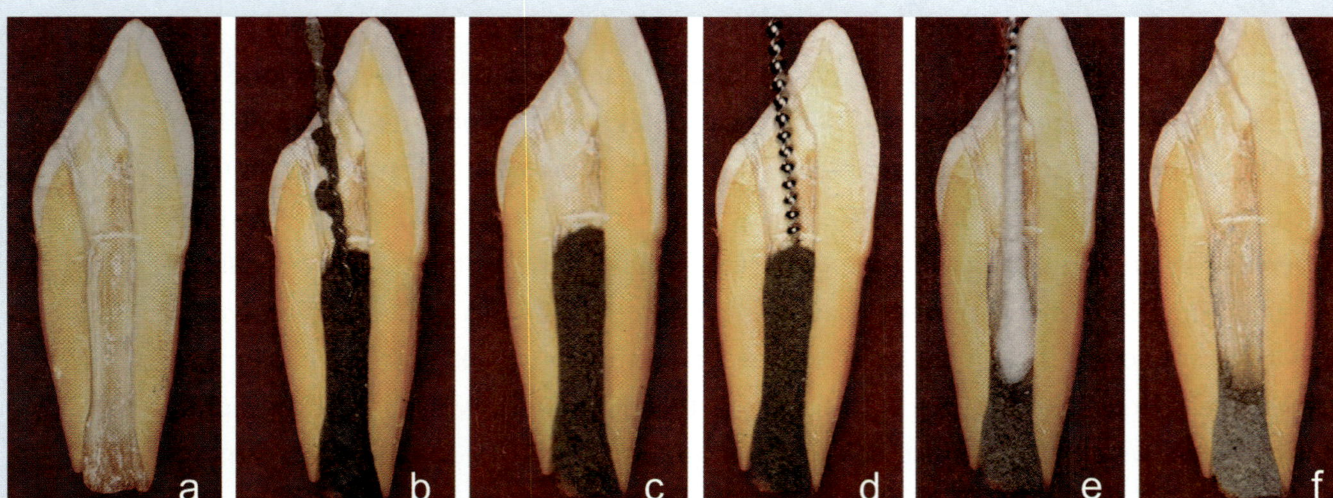

FIGS. 2.XI-15A-F

Making the plug by filling the entire canal with MTA.

in the canal and removed later, it would have set, making it difficult, if not impossible to remove. Ideally the apical plug should be 5 mm long, but it can be longer, depending on the degree of development of the root.

If the plug offers adequate resistance, the root canal filling can be done in the same session, otherwise, the remainder of the canal must be filled with calcium hydroxide paste (Calen), leaving the filling to be done in another session, thus promoting complete hardening of the MTA. It is not recommended to leave a moist cotton pellet over the MTA inside the canal, as this will influence the setting of the material.

Figure 2.XI-16 shows the treatment of a tooth with incompletely formed apices, in which an apical plug of MTA was placed and the reainder of the canal was filled with gutta-percha cones and a sealer cement.

Moroto et al.[115] observed complete apical dvelopment after the canal had been sealed with MTA. The same result was observed by other authors in teeth with incompletely formed apices [9,12,52,58,62,69,73,89,106,112,127,129].

Figure 2.XI-17 shows apical sealing with mineralized tissue in a tooth with incompletely formed apices, in which the canal was completely filled with MTA.

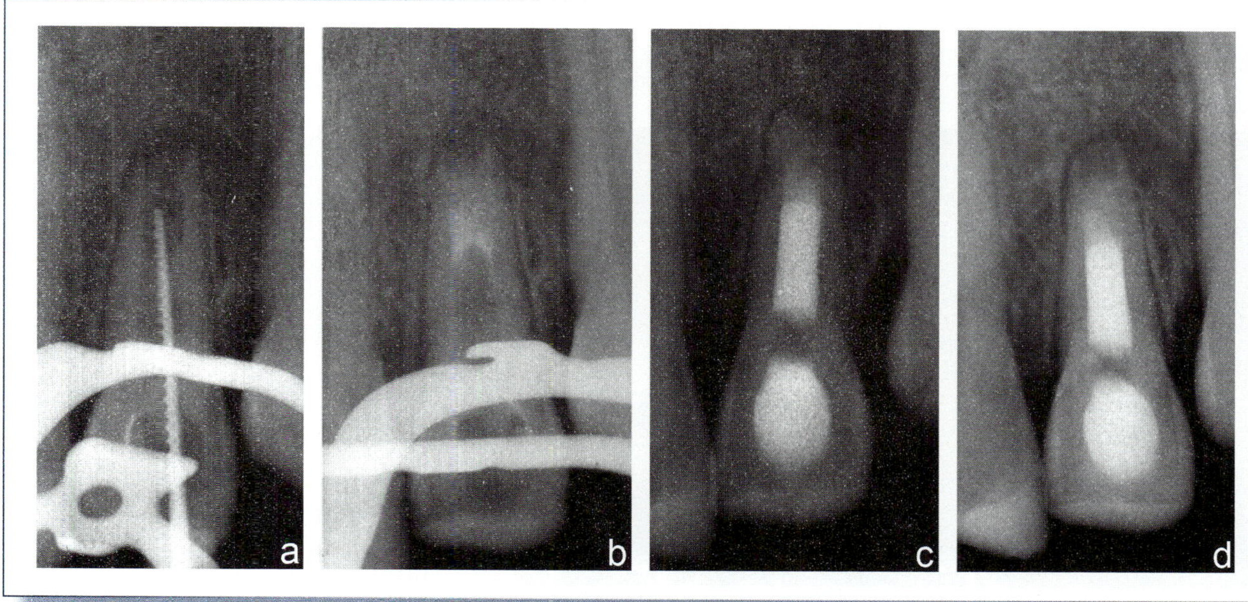

FIGS. 2.XI-16A-D

Incompletely formed apices, treated with MTA plug.

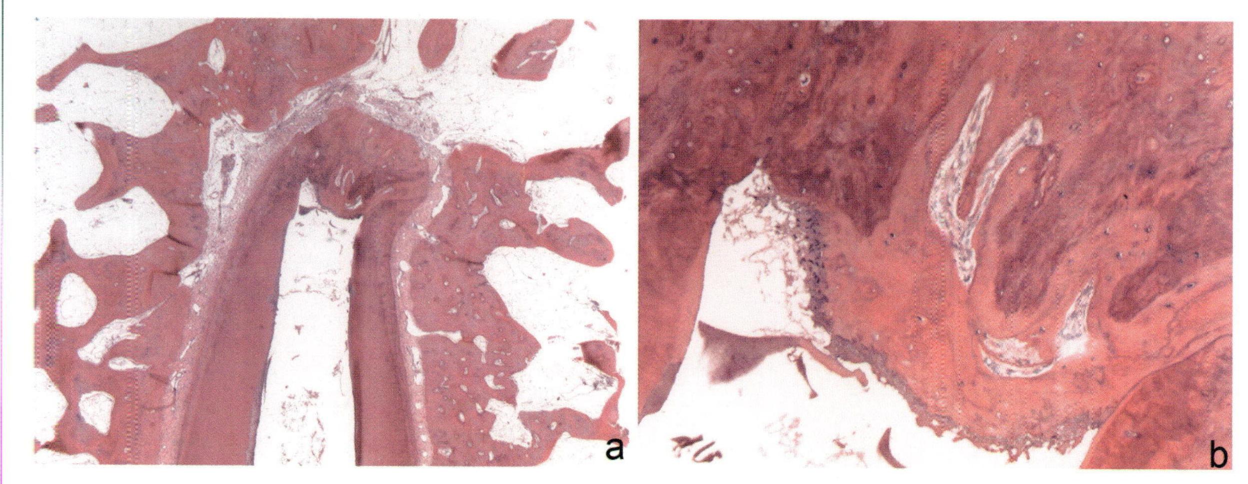

FIGS. 2.XI-17A-B

Apical sealing of tooth with Incompletely formed apices, treated with MTA.

If the apical region is not conducive for MTA placement without the risk of extravasation, a collagen matrix can be used (Fig. 2.XI-18), which is placed at the apex through the canal. After the canal has been completely prepared (Fig. 2.XI-19A), select collagen of a size that is compatible with the foraminal opening (Fig. 2.XI-19B). With the aid of a Paiva gutta-percha condenser, the collagen is inserted until it reaches the apical area where it is compacted (Figs. 2.XI-19C-D). Once compacted, MTA is inserted in the canal with a Lentulo spiral (Fig 2.XI-19E), which is condensed against the matrix with a type K file wrapped in cotton (Fig. 2.XI-19F), thus obtaining the apical plug (Fig. 2.XI-19G). Subsquently the root canal is filled with gutta-percha cones and a sealer cement (Fig. 2.XI-19H). Figure 2.XI-20 shows the clinical sequence of making the apical matrix with collagen.

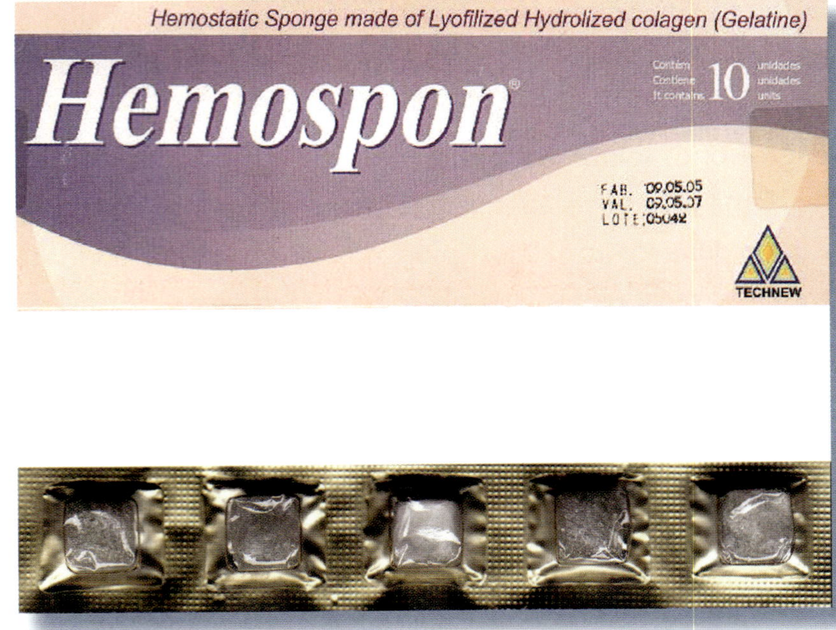

FIG. 2.XI-18

Collagen (Hemospon) used as apical matrix in a tooth with Incompletely formed apices.

FIGS. 2.XI-19A-H

Sequence for making apical matrix with collagen, making the MTA plug and filling the canal.

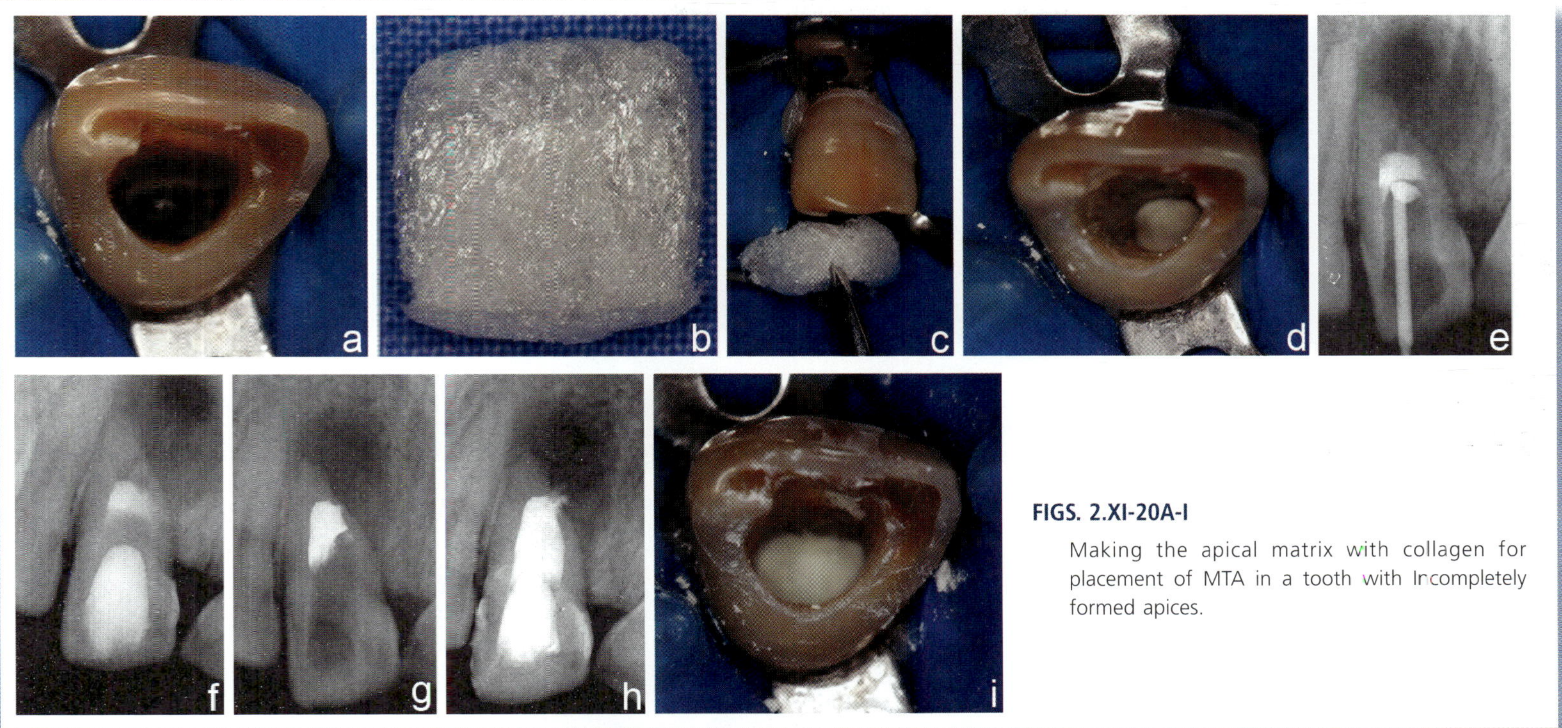

FIGS. 2.XI-20A-I

Making the apical matrix with collagen for placement of MTA in a tooth with Incompletely formed apices.

d. Perforation

Perforation is a communication between the pulp space and the external surface of the tooth, which can occur at any time during endodontic treatment. It can be at the level of the pulp chamber or root canal[33].

The treatment of a perforation with MTA, as with calcium hydroxide, should only be indicated in intraosseous perforations. When perforation occurs, the sooner treatment is performed, the greater the possibility of success. When a perforation is at the pulp chamber level, the perforation area must be cleaned by irrigating with physiological saline. When hemorrhage is controlled MTA is applied a sufficient quantity of material is used to seal the perforation and it is compacted with a small cotton pellet. If the tooth was exposed to the oral cavity and the area is contaminated, then after cleaning the pulp chamber, it is important to place antiseptic medication (camphorated paramonochlorophenol) to seal the tooth. In the next session, the medication is removed, the chamber irrigated and an aqueous calcium hydroxide paste is placed in the perforation. During the third session MTA is placed (Figs. 2.XI-21 and 2.XI-22), followed by completion of the treatment as described above.

If the perforation is in the root, cleaning and instrumentation, is followed by placement of calcium hydroxide paste (Calen), which remains in place as medication. During the subsequent session, the paste is removed from the canal and the root is filled. Subsquently at a later session, this filling is carefully removed, exposing the location of the perforation; MTA is prepared and placed with a Lentulo spiral or a type K file. With a Paiva gutta percha condenser or similar instrument, the MTA is condensed against the perforation, while at the same time excess should be removed from the canal.

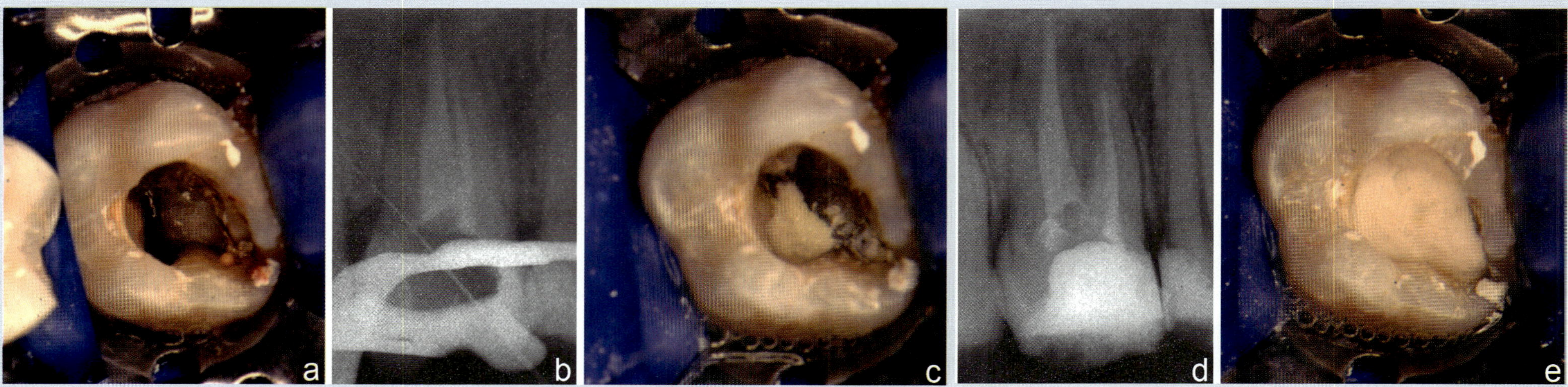

FIGS. 2.XI-21A-E

Perforation in pulp chamber in maxillary first molar, sealed with MTA.

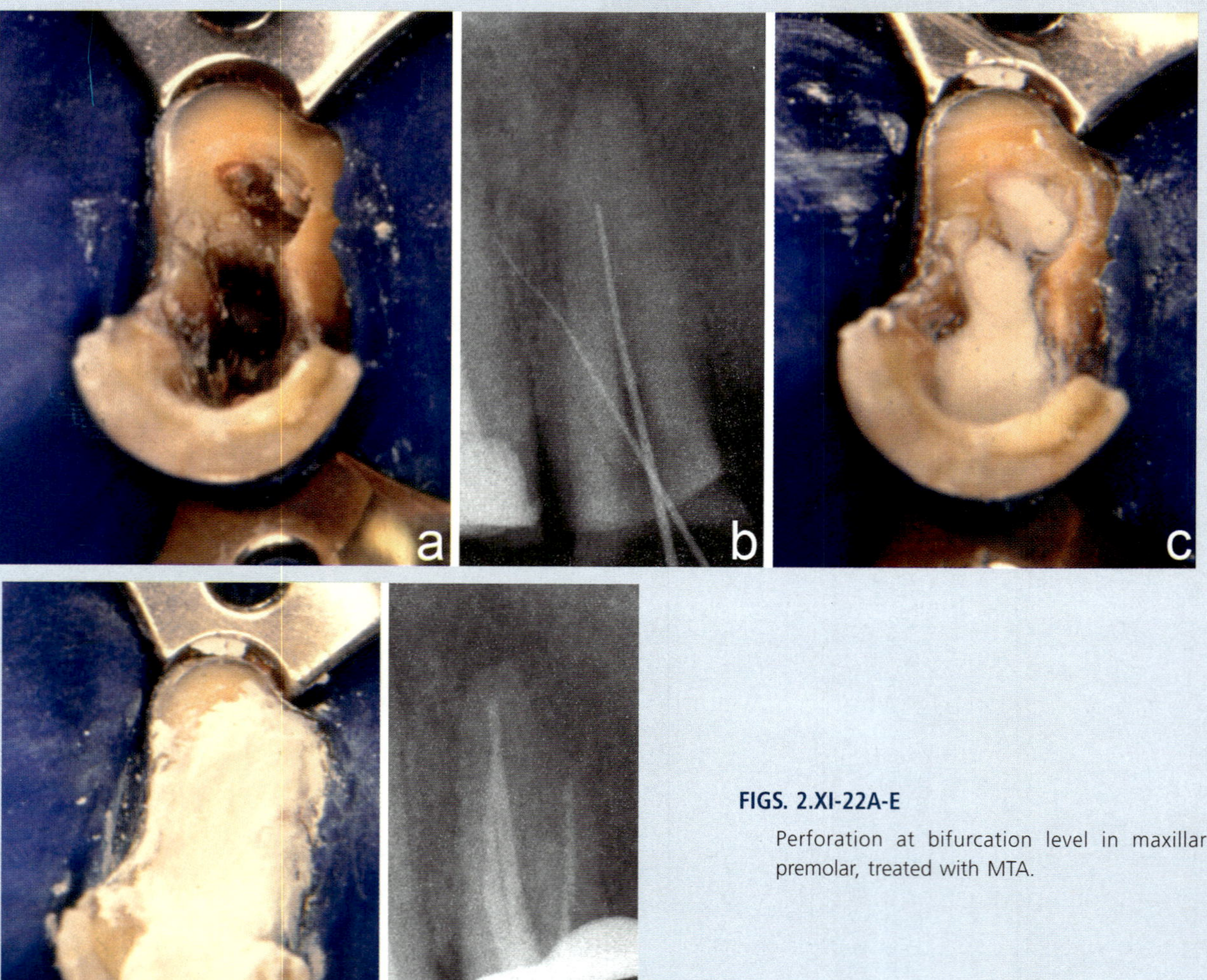

FIGS. 2.XI-22A-E

Perforation at bifurcation level in maxillary premolar, treated with MTA.

Figure 2.XII-23 shows a perforated mandibular premolar with an intracoronal post. The post was removed with ultrasound and the perforation sealed with MTA.

In Figure 2.XI-24 note the extrusion of gutta-percha cone from the perforation in the maxillary lateral incisor that had a fixed restoration and a core. The core was removed with ultrasound, the canal re-treated and the perforation sealed with MTA. A follow-up radiograph shows the repair of the area.

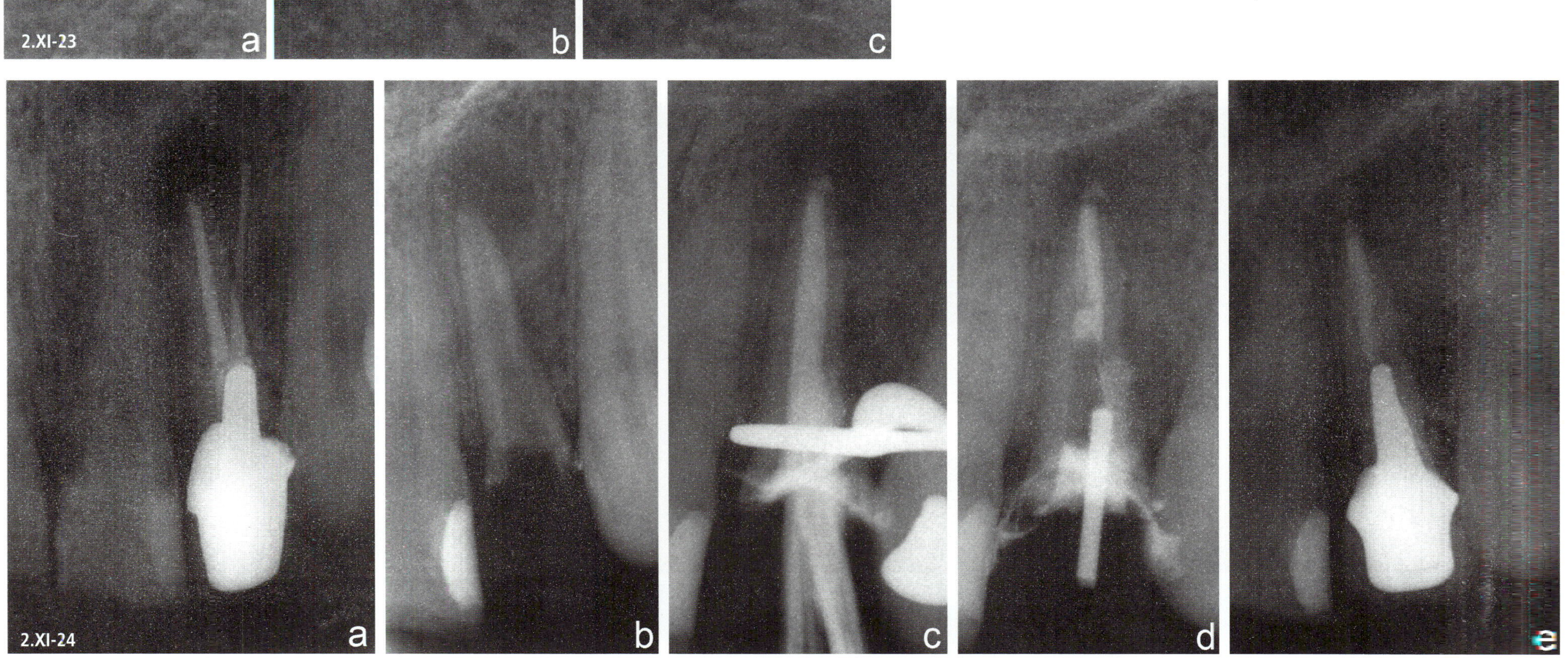

FIGS. 2.XI-23A-C

Perforation in mandibular premolar, treated with MTA (note the repaired area).

FIGS. 2.XI-24A-E

Maxillary left lateral incisor with post and core and gutta-percha cones coming out of the perforation. After removing the post and gutta-percha, and correctly filling the canal, the perforation was sealed with MTA (CPM).

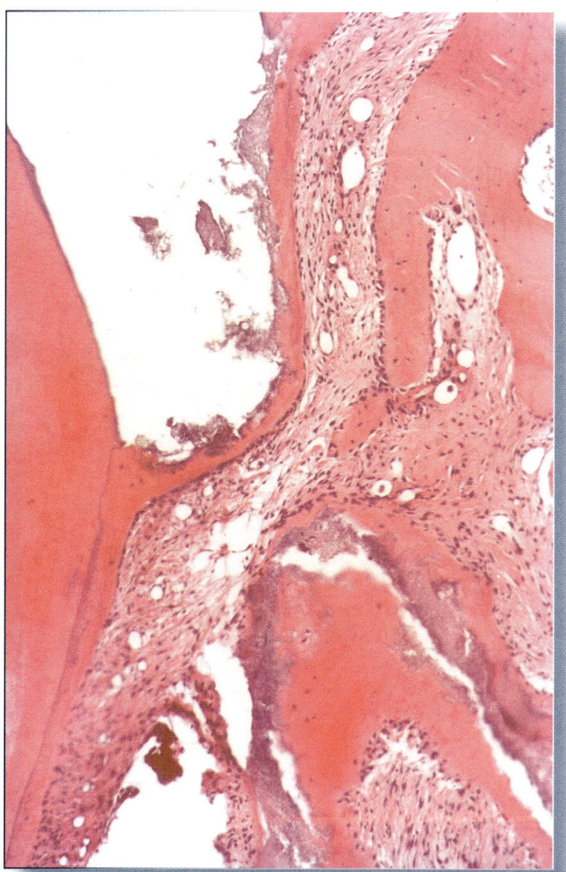

FIG. 2.XI-25

Sealing with mineralized tissue of perforation treated with MTA.

Repair of a perforation occurs with the formation of mineralized tissue (cement), sealing it, new bone tissue formation and regeneration of the periodontal ligament[5,15,38,41,42,43,63,70,72,75,99,103,108,116,144,149] (Fig. 2.XI-25).

With a large perforation MTA placement can cause extravasation in the periodontium, which may make it difficult for the repair process to occur. In this case, it is recommended to use a matrix, placed in the bone cavity at the perforation. This matrix can be made with calcium hydroxide, calcium sulphate or collagen (Fig. 2.XI-26). After hemorrhage in the location has been contained and the perforation cleaned (Fig. 2.XI-26A), the material used for the matrix is placed via the perforation, and compressed with a cotton pellet, so that it exits to the external surface, until it forms a protective barrier inside the bone cavity (Fig. 2.XI-26B). This is followed by removing excess matrix material from the perforation with a type K file that matches the diameter of the perforation (Fig. 2.XI-26c). Then the MTA is placed (Fig. 2.XI-26D). Thus, the matrix inserted into the bone cavity allows for better control of placing the MTA (Fig. 2.XI-26E). Fig. 2.XI-27 shows a perforation treated with a calcium sulphate matrix and MTA.

The importance using a matrix was pointed out by Alhadainy & Himel[6] (1994), Mesimeris, Sade, Baer[109] (1996), Jantarat, Daspher, Messer[85] (1999), Rafter et al.[125] (2002), Bargholz[18] (2005), Broon et al.[43] (2006), Hamad et al.[71] (2006), Al-Daafas & Al Nazhan[5] (2007), Bramante et al.[37] (2007) and Holland et al.[74] (2007).

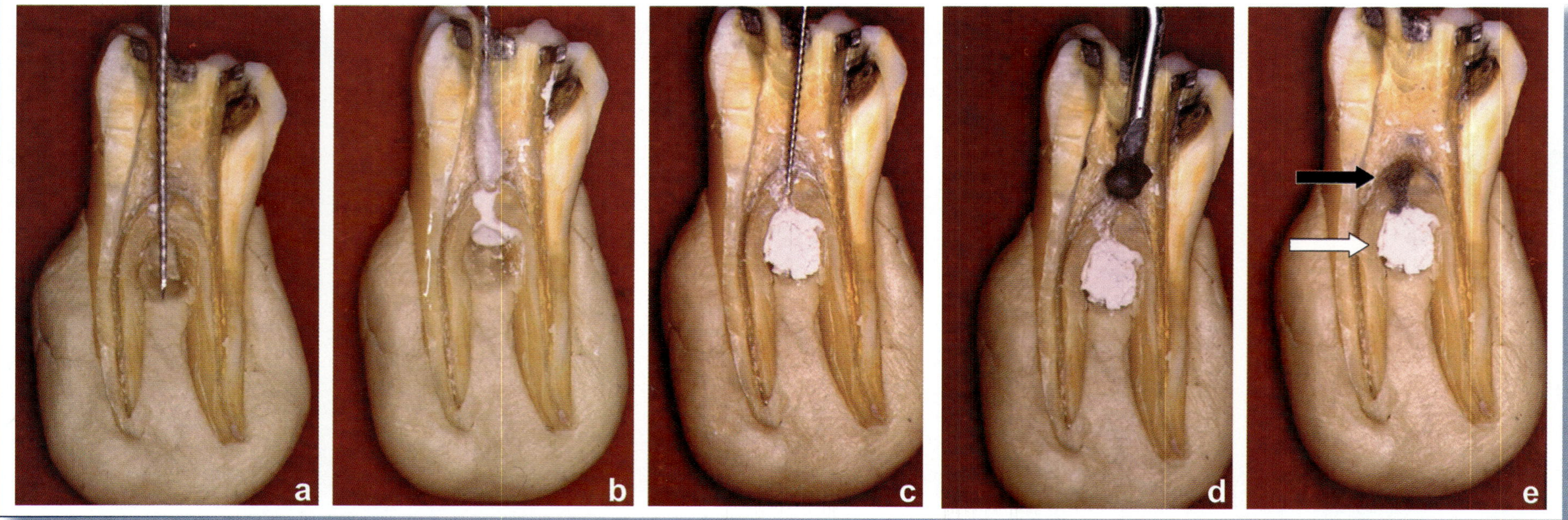

FIGS. 2.XI-26A-E

Perforation in the furcation area and placement of calcium sulphate as matrix.

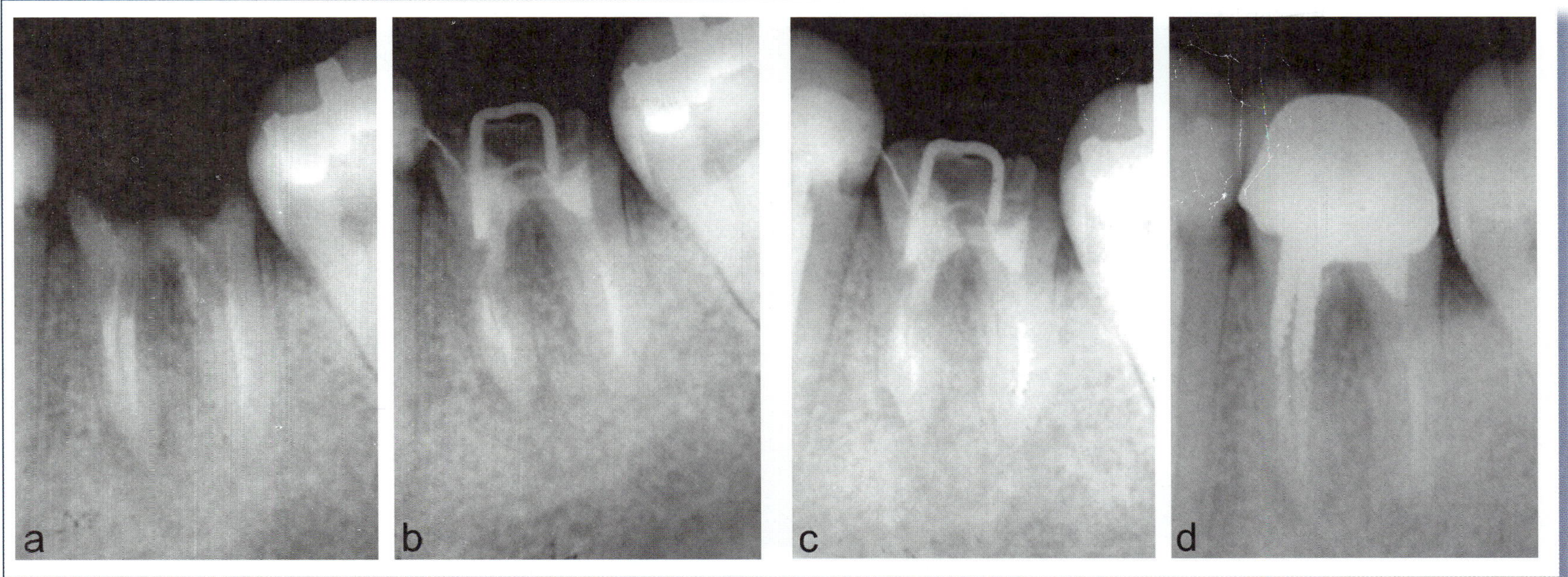

FIGS. 2.XI-27A-D

Treatment of perforation with calcium sulphate matrix and MTA.

e. Root Canal Filling

When overinstrumentation of the root canal happens, causing perforation of the foramen, it may be difficult to control the level of the filling. Attempting to perform a conventional filling may result extrusion of the filling material. One can use an MTA plug, similar to the technique described for a tooth with incompletely formed apices[39,49,96,102,119]. When root canal preparation has been completed, the MTA is carried to the apical region with a Lentulo spiral and the apical plug is made. A file wrapped in cotton is used to compact the plug, and to clean the canal walls.

An alternative method for making the plug is to completely fill the root canal with MTA (Fig. 2.XI-28B), and to subsequently remove part of the filling, leaving only the portion required for the plug (Fig. 2.XI-28C), which must be at least 3 mm. The larger the diameter of the instrument that ruptured the foramen, the thicker the plug must be. Canal filling can be done during the same session, or in a next one, depending on the consistency and resistance of the plug. At the time of filling, the gutta-percha cone must be well adapted to the canal walls, so that it does not cause undue pressure on the plug during lateral condensation (Fig. 2.XI-28D). One can also mold the cone to achieve better adaptation.

Figs. 2.XI-29 and 2.XI-30 show the use of an apical plug with MTA in an overinstrumented canal.

The thickness of the plug when filling an overinstrumented root canal must be at least 3 mm, in order to support the condensation pressure of the filling and allow apical sealing (Kwak, Park, Oh[96], 2000; Al-Kahtani et al.[9], 2003; Lamb et al.[97], 2003; Bramante, Bortoluzzi, Broon[39], 2004; Coneglian et al.[49], 2007).

The root canal can also be filled with gutta-percha cones and MTA-based cements, such as Endo CPM Sealer and MTA Obtura, which have vehicles that enhance their plasticity.

The powder/liquid ratio of this cement can vary according to the need for more or less fluidity. This does not alter or modify its chemical or biological behavior, its capacity to bond or its three dimensional sealing property.

In a manner similar to that of conventional treatment, the entire canal preparation sequence and cone selection is performed. The Endo CPM Sealer or MTA Obtura is mixed with the provided liquid, and a paste with of creamy consistency is obtained. It is recommended to wait a few minutes for the powder to get incorporated in the liquid, and to then mix it again with a spatula to obtain the desired consistency.

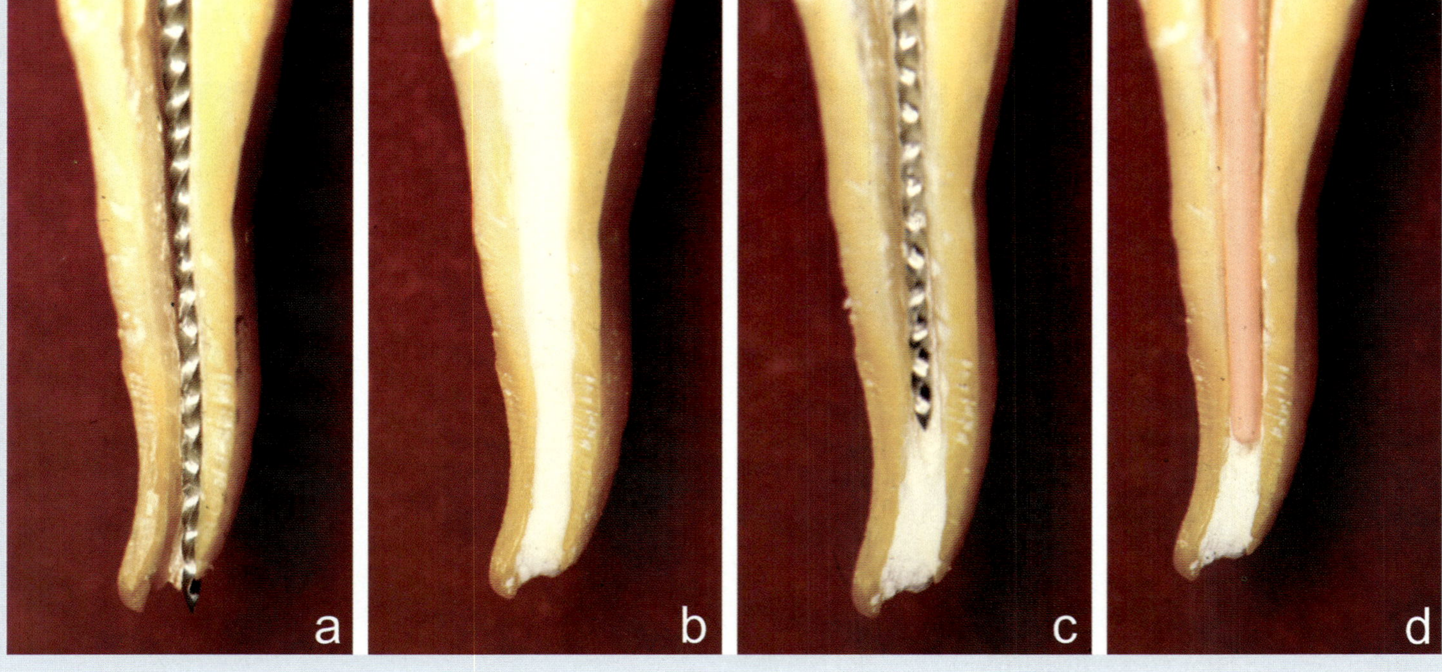

FIGS. 2.XI-28A-D

Making apical plug with MTA for filling the canal.

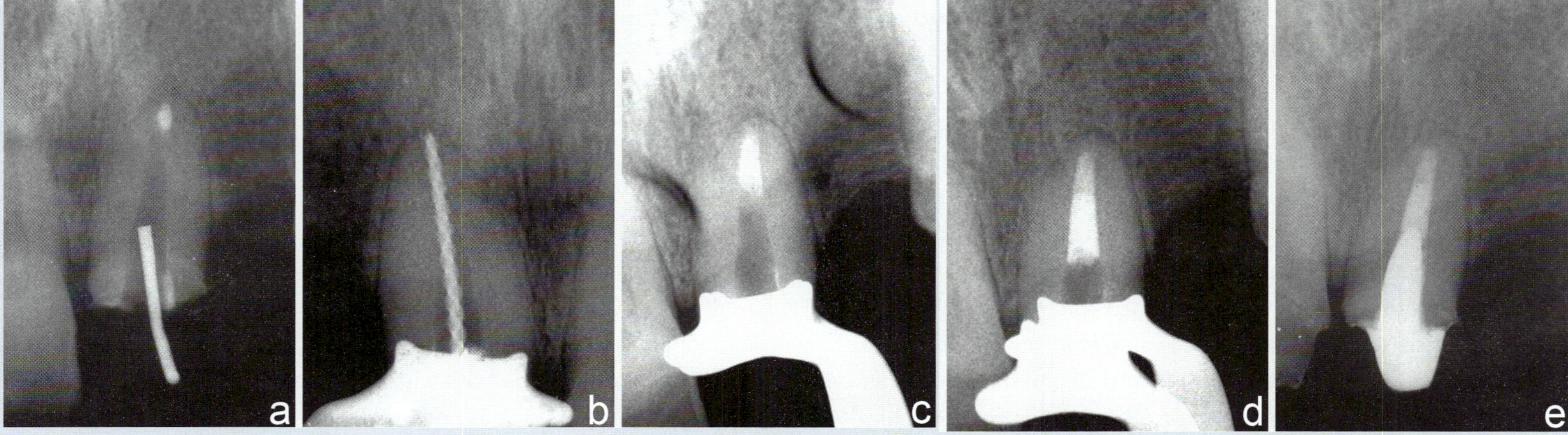

FIGS. 2.XI-29A-E

Use of apical plug with MTA and filling the canal with gutta-percha and sealer cement.

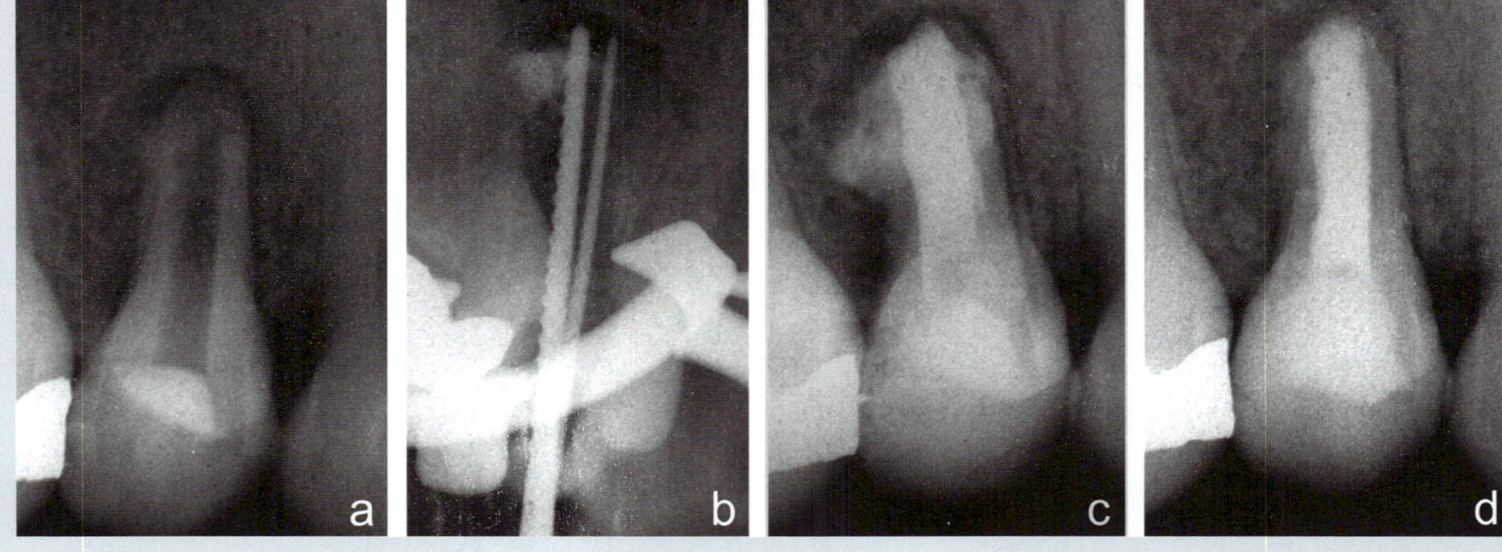

FIGS. 2.XI-30A-D

MTA plug in premolar with overinstrumented canals.

If the biological filling technique is used, the gutta-percha cone is coated with the MTA cement, introduced into the canal and lateral condensation is performed. If the classical technique is used, the cement can be placed with a Lentulo spiral or with a type K file, turning it in a counter-clockwise direction with an up-and- down movement. After seating the master cone, auxiliary cones are inserted, and lateral condensation is performed until the canal filling has been completed (Figs. 2.XI-31, 2.XI-32 and 2.XI-33).

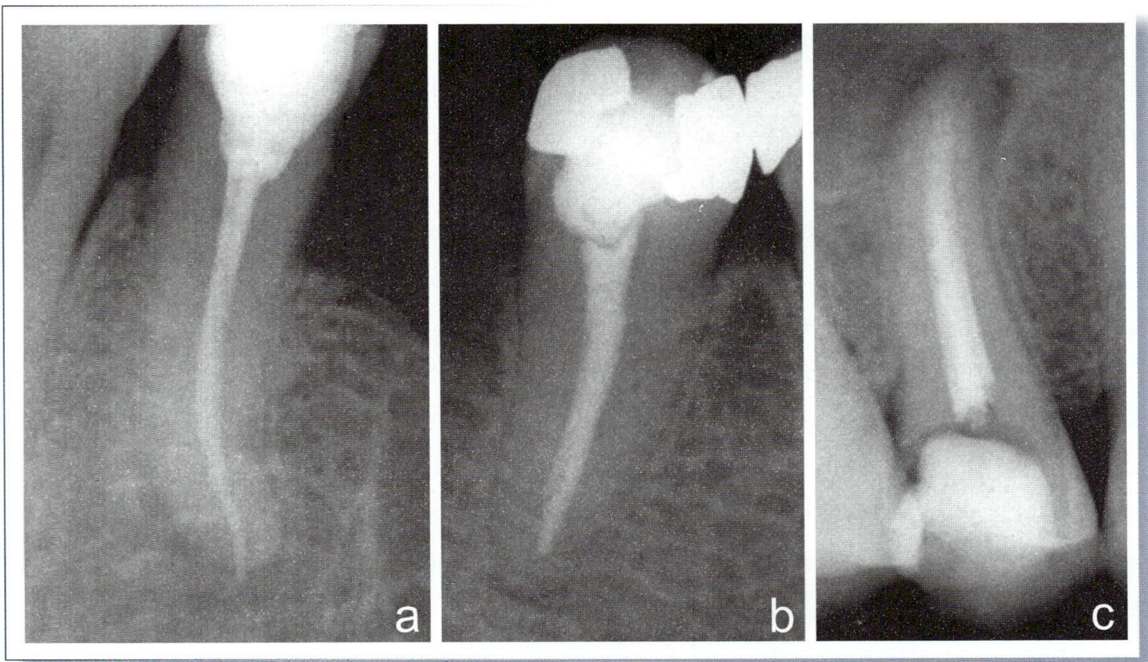

FIGS. 2.XI-31A-C
Root canals filled with gutta-percha cones and Endo CPM Sealer.

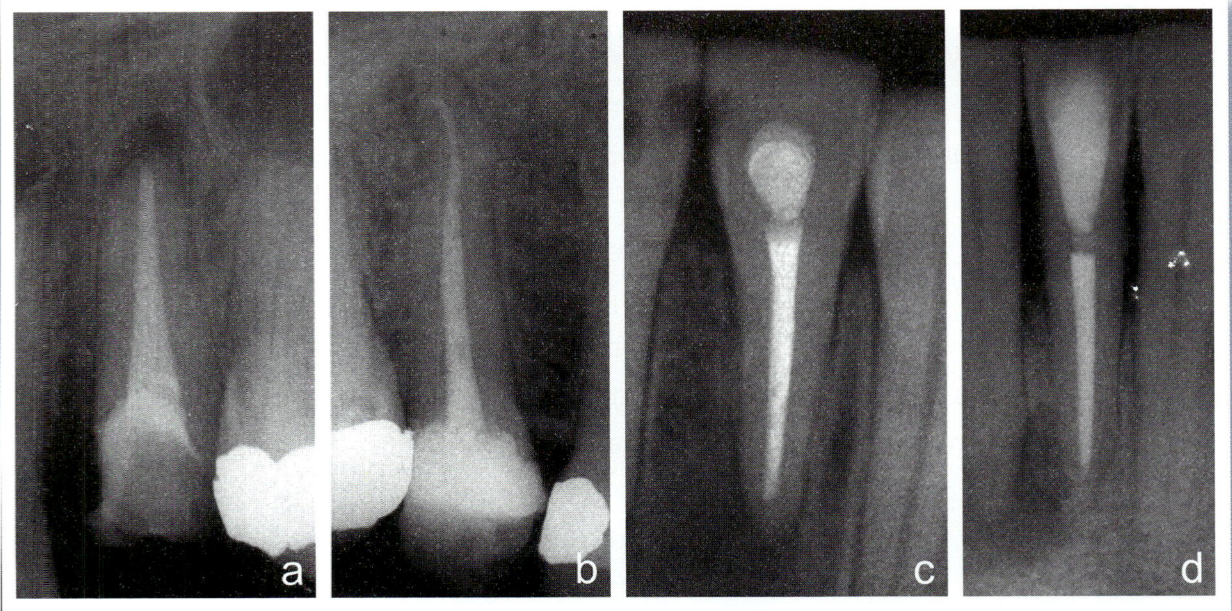

FIGS. 2.XI-32A-D
Root canal filled with gutta-percha cones and Endo CPM Sealer.

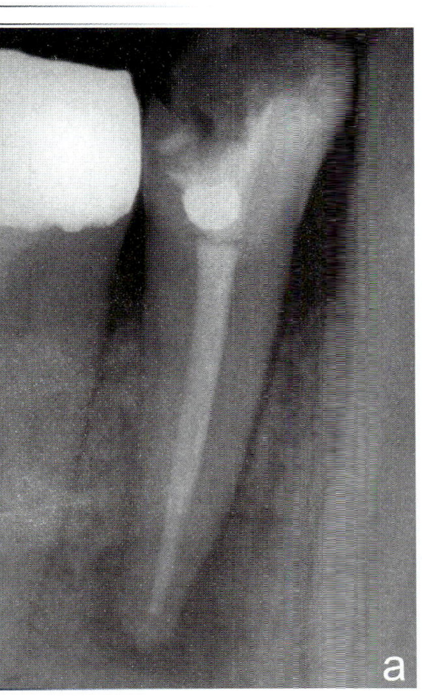

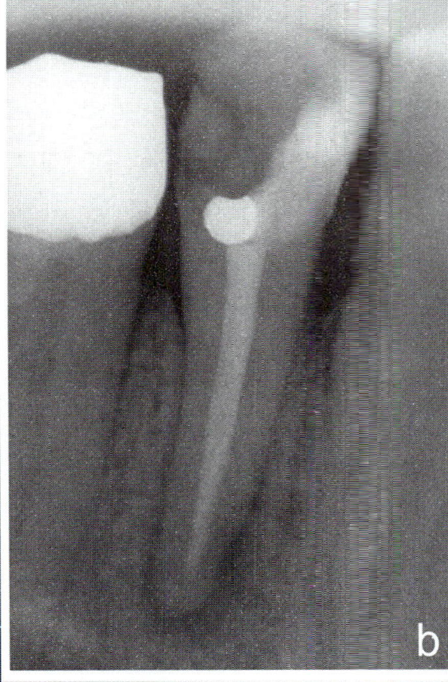

FIG. 2.XI-33A-B
Root canals filled with gutta-percha cones and MTA Obtura

MTA has been shown to be effective from a physical and biological point of view, when used in filling canals with and without gutta percha[74,77,79,80,146].

f. Apical Surgery

When endodontic treatment fails, or when it is not been possible to re-treat, apical surgery is indicated. Among the different surgical modalities there is the retrograde filling, which consists of preparing an apical cavity in the lumen of the root canal and filling it with a retro-filling material [24,34]. Various materials can be used for this purpose, among them, MTA is outstanding[3,11,13,17,20,22,23,47,48,57,64,97].

The apical cavity can be prepared with ultrasound and has to follow the direction of the canal, have a depth of 3 to 5 mm, be retentive, and be regular. After the cavity has been prepared, MTA is prepared and inserted[10]. Insertion can be done with a chisel, Hollenback instrument, micro MTA tip or micro amalgam tip. The MTA must have a heavier consistency to allow it to be inserted into the cavity. Excess material on the root surface needs to be removed with a curette and the material must be burnished with a smooth instrument. The surgical cavity can not be irrigated after placing the MTA, as it will be removed from the retro grade cavity. If it is necessary to remove excess MTA from the surgical cavity, this must be done with a curette and gauze.

Figures 2.XI-34 and 2.XI-35 show retrograde fillings with MTA.

g. Resorption

This is a pathology that has distinct origins and can even cause loss of a tooth. Resorption can be internal or external, and the etiologic factor of a large majority of resorptions is dental trauma, however, pulp necrosis, orthodontic movement and tooth bleaching may also be the cause. When there is communication between the root canal and the periodontium, resorption causes perforation, and consequently, its treatment is more complicated. In general, treatment of resorption, particularly external resorption, is treated with a calcium hydroxide paste (Calen). This will counteract resorption and initiate repair. Another option is to use MTA[35,84,118,120,150].

If the resorption is internal and communicates with the periodontium, one first has to eliminate the granulation tissue found in the area of resorption. This is achieved with a type K file with a curved tip, and irrigation with a 1% sodium hypochlorite solution. Calcium hydroxide dressing (Calen) can also be used as it also facilitates elimination of granulation tissue, as the necrosis it causes allows the irrigation and the instrumentation itself to make it very easy to remove. Therefore, it is important to use a medication, such as calcium hydroxide, between sessions until granulation tissue from the resorption area can completely be removed.

Initially, the canal itself can have granulation tissue (Fig. 2.XII-36A), which needs to be instrumented. An attempt should be made to remove the maximum possible amount of tissue (Figs. 2.XI-36B-C). Once instrumentation has been completed (Fig. 2.XI-36D), the canal is filled with calcium hydroxide paste (Calen), while exerting pressure, so that it occupies most of the resorption area (Fig. 2.XI-36E). Periodical changes are performed (monthly), until the granulation tissue is eliminated from the resorption area (Figs. 2.XI-36F-J). Once this has been achieved, MTA is placed in the canal with a Lentulo spiral, and with a type K file wrapped in cotton, it is condensed until it fills the entire resorpted area (Figs. 2.XI-36K-L). Figure 2.XI-37 shows a perforating internal resorption in the middle third of a mandibular premolar root canal, treated with MTA.

Figure 2.XI-38 presents the sequence of treatment for perforating resorption with the use of MTA. Figure 2.XI-39 shows cervical resorption in the maxillary central incisor, treated with MTA.

When the resorption is at the apical level of the root canal, MTA can be used in the form of a *plug*, before filling the

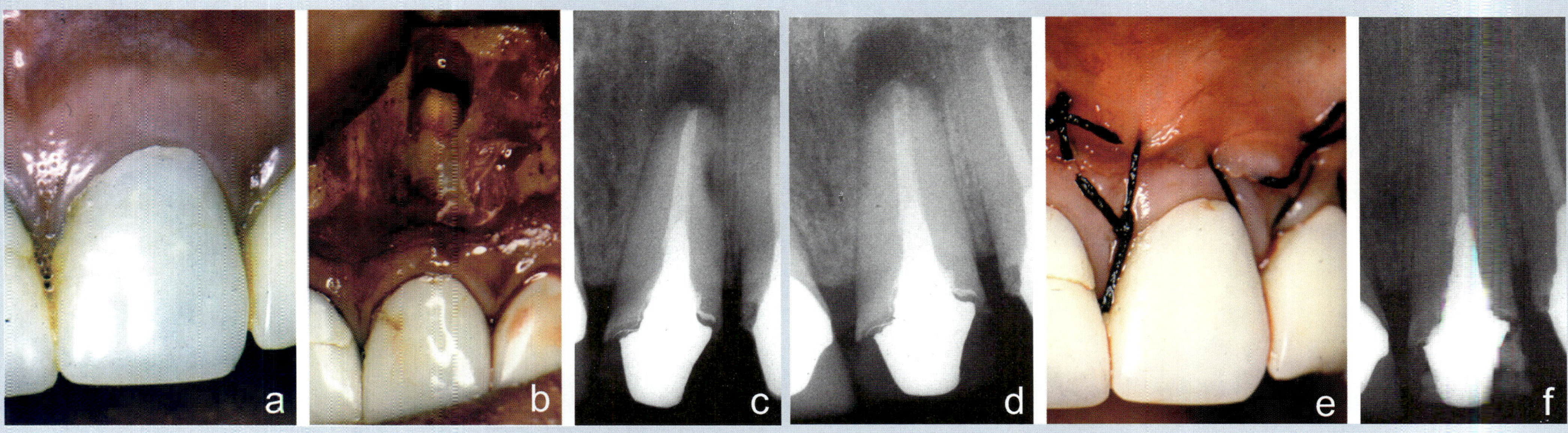

FIGS. 2.XI-34A-F

Retrograde filling in a maxillary central incisor using MTA.

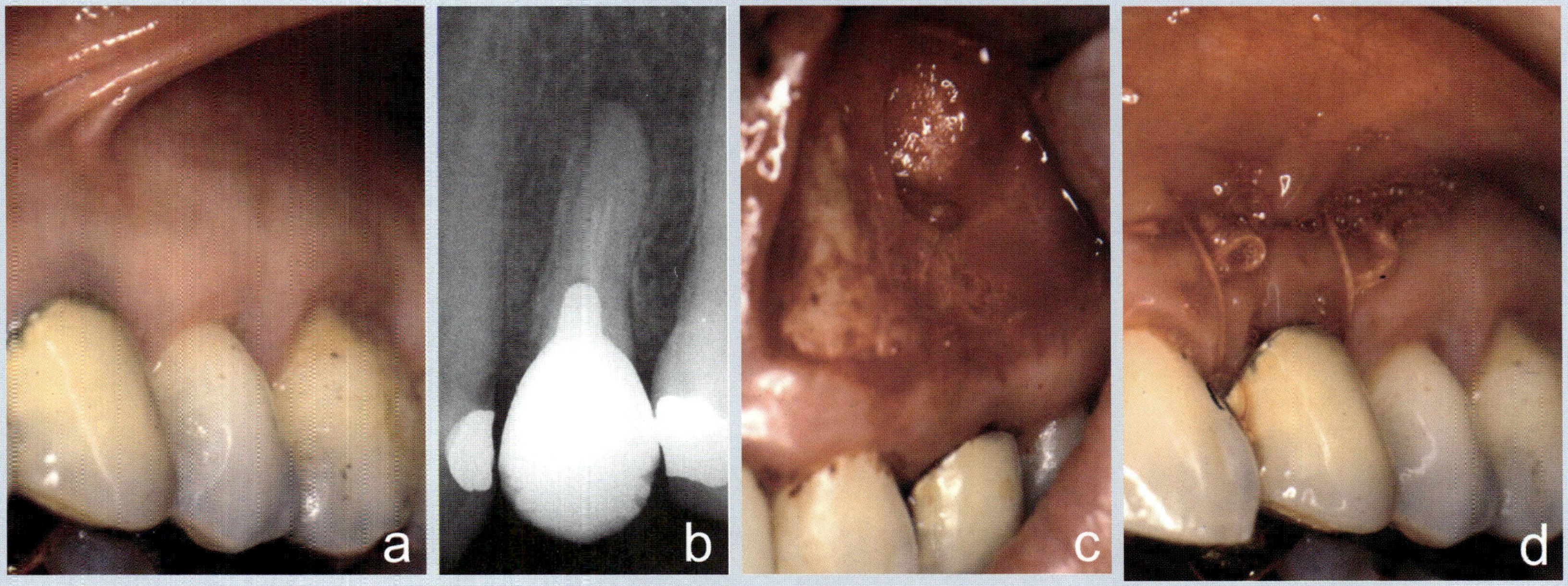

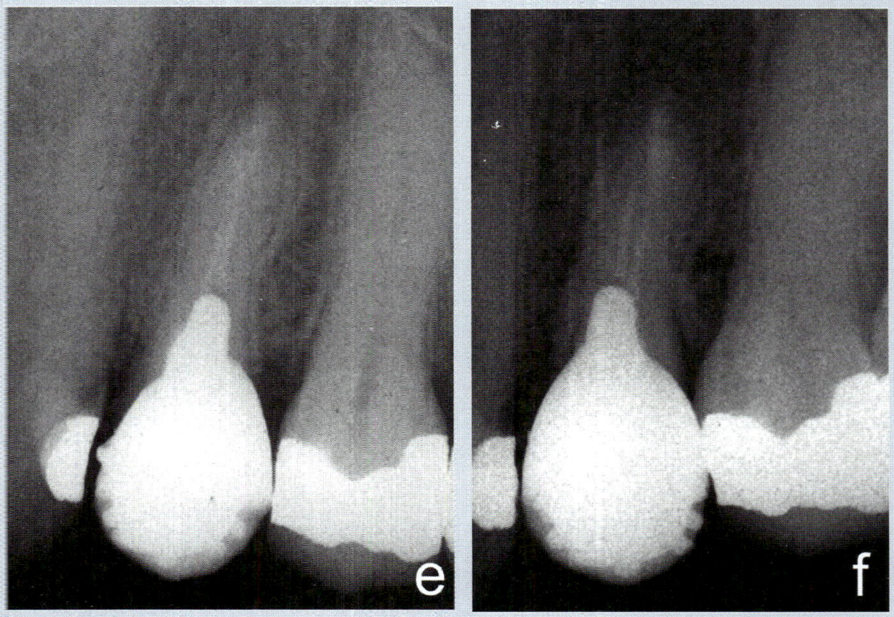

FIGS. 2.XI-35A-F

Retrograde filling in a maxillary first premolar, performed with MTA.

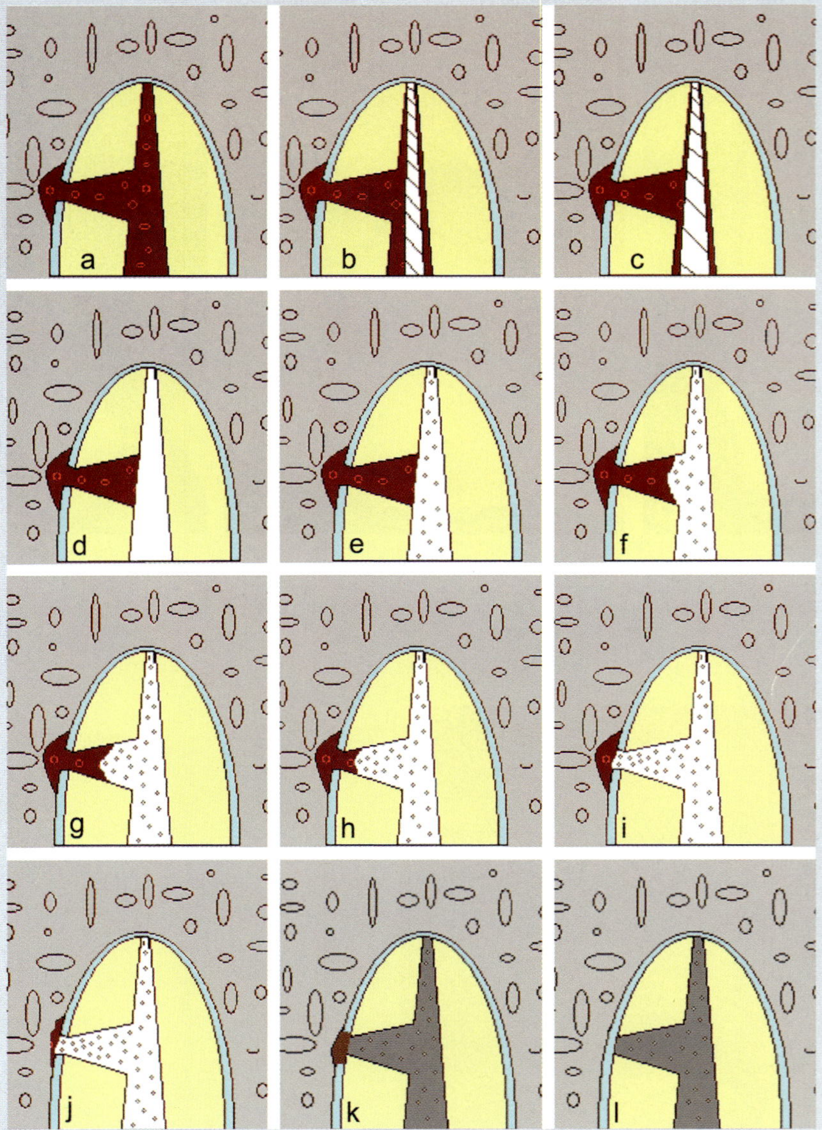

FIGS. 2.XI-36A-L

Diagram of treatment of perforating resorption treated with MTA, according to the text.

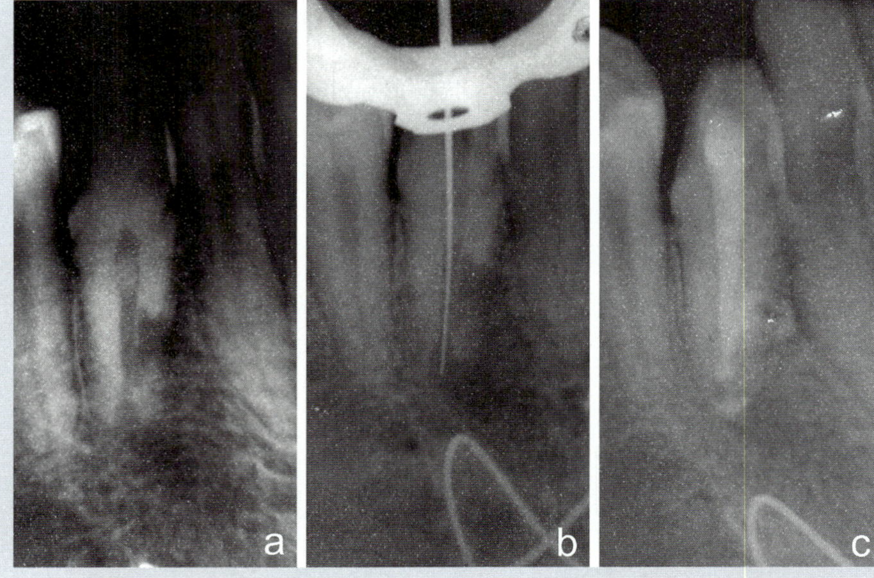

FIGS. 2.XI-37A-C

Perforating internal resorption in the middle third of the premolar root canal, treated with MTA.

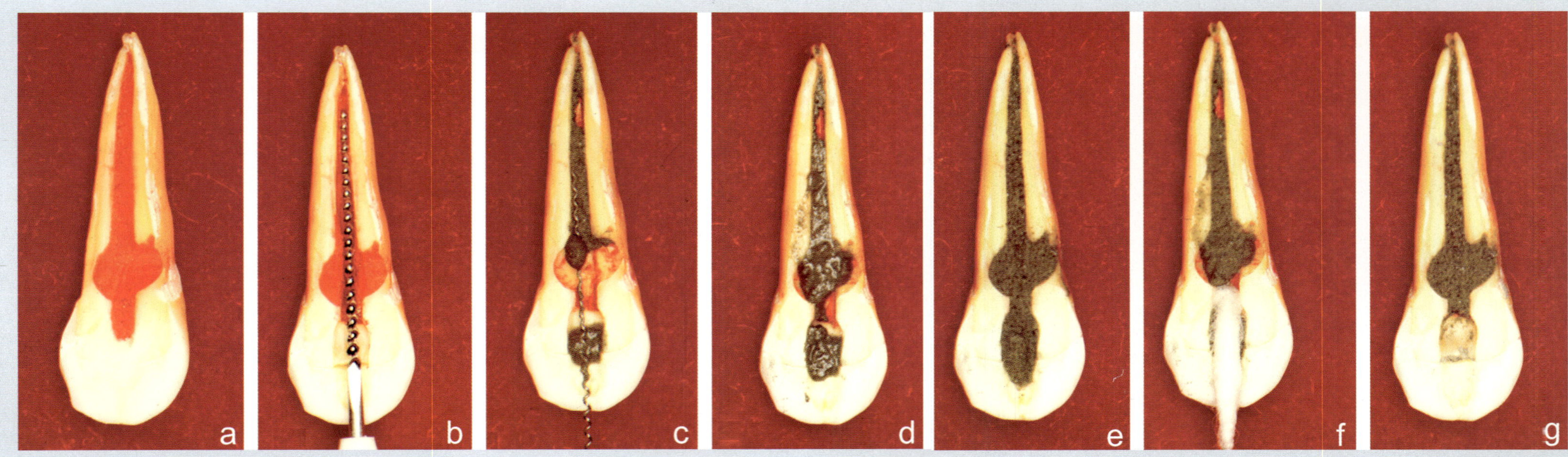

FIGS. 2.XI-38A-G

Treatment sequence of cervical resorption treated with MTA, according to the text.

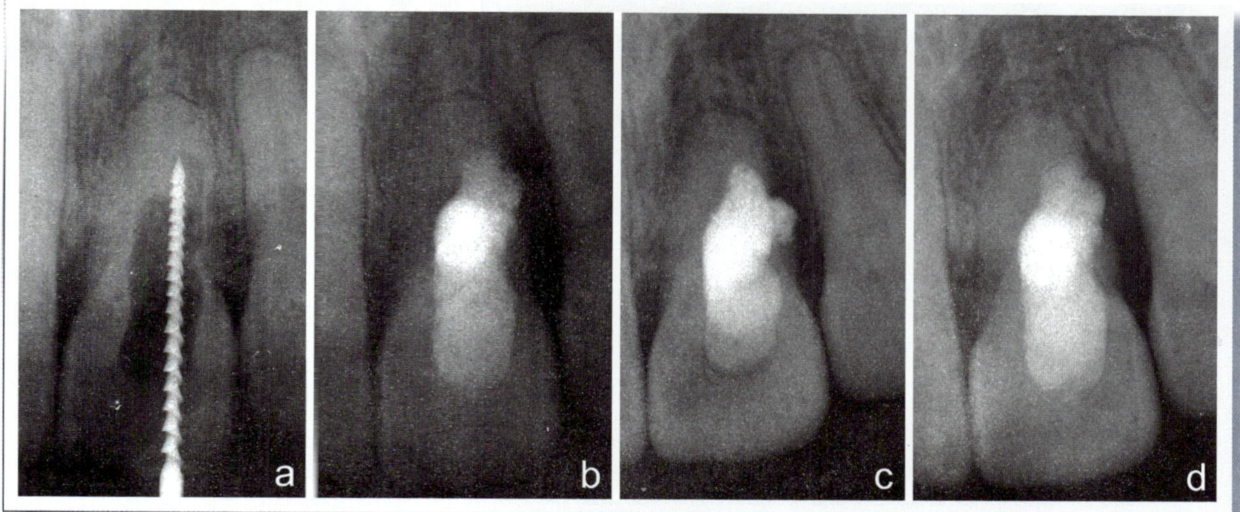

FIGS. 2.XI-39A-D

Cervical resorption treated with MTA.

root canal. The root canal procedures are the conventional ones. With a Lentulo spiral or type K file, an apical plug is made, following which the canal is filled with gutta-percha and sealer cement (Fig. 2.XI-40).

If there is external resorption and the treatment with calcium hydroxide does not produce a satisfactory result, MTA can be used. Initially, it should be attempted to prevent further resorption with a calcium hydroxide dressings, as this medication, in case it is of a perforating type, also promotes removal of granulation tissue at the site of the resorpted area. This is achieved by making periodic changes of the calcium hydroxide, until it is possible to place the MTA, attaempting to completely fill the resorpted area. Care must be taken to prevent extravasation of the material. For this purpose, MTA is prepared in a firmer consistency and condensed carefully (Fig. 2.XI-41).

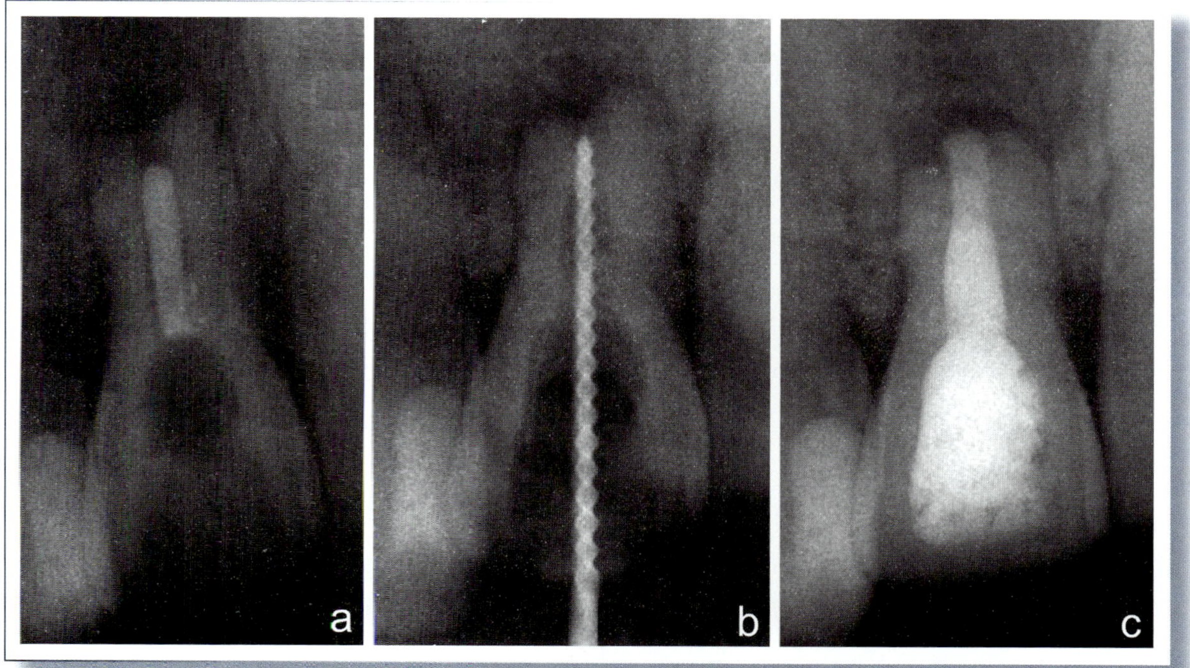

FIGS. 2.XI-40A-C

Apical plug with MTA and filling the root canal with gutta-percha cones and cement, in an apical resorption case.

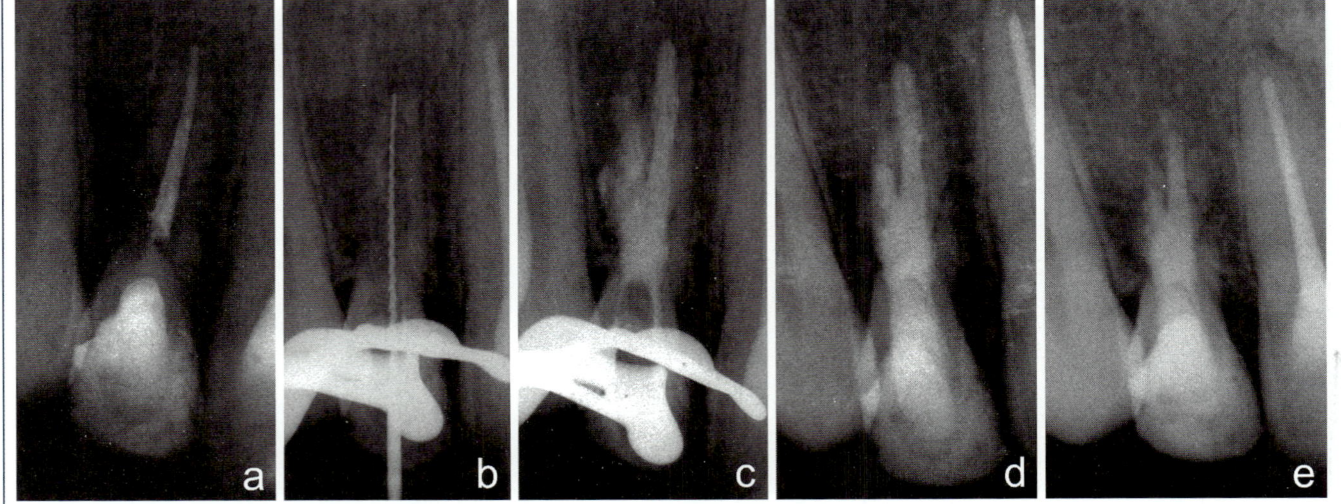

FIGS. 2.XI-41A-E

Perforating external resorption treated with MTA.

h. Root Fracture

Generally resulting from blows, the fractures can be in the crown, root or crown/root. When they are in the root, they can be located in the cervical, middle or apical thirds. Root fracture located in the cervical and middle thirds are more difficult to treat, as it is not easy to keep the tooth immobilized, which harms repair. For these cases, it is possible to reinforce the tooth with an intracanal post cemented with MTA (Bramante et al.[36]).

Initially, the canal is prepared in the conventional manner, performing final irrigation with physiological solution. After this, an apical plug is made using MTA, and a metal post is selected, so that it is lightly adjusted in the root canal. After the root canal is filled with MTA, the pin is seated inside it. Thus the root is reinforced, preventing mobility of the coronal segment (Fig. 2.XII-42).

OTHER APPLICATIONS

In addition to the applications presented above, MTA can also be used in cases of teeth with *Dens in dente* and for maintaining primary teeth.

Dens in dente is an anomaly that consists of invagination of enamel and dentin into the pulp cavity, completely changing its anatomy, and consequently, making it difficult to perform endodontic treatment. It occurs most commonly in maxillary lateral incisors, but it can be found in other teeth as well. Invagination can affect all third portions of a tooth, from the cervical to the apical third,

In view of the special anatomy of this anomaly, communication between the pulp cavity and the external environment can easily occur. Thus, the onset of a caries can easily cause exposure of the pulp. When the presence of a *Dens in dente* is clinically and radiographically diagnosed, and if possible, prophylactic treatment should be performed, which will prevent the appearance or progression of the lesion. If the pulp is already necrotic, proceed with cleaning the canal after removing the invagination, and treatment with MTA, either in the form of a *plug* or by filling the entire canal (Koh et al.[94], 2001 e Lima et al.[101],2007). Figure 2.XI-43 shows the treatment of a *Dens in dente* with the use of the MTA *plug*.

Another use of MTA is in primary teeth. When a primary tooth has no permanent replacement, it is very important to maintain the primary tooth to preserve the patient's occlusal harmony. As the internal anatomy of these teeth is variable, frequently with root resorption that is difficult to locate, one of the alternatives is to fill the entire canal with MTA. This must be done carefully and the canal cleaned as thorough as possible using endodontic instruments and irrigation solutions (1% sodium hypochlorite solution). After completion of the preparation, proceed with irrigation with physiological saline, drying the canal and filling it with MTA. This has to be prepared in a more fluid consistency, to allow placement in the entire canal with a Lentulo spiral or a type K file, taking care not to cause extravasation. O'Sulivan & Hartwell[117] (2001) and Araújo et al.[14] (2006) successfully used MTA for maintaining primary teeth.

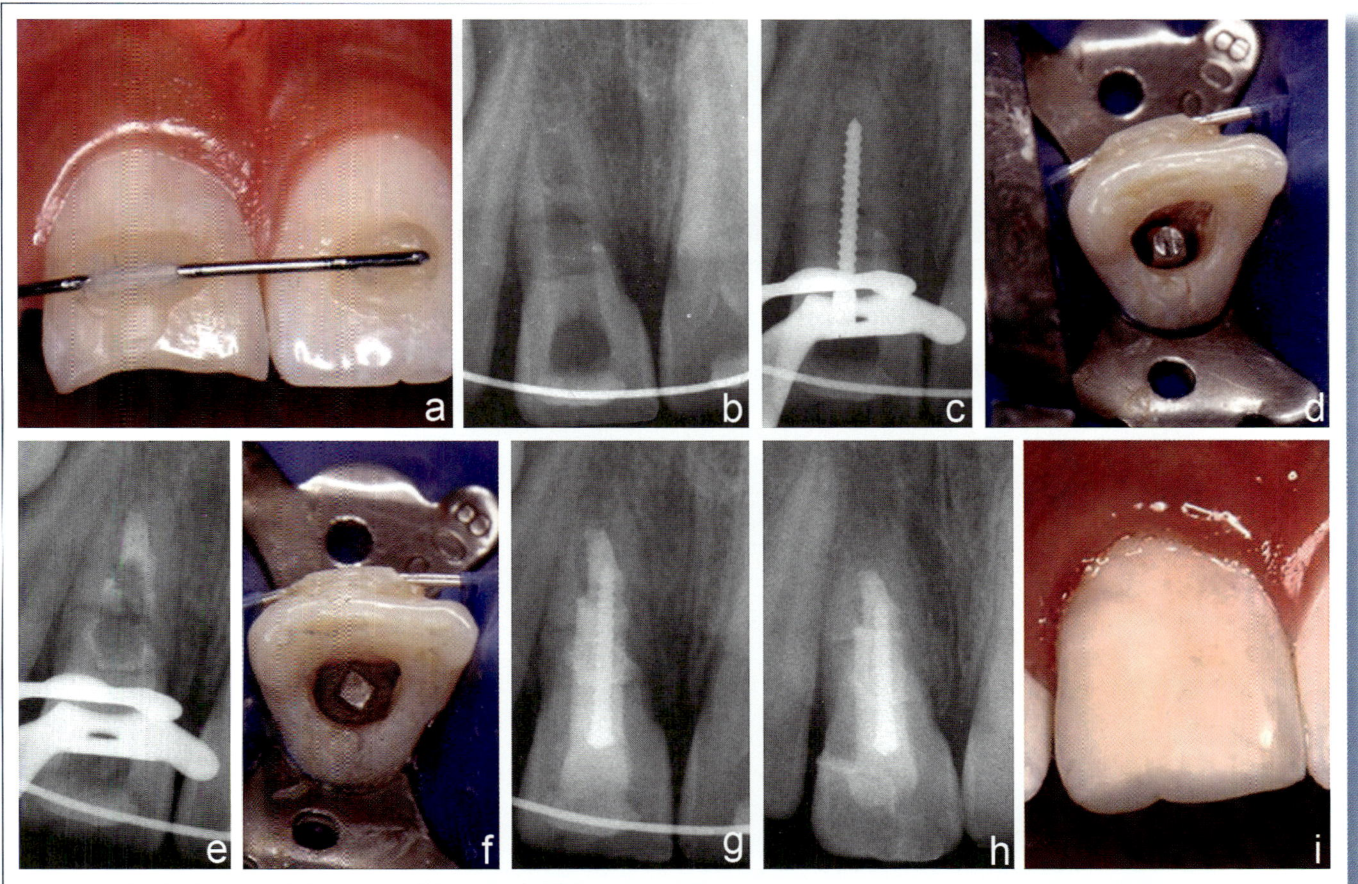

FIGS. 2.XI-42A-I

Root fracture treatment with MTA, reinforced with intracanal post.

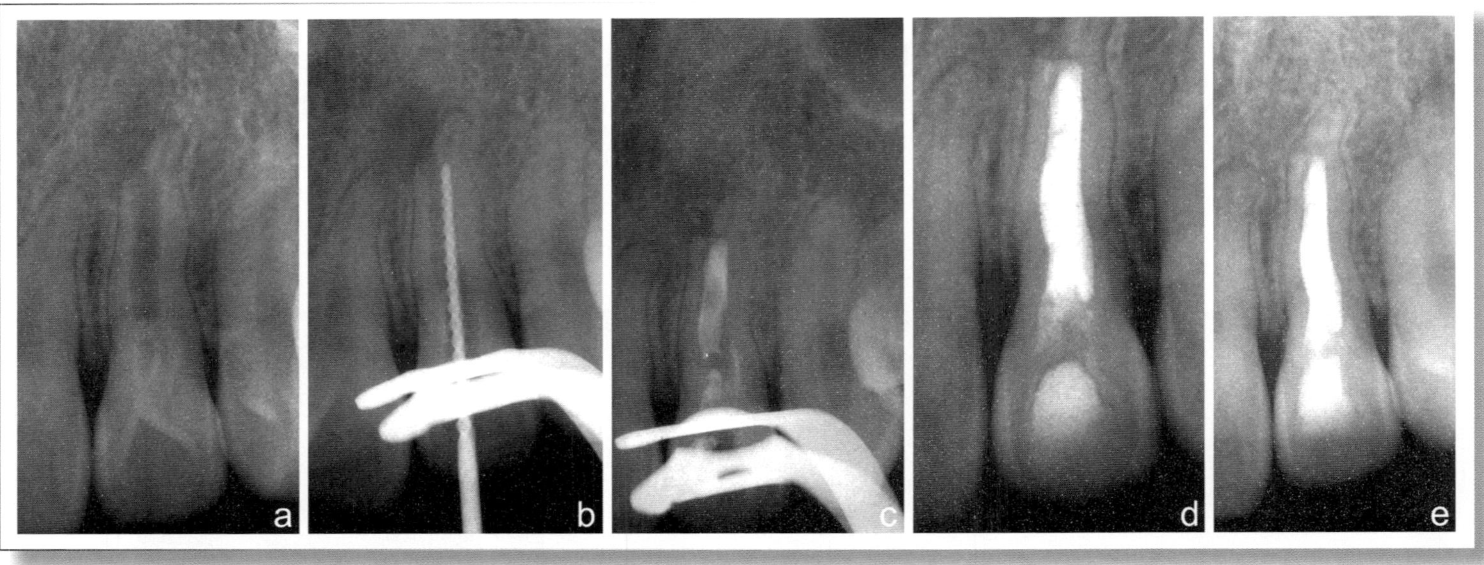

FIGS. 2.XI-43A-E

Dens in dente treated with MTA plug and filling the root canal with gutta-percha cones and sealer cement.

FINAL CONSIDERATIONS

Currently, with the availability of mineral trioxide aggregate (MTA), many situations that used to condemn a tooth can now be treated via the root canal without the need for apiectomy surgery or extracting the tooth. A prime requirement is a correct diagnosis and treatment plan in order to ensure successful treatment. This is the practitioner's responsibility, and allows evaluation of the treatment alternatives. With regard to the use of MTA, some requisites must be considered:

a. The powder/liquid ratio can be altered with the objective to use the desired consistency of the cement in view of the location where it has to be placed.
b. A very thick or fluid consistency makes it more difficult to work with the material.
c. Avoid excessive extravasation of the material into the periodontium, as it will set before resorption occurs.
d. If there is risk of extravasation, a calcium hydroxide, calcium sulphate or collagen matrix should be used.
e. There is no need to place small moist cotton pellets on the material in the pulp chamber or root canal, as too much moisture prevents the material from hardening completely. If necessary, an aqueous calcium hydroxide paste can be placed over the MTA, but with the least possible amount of liquid.
f. Avoid having the material in the pulp chamber, as it can cause changes in the color of the tooth (Bortoluzzi et al.[28], 2007).
g. Cement residue must immediately be removed from inside the canal, since after setting it will be
difficult, or cannot be removed at all.
h. When it is used as a retrograde filling, the excess must be removed with curettes, or gauze moistened with physiological saline. If irrigation is used, all the material will be removed, including what was placed in the retrograde cavity.
i. White MTA has better viscosity and is easier to use than the gray MTA.

References

1. Abedi HR, Torabinejad M, Pitt Ford TR, Bakland LK. The use of mineral trioxide aggregate cement (MTA) as a direct pulp capping agent. J Endod, v.22, p.199, Abstract n.44, 1996.
2. Accorinte MLR, Holland R, Reis A, Bortoluzzi M, Murata SS, Dezan Jr E, Souza V, Alessandro LD. Evaluation of mineral trióxide aggregate and calcium hydroxide cement as pulp-capping agents in human teeth. J Endod, v.34, p.1-6, 2008.
3. Adamo HL, Buruiana R, Schertzer L, Boylan RJ. A comparison of MTA, super EBA, composite and amalgam as root-end filling materials using bacterial microleakage model. Int Endod J, v.32, p.197-203, 1999.
4. Aeinehchi M, Eslami B, Ghanbariha M, Saffar AS. Mineral trioxide aggregate (MTA) and calcium hydroxide as pulp-capping agents in human teeth: a preliminary report. Int Endod J, v.36, p.225-231, 2003.
5. Al-Daafas A, Al Nazhan S. Histological evaluation of contaminated furcal perforation in dogs teeth repaired by MTA with or without internal matrix. Oral Surg Oral Med Oral Pathol Oral Radiol Endod, v.103, p.92-99, 2007.
6. Alhadainy HA, Himel VT. An in vitro evaluation of plaster of Paris barriers used under amalgam and glass ionomer to repair furcation perforation. J Endod, v.20, p.449-452, 1994.
7. Al-Hezaimi K, Al-Shalan TA, Naghsbandi J, Oglesby S, Simon JHS, Rostetein I. Antibacterial effect of two mineral trioxide aggregate (MTA) preparations against Enterococcus faecalis and Streptococcus sanguis in vitro. J Endod, v.32, n.11, p.1.053-1.056, 2006.
8. Al-Hezaimi K, Naghshbandi J, Oglesby S, Simon JHS, Rotstein I. Human saliva penetration of root canals obturated with two types of mineral trioxide aggregate cements. J Endod, v.31, n.6, p.453-456, 2005.
9. Al-Kahtani A, Shostad S, Schifferle R, Bhambhani S. In vitro evaluation of microleakage of an orthograde apical plug of mineral trioxide aggregate in permanent with simulated immature apices. J Endod, v.31, p.117-119, 2005.
10. Aminoshariae A, Hartwell GR, Moon PC. Placement of mineral trioxide aggregate using two different techniques. J Endod, v.29, n.10, p.679-682, 2003.
11. Andelin WE, Browning DF, Hsu HR, Roland DD, Torabinejad M. Microleakage of resected MTA. J Endod, v.28, p.573-574, 2002.
12. Andreasen JO, Munksgaard EC, Bakland LK. Comparison of fracture resistance in root canals of immature sheep teeth after filling with calcium hydroxide or MTA. Dental Traum, v.22, p.154-156, 2006.
13. Aqrabawi J. Sealing ability of amalgam, super EBA cement, and MTA when used as retrograde filling materials. Br Dent J, v.188, p.266-268, 2000.
14. Araújo RA, Occhiuto VAR, Marques BA, Bengtson AL, Pinheiro SL. Pulpoterapia odontopediátrica utilizando o agregado trióxido mineral. J Brás Endod, v.6, n.26, p.223-229, 2006.
15. Arens DE, Torabinejad M. Repair of furcal perforations with mineral trioxide aggregate – two cases reports. Oral Surg Oral Med Oral Pathol Oral Radiol, v.82, p.84-88, 1996.
16. Asgary S, Parirokh M, Eghbal MJ, Brink F. Chemical differences between white and gray mineral trioxide aggregate. J Endod, v.31, p.101-103, 2005.
17. Baek SH, Plenk H, Kiom S. Periapical tissue responses and cement regeneration with amalgam, super EBA and MTA as root-end filling materials. J Endod, v.31, p.444-449, 2005.
18. Bargholz C. Perforation repair with mineral trioxide aggregate a modified matrix concept. Int Endod J, v.38, p.59-69, 2005.
19. Barrieshi-Nusair KM, Qudeimat MA. A prospective clinical study of mineral trioxide aggregate for partial pulpotomy in cariously exposed permanent teeth. J Endod, v.32, n.80, p.731-735, 2006.
20. Bates CF, Carnes DL, Del Rio CE. Longitudinal sealing ability of mineral trioxide aggregate as a root-end filling material. J Endod, v.22, p.575-578, 1996.
21. Berástegui Jimeno EM. Actualización sobre el ProRoot-MTA en el a–o 2002. Endodoncia, v.21, p.36-49, 2003.
22. Bernabé PFE, Gomes-Filho JE, Rocha WC, Nery MJ, Otoboni Filho JA, Dezan Junior E. Histological evaluation of MTA as a root-end filling material. Int Endod J, v.40, p.758-765, 2007.
23. Bernabé PFE, Holland R, Morandi R, Souza V, Nery MJ, Otoboni Filho JA, Dezan Junior E, Gomes-Filho JE. Comparative study of MTA and other materials in retrofilling of pulpless dogs' teeth. Braz Dent J, v.16, n.2, p.149-155, 2005.
24. Bernabé PFE, Holland R. Cirurgia parendodôntica: quando indicar e como realizá-la. In: Gonçalves EA, Feller C. Atualização na clínica odontológica: a prática da clínica geral. São Paulo: Artes Médicas, p.217-254, 1998.
25. Bernabé PFE, Holland R. MTA e cimento Portland: considerações sobre as propriedades físicas, químicas e biológicas. In: Cardoso RJA, Machado MEL. Odontologia Arte e Conhecimento. São Paulo: Artes Médicas Ltda., v.1, p.225-264, Cap.11, 2003.
26. Bidar M, Moradi S, Jafarzadeh H, Biddad S. Comparative SEM study of the marginal adaptation of white and grey MTA and Portland cement. Aust Endod J, v.33, p.2-6, 2007.
27. Boletin informativo sobre el CPM y Endo CPM sealer. www.cpmodontologia.com
28. Bortoluzzi EA, Araújo GS, Tanomaru JMG, Tanomaru Filho M. Marginal gingiva discoloration by gray MTA: a case report. J Endod, v.33, p.325-327, 2007.
29. Bortoluzzi EA, Broon NJ, Bramante CM, Consolaro A, Garcia RB, Moraes IG, Bernardineli N. Mineral Trioxide Aggregate with or without calcium chloride in pulpotomy. J Endod, v.34, n.2, p.172-175, 2008.
30. Bortoluzzi EA, Broon NJ, Bramante CM, Garcia RB, Moraes IG, Bernardineli N. Sealing ability of MTA and radiopaque Portland cement with or without calcium chloride for root-end filling. J Endod, v.32, p.897-900, 2006.
31. Bortoluzzi EA, Broon NJ, Duarte MAH, Dermachi ACCO, Bramante CM. The use of a setting accelerator and its effect on pH and calcium ion release of mineral trioxide aggregate and white Portland cement. J Endod, v.32, p.1194-1197, 2006.
32. Bortoluzzi EA, Broon NJ, Bramante CM. Avaliação da capacidade seladora do MTA e cimento Portland com ou sem cloreto de cálcio em obturações retrógradas. Braz Oral Res, v.18, p.213/ Abstract n.Pc082, 2004.
33. Bramante CM, Berbert A, Bernardineli N, Moraes IG, Garcia RB. Acidentes e complicações no tratamento endodôntico – soluções clínicas. 2.ª ed., Editora Santos: São Paulo, 2004.
34. Bramante CM, Berbert A. Cirurgia Parendodôntica, Ed. Santos: São Paulo, 2000.

35. Bramante CM, Bramante AS, Moraes IG, Bernardineli N, Garcia RB. CPM y Endo CPM Sealer – Nuevos materiales de uso em endodoncia. Endodoncia, v.26, n.1, 2008.

36. Bramante CM, Menezes RS, Moraes IG, Bernardineli N, Garcia RB, Letra A. Use of MTA and intracanal post reinforcement in a horizontally fractured tooth: a case report. Dent Traumat, v.22, p.275-278, 2006.

37. Bramante CM, Moraes IG, Bernardineli N, Garcia RB, Broon N, Bramante AS. Is a matrix required for treatment of root perforation with MTA? ENDO-Endodontic Practice today, v.1, p.295-300, 2007.

38. Bramante CM, Tello LYA, Broon NJ, Bernardineli N, Moraes IG, Garcia RB. Tratamiento de una perforación radicular con trióxido mineral agregado (CPM). Rev As Odon Argentina, v.94 p.23-26, 2006.

39. Bramante CM, Bortoluzzi EA, Broon NJ. Agregado Trióxido Mineral (MTA) como plug para la obturación de conductos radiculares: descripción de la técnica y caso clínico. Endodoncia, v.22, p.155-161, 2004.

40. Broon N, Bortoluzzi EA, Bramante CM, Bernardineli N, Moraes IG, Garcia RB. Evaluación de la capacidad selladora del agregado trióxido mineral blanco de dos marcas comerciales y cemento Portland blanco en obturación retrógrada. Méd Oral, v.6, n.2, p.41-46, 2004.

41. Broon NJ, Bortoluzzi EA, Bramante CM, Assis GF, Bernardineli N, Moraes IG, Garcia RB. Tratamiento de perforaciones radiculares con agregado trióxido mineral (MTA) y cemento Portland blanco con cloruro de cálcio al 10% en dientes de perros. Rev Sanid Milit Mex, v.60, n.2, p.94-102, 2006.

42. Broon NJ, Bramante CM, Assis GF, Bortoluzzi EA, Bernardineli N, Moraes IG, Garcia RB. Tratamiento de perforaciones radiculares en dientes de perros con dos marcas comerciales de agregado trióxido minerales (MTA) Endodoncia, v.23, p.165-170, 2005.

43. Broon NJ, Bramante CM, Assis GF, Bortoluzzi EA, Bernardineli N, Moraes IG, Garcia RB. Healing of root perforations treated with mineral trioxide aggregate (MTA) and Portland cement. J Appl Oral Sci, v.14, p.305-311, 2006.

44. Calderon Farfan PS, Espinoza ReyesI, Villalobos Domínguez EI, Vásquez Espinosa E. Utilización de MTA (agregado trioxido mineral) para recubrimientos pulpares directos en dientes permanentes jovenes. Reporte de nueve casos. Medicina Oral, v.4, n.3, p.69-77, 2002.

45. Camilleri J, Montesi FE, DiSilvio L, Pitt Fotd TR. The chemical constitution and biocompatibility of accelerat (accelerate?) Portland cement for endodontic use. Int Endod J, v.38, p.834-842, 2005.

46. Camilleri J. Hydration mechanisms of mineral trioxide aggregate. Int Endod J, v.40, p.462-470, 2007.

47. Chong BS, Pitt Ford TR, Hudson MB. A prospective clinical study of Mineral Trioxide Aggregate and IRM when used as root-end filling materials in endodontic surgery. Int Endod J, v.36, p.520-526, 2003.

48. Cintra LT, Moraes IG, Bernabé PFE, Gomes-Filho JE, Bramante CM, Garcia RB, Bernardineli N. Evaluation of the tissue response to MTA and MBPc. Microscopic analysis of implants in alveolar bone of rats. J Endod, v.32, p.556-559, 2006.

49. Coneglian PZA, Orosco FA, Bramante CM, Moraes IG, Garcia RB, Bernardineli N. In vitro sealing ability or white and gray mineral trioxide aggregate (MTA) and white Portland cement used as apical plug. J Appl Oral Scien, v.15, p.181-185, 2007.

50. Costa MMTM. Avaliação da resposta tecidual frente aos cimentos MTA Angelus cinza e um MTA fotopolimerizável experimental. Análise microscópica de implantes realizados em alvéolo de ratos. Araçatuba, 2008, 107p Tese (doutorado). Faculdade de Odontologia de Araçatuba – Unesp 2008.

51. Cunha AMSR. Resposta pulpar e periapical de dentes de cães após a utilização do MTA (Agregado Trióxido Mineral). Estudo histopatológico e radiográfico, 2002. 159p. Dissertação (mestrado) – Faculdade de Odontologia de Ribeirão Preto, Universidade de São Paulo, Ribeirão Preto, SP, Brasil.

52. D'Arcângelo C, D'Amario M. Use of MTA for orthograde obturation of nonvital teeth with open apices: report of two cases. Oral Surg. Oral Méd. Oral Pathol. Oral Radiol Endod, v.104, p.e98-e101, 2007.

53. DeDeus G, Coutinho Filho T. The use of white Portland cement as an apical plug in the tooth with a necrotic pulp and wide-open apex: a case report. Int Endod J, v.40, p.653-660, 2007.

54. DeDeus G, Reis C, Brandão C, Fidel S, Fidel RAS. The ability of Portland cement, MTA and MTA Bio to prevent through-and Through (??) fluid movement in repaired furcal perforations. J Endod, v.33, p.1374-1377, 2007.

55. Diamanti E, Kerezoudis NP, Gakis DB, Tsatsas V. Chemical composition and surface characteristics of grey and new white ProRoot MTA. Int Endod J, v.36, p.946 / Abstract. R81, 2003.

56. Dumsha TC, Holt GM. Biocompatibility of bone cement, ProRoot and Super-EBA in ferret canines. J Endod, v.26, p.554/Abstract.8, 2000.

57. Economides N, Pantelidou O, Kokkas A, Tziafas D. Short-term periradicular tissue response to mineral trioxide aggregate (MTA) as root-end filling material. Int Endod J, v.36, p.44-48, 2003.

58. El Meligy OAS, Avery DR. Comparison of apexification with mineral trioxide aggregate and calcium hydroxide. Pediatric Dentistry, v.28, n.3, p.248-253, 2006.

59. Estrela C, Bahmann LL, Estrela CRA, Silva RS, Pécora JD. Antimicrobial and chemical study of MTA, Portland cement, calcium hydroxide paste, Sealapex and Dycal. Braz Dent J, v.11, p.3-9, 2000.

60. Faraco Júnior IM, Holland R. Response of the pulp of dogs to capping with mineral trioxide aggregate or a calcium hydroxide cement. Dent. Traumatol., v.17, p.163-166, 2001.

61. Faria MD. Avaliação quantitativa e qualitativa da resposta tecidual frente aos cimentos MTA Angelus cinza e MTA fotopolimerizável experimental. Análise microscópica de implantes realizados em subcutâneo (??) de ratos. Araçatuba 2006;87p. Dissertação (mestrado). Faculdade de Odontologia de Araçatuba, Unesp.

62. Felippe WT, Felippe MCS, Rocha MJC. The effect of mineral trioxide aggregate on the apexifixation and periapical healing of teeth with incomplete root formation. Int Endod J, v.39, p.2-9, 2006.

63. Ferris DM, Baumgartner JC. Perforation repair comparing two types of mineral trioxide aggregate. J Endod, v.30, p.422-424, 2004.

64. Fischer EJ, Arens DA, Miller CH. Bacterial leakage of mineral trioxide aggregate as compared with zinc-free amalgam, intermediate restorative material, and super-EBA as a root-end filling material. J Endod, v.24, p.176-179, 1998.

65. Fridland M, Rosado R. Mineral trioxide aggregate (MTA) solubility and porosity with different water-to-powder ratios. J Endod, v.29, p.814-817, 2003.

66. Gandolfi MG, Perut F, Ciapetti G, Mongiorgi R, Prati C. New Portland cement-based material for endodontic mixed with articaine solution: A study of cellular response. J Endod, v.34, p.39-44, 2008.

67. Gomes Filho JE, Faria MD, Bernabé PFE, Nery MJ, Otoboni Filho JA, Dezan Junior E, Costa MMTM, Cannon M. Mineral trioxide aggregate but not light-cure mineral trioxide aggregate stimulated mineralization. J Endod, v.3, p.62-55, 2008. (favor verificar; mudei porque o 68 começava em OTOBONI... e o item anterior terminava em M.J., sem indicação de obra)

68. Guarienti D, Osinaga PWR, Figueiredo JAP. Avaliação química e estrutural comparativa entre o cimento Portland e o MTA. Braz. Oral Res, v.16, p.190/Abstract, 2002.

69. Ham KA, Witherspoon DE, Gutmann JL, Ravindranath Gait TC, Opperman LA. Preliminary evaluation of BMP-2 expression and histological characteristics during apexification with calcium hydroxide and mineral trioxide aggregate. J Endod, v.31, p.275-279, 2005.

70. Hamad HA, Tordik PA, Mcclanahan SB. Furcation perforation repair comparing gray and white MTA: a dye extraction study. J Endod, v.32, p.337-340, 2006.

71. Hardy I, Lieweehr FR, Joyce AP, Agee K, Pashley DH. Sealing ability of one-up bond and MTA with and without a secondary seal as furcation perforation repair materials. J Endod, v.30, p.658-661, 2004.

72. Hashem AAR, Hassanien EE. ProRoot MTA, MTA-Angelus and IRM used to repair large furcation perforations: Sealability study. J Endod, v.34, p.59-61, 2008.

73. Hayashi M, Shimizu A, Ebisu S. MTA for obturation of mandibular central incisors with open apices: case report. J Endod, v.30, n.2, p.120-122, 2004.

74. Holland R, Mazuqueli L, Souza V, Murata SS, Dezan Junior E. Influence of the type of vehicle and limit of obturation on apical and periapical tissue response in dogs teeth after root filling with mineral trioxide aggregate. J Endod, v.33, p.693-697, 2007.

75. Holland R, Otoboni Filho JA, Souza V, Nery MJ, Bernabé PFE, Dezan Junior E. Mineral trioxide aggregate repair of lateral root perforations. J Endod, v.27, p.281-284, 2001.

76. Holland R, Souza V, Murata SS, Nery MJ, Bernabé PFE, Otoboni Filho JA. Healing process of dog dental pulp after pulpotomy and pulp covering with mineral trioxide aggregate or Portland cement. Braz Dent J, v.12, p.109-113, 2001.

77. Holland R, Souza V, Nery MJ, Otoboni Filho JA, Bernabé PFE, Dezan Junior E. Reaction of dog's teeth to root canal filling with mineral trioxide aggregate or a glass ionomer sealer. J Endod, v.25, p.728-730, 1999.

78. Holland R, Souza V, Nery MJ, Otoboni Filho JA, Bernabé PFE, Dezan Junior E. Reaction of rat connective tissue to implanted dentin tubes filled with mineral trioxide aggregate or calcium hydroxide. J Endod, v.25, p.161-166, 1999.

79. Holland R, Souza V, Nery MJ, Otoboni Filho JA, Bernabé PFE, Dezan Junior E. Reaction of dog's teeth to root canal filling with mineral trioxide aggregate or a glass ionomer sealer. J Endod, v.25, p.728-730, 1999.

80. Holland R, Souza V, Nery MJ, Otoboni Filho JA, Bernabé PFE, Dezan Junior E. Agregado de trióxido mineral y cemento Portland en la obturación de conductos radiculares de perro. Endodoncia, v.19, p.275-280, 2001.

81. Holland R. Agregado de trióxido mineral (MTA): Composição, mecanismo de ação, comportamento biológico e emprego clínico. Rev Ciênc Odontol, v.5, p.7-21, 2002.

82. Holland R. Histochemical response of the pulp of dogs to capping with mineral trioxide aggregate or a calcium hydroxide cement. Dent Traumatol, v.17, p.163-166, 2001.

83. Hong ST, Bae KS, Baek SH, Kum KY, Lee WC. Microleakage of accelerated Mineral Trioxide Aggregate and Portland cement an in vitro apexification model. J Endod, v.34, p.56-58, 2008.

84. Hsien H, Cheng YA, Lee YL, Lan NH, Lin CP. Repair of perforating internal resorption with mineral trioxide aggregate: a case report. J Endod, v.29, p.538-539, 2003.

85. Jantarat J, Daspher SJ, Messer HH. Effect of matrix placement on furcation perforation repair. J Endod, v.25, p.192-195, 1999.

86. Junn DJ, Mc Millan P, Bakland LK, Torabinejad M. Quantitative assessment of dentin bridge formation following pulp capping with mineral trioxide aggregate (MTA). J Endod, v.24, p.278/ Abstract 29, 1998.

87. Karabucak B, Li L, Lim J, Iqbal M. Vital pulp therapy with mineral trioxide aggregate. Dent Traumat, v.21, p.240-243, 2005.

88. Karimjee CK, Koka S, Rallis DM, Gound TG. Cellular toxicity of mineral trioxide aggregate mixed with an alternative delivery vehicle. Oral Surg Oral Méd Oral Pathol Oral Radiol Endod, v.102, p.e115-e120, 2006.

89. Karp J, Bryk J, Menke E, McTigue D. The complete endodontic obturation of an immature permanent incisor with mineral trioxide aggregate: a case report. Pediatric Dentistry, v.28, p.273-278, 2006.

90. Keiser K, Johnson CC, Tipton DA. Cytotoxicity of mineral trioxide aggregate using human periodontal ligament fibroblasts. J Endod, v.26, p.288-291, 2000.

91. Kettering JD, Torabinejad M. Investigation of mutagenicity of mineral trioxide aggregate and other commonly used root-end filling materials. J Endod, v.21, p.537-539, 1995.

92. Kogan P, HEJ, Glickman GN, Watanabe I. The effects of various additives on setting properties of MTA. J Endod, v.32, p.569-572, 2006.

93. Koh ET, McDonald F, Pitt Ford TR, Torabinejad M. Cellular response to mineral trioxide aggregate. J Endod, v.24, p.543-547, 1998.

94. Koh ET, Pitt Ford TR, Kariyawasam SP, Chen NN, Torabinejad M. Prophylactic treatment of dens evaginatus using mineral trioxide aggregate. J Endod, v.27, p.540-542, 2001.

95. Komabayashi T, Spangberg LSW. Comparative analysis of the particle size and shape of commercially available mineral trioxide aggregates and Portland cement: a study with a flow particle image analyzer. J Endod, v.34, 94-98, 2008.

96. Kwak KI, Park DS, Oh S. The effect of obturation timing and thickness of mineral trioxide aggregate matrix on sealing ability. (abstract) J Endod, v.26, p.557, 2000.

97. Lamb EL, Loushine RJ, Weller RN, Kimbrough WF, Pashley DH. Effect of resection on the apical sealing ability of mineral trioxide aggregate. Oral Surg Oral Med Oral Pathol Oral Radiol Endod, v.95, p.732-735, 2003.

98. Lee ES. A new mineral trioxide aggregate root-end filling technique. J Endod, v.26, p.764-765, 2000.

99. Lee SJ, Monsef M, Torabinejad M. Sealing ability of a mineral trioxide aggregate for repair of lateral root perforations. J Endod, v.19, p.541-544, 1993.

100. Leonhardt AM, Paduli NR. Evaluación de la capacidad selladora de un cemento endodóntico experimental a base de polvo del Proroot (MTA) con una resina de base acuosa como vehículo. RAOA, v.95, p.259-264, 2007.

101. Lima MV, Bramante CM, Garcia RB, Moraes IG, Bernardineli N. Endodontic treatment of dens in dente associated with a chronic periapical lesion using an apical plug of mineral trioxide aggregate. Quintessence Int, v.38, p.41-45, 2007.

102. Mah T, Basani B, Santos JM, Pascon EA, Tjadrhane L, Yared G, Lawrence HP, Friedman S. Periapical inflammation affecting coronally-inoculated dog teeth with root filling augmented by white MTA orifice plugs. J Endod, v.29, p.442-446, 2003.

103. Main C, Mirzayan N, Shabahang S, Torabinejad M. Repair of root perforations using mineral trioxide aggregate: a long-term study. J Endod, v.30, p.80-83, 2004.

104. Martell B, Chandler NP. Electrical and dye leakage comparison of MTA, super EBA and IRM. J Endod, v.26, p.545/Abstracts 39, 2000.

105. Martin RL, Monticelli F, Brackett WW, Loushine RJ, Rockman RA, Ferrari M, Pashley DH, Tay FR. Sealing properties of mineral trioxide aggregate orthograde apical plugs and root filling an in vitro apexification model. J Endod, v.33, p.272-275, 2007.

106. Mendoza AM, Reina ES, Luque F. Cierre apical mediante agregado de trióxido mineral (MTA). Endodoncia, v.2, p.28-38, 2002.

107. Menezes RS, Bramante CM, Letra A, Carvalho VGG, Garcia RB. Histologic evaluation of pulpotomies in dog using two types of mineral trioxide aggregate and regular and white Portland cement as wound dressings. Oral Surg Oral Med Oral Pathol Oral Radiol Endod, v.98, p.376-379, 2004.

108. Menezes RS, Silva Neto UX, Carneiro E, Letra A, Bramante CM, Bernardineli N. MTA repair of a subcrestal perforation: a case report. J. Endod., v.31, p.212-214, 2005.

109. Mesimeris V, Sade E, Baer PN. Calcium sulfate as a biodegradable barrier membrane: a preliminary report on the Surgplat technique. Periodontol Clin Invest, v.17, p.13-16, 1996.

110. Mitchell PJC, Pitt Ford TR, Torabinejad M, McDonald F. Osteoblast biocompatibility of mineral trioxide aggregate. Biomaterials, v.20, p.167-173, 1999.

111. Mohammadi Z, Modaresi J, Yazdizadeh M. Evaluation of the antifungal effects of mineral trioxide aggregate material. Australian Endod J, v.32, p.120-122, 2006.

112. Mooney GC, North S. The current opinions and use of MTA for apical barrier formation of non-vital immature permanent incisors by consultants in pediatric dentistry in the UK. Dent Traumatol, v.24, p.65-69, 2008.

113. Morais CAH, Bernardineli N, Garcia RB, Duarte MAH, Guerisoli DMZ. Evaluation of tissue response to MTA and Portland cement with iodoform. Oral Surg Oral Med Oral Pathol Oral Radiol Endod, v.102, p.417-421, 2006.

114. Moretton TR, Brown CE, Legan JJ, Kafrawwy AH. Tissue reactions after subcutaneous and intraosseous implantation of mineral trioxide aggregate and ethoxybenzoic acid cement. J Biom Mat Res, v.52, p.528-533, 2000.

115. Moroto M, Barberia E, Planells P, Vera V. Treatment of a non-vital immature incisor with mineral trioxide aggregate (MTA). Dent. Traumatol., v.19, p.165-169, 2003.

116. Nakata TT, Bae KS, Baumgartner JC. Perforation repair comparing mineral trioxide aggregate and amalgam using an anaerobic bacterial leakage model. J Endod, v.3, p.184-186, 1998.

117. O'Sullivan SM, Hartwell GR. Obturation of retained primary mandibular second molar using mineral trioxide aggregate: a case report. J Endod, v.27, p.703-705, 2001.

118. Ozdemir HO, Ozçelik B, Karabucak, Cehreli ZC. Calcium ion diffusion from mineral trioxide aggregate through simulated root resorption defects. Dent Traumatol, v.24, p.70-73, 2008.

119. Pace R, Giuliani V, Lini Prato L, Bacceti T, Pagavino G. Apical plug technique using mineral trioxide aggregate; results from a case series. Int Endod J, v.40, p.478-484, 2007.

120. Panzarini SR, Holland R, Souza V, Poi WR, Sonoda CK, Pedrini D. Mineral trioxide aggregate as a root canal filling material in reimplanted teeth. Microscopic analysis in monkeys. Dent Traumatol, v.23, p.265-272, 2007.

121. Pariroki M, Asgary S, Eghbal MJ, Stowe S, Eslami B, Eskandarizade A, Shabahang S. A comparative study of white and grey mineral trioxide aggregate as pulp capping agents in dog's teeth. Dent Traumatol, v.21, p.150-154, 2005.

122. Pelliccioni GA, Vellani CP, Gatto MRA, Gandolfi MG, Marchetti C, Prati. Proroot mineral trioxide aggregate cement used as retrograde filling without addition of water: An in vitro evaluation of its microleakage. J Endod, v.33, p.1082-1085, 2007.

123. Pitt Ford TR, Torabinejad M, McKendry DJ, Hong CU, Kariyawasam SP. Use of mineral trioxide aggregate for repair of furcal perforations. Oral Surg Oral Méd Oral Pathol Oral Radiol Endod, v.79, p.756-763, 1995.

124. Queiroz AM, Assed S, Leonardo MR, Nelson Filho P, Silva LAB. MTA and calcium hydroxide for pulp capping. J Appl Oral Sci, v.13, p.126-130, 2005.

125. Rafter M, Baker M, Alves M, Daniel J, Remeikis N. Evaluation of healing with use of an internal matrix to repair furcation perforations. Int Endod J, v.36, p.775-783, 2002.

126. Sarkar NK, Caicedo R, Ritwik P, Moiseyeva R, Kawashima I. Physicochemical basis of the biologic properties of mineral trioxide aggregate. J Endod, v.31, p.97-100, 2005.

127. Sarris S, Tahmassebi JF, Duggal MS, Croos IA. A clinical evaluation of mineral trioxide aggregate for root-end closure of non vital immature permanent incisors in children-a pilot study. Dent Traumatol, v.24, p.79-85, 2008.

128. Shahi S, Rahimi S, Yavari HR, Shakouie S, Nezafati S, Abdolrahimi M. Sealing ability of white and gray mineral trioxide aggregate mixed with distilled water and 0.12% Chlorhexidine gluconate when used as root end filling materials. J Endod, v.33, p.1429-1432, 2007.

129. Simon S, Rilliard F, Berdal A, Machtou P. The use of mineral trioxide aggregate in one-visit apexification treatment: a prospective study. Int Endod J, v.40, p.186-197, 2007.

130. Soares IML. Reposta pulpar ao MTA, agregado trióxido mineral, comparado ao hidróxido de cálcio em pulpotomia. Estudo histológico em dentes de cães. (Tese) – Faculdade de Odontologia de Florianópolis, UFSC, Florianópolis, Santa Catarina, 1996.

131. Storm B, Eichmiller FC, Tordik P, Goodell GG. Setting expansion of gray and white mineral trioxide aggregate and Portland cement. J Endod, v.34, p.80-82, 2008.

132. Summer M, Muglali M, Bodrumlu E, Guvenc T. Reaction of connective tissue to amalgam, intermediate restorative material, mineral trioxide aggregate, and mineral trioxide aggregate mixed with chlorhexidine. J Endod, v.32, p.1094-1096, 2006.

133. Title K, Farley J, Linkhardt T, Torabinejad M. Apical closure induction using bone growth factors and mineral trioxide aggregate. (abstract) J Endod, v.22, p.198, 1996.

134. Torabinejad M, Chivian N. Clinical applications of mineral trioxide aggregate. J Endod, v.25, p.197-205, 1999.

135. Torabinejad M, Hong CU, Lee SJ, Monsef M, Pitt Ford TR. Investigation of mineral trioxide aggregate for root-end filling in dogs. J Endod, v.21, p.603-608, 1995.

136. Torabinejad M, Hong CU, McDonald F, Pitt Ford TR. Physical and chemical properties of a new root-end filling material. J Endod, v.21, p.349-353, 1995.

137. Torabinejad M, Hong CU, Pitt Ford TR, Kettering JD. Antibacterial effects of some root-end filling materials. J Endod, v.21, p.403-406, 1995.

138. Torabinejad M, Lee SJ, Hong UC. Apical marginal adaptation of orthograde and retrograde root-end fillings: a dye leakage and scanning electron microscopie study. J Endod, v.20, p.402-407, 1994.

139. Torabinejad M, Pitt Ford TR, McKendry DJ, Abedi HR, Miller DA, Kariyawasam SP. Histologic assessment of mineral trioxide aggregate as a root end filling in monkeys. J Endod, v.23, p.225-228, 1997.

140. Torabinejad M, Watson TF, Pitt Ford TR. Sealing ability of a mineral trioxide aggregate when used as a root-end filling material. J Endod. v.19, p.591-595, 1993.

141. Tziafas D, Pantelidou O, Alvanou A, Belibasakis G, Papadimitriou S. The dentinogenic effect of mineral trioxide aggregae (MTA) in short-term capping experiments. Int. Endod. J., v.35, p.245-254, 2002.

142. Valois CRA, Costa ED. Influence of the thickness of mineral trioxide aggregate on sealing ability of root-end fillings in vitro. Oral Surg Oral Med Oral Pathol Oral Radiol Endod, v.97, p.108-111, 2004.

143. Vander-Weele RA, Schwartz SA, Beeson TJ. Effect of blood contamination on retention characteristics of MTA when mixed with different liquids. J Endod, v.32, p.421-424, 2006.

144. Weldon JK, Pashley DH, Loushine RJ, Weller RN, Kimbrough F. Sealing ability of mineral trioxide aggregate and Super-EBA when used as furcation repair materials: a longitudinal study. J Endod, v.28, p.467-470, 2002.

145. Westphalen FH. et al. Análise comparativa da radiopacidade de cimentos Portland e MTA. Braz. Oral Res, v.17, p.182, Supplement Abstract n.Pb192, 2003.

146. Vizgirda PJ, Liewehr FR, Patton WR, McPherson JC, Buxton, TB Comparison of laterally condensed gutta-percha, thermoplasticized gutta-percha and mineral trioxide aggregate as root canal filling materials. J Endod, v.30, p.103-106, 2004.

147. Wucherpfenning AL, Green DB. Mineral trioxide vs. Portland cement: two biocompatible filling materials. J Endod, v.25, p.308, Abstract n.40, 1999.

148. Yaltirik M, Ozbas H, Bilgic B, Issever H. Reaction of connective tissue to mineral trioxide aggregate and amalgam. J Endod, v.30, p.95-99, 2004.

149. Yildrim T, Gençoglu N, Firat I, Guzel O. Histologic study of furcation perforation treated with MTA or Super EBA in dog teeth. Oral Surg Oral Med Oral Pathol Oral Radiol Endod, v.100, p.120-124, 2005.

150. Zoletti GO, Araújo MCP, Gusman H. Utilização do MTA como obturador de lesão reabsortiva: relato de caso clínico. J Bras Endod, v.5, p.416-421, 2005.

2.XII

Digital radiography in Endodontics

Andréa Gonçalves
Marcelo Gonçalves

A conventional intra-oral radiograph, one in which an image is created in the silver halide emulsion of the film, is of recognized value and importance, and is the most used in Endodontics, as it provides an image of good quality at low cost. Nevertheless, radiographic film has some disadvantages. For instance it is inefficient as a photon detector, because it absorbs only a small percentage of the total of photons that strike it. It provides a static image that cannot be significantly altered and it requires processing that may lead to loss of information, especially if it is not carried out under ideal conditions. Processing requires chemical solutions that may cause allergic reactions and pollute the environment. The film requires a relatively high dose of radiation and is sensitive to variations in exposure time.

With the development of computerized radiography technology, there is ongoing research in several areas of dentistry seeking means to improve the precision of interpretation and reduce the radiation dose. There has been considerable advancement in the field of digital radiographic imaging, and it has been noted that the digital system of intra-oral radiographs offers great potential for a radical change in the manner in which dentists diagnose and treat dental pathologies. While the intra-oral film records, stores, and displays the image in the conventional technique, in digital radiography these same tasks are carried out separately: the digital sensor records the image, the monitor displays it and the computer stores it. The speed of the technology and benefits of using it, have forced practitioners to stay up to date and seek innovations that improve with amazing speed, so that they are an important part of today's practice, and have become indispensable in numerous dental clinics and clinical practices.

The digital image is one that can be recorded by a sensor, instead of a radiographic film. After the sensor is sensitized by X-rays, it captures the image and transfers it to a computer, where it is stored, analyzed, manipulated and quantified. The first digital image system introduced in Dentistry was RadioVisioGraphy (Trophy-France), which received full approval from the FDA for use in intra-oral radiography, in 1989. The system has a device called CCD (charge couple device) as a receptor.

Considering that Endodontics is a highly critical specialty, in which the limits of therapy are determined by radiographic images obtained during operative procedures, it is sometimes necessary to make a large number of images. This enables the practitioner to better control his/her endodontic procedures or confirms a diagnosis in more specific situations, such as root fractures, external and internal resorptions, follow-up of periapical lesions, dental trauma and periapical surgeries. It should be pointed out that the radiographic image is a two dimensional view of three dimensional structures, and that various factors, such as the positioning and inclination of the tooth in the arch, as well as the superimpositions of bone structures influence the final image, causing alterations and producing possible artifacts in interpretation. The use of digital radiographs offers a means to optimize the working time at a reduced exposure time, enabling faster diagnosis, as the images to be analyzed are displayed almost instantaneously without requiring chemical processing.

SENSORS AND RESOLUTION

For better understanding of the sensor/resolution binomial, it is necessary to discuss the initial investigation of Nelvig et al. (1992)[31], who stated that the CCD sensor was inefficient as a direct detector of the X-rays, because of its inability to capture photons with energy higher than 20 KeV. They therefore proposed the use of a plate image intensifier that converts the incident radiation into light. This resulted in the intra-oral sensor (Figs. 2.XII-1A-B) which consists of a scintillation plate measuring approximately 18 x 26 millimeters, optical fibers and a CCD device, incorporated in a plastic housing. When the X-ray photons strike the scintillation plate, it fluoresces. The optic fibers then conduct the light to the CCD and it is transformed into electric signals, which are received by the data processing unit. An analog-to-digital converter converts the signal into a digitized image, which is stored and can be displayed on a monitor almost immediately after the sensor is exposed to radiation.

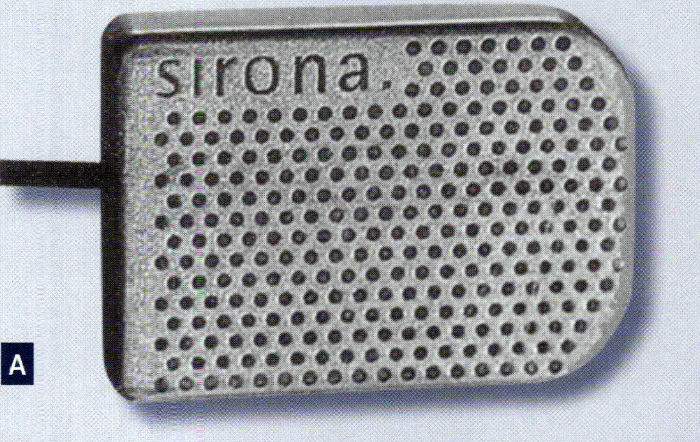

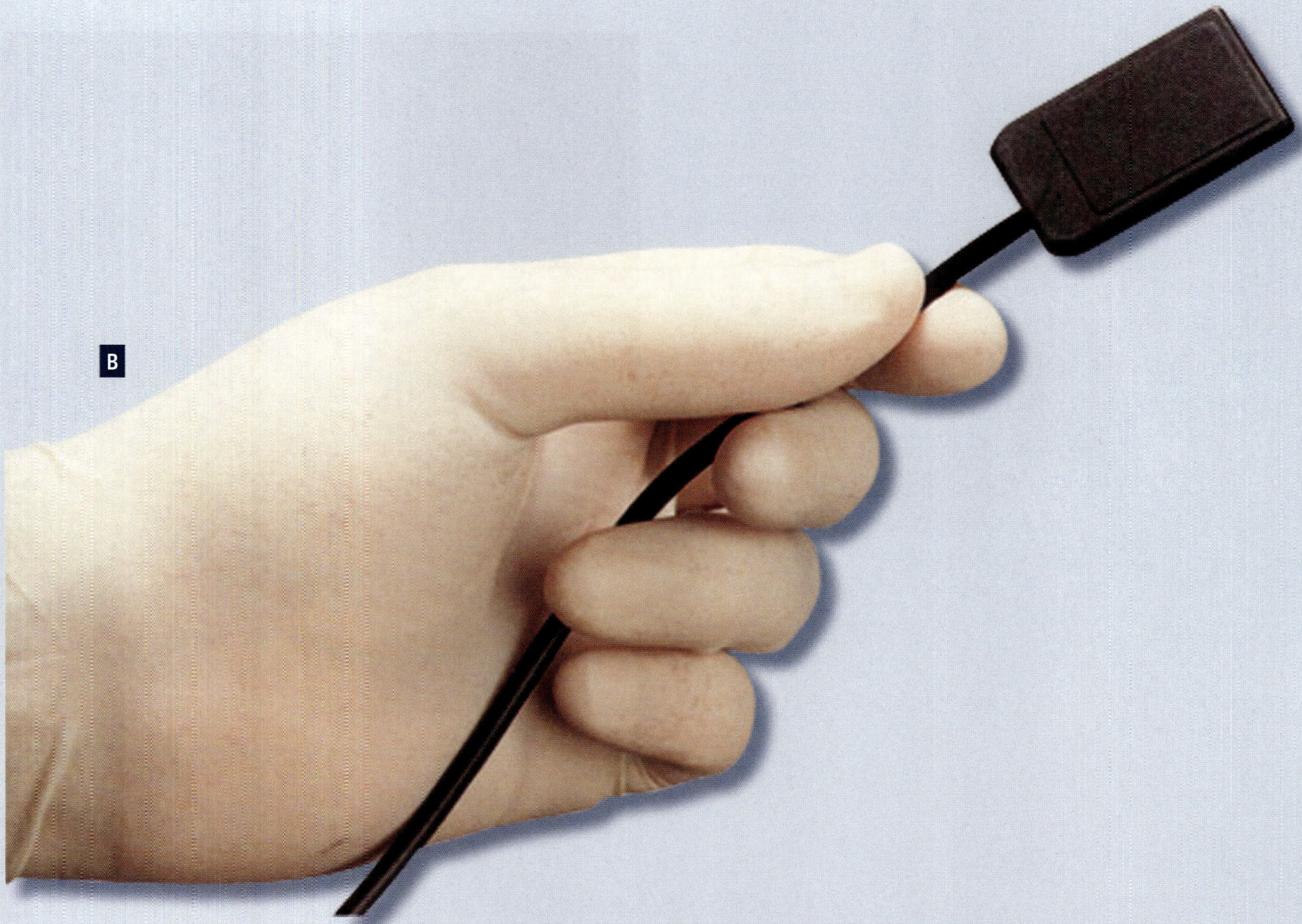

B

FIGS. 2.XII-1A-B

Sensor of the type CCD from Sirona with a connecting optic fiber cable

During digital conversion, the information contained in the image is broken down into bits (binary digits), arranged in rows and columns called a matrix, which contains dots, called pixels, which are the smallest units of information into which an image can be broken down. The pixel size is responsible for the spatial resolution of the image; therefore, the smaller it is, the higher the resolution and the more details will be displayed. Consequently, the quality of the image improves according to the number of pixels per unit of surface.

The increase in detail of the image can be achieved by reducing the size and the number of pixels per unit of surface, which is done by changing the spatial resolution of the video monitor. In other words, the digital image is totally described by the numeric address of each pixel and by the numeric value of its intensity, which assume a digital value corresponding to a shade of grey. The number of grey shades available in the digital system determines the density of the resulting image. In general, the standard for intra-oral radiography is the digitization of the image into 256 shades of grey.

Studies by Horner et al. (1990) and Shearer et al. (1990)[37] suggest that the digital system is of importance, particularly in endodontic treatment. The ability of this system to output instant images eliminates the time involved in processing the conventional film, while the small sized sensor is particularly appropriate for displaying single teeth. Nevertheless, it is necessary to express some reservations with respect to the correct positioning of the sensor in the mouth, due to the fiber optic cable. As the CCD sensor has a smaller active (sensitive) area for image capture, this may require a larger number of radiographs to be taken, potentially reducing the advantage of diminishing exposure to radiation, in comparison with the conventional film.

According to research by Horner et al. (1990)[19], 25% of digital system images evaluated by observers were rejected because they were unable to fit the area of interest on the receptor. This was attributed to a lack of familiarity with the system or to a lack of professional training in the use of the digital system. Today's sensors (Fig. 2.XII-2) have similar dimensions to conventional films, comprising a larger area, with the main objective of reducing the incidence of X-radiation.

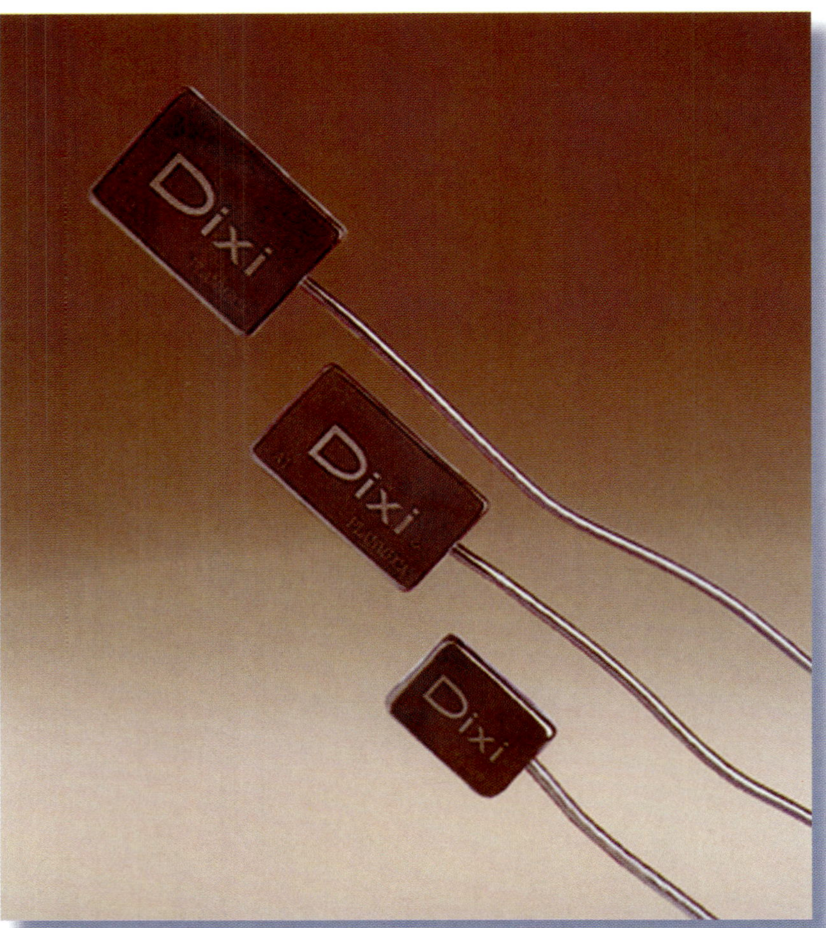

FIG. 2.XII-2

Different sizes of CCD sensors.

With the use of the CCD capture system, the images are taken without the need to remove the sensors from the oral cavity. This allows the head of the X-ray unit to be repositioned at a different angulation, while the sensor can remain in its original position.

The digital system can have a lower or higher resolution than the conventional radiographic film (12 to 14 pairs of lines per millimeter), depending on the model analyzed, which can reduce the efficiency of this system in showing small structures, for instance thin endodontic files. In some cases, the high resolution of the conventional radiographic films allows for better visualization of the image of endodontic instruments inside the root canals. Consequently, any alternative image system has to be evaluated, and has to be at least equally efficient and convenient for the procedures that need to be done.

Based on the characteristics of image resolution, it is clear that only some sensors are capable of detecting thinner files. The presence of noise*, which is the interference captured during the image acquisition process, reduces the contrast of the files in relation to the surrounding structures, which results in an unacceptable loss of image quality during radiographic interpretation.

More recently, digital image systems have been introduced, which unlike the CCD systems, do not use an image receptor connected by fiber optics (Figs. 2.XII-3 and 2.XII-4). The Digora system (Soderex, Finland) and the DenOptix system (Gendex, Italy) capture images by means of a reusable optical plate coated with phosphor, which does not require a cable connection. The plate has similar dimensions to those of standard radiographic films, both in size (30 mm x 40 mm) and in thickness (1 mm). In comparison with the CCD systems, the phosphor coated sensors are easy to place in the oral cavity, resulting in greater comfort to the patient, due to the absence of a wire and avoiding the need for a larger number of radiographs when a more extensive area requires examination. When the optical plate is irradiated, a certain amount of energy from the X-rays is stored on its surface, thus forming the latent image. After the radiographic procedure is finished, a laser reads the latent image by means of a specific device provided by the manufacturer (Figs. 2.XII-5 and 2.XII-6). After reading, the image is sent to a computer, which, after the digitization process displays the image on a monitor. After examination of the image it can be filed and manipulated by means of a variety of resources available for this system.

* Intrinsic noise of the digital system and structured noise of the bone anatomy and soft tissues.

2.XII-3

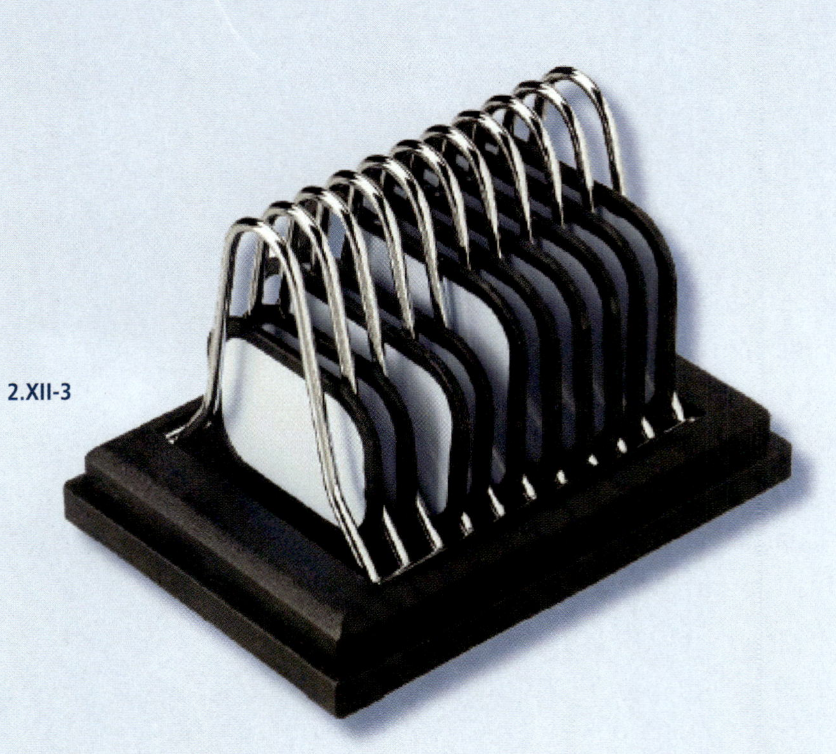

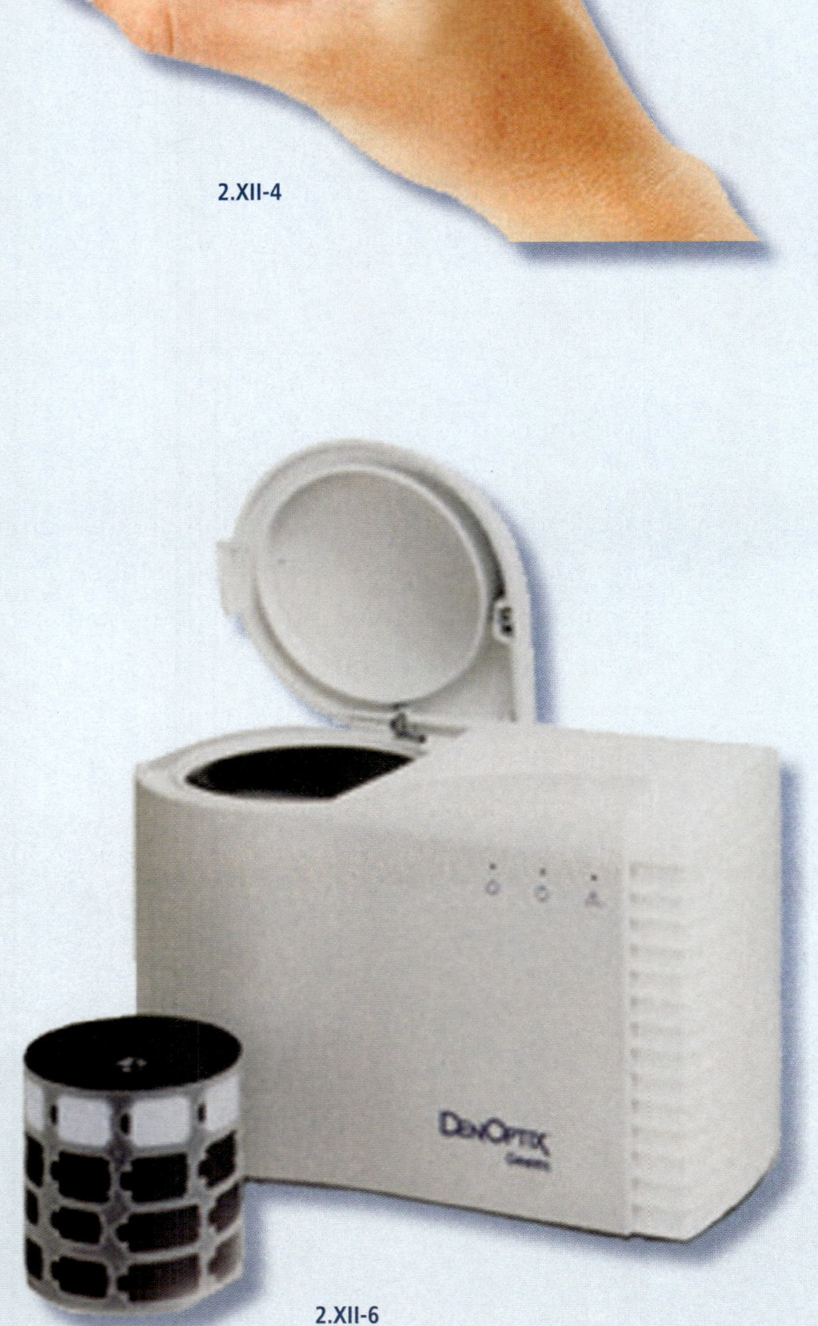

2.XII-4

FIG. 2.XII-3
Reusable phosphor coated sensors from Digora system.

FIG. 2.XII-4
Malleable phosphor sensors from DenOptix system.

FIG. 2.XII-5
Latent image reading scanner from Digora system.

FIG. 2.XII-6
Latent image reading scanner from Denoptix system.

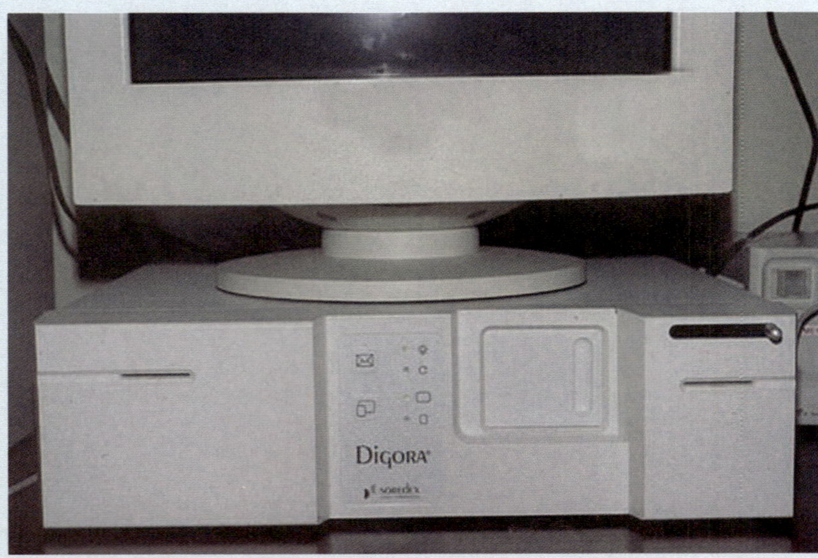

2.XII-5

2.XII-6

Schick Technologies has developed a system called CDR Wireless, which makes use of a phosphor coated plate without a fiber optic cable connection, in which the images formed by the pixels are transmitted through radiofrequency waves to an interface station, which decodes the images and sends them to a computer which displays them on a monitor (Fig. 2.XII-7).

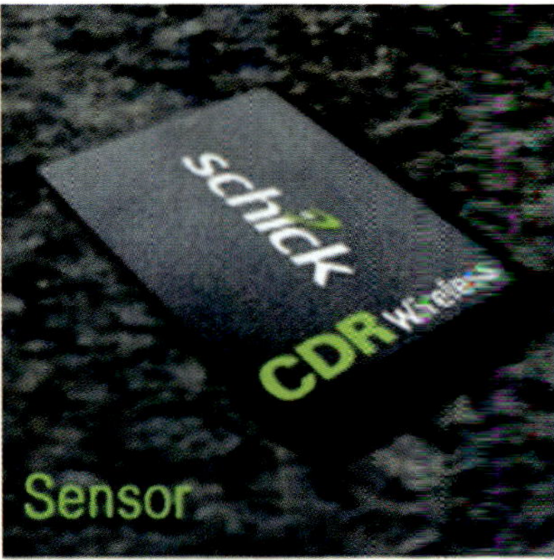

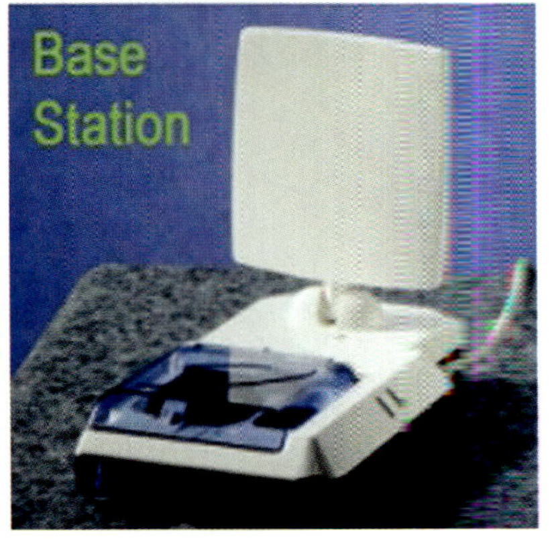

FIG. 2.XII-7
CDR Wireless with sensor and interface with a radiofrequency antenna.

RADIATION DOSE

Every time a radiograph is made, there should be concern about determining the radiation dose to which a patient is being submitted. Therefore radiology and its components, such as films and intensifier plates, have undergone rapid development in recent times. Over the last decade, intra-oral radiographic films have become more sensitive and faster, at the expense of the format and disposition of the halogenated silver salt crystals, which have greatly minimized the dose of radiation required to produce images of diagnostic quality.

Recent research has shown that with a digital system, the resultant dose of radiation is much lower compared to conventional films. Research on radiation doses have verified that with digital systems there is a reduction of around 40 to 90% in comparison to conventional films of the sensitivity groups D, E and F*.

SOFTWARE APPLICATIONS AND THEIR TOOLS

With the image acquisition software supplied by the manufacturer digital systems have computer tools that allow images to be modified, which are useful for several dental applications and of immense applicability in endodontics.

An image on the monitor can be magnified between 2X and 4X, over and above the standard pre-established by the software manufacturer, (Figs. 2.XII-8A-C). With the use of magnification, practitioners are able to obtain an enlargement of the image, although this does not mean that more details can be seen, in comparison with the original image. This is based on the fact that the greater the magnification of the image, the greater the magnification of the pixels, which results in a distorted and grainy image. Griffiths et al. (1992)[15] reported that the magnified images shown on the monitor offer a better quality than printed images. In endodontics, the image magnification tool can be used to determine the working length, assess the quality of root canal filling, determine the presence of accessory canals and root dilacerations.

* Sensitivity is the capability of the radiographic film to produce images with greater or less amount of radiation. The faster films are those from group F, which require 50% less than group E, and so on, subsequenty.

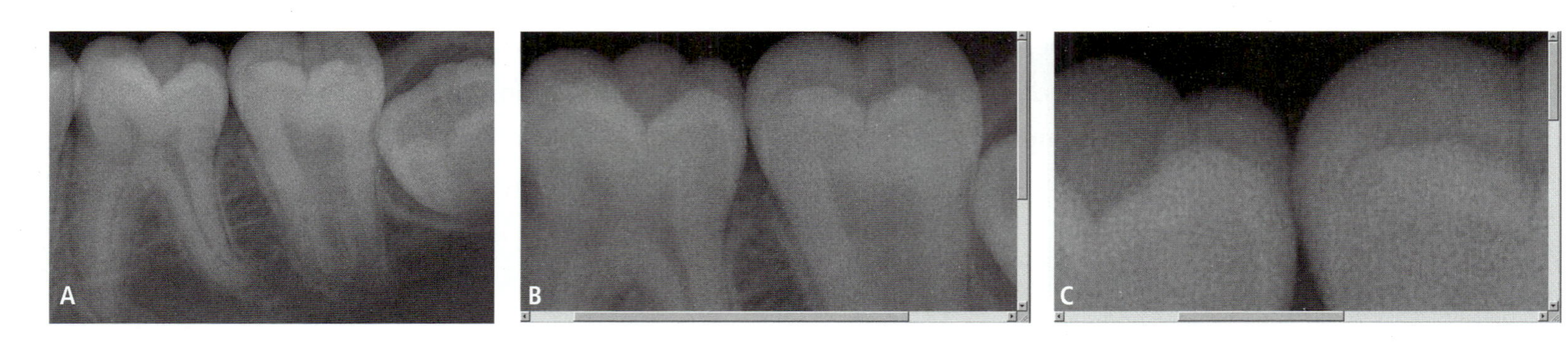

FIGS. 2.XII-8A-C

A – Original size image.
B – 2 X magnified size image.
C – 4 X magnified size image.

When there is an omission in the adjustment of exposure time the resultant image can be lighter or darker than the ideal one. Up to a certain point, digital systems are capable of compensating for these errors by altering the brightness and contrast of the image (Figs. 2.XII-9A-E).

In some areas of the mouth, the CCD type sensor captures the image in an inverted position; that is, the structures are rotated 180º in relation to the horizontal plane. Rotation of the digital image is a basic tool of the software program and does not affect the quality (Fig. 2.XII-10).

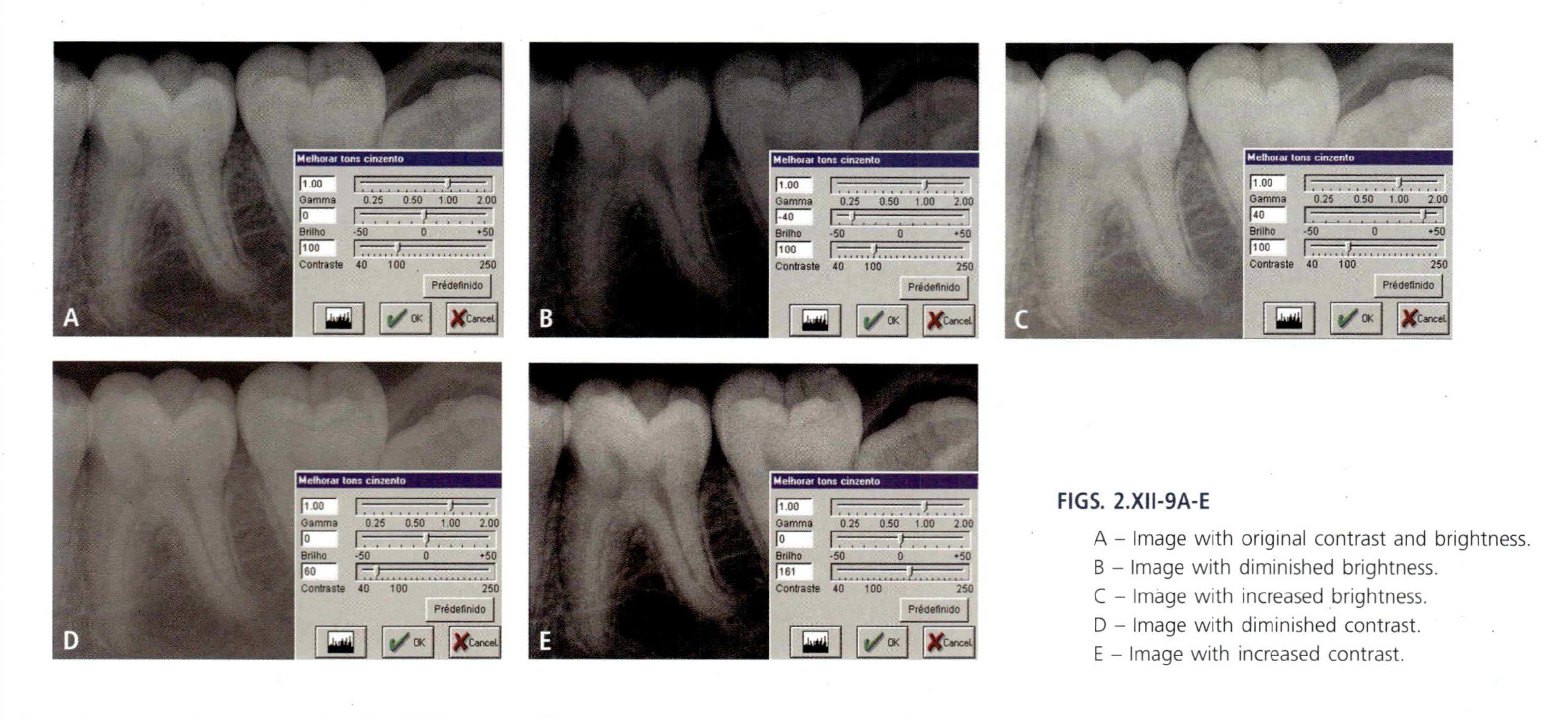

FIGS. 2.XII-9A-E

A – Image with original contrast and brightness.
B – Image with diminished brightness.
C – Image with increased brightness.
D – Image with diminished contrast.
E – Image with increased contrast.

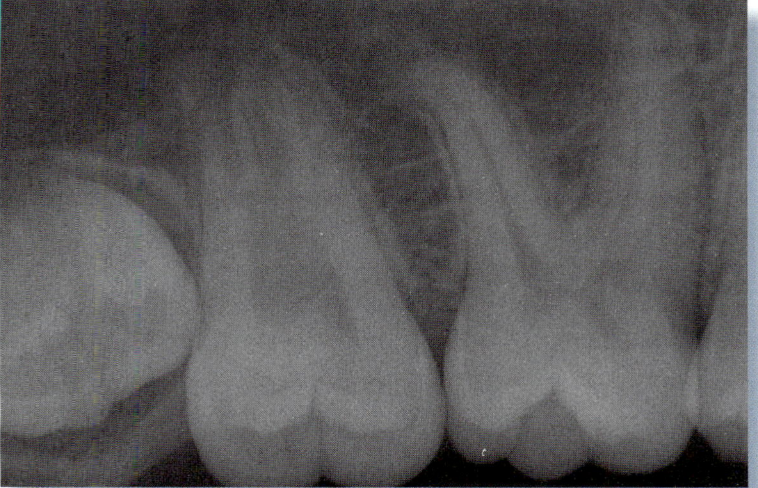

FIG. 2.XII-10
180° rotation of original image.

The digital image can also be observed in an inverse relationship; that is, structures that appeared radiopaque in the original image will now appear radiolucent in the modified image. This tool is known as "negative image", similar to the negatives of hard copy photographs (Fig. 2.XII-11). The main indication for the use of this tool is during working length determination, to observe endodontic files beyond the apical foramen or in cases of overfilling.

Some software applications are capable of altering digital images, modifying the pixel disposition and giving the human eye the impression that it is seeing the third dimension image (depth), whereas in reality software continues to show only the height and width of structures. This type of modification is known as "relief image", and according to some software manufacturers, its purpose is to increase the precision for visualizing instruments inside root canals (Fig. 2.XII-12).

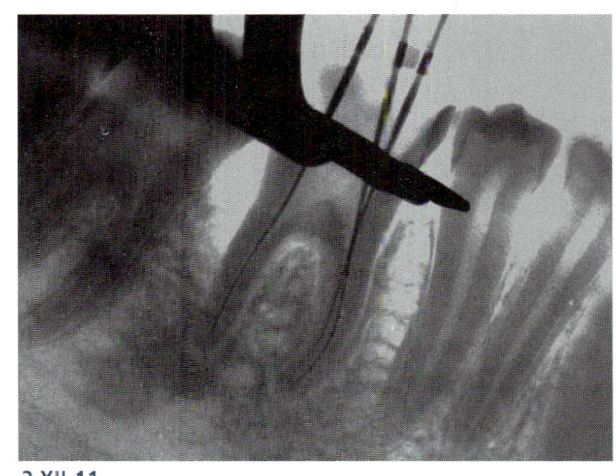

2.XII-11

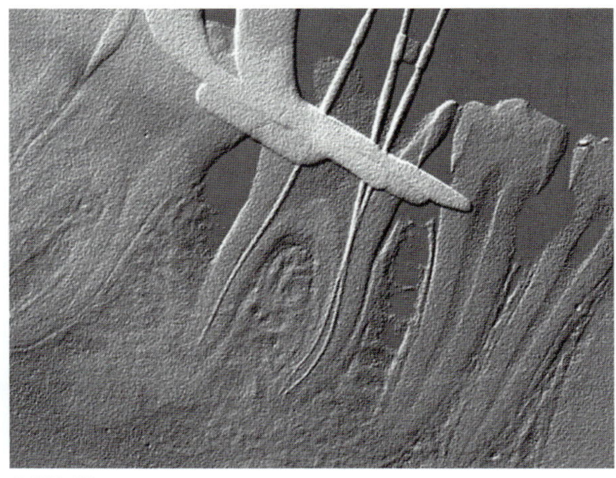

2.XII-12

FIG. 2.XII-11
Negative image of working length determination of a mandibular molar (image courtesy of Prof. Dr. Daniel Pinto de Oliveira).

FIG. 2.XII-12
Relief image of working length measurement of a mandibular molar (image courtesy of Prof. Dr. Daniel Pinto de Oliveira).

The software can easily transform an image captured in the gray scale into an image in color. Furthermore there is a tool known as "color image", which transforms the image in tones of color that are in the range of the visible light spectrum, with all the intermediate nuances representing the degree of density of the image (Figs. 2.XII-13A-B). Its main application is for observing early periapical lesions. Wenzel (1993)[50] mentions that Van der Stelt (1979) showed that periapical bone lesions were perceived earlier with a color radiographic image than with a traditional radiograph.

The radiographic density of filling materials has frequently been investigated. The digital system is capable of detecting areas that have the same density in radiographs. According to Tanomaru Filho et al. (2008)[41], this allows evaluation of filling material homogenization, bubbles inside cements and the comparison of radiographic density of filling cements as indicators of excellence (Fig. 2.XII-14). Tanomaru Filho et al. (2007)[42] reported that the assessment of radiopacity of dental materials is an important requisite of filling materials, as the image obtained by means of X-rays, either conventionally or by means of a digitized image, is the only available means of assessing root canal filling quality. The canal filling material must have radiopacity in order for the filling to provide a clear and homogenous radiographic image to its fullest extent. According to the ADA Specification No 57, the radiopacity of a cement must be equivalent to not less than 4 millimeters of aluminum. The inclusion of the aluminum scale image in radiographic films or sensors has made it possible to transform the light transmission readings into aluminum thickness (Fig. 2.XII-15).

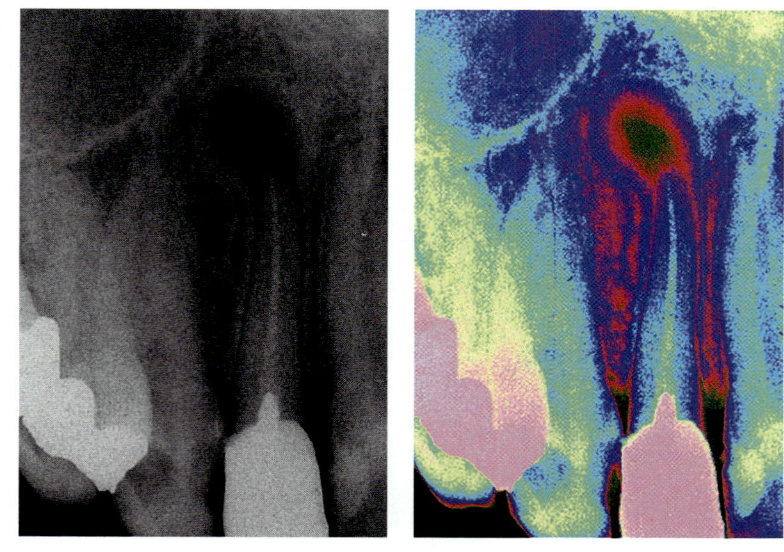

FIGS. 2.XII-13A-B

A – Original image.
B – Radiographic image showing different nuances of color.

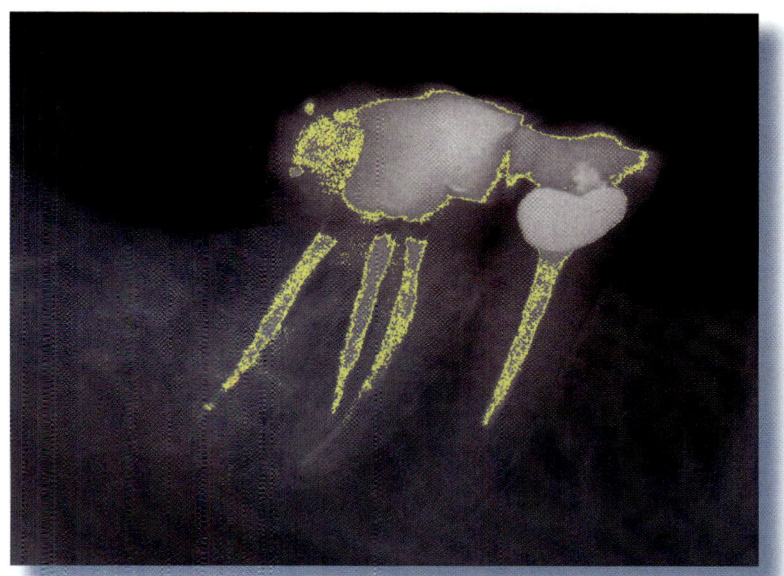

FIG. 2.XII-14

Radiographic image of endodontically treated teeth showing the presence of internal irregularities of the filling material, represented by the difference in density.

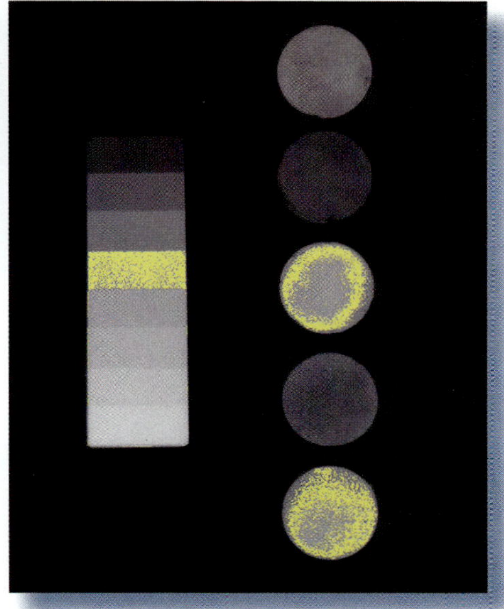

FIG. 2.XII-15

Image of 5 test specimens made with endodontic filling cements (right) and scale of aluminum (left) showing which degree of scale is compatible with the radiopacity of the selected cements (each degree equals 2 mm of aluminum, from top to bottom).

A digital radiography tool that is widely used in endodontics is the measurement of distances. One can determine the length of a tooth by tracing a line that runs from a coronal reference point to the radiographic vertex of the apex and the program will instantly provide a measurement in millimeters, so that the practitioner has a reading on which to base the working length (Fig. 2.XII-16). In curved roots, one can trace various straight segments joined by points, and the total length will be supplied by the program by adding up the marked segments (Fig. 2.XII-17).

Radiographic follow-up of endodontically treated teeth for the purpose of verifying the regression of a periapical bone lesion, can be done by measuring the total area of rarefaction. The digital system can count the number of pixels that are present inside an area outlined by the practitioner (Fig. 2.XII-18), thus providing evidence of repair when the number diminishes from the baseline to the follow-up evaluation.

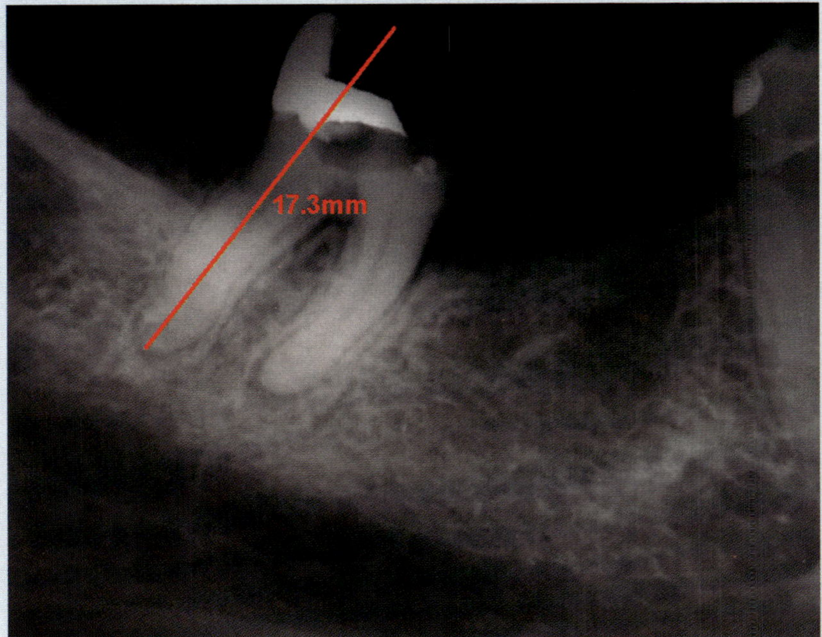

FIG. 2.XII-16

Total length of tooth measured with the software tool from the digital system.

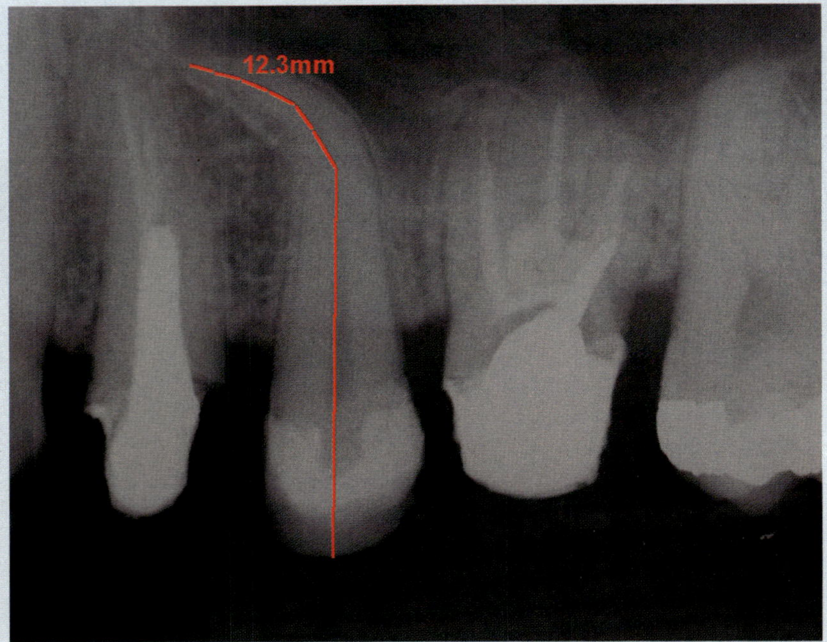

FIG. 2.XII-17

Total length of tooth measured in several sequential segments.

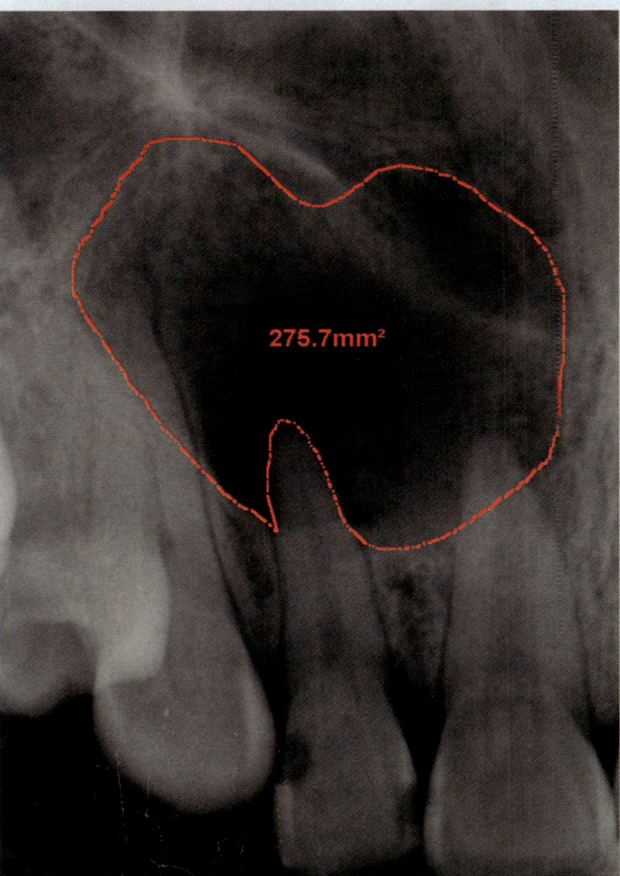

FIG. 2.XII-18

External outline of the lesion of tooth 1.2 and total measured area.

ADVANTAGES AND DISADVANTAGES

The innumerable advantages when using a digital image system include: reduction in the amount of radiation; good image quality; dispenses with the use of radiographic film, processing solutions, darkroom and automatic processors; rapid image acquisition with the image appearing almost instantaneously on the monitor, without requiring the developing and fixation process, which require time. The optimization of working time provided by digital radiography is enormous. While one spends several valuable minutes when processing a radiograph by the conventional technique, one is able to proceed with treatment when using the digital technique. Since on average five to six radiographs are needed for endodontic treatment, there is a considerable time saving of about 30 minutes. Nevertheless, as pointed out before, as it is easy to exhibit an image immediately after it is taken, this can also be abused, as the dentist may be encouraged to make additional exposures, of which some may be unnecessary.

Other advantages are directly related to the digital system, such as: filing, magnification and manipulation, altering density and contrast; wide scale of exposure time; measurements of anatomical features or pathologic entities; ease of electronically sending a digital radiograph to other locations; working with an image that has 256 tones of gray in stead of 25 (naked eye) of traditional radiographs, which allows a greater range of variations in observable tones of gray.

Undoubtedly, the greatest disadvantage of the digital system for image acquisition is the high cost of the equipment. Although these systems appeared in the 1990s, in Brazil the cost of purchasing is still high, requiring an initial investment of around 5 - 10 thousand dollars. The delay in the return of this investment may be a decisive factor at the time of buying the equipment.

It is generally acknowledged that the use of this system requires the operator to undergo prior training and acquire additional manual and computer skills.

LEGAL ASPECT

Because of the possibilities of editing and/or manipulating digital images, the system can be abused to justify possible iatrogenic performances in clinics or dental offices. With an increase in legal processes against professionals in the health care profession, digital radiography is an important component in the trials of these cases, and if fraudulently manipulated, it represents a dishonest manner to justify treatments. Therefore, manufacturers of software for the purpose of editing and/or manipulating radiographic images, must be warned of the importance of developing mechanisms of protection against abusive use or it may be necessary to restrict the use of computerized radiography.

Holmes (2000)[18] outlined the legal aspects of radiography and digital images in general, including the reports on which they were based. He also investigated the medical-legal aspects inherent to the manipulation of images, and concluded that they can be useful during a legal evaluation and in the event that they have gone astray, the report made by the practitioner could be used during the process. He suggested that strict measures should be taken to limit possible abuse in electronic manipulation of images in scientific publications, and established guidelines for the reproduction of radiographic images.

Furthermore, it should be reported that in Brazil, the validity of digital radiography as material proof in legal processes is under discussion at present. Manufacturers seek new ways of adapting their products to national resolutions, including the implementation of symbols that appear on modified digital images, to differentiate them from the originals. Moreover, in dental radiography, a mechanism is being introduced for the certification of images issued by specialized clinics and institutes, to attest to their originality.

APPLICATIONS IN ENDODONTICS

Determining the real working length is of fundamental importance for the success of endodontic therapy, because it establishes the apical limit of the preparation and it allows the creation of an apical stop. It also allows necrotic remnants to be removed from the canal without being transported beyond the apex, thus avoiding trauma to the periapical tissues or damage of the root apex anatomy. Success of conventional endodontic treatment has been correlated to the extent of the end of the root canal filling. In spite of the introduction of electronic apex locators, determining working length still depends on the use of a diagnostic file and radiography, particularly the intra-oral technique that use conventional films, a system that is a economical and practical.

Curently, the digital radiograph systems present better resolution, and can be used safely, practically and efficiently in determining the working length, as well as during all stages of conventional endodontic treatment.

On the other hand, it has been demonstrated that the diameter of endodontic files introduced into root canals may play a role in the accuracy of the digital systems. For this reason, Sanderink et al. (1994)[34] compared five different intra-oral digital sensors with conventional films of E sensitivity in the detection of endodontic files, and reported that the digital systems are comparable with conventional films only in images that were made with files No 15, and not for files smaller than No 10. Addressing a similar issue, Shearer et al. (1991)[36] compared working length measurements obtained with a conventional film with digital radiography and concluded that the appearance of file No 15 was better visible in conventional films than in digital images. However, when the digital images underwent a change in contrast, significant differences were no longer observed between the images. The authors confirmed that the resolution of the digital systems is inferior, and therefore its efficacy in reproducing small structures, such as thin files, is limited. Furthermore, they suggested the use of software tools that are available in digital radiography, to replace conventional films for determining the working length. According to Kal *et al* (2007)[23], image inversion, contrast/brightness changes, modifying the "relief image", are techniques that can be recommended for measuring the file length precisely. In a study recently conducted by Heo et al. (2008)[17], the effects of ambient light and depth of bits of digital radiography was conducted when an observer determined the position of the endodontic file inside root canals. They demonstrated that there was greater precision with 12 bits images; moreover, the time of interpretation was much longer in ambient light and with images of 8 bits.

BONE LESIONS

Endodontics offers excellent opportunities for comparative studies between digital and traditional radiography because it is a specialty that depends preponderantly on radiography. It is a very important tool in the evaluation of periapical lesions, as well as evaluation of completed treatments, because it is by observing that we analyze the cahnges of structure and the shape of bone tissues. However, in spite of the importance of radiography in endodontics, frequently some limitations restrict the capability of arriving at a precise diagnosis. Several authors, among them Bender & Seltzer (1961)[2], have emphasized that small defects in the alveolar bone may not be detected radiographically. Another study, Theilade (1960)[43], reported that radiography tends to show a bone lesion smaller than it actually is. Alterations in bone density are the most consistent aspects of progression or resolution of a periapical rarefaction. In order for these to be detected on a radiograph by the human eye, a change of approximately 30% in mineralization is necessary.

The accuracy of a diagnosis by means of radiography can be increased by using resources that supplement the faculties of a human observer. The use of a computer, as an auxiliary, offers these advantages.

When a digital system is compared with a conventional film in detecting periapical bone rarefactions, the literature has shown that the digital system has a high degree of objectivity. On the other hand, in spite of the innumerable advantages of the digital image, its capability to detect periapical bone lesions is limited when compared to conventional radiography. These problems can be overcome by the cone-beam computerized tomography (Stavropoulos & Wenzel, 2007)[39].

Radiography of digital subtraction has shown to be more sensitive than conventional radiography in detecting small dimension periapical bone alterations. The use of this image modality has shown to be a reliable indicator to assess treatment of root canal(s) in teeth with periapical lesions.

A study conducted by Shrout et al. (1993)[38], indicated that differences among pathological conditions, cysts and granulomas, by means of standard of distributions of the scale of gray of the digitalized radiographic images can be obtained.

References

1. ΦrstavIk D. Radiographic evaluation of apical periodontitis and endodontic treatment results: a computer approach. Int Dent J, London, v.41, n.2, p.89-98, Apr. 1991.
2. Bender I, Seltzer S. Roentgenographic and direct observation of experimental lesions in bone. J Am Dent Assoc, Chicago, v.62,p.708-716,1961.
3. Borg E, Gröndahl HG. On the dynamic range of different X-ray photon detectors in intra-oral radiography. A comparison of image quality in film, charge-coupled device and storage phosphor systems. Dentomaxillofac Radiol, Houndsmills, v.25,n.2,p.82-88,Abr.1996.
4. Bragger U et al. Computer-assisted densitometric image analysis in periodontal radiography. A methodological study. J Clin Periodontol, Copenhagen, v.15,n.1,p.27-37,Jan.1988.
5. Coleman S, Davis S. Computer-aided diagnosis and treatment planning. Curr Opin Cosmet Dent, Philadelphia, p.113-122,1994.
6. Conover GL, Hildebolt CF, Yokoyama-Crothers N. Comparison of linear measurements made from storage phosphor and dental radiographs. Dentomaxillofac Radiol, Houndsmills, v.25,n.5,p.268-273,Nov.1996.
7. Costa RF, Scelza MFZ, Costa AJO. Radiopacidade de cimentos endodônticos: avaliação pela intensidade pixel. J Bras Clin Odontol Int, Curitiba, v.6,n.32,p.137-139,Mar./Abr.2002.
8. Delano EO et al. Quantitative radiographic follow-up of apical surgery: a radiometric and histological correlation. J Endod, Baltimore, v.24,n.6,p.420-426,Jun.1998.
9. Delano EO et al. Comparison between PAI and quantitative digital radiographic assessment of apical healing after endodontic treatment. Oral Surg Oral Med Oral Pathol Oral Radiol Endod, St. Louis, v.92,n.1,p.108-115,July2001.
10. Digora Instruction Manual, Soredex, Finlândia, 1994.
11. Dunn SM, Kantor ML. Digital Radiology – facts and fictions. J Am Dent Assoc, Chicago, v.124,n.12,p.38-47,Dec.1993.
12. Ferreira RA. Odontologia em imagens. Revista da APCD, São Paulo, v.50,n.3,p.218-228,Mai/Jun.1996.
13. Furkart AJ et al. Direct digital radiography for the detection of periodontal bone lesions. Oral Surg Oral Med Oral Pathol, St. Louis, v.74,n.5,p.652-660,Nov.1992.
14. Goaz PW, White SC. Oral Radiology – Principles and Interpretation. 3. ed. Mosby, p. 272-290, 1994.
15. Griffiths BM et al. Comparison of three imaging techniques for assessing endodontic working length. Int Endod J, Oxford, v.25,n.6,p.279-287,Nov.1992.
16. Hayakawa Y et al. Optimum exposure ranges for computed dental radiography. Dentomaxillofac Radiol, Houndsmills, v.25,n.2,p.71-75,Abr.1996.
17. Heo MS, Han DH, An BM, Huh KH, Yi WJ, Lee SS, Choi SC. Effect of ambient light and bit depth of digital radiograph on observer performance in determination of endodontic file positioning. Oral Surg Oral Med Oral Pathol Oral Radiol Endod, St. Louis, v.105,n.2,p.239-44,Feb.2008.
18. Holmes S. Medicolegal issues relating to retention, ownership and transmission of images and image reports. Imaging, Stanford, v.12,n.4,p.292-297,2000.
19. Horner K et al. RadioVisioGraphy: an initial revolution. Br Dent J, London, v.168,n.6,p.244-248,1990.
20. Horner K, Brettle DS, Rushton VE. The potential medico-legal implications of computed radiography. Br Dent J, London, v.180,n.7,p.271-273,Abr.1996.
21. Horner K, Hirschmann PN. Dose reduction in dental radiography. J Dent, Guildford, v.18,n.4,p.171-184,Aug.1990.
22. Jeffcoat MK. Radiographic methods for detection of progressive alveolar bone loss. J Periodontol, Chicago, v.63,n.4,p.367-372,Apr.1992.
23. Kal BI, Baksi BG, Dündar N, Şen BH. Effect of various digital processing algorithms on the measurement accuracy of endodontic file length. Oral Surg Oral Med Oral Pathol Oral Radiol Endod, St. Louis, v.103,n.2,p.280-284,Feb.2007.
24. Kullendorf B et al. Subtraction radiography for diagnosis of periapical bone lesions. Endod Dent Traumatol, Copenhagen, v.4,n.6,p.253-259,Dec.1988.
25. Kullendorff B, Nilsson M. Diagnostic accuracy of direct digital dental radiography for the detection of periapical bone lesions. II Effects on diagnostic accuracy after application of image processing. Oral Surg Oral Med Oral Pathol, St. Louis, v.82,n.5,p.585-589,Nov.1996.
26. Lavelle CL, Wu CJ. Digital radiographic images will benefit endodontic services. Endod Dent Traumatol, Copenhagen, v.11,n.6,p.253-260,Dez.1995.
27. Lim KF, Loh EEM, Hong YH. Intra-oral computed radiography – an in vitro evaluation. J Dent, Guildford, v.24,n.5,p.359-364,Sep.1996.
28. MØystad A et al. Detection of approximal caries with a storage phosphor system. A comparison of enhanced digital images with dental X-ray film. Dentomaxillofac Radiol, Houndsmills, v.25,n.4,p.202-206,Set.1996.
29. Mistak EJ et al. Interpretation of periapical lesions comparing conventional, direct digital, and telephonically transmitted radiographic images. J Endod, Baltimore, v.24,n.4,p.262-266,Apr.1998.
30. Mol A, Van Der Stelt PF. Application of digital image analysis in dental radiography for the description of periapical bone lesions: a preliminary study. IEEE Trans Biomed Eng, New York, v.38,n.4,p.357-359,Abr.1991.
31. Nelvig P, Wing K, Welander U. Sens-A-Ray. A new system for digital intra oral radiography. Oral Surg Oral Med Oral Pathol, St. Louis, v.74,n.6,p.818-823,Dec.1992.
32. Nicopoulou-Karayianni K et al. Image processing for enhanced observer agreement in the evaluation of periapical bone changes. Int Endod J, Oxford, v.35,n.7,p.615-622,July.2002.
33. Razmus TF. Caries, periodontal disease and periapical changes. Dent Clin North Am, Philadelphia, v.38,n.1,p.13-31,Jan.1994.
34. Sanderink GC. Image quality of direct digital intraoral X-ray sensors in assessing root canal length. The RadioVisioGraphy, Visualix/VIXA, Sens-A-Ray, and Flash Dent systems compared with Ektaspeed films. Oral Surg Oral Med Oral Pathol Oral Radiol Endod, St. Louis, v.78,n.1,p.125-132,July1994.

35. Scarfe WC et al. In vivo accuracy and reliability of color-coded image enhancements for the assessment of periradicular lesion dimensions. Oral Surg Oral Med Oral Pathol Oral Radiol Endod, St. Louis, v.88,n.5,p.603-611,Nov.1999.
36. Shearer AC. Radiovisiography for length estimation in root canal treatment: an in-vitro comparison with conventional radiography. Int Endod J., Oxford, v.24, n.5. p.233-239, Sep. 1991.
37. Shearer AC, Horner K, Wilson NHF. RadioVisioGraphy for imaging root canals: an in vitro comparison with conventional radiography. Quintessence Int, Illinois, v.21,n.10,p.789-794,Oct.1990.
38. Shrout MK, Hall JM, Hildebolt CE. Differentiation of periapical granulomas and radicular cysts by digital radiometric analysis. Oral Surg Oral Med Oral Pathol, St. Louis, v.76,n.3,p.356-361,Set.1993.
39. Stavropoulos A, Wenzel A. Accuracy of cone beam dental CT, intraoral digital and conventional film radiography for the detection of periapical lesions. An ex vivo study in pig jaws. Clin Oral Invest, Heidelberg, v.11,n.1,p.101-105,Mar.2007.
40. Sullivan JE Jr, Di Fiore PM, Koerber A. RadioVisiography in the detections of periapical lesions. J Endod, Baltimore, v.26,n.1,p.32-35,Jan.2000.
41. Tanomaru Filho M et al. Evaluation of the radiopacity of calcium hydroxide-and glass-ionomer-based root canal sealers. Int Endod J, Oxford, v.41,n.1,p.50-53,Jan.2008.
42. Tanomaru Filho M et al. Radiopacity evaluation of new root canal filling materials by digitalization of images. J Endod, Baltimore,v.33,n.3,p.249-251,Mar.2007.
43. Theilad J. An evaluation of the reability of radiographs in the measurement of bone loss in periodontal disease. J Periodontol, Chicago, v.31,p.143-153,1960.
44. Tirrell BC et al. Interpretation of chemically created lesions using direct digital imaging. J Endod, Baltimore, v.22,n.2,p.74-78,Feb.1996.
45. Tyndall DA, Kapa SF, Bagnell CP. Digital subtraction radiography for detecting cortical and cancellous bone changes in the periapical region. J Endod, Baltimore, v.16,n.4,p.173-178,Apr.1990.
46. Van der Stelt PF et al. Digitized pattern recognition in the diagnosis of periodontal bone defects. J Clin Periodontol, Copenhagen, v.12,n.10,p.822-827,Nov.1985.
47. Van der Stelt PF, Geraets WG. Computer-aided interpretation and quantification of angular periodontal bone defects on dental radiographs. IEEE Trans Biomed Eng, New York, v.38,n.4,p.334-338,Apr.1991.
48. Vandre RH, Webber RL. Future trends in dental radiology. Oral Surg Oral Med Oral Pathol Oral Radiol Endod, St. Louis, v.80,n.4,p.471-478,Oct.1995.
49. Wallace JA et al. A comparative evaluation of the diagnostic efficacy of film and digital sensors for detection of simulated periapical lesions. Oral Surg Oral Med Oral Pathol Oral Radiol Endod, St. Louis, v.92,n.1,p.93-97,July 2001.
50. Wenzel A. Computer-aided image manipulation of intraoral radiographs to enhance diagnosis in dental practice: a review. Int Dent J, London, v.43,n.2,p.99-108,Apr.1993.
51. Wenzel A et al. Accuracy of caries diagnosis in digital images from charge-coupled device and storage phosphor systems: an in vitro study. Dentomaxillofac Radiol, Houndsmills, v.24,n.4,p.250-254,Nov.1995.
52. Yokota ET et al. Interpretation of periapical lesions using Radiovisiography. J Endod, Baltimore, v.20,n.10,p.490-494,Oct.1994.

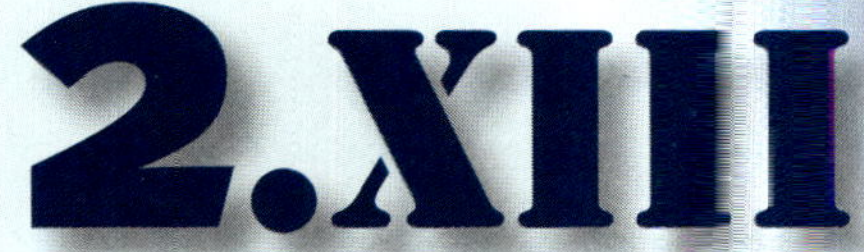

The reappearance of ultrasound in Endodontics

(Operating and surgical microscope)

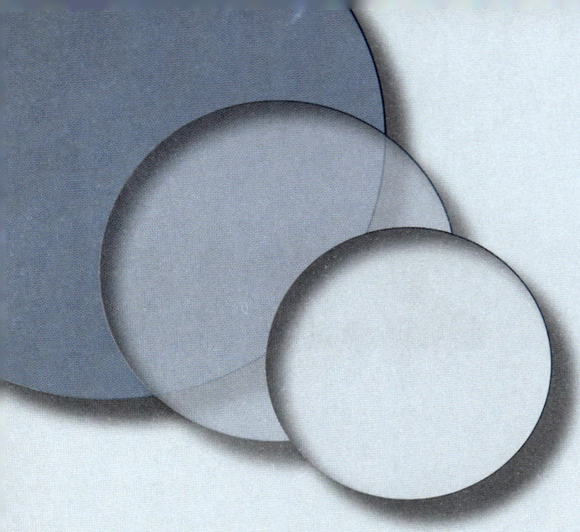

Carlos Alberto Ferreira Murgel

The aim of this chapter is to present a historical overview of the use of ultrasound in endodontics, from the time of its introduction until the present time. This very useful piece of equipment, today indispensable in any endodontic practice was not always unanimously accepted. This chapter will explain how an item with revolutionary technology can almost disappear when its use is recommended focusing on only one aspect and the promised results are not achieved.

In general, industries create enormous expectations with regard to the use of new technology and equipment, however, mostly it is not based on scientific principles. It is the responsibility of the clinician to carefully evaluate new technological releases, and to evaluate the merits of independent and impartial publications.

It is imperative that we set aside the passive image of just being a consumer, and that we do not succumb to aggressive marketing, rather question the true feasibility and utility of new technologies. Ultrasound is a classical case of mistaken marketing strategy, and it is very important for us not to repeat the errors of judgment of the past.

This chapter has been divided into topics to make it easier to read and understand. These topics cover specific periods of the use of ultrasound and enable an overview of the literature, linking the past to the present and creating a bridge to the future.

This chapter has specifically been written for general practitioners involved in endodontics and specialists, with the aim to demonstrate by means of the literature and clinical cases, how this technology became indispensable in present-day practices and clinics. It demonstrates how the incorporation of the operating microscope created new methods of using ultrasound, making it reappear "like a phoenix rising from the ashes". It is no longer a practically abandoned technology. It has been transformed into the prime modus operandi of both conventional and surgical endodontics. The future appears to be even more promising, as ultrasound is being investigated in great detail, used in surgery, particularly in implants, to perform osteotomies, bone preparations, to elevate the maxillary sinus, and for many other applications.

THE RISE AND FALL OF THE USE OF ULTRASOUND IN ENDODONTICS

Since the innovative proposal of Richman, in 1957[1], the use of ultrasound in endodontics for cleaning and shaping the root canal system and for root resection, many scientific studies have been conducted to verify its feasibility. No technology had received so much attention and had initial acceptance so quickly as ultrasound. However, in only a short period of time it went from being the purported miracle equipment that would solve all clinical problems to complete disuse and abandonment. Since then it has gone through various periods of interest and ultimately it established itself as an indispensable piece of equipment in modern endodontic practice.

The first wave of interest of ultrasound in endodontics occurred in the early 1980s as a result of the publication of several positive scientific articles, which appeared over a short period of time, by Martin & Cunningham and co-workers[3,4,5,6,7,8]. They presented encouraging results with respect to the various possible advantages of this technology, when compared with the manual technique for root canal instrumentation, among which were the faster removal of dentin[2]; use of more efficient ultrasonic diamond files[3]; greater cleanliness of the root canal system[4,5]; less apical extrusion of dentin debris[6]; less post-operative pain[7]; greater capability to eliminate bacteria from infected canals[8].

It was the magic word everyone wanted to hear about a piece of equipment that would definitively simplify instrumentation of the root canal system, facilitating the very tiring and difficult art of cleaning and shaping canals. In addition, an enormous amount of resources were allocated to promote this marvel, pressuring dentists to buy it. From then on, concepts such as cavitation, synergy, speed, ease of use, less stress, less fatigue became synonymous with ultrasound in endodontics.

The equipment quickly became a must among consumers, particularly among endodontists, and everybody appeared satisfied with this technological marvel. During the early years, the only equipment available abroad was the *Cavi-Endo* (Dentsply-USA), and in Brazil, the *Profi-Endo* (Dabi-Atlante-Brazil). The system had a magnetostrictive transducer, with a vibration frequency of approximately 25 kHz, optional periodontal points and an adaptor for endodontic files.

Subsequently studies by independent researchers appeared reporting the true capabilities, and particularly the safety of ultrasound for instrumentation and the results were discouraging. Almost all claims that were attributed to ultrasound were refuted.

Ahmad et al.[9] demonstrated that in reality the much heralded cavitation did not occur inside the canals, and that there was only an acoustic wave that moved the liquid inside the canal, provided the file was not firmly pressed against the walls.

The power generation system of the standard equipment, at that time the *Cavi-Endo* (Dentsply-USA) and *Profi-Endo* (Dabi-Atlante-Brazil), used a magnetostrictive transducer (energy produced by the vibration of metal plates), was essentially rendered obsolete when equipment with a piezoelectric transducer appeared. The later used quartz crystals, were more compact and efficient and produced higher vibrations in the range of 30 kHz[10].

At that time questions were raised whether there was a standard among the different types of ultrasound generators and transducers that the different manufacturers marketed. Research clearly demonstrated that there was a considerable variation in the frecuency of energy that was generated among different pieces of equipment. Therefore there was a need for equipment to calibrate the energy output, so that operators would always be working using a maximum frequency[11].

Another problem caused by ultrasound was the incidence of file fractures. Ahamad & Roy[12], investigated the incidence of type K file fractures, and observed that, when activated without irrigation solution and outside the canal, fractures easily occurred, but when activated inside the canal with light support of the walls, this did not happen.

Due to the nature of the oscillatory pattern of the ultrasonically activated files (formation of node and antinode) inside the canals, they produced non-uniform longitudinal grooves, a faithful copy of the active part of the instrument used[13].

Murgel et al.[14], using scanning electronic microscopy, reported that the at that time most used *step back* instrumentation technique, produced more dentin debris in the apical region, when compared with the *step down* technique. The authors concluded that this possibly occurred, due to the fact that the ultrasonic file was more firmly fixed inside the canals in the *step back* technique (without previous cervical preparation) than in the *step down* technique (with previous cervical preparation), which prevented it from moving freely.

Schulz-Bongert et al.[15] concluded that ultrasonic instrumentation of curved canals was not indicated, due severe straightening of the curvature, perforations and formation of apical steps, and recommended their use only in straight canals or in the straight portion of curved root canals.

The above referenced publications are only a few examples of the extensive early literature that clearly contradict the supposedly unsurpassed qualities of ultrasound for canal instrumentation. Science had proven that ultrasound was not suitable for the instrumentation of root canals, and that the equipment (magnetostrictive system) was not living up to the expectations. As a result, interest in this technology slowly dwindled, and practitioners gave up on their equipment. The ultrasonic systems were soon complete discredited.

STAGE OF DIVERSIFICATION

In spite of the initial setback, some clinicians and outstanding researchers, seeing the great potential, began to seek new applications for ultrasound. There are a few reports that suggested different applications for the equipment.

In this further stage of development, we can point out some of the proposals for expanding the clinical use of ultrasonic energy, such as: removal of silver cones in complex cases[16]; retreatment of root canals with filling pastes[17]; removal of fractured cast posts[18]; removal of bonded prostheses with modified periodontal tips[19]; activation of 1% sodium hypochlorite solution for cleaning the dentinal tubules before internal bleaching[20]; heated lateral condensation with ultrasonically activated spacer[21]; clinical and surgical treatment of *dens invaginatus*[22].

This stage was extremely important, as after the considerable initial interest, the majority of practitioners showed little interest in ultrasound. After the publication of the studies that pioneered these new concepts, ultrasound slowly began to be seen in a favorable light again and considered a feasible technology for dentistry.

At that time, the greatest impediment of the technology was the lack of specific tips, suitable for the many different clinical situations to make optimum use of the energy generated. Another factor to consider was the lack of magnification of the operating field, which did not allow details to be seen in full. In the next stage we shall explain how magnification with an **operating and surgical microscope** promoted the reappearance of ultrasound and generated new interest, allowing for the development of new very precise and conservative instruments and techniques.

STAGE OF SYNERGY BETWEEN ULTRASOUND AND THE OPERATING AND SURGICAL MICROSCOPE

We can with a fair amount of certainty state that a new era in endodontics began when in 1992[23], Gary Carr published a classical article showing the possibilities of using the operating microscope with ultrasonics employing new tips for multiple use. Subsequently, in addition to the new tips, he introduced specific tips and concepts for endodontic microsurgeries, completely revolutionizing the field[24]. From then on, ultrasound combined with magnification increased and various articles were published, proposing new and innovative applications for the technology.

Ruddle[25] presented revolutionary techniques for performing non-surgical endodontic retreatments, showing how the incorporation of ultrasound and the operating microscope could make a significant contribution to the predictability of these procedures.

Lea & Walmsley[26] emphasized the ample availability of ultrasonic tips, that made it possible to access difficult locations in the oral cavity, and which depended on the procedures to be performed.

In 2004, Rubenstein & Torabinejad[27] asserted that in the previous decade, with the interaction of the operating microscope and ultrasound, advancement in endodontic surgery had been extraordinary, making it possible to save teeth, which would traditionally have been extracted.

In spite of the development of new equipment and techniques, Clark, in 2004[28], emphasized that these new technologies could only be used to their full potential when they were associated with the operating microscope.

Reaffirming the synergy between ultrasound and the operating microscope, Plotino et al.[29] concluded that this technology made it possible to treat complex cases, such as calcified canals, perforations, endodontic surgery and removal of intra-radicular obstructions with greater predictability and safety.

In spite of being very useful and efficient, ultrasound has to be used with caution and precision, since contact of the tips with root structure produces heat. This is very important, particularly when the intent of the tips is to vibrate metal, since it rapidly transmits heat to the periodontium. Therefore irrigation is required and needs to be continuous and copious, with intermittent vibration, while being applied with light pressure[30].

There are reports in the literature, reporting the detrimental effect of excessive heat generated by ultrasonic tips to tooth structure, soft tissue and bone. The sequelae range from tissue burns, necrosis of soft tissues and bone, to extraction of the tooth that was treated[31,32].

CURRENT STATUS OF ULTRASOUND POINTS

At present, ultrasound is well established in endodontics, and now makes inroads into other dental specialties, such as prosthodontics and general dentistry[28]. The current trend is to wards the development of new equipment and new tips, with innovative materials and new abrasive agents on the active portion of the tips.

The equipment itself has remained relatively stable, since the overwhelming majority of practitioners use the piezoelectric type of transducer, with a vibratory frequency of approximately 30 kHz. This technology is already well known, also in Brazil, and various manufacturers are producing excellent equipment at a very reasonable price.

Concerning the equipment, it is important to know what kind of coupling the transducer has (male, female, thread pitch, etc.), since this can limit the possibility of using tips from different manufacturers. The more compatible the equipment, the greater the interchangeability of the different tips. The true development in fact occurred in the tips, which today are offered in diversity of shapes, diameters, sizes, tapers and angles in relation to the transducer and handle of the instrument. This diversity allows for a greater number of clinical applications in teeth in the oral cavity.

One has to pay special attention to the active tips parts of the new instruments, since they determine the area and the substrate we work on, as well as the type of action we expect. This is important to maximize the vibratory action of the instruments.

The shape of the tip is important, as it will determine the type of reduction that will be produced, particularly in dentin. To locate calcified canals and secondary anatomy (superficial or deep), it is recommended to use rhomboid shaped tips without a sharp active part, since this causes surface microcavities that frequently confuse us.

Tips without abrasives on the active part are indicated for removing filling materials, gutta-percha, fractured instruments, cores, crowns, and intra-radicular obstructions. They should not be used to remove tooth structure as they can cause superficial burns.

Tips with abrasives are indicated for removing restorative materials (resin, glass ionomers, silver amalgam), enamel, dentin, and gutta-percha. They should not be used on metals, as the abrasives will wear off.

Traditionally, ultrasonic points are made of stainless steel, but Bahcall & Olsen[33] reported on the development of polymers and plastic for disposable points. The use of disposable points would be very useful, particularly considering the growing problems of cross-infection.

As an abrasive agent diamond particles have traditionally been used, however, newer materials include, zirconium nitrite and CVD technology (Chemical vapor deposition)[34,35].

There is still no consensus as to the best and most durable tip. It is important to use a system (set of tips) that has broad clinical application (for conventional endodontics, retreatment, core removal, and surgery), durability, efficiency, availability and that are cost-effective. Each practitioner has to choose the system that best suits his/her clinical need(s). Tips are manufactured in Brazil and abroad and each system has advantages and disadvantages.

The following is an example of ultrasonic tips showing their shapes and the functions thereof.

To make it easier to understand we have discussed only tips from one manufacturer (www.eie2.com), which clearly show the differences between the various models and their specific functions. It is important to point out that the best system is the one that we know and master, as it allows us to use our investment to maximum advantage.

The tips available from this manufacture are the following: Ball-D; Pear-D; UT4; UT4-D; CT4; CT4-D; CKT1; CKT2; CKT3; CKT1-D; CKT2-D; CKT3-D; SP1 and SP2. The letter D at the end of the name of the tip refers to a abrasive diamond active tip (for dentin or enamel reduction). This is followed by showing each tip or family of tips in detail (same shape, with or without diamond on the active portion and/or different diameters of tips).

Ball-D

FUNCTION	LOCATION OF ACTION	POWER FOR USE
Refinement of access	Enamel and Dentin	Intermediate
Restorative material removal	Pulp Chamber	High
Gutta-Percha removal	Pulp Chamber	Intermediat

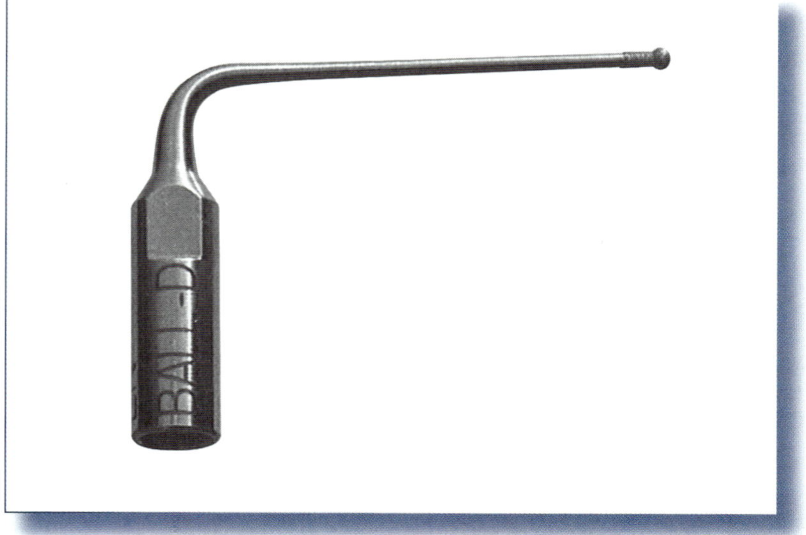

FIG. 2.XIII-1

Ball-D with thin rod allowing changes of angles to access difficult-to-reach areas.

Pear-D

FUNCTION	LOCATION OF ACTION	POWER FOR USE
Refinement of access	Enamel and Dentin	Intermediate
Restorative material removal	Pulp Chamber	High
Gutta-Percha removal	Pulp Chamber	Intermediate
Location of anatomy	Pulp chamber floor	Intermediate
Fracture diagnosis	Extra-radicular dentin	Intermediate

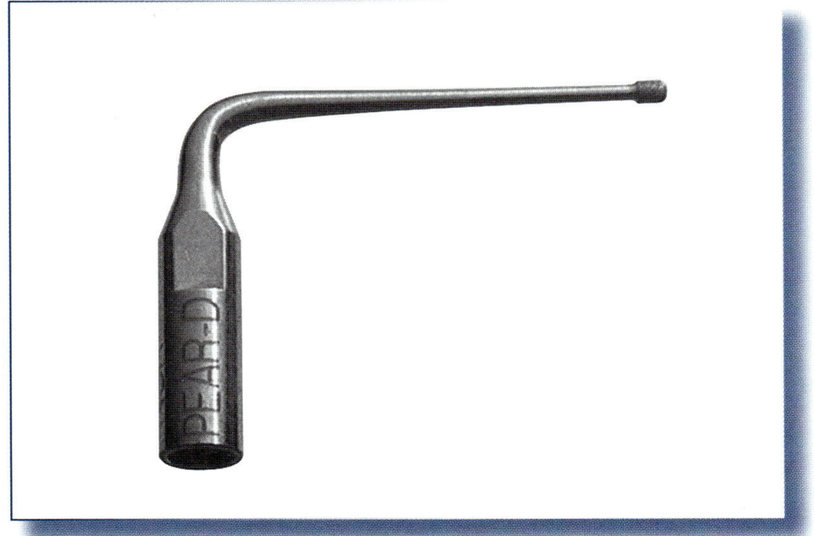

FIG. 2.XIII-2

Pear-D, a true multi-utility, extremely resistant point.

UT4 and UT4-D

FUNCTION	LOCATION OF ACTION	POWER FOR USE
Isthmus Cleaning	Coronal and root dentin	Intermediate
Restorative material removal	Middle third	Low
Gutta-Percha removal	Middle third	Intermediate
Deep anatomy location	Middle third	Low
Fractured instrument removal	Cervical and middle third	Low
Core removal	Cementation line	Intermediate

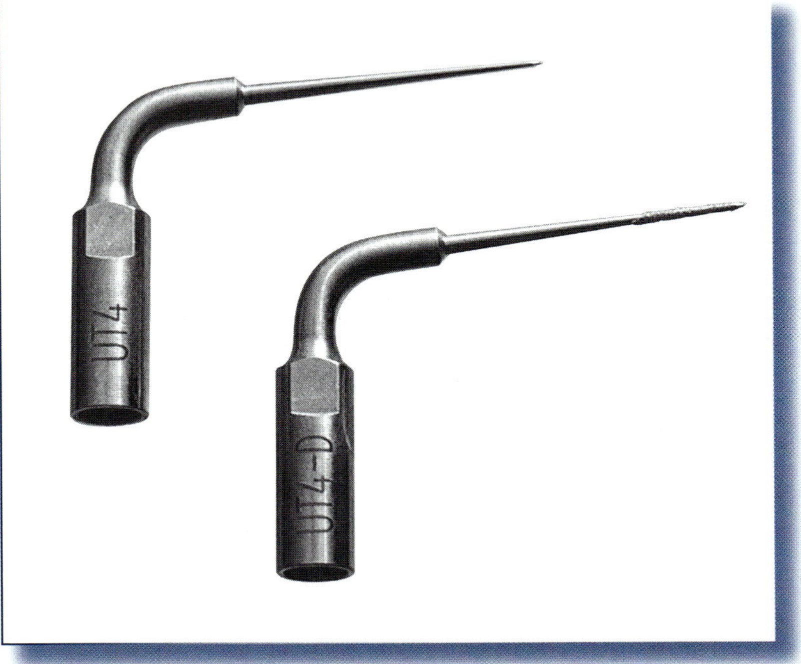

FIG. 2.XIII-3

UT4 and UT4-D, very thin, and practically without taper, allowing excellent intracanal visualization as well as of the isthmus region.

CT4 and CT4-D

FUNCTION	LOCATION OF ACTION	POWER FOR USE
Refinement of access	Enamel and Dentin	Intermediate
Restorative material removal	Pulp Chamber	Intermediate
Gutta-Percha removal	Pulp Chamber	Intermediate
Location of anatomy	Middle third	Intermediate
Apical surgery (customize angle for each situation)	Apex	Intermediate
Fractured instrument removal	Cervical Third	Low
Core removal	Cementation line	High

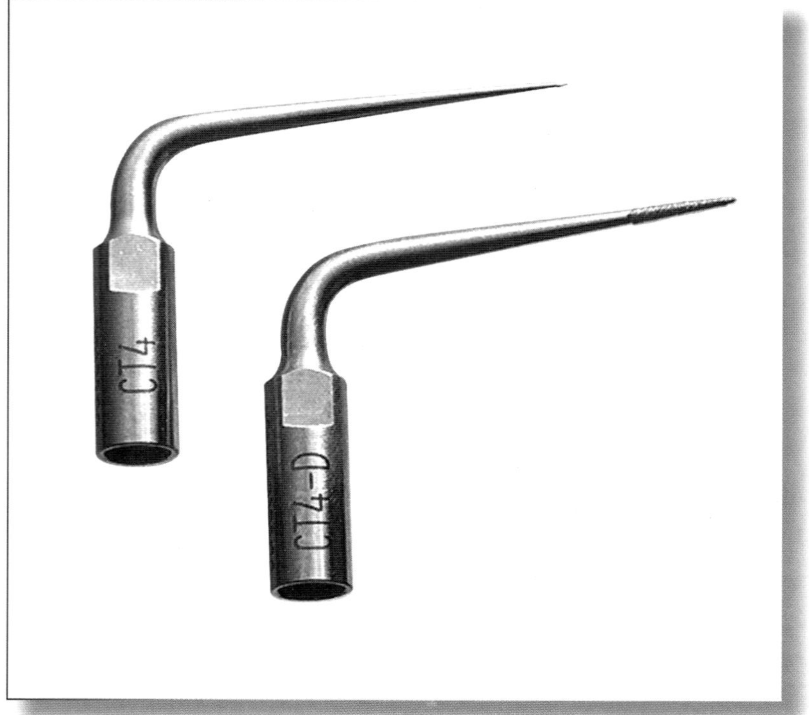

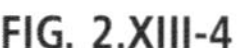
FIG. 2.XIII-4

CT4 and CT4-D, more tapered and with excellent energy transmission. Excellent t tips for surgery and working in the cervical third of root canals.

CKT1, CKT2, CKT3

Functions similar to those of UT4 and CT4, but with different diameters and angles, facilitating access to more difficult and deeper areas (Fig. 2.XIII-5).

CKT1-D, CKT2-D, CKT3-D

Functions similar to those of UT4-D and CT4-D, but with different diameters and angles, facilitating access to more difficult and deeper areas (Fig. 2.XIII-6).

SP1 and SP2

These are dedicated tips for the removal of fractured instruments in the apical third of straight canals or obstructions in longer roots. They cut well, and must be used at low power, and never without magnification, as they can cause perforations, steps and other iatrogenic procedures (Fig. 2.XIII-7).

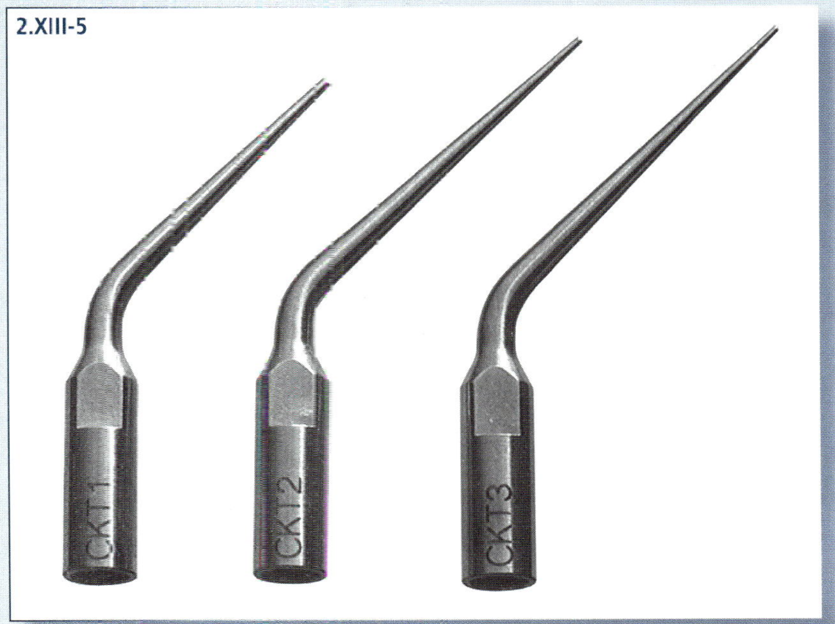

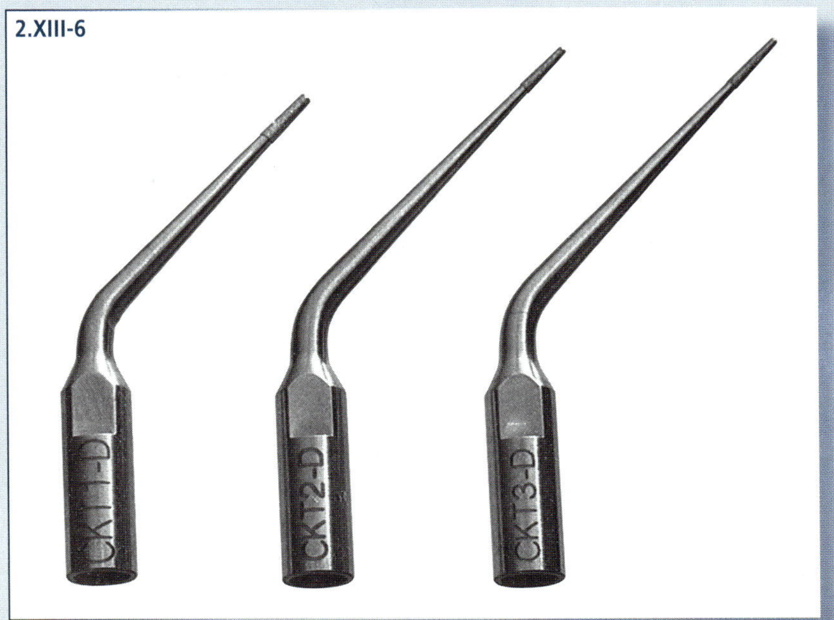

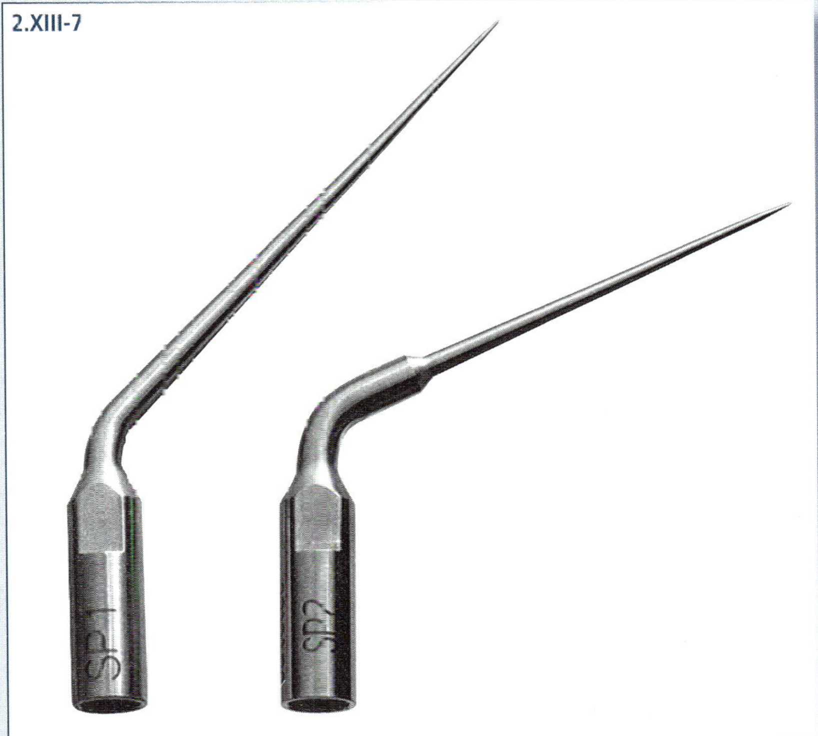

FIG. 2.XIII-5
CKT1, CKT2, CKT3, with various diameters and opening angles for access to difficult-to-reach areas.

FIG. 2.XIII-6
CKT1-D, CKT2-D, CKT3-D, with various diameters and opening angles, for access to difficult-to-reach areas.

FIG. 2.XIII-7
SP1 and SP2, with minimal taper, allowing excellent visualization in deep areas of the canal, extremely customizable and sharp.

The following is a brief description of how the author uses and teaches this system, maximizing the use of the operating microscope and ultrasound. This does not mean that other techniques are not efficient – only that it seems that the one we recommend is more suitable. We remind you of the importance of planning before the acquisition of any technology, in order to make full use of it and obtain the intended results.

TOTAL DIGITAL OFFICE (TDO) SYSTEM

Usually when one implements an operating microscope or other new piece of equipment in an operatory, it is common to mimic the standard operating room of the XVIII century, consisting of many cupboards, dental spittoon, drawers, and sinks, transforming it into a place that perfectly reproduces and perpetuates old established concepts and dogmas. Invariably the operatory is a copy of the established ordinary, with perhaps small superficial esthetic changes. In reality, one generally may spend a great deal of money, resulting in an inefficient operatory that is unsuitable for new equipment.

Gary Carr[23 24], considered the father of microdentistry in endodontics, and who introduced the operating microscope, created a working environment in which the operating microscope became the center of all activities (ergonomics). Since 2002, in collaboration with Dr. Carr, we developed the *Total Digital Office System* (*TDO System*) concept, entirely redesigning the dental office, in search of maximum efficiency, productivity and rationalization of actions.

Everything was geared to maximize efficiency, both in operating procedures and in the use of the most modern technology, as in these cases the practitioner constantly works with magnification. It is also important for the assistant to work with an assistant microscope, to share the view of the magnified and illuminated operating field.

This new dental environment must be as spacious and uncluttered as possible, so that the dental surgeon can perform the scheduled clinical procedures using only the materials and instruments that are required, thus eliminating the need for innumerable cupboards and drawers.

According to this modern concept of an operating theater, there must be reverse planning, starting with the operating microscope rather than the dental chair, as was traditionally the case, which will be the center of the design while the rest will be designed around it (exactly opposite to what we did when we acquired equipment and tried to introduce it into the traditional operatory).

It is important that when the new operatory is planned, all existing as well as potential future technology is taking into consideration, leaving open space available and that interaction with computers is planned, while being as simple and economical as possible, yet offering an efficient and organized environment.

Concepts such as size, shape, furniture, dental equipment and peripherals must be reviewed and modified to accommodate the operating microscope and its supporting technologies, taking into account the new necessities of efficiency and ergonomics that dentistry requires. These are significant and important changes that we must face if we wish to attain higher levels of proficiency when practicing new endodontics, working with magnification all the time, and working as a team with the auxiliary staff (Fig. 2.XIII-8).

CLINICAL USE OF ULTRASOUND AND THE OPERATING MICROSCOPE

Here only our imagination is the limit, since new suggestions for the joint use of these complementary technologies appear all the time. Dentists are known for their enormous creativity, and with magnification that the operating microscope offers, they are more inventive by the day.

At present, a number of recommendations have appeared in the literature, such as: disinfection of the root canal system with passive ultrasonic irrigation[36]; cleaning the isthmus and root recesses[37]; locating canals[38]; apical preparations[39]; MTA compaction in the apical third[40]; lateral condensation[41,42]; placing calcium hydroxide inside the canals[43]; removing calcium hydroxide from inside the canals[44]; treating complex calcified cases[45]; removing dentin debris[46]; removing fractured instruments [47].

We could continue and add more to the list of possibilities, but we prefer to show how the techniques are applied clinically, thus demonstrating the numerous possibility of ultrasound and the operating microscope in endodontics. It should be emphasized that all photographs presented here were taken with the operating microscope, and that when working with the operating microscope all the time is only possible with prior training and with a change in the very deep-rooted paradigms.

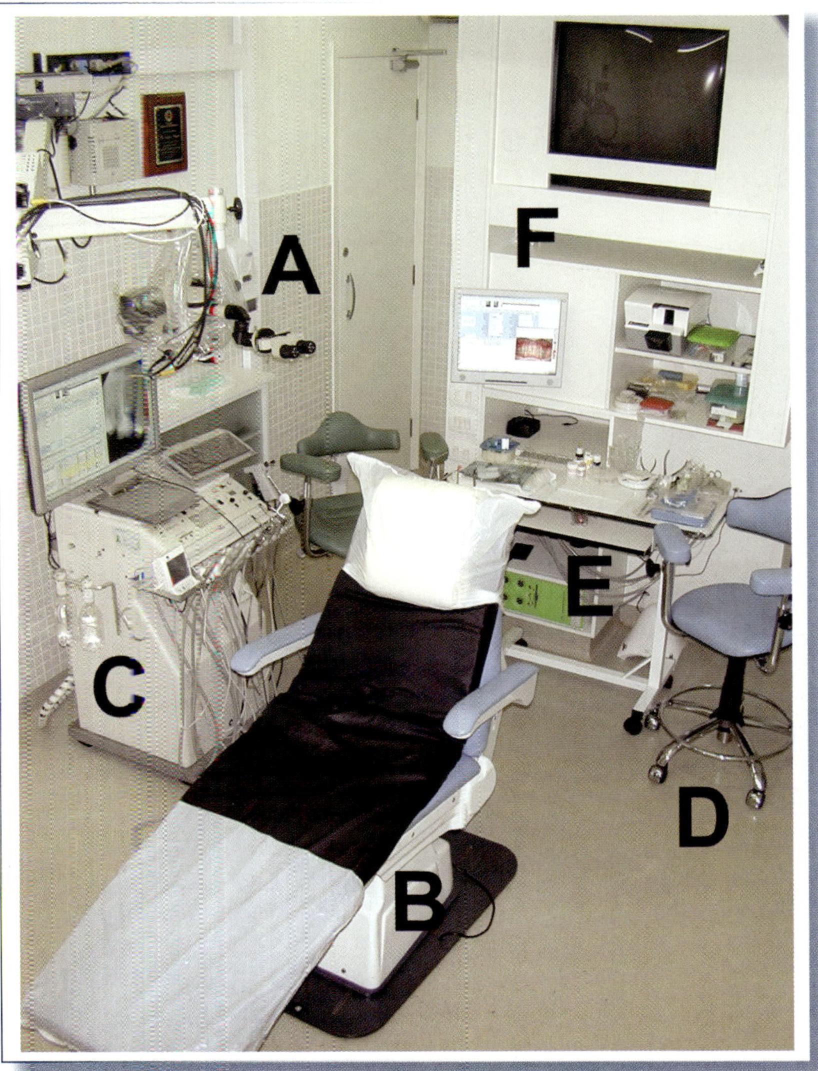

FIG. 2.XIII-8

Dental office designed according to the concepts of the TDO System (version 4):
A – Operating Microscope fixed to the wall with digital photographic equipment and auxiliary microscope (Carona).
B – Swivel chair with vertical lift developed for the operating microscope (Murgel&Carr).
C – Mobile cart concentrating all the technologies (Carr&Murgel).
D – Stool with armrest both for dentist and assistant (Murgel&Carr).
E – Auxiliary mobile table, providing materials and equipment (suction tips, triple syringe) required for assistant (Murgel&Carr).
F – Back wall designed to accommodate the wireless technologies (Carr&Murgel).

DIAGNOSIS OF VERTICAL ROOT FRACTURE

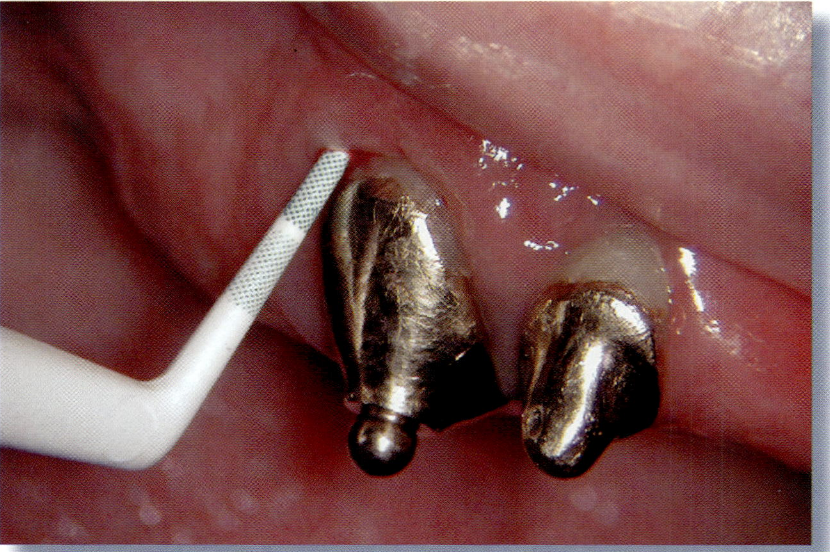

FIG. 2.XIII-9

Tooth 1.3 with isolated periodontal pocket in the buccal region; patient had painful symptoms, and suspected vertical root fracture. On the buccal margin, a resin composite restoration can be seen that needs to be removed.

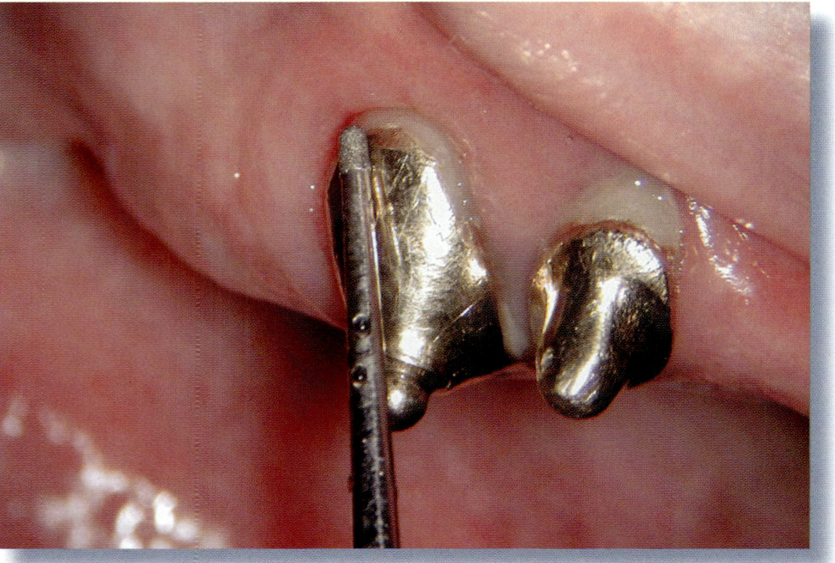

FIG. 2.XIII-10

Detail of the Pearl-D ultrasonic tip, showing its dimension, compared with the buccal gingival margin restored with resin composite. Note how important it is to have an enlarged operating field in order to be precise.

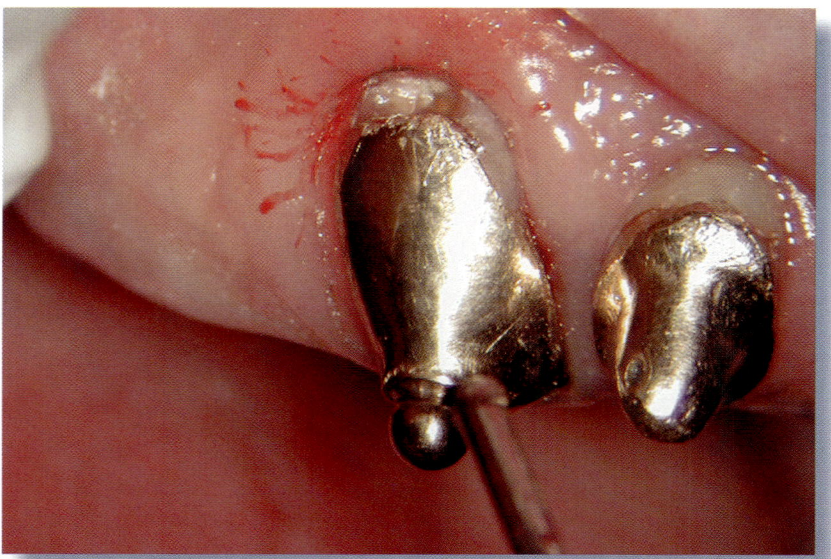

FIG. 2.XIII-11

Detail of the buccal margin, exposed after removal of the resin composite restoration. It is still not possible to make a definitive diagnosis as to whether there is a fracture.

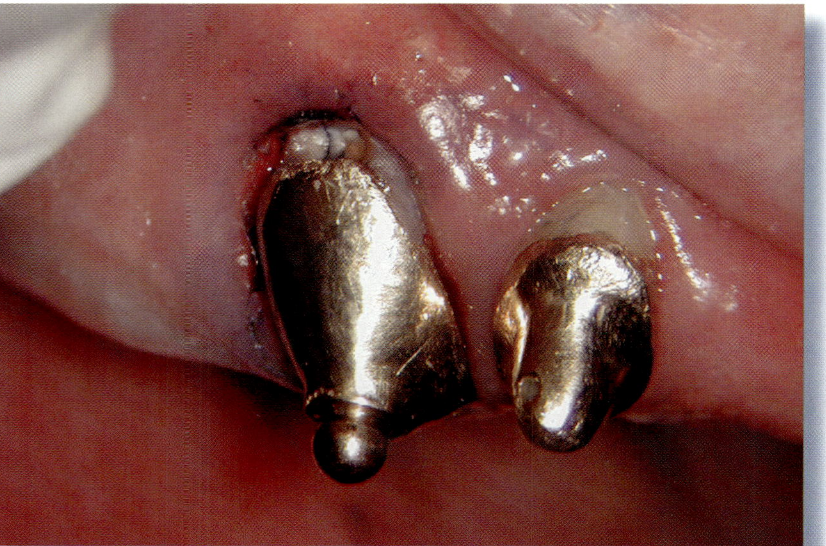

FIG. 2.XIII-12

Detail of the buccal margin stained with methylene blue. Even at an intermediate level of magnification, the vertical fracture of the root is evident.

REFINEMENT OF ACCESS

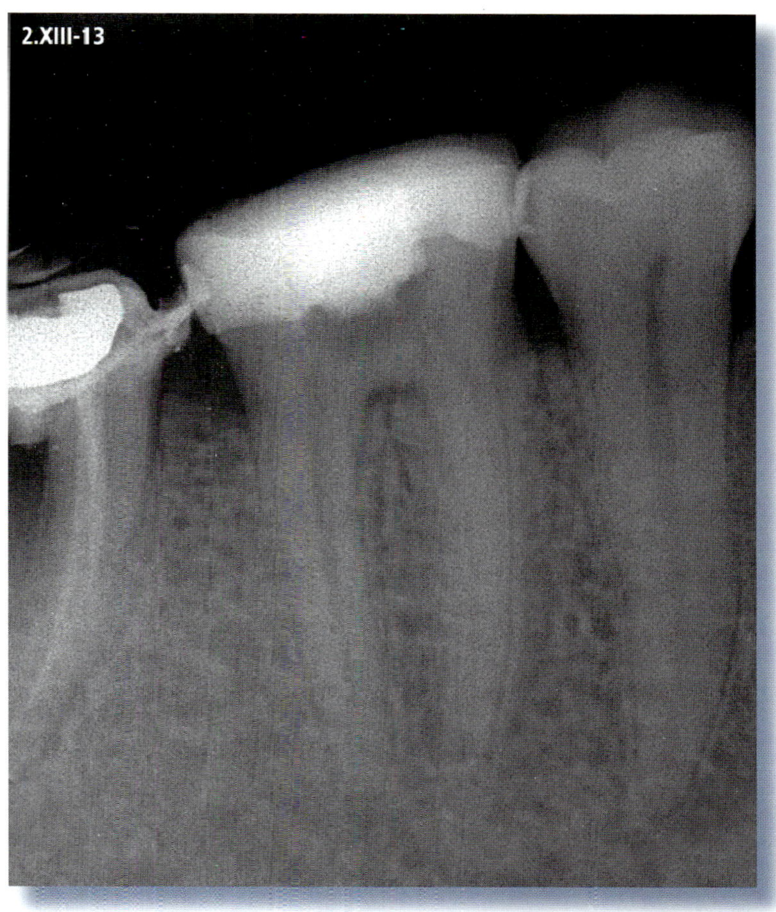

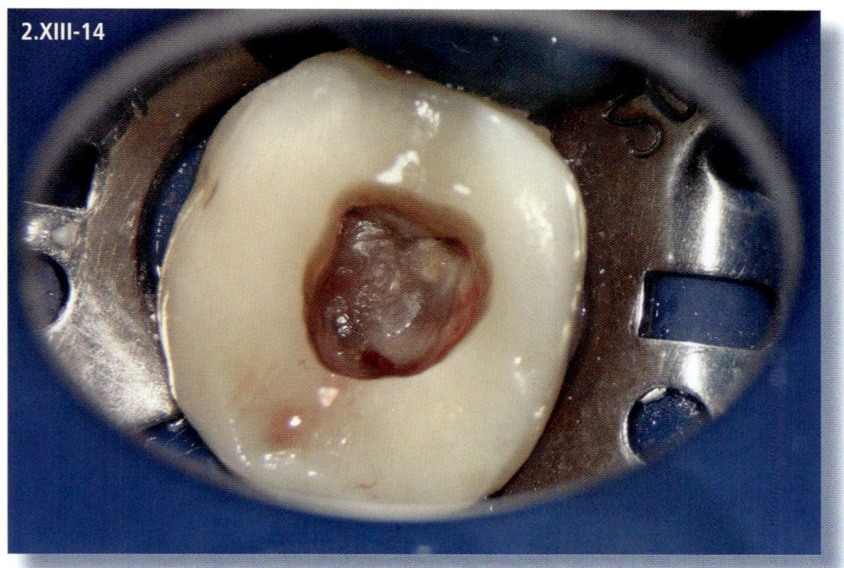

FIG. 2.XIII-13

Preoperative radiograph showing access that had been made by another practitioner.

FIG. 2.XIII-14

Clinical image showing previous access with location of some canals. Note the translucency of the dentin.

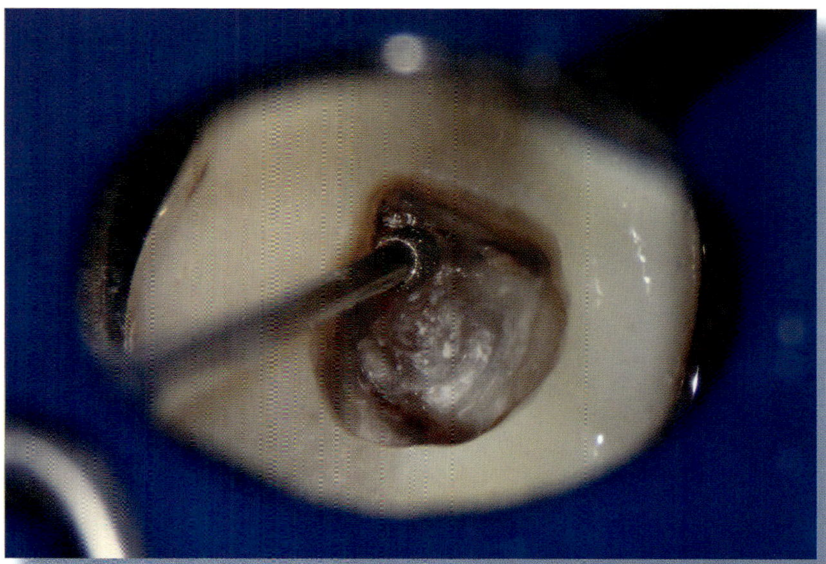

FIG. 2.XIII-15

Clinical image showing the Pearl-D ultrasonic tip definitively removing the roof of the pulp chamber.

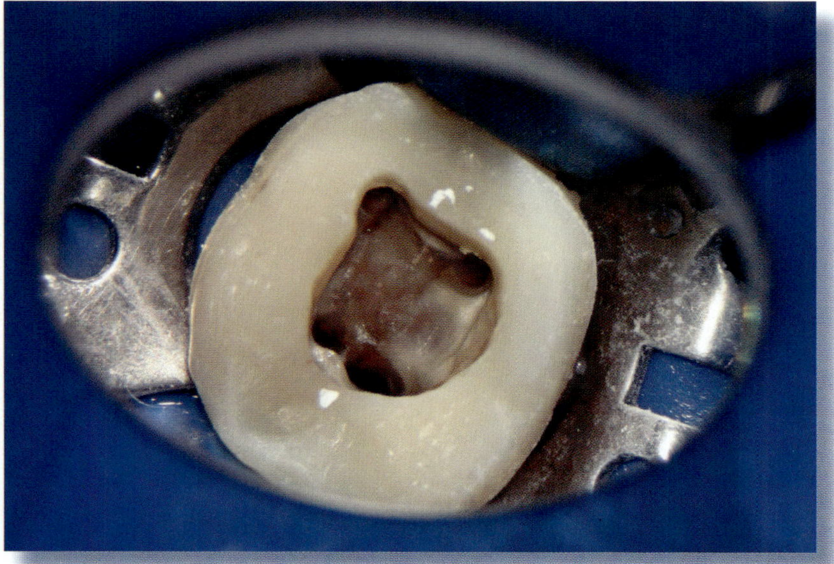

FIG. 2.XIII-16

Clinical image of completed access locating four canals. Note cleanliness and definition of the access.

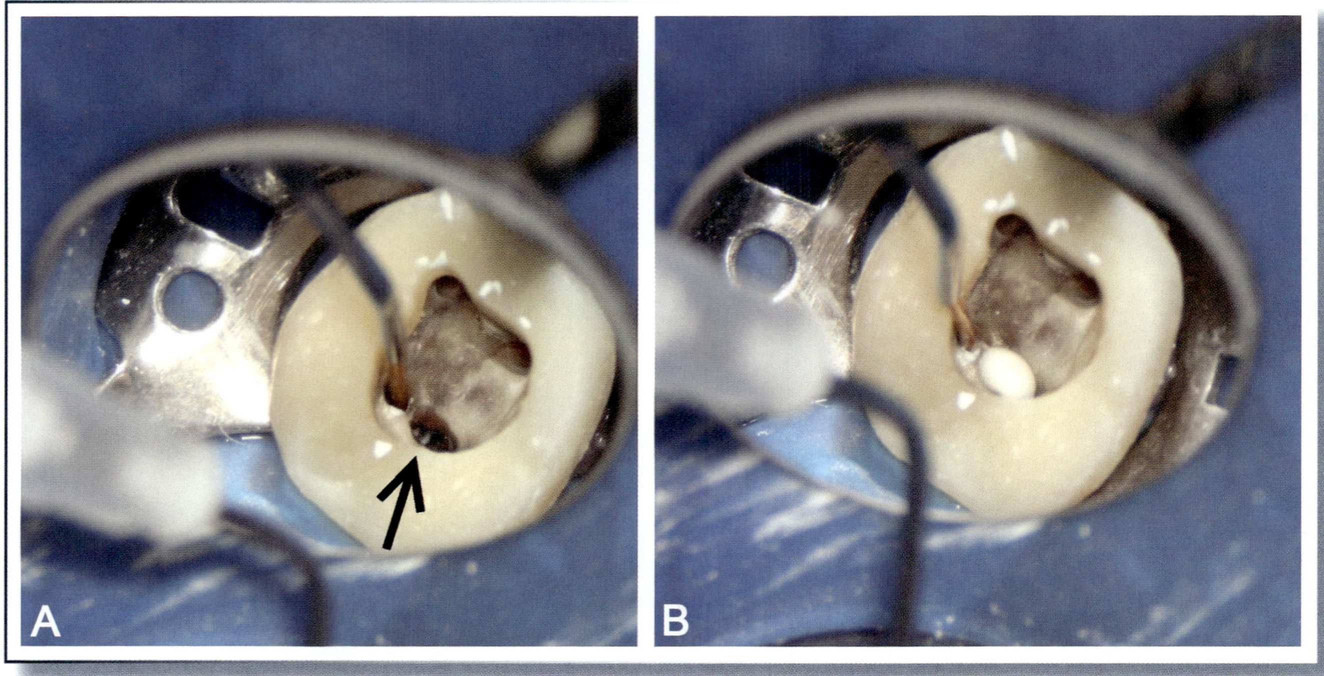

FIGS. 2.XIII-17A-B

Clinical images of insertion of intracanal medication (CaOH2). Note how the medication is being inserted into the disto-buccal canal, and traveled to the disto-lingual canal (arrow) demonstrating that the distal canals were confluent.

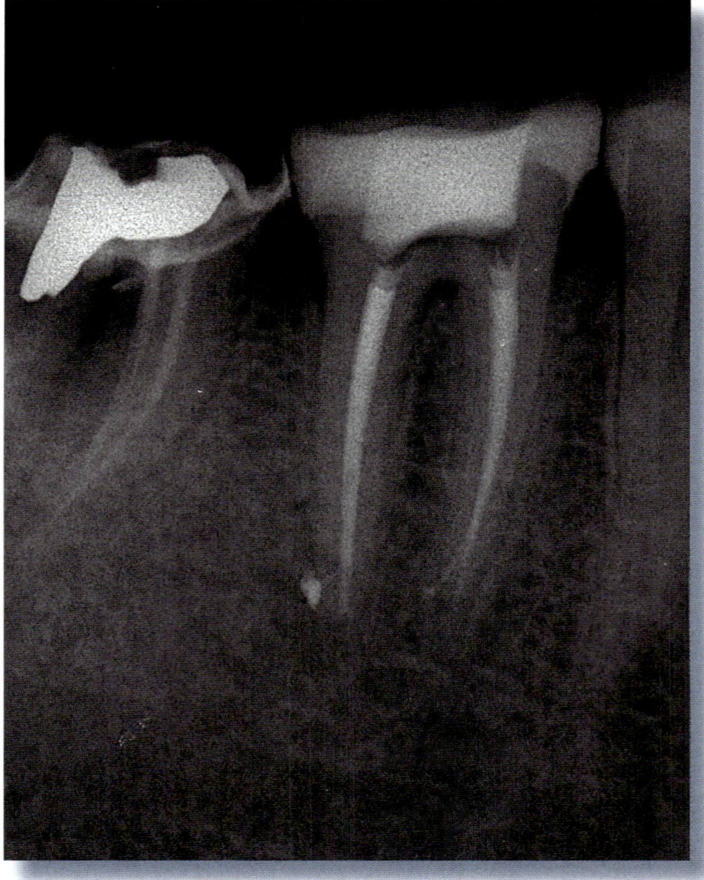

FIG. 2.XIII-18

Final radiograph, showing complete filling of the root canal system, including a lateral canal in the distal root.

LOCATION OF SUPERFICIAL SECONDARY ANATOMY

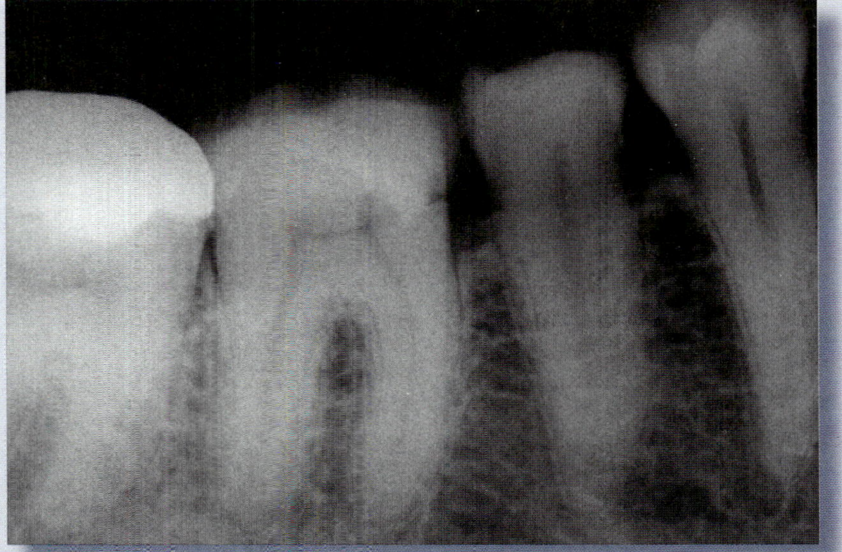

FIG. 2.XIII-19

Preoperative radiograph of tooth 4.6, indicated for endodontic treatment, due symptoms of irreversible pulp inflammation. Note the calcification in the pulp chamber region and canals of both roots.

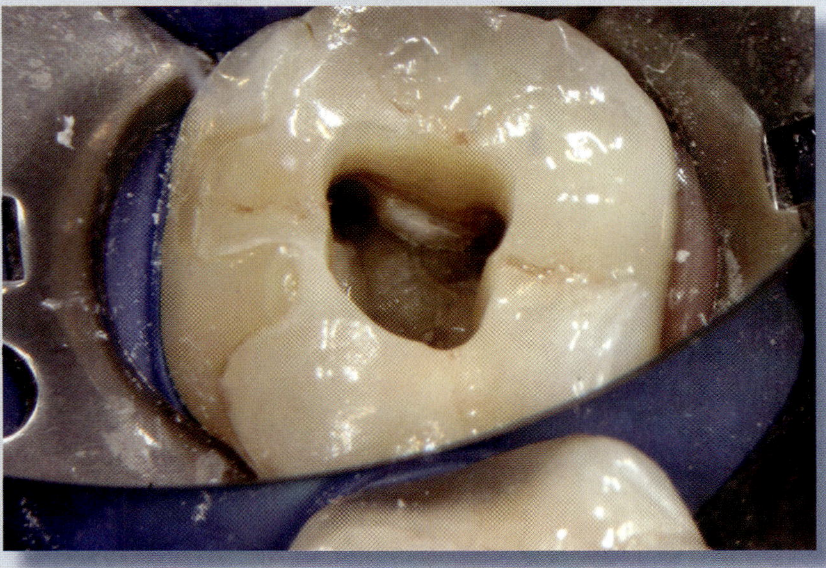

FIG. 2.XIII-20

Clinical image of access, showing the region between the mesial canals. Note the difference in dentin color in the region to be worked on (between the mesial canals).

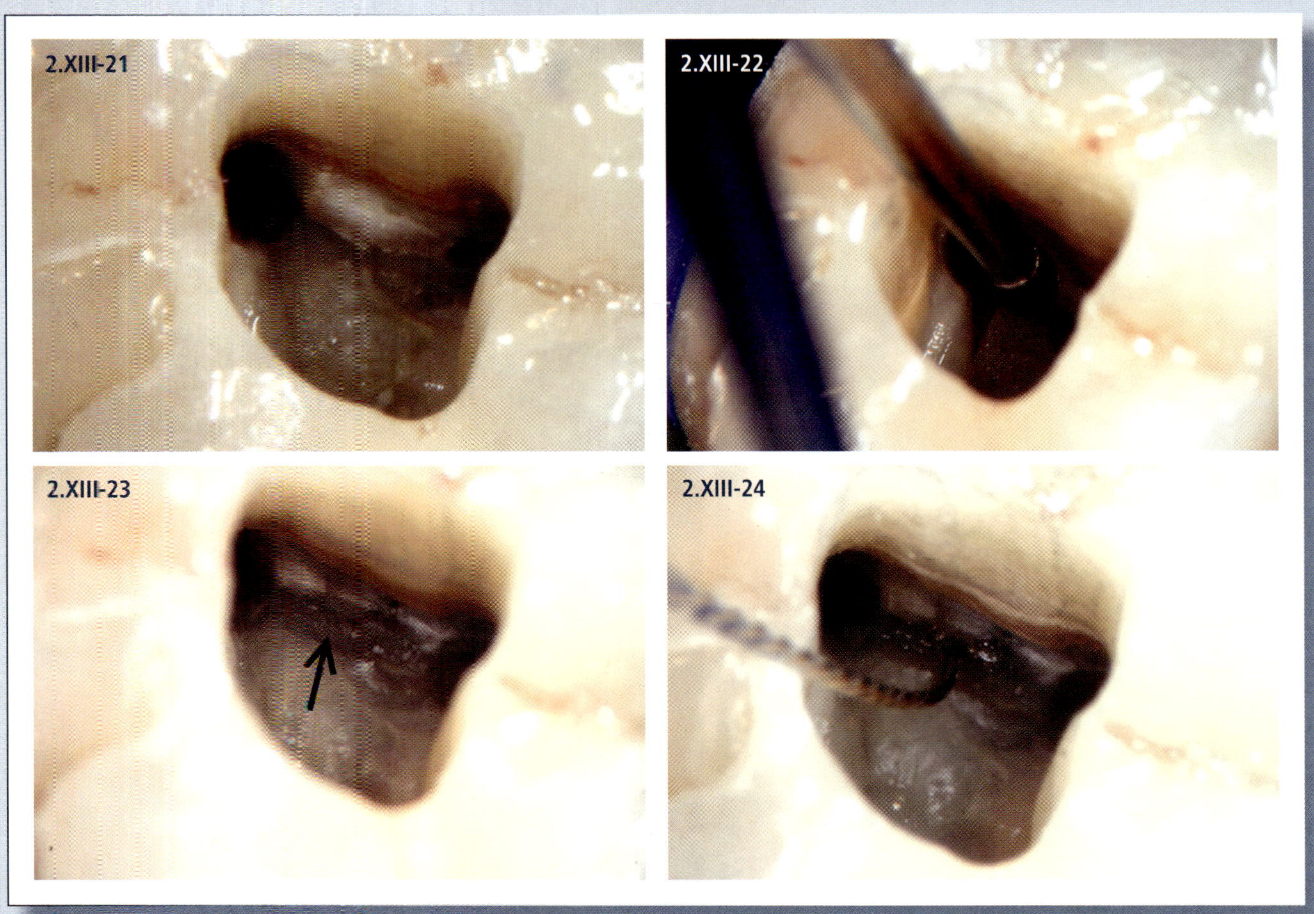

FIG. 2.XIII-21

Clinical image of access, showing the region between the mesial canals at higher magnification. Note the difference in dentin color in the region to be worked on (between the mesial canals).

FIG. 2.XIII-22

Clinical image of the Pearl-D ultrasonic tip ready to be activated in the desired area. Note how important magnification is in order to obtain the much needed operating precision.

FIG. 2.XIII-23

Clinical image of the region between the mesial canals after removal of whitened dentin that covered the isthmus. Note the possible entry of a mesio-mesial canal (arrow).

FIG. 2.XIII-24

Clinical image of the region between the mesial canals with the insertion of a type K file 06. Note the precision obtained with magnification.

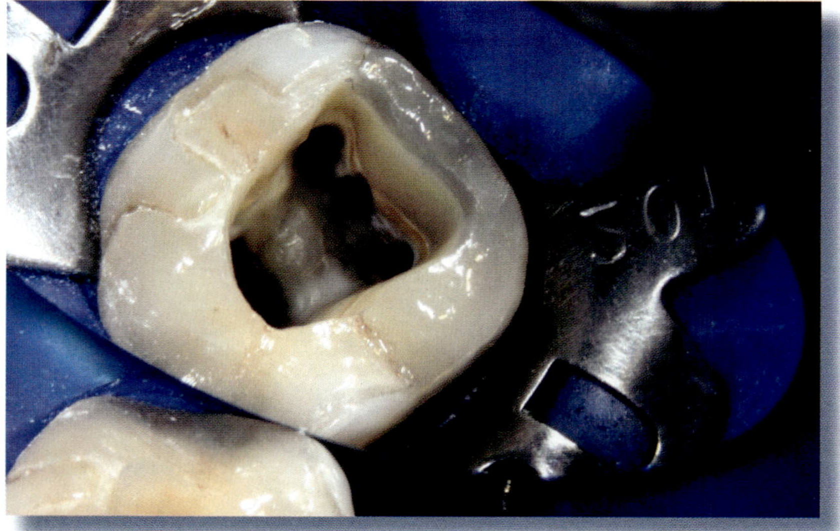

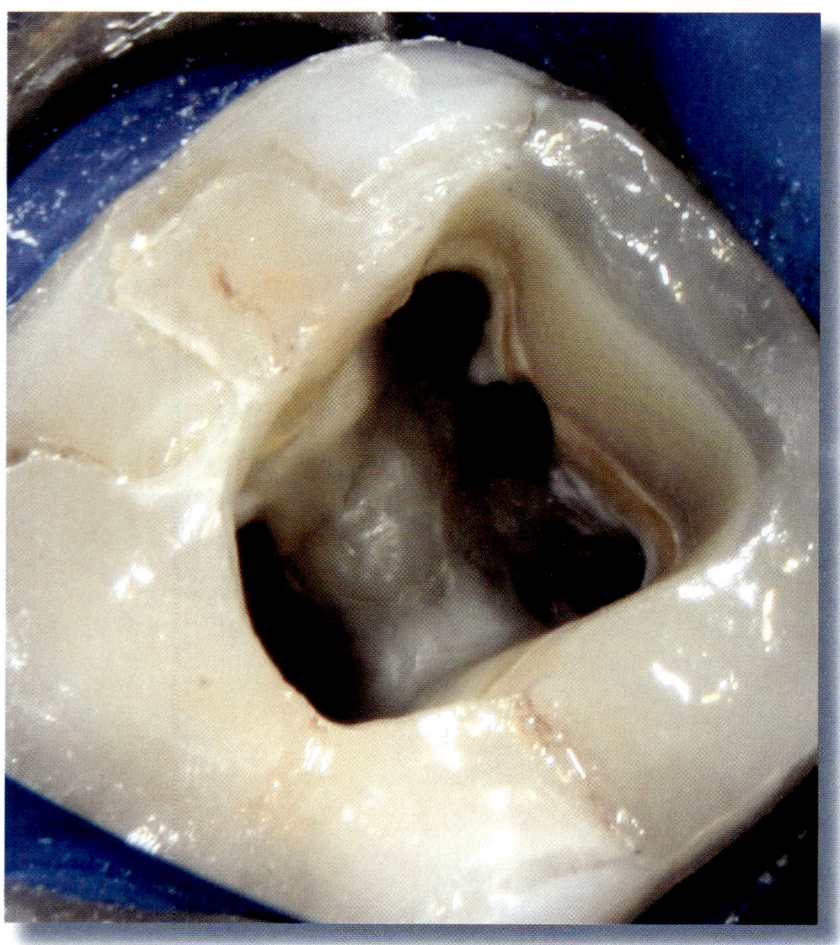

FIG. 2.XIII-25

Clinical image of the three mesial canals after instrumentation.

FIG. 2.XIII-26

Clinical view of the three mesial canals after instrumentation at higher magnification, at the suitable time for filling. Note the cleanliness of the pulp chamber and absence of tissue rests.

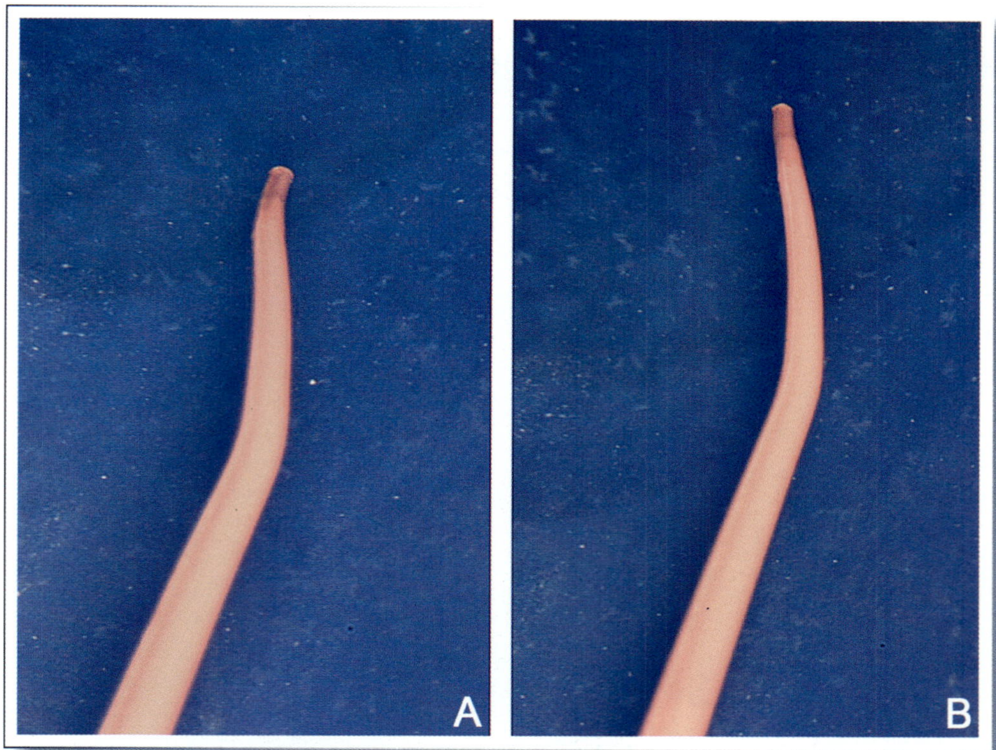

FIGS. 2.XIII-27A-B

Clinical images of the Gutta-Percha cone that was removed from the mesio-mesial canal, seen from different angles. It is completely deformed by the curvatures in the middle and apical thirds. Note the importance of "reading" the Gutta-Percha cones, before the filling procedure.

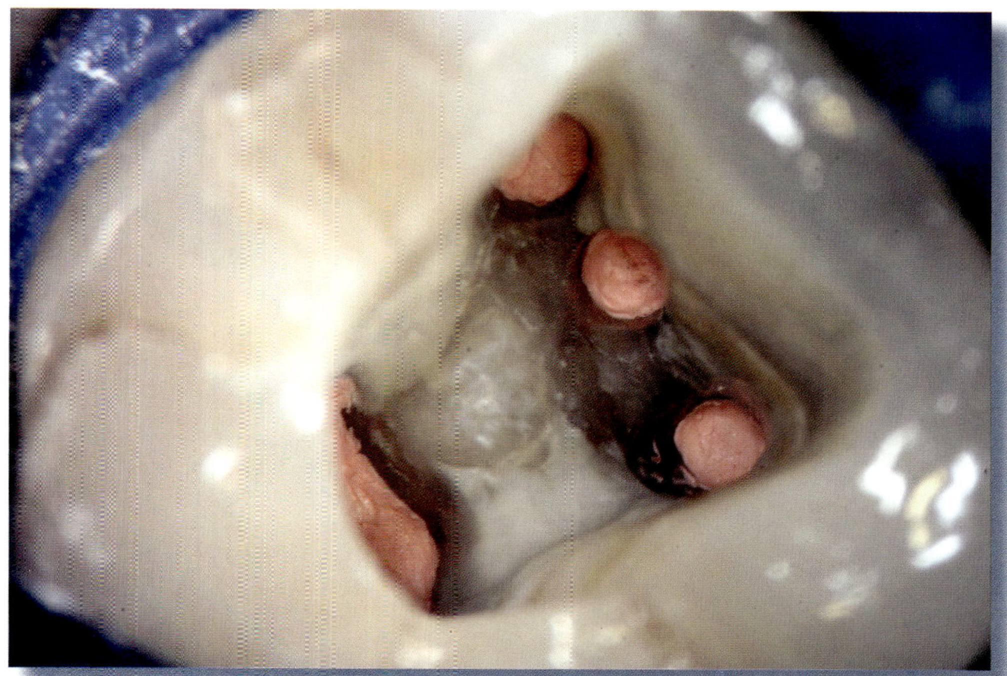

FIG. 2.XIII-28

Clinical image of the three filled mesial canals and distal canal. Note the cleanliness of the pulp chamber as well as the correct filling of all the canals.

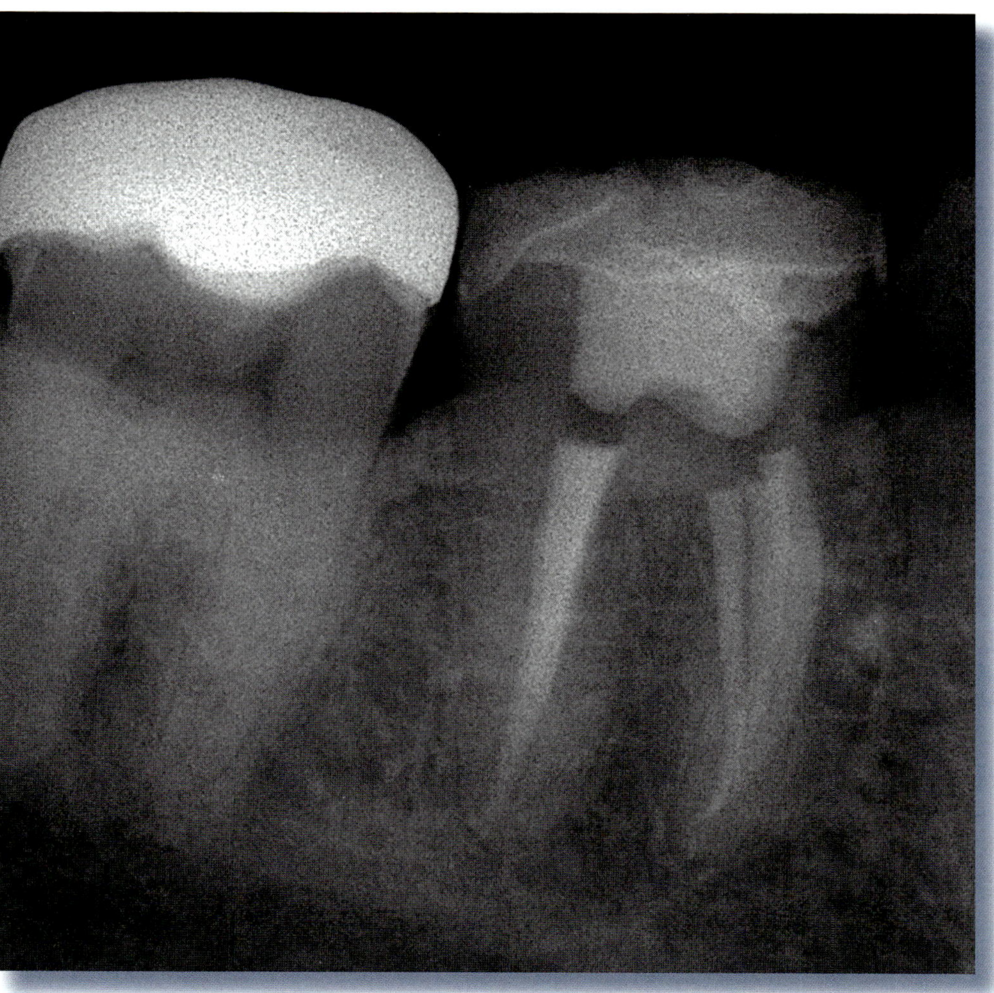

FIG. 2.XIII-29

Postoperative radiograph of tooth 4.6 three years after completion of treatment. Note the perfect filling of the root canal system, both in the mesial and distal roots, with complete integrity of the peri-radicular region.

LOCATION OF SUPERFICIAL SECONDARY ANATOMY

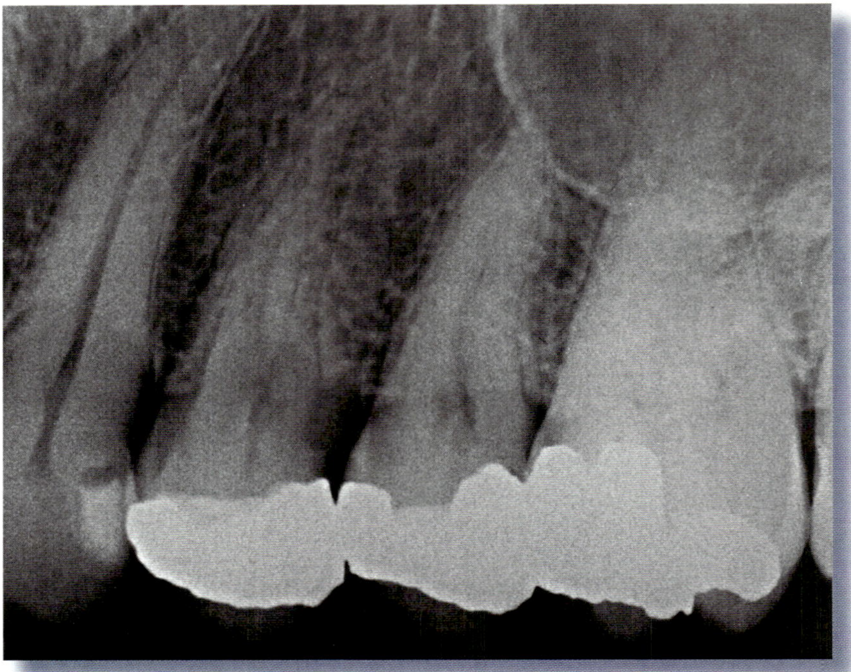

FIG. 2.XIII-30

Preoperative radiograph showing suspected anatomic anomaly in tooth 2.4 (periodontal ligament without clear definition).

FIG. 2.XIII-31

Clinical image of initial access clearly showing the existence of the pulp chamber roof as well as tissue remnants.

FIG. 2.XIII-32

Clinical image of access being refined with Pearl-D ultrasonic tip.

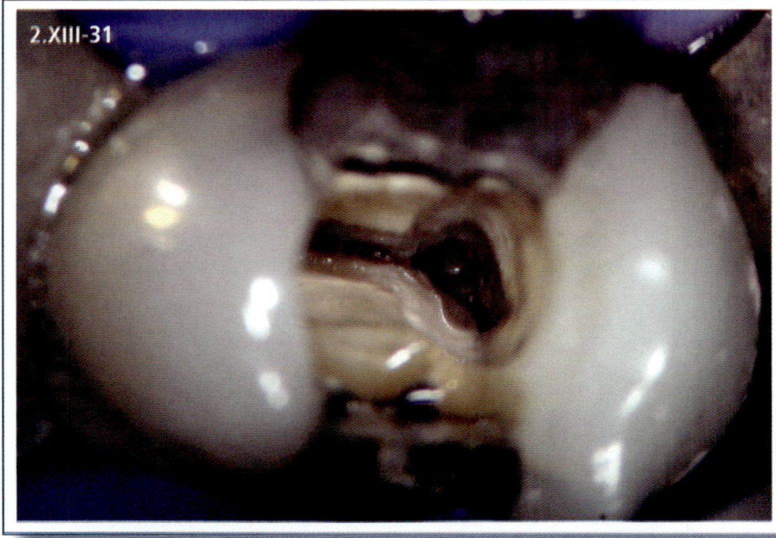

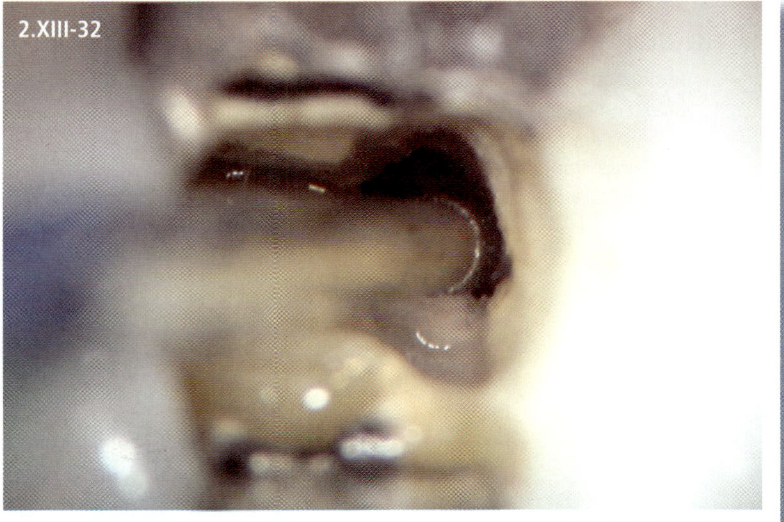

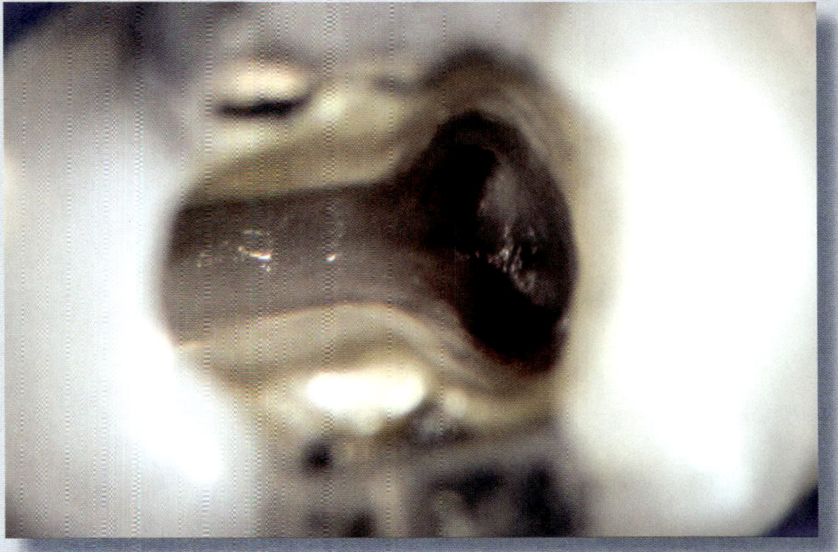

FIG. 2.XIII-33

Clinical image of access showing two buccal canals and a third canal in between. Note how easily the canals are identified, as well as the clear difference between the dentin color of the various areas.

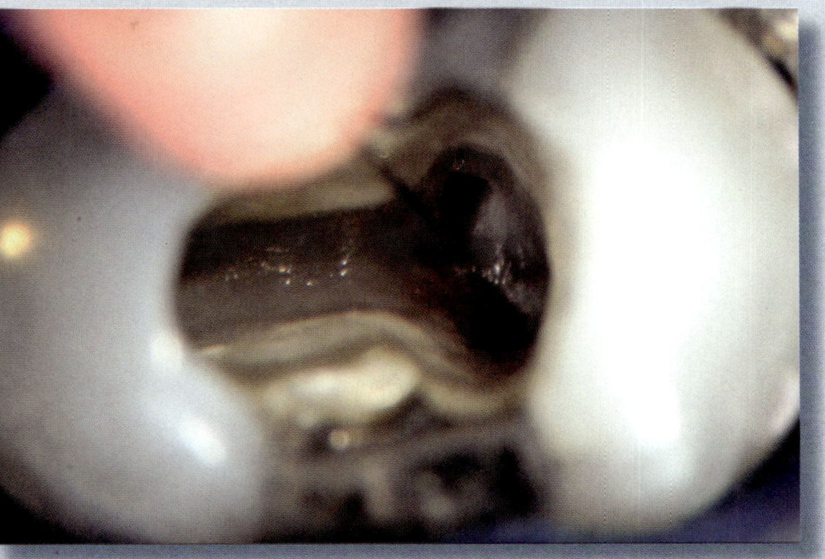

FIG. 2.XIII-34

Clinical image of access showing a type K file 06 inserted in the third buccal canal.

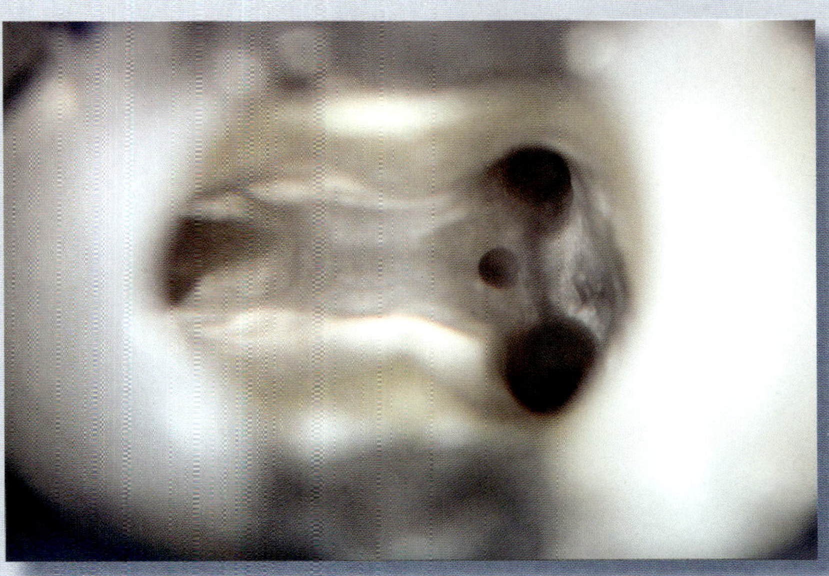

FIG. 2.XIII-35

Clinical image of the three buccal canals after instrumentation, as well as the palatal canal. Note the cleanliness of the pulp chamber, and absence of tissue remnants.

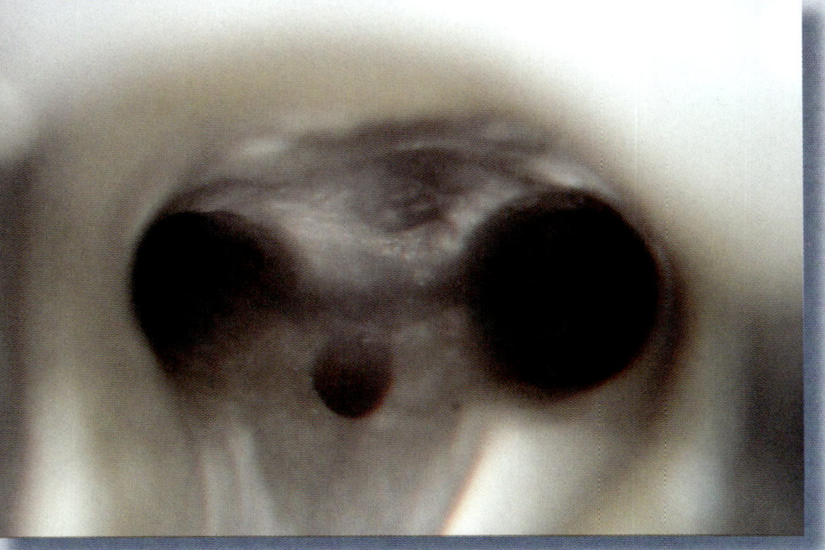

FIG. 2.XIII-36

Clinical image at high magnification of the three mesial canals after instrumentation. Note the cleanliness of the pulp chamber, and absence of tissue remnants.

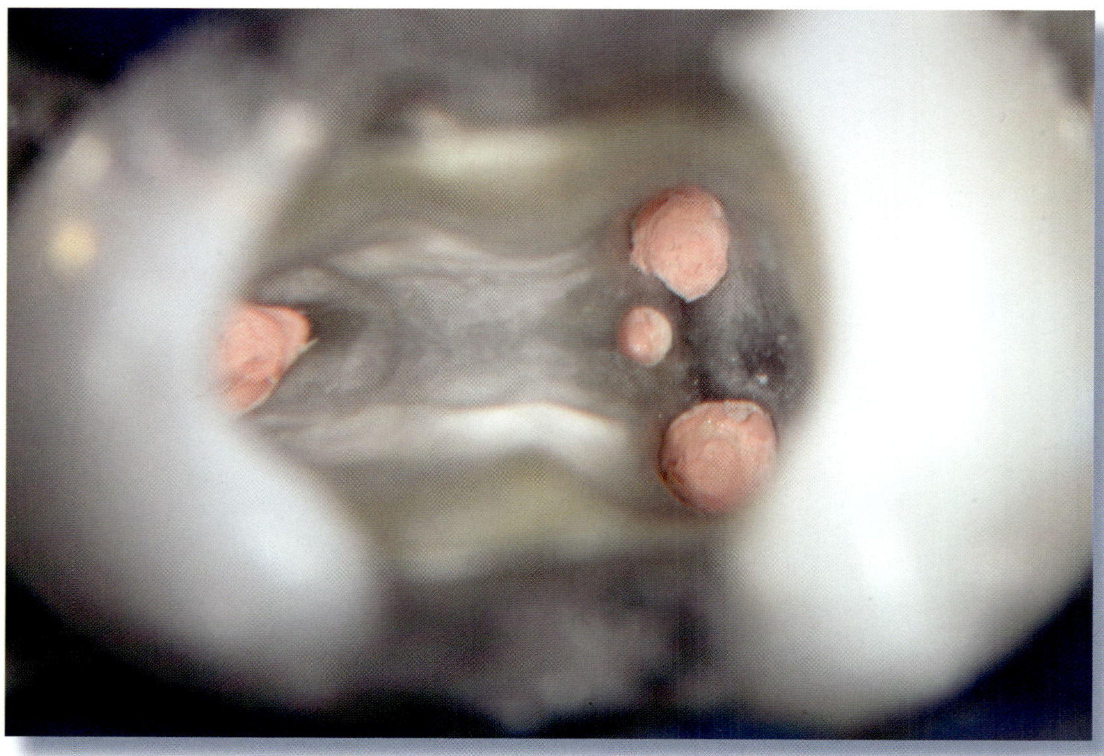

FIG. 2.XIII-37

Clinical image of the three filled mesial canals and palatal canal. Note the cleanliness of the pulp chamber as well as the correct filling of all canals.

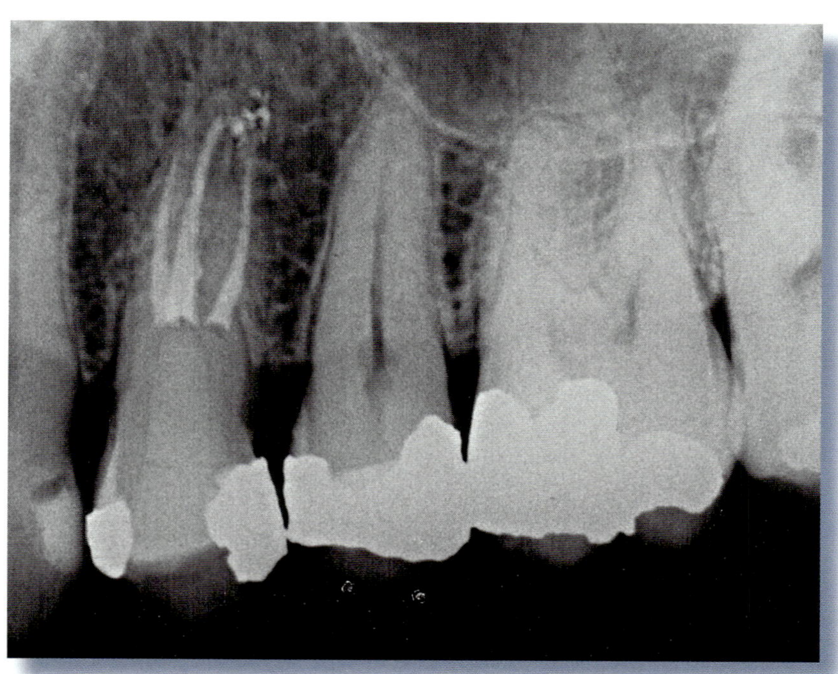

FIG. 2.XIII-38

Postoperative radiograph of tooth 2.4. Note perfect filling of the root canal system, both in the buccal roots and in the palatal root.

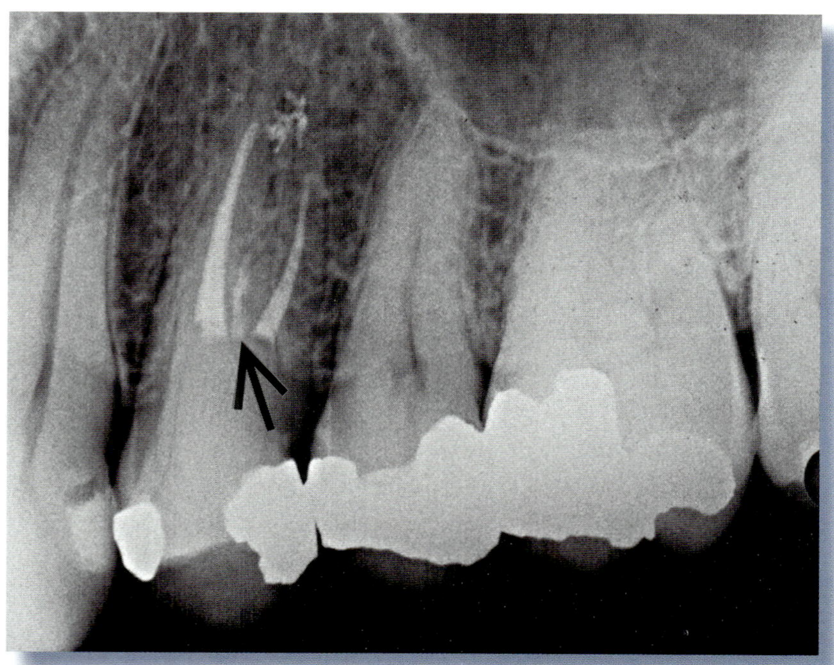

FIG. 2.XIII-39

Postoperative radiograph of tooth 2.4. Note the perfect filling of the third canal of the buccal root (arrow) and its discrepancy in size compared to the other roots.

LOCATION OF DEEP SECONDARY ANATOMY

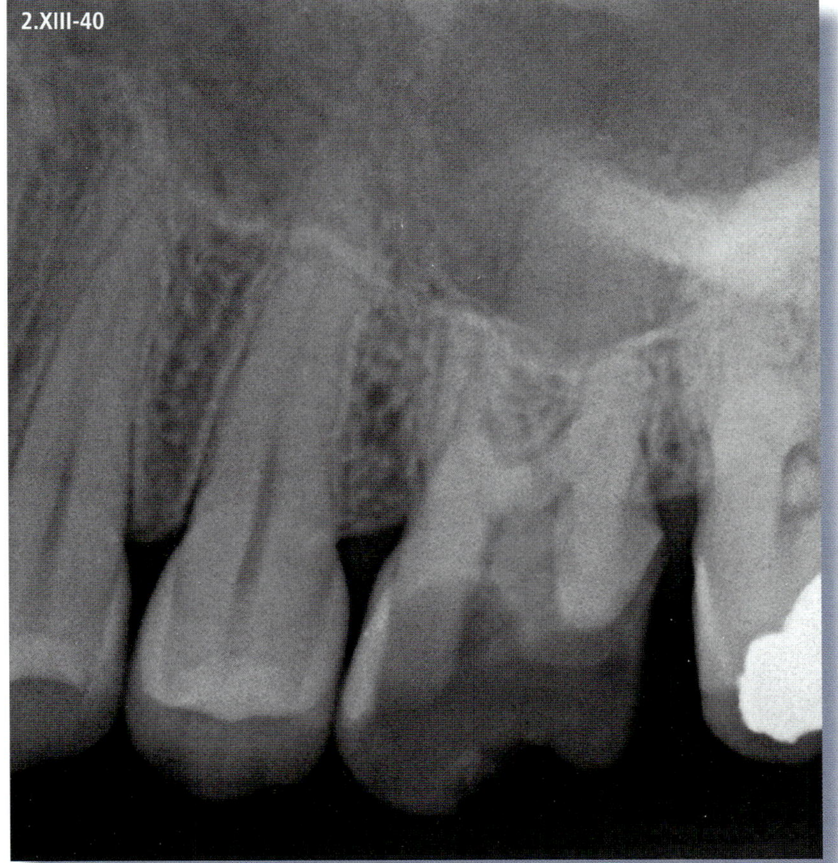

FIG. 2.XIII-40

Preoperative radiograph showing suspected anatomic anomaly in tooth 2.6.

FIG. 2.XIII-41

Clinical image of access seeking deep anatomy with CKT3-D ultrasonic point.

FIG. 2.XIII-42

Clinical image of access at high magnification, showing the filling of the 3 mesio-buccal root canals. Note the depth at which the bifurcation occurs.

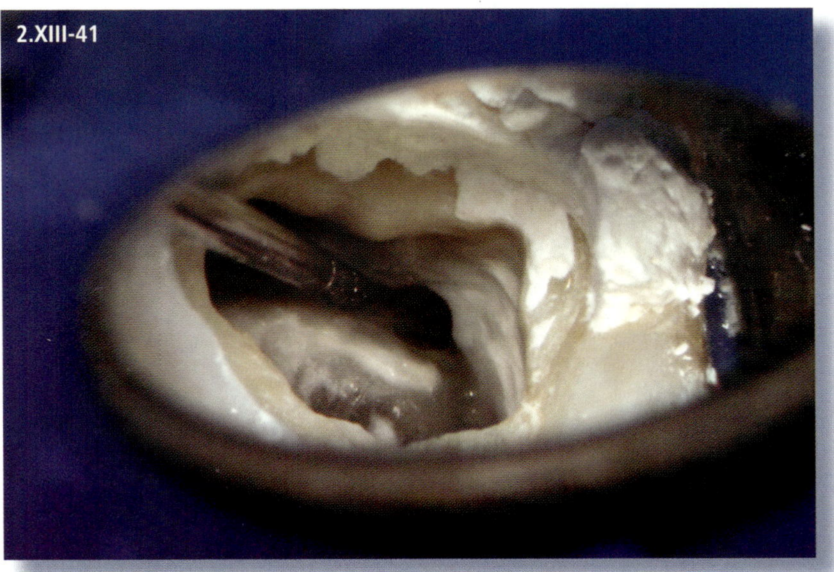

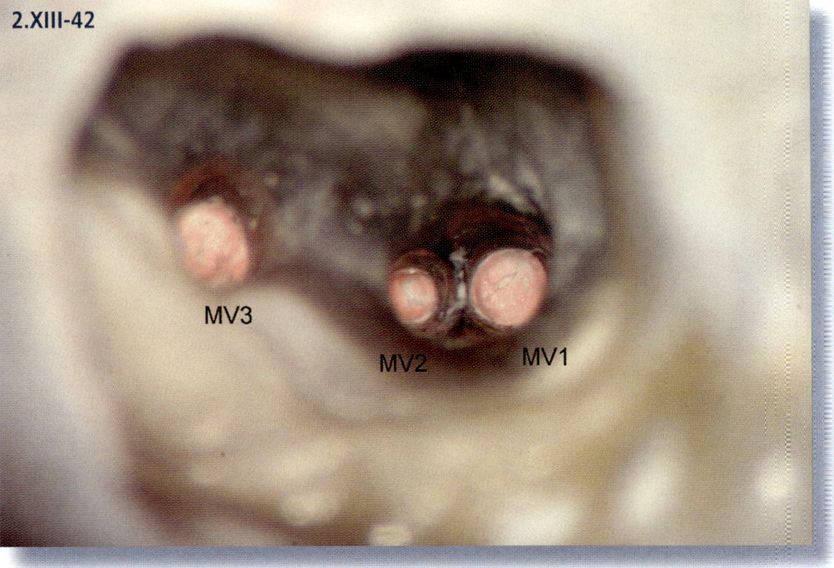

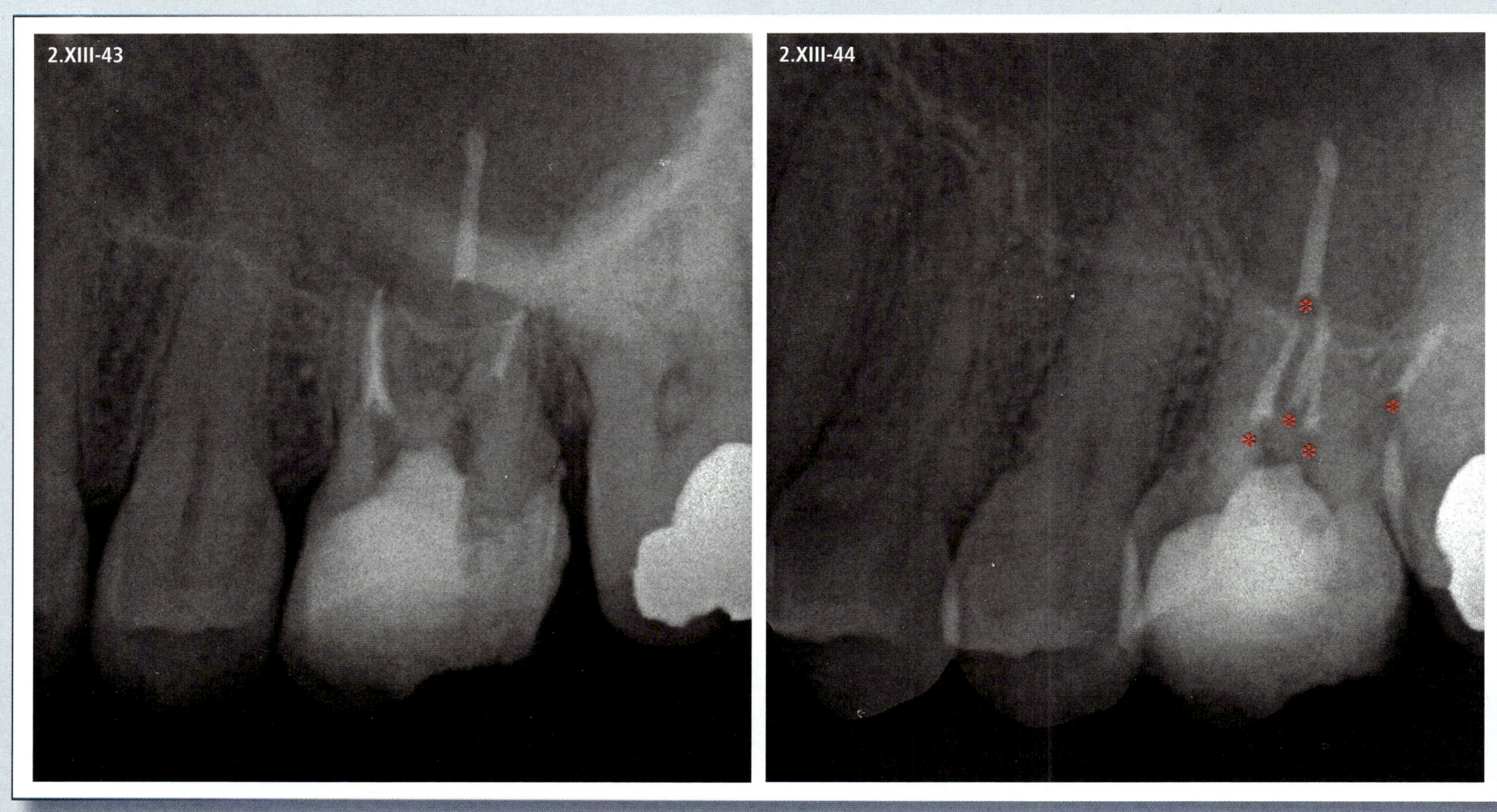

FIG. 2.XIII-43

Postoperative radiograph of tooth 2.6. Note perfect filling of the root canal system, both in the buccal roots and palatal roots.

FIG. 2.XIII-44

Postoperative radiograph of tooth 2.6, with distalized horizontal angulation. Note the perfect filling of the five canals.

RETREATMENT AND REMOVAL OF FRACTURED INSTRUMENTS

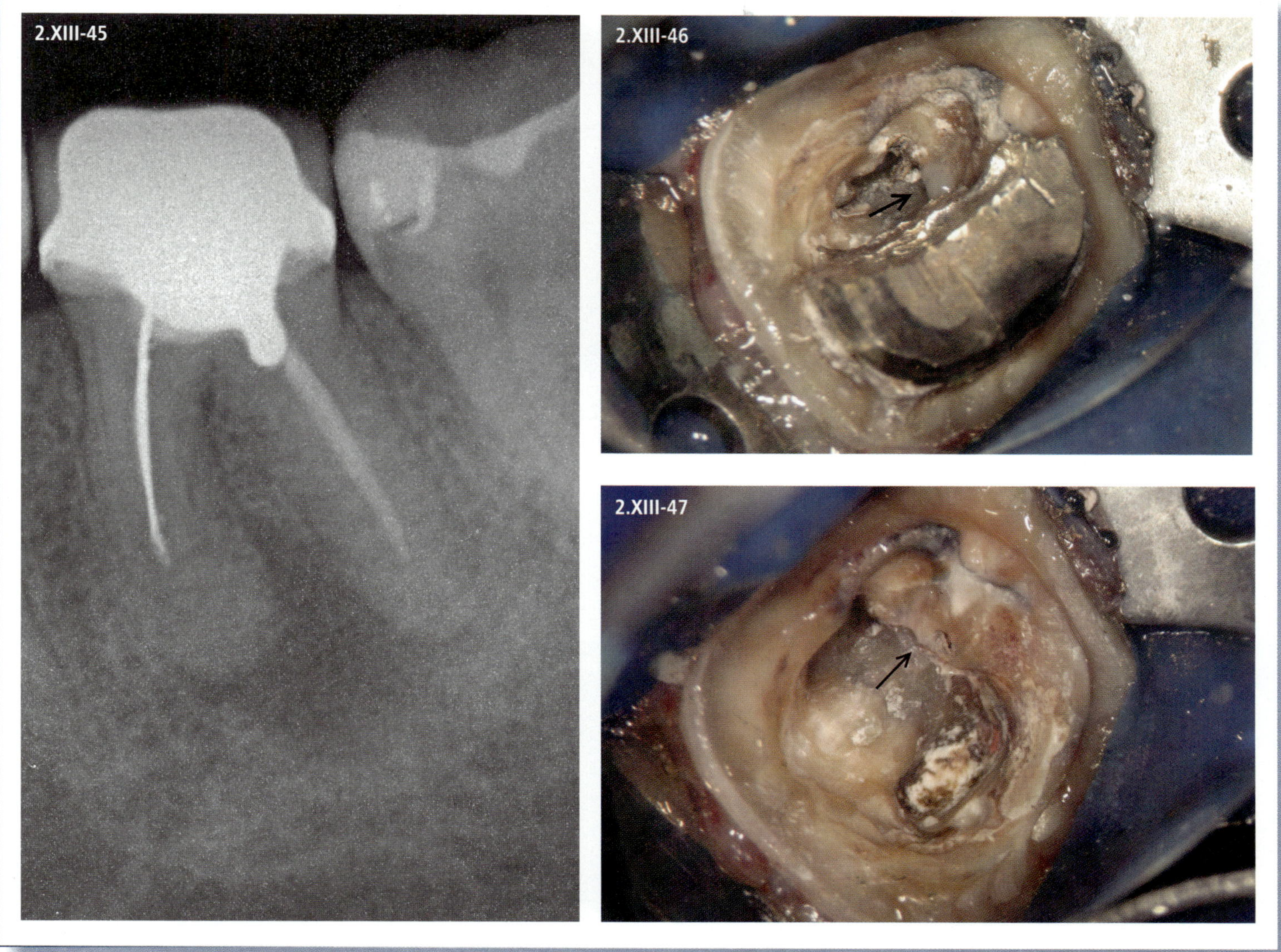

FIG. 2.XIII-45

Preoperative radiograph showing a tooth with a silver cone, or fractured instruments in the mesial root, cast core in the distal root and extensive lesion in the mesial root of tooth 3.6.

FIG. 2.XIII-46

Clinical image of partial access after core was sectioned in a bucco-lingual direction (at all times performed under complete isolation to narrow the field of view). Note the presence of a purulent exudate in the mesio-lingual area (arrow).

FIG. 2.XIII-47

Clinical image of access after complete removal of the core. Note the presence of the roof in the mesio-lingual area where the exudate was coming out (arrow).

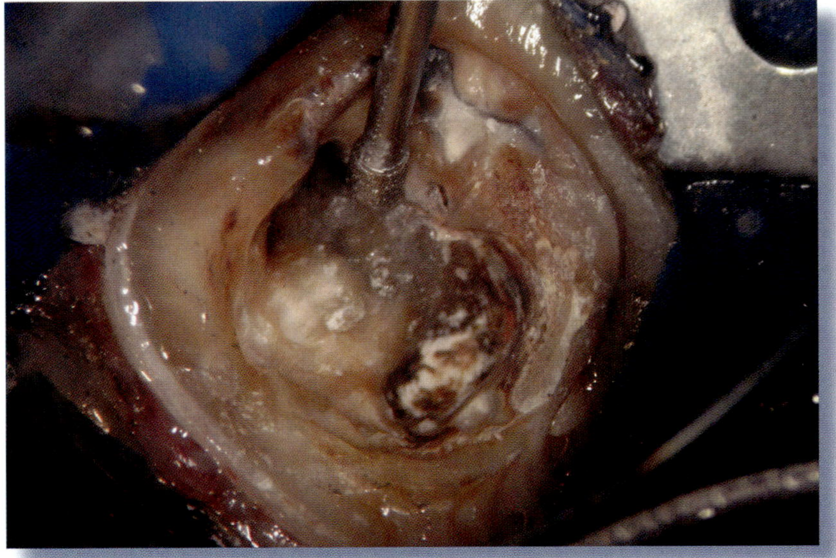

FIG. 2.XIII-48

Clinical image of access with a Pearl-D ultrasonic tip, used for the removal of the remainder of the roof.

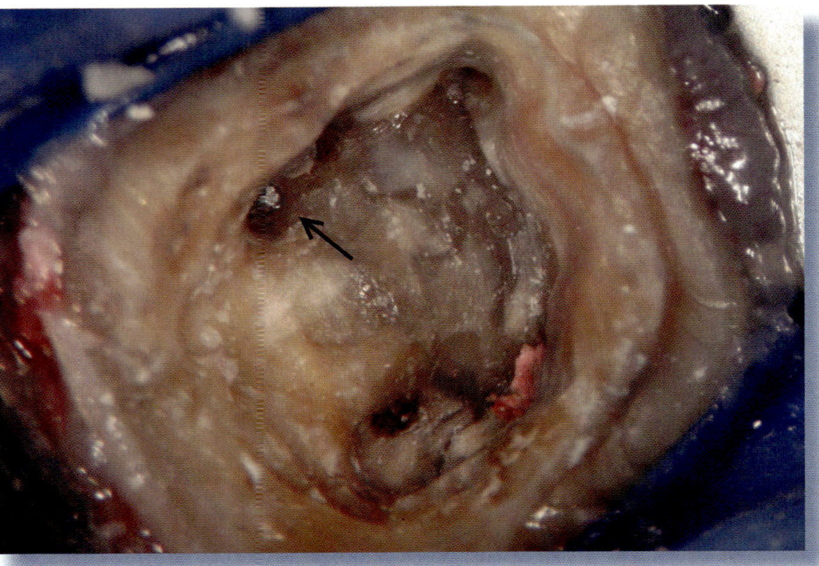

FIG. 2.XIII-49

Clinical image of completed access showing location of 3 canals in the mesial root (mesio-lingual canal had not been located in previous treatment. Note the presence of a silver cone in the mesio-buccal canal (arrow).

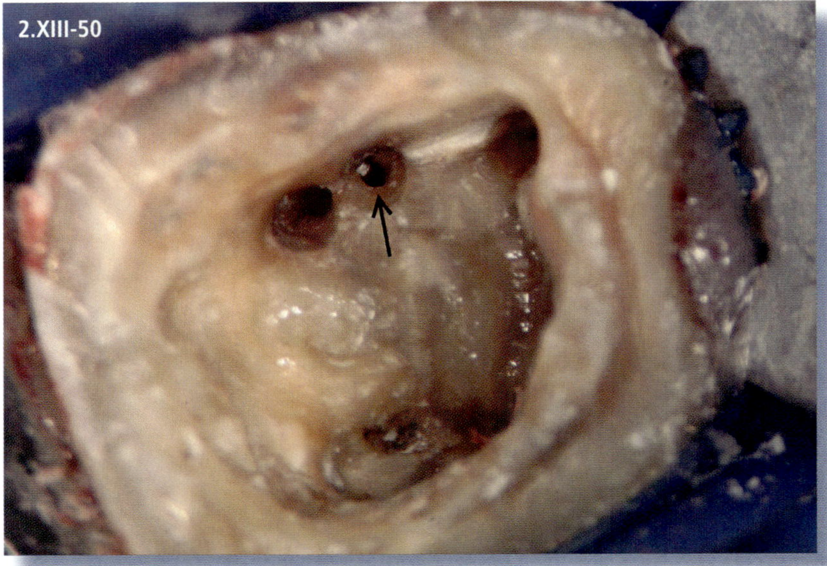

FIG. 2.XIII-50

Clinical image of access showing the mesio-buccal canal without the silver cone. Note the fractured instrument in the mesio-mesial canal (arrow).

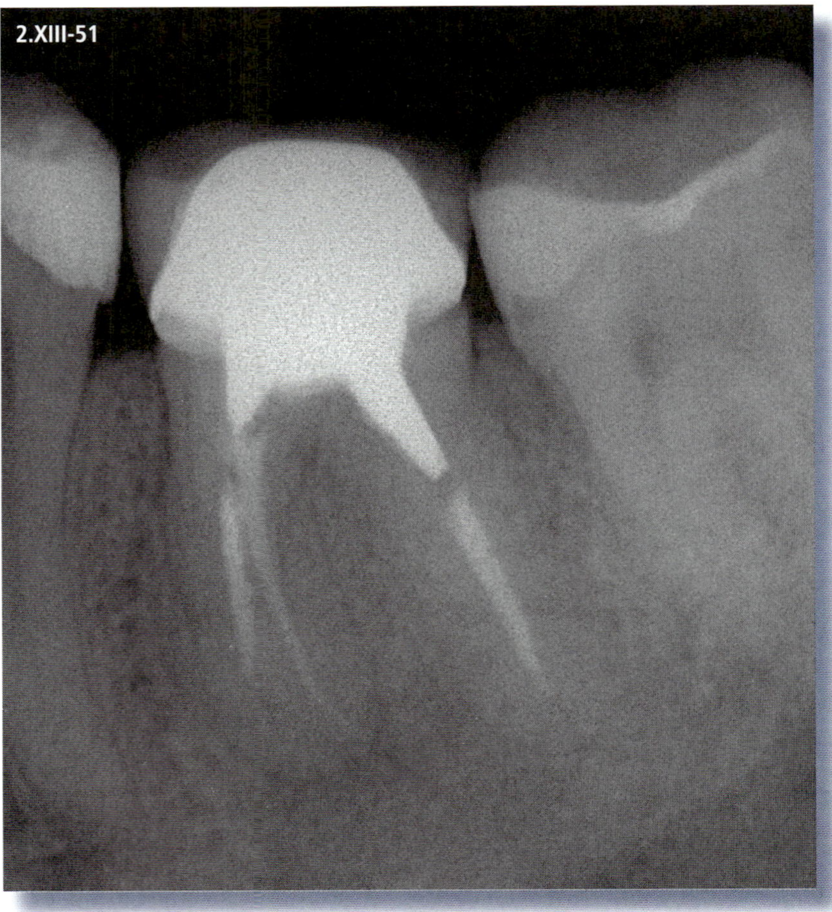

FIG. 2.XIII-51

Postoperative radiograph of tooth 3.6 one year after completion of treatment. Note the almost complete resolution of the lesion, in spite of the mesio-buccal and mesio-distal canals being blocked due to the presence of insuperable steps.

LOCATION OF CALCIFIED CANAL AND REMOVAL OF FRACTURED INSTRUMENT

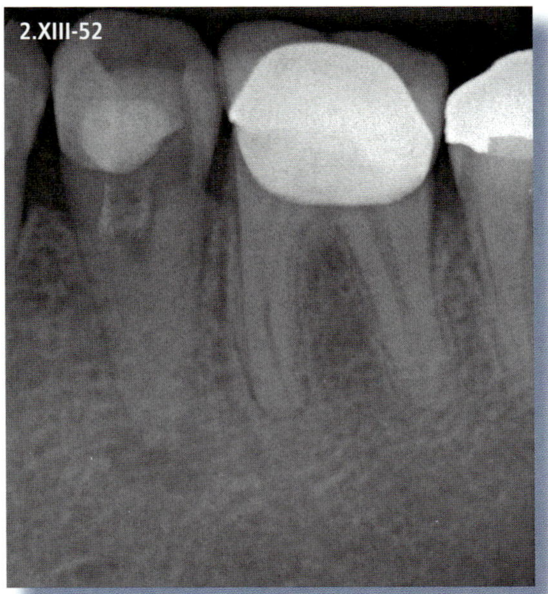

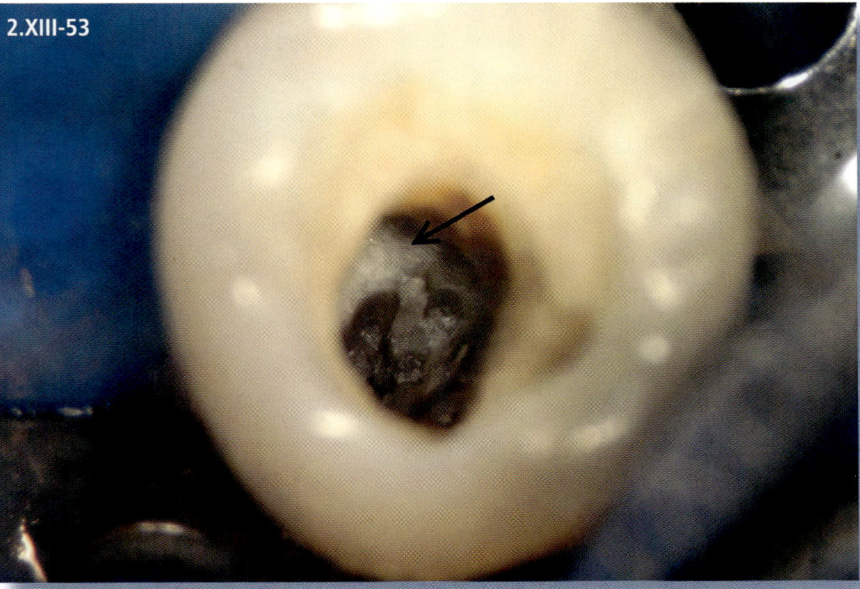

FIG. 2.XIII-52

Preoperative radiograph showing tooth 3.5 with extensive coronal wear, after numerous frustrated attempts to locate the calcified canal with low speed spherical burs (report by colleague). Note the presence of peri-radicular lesion; that is, an anatomic canal containing irritants is present.

FIG. 2.XIII-53

Clinical image of partial access, showing large quantity of dentin removed (during previous attempts to locate the calcified canal), hampering location of the anatomical canal. Note excessive ground area in the mesial aspect (arrow).

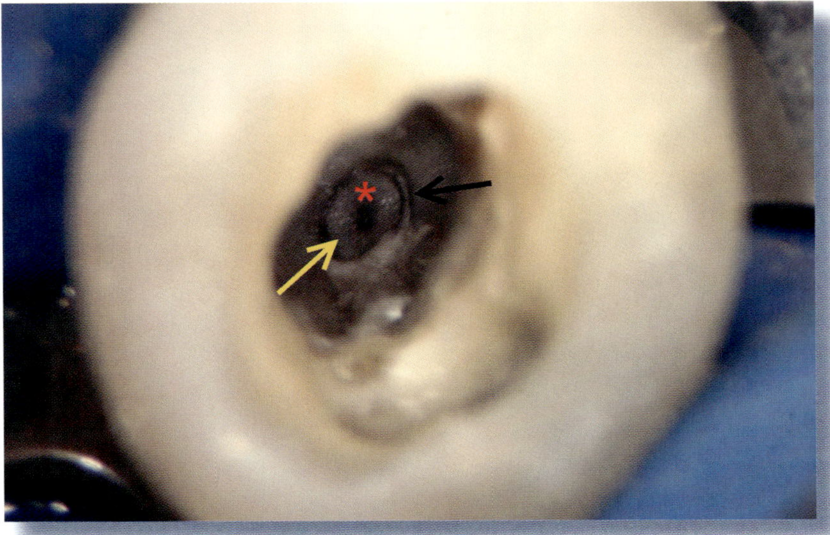

FIG. 2.XIII-54

Clinical image of partial access, showing the clarity of definition of the location of the canal after the use of the ultrasonic tip CKT2-D. Note the canal in center of the image (red asterisk), calcification of the canal (yellow arrow) and original limit or the anatomic canal (black arrow).

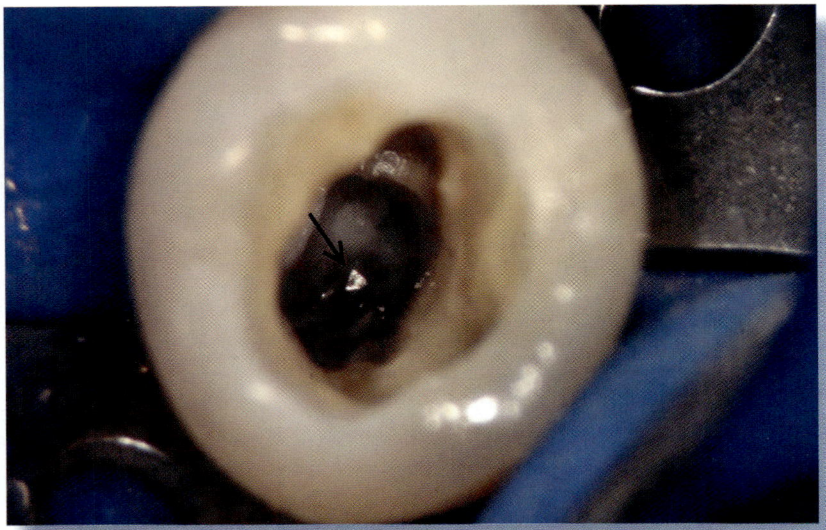

FIG. 2.XIII-55

Clinical image of access with fractured instrument. Note the many details that can be seen, such as the fractured instrument, which appears as a triangular ccrossection (arrow).

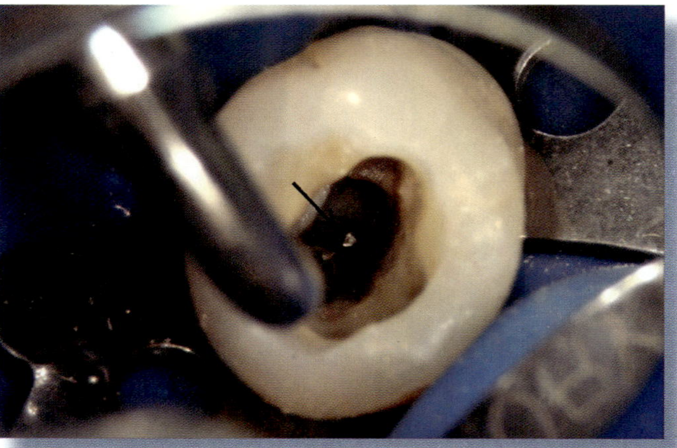

FIG. 2.XIII-56

Clinical image of the use of ultrasonic tip UT4. Note that the ultrasound tip vibrates at the side of the fractured instrument, moving it in an counter-clockwise direction (arrow).

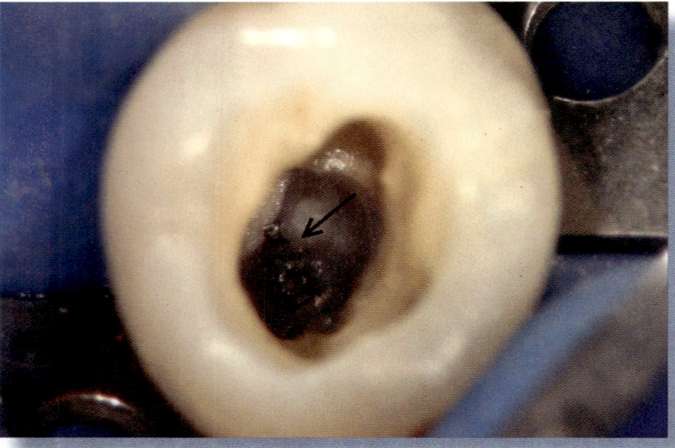

FIG. 2.XIII-57

Clinical image of access after the fractured instrument had been removed. Note the integrity of the instrument. The ultrasonic energy only promoted retrieval, without destroying it (arrow).

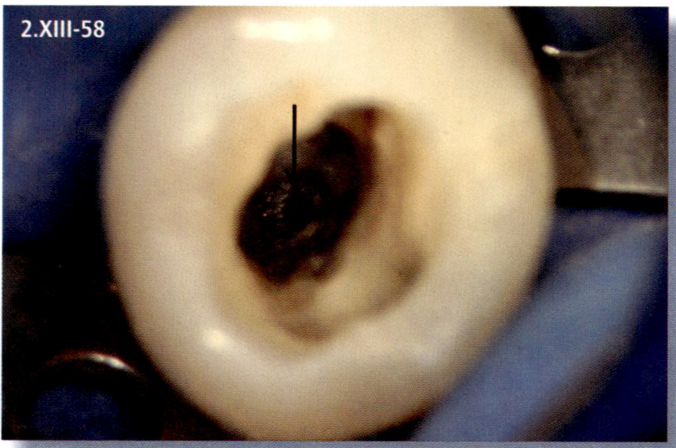

FIG. 2.XIII-58

Clinical image of access showing the canal after removal of the fractured instrument. Note the integrity of the canal opening without unnecessary removal of surrounding dentin (arrow).

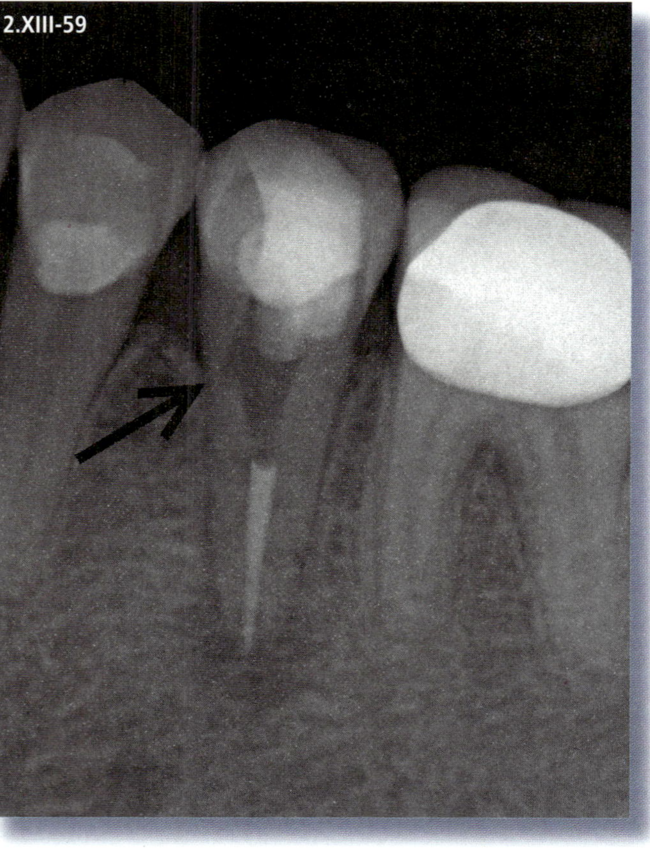

FIG. 2.XIII-59

Postoperative radiograph of tooth 3.5, with canal prepared for a filling with adhesive restorative material (root reinforcement). Note excessive coronal grinding from round burs to locate the calcified canal, almost causing a lateral perforation (arrow).

REMOVAL OF SILVER CONE AND LOCATION OF DEEP ANATOMY

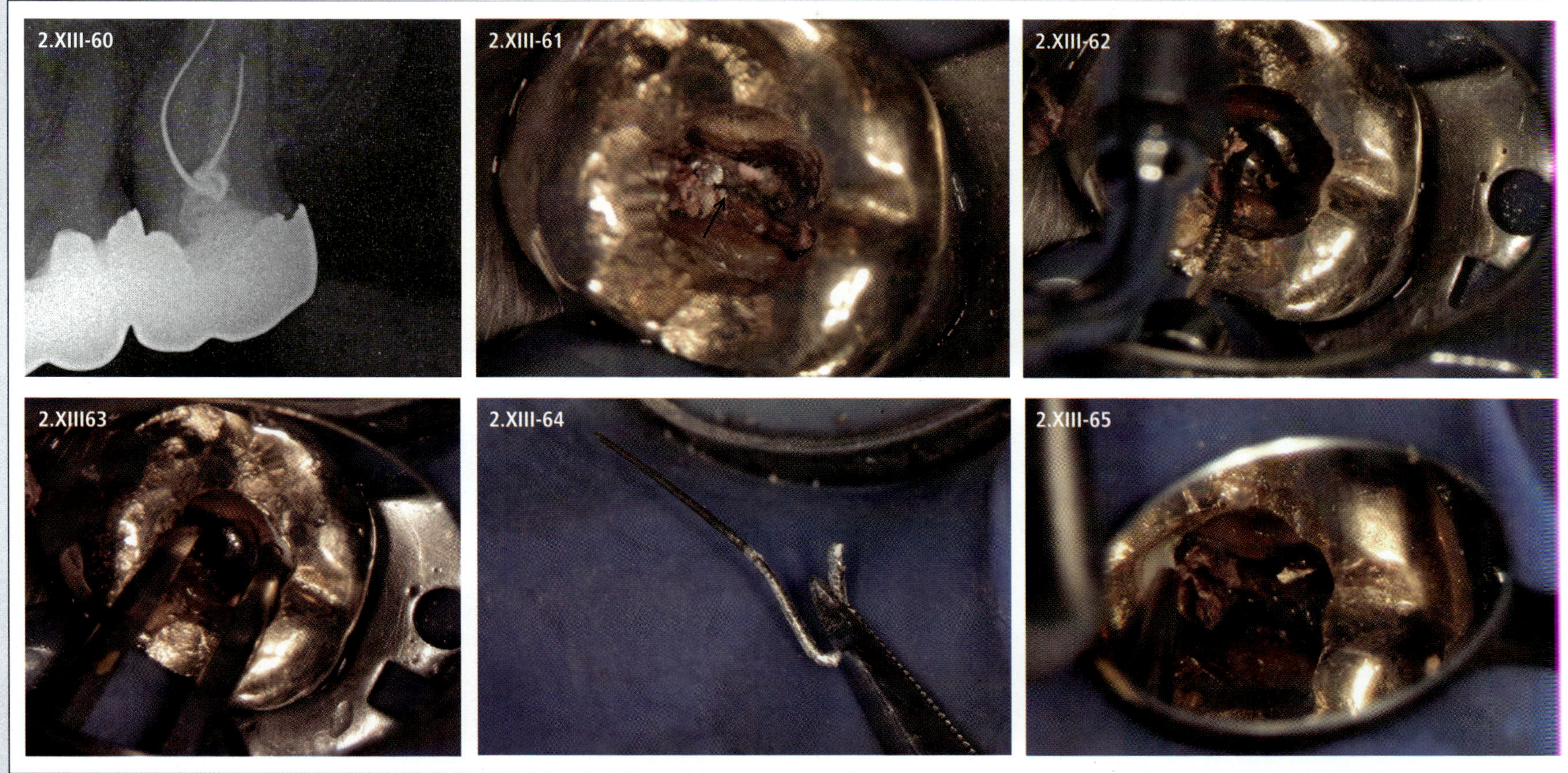

FIG. 2.XIII-60

Preoperative radiograph showing tooth 2.7 with an endo-perio lesion and silver cones filling the buccal canals, with gutta-percha in the palatal canal. Note – Diagnosis if essential for the predictability of the treatment.

FIG. 2.XIII-61

Clinical image of partial access, showing the large quantity of filling material in the pulp chamber. Note also a silver cone in the filling material, and its integrity after access to the metal restoration had been completed (arrow).

FIG. 2.XIII-62

Clinical image of partial access, showing the use of an ultrasonic type K 15 file, enabling cleaning around the silver cone. Note the complete visualization of the operating field, even in a maxillary left second molar.

FIG. 2.XIII-63

Clinical image of partial access, showing the use of a special forceps for removing the silver cones.

FIG. 2.XIII-64

Image of the silver after removal. Note the complete oxidization of the portion that was in the canal.

FIG. 2.XIII-65

Clinical image of the use of an ultrasonic point CKT2, to remove the restorative material and gutta-percha from inside the cervical and middle thirds of the canal. Note the complete visualization of the operating field.

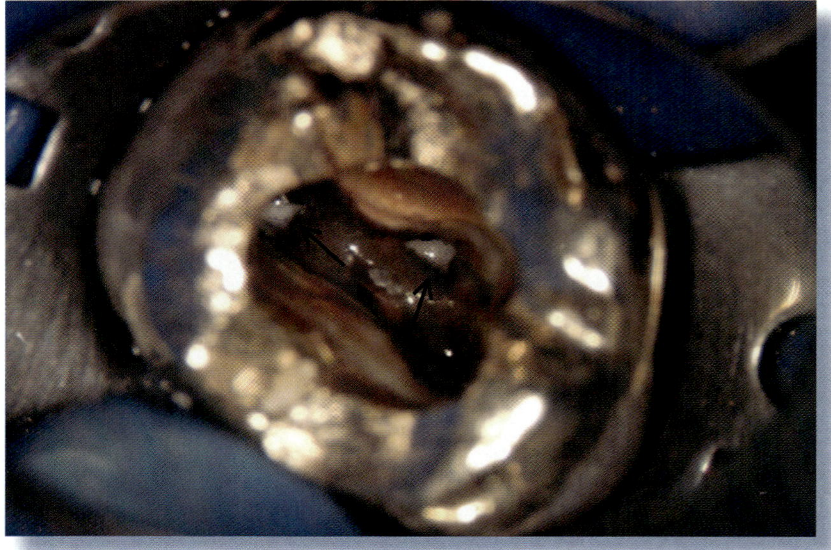

FIG. 2.XIII-66

Clinical image after removal of obstructions in the canals and cleaning of the pulp chamber. Note the effect of release of nascent oxygen of the sodium hypochlorite (arrows).

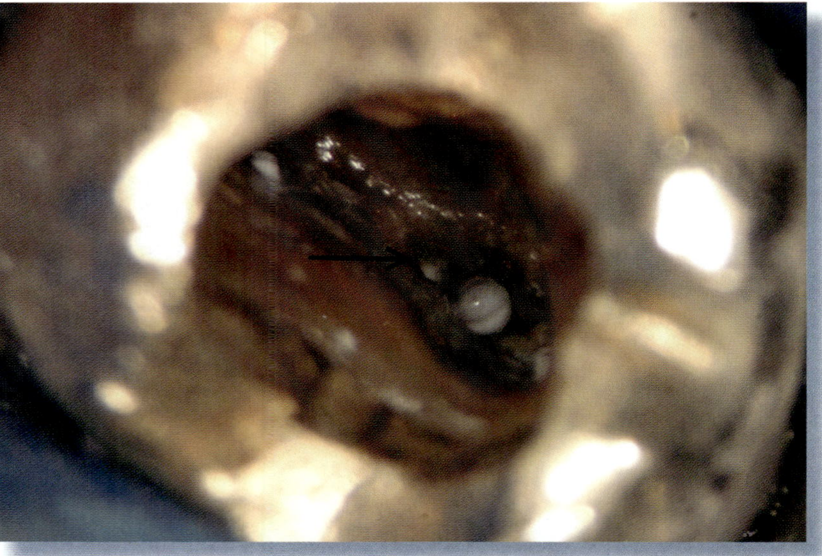

FIG. 2.XIII-67

Clinical image after placing calcium hydroxide. Note that at the side of the mesio-buccal canal, there is a small white area indicating the presence of an isthmus (arrow).

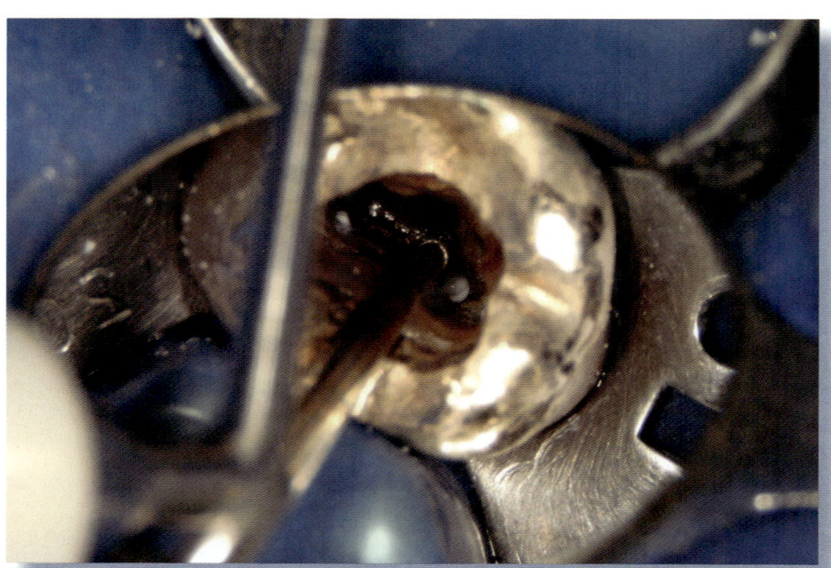

FIG. 2.XIII-68

Clinical image of a Pearl-D ultrasonic tip to locate the superficial secondary anatomy.

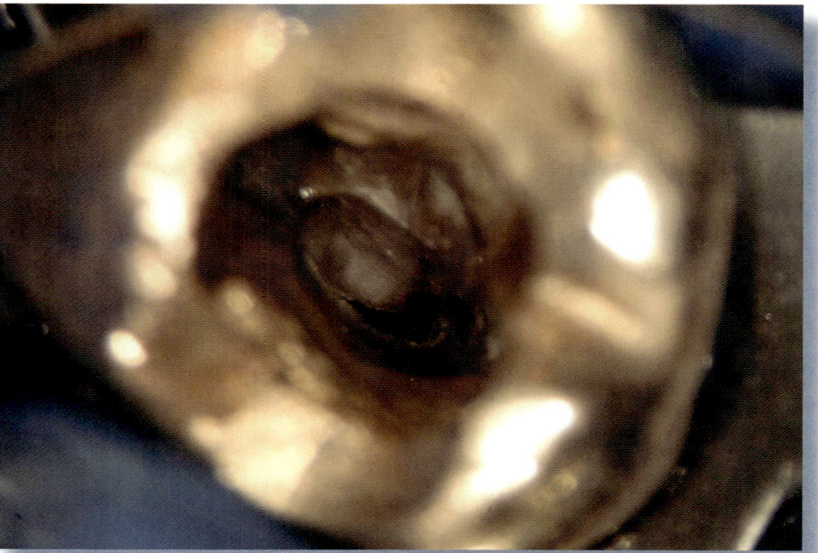

FIG. 2.XIII-69

Clinical image of the mesio-buccal canal and isthmus region. Note the perfect visualization of the isthmus, but making it impossible to locate the mesio-buccal canal 2.

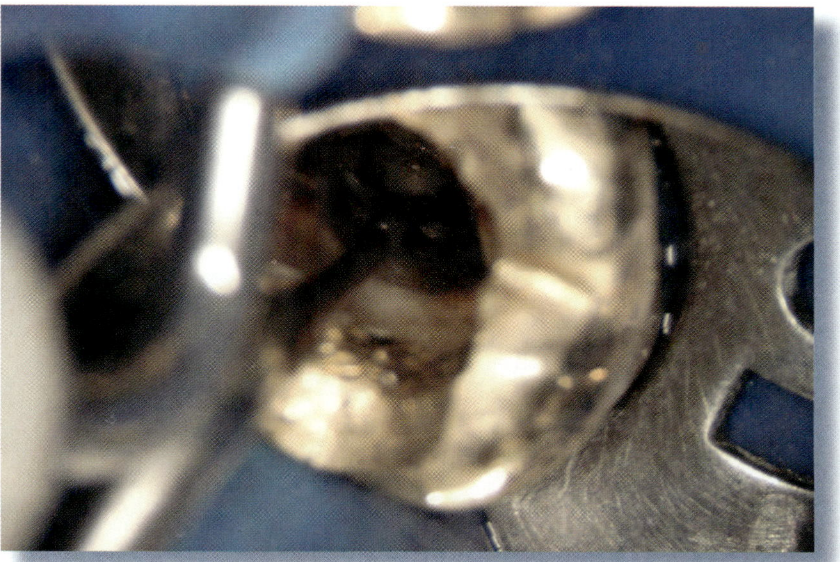

FIG. 2.XIII-70

Clinical image of a UT4-D ultrasonic tip to locate the deep secondary anatomy.

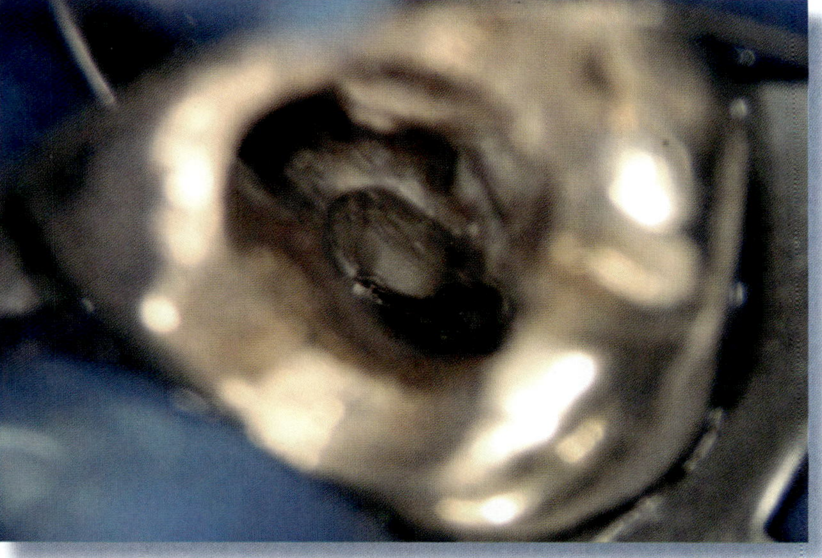

FIG. 2.XIII-71

Clinical image of the mesio-buccal canal and isthmus region. Note the perfect visualization of the isthmus, now enabling the mesio-buccal canal 2 to be located.

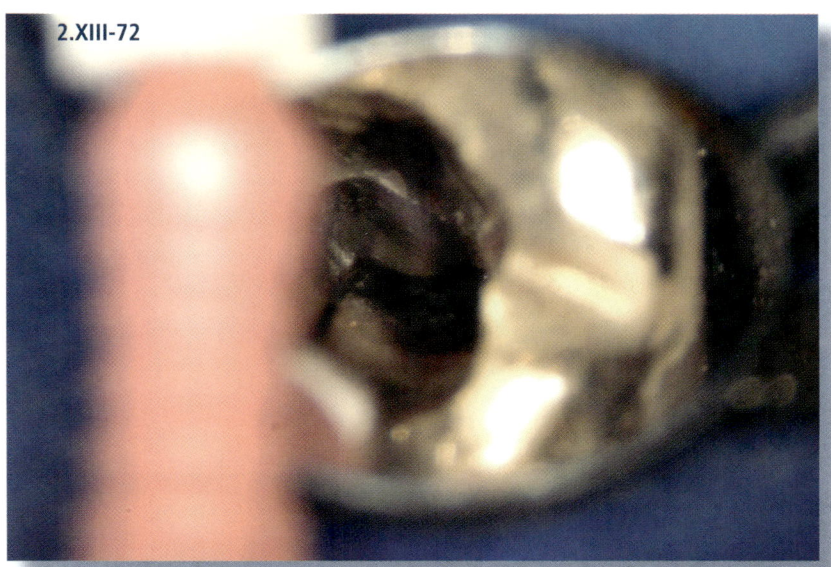

FIG. 2.XIII-72

Clinical image of the mesio-buccal canal 2, with a type K 06 file and the isthmus.

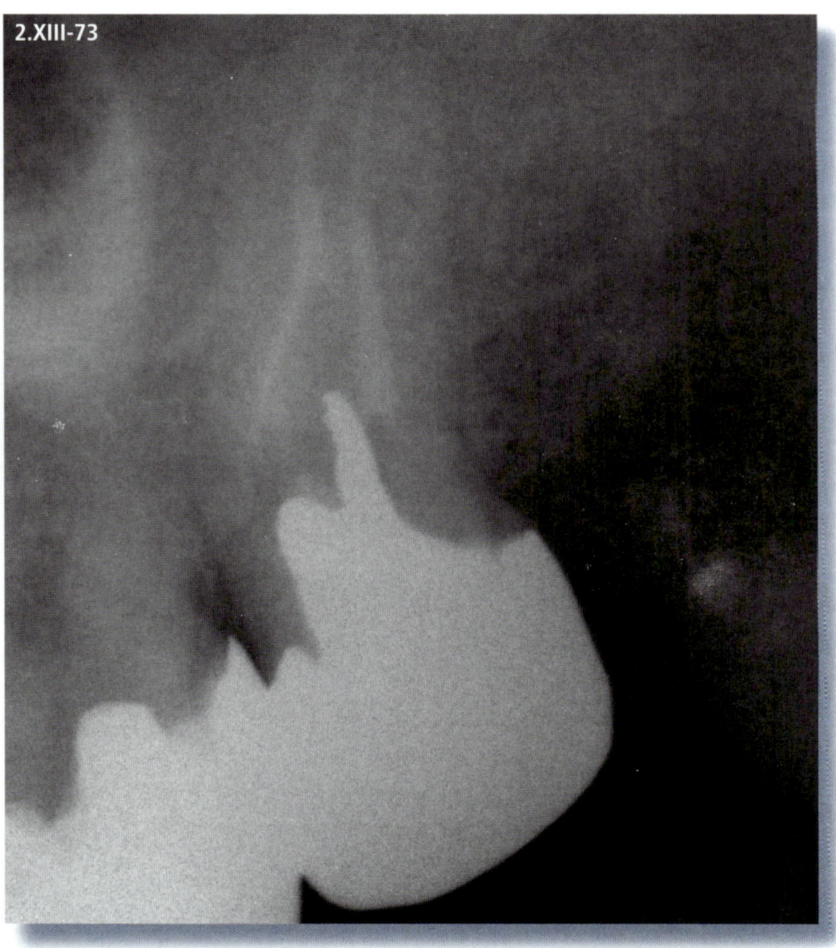

FIG. 2.XIII-73

Follow-up radiograph of tooth 2.7, three years after completion of treatment showing complete resolution of the lesion. A case like this one makes endodontics a unique specialty, since we are able of initiating regeneration of compromised tissues while preserving the affected teeth.

ENDODONTIC SURGERY IN TOOTH 16 INCLUDING PALATAL ROOT

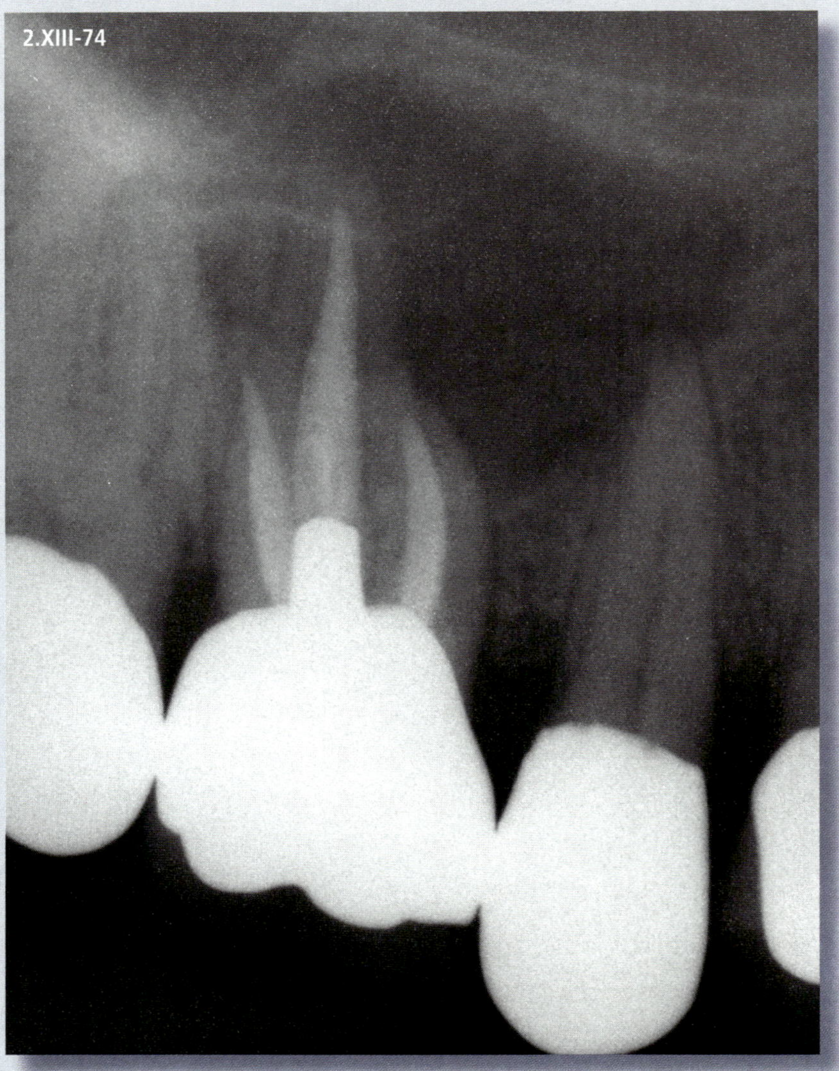

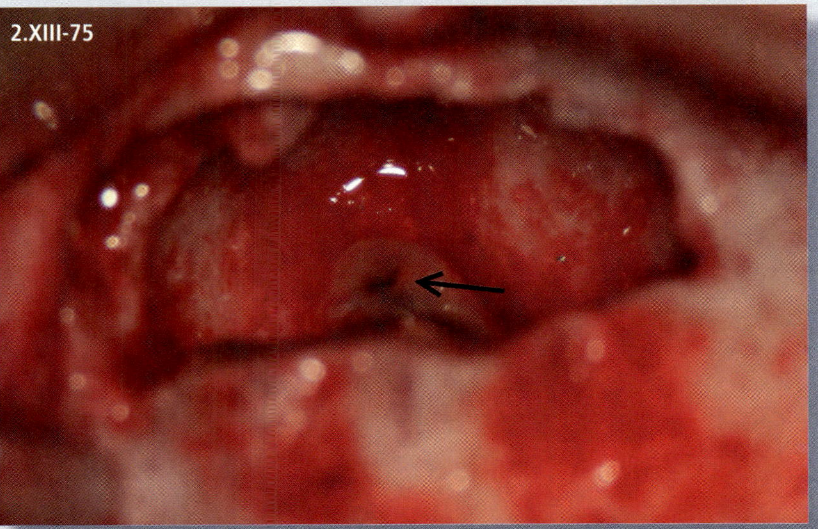

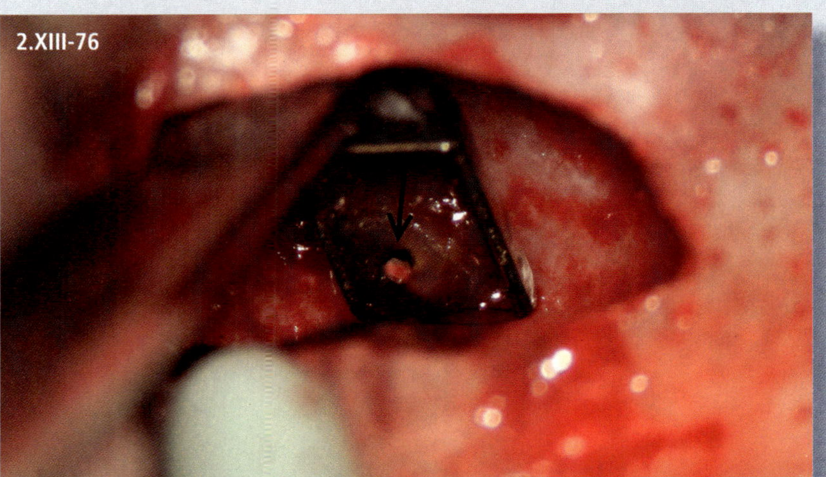

FIG. 2.XIII-74

Preoperative radiograph, showing tooth 1.6 with an extensive lesion of endodontic origin, with possible involvement of tooth 1.5.

FIG. 2.XIII-75

Clinical aspect of the bone recess after removal of the lesion and apicectomy in the vestibular roots. Note the detail of the palatal root apex with darkened aspect, probably apical biofilm (arrow).

FIG. 2.XIII-76

Clinical aspect of the palatal root after apicectomy was performed (mirror view). Note the detail of the palatal root apex with dark area, probably apical biofilm (arrow).

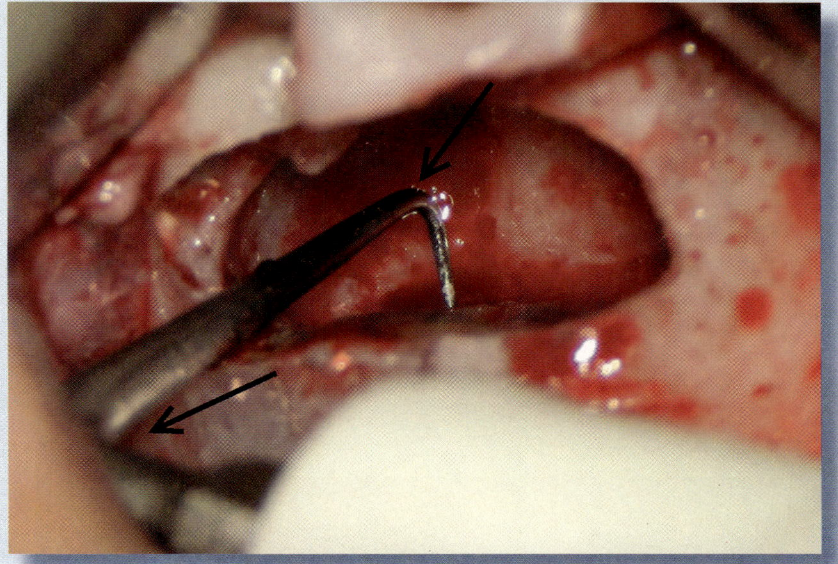

FIG. 2.XIII-77

Clinical aspect of a direct view of the palatal root apex being prepared with a customized CT4 ultrasonic tip. Note the angles of the tip, which was customized for this case (arrows).

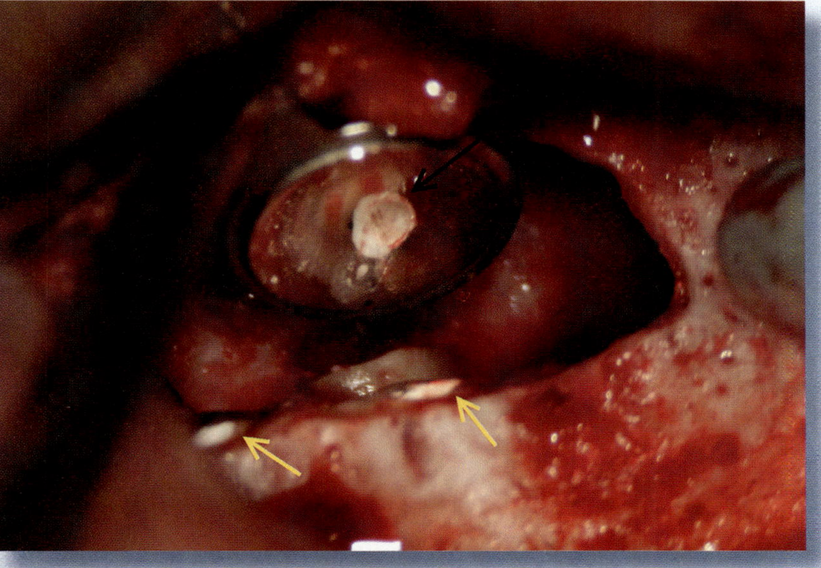

FIG. 2.XIII-78

Clinical aspect of the palatal root after backfilling with IRM (mirror image). Note the detail of the filled apex with excellent adaptation of the material (arrow), and the apexes of the vestibular roots (out of focus, because the surgical microscope was focused on the palatal root) also backfilled with the same material (yellow arrows).

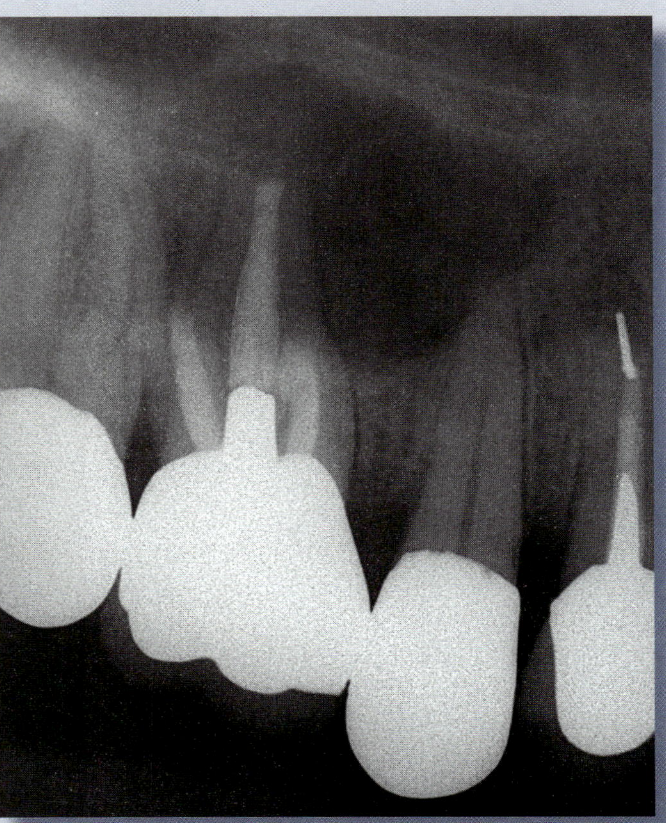

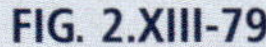

FIG. 2.XIII-79

Postoperative radiograph of tooth 1.6 showing apicectomy and backfilling of all roots.

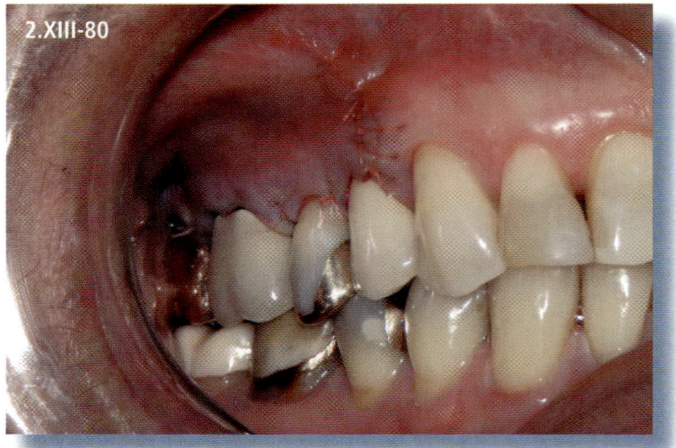

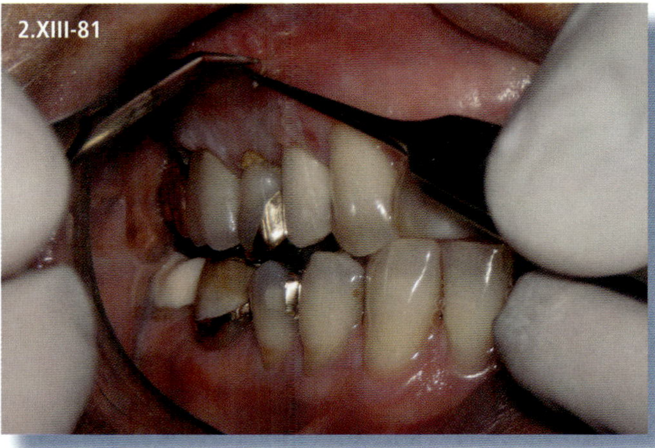

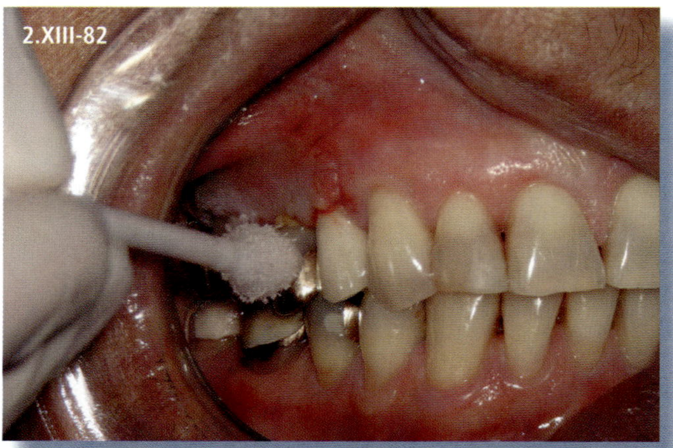

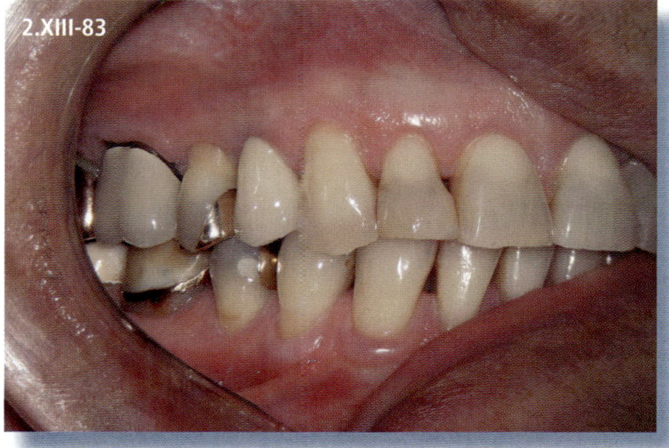

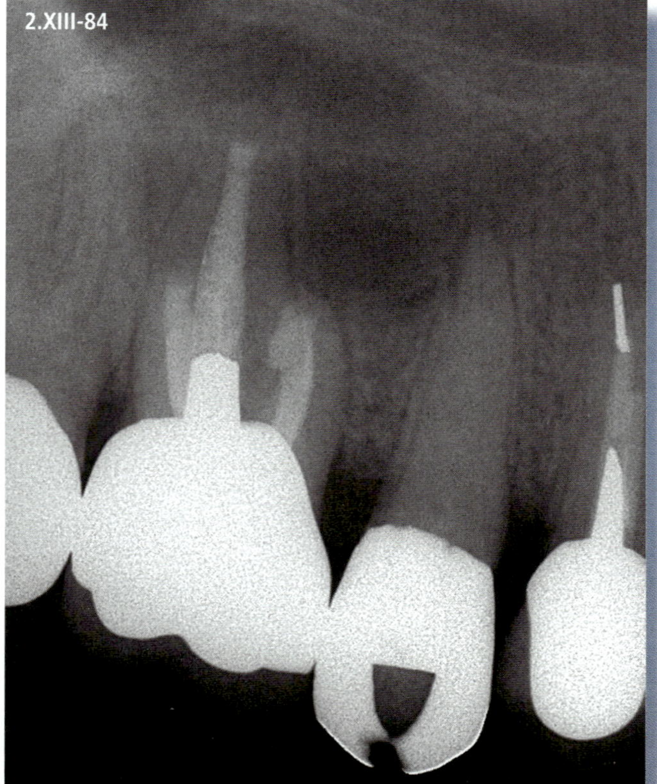

FIG. 2.XIII-80

Clinical view immediately after suturing (6/0 Vicryl thread). Note the minimal tissue trauma and the perfect adaptation of the flap.

FIG. 2.XIII-81

Clinical view 5 days after surgery Note the very favorable tissue response and use of micro instruments to remove the small suture thread under magnification.

FIG. 2.XIII-82

Clinical view 5 days after surgery. A pulp vitality test was performed on tooth 1.5 using dry ice. It elicited a negative response. The patient was advised to return to the endodontist who had referred the patient to us for conventional endodontic treatment.

FIG. 2.XIII-83

Clinical view 3 months after surgery. Note the complete tissue healing and almost total absence of scar tissue, which was significant considering the short period of time of healing.

FIG. 2.XIII-84

Postoperative radiograph of tooth 1.6, three months after completion of treatment, showing the resolution of the repair process in progress (patient is asymptomatic). Note that tooth 1.5 contains intracanal medication ($CaOH_2$), and has not yet been definitively completed.

REMOVAL OF FRACTURED CORE IN THE APICAL REGION

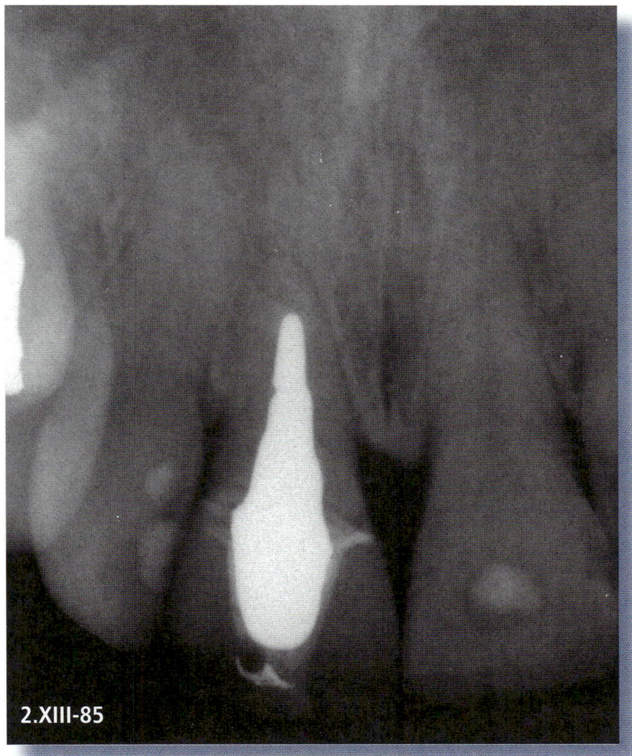

FIG. 2.XIII-85

Preoperative radiograph, showing tooth 1.1 with an oversized post and core, which has a fracture in the apical portion, with slight apical deviation (possible lateral perforation of the root due to the core diameter). The patient was referred to us for removal of the core by an endodontist who did not feel comfortable treating the case as he was not equipped with an operating microscope.

FIG. 2.XIII-86

Clinical view of access opening (low magnification) showing the remnant of the fractured core. With an absence of isolation an operating field exists that has many distractions. (whenever possible we recommend to remove cores under absolute isolation).

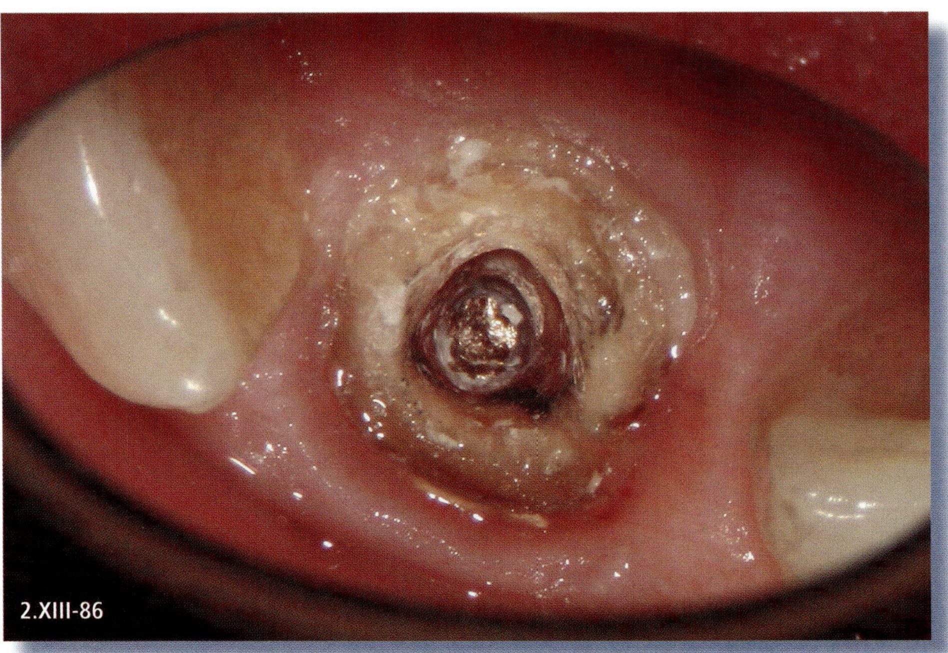

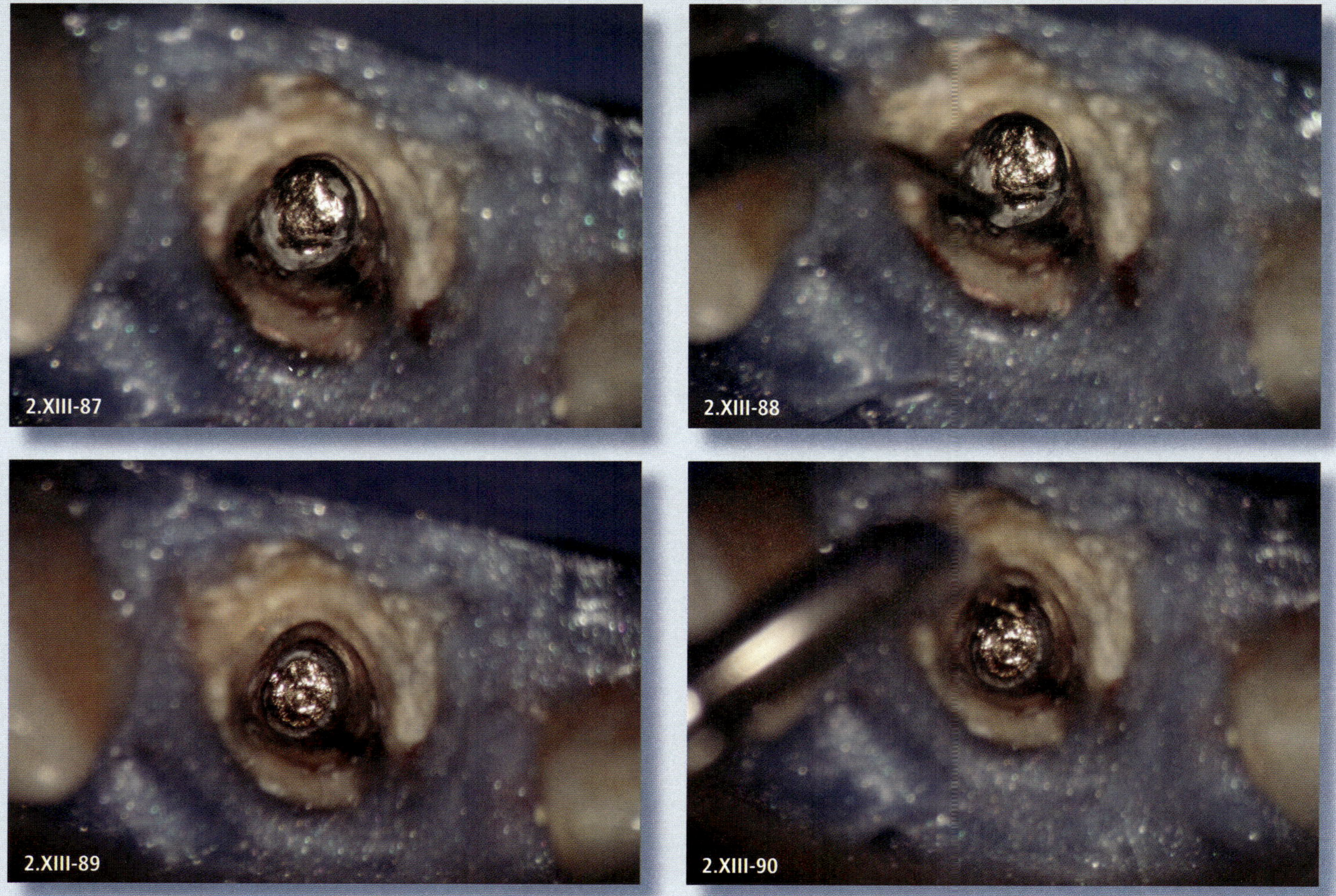

FIG. 2.XIII-87

Clinical image of access opening (medium magnification) showing the fractured core note the cementation line). Note how absolute isolation (a light curing resin dam was used for isolation) produces an uncluttered operating field free of visual interferences.

FIG. 2.XIII-88

Clinical image of access opening (high magnification) showing the fractured core with the ultrasonic point CT4 ready to be activated on the cement line. Note the thin end of the tip, allowing complete visualization of the operating field, in spite of the fact that it is in the canal.

FIG. 2.XIII-89

Clinical image of access opening (high magnification) after the initial use of the ultrasonic point UT4. The cement has been removed around the periphery of the post without removing dentin, leaving the coronal portion of the core exposed.

FIG. 2.XIII-90

Clinical image of access opening (high magnification), showing the fractured core with the ultrasonic point CT4 ready to be activated on the core (vibrating it to break the remainder of the cement seal). Note the complete mastery of the operating field achieved through the operating microscope.

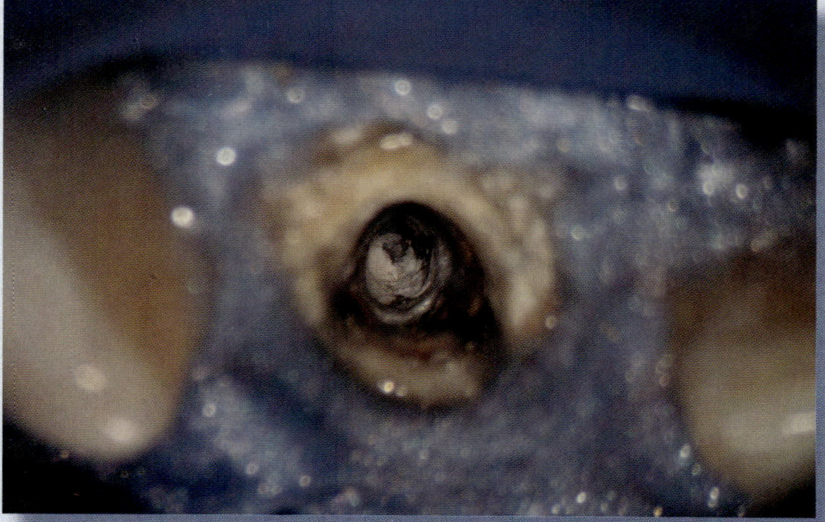

FIG. 2.XIII-91

Clinical image of access (high magnification) after removal of the fractured portion of the core. Note the presence of cement remnants in the apical third of the canal.

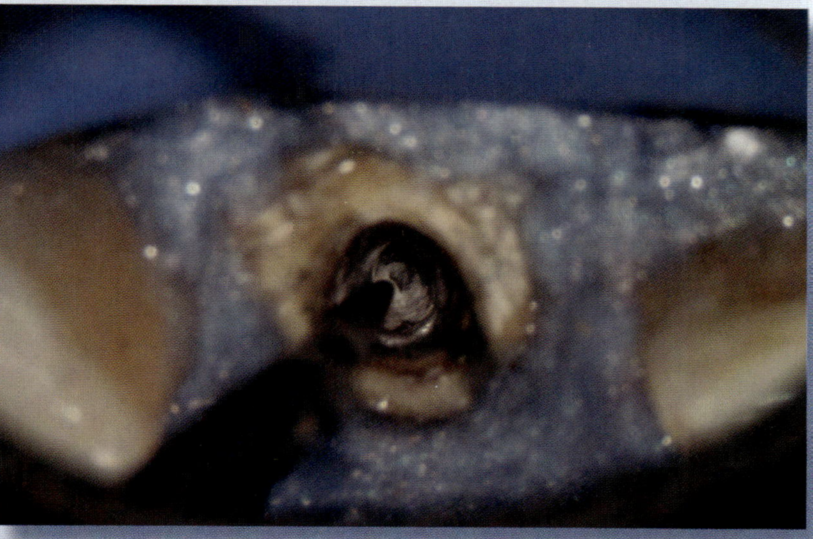

FIG. 2.XIII-92

Clinical image of access opening (intermediate magnification) showing a CKT2-D ultrasonic tip used for the removal of the remainder of the cement. Note a change of the ultrasonic CT4 point (Fig. 2.XIII-3), which is sharp and may cause perforation of the root, to a CKT2-D, a diamond-covered rhomboid shaped tip (Fig. 2.XIII-6).

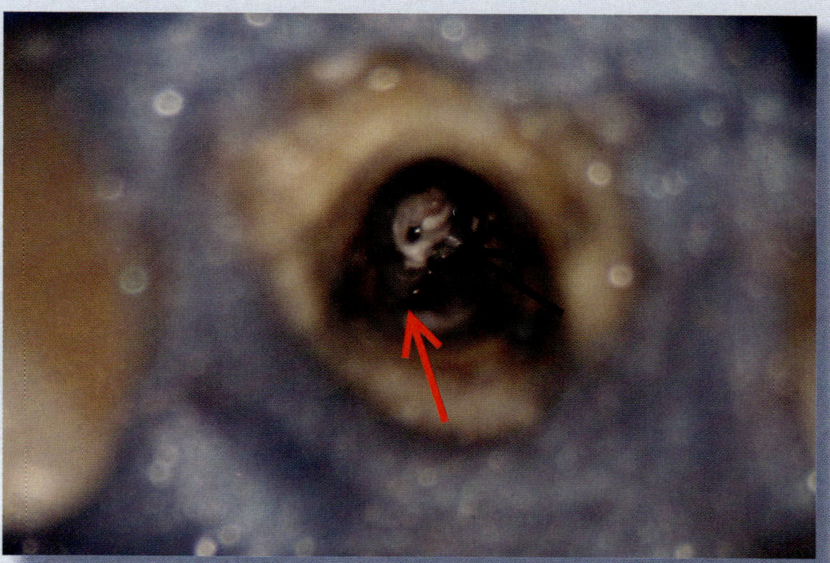

FIG. 2.XIII-93

Clinical image of access opening (high magnification) showing gutta-percha remnants in the apical third (black arrow). An apical perforation may be present (caused at the time of placing the core), with invagination of granulation tissue inside the canal and an absence of bleeding (red arrow).

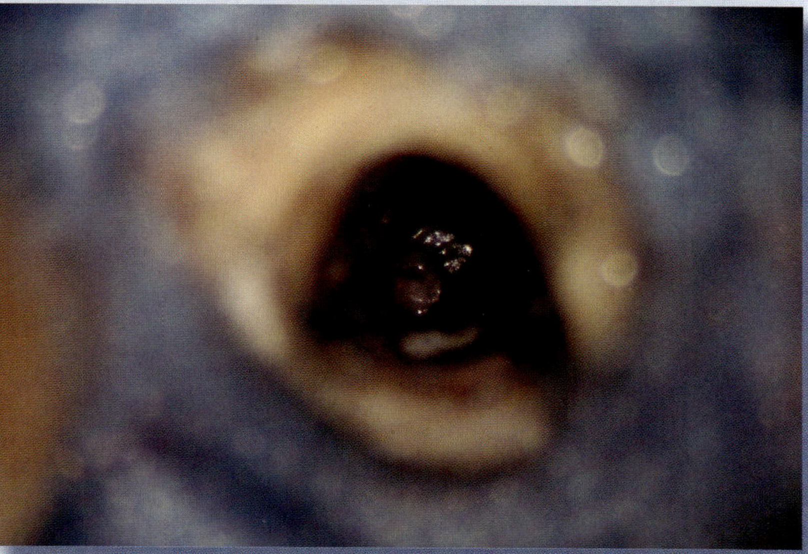

FIG. 2.XIII-94

Clinical image of access opening (high magnification) clearly showing the lateral perforation of the root (disto-buccal surface). Note how the operating microscope enables all the details of the perforation to be verified: location, shape, type and tissue present, and so on.

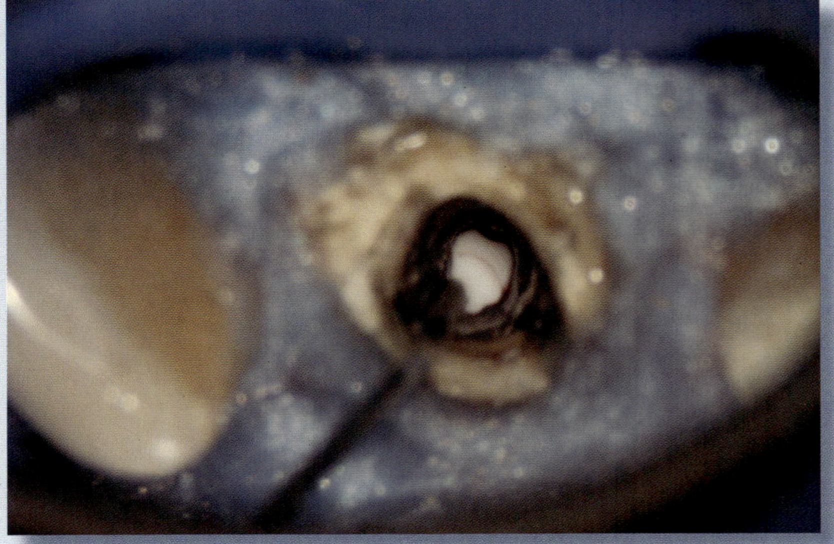

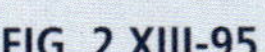

FIG. 2.XIII-95

Clinical image of access opening (intermediate magnification) showing the insertion of intracanal medication ($CaOH_2$). Using magnification it is possible to insert the medication in a controlled manner and only in the location of the perforation, without excess material.

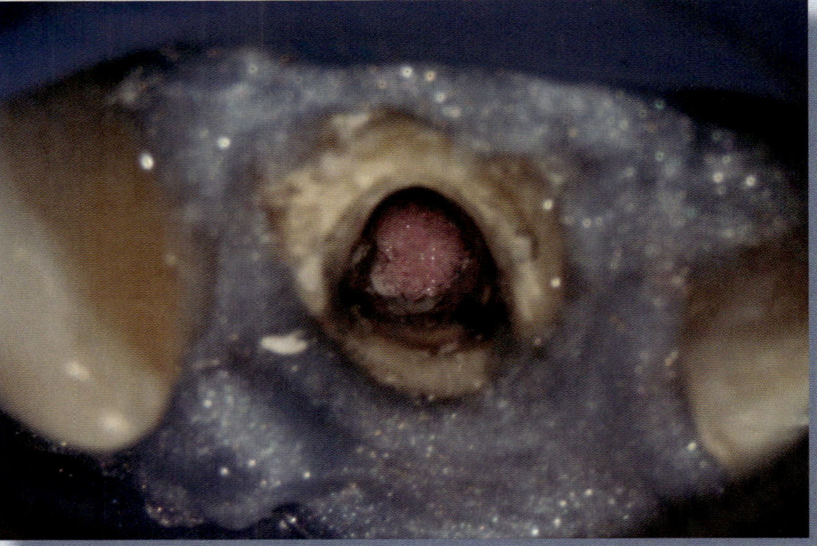

FIG. 2.XIII-96

Clinical image of access (intermediate magnification) showing a sterile sponge over the intracanal medication ($CaOH_2$). Note total control and cleanliness of the operating field.

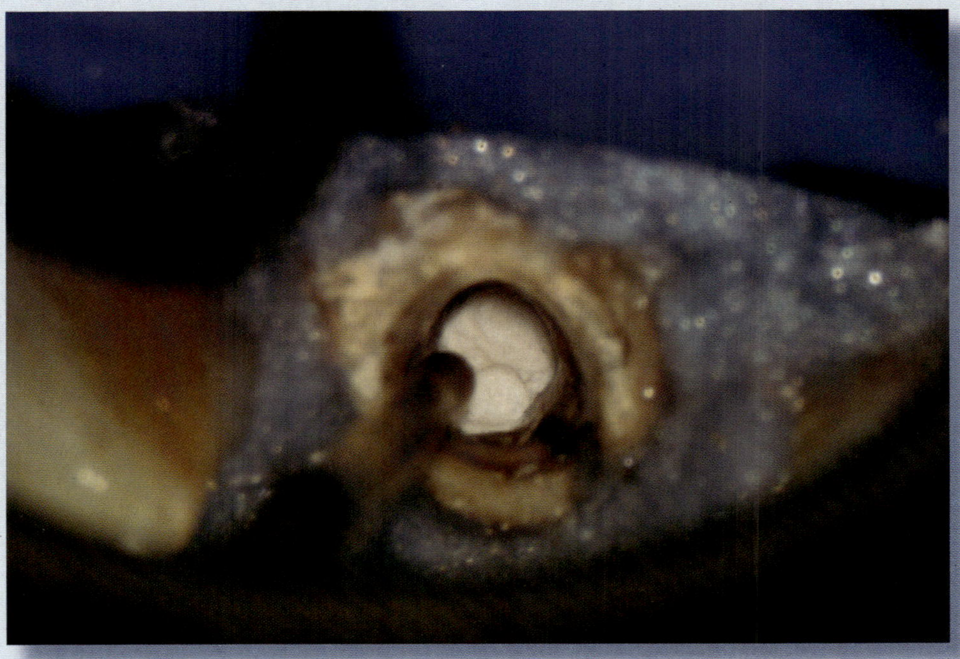

FIG. 2.XIII-97

Clinical image of access opening (intermediate magnification) showing temporary seal placed over the sponge. This is a crucial step to prevent coronal microleakage from a temporary restoration.

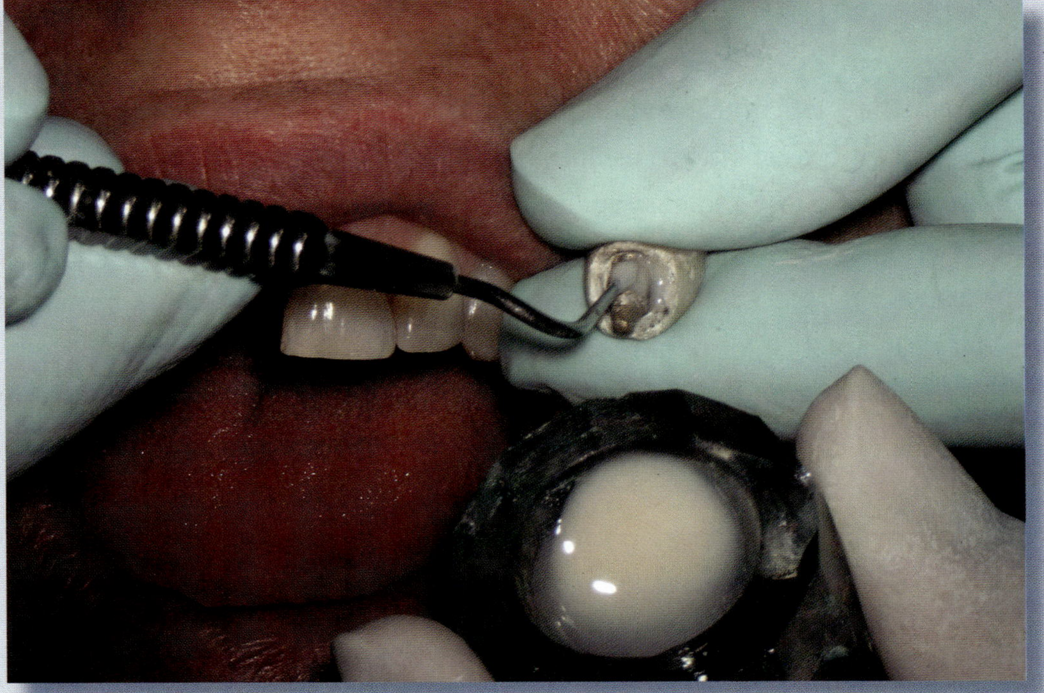

FIG. 2.XIII-98

Clinical image of lining the temporary restoration. Note that even during this step we are also working with the operating microscope for greater precision. The ideal operating microscope offers the possibility of a low magnification of 2.5x and 9.5x on the high end. This allows us to perform a broad number of clinical procedures under various magnifications. Note that the intact portion of the post and core and crown was used as a provisional restorative material.

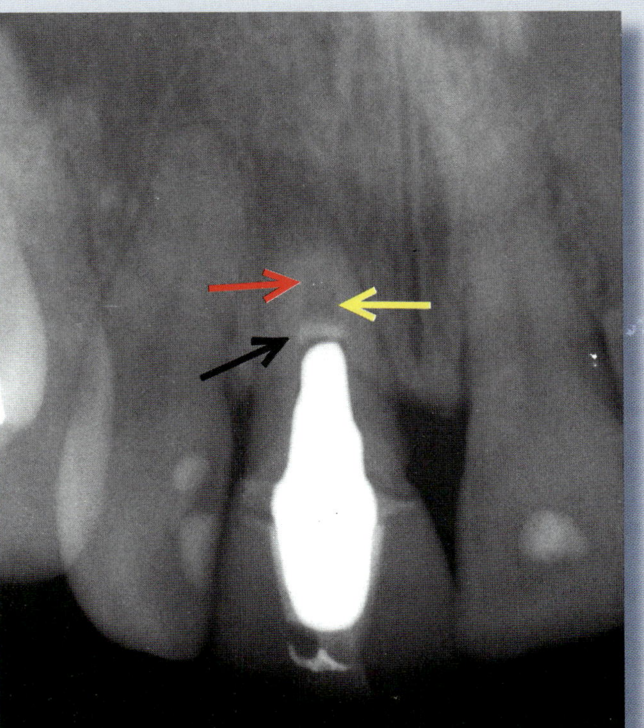

FIG. 2.XIII-99

Postoperative radiograph after completion of the removal of the fractured apical portion of the core. Note the presence of root buffer (black arrow), radiolucent space occupied by the sterile sponge (yellow arrow) and radiopaque space occupied by $CaOH_2$ (red arrow).

CONCLUSIONS

We are certain that with the incorporation of the operating microscope and ultrasound in endodontics, we were more capable to perform our difficult clinical work. Endodontics, contrary to what is being said, is not a fast and easy specialty.

There still is no substitute, and there probably never will be, for human talent in this noble art. But there are several pieces of equipment, such as those discussed here, that are excellent synergists in the daily practice for dental surgeons and endodontists.

Indeed, the true revolution that is necessary is the increased awareness of our view as health professionals. Dental surgeons like ourselves have been trained to see only the teeth and their restorative, functional and esthetic requirements.

To be sure, magnification (operating microscope) and ultrasound are indispensable working tools enabling us to accomplish excellence in dentistry. When we expand our visualization capabilities, we broaden our horizons.

The quest for excellence is an endless road, and it is up to health professionals to tread it with perseverance and wisdom. When we see things in greater detail, we are capable of performing our work with considerable more proficiency and assurance. With magnification, excellence is a mandatory path that transforms vision into quality[48].

References

1. Richman MJ. The use of ultrasonics in root canal therapy and root resection. J Dent Med 1957;12:12–8.
2. Martin H, Cunningham WT, Norris JP, Cotton WR. Ultrasonic versus hand filing of dentin: a quantitative study. Oral Surg Oral Med Oral Pathol. 1980;49(1):79-81.
3. Martin H, Cunningham WT, Norris JP. A quantitative comparison of the ability of diamond and K-type files to remove dentin. Oral Surg Oral Med Oral Pathol. 1980 Dec;50(6):566-8.
4. Cunningham WT, Martin H, Forrest WR. Evaluation of root canal débridement by the endosonic ultrasonic synergistic system. Oral Surg Oral Med Oral Pathol. 1982 Apr;53(4):401-4.
5. Cunningham WT, Martin H. A scanning electron microscope evaluation of root canal débridement with the endosonic ultrasonic synergistic system. Oral Surg Oral Med Oral Pathol. 1982 May;53(5):527-31.
6. Martin H, Cunningham WT. The effect of endosonic and hand manipulation on the amount of root canal material extruded. Oral Surg Oral Med Oral Pathol. 1982 Jun;53(6):611-3.
7. Martin H, Cunningham WT. An evaluation of postoperative pain incidence following endosonic and conventional root canal therapy. Oral Surg Oral Med Oral Pathol. 1982 Jul;54(1):74-6.
8. Cunningham WT, Martin H, Pelleu GB Jr, Stoops DE. A comparison of antimicrobial effectiveness of endosonic and hand root canal therapy. Oral Surg Oral Med Oral Pathol. 1982 Aug;54(2):238-41.
9. Ahmad M, Roy RA, Kamarudin AG. Observations of acoustic streaming fields around an oscillating ultrasonic file. Endod Dent Traumatol. 1992 Oct;8(5):189-94.
10. Ahmad M, Roy RA, Kamarudin AG, Safar M. The vibratory pattern of ultrasonic files driven piezoelectrically. Int Endod J. 1993 Mar;26(2):120-4.
11. Ahmad M, Roy RA, Kamarudin AG. Variations in power output of the Piezon-Master 400 ultrasonic endodontic unit. Int Endod J. 1994 Jan;27(1):26-31.
12. Ahmad M, Roy RA. Some observations on the breakage of ultrasonic files driven piezoelectrically. Endod Dent Traumatol. 1994 Apr;10(2):71-6.
13. Walmsley AD, Murgel C, Krell KV. Canal markings produced by endosonic instruments. Endod Dent Traumatol. 1991 Apr;7(2):84-9.
14. Murgel C, Walmsley AD, Walton RE. The efficacy of step-down procedures during endosonic instrumentation. J Endod. 1991 Mar;17(3):111-5.
15. Schulz-Bongert U, Weine FS, Schulz-Bongert J. Preparation of curved canals using a combined hand-filing, ultrasonic technique. Compend Contin Educ Dent. 1995 Mar;16(3):270, 272, 274.
16. Krell KV, Fuller MW, Scott GL. The conservative retrieval of silver cones in difficult cases. J Endod. 1984 Jun;10(6):269-73.
17. Krell KV, Neo J. The use of ultrasonic endodontic instrumentation in the re-treatment of a paste-filled endodontic tooth. Oral Surg Oral Med Oral Pathol. 1985 Jul;60(1):100-2.
18. Krell KV, Jordan RD, Madison S, Aquilino S. Using ultrasonic scalers to remove fractured root posts. J Prosthet Dent. 1986 Jan;55(1):46-9.
19. Krell KV, Jordan RD. Removal of acid-etched fixed partial dentures with modified ultrasonic scaler tips. J Am Dent Assoc. 1986 Apr;112(4):505-7.
20. Nishiyama CK, Lacerda AG, Souza MH Jr, Franciscchone CE, Ishikiriama A, Berbert A. Bleaching of devitalized teeth with ultrasonic assistance. Rev Fr Endod. 1989 Mar;8(1):43-7.
21. Baumgardner KR, Krell KV. Ultrasonic condensation of gutta-percha: an in vitro dye penetration and scanning electron microscopic study. J Endod. 1990 Jun;16(6):253-9.
22. Skoner JR, Wallace JA. Dens invaginatus: another use for the ultrasonic. J Endod. 1994 Mar;20(3):138-40.
23. Carr GB. Microscopes in Endodontics. J. Calif Dent Assoc. 1992, v20, n11, p 55-61.
24. Carr GB. Ultrasonic root end preparation. Dent Clin North Am. 1997 Jul;41(3):541-54.
25. Ruddle CJ. Micro-endodontic nonsurgical retreatment. Dent Clin North Am. 1997 Jul;41(3):429-54.
26. Lea SC, Walmsley AD. Technology, ultrasonics and dentistry. Dent Update. 2002 Oct;29(8):390-5.
27. Rubinstein R, Torabinejad M. Contemporary endodontic surgery. J Calif Dent Assoc. 2004 Jun;32(6):485-92.
28. Clark D. The operating microscope and ultrasonics; a perfect marriage. Dent Today. 2004 Jun;23(6):74-6, 78-81.
29. Plotino G, Pameijer CH, Grande NM, Somma F. Ultrasonics in endodontics: a review of the literature. J Endod. 2007 Feb;33(2):81-95.
30. Ettrich CA, Labossière PE, Pitts DL, Johnson JD. An investigation of the heat induced during ultrasonic post removal. J Endod. 2007 Oct;33(10):1222-6.
31. Gluskin AH, Ruddle CJ, Zinman EJ. Thermal injury through intraradicular heat transfer using ultrasonic devices: precautions and practical preventive strategies. J Am Dent Assoc. 2005 Sep;136(9):1286-93.
32. Walters JD, Rawal SY. Severe periodontal damage by an ultrasonic endodontic device: a case report. Dent Traumatol. 2007 Apr;23(2):123-7.
33. Bahcall JK, Olsen EK. Integrating ultrasonic tips into the endodontic treatment armamentarium. Dent Today. 2007 May;26(5):120, 122-3.
34. Lin YH, Mickel AK, Jones JJ, Montagnese TA, González AF. Evaluation of cutting efficiency of ultrasonic tips used in orthograde endodontic treatment. J Endod. 2006 Apr;32(4):359-61.
35. Carvalho CA, Fagundes TC, Barata TJ, Trava-Airoldi VJ, Navarro MF. The use of CVD diamond burs for ultraconservative cavity preparations: a report of two cases. J Esthet Restor Dent. 2007;19(1):19-28.
36. Carver K, Nusstein J, Reader A, Beck M. In vivo antibacterial efficacy of ultrasound after hand and rotary instrumentation in human mandibular molars. J Endod. 2007 Sep;33(9):1038-43.
37. Burleson A, Nusstein J, Reader A, Beck M. The in vivo evaluation of hand/rotary/ultrasound instrumentation in necrotic human mandibular molars. J Endod. 2007 Jul;33(7):782-7.
38. Buhrley LJ, Barrows MJ, BeGole EA, Wenckus CS. Effect of magnification on locating the MB2 canal in maxillary molars. J Endod. 2002 Apr;28(4):324-7.
39. Bernardes RA, de Moraes IG, Garcia RB, Bernardineli N, Baldi JV, Victorino FR, Vasconcelos BC, Duarte MA, Bramante CM. Evaluation of apical cavity preparation with a new type of ultrasonic diamond tip. J Endod. 2007 Apr;33(4):484-7.

40. Lawley GR, Schindler WG, Walker WA 3rd, Kolodrubetz D. Evaluation of ultrasonically placed MTA and fracture resistance with intracanal composite resin in a model of apexification. J Endod. 2004 Mar;30(3):167-72.

41. Bailey GC, Cunnington SA, Ng YL, Gulabivala K, Setchell DJ. Ultrasonic condensation of gutta-percha: the effect of power setting and activation time on temperature rise at the root surface – an in vitro study. Int Endod J. 2004 Jul;37(7):447-54.

42. Bailey GC, Ng YL, Cunnington SA, Barber P, Gulabivala K, Setchell DJ. Root canal obturation by ultrasonic condensation of gutta-percha. Part II: an in vitro investigation of the quality of obturation. Int Endod J. 2004 Oct;37(10):694-8.

43. Deveaux E, Dufour D, Boniface B. Five methods of calcium hydroxide intracanal placement: an in vitro evaluation. Oral Surg Oral Med Oral Pathol Oral Radiol Endod. 2000 Mar;89(3):349-55.

44. van der Sluis LW, Wu MK, Wesselink PR. The evaluation of removal of calcium hydroxide paste from an artificial standardized groove in the apical root canal using different irrigation methodologies. Int Endod J. 2007 Jan;40(1):52-7.

45. Yao LL, Gao YS, Niu F, Wang Y, Zhang FH. Evaluation of the use of dental operating microscope in the management of blocked canals. Shanghai Kou Qiang Yi Xue. 2007 Aug;16(4):395-8.

46. van der Sluis LW, Wu MK, Wesselink PR. A comparison between a smooth wire and a K-file in removing artificially placed dentine debris from root canals in resin blocks during ultrasonic irrigation. Int Endod J. 2005 Sep;38(9):593-6.

47. Souter NJ, Messer HH. Complications associated with fractured file removal using an ultrasonic technique. J Endod. 2005 Jun;31(6):450-2.

48. Murgel CAF, Gondim EJR, Souza Filho FJ. Microscópio Cirúrgico: a busca da excelência na Clínica Odontológica. Rev da APCD. v51, p31-35, 1997.

2.XIV

Computed tomography in Endodontics

Marco Aurélio Gagliardi Borges

In November of 1895, Röentgen discovered the X-ray, and this event was responsible for the appearance of Radiology, the science that studies the inside of the human body by means of images. This invention enabled an advance in clinical diagnosis for the entire medical profession, reaffirming the Hippocratic motto "Something that is well diagnosed can be cured well" [6].

For good diagnosis in endodontics, one must comply with a routine. It is not enough to establish the condition of the root canal; it is necessary to know the patient as a whole, respecting the general conditions that govern his/her being. A practitioner can perform any clinical procedure to perfection, but if the necessary steps for a correct diagnosis are ignored, serious errors in implementing the chosen therapy can occur, which will certainly lead to clinical failure.

In endodontics, diagnosis is achieved simultaneously by *subjective* examinations through data supplied by the patient, by anamnesis and by *objective* examinations through data collected from the patient by the practitioner. Objective examinations consists of physical examination of the oral cavity, percussion test, thermal pulp sensitivity tests (hot and cold), mobility test, and lastly, complementary or laboratory examinations, and in the case of endodontics, radiography.

Anamnesis, based on the medical history, main complaint and current dental condition, added to clinical and radiographic examination, frequently allows a precise diagnosis of dental pathologies. However, root fractures and periapical lesions and some anatomic anomalies are difficult to visualize[3,4,5] and therefore require a clinical and radiographic diagnosis. Consequently, errors or even treatment failure may occur. Undoubtedly radiographs, widely used by dentists, play an important role in obtaining diagnostic data. However, we also know that although it is indispensable, in endodontics it has a suggestive value, not in the sense that it can be dispensed with, but because "the absence of a radiographic image does not necessarily mean that disease is not present". Conventional as well as digital radiography, present the same limitations because both supply two-dimensional images, images in a single plane, and in cases of superimposition, images of anatomic structures that are apparently healthy, may mask or even hide pathologies[8,12,17,53,64].

In Medicine, diagnosis through imaging has developed a great deal over the last few years, particularly with the introduction of magnetic resonance (MRI), which permits visualization of soft tissues and tissues rich in water and computed tomography, which makes it possible to visualize hard tissues. The latter, due to the richness of details and the possibility of visualization in different planes in a single examination is complementary in the diagnosis of pathologies that affect the stomatognathic system[26,29].

Computed tomography inventors Allan M. Cormack, an American physicist, and Godfrey M. Hounsfield, a British engineer were awarded the Nobel Prize in Medicine in 1979[56]. Since then, computed tomography has evolved and the technique has found application in several medical specialties. Already in 1989, periapical lesions in humans were evaluated by computerized tomography in order to ascertain if this non invasive method would be useful for distinguishing between periapical cysts and granulomas[57]. A marked difference in density between the content of a cyst cavity and granulation tissue permitted disease identification confirmed by histopathological analysis. Subsequently, further interest in finding suitable applications for computerized tomography in endodontics was expressed[54].

The increased application of CT Scan is due to the fact that this technology is superior to conventional radiographs. Disadvantages of conventional radiographs can be overcome by CT scans. An X-ray provides a two dimensional image which does not permit the evaluation of bone thickness, precise mandibular canal localization, and determining the size and localization of a periapical lesions. The conventional periapical radiograph provides information in a mesio-distal orientation, but a bucco-lingual evaluation is not possible[50,62]. Structures situated along the X-ray beam are projected in the same position on the radiographic film. Buccal and lingual root canals cannot be differentiated in a radiograph since they are superimposed. A mandibular canal can be projected over the apex of a tooth or over periapical disease, even if they are not in close proximity[27,61,62].

Currently, different methods of tomography are being used for diagnosis in Endodontics, especially conventional helical tomography and cone beam computed scans[10,39].

HELICAL COMPUTED TOMOGRAPHY (HCT)

The helical computed tomography[25] (Fig. 2.XIV-1) consists of three major components: (1) a table to accommodate the patient which permits cranial-caudal movement and an anatomic area selection in the exact plane of cut; (2) a Gantry which is a unit composed of a tube emitting ionizing radiation, detectors and the data acquisition system; and (3) a computer for image reconstruction, although only partial control of functions are possible.

Dental evaluation from images acquired by helical computerized tomography requires that the entire dental arch must be scanned, including the teeth to be analyzed. Then, the images have to be transferred to the *diagnostic workstation* (Fig. 2.XIV-2), which has a storage capacity of up to 40 Giga bytes. At this time all the teeth and their adjacent structures can be evaluated. During the next step, the selected images need to be properly manipulated according to the following steps:

1. **Adaptation of the image pattern:** the aim of this procedure is to improve definition of the anatomic and pathologic structures of the area being visualized, by means of adjusting the brightness and contrast to the pattern condition of the equipment.
2. **Identification of the pathology:** images are reconstructed in multiple planes (MPR) which allows reconstruction in two-dimensions, a condition in which each image can only be observed in one of the three planes (axial, sagittal, or coronal). During this step it

is already possible to detect the pathology, although diagnosis is only considered definitive when it is detected in at least three serial cuts and two different planes.

3. **Selection of images:** magnification of representative images of the location and type of pathology are made to obtain better visualization.

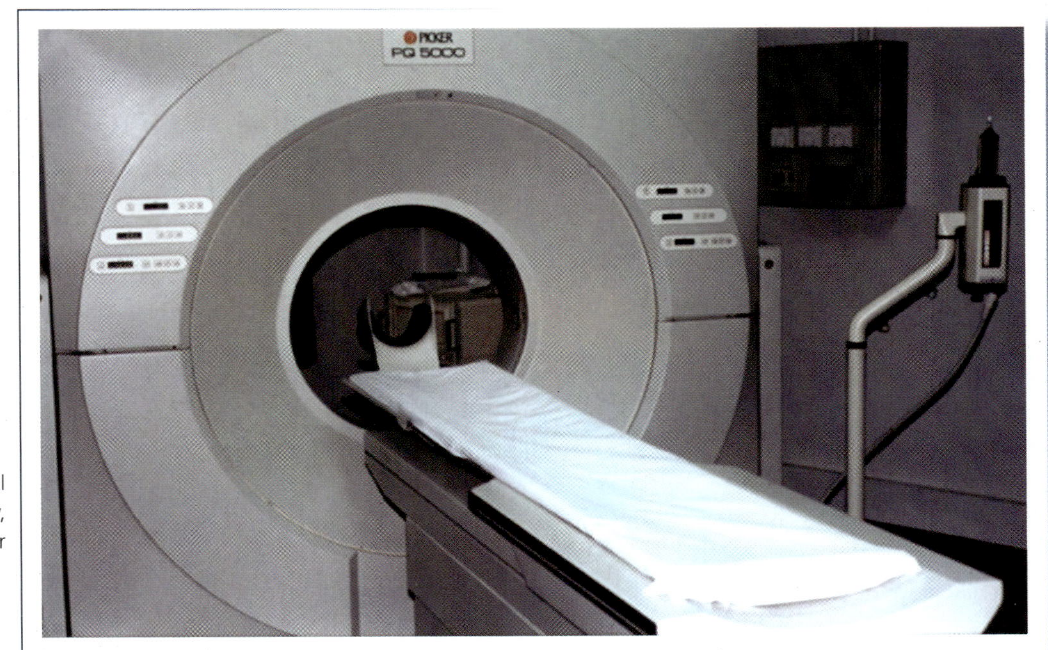

FIG. 2.XIV-1
Fourth generation helical computerized tomography, Picker 5000 from Picker – USA.

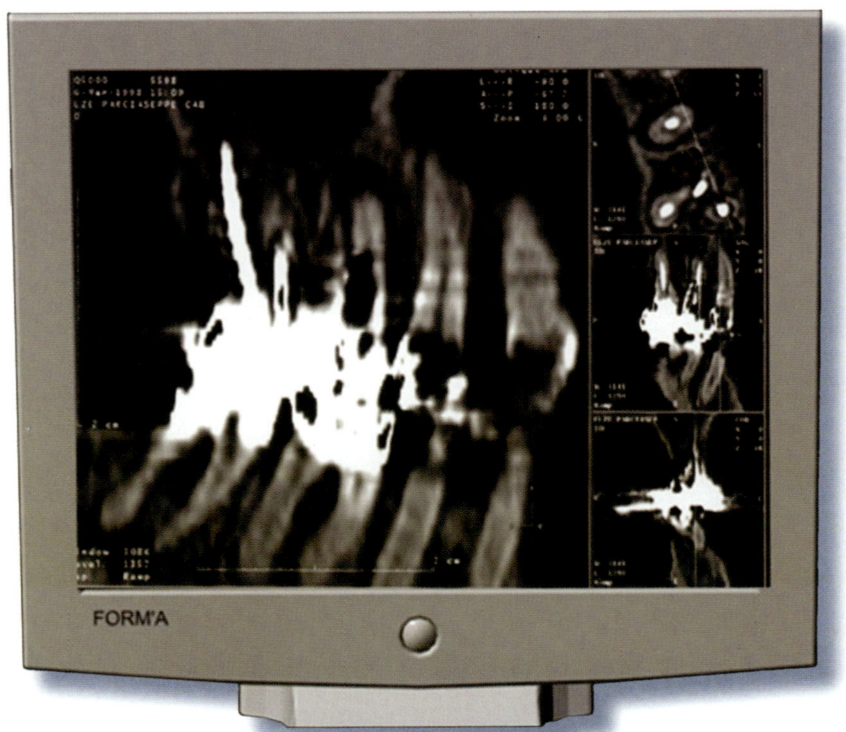

FIG. 2.XIV-2
HCT workstation.

The HCT exam presents the following advantages over conventional radiographs[11,16,19,24,36,58,60,66]:

1. **Richness of details of anatomy and pathological lesions.** In an exam performed with HCT, the oral cavity is scanned in helical cuts, 2.5 mm thick with interpolation of 0.25 mm, in a cranial-caudal direction, which characterizes a reconstruction for hard tissues, called reconstruction of the bone type. For each arch, 70 to 120 cuts are made, which will then be reprocessed for 3D and 4D reconstructions by using volumetric reconstruction algorithms that allow visualization of details of the anatomic structure without any superimposition, allowing one to see, for example, incipient periapical lesions that did not reach the cortical bone.
2. **Visualization of all the dental surfaces.** Unlike conventional radiographs, which provide images in a single plane (anterior teeth can only be seen in a mesio-distal direction), HCT permits visualization in simultaneous multiple planes in a single exam. Teeth can be examined in a mesio distal, bucco-lingual and transverse direction, along the axis of the tooth; and the tooth can also be divided into several fractions, in order to study them one by one.
3. **Reconstructions in 3D (three-dimensions).** The examination performed in HCT allows three-dimensional reconstruction of anatomical features, whether they are soft (muscles, organs, arteries) or hard tissues (bone, tooth). The three-dimensional models are faithful at the external surface of the structure studied; the images do not allow visualization of the interior of anatomical structures, but they are very important for surgical planning, because they provide real images of a specific structure, showing the relationship of the pathology with the healthy adjacent anatomic structures.
4. **4D-Angio Reconstructions.** As with reconstruction in 3D, 4D-Angio reconstruction allows the three dimensional, but transparent visualization of an anatomic structure, which allows the visualization of other internal hidden anatomical structures.
5. **Visualization by kinetic means.** With HCT, the anatomic structures can be observed in movement; that is, it is possible to go on a "virtual trip" through the structures to be analyzed, and in addition to obtaining richness of details, it is a true surgical guide for the treatment to be performed.

Helical computerized tomography was used in the diagnosis of vertical root fractures for the first time in 1999[66]. Thirty-seven patients presenting 42 teeth with suspicion of root fractures were examined by computed tomography and were submitted to exploratory endodontic surgery. Twenty-eight root fractures were identified by exploratory surgery, and of these, 20 root fractures had been diagnostically identified by computed tomography.

Conventional radiography, indirect digital radiography and helical computerized tomography (HCT) were used to compare diagnosis of root fractures in endodontics in 20 patients who presented with questionable clinical diagnosis of[6]. All patients had radiographic and tomography examinations performed, after which they were submitted to exploratory surgery. Root fractures were best observed with the helical computed tomography, followed by digital radiography and lastly with conventional radiography.

Conventional spiral tomography (Scanora) is adequate to detect periapical lesions on premolar and molar teeth[55]. The use of computed tomography provides additional, beneficial information not available from dental radiographs for treatment planning in apical surgery of mandibular premolars and molars especially when the mandibular canal cannot be detected in dental radiographs or is in close proximity to the lesion or root apex. In those cases, CT should be considered before endodontic surgery, especially because the presence, extent, and location of the lesion and its relation to the mandibular canal can be predictably evaluated in a CT scan of the area[61].

Other applications for CT Scan in endodontics include: follow-up of extensive periapical lesions to evaluate the degree of bone repair[9], evaluation of root canal filling associated with persistent pain not identified by radiographic evaluation[7], and to evaluate the extent of external radicular resorption[28].

As with any other means of diagnosis, HCT has the disadvantage of a high effective dose of absorption, which may reach 1,160 µSv for both arches or 514 µSv for the mandible[20,21]. This effective dose of absorption has led industries to create a new type of tomography, just for dentistry, named cone-beam computerized tomography (CBCT) or volumetric computerized tomography (VCT).

CONE-BEAM COMPUTED TOMOGRAPHY (CBCT)

The first reports in the literature about cone-beam computerized tomography for dentistry appeared very recently towards the end of the 20th century. This new technology was pioneered in Italy by Mozzo et al.[38], from the University of Verona who, in 1998, presented the preliminary results of a "new volumetric CT appliance for dental images, based on the cone-shaped beam technique (*cone-beam technique*)", named NewTom-9000. Prior to that, cone-beam technique had already been used for radiotherapy, vascular imaginology and microtomography of small specimens with biomedical or industrial applicability.

The CBCT (Fig. 2.XIV-3) is very compact and resembles panoramic radiography equipment. It has two main components, placed at opposite ends of the patient's head: a source or X-ray tube, which emits a cone-shaped beam and an X-ray detector. The tube-detector system makes only one 360 degree turn around the patient's head and at each determined degree of turn (usually at every 1 degree), the appliance acquires a base-image of the patient's head, very similar to a teleradiograph, from different angles or perspectives. At the end of the examination, this sequence of base images (raw data) is reconstructed to generate a volumetric 3D image, by means of dedicated software, with a sophisticated algorithm program installed in a conventional computer coupled to the tomograph. The examination time may range from 10 to 70 seconds (a complete turn of the system), but effective time of exposure to the X-rays is much lower, up to 7 seconds[30].

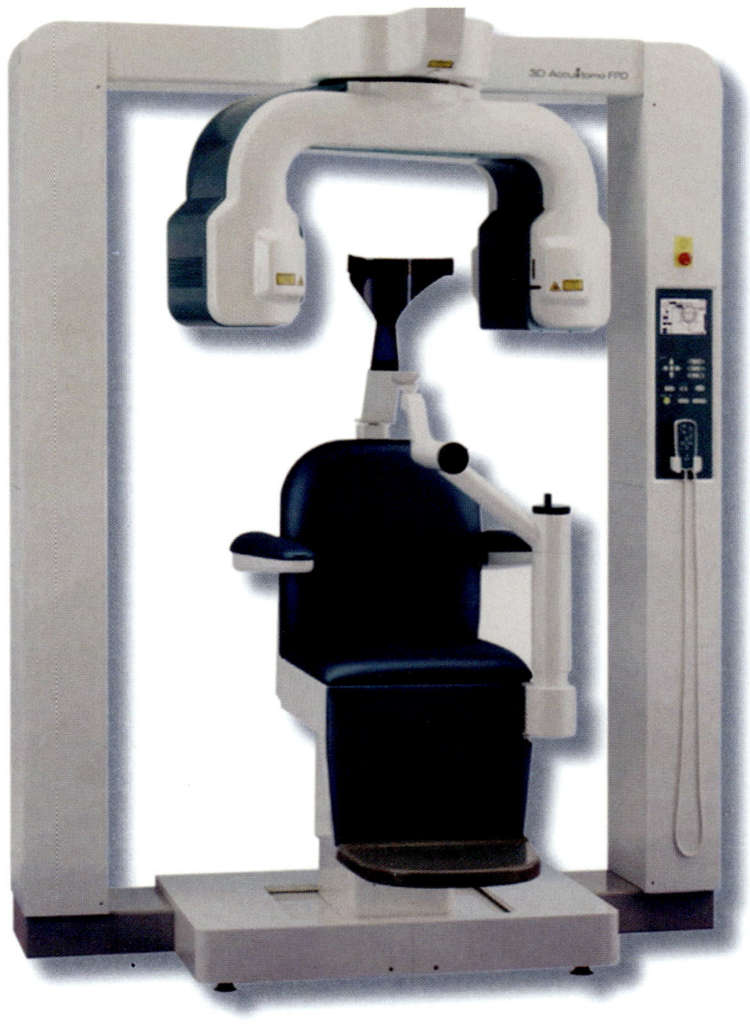

FIG. 2.XIV-3

Cone-beam computerized tomography, 3D Accuitomo, J. Morita – Japan.

The image reconstruction in CBCT does not require a workstation, as the conventional tomographs do – the images can be manipulated on a personal computer, making image processing easy and allowing multiplanar reconstruction of the scanned volume; that is, visualization of axial, coronal, sagittal and oblique images as well as 3D reconstruction.

The CBCT systems can be classified by their scanning area, such as limited dental or regional CBCT and complete CBCT, but both present isometric *voxel*, that is, height, length and depth of equal dimensions[15], allowing perfect distinction of the enamel, dentin, pulp cavity, and cortical alveolar bone. The artifacts produced by metal restorations are much less significant than those produced in traditional computed tomography[10].

The advantages of CBCT are the same as HCT, but CBCT presents the additional advantage of a low effective absorbed dose, which may range from 30 μSv to 88 μSv[33,58].

The use of computerized tomography (CBCT or HCT) should be carefully indicated. In most cases, a thorough clinical examination, together with anamnesis and radiographic evaluation, is sufficient to obtain the correct diagnosis. However, sometimes we cannot obtain sufficient data for a correct diagnosis. The majority of discussions with regards to the definition of a diagnosis in endodontics are related to bone resorption, dentin and cement lesions and dental fractures. As it has been widely reported in the literature, the major difficulty in diagnosis occurs with root fractures, particularly longitudinal ones, while horizontal fractures are related to traumatic injuries and are relatively easy to detect. Nevertheless, vertical fractures are difficult to diagnose and are usually related to iatrogenic dentistry. Early detection of vertical root fracture is clinically important, because an infection may occur through the fracture line when it originates at the gingival margin, causing adjacent bone destruction, in addition to chronic periradicular or periapical inflammation as well as the formation of a periapical cyst. When HCT or CBCT is used, these lesios, even though incipient, can be detected because superimposition of anatomic structure images is diminished[24,59].

The major indications for CBCT are the following:

1. Assess bone or dental resorption abnormalaties of unknown origin[14,30,34,41,43,49,52,57].
2. Cases in which diagnosis by conventional means was inconclusive[35,37].
3. Patients with a history of facial or dental trauma[43,45,63].
4. For diagnosis and location of bone pathology[31,32,51].
5. For detection of root fractures[6,22].
6. For follow-up of root canal treatment in teeth with periapical lesions[46,47].
7. For pretreatement anatomic assessment, such as identification of root canal anatomy and isolation of each root canal of a multi-rooted tooth to determine from which one the periapical lesion originates[10,35,40].
8. To evaluate the quality of root canal filling in order to provide information in re-treatment decisions[23].

Clinically we detected a fistula in the cervical area close to the region of the furcation after root canal treatment in a 40-year-old patient (Fig. 2.XIV-4).

RADIOGRAPHIC ANALYSIS

In the radiograph (Fig. 2.XIV-4) we can note the following radiographic aspects:

1. Teeth #3.5, 3.6 and 3.7 present with restorations;
2. Tooth #3.6 has been root canal treated;
3. Tooth 3.7 presents with dilaceration;
4. The radiolucent image of the cervical third of the distal root of tooth 3.6 indicates fracture.

Even with the aid of several radiographs, including a digital one, it was not possible to establish a conclusive diagnosis.

With the tomography analysis, we obtained a more accurate diagnosis (Fig. 2.XIV-5).

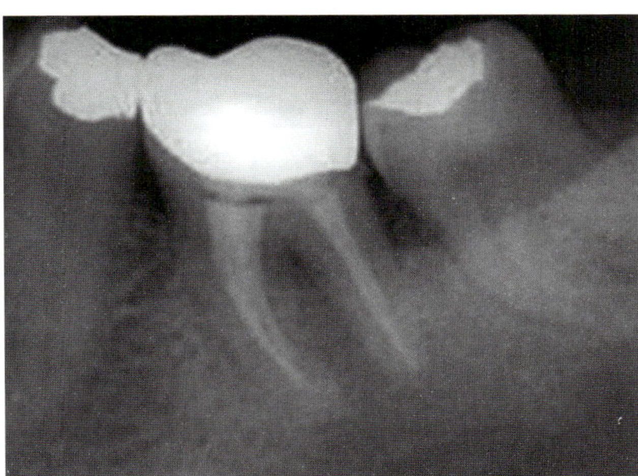

FIG. 2.XIV-4

FIG. 2.XIV-4
Radiographic image of tooth 3.6, described in the text.

FIG. 2.XIV-5
Tomographic images of tooth 3.6, described in the text.

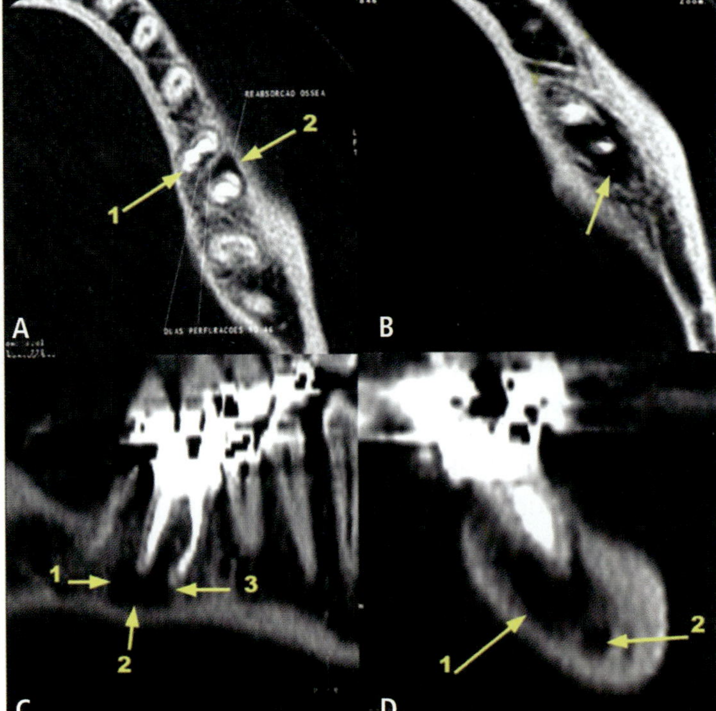

FIG. 2.XIV-5

A. Axial cut; arrow number 1 shows two perforations, arrow number 2 indicates a periapical lesion, all in tooth 3.6.

B. Axial cut showing periapical lesion in the distal root of tooth 3.6.

C. Sagittal cut showing periphery of periapical lesion in tooth 3.6 (arrows 1, 2 and 3).

D. Coronal cut indicating the periapical lesion in tooth 3.6 (arrow 1) and mandibular canal (arrow 2).

Therefore, the diagnostic hypothesis by tomography was chronic periapical lesion involving the distal root, 1.5 cm in extent, which was confirmed by macroscopic examination.

Conventional as well as digital radiographic diagnoses were not conclusive. Tomographic evaluation did not establish a correlation with conventional and digital radiography, but it did coincide with the macroscopic findings of a chronic periapical lesion observed during endodontic surgery. As mentioned previously, periapical bone lesions are only diagnosed radiographically when there is rupture of the cortical bone, whether in a buccal or lingual direction. Therefore, it is a lesion of long duration, and due to superimposition of the anatomic structures, it would be difficult to reach a diagnostic conclusion; therefore complementary diagnosis by means of HCT or CBCT was necessary.

Computerized tomography, both HCT and CBCT, are important additional resources for diagnosing several dental pathologies, particularly those not detected by conventional radiographic examinations which include vertical or longitudinal fractures, root perforations, root resorption of buccal and lingual walls and periapical lesions of different sizes. Additionally, CT Scan can be considered a non-invasive diagnostic tool for differentiating periapical cysts from granulomas[1].

For a long time, absence of periapical radiolucency diagnosed by periapical radiography has been used to diagnose a healthy periapex. However, the periapical radiographic image corresponds to a 2-dimensional aspect of a 3-dimensional structure. Periapical lesions confined within the cancellous bone are usually not detected[48]. A lesion of a certain size can be detected in a region covered by a thin cortex, whereas the same size lesion cannot be detected in a region covered by thicker cortex[65].

It has been demonstrated that CBCT can detect more accurately periapical lesions refractory to root canal therapy compared to conventional periapical radiographs[46,47]. Favorable outcomes (lesion reduced or absent) was demonstrated in 57 (79%) roots which presented periapical lesions and were submitted to root canal treatment when determined by PR, but in only 25 (35%) roots when determined by CBCT. Unfavorable outcomes occurred more frequently after one-visit therapy than two-visit therapy when determined by CBCT. However, the difference was not significant when determined by PR[47]. Furthermore, the periapical lesions extended in a more mesio-distal direction if compared to conventional radiographs, either 45 days after root canal contamination or 180 days after root canal filling. This difference between CT Scan and radiography is probably related to the superimposition of anatomical structures in a periapical radiograph that can mask the true size of the lesion. In addition, when using CT Scan it is possible to perform thin serial sections in order to access different areas of the lesion.

The higher accuracy of CBCT compared to conventional periapical radiographs for detecting periapical lesions has been frequently reported[13,14,44-47,52]. Periapical lesions identified in nearly 40% of the cases by periapical radiographs are identified in almost 61% of the cases by CBCT scans[14]. These results opened the door to a proposal of a new periapical index based on cone beam computed tomography[13]. The new periapical index has some advantages for clinical applications. The scores used for evaluation are calculated by 3-D analysis of the lesion, the measurement of the lesion depth contributes to an improved prognosis, the evaluation of the cortical bone destruction or expansion permits distinguishing those conditions that may affect the outcome.

MICRO-COMPUTED TOMOGRAPHY

Currently, a novel imaging technique is available for research, namely micro-computed tomography (μ-CT). μ-CT acquisition system is similar to CBCT and produces true 3-D reconstruction of the object with cubic voxels and isotropic resolution. The advantage of this method over the other is that it provides images which are closely compared with those obtained by histology. In endodontics, μ-CT has been used for assessing the severity of dental root resorption[2], 3-D quantification of periradicular bone destruction[42,62], and for quantification of new bone formation and graft modeling in artificial bone defects[18].

References

1. Aggarwal V, Logani A, Shab N. The evaluation of computed tomography scans and ultrasounds in the differential diagnosis of periapical lesions. J Endod 2008;34:1312-5.
2. Balto K, White R, Mueller R, Stashenko P. A mouse model of inflammatory root resorption induced by pulpal infection Oral Surg Oral Med Oral Pathol Oral Radiol Endod 2002;93:461-8.
3. Bender IB, Seltzer S. Roentgenographic and direct observation of experimental lesions in bone: I. J Am Dent Assoc 1961;62:152-60.
4. Bender IB, Seltzer S. Roentgenographic and direct observation of experimental lesions in bone: II. J Am Dent Assoc 1961;62:708-16.
5. Borg E, Källqvist A, Gröndahl K, Gröndahl HG. Film and digital radiography for detection of simulated root resorption cavities. Oral Surg Oral Med Oral Pathol Oral Radiol Endod 1998;86(1):110-4.
6. Borges MAG. Avaliação comparativa de três meios para diagnóstico em endodontia. Araraquara. 2002. 133p. Dissertação (mestrado em Endodontia) – Faculdade de Odontologia, Universidade Estadual Paulista "Julio de Mesquita Filho", Araraquara, 2002.
7. Boucher Y, Sobel M, Sauveur G. Persistent pain related to root canal filling and apical fenestration: a case report. J Endod 2000;28:242-4.
8. Campos HF. La radiografía, nos dice todo lo que queremos saber? Endodoncia 1998;4:211-7.
9. Cotti E, Vargiu P, Dettori C, Mallarini G. Computadorized tomography in the management and follow-up of extensive periapical lesion. Endod Dent Traumatol 1999;15:186-9.
10. Cotton TP, Geisler TM, Holden DT, Schwartz SA, Schindler WG. Endodontic applications of cone-beam volumetric tomography. J Endod 2007;33:1121-32.
11. Danforth RA, Dus I, Mah I. 3-D volume imaging for dentistry: a new dimension. J Calif Dent Assoc 2003;31:817-23.
12. Duinkerke ASH, van de Poel, ACM Doesburg WH. Variations in the interpretation of periapical radiolucencies. Oral Surg 1975;40:414-21.
13. Estrela C, Bueno MR, Azevedo BC, Azevedo JR, Pécora JD. A new periapical index based on cone beam computed tomography. J Endod 2008;34:1325–31.
14. Estrela C, Bueno MR, Leles CR, Azevedo JR. Accuracy of cone beam computed tomography and panoramic and periapical radiography for detection of apical periodontitis. J Endod 2008;34:273-9.
15. Farman AG, Scarfe WC. Development of imaging selection criteria and procedures should precede cephalometric assessment with cone-beam computed tomography. Am J Orthod Dentofacial Orthop 2006;130:257-65.
16. Friedland B, Faiella RA, Bianchi J. Use of rotational tomography for assessing internal resorption. J Endod 2001;27:797-99.
17. Gegler A, Mahl C Fontanella V. Reproducibility of and file format effect on digital subtraction radiography of simulated external root resorptions. Dentomaxillofac Radiol 2006;35:10-3.
18. Gielkens PF, Schortinghuis J, de Jong JR, Huysmans MC, Leeuwen MB, Raghoebar GM, Bos RR, Stegenga B. A comparison of micro-CT, microradiography and histomorphometry in bone research. Arch Oral Biol 2008;53:558-66
19. Hashimoto K, Arai Y, Araki M. A comparison of a new limited cone beam computed tomography machine for dental use with a multidetector row helicoidal CT machine. Oral Surg Oral Med Oral Pathol Oral Radiol Endod 2003;95:371-7.
20. Hashimoto K, Kawashima S, Araki M, Iwai K, Sawada K. Comparison of image performance between cone beam computed tomography for dental use and four-row multidetector helical CT. J Oral Sci 2006;48:27-34.
21. Hashimoto K, Kawashima S, Kameoka K, Akiyama Y, Honjova T, Ejima K, Sawada K. Comparison of image validity between cone beam computed tomography for dental use and multidetector row helical computed tomography. Dentomaxillofac Radiol 2007;36:465-71.
22. Hassan B, Metska ME, Ozok AR, van der Stelt P, Wesselink PR. Detection of vertical root fractures in endodontically treated teeth by a cone beam computed tomography scan. J Endod 2009;35:719-22.
23. Huumonen S, Kvist T, Gröndahl K, Molander A. Diagnostic value of computed tomography in re-treatment of root fillings in maxillary molars. Int Endod J 2006;39:827-33.
24. Jorge EG, Tanomaru-Filho M, Gonçalves M, Tanomaru JM. Detection of periapical lesion development by conventional radiography or computed tomography. Oral Surg Oral Med Oral Pathol Oral Radiol Endod 2008;106(1):e56-61.
25. Kachelriess M, Watzke O, Kalender WO. Generalized multi-dimensional adaptive flitering for conventional and spiral singleslice, multi-slice and cone-beam CT. Med Phys 2001;28:475-90.
26. Kamatana A, Ariji Y, Langlais RP. Three-dimensional computed tomography imaging in dentistry. Dent Clin North Am 2000;44:395-410.
27. Kassebaum DK, Reaedr CM, Kleier DJ, Averbach RE. Localization of anatomic structures before endodontic surgery with tomograms. Oral Surg Oral Med Oral Pathol 1991;72:610-3.
28. Kim E, Kim K-D, Roh B-D, Cho Y-S, Lee S-J. Computed tomography as a diagnostic aid for extracanal invasive resorption. J Endod 2003;29:463-5.
29. Kullendorff B, Nilson M, Rohlin M. Diagnostic accuracy of direct digital dental radiography for the detection of periapical bone lesions. Overall comparison between conventional and direct digital radiography. Oral Surg Oral Med Oral Pathol Oral Radiol Endod 1996;82:334-50.
30. Liedke GS, Silveira HED, Silveira HLD, Dutra V, Figueiredo JAP. Influence of voxel size in the diagnostic ability of cone beam tomography to evaluate simulated external root resorption. J Endod 2009;35:233-5.
31. Lofthag-Hasen S, Huumonen S, Gröndahl K, Gröndahl HG. Limeted cone-beam CT and intraoral for diagnosis of periapical pathology. Oral Surg Oral Med Oral Pathol 2007;103:114-9.
32. Loubele M, Maes F, Schutyser F, Marchal G, Jacobs R, Suetens P. Assessment of bone segmentation quality of cone-beam CT versus multislice spiral CT: a pilot study. Oral Surg Oral Med Oral Pathol Oral Radiol Endod 2006;102:225-34.
33. Ludlow JD, Ludlow LE, Brooks SL, Howerton WB. Dosimetry of 3 CBCT devices for oral and maxillofacial radiology: CB Mercuray, NewTom 3G and i-CAT. Dentomaxillofac Radiol 2006;35:219-26.
34. Maini A, Durning P, Drage N. Resorption: within or without? The benefit of cone-beam computed tomography when diagnosing a case of an internal / external resorption defect. Br Dent J 2008;9:135-7.
35. Matherne RP, Angelopoulos C, Kulild JC, Tira D. Use of cone-beam computed tomography to indentify root canal systems in vitro. J Endod 2008;34:87-9.
36. Melcher AH, Holowka S, Pharoah M, Lewin PK. Non-invasive computed tomography and three-dimensional reconstruction of the dentition

of a 2800 year old Egyptian mummy exhibiting extensive dental disease. Am J P Anthr 1997;103:329-40.

37. Misch KA, Yi ES, Sarment DP. Accuracy of cone beam computed tomography for periodontal defect. J Periodontol 2006;77:1261-6.
38. Mozzo P, Procacci C, Tacconi A, Martini PT, Andreis IA. A new volumetric CT machine for dental imaging based on the cone-beam technique: preliminary results. Eur Radiol 1998;8(9):1558-64.
39. Nair MK, Nair UP. Digital and advanced imaging in endodontics. J Endod 2007;33:1-6.
40. Nakata K, Naitoh M, Izumi M, Inamoto K, Ariji E, Nakamura H. Effectiveness of dental computed tomography in diagnostic imaging of periradicular lesion of each root of a multirooted tooth: a case report. J Endod 2006;32:583-7.
41. Nance RS, Tyndall D, Levin LG, Trope M. Diagnosis of external root resorption using TACT. Endod Dent Traumatol 2000;16:24-8.
42. Park CH, Abramson ZR, Taba M Jr, Jin Q, Chang J, Kreider JM, Goldstein SA, Giannobile WV. Three-dimensional micro-computed tomographic imaging of alveolar bone in experimental bone loss or repair. J Periodontol 2007;78(2):273-81.
43. Patel S, Dawood A, Ford TP, Whaites E. The potential applications of cone beam computed tomography in the management of endodontic problems. Int Endod J 2007; 40:818-30.
44. Patel S, Dawood A. The use of cone beam computed tomography in the management of external cervical resorption lesions. Int Endod J 2007;40:730-7.
45. Patel S. New dimensions in endodontic imaging: part 2. Cone beam computed tomography. Int Endod J 2009. In press.
46. Paula-Silva FWG, Hassan B, Silva LAB, Leonardo MR, Wu M-K. Outcome of root canal treatment in dogs determined by periapical radiography and cone-beam computed tomography scans. J Endod 2009;35:723-6.
47. Paula-Silva FWG, Wu M-K, Silva LAB, Leonardo MR, Wesselink PR. Accuracy of periapical radiography and cone-beam computed tomography in diagnosing apical periodontitis using histopathological findings as a gold standard. J Endod 2009. In press.
48. Ricucci D, Bergenholtz G. Bacterial status in root-filled teeth exposed to the oral environment by loss of restoration and fracture or caries – a histobacteriological study of treated cases. Int Endod J 2003;36:787–802.
49. Scarfe WC, Farman AG, Sukovic P. Clinical applications of cone beam computed tomography in dental practice. J Can Dent Assoc 2005;72:75-80.
50. Schwarz MS, Rothman SLG, Rhodes ML, Chafetz N. Computed tomography: part 1. Preoperative assessment of the mandible for endosseous implant surgery. Int J Oral Maxillofac Implants 1987;2:137-41.
51. Simon JHS, Enciso R, Malfaz JM, Roges R, Bailey-Perry M, Patel A. Differential diagnosis of large periapical lesions using cone-beam computed tomography measurements and biopsy. J Endod 2006;32:833-7.
52. Stavropoulos A, Wenzel A. Accuracy of cone beam dental CT, intraoral digital and conventional film radiography for detection of periapical lesions. An ex vivo study in pig jaws. Clin Oral Investing 2007;11:101-6.
53. Sullivan JE, Di Fiore PM, Koerber A. Radiovisiography in the detection of periapical lesions. J Endod 2000;26:32-5.
54. Tachibana H, Matsumoto K. Applicability of x-ray computerized tomography in endodontics. Endod Dent Traumatol 1990;6:16-20.
55. Tammisalo T, Luostarinen T, Vähätalo K, Neva M. Detailed tomography of periapical and periodontal lesions. Diagnostic accuracy compared with periapical radiography. Dentomaxillofac Radiol 1996;25:89-96.
56. The Nobel Foundation. Available in http://nobelprize.org/nobel_prizes/medicine/laureates/1979/index.html. Accessed in 05/07/2009.
57. Trope M, Pettigrew JP, Barnett F, Tronstad L. Differentiation of radicular cyst and granulomas using computerized tomography. Endod Dent Traumatol 1989;5:69-72.
58. Tsiklakis K, Donta C, Gavala S, Karayianni K, Kamenopoulou V, Hourdakis CJ. Dose reduction in maxillofacial imaging using low dose Cone Beam CT. Eur J Radiol 2005;56:413-7.
59. Tyndall DA, Rathore S. Cone-Beam CT diagnostic applications: caries, periodontal bone assessment, and endodontic applications. Dent Clin N Am 2008;52:825-41.
60. Vannier MW, Hildebolt CF, Conover G, Knapp RH, Wang G. Three-dimensional dental imaging by spiral CT. Oral Surg Oral Med Oral Pathol 1997;84:561-70.
61. Velvart P, Hecker H, Tililinger G. Detection of the apical lesions and the mandibular canal in conventional radiography and computed tomography. Oral Surg Oral Med Oral Pathol Oral Radiol Endod 2001;92:682-8.
62. von Stechow D, Balto K, Stashenko P, Müller R. Three-dimensional quantitation of periradicular bone destruction by micro-computed tomography. J Endod 2003;29:252.
63. Walter L, Enciso R, Mah J. Three-dimensional localization of maxillary canines with cone-beam computed tomography. Am J Orthod Dentofacial Orthop 2005;128:418-23.
64. Wengraf AM. Angulation in periapical radiography. Br Dent J 1965;15:528-31.
65. Wu M-K, Dummer PMH, Wesselink PR. Consequences of and strategies to deal with residual post-treatment root canal infection. Int Endod J 2006;39:343–56.
66. Youssefzadelh S, Gahleitner A, Dorffner R, Bernhart T, Kainberger FM. Dental vertical root fractures: value of Ct in detection. Radio 1999;210:545-9.

2.XV

Clinical Microscope in Contemporary Endodontics

Why keep on "seeing with one's fingers"?

Francisco José de Souza Filho
Adriana de Jesus Soares

The

technological advances and innovations of the last decade have drastically influenced endodontic clinical procedures. Results previously considered unattainable are now possible to achieve. Files made of nickel-titanium alloys, rotary, oscillatory and ultrasound systems and instruments, thermoplastic filling techniques, electronic apex locators, in addition broader knowledge of the biological aspects of the root canal systems and different chemical-mechanical preparation protocols, exemplify this development. However, the introduction of the clinical microscope in endodontic therapy was undoubtedly the most significant event that affected the protocols until then adopted and consequently, the results and prognoses.

Innumerable benefits have arisen with the use of the clinical microscope in endodontics. The fascination of the results achieved is exclusively based on the operator's ability to visualize, that what previously depended on tactile sense, experience, imagination and perseverance. The alternative has led to changes, often radical, of the previously recommended conventional and surgical techniques, fundamentally governed by the enlargement/illumination binomial, which intensity and quality cannot be compared with the classical methods. The benefit achieved is very clear, considering that the microscope allows the dentist to see better, feel better and to think better, achieving greater level of precision and a potential excellence in clinical procedures (West[11], 2006). Why then, keep on "seeing with one's fingers"?

OPERATING MICROSCOPE

Completely adaptable to the dental office, the microscope is a simple instrument that is easy to handle, and within in a short time of daily use allows great improvement in the quality of clinical work and in the operator's ergonomic position (Fig. 2.XV-1A). To use the operating microscope, the dentist will need the help of one or two assistants, depending on the procedure to be performed. During the entire intervention, the dentist must keep his/her eyes on the binocular and hands in the operating field – the necessary instruments are handed to him/her by the assistant, who is seated facing the dentist, when non surgical procedures are performed (Fig. 2.XV-1B). The entire procedure is performed with the aid of an intra oral mirror, which directs the light, and therefore is held by the dentist to control the distance between the tooth and mirror considering the size of the instrument that is used. Surgical procedures require a second assistant, who stands on the right side of the dentist and follows the procedure by means of a monitor. During these procedures, the first assistant is in charge of keeping the operating field free from bleeding at all times, so that visibility is not impaired.

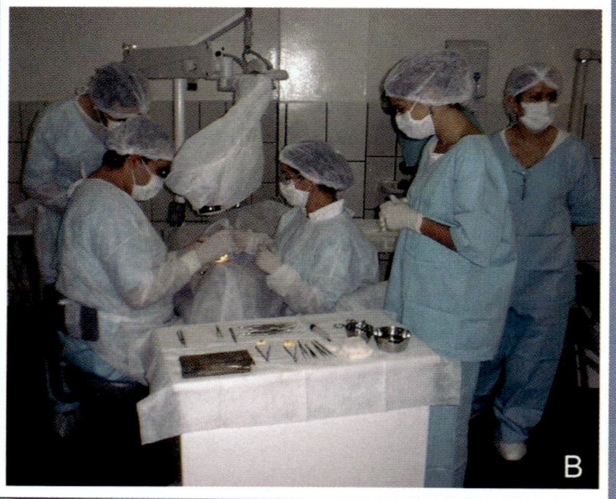

FIGS. 2.XV-1A-B
In clinical procedures performed with the aid of the microscope, note the ergonomic position of the operators, which is determined by the operating microscope.

Image magnification provided by the clinical microscope is far superior to that of magnification loupes. Furthermore, the greater the magnification capacity of loupes, the heavier and more uncomfortable they become. In addition to the magnification power, lighting is one of the most important characteristics of the microscope. The energy source generates light which is coaxial, a characteristic that eliminates shadows and enables illumination of the deeper portions of the root canal. The light source can be halogen or xenon. Yellow light does not allow for quality documentation, that is why white light is recommended. Fiber optic cables connect the light source to the microscope and light intensity is controlled by a rheostat.

As with any other equipment, command of its operation demands time and training. Evidently, until the dentist gets used to this different way of practicing, his/her performance may initially be slower. In order for the beginning not to become frustrating, correct guidance is necessary, so that the convenience of using the microscope and mastery of the technique gradually increase.

- In the laboratory, one is trained to handle the hinging arms, adjust the binocular at the interpupillary distance, adjust the focus by means of the objective lens setting, adjust the focal distance and the best adaptation to the intense coaxial light. Training can be performed on extracted teeth.

- The practitioner has to apply what has been learned in the laboratory to actual patients. It is recommended to begin by performing the simplest procedures, such as clinical observations, visualization of easy access preparations, etc.
- More complex cases, especially surgical cases, should only be performed when the operator has gained expertise using the microscope.
- Ideally as time passes, routine use of the microscope to perform any clinical procedure should become second nature.

APPLICATIONS OF THE CLINICAL MICROSCOPE IN CONVENTIONAL ENDODONTIC TREATMENT

In non-surgical endodontic procedures, that is treatment and re-treatment of root canals, the operating microscope allows for better execution of clinical procedures, thanks to an increase in visibility provided by the coaxial light. Important steps such as access opening preparation, complete removal of caries and remaining restorative material can easily be performed by the operator. Removal of the roof of the pulp chamber and cleaning and shaping of the cavity walls can be performed with confidence, even when there are calcifications or perforations on the pulp chamber floor, anatomical anomalies that make procedures difficult and can lead to errors and accidents. With the aid of the microscope, the orifices of the root canal entrances are easily identified, particularly when observing the darker color of the natural dentin on the pulp chamber floor in contrast to the lighter tertiary dentin (Figs. 2.XV-2A-C). Thus, the preparation of the root canal entrance can be performed without removing unnecessary tooth structure, as these procedures are visually under control.

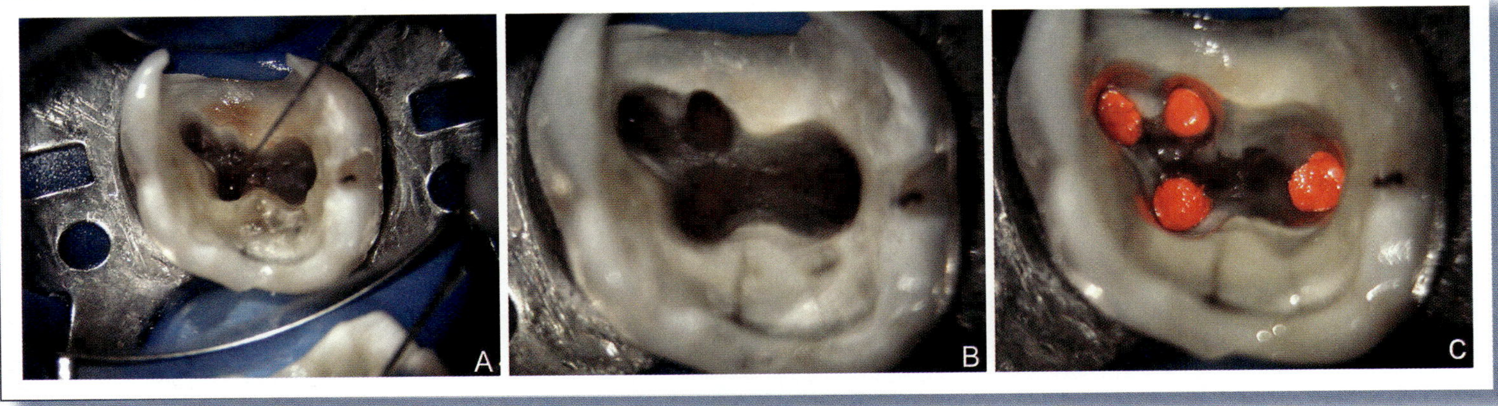

FIGS. 2.XV-2A-C

Clinical sequence showing the details of coronal opening and location of the fourth canal in the maxillary first molar. In Figure B, there are details of the preparation of the entrance of root canals and in C, the filling material can be seen in the entrance of the root canals, as well as the complete removal of the caries tissue and adaptation of contour and convenience shape of the access cavity. (Courtesy of Dr. Patrick Baltieri – Specialist in Endodontics).

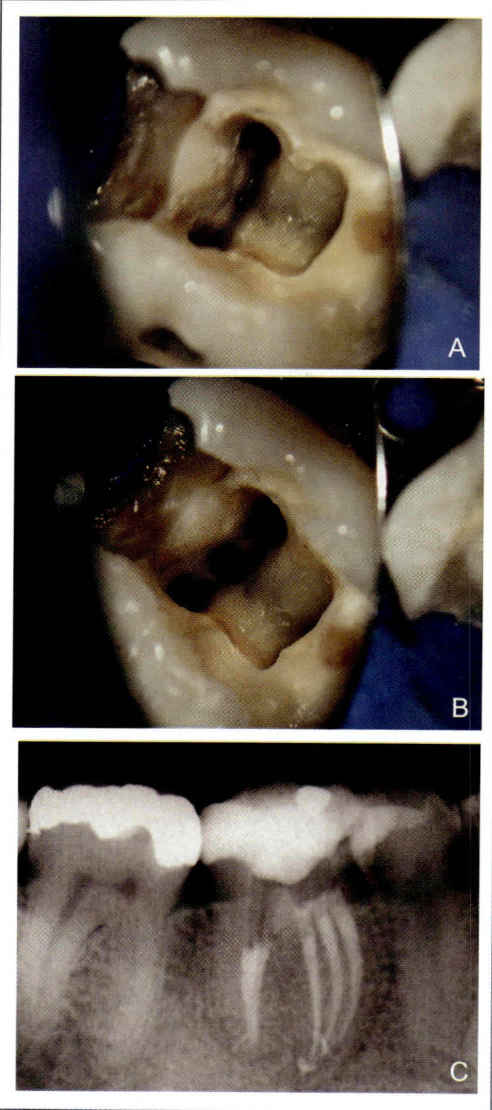

FIGS. 2.XV-3A-C

Clinical sequence and final radiograph of location and endodontic treatment of extra canal in the mesial root of the mandibular first molar. (Courtesy of Dr. Ricardo Ferreira – Endodontics at Univalli).

Other difficulties that can be minimized during the coronal access opening sequence are identifying extra canals in the pulp chamber of molars or in flattened canals, which tend to duplicate (Figs. 2.XV-3A-C and 2.XV-4A-B). The microscope facilitates visual identification of the isthmus and reentries, mainly located in the cervical and middle third of root canals, enabling mechanical removal of organic remnants that are present in these anatomic variations of root canals.

Other difficulties that are frequently associated with unsuccessful endodontic treatment may be easily overcome with the aid of the clinical microscope. Among them, sealing of accidental perforations located on the pulp chamber floor or dentinal walls of the roots (Figs. 2.XV-5A-D), and pathological perforations caused by internal root resorption are some examples. In these cases, magnification and light provide visual access to the location of the perforation, allowing the operator to have greater command of the clinical procedures for inserting the sealing material, which promote results that are far more reliable.

Endodontic treatment of teeth with incompletely formed apices (Fig. 2.XV-6A-C), endodontic treatment of teeth with unusual anatomy, such as *dens-in-dente* and C-shaped roots, which can be accessed and prepared with greater predictability with the aid of the microscope, must also be considered. Among the more difficult problems, endodontic re-treatments have a serious impact on clinical results. The difficulty of completely removing the sealer and filling material that adhere to the recesses of root canals can lead to unsuccessful endodontic re-treatment (Figs. 2.XV-7A-B). There is greater precision in visualizing and identifying the remaining material, which can be removed easier when using an operation microscope.

Another example is the visualization of fractured instruments inside a root canal. The microscope allows precise removal of dentin around the instrument enabling retrieval with minimum damage (Figs. 2.XV-8A-B).

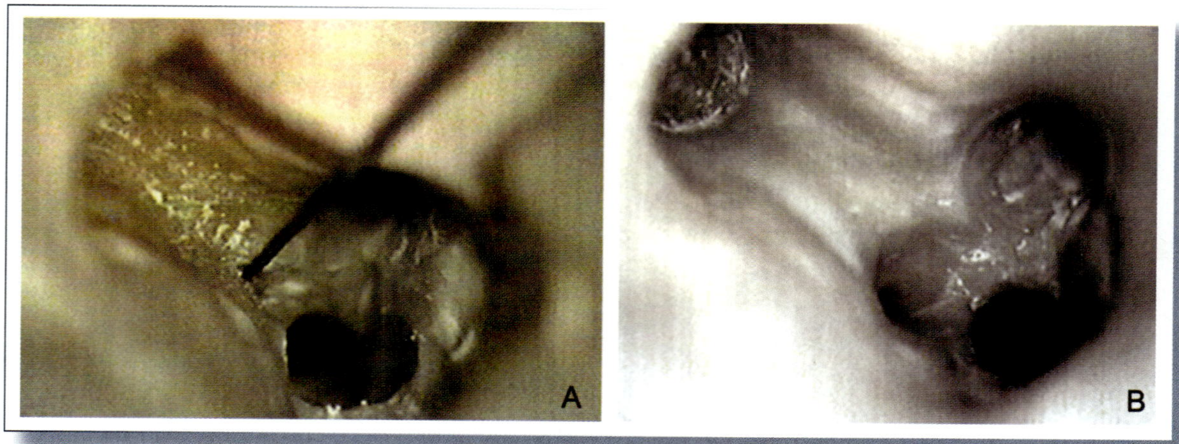

FIGS. 2.XV-4A-B

Visualization of the fourth canal in the mesial root of the maxillary molar (A). Preparation of the orifices of the root canals showing difference in color of dentin in the pulp chamber floor (B).

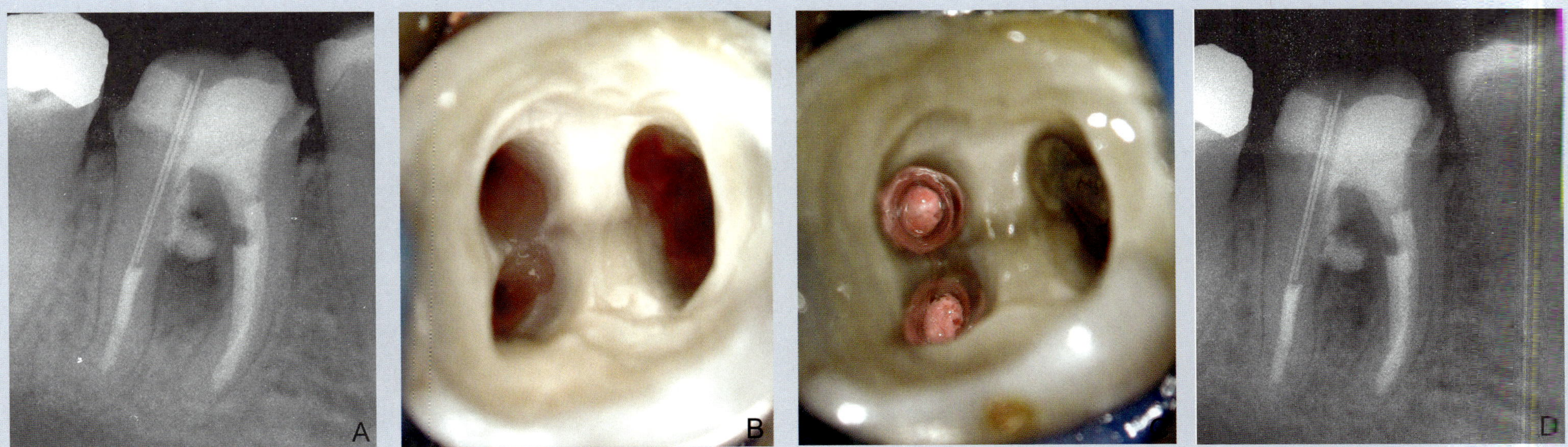

FIGS. 2.XV-5A-D

A periapical radiograph (A) shows the radiolucent area in the region of the furcation of tooth 4.6, resulting from perforation located in the root wall of the distal root (B). The perforation site was filled with MTA (C) and in Figure D, note the radiographic signs of repair eight months after the clinical procedures were performed. (Courtesy of Dr. Antonio Batista – Endodontics at UFPF).

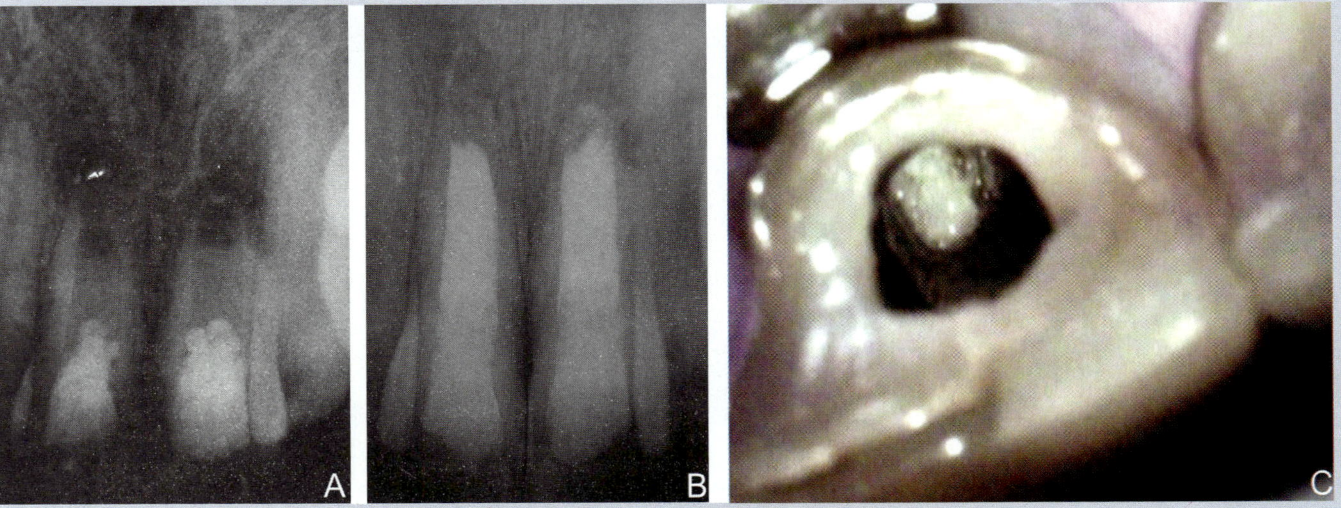

FIG.S 2-XV-6A-C

Radiographic aspect of the maxillary central incisors with incompletely formed apices, showing evidence of periapical lesion resulting from trauma (A); radiograph showing the closing of the root apexes after use of intracanal medication for a period of nine months (B), and clinical photograph obtained after this period, revealing the apical barrier that was formed (20x magnification). (Courtesy of Prof. Alexandre Augusto Zaia – Endodontics at Unicamp).

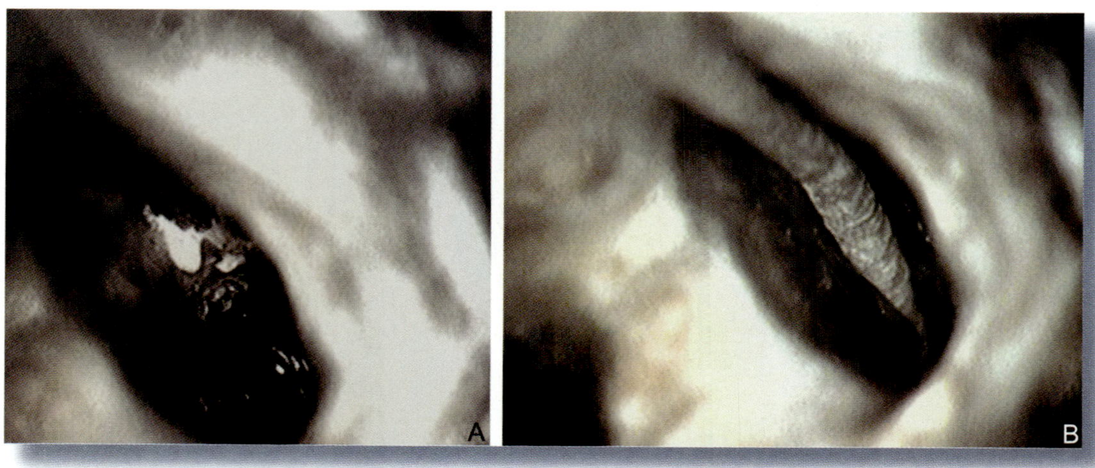

FIGS. 2.XV-7A-B

Interior view of the root canal at 30x magnification, showing cement and filling material remnants adhering to the recesses of the root walls during endodontic re-treatment (A). In Figure B, we can see the canal free from filling material residues being dried with a paper point. (Courtesy of Dr. Noboru Imura – Endodontics at EAP-APCD/ABCD-SP).

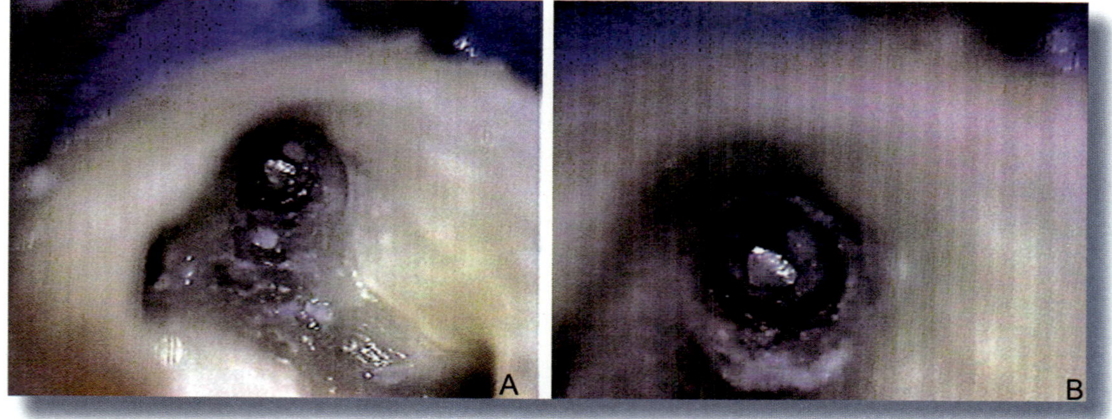

FIGS. 2.XV-8A-B

Endodontic instrument fractured inside the root canal seen at different magnifications A, 12x and Fig. B, 20x.

Furthermore, identification of cracks and root fractures is much easier with the aid of the microscope, which promotes a diagnostic and prognostic precision of clinical cases (Figs. 2.XV-9A-B).

A further example is the removal of a resin posts from a root canal by grinding, which can be done with more predictability when it is performed with the aid of the microscope. This makes these procedures safer and more controlled, offering more predictable success (Fig. 2.XV-10). The removal of metal cores and preserving the surrounding dentin can also more precisely performed with the aid of the microscope.

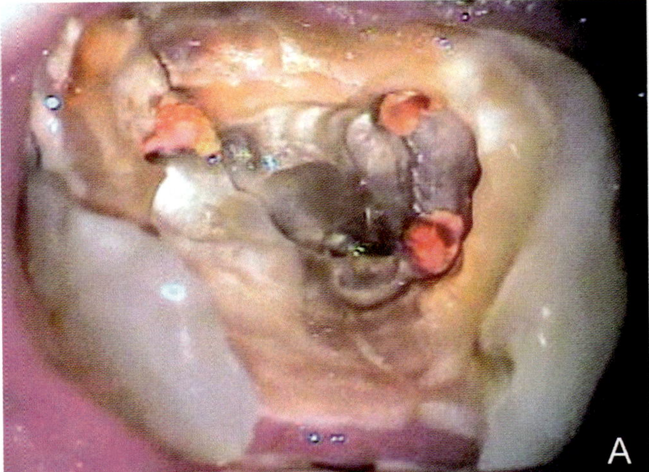

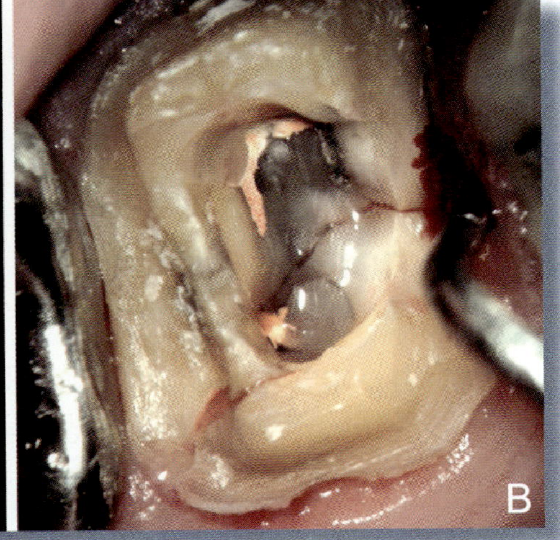

FIGS. 2.XV-9A-B

In Figure A, crack identified in the pulp chamber floor of the mandibular molar at 20x magnification. In Figure B, note the fracture line from the mesial to the distal region in the floor of the maxillary molar (20x).

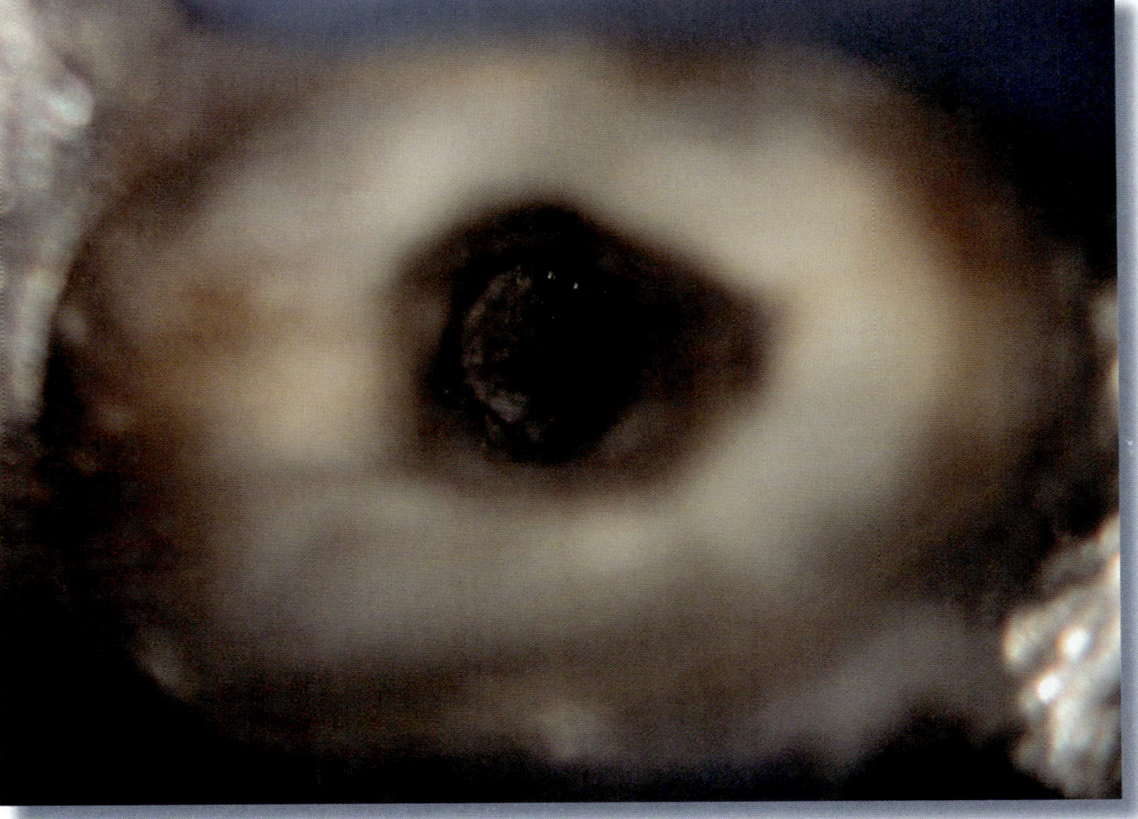

FIG. 2.XV-10

Interior view of a root canal during the process of removing a fiber glass post by means of grinding. (Courtesy of Dr. Patrick Baltieri – Specialist in Endodontics).

DOCUMENTATION, COMMUNICATION AND MARKETING

The dental clinical microscope also provides another extremely valuable application: the documentation of clinical cases. Storage and filing of data and clinical procedures can be done by means of peripherals connected to the microscope, such as video and photographic cameras. Recordings of procedures can be used for education and documentation for legal purposes.

Visual demonstrations are easily understood by patients, which makes it useful to show caries, restoration failures, fractures, presence of plaque, calculus, etc. on the video monitor.

At the same time as we are teaching, educating and guiding patients by means of the microscope, another no less important aspect appears; marketing. Patients watching a comprehensive demonstration of the application of up-to-date technology that produces results will act as agents promoting the product.

FINAL CONSIDERATIONS

While the use of the operating microscope is important in specialties such as periodontics, general dentistry, prosthodontics and for small cases in oral surgery, in endodontics it is essential in order for the outcome of the treatment to be predictable, successful and long lasting. The Brazilian dental profession has become increasingly more aware of the need to use a clinical microscope. According to West (2006)[11], "in the United States and Canada, post-graduate students in Endodontics have been trained to use the operating microscope expertly since 1997. It is estimated that 76% of American endodontists have a microscope in their private dental office. On the other hand, the percentage of general dentists who use a microscope is estimated at only 1%. The University of Washington, School of Dentistry, Seattle, was the first university in the United States and in the world to teach their undergraduate students the use of a clinical microscope, predicting that these students would be the first generation of dentists who were trained to practice dentistry with the operating microscope".

In Brazil, at the University of Campinas (Unicamp), Dental Faculty of Piracicaba was the pioneer in teaching the endodontic course using microscopy, and created the Center of Oral Microscopy Studies (Cemo) at the end of 1995. Since then, in addition to the courses offered by the Professors of Endodontics and other dentists, the program includes clinical microscopy in the Endodontic post-graduate courses (specialization, masters and doctorate level) for conventional as well as surgical procedures.

Other schools in Brazil have introduced teaching the operating microscopy in their specialization courses. Soon, clinical microscopy will be a mandatory requirement for all dental courses because it has demonstrated to be an extraordinary adjunct for the advancement of Endodontics. In this respect the words of West (2006) are appropriate: ... "the use of the microscope will not transform a good dentist into a brilliant one, but it will make both better because they can see better".

References

1. Carr GB. Microscopes in Endodontics. CDA Journal, V.20, P.55-61, 1992.
2. De Moor RJ, Calberson FL. Root canal treatment in a mandibular second premolar with three root canals. J Endod, v.31, n.4, p.310-313, 2005.
3. Jung M. Endodontic treatment of dens invaginatus type III with three root canals and open apical foramen. Int Endod J, v.37, n.3, p.205-213, 2004.
4. Khayat BG. The use of magnification in endodontic therapy: the operating microscope. Review. Pract. Periodontics Aesthet Dent, v.10, n.1, p.137-144, 1998.
5. Kulid JC, Peters DD. Incidence and configuration of canal systems in the mesiobuccal root of maxillary first and second molars. J Endod, v.16, p.311, 1990.
6. Mounce R. Surgical Operating Microscope in Endodontics; The Paradigm Shift. General Dentistry, v.43, p.346-349, 1995.
7. Murgel CAF, Gondim Jr E, Souza Filho FJ. Microscópio cirúrgico: a busca da excelência na clínica odontológica. Rev. Assoc. Paul. Cir Dent, v.51, n.1, p.31-34, 1997.
8. Ruddle CJ. Non-Surgical Endodontic Retreatment. CDA Journal, v.25, n.11, p.769-799, 1997.
9. Saunders WP, Saunders EM. Conventional endodontics and the operating microscope. Dent Clin North Am, v.41, n.3, p.415-428, 1997.
10. Souza Filho FJ. Microscópio clínico odontológico na endodontia. In: Dotto CA, Antoniazzi, J.H. Opinion makers: tecnologia e informática. São Paulo: VM Comunicações, p.62-63, 2002.
11. West J. Endodontic Update 2006. Journal of Esthetic and Restorative Dentistry, v.18, n.5, p.280-300, 2006.

Pain control in Endodontics (ANESTHETICS)

Ricardo M. Oliveira-Filho

The technological advancements in Pharmacology, notably the development of new groups of anesthetics, has benefitted Endodontics, mainly because the improvement in application techniques has led to root canal treatment becoming an almost painless operative procedure.

With new anesthetics and new accurate application techniques, the old belief that endodontic treatment was synonymous with pain has been replaced by the certainty of a more comfortable treatment for the patient and much less stressful for both patient and practitioner. The technique of administering these anesthetics can be reviewed in specialized text books.

In 1940, with the synthesis of lidocaine, a new chemical group of anesthetics – the amides – replaced the ester group of anesthetics to great advantage. Of the amide group, the main salts available in Brazil are lidocaine, prilocaine, bupivacaine, mepivacaine and articaine. They are offered in different concentrations, usually between 2 and 4 % with or without vasoconstrictor.

In 2000, Malamed et al.[12] published *a report* in the *Journal of the American Dental Association, on the efficacy of articaine as a new anesthetic amide for local use, revolutionizing pain control in dentistry.*

ARTICAINE

Articaine is the methyl ester of 4-methyl-3-[1-oxo-2-(propylaminopropanoylamino]-thiophene-2-carboxylate acid, and was synthesized in 1969 by Rusching et al., apud Ferger & Marxkors[1], and initially named "carticaine". When it was introduced in clinical practice in German in 1976 the name was changed to articaine. Under the new name the anesthetic was gradually adopted in other countries, such as Canada (1983); and the United Kingdom and Brazil in 1998. In the United States of America it was adopted in 2000[12] and sold under the label of Septocaine (Septodont Inc, New Castle, DE, EUA), and in Brazil under the label of Septanest (Septodont do Brasil Imp. Ltda, Barueri, São Paulo, Brazil).

The substance is prepared in the form of a racemic mixture; its oil-water partition coefficient is 17.

From a chemical point of view, the articaine molecule has two distinctive peculiarities. Firstly, it is the only local anesthetic of the amide type that has a thiophene ring, which accounts for its increased potency (this is why it is classified among the amides as a thiophene (Fig. 2.XVI-1). Also present in the chemical structure of the sulfa drugs, the thiophene ring is mentioned as being responsible for the contraindication of articaine, because it may cause cross-allergy with these anti-bacterial agents. Secondly, in addition to the amide link in the intermediary chain, it has an ester link attached to the ring, which is the primary target of plasmatic metabolism, allowing fast hydrolysis through the plasmatic cholinesterases, which accounts for its low systemic toxicity.

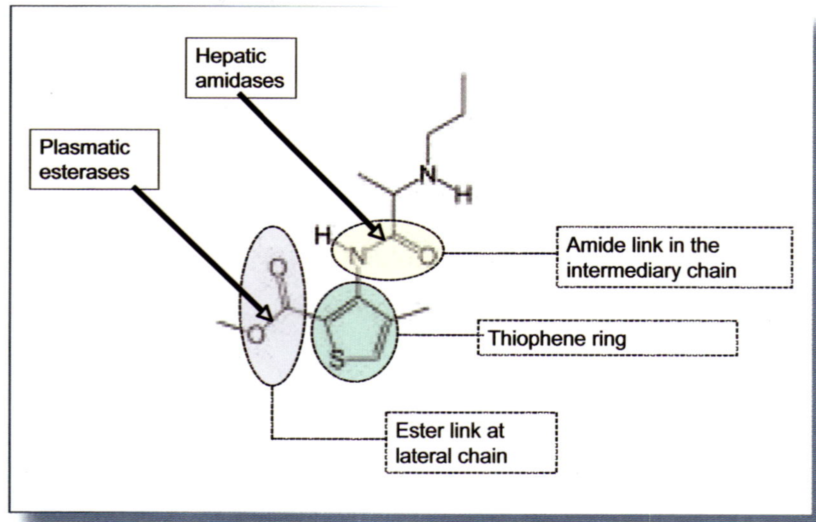

FIG. 2.XVI-1

Articaine structure, showing two rupture points by the action of metabolic enzymes.

Approximately 60 to 80% of articaine that enters the bloodstream binds to albumin and to γ-globulin. The drug is quickly metabolized by a plasmatic esterase (carboxiesterase), creating the primary metabolic articainic acid, which is inactive. A small fraction (5-10%) is also metabolized in the liver (P450 system), with the formation of articainic acid glucoronide, also inactive. The elimination half-life for articaine is approximately 1.8h[24].

Articaine does not differ from other local anesthetic agents with respect to the action mechanism. Nevertheless, variations in physical-chemical parameters (liposolubility, pKa, etc.) impose certain differences in pharmacologic properties in comparison to other drugs of the group (Table 2.XVI-1). Its low pKa in comparison with bupivacaine, makes it act faster, whereas, the pKa value combined with the presence of a vasoconstrictor and the percentage of protein binding, make the depth and duration of its effect convenient for endodontics.

Several clinical studies have indicated that articaine is a safe and efficient anesthetic with few side effects[11,15,27].

Over the past few years, the use of articaine/adrenalin (AA) has increased considerably in Europe and in the United States[9]. Placebo-controlled double-blind clinical research under strict scientific resources are necessary to determine the true difference in the effectiveness and safety of this anesthetic, in comparison to other anesthetics available[25].

Schertzer & Malamed[23] reported that articaine produced a better anesthetic effect in comparison with lidocaine. Several well-controlled studies have, however, been unable to show a clinically appreciable difference between articaine and other local anesthetics commonly used in dentistry, such as lidocaine, mepivacaine or prilocaine.

Table 2-XVI-1 – Physical-chemical and clinical data of articaine in comparison with other local anesthetics

LOCAL ANESTHETIC	VASOCONSTRICTOR	COMMERCIAL BRAND	PKA	LIPOSOLUBILITY[1*]	PROTEIN BINDING	START OF THE EFFECT	DURATION OF EFFECT	WARNINGS
4% articaine	Adrenalin 1:100,000	Septanest®-Articaine	7.8	1.5	95%	fast	Intermediate[2**]	AVOID: allergic to sulfa drugs[21].
4% articaine	Adrenalin 1:200,000	Septanest®-Articaine	7.8	1.5	95%	fast	Intermediate	AVOID: allergic to sulfas[21].
5% Bupivacaine	Adrenalin 1:200,000	Neocaine®	8.1	30	95%	moderate	prolonged	AVOID: Pregnant. Children.
2% Lidocaine	Adrenalin 1:100,000	Alphacaine 100® Xylocaine® Lidostesin 100®	7.8	4	65%	fast	Intermediate	AVOID[4,21,22]: Arterial hypertension. Persons with increased respiratory frequency. Patients with hepatic and renal diseases.
2% Lidocaine	phenylephrine 1:2500	Biocaine® Novocol®	7.8	4	65%	fast	Intermediate	
2% Mepivacaine	Adrenalin 1:100,000	Scandicaine® Mepivalen AD®	7.7	1	75%	fast	Intermediate	AVOID: Pregnant[20].
3% Prilocaine	Felypressin 0.03UI/ml	Citanest® Biopressin® Citocaine® Prilonest®	7.9	1.5	55%	fast	Intermediate	AVOID: Anemic Patients. Pregnant. Respiratory diseases.

(*) on the basis of procaine as reference (=1.0)

* taking procaine as a reference (=1.0)
** Articaine A (AA) determines pulp anesthesia for 60-75 minutes[9]

Sherman et al.[25], 2008, in a randomized double-blind study, evaluated the anesthetic efficiency of 4% articaine (AA), with 1:100.000 adrenalin, in comparison with 2% lidocaine (LA), also with adrenaline of the same concentration, by Gow-Gates[2] injection and infiltration in the maxillae of patients with irreversible acute pulpitis in posterior teeth. The overall anesthetic success was 87.5%. The association of AA proved to be very efficient, but not superior to LA.

The possibility of a greater neurotoxicity of these drugs when compared with others has drawn attention in recent years. A very small fraction of patients reported temporary or permanent impairment of sensory function after a mandibular block with the local anesthetics. The estimates point towards a prevalence of temporary lack of sensory function[5,8] in the range of 0.15-0.54%, and much less frequent for permanent damage (0.0001-0.01%)[5,8].

Several articles appeared in the literature after a publication by Haas & Lennon[3] who emphasized the dramatic increase in reports on paresthesia after the administration of local anesthetics, coinciding with the introduction of articaine in clinical dental practice in Ontario, Canada[3]. Various other articles appeared, confirming[6,13,17,26] or raising doubts about this[7,10,14]. In view of the present status of this concern, when using articaine, it is prudent and advisable to pay special attention to the technique that is used, especially with regards to the time of application (properly prolonged), doses (which should be in accordance with recommended limits) and the post-anesthetic period.

The effect of the addition of tramadol (an opiate analgesic) to articaine solution used for difficult extractions (e.g. impacted mandibular third molars) has also aroused interest. A recent, randomized, double-blind and placebo controlled study has shown[19] that the level and duration of the analgesic effect of this combination were superior to those obtained with articaine alone. The use of this strategy in endodontic practice apparently involves promising aspects for the efficient control of trans- and post-operative pain.

PRESENTATIONS

In Brazil, Articaine for endodontic use is marketed in carpules in the form of 4% chloride, with adrenalin 1:100.000 (Septanest 1:100.000 and Articaine 100) (Fig. 2.XVI-2) or adrenalin 1:200.000 (Septanest 1:200.000 and Articaine 200) (Septodont do Brasil Imp. Ltda, Barueri, São Paulo, Brazil).

In 2003, the American Dental Association specified a uniform mandatory color code to identify anesthetic carpules, in accordance with the commercial brand (www.ada.org/prof/resources/topics/color.asp). The color code for the 4% articaine carpule is gold.

The maximum recommended dose for 4% articaine is 7mg/kg (maximum of 500mg) for adults and 5mg/kg for children; that is, 7 carpules for adults (typical maximum dose for endodontic interventions) and 3 carpules for children[21].

Adrenalin, a potent and efficient vasoconstrictor, is well tolerated by healthy patients at the recommended doses. With regards to cardiovascular compromised patients, Neves et al.[16] recently evaluated the electrocardiograms and blood pressure parameters of 62 patients with coronary arterial diseases, during dental procedures, under local anesthesia, with and without vasoconstrictor (adrenalin-1:100.000). They concluded that there was no difference between the two groups with respect to blood pressure and heart rate, nor evidence of ischemia and arrhythmias. The use of this vasoconstrictor has been shown to be safe within the limits of the study.

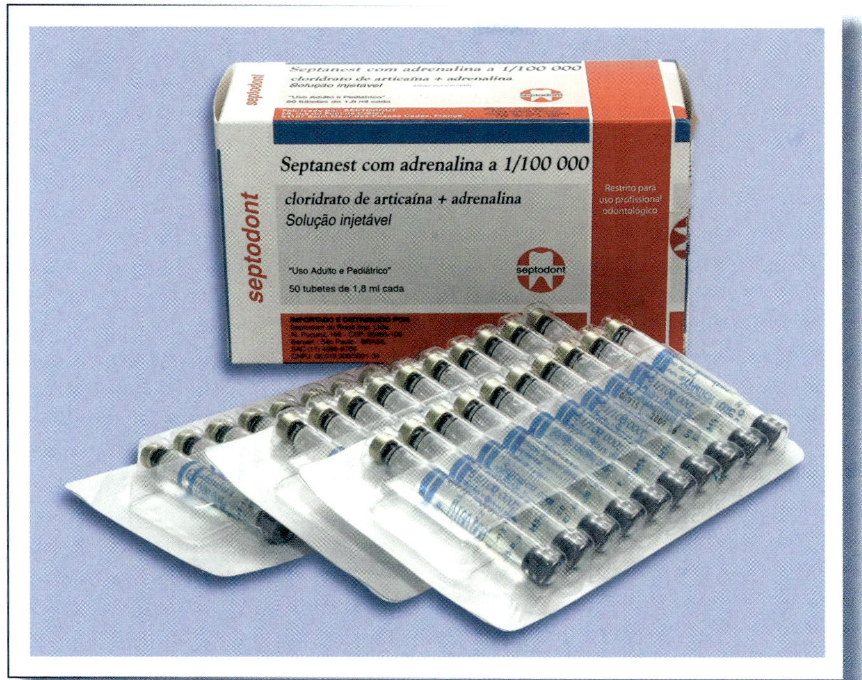

FIG. 2.XVI-2

4% Articaine chloride-based injectable anesthetic. Septanest with adrenalin at 1:100,000 – Septodont do Brasil, Imp. Ltda, São Paulo, Brazil).

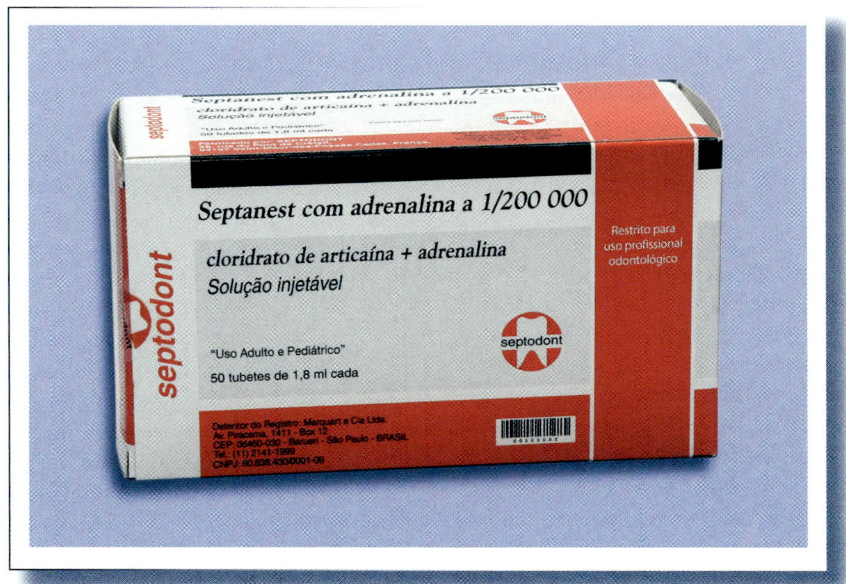

FIG. 2.XVI-3

4% Articaine chloride-based injectable anesthetic. Septanest with adrenalin at 1:200,000 – Septodont do Brasil, Imp. Ltda, Barueri, São Paulo, Brazil).

References

1. Ferger P, Marxkors R. Ein neues anasthetikum in der zahnarztlichen prosthetik. Dtsch Zahnarztl Z, v.28, p.87-89, 1973.
2. Gow-Gates GA. Mandibular conduction anesthesia: a new technique using extraoral landmarks. Oral Surg Oral Med Oral Pathol, v.36, p.321-328, 1973.
3. Haas DA, Lennon DA. A 21-year retrospective study of reports of paresthesia following local anaesthetic administration. J Can Dent Assoc, v.61, p.319-330, 1995.
4. Haase A, Heng M, Garret N. Blood pressure and electrocardiographic response to dental treatment with use of local anesthesia. J Am Dent Assoc, v.113, p.639, 1986.
5. Harn SD, Durham TM. Incidence of lingual nerve trauma and postinjection complications in conventional mandibular block anaesthesia. J Am Dent Assoc, v.121, p.519-523, 1990.
6. Hillerup S, Jensen R. Nerve injury caused by mandibular block analgesia. Int J Oral Maxillofac Surg, v.35, p.437-443, 2006.
7. Hoffmeister B. Morphologic changes in peripheral nerves following intraneural injection of local anesthetic. Dtsch Zahnaerzl Z, v.46, p.126-132, 1991.
8. Krafft TC, Hickel R. Clinical investigation into the incidence of direct damage to the lingual nerve caused by local anesthesia. J Craniomaxillofac Surg, v.22, p.294-296, 1994.
9. Malamed SF. Handbook of local anesthesia. 5th ed. St. Louis: Mosby, 2004.
10. Malamed SF. Nerve injury caused by mandibular block analgesia. Int J Oral Maxillofac Surg, v.35, p.876-877, 2006.
11. Malamed SF, Gagnon S, Leblanc D. A comparison between articaine HCl and lidocaine HCl in pediatric dental patients. Pediatr Dent, v.22, p.309-311, 2000.
12. Malamed SF, Gagnon S, Leblanc D. Efficacy of articaine: a new amide local anesthetic. J Am Dent Assoc, v.131, p.635-642, 2000.
13. Meechan JG. Prolonged paraesthesia following inferior alveolar nerve block using articaine. Brit J Oral Maxillofac Surg, v.41, p.201, 2003.
14. Missika P, Khoury G. Paresthesia and local infiltration or block anesthesia. L´Inform Dent, v.87, p.2.731-2.736, 2005.
15. Moller RA, Covino BG. Cardiac electrophysiologic effects of articaine compared with bupivacaine and lidocaine. Anesth Analg, v.76, p.1.266-1.273, 1993.
16. Neves RS, Neves IL, Giorgi DM, Grupi CJ, César LA, Hueb W, Grinberg M. Effects of epinephrine in local dental anesthesia in patients with coronary artery disease. Arq Bras Cardiol, v.88, n.5, p.545-551, 2007.
17. Pedlar J. Prolonged paraesthesia. Brit Dent J, v.195, p.119, 2003.
18. Pogrel MA, Thamby S. Permanent nerve involvement resulting from inferior alveolar nerve blocks. J Am Dent Assoc, v.131, p.901-907, 2004.
19. Pozos AJ, Martinez R, Aguirre P, Perez J. The effects of tramadol added to articaine on anesthesia duration. Oral Surg Oral Med Oral Pathol Oral Radiol Endod, v.102, p.614-617, 2006.
20. Ramacciato JC, Groppo FC. Anestésicos locais. Caderno de Farmacologia, v.II, n.2, Cap.3, p.45-49, Ed. Implantnews: Campinas.
21. Reader A, Nusstein J, Hargreaves KM. Anestesia local em Endodontia. Cap.19. In: Cohen S, Hargreaves KM. Caminhos da polpa. 9.ª ed. Elsevier Ed. Ltda.: Rio de Janeiro, 2007. p.691-723.
22. Salomen M, Forsell H, Sceinin M. Local dental anesthesia with lidocaine and adrenalin: effects on plasma catecholamines, heart rate, and blood pressure. Int Oral Maxilofac Surg, v.17, p.392, 1988.
23. Schertzer E, Malamed S. Articaine vs Lidocaine. J Am Dent Assoc, v.131, p.1248, 2000.
24. Septocaine Information, in: http://dailymed.nlm.nih.gov/dailymed/fda/fdaDrugXsl.cfm?id=5131&type=display (acessado em 25-2-2008).
25. Sherman MG, Flax M, Namerow K, Murray PE. Anesthetic efficacy of the Gow-Gates injection and maxillary infiltration with Articaine and Lidocaine for irreversible pulpitis. J Endod, v.34, n.6, p.656-659, 2008.
26. Vaneeden SP, Patel MF. Prolonged paraesthesia following inferior alveolar nerve block using articaine. Brit J Oral Maxillofac Surg, v.40, p.519-520, 2002.
27. Wright GZ, Weinberger SJ, Friedman CS, Plotzke OB. The use of articaine local anesthesia in children under 4 years of age: a retrospective report. Anesth Prog, v.36, p.268-271, 1989.

2.XVII

Detoxification of septic/toxic contents (Endotoxins) in root canals of teeth with pulp necrosis and evident periapical lesions (Apical Periodontitis)

Mario Roberto Leonardo
Lea Assed Bezerra da Silva

Root

canal treatment of teeth with pulp necrosis (gangrene) without radiographically visible periapical lesions or with evident chronic periapical lesions are subsequently called by us as necropulpectomy I and necropulpectomy II. They occur because of the precarious dental caries prevention programs in our country (Brazil) and therefore continue to be a routine procedure for the endodontist.

Due to a rise in awareness of dental health of our population, extraction is now considered a last resort option, as value is placed on preservation of the dentition. Consequently root canal treatment has become more of a routine treatment and priority in dental health care.

The concepts discussed in Chapter 1, as well as the systemic implications of an infectious nature, particularly in the case of treatment of infected pulpless teeth with evident chronic periapical lesion (necropulpectomy II), are closely related to the importance of this chapter; that is, detoxification of the septic/toxic contents of root canals, performed in a crown/apex direction without pressure. Treatment techniques that use this detoxification protocol follow the crown/down principle, which was first published in the endodontic literature by Marshall & Pappin[5], in 1980.

As was described in Chapter 2-I, this new technique initially caused an impact among endodontists because of the successive use of gradually larger diameter instruments, first in the coronal and posterior thirds, followed by the use of smaller diameter instruments until the real tooth length (RTL) is reached, in cases of necropulpectomies II and/or real working length (RWL), in cases of necropulpectomies I. According to this sequence, when the instruments reach the apical third, most of the septic/toxic contents of the root canal has already mechanically been removed and neutralized by the action of the irrigation solutions, since the higher concentration of these toxic contents is found in the coronal and middle thirds.

The technique used for 160 years – until 1980, practiced in an apex/crown direction, was mainly responsible for post-operative pain and acute apical periodontitis, and also for the unpleasant Fenix abscesses (*flare-up*).

In cases of necropulpectomies II, the high incidence (predominance) of anaerobes, especially Gram-negative bacteria[1,14], high concentrations of endotoxins in the periapex and their implications [2,9], as well as aerobic, microaerophilic and Gram-positive bacteria (exotoxins)[6,7,8,9] also involved in this infectious process, demand that the treatment technique progressively neutralizes the septic/toxic contents of the root canal, which precedes the biomechanical preparation.

The gram-negative anaerobes, predominant in these cases, in addition to having different virulence, release toxic products and byproducts, particularly endotoxins (LPS) (Fig. 2.XVII-1), constituents of cell walls of these bacteria which, if taken to the periapical region in excess may, from a clinical point of view, result in the so-called Fenix abscess (*flare-up*). These may be responsible for systemic problems, and even be fatal in patients who already have some prior organic problems, in addition to causing exacerbated pain and rapid development of edema. All these factors have a decisively negative impact on the reputation of the profession.

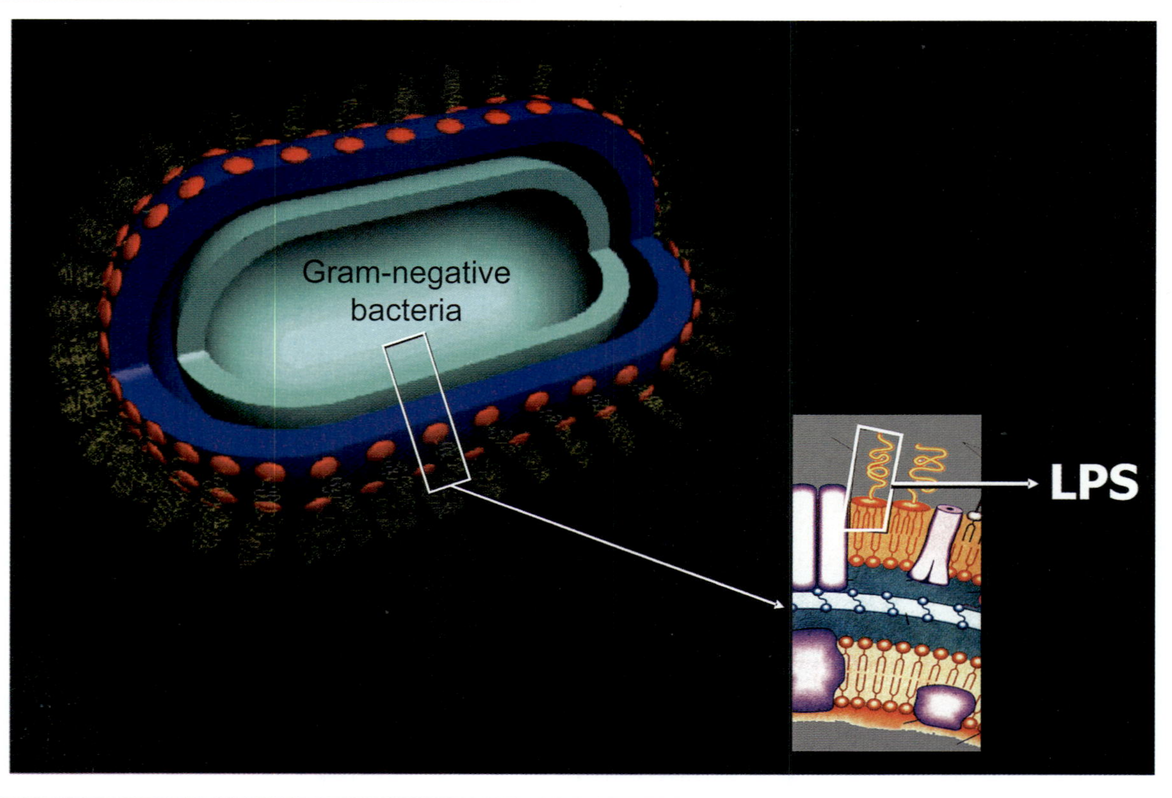

FIG. 2.XVII-1

Diagrammatic illustration of bacterial LPS – endotoxins[4].

This knowledge is especially important, since the endotoxins composed of lipopolysaccharides (LPS) exert a series of harmful biological effects on the body (system effect), particularly in humans, who are the most sensitive among all animals[7].

The toxicity of endotoxins is found in the molecule corresponding to the lipid A. Thus, the endotoxin of living or dead bacteria, whether whole or in fragments, acting on the macrophages, neutrophils and fibroblasts, sets of the release of a large number of bioactive or cytokin inflammatory chemical mediators. The LPS activate the Hageman factor, potentiating the painful effects of the kinins as well as contributing to the release of vasoactive and neurotransmitter substances in the periapical tissue nerve endings, leading to pain[4,13].

These properties are responsible for the intense pain the patient experiences and also for the rapid development of edema, in cases of Fenix abscesses (*flare-up*)[10] (Figs. 2.XVII-2A-G).

In addition to activating the release of mediators responsible for the inflammatory reaction, the LPS irreversibly adhere to the resorbed mineralized tissues of the apical and periapical regions (bone and apical cement), in cases of teeth with evident periapical lesion, perpetuating the inflammatory reaction[4].

Therefore, it is important for the endodontist and general clinician who practice endodontics to know that when gram-negative bacteria are stressed, or during multiplication and after their death, they release endotoxins (LPS) which, as we have seen, irreversibly adhere to the reabsorbed hard tissues, such as the apical cement and periapical alveolar bone, sustaining their deleterious effects until they are surgically removed or chemically inactivated[1,8,12] by the action of calcium hydroxide (Calen) used as a temporary dressing.

With the aim of assessing the capacity of detoxifying endotoxin during the stage of neutralizing the septic/toxic content of the root canal in the crown/apex direction in cases of necropulpectomies II, Silva *et al.*[11], in 2002, in a study in dog's teeth published in 2004, used different irrigation solutions. LPS was introduced into the root canals and left for a period of 10 days followed by various irrigation solutions, with protocols applying the crown/apex principle.

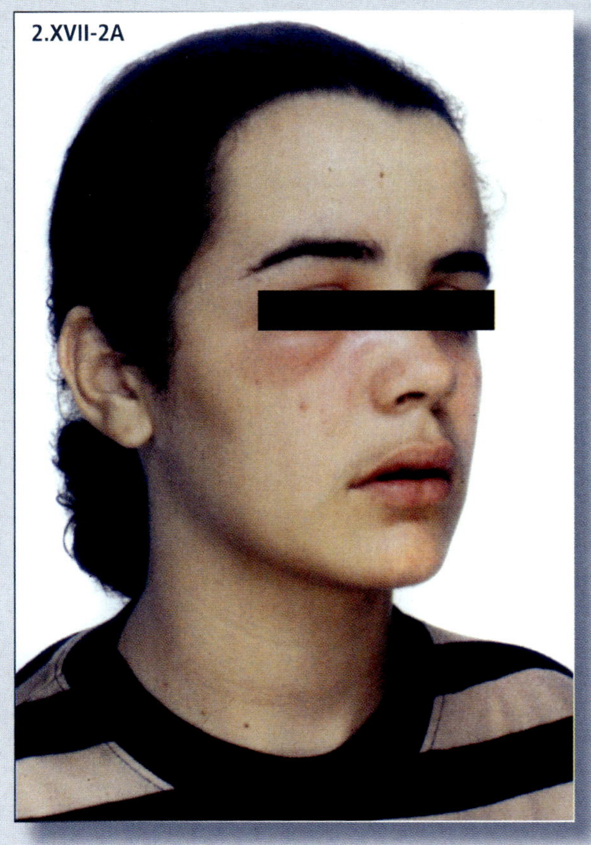
2.XVII-2A

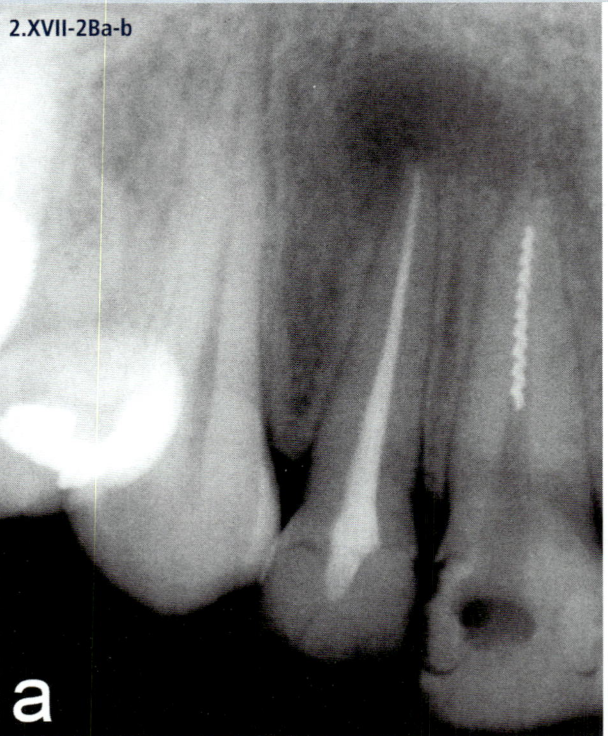
2.XVII-2Ba-b
a

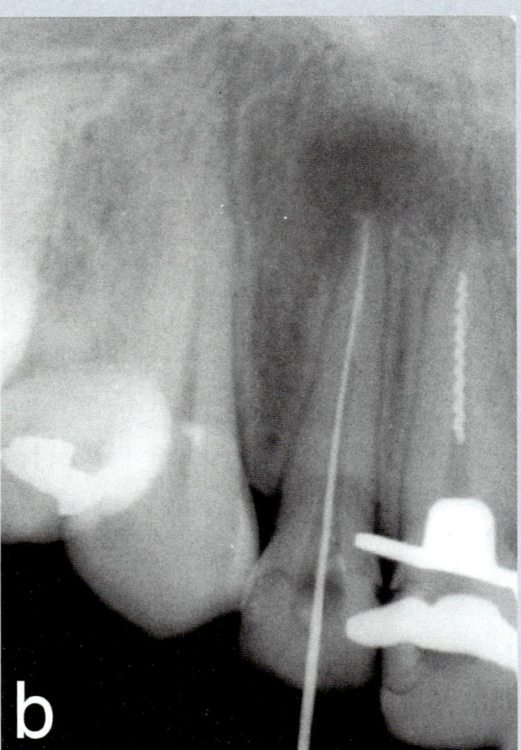
b

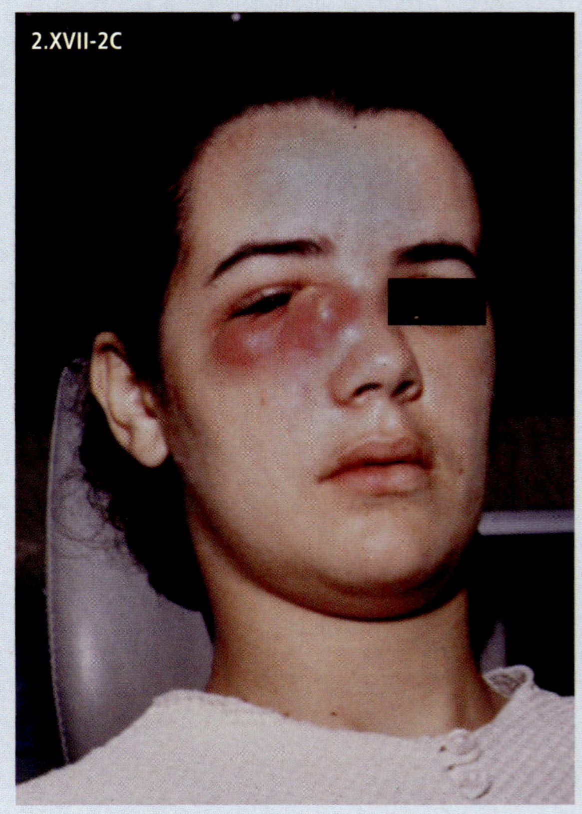
2.XVII-2C

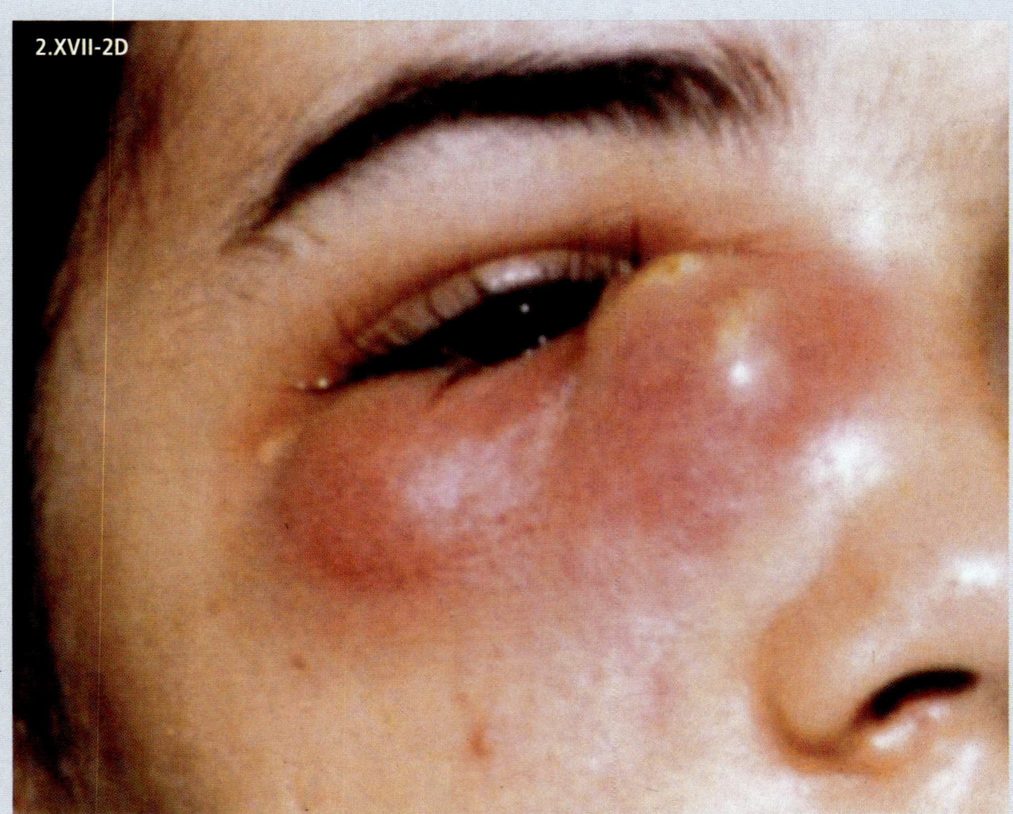
2.XVII-2D

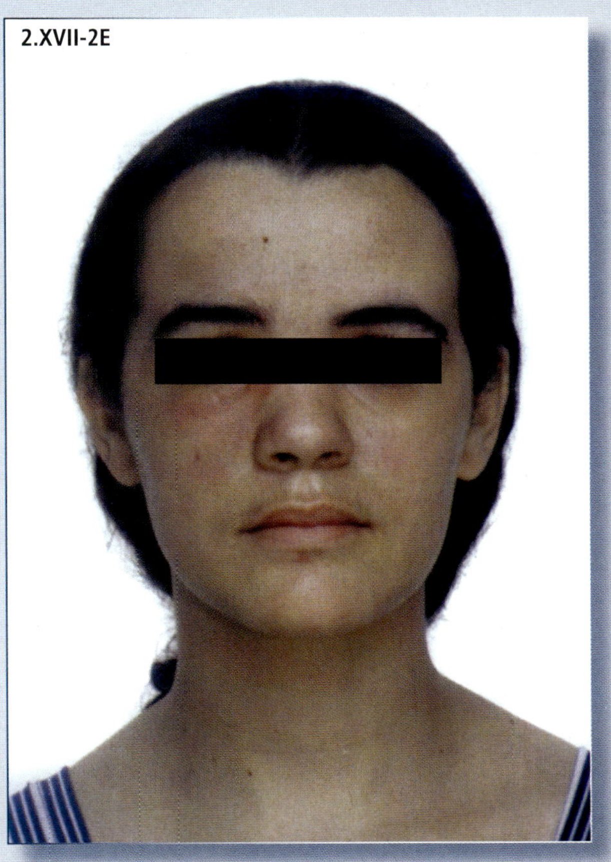
2.XVII-2E

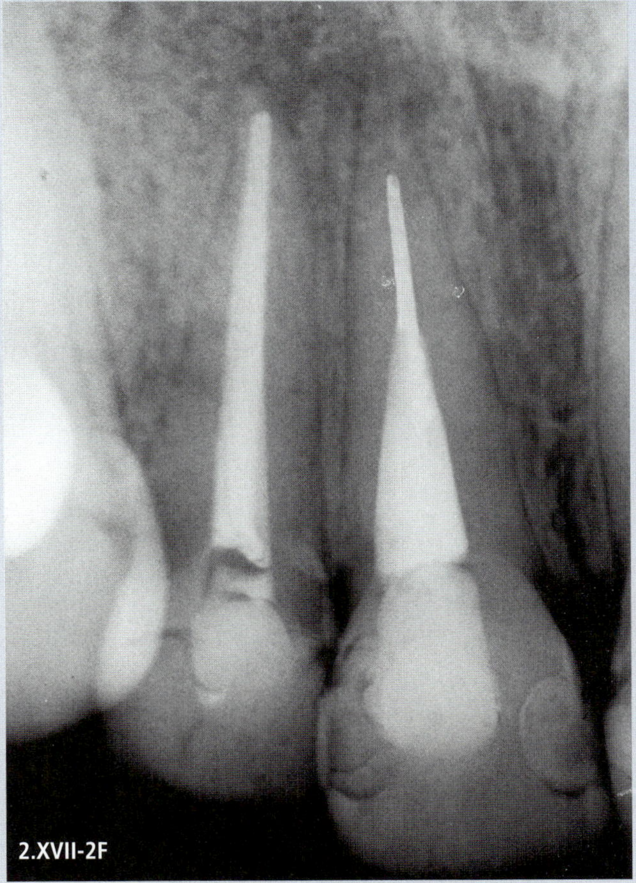
2.XVII-2F

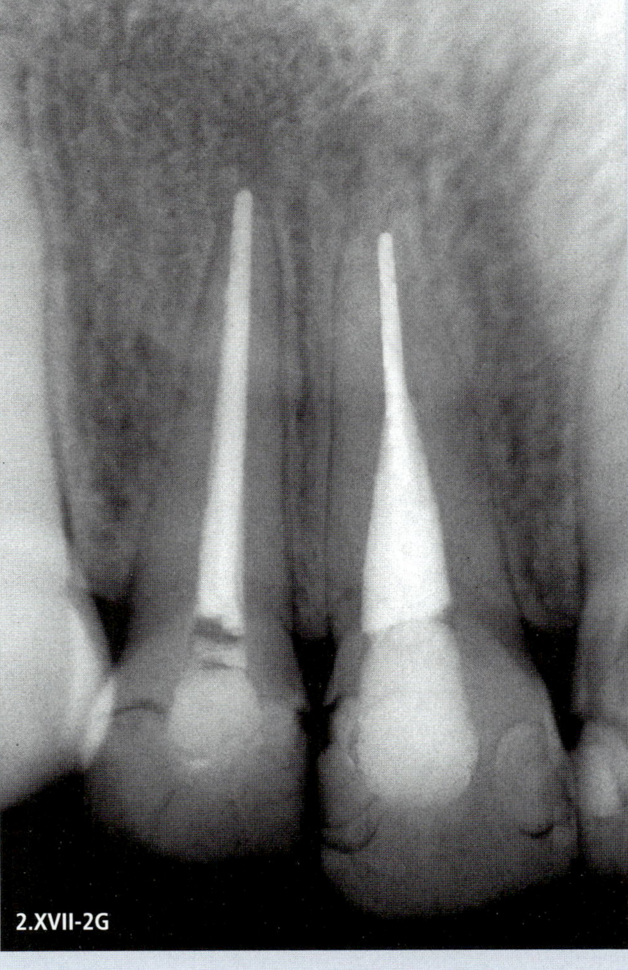
2.XVII-2G

FIGS. 2.XVII-2A-G

A – Clinical aspect of the patient J.F.S., with clinical/radiographic diagnosis of Fenix abscess in the developmental stage (***flare-up***), approximately 6 hours after root canal filling of tooth 1.2, in a single session[10].

Ba – Periapical radiograph of tooth 1.2, showing diffuse rarefaction osteitis, suggesting chronic dentoalveolar abscess that became acute during operative procedures. Note the root canal filling, performed in the same treatment session (29/7/1998 at approximately 10 o'clock).

Bb – Periapical radiograph of tooth 1.2. Removal of obstruction to drain the abscess via the root canal (29/7/1998 at 16 o'clock).

C – Clinical view of the patient J.F.S., the day after emergency treatment (30/7/1998 at 8 o'clock) with diagnosis of a developed Fenix abscess (***flare-up***), in spite of local emergency treatment and systemic medication prescribed the day before.

D – Higher magnification of the clinical features of the previous figure.

E – Clinical view of the patient 72 hours after emergency treatment and systemic medication (Clavulin, 500 mg tabs, every 8 hours, for seven days). Note that the edema, pathognomonic sign of the Fenix abscess, has practically disappeared. At this time the treatment we call necropulpectomy II was started.

F – Radiographic check-up, one year after root canal retreatment of tooth 1.2. Note radiographic repair of previous periapical lesion.

G – Radiographic check-up, two years after root canal filling of tooth 1.2. Note complete repair of the periapical lesion.

EXPERIMENTAL GROUPS

GROUP I – LPS during all the entire experimental period (60 days) (positive control) (Figs. 2.XVII-3A-D).

GROUP II – 1% sodium hypochlorite solution (Fig. 2.XVII-4).

GROUP III – 2.5% sodium hypochlorite solution (Labarraque solution) (Figs. 2.XVII-5 A-B).

GROUP IV – 5.25% sodium hypochlorite solution (USP standard solution) (Figs. 2.XVII-6A-B).

GROUP V – 2% chlorhexidine gluconate solution (Fig. 2.XVII-7).

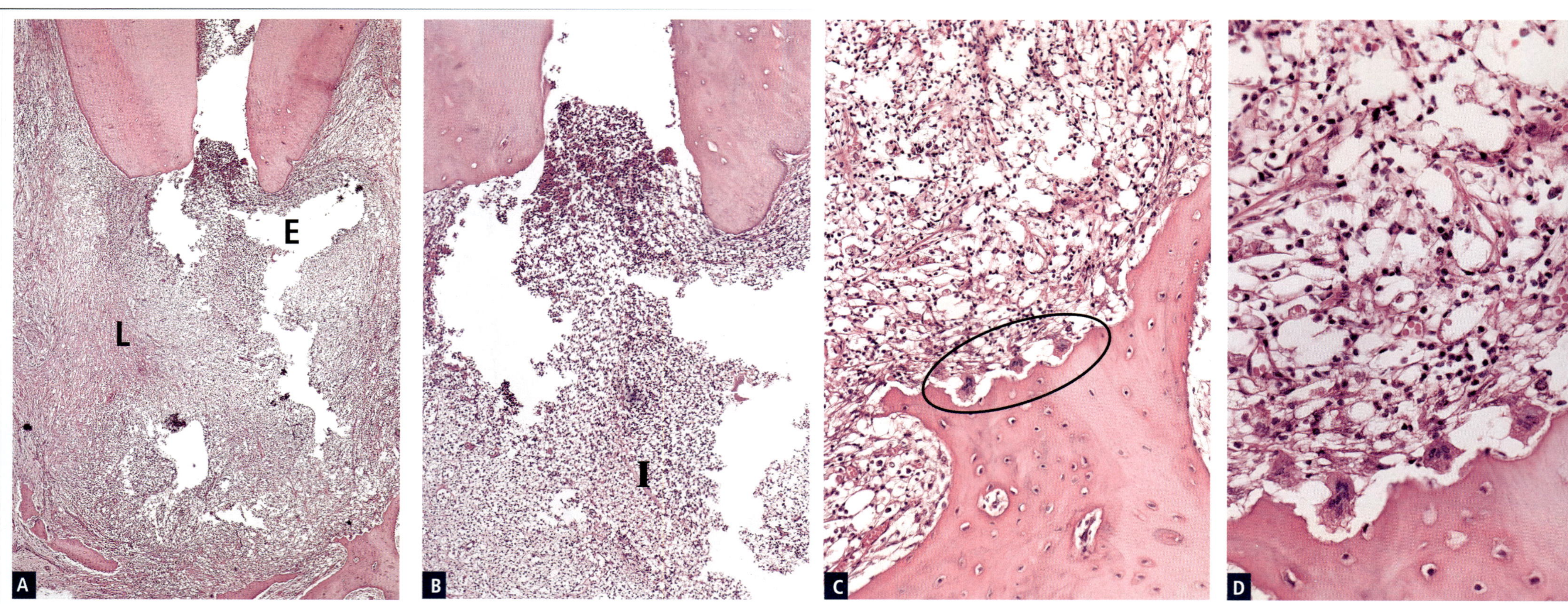

FIGS. 2.XVII-3A-D

A – Group I bacterial LPS (positive control) – Histological section of periapical and apical region of a dog tooth, 60 days after placing bacterial LPS (Escherichia coli-LPS) for 10 days. Note resorption of apical cement, severe mixed inflammatory infiltrate, diffused and abscessed areas (E). Periodontal ligament (L) severely thickened. (H&E stain 40X)

B – Detail of previous figure, highlighting intense inflammatory infiltrate (I) in the periapical region. (H&E stain 100X)

C – Detail of previous figure (circle), showing areas of bone resorption, with emphasis on the osteoclasts in activity. (H&E stain 200X).

D – Higher magnification of the previous figure (circle), highlighting the activated osteoclasts near the resorption area. (H&E stain 400X)[11].

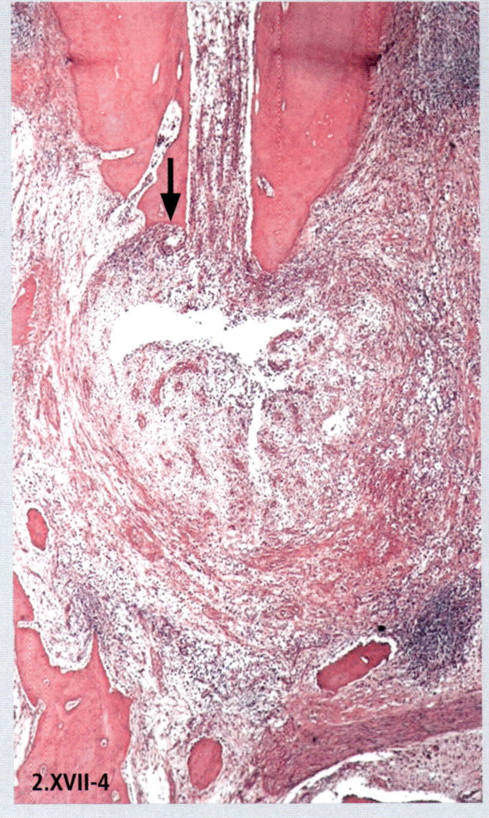

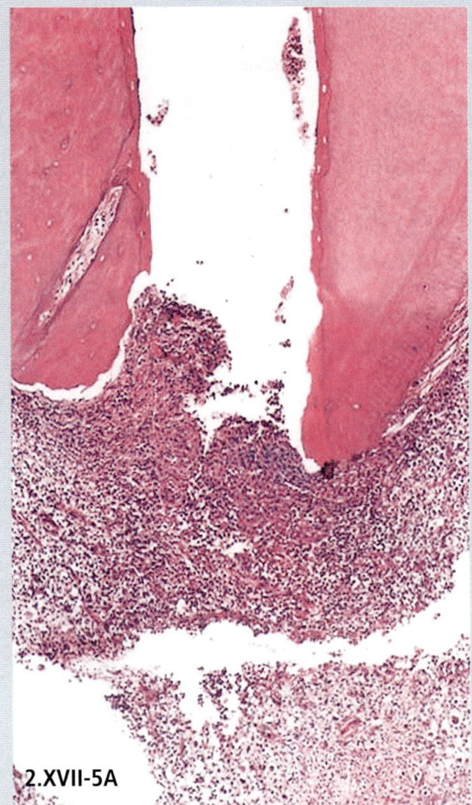

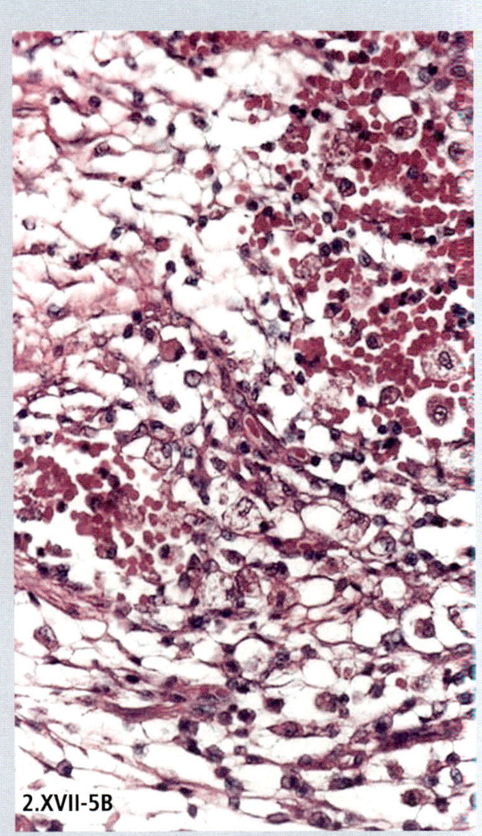

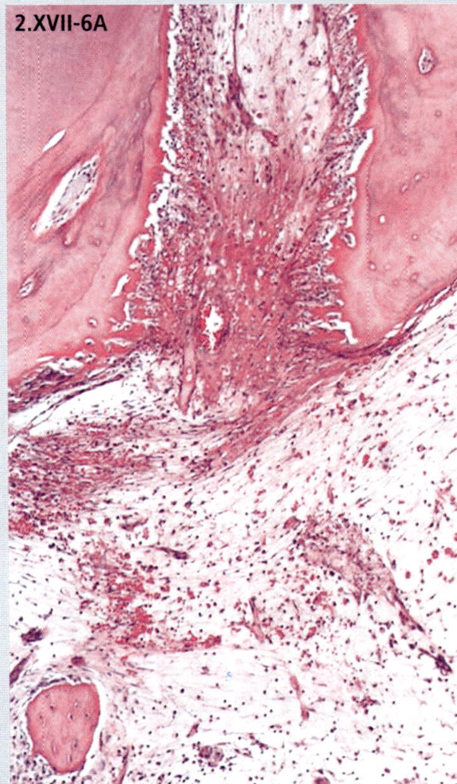

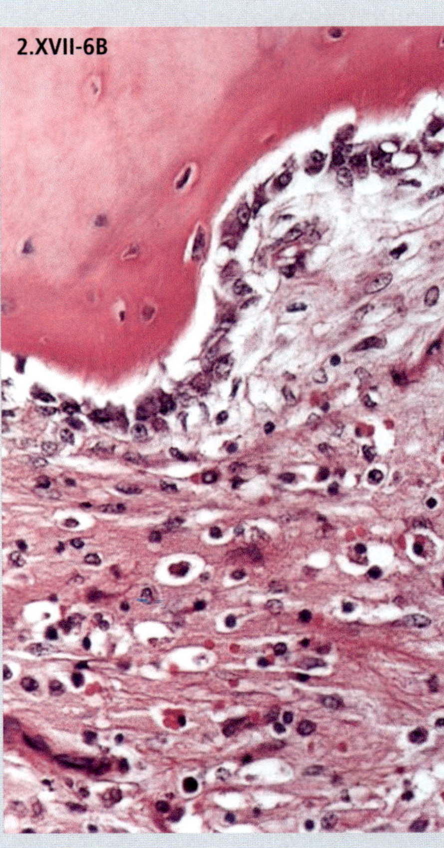

FIG. 2.XVII-4

Group II – 1% sodium hypochlorite solution – Histological section of the periapical and apical region of a dog tooth root canal obtained after 60 days during which time bacterial LPS remained for 10 days. It was then irrigated with 1% sodium hypochlorite solution. Note resorption of apical cement (arrow), with severe thickening of apical periodontal ligament, with extensive mixed diffused inflammatory infiltrate. (H&E stain 40X)[11].

FIGS. 2.XVII-5A-B

A – Group III – 2.5% sodium hypochlorite solution (Labarraque solution – 60 days of observation) – Histologic section of periapical and apical regions of a dog tooth in which the bacterial LPS remained in the root canal for 10 days. After irrigation with 2.5% sodium hypochlorite solution was performed. Note areas of resorption of apical cement and at the foramen, as well as a severe inflammatory infiltrate. Thickening of apical periodontal ligament. (H&E stain 40)
B – Magnification of previous figure, showing inflammatory cells and collagen fibers at a distance from the foramen. (H&E stain 100X[11])

FIGS. 2.XVII-6A-B

A – Group IV – 5.25% sodium hypochlorite solution (USP – 60 days of observation) – Histological section of periapical and apical region of the dog tooth in which bacterial LPS remained for 10 days and after irrigating the root canal with 5.25% sodium hypochlorite solution (USP). Note apical region with moderate inflammatory infiltrate of the mononuclear type. Presence of collagen fiber matrix with few inflammatory cells, at a distance from apical foramen. (H&E stain 40X)
B – Higher magnification of the previous figure, showing moderate inflammatory infiltrate in the periapical region. (H&E Stain100X[11])

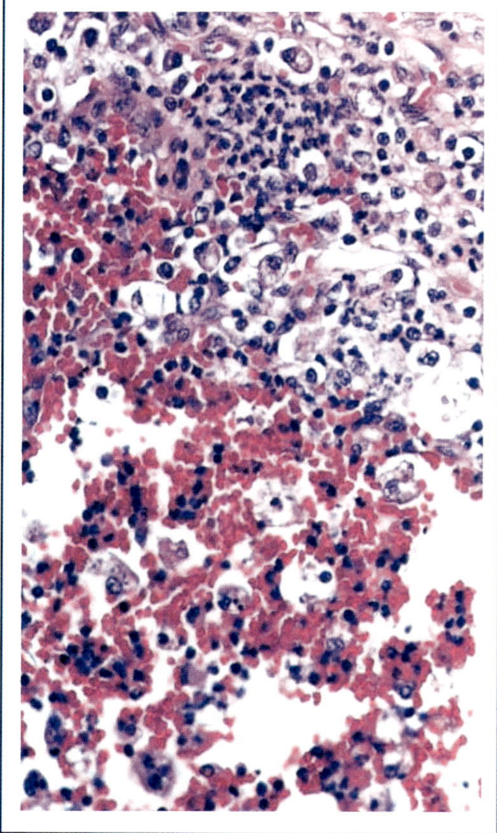

FIG. 2.XVII-7

Group V – 2% chlorhexidine gluconate solution (USP) – Histological section of periapical and apical region of the dog tooth in which bacterial LPS remained for 10 days and after irrigating the root canal with 2% chlorhexidine gluconate solution. Note apical and periapical region with inflammatory infiltrate of moderate to severe intensity. (H&E stain 100X[11])

After irrigation of the root canals with the above-mentioned solutions, the canals were dried, first by means of aspiration and next with sterile paper points. The coronal openings were restored with glass ionomer and silver amalgam.

After the experimental period (60 days), the animals were killed with an anesthetic overdose and routine laboratory procedures were used to obtain serial histologic sections of the apical and periapical region, which were stained with hematoxylin and eosin.

The comparative histopathological evaluation showed that only in the group in which a concentrated solution of 5.25% sodium hypochlorite was used (USP)the inflammatory infiltrate of the periapical region was less intense and that repair collagen fibers were already present.

In 2003, Tanomaru *et al.*[15] also conducted a comparative study of the action of different irrigation solutions and confirmed the results reported by SILVA *et al.*[11]. In this *in vivo* study, which was also conducted in dog's teeth, after pulp removal and irrigation with physiological saline, the canals were filled with bacterial LPS, left in for a week and were then submitted to the detoxification techniques in a crown/apex direction, without pressure, using the following irrigation solutions:

GROUP I - 1% sodium hypochlorite solution.
GROUP II - 2.5% sodium hypochlorite solution (Labarraque solution).
GROUP III - Sodium hypochlorite solution at a concentration of 5%.
GROUP IV - 2% chlorhexidine gluconate solution.
GROUP V - (positive control) – Physiological solution.

Note: After the endodontic operative procedure, using the different irrigant solutions mentioned, the coronal openings were sealed with glass ionomer and restored with silver amalgam. After histopathological analysis of the periapical and apical region, 60 days after the operative procedure, the authors concluded that the different irrigant solutions were not capable of completely inactivating LPS, but the concentrated solution of 5% sodium hypochlorite offered the best results (Figs. 2.XVII-8, 2.XVII-9A-B and 2.XVII-10A-B).

Therefore, based on the favorable results obtained with the concentrated solution of 5.25% sodium hypochlorite (USP), it became the irrigation solution indicated by us in the technique for detoxify the septic/toxic content of the root canal in cases of necropulpectomies II. It should be emphasized that at this stage, we do not indicate the use of physiological saline, distilled water or Dakin solution (0,5% sodium hypochlorite solution). The latter is no longer recommended due to its very limited shelf life.

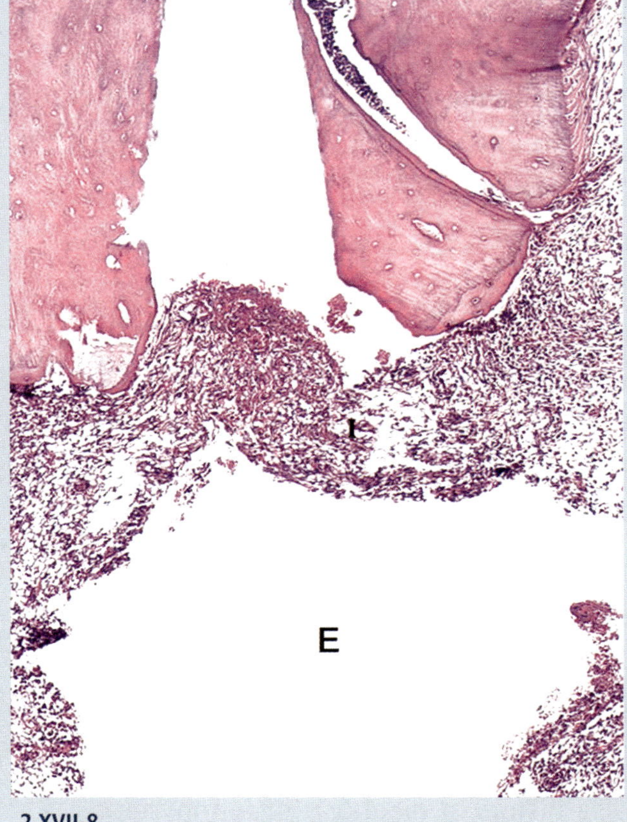

2.XVII-8

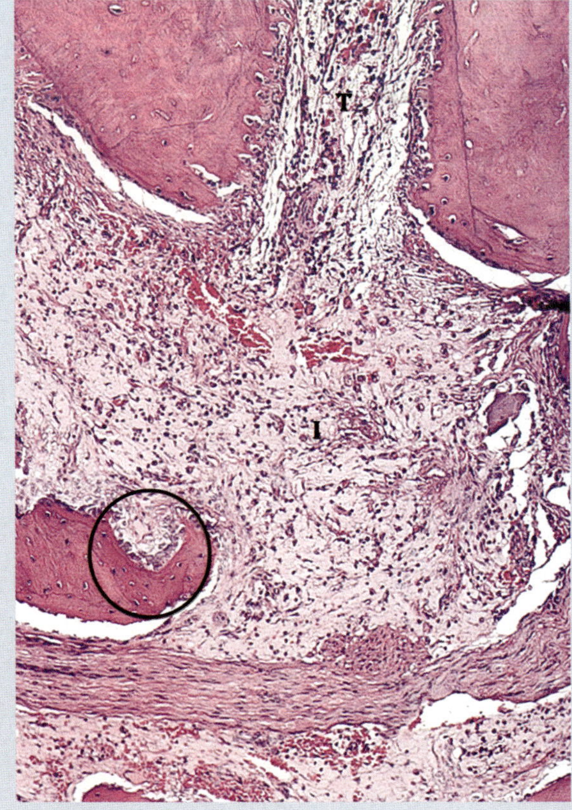

2.XVII-9A

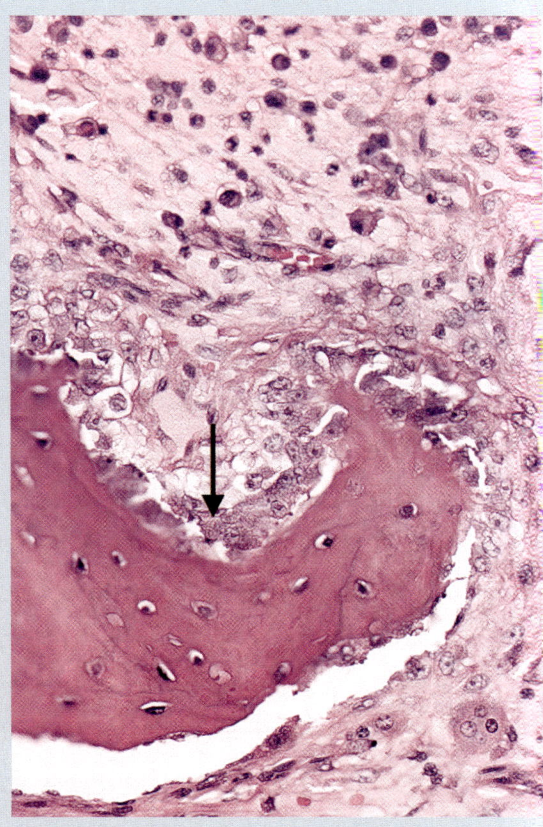

2.XVII-9B

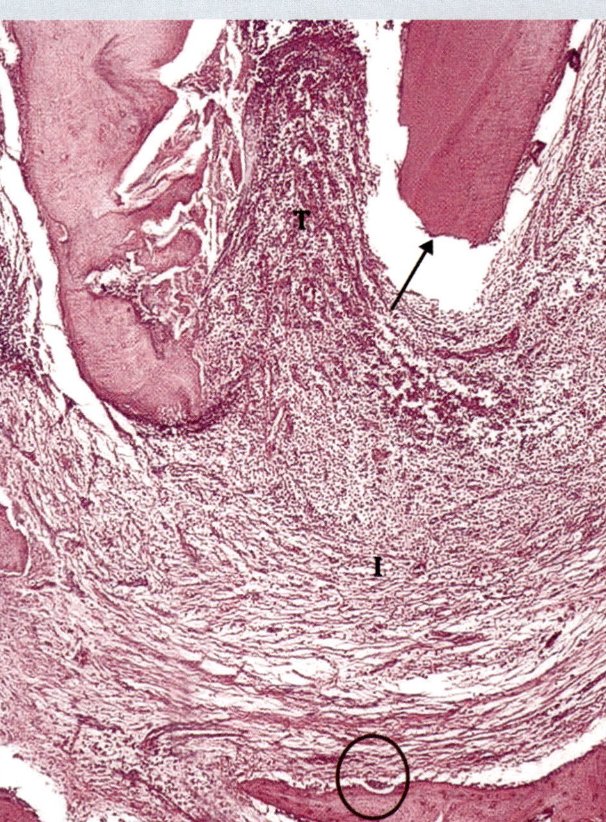

2.XVII-10A

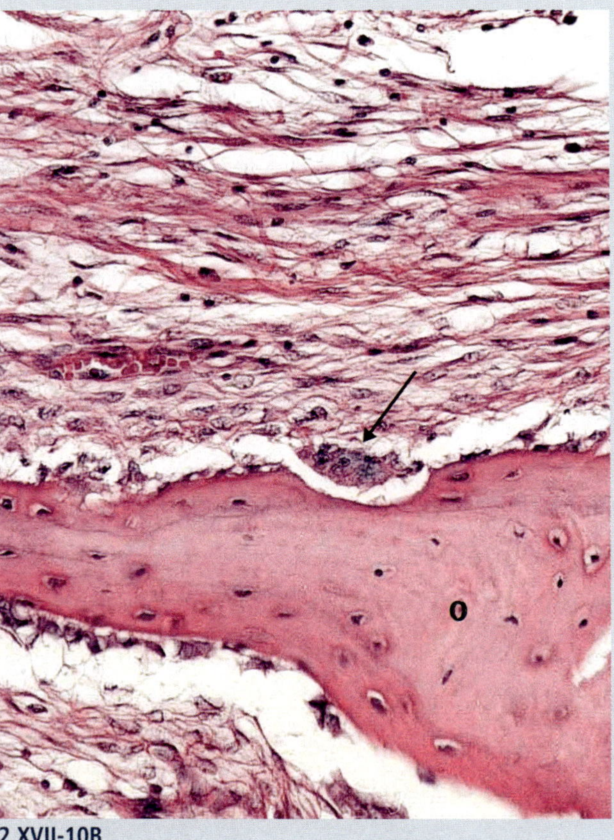

2.XVII-10B

FIG. 2.XVII-8

Group II – 2.5% sodium hypochlorite solution (Labarraque solution) – Histological section of periapical and apical region of the dog in which bacterial LPS remained in the root canal for a week and after irrigation with 2.5% sodium hypochlorite solution, showing severe and intense inflammatory infiltrate (I). Generalized edema (E). (H&E stain 40X[15])

FIGS. 2.XVII-9A-B

A – Group III – 5% sodium hypochlorite solution – Histological section of periapical and apical region of the dog in which bacterial LPS remained for one week and after irrigating the root canal with 5% sodium hypochlorite solution. Note moderate inflammatory reaction (I) and presence of collagen fibers (T) outlining the inflammatory process. (H&E stain 40X)

B – Magnification of the previous figure (circle), showing moderate mononuclear inflammatory infiltrate. Areas of bone resorption (arrow)[15].

FIGS. 2.XVII-10A-B

A – Group IV – 2% chlorhexidine gluconate solution – Histological section of periapical and apical region of the dog tooth in which bacterial LPS remained for one week and after irrigating the root canal with 2% chlorhexidine gluconate solution. Note apical periodontal ligament, containing mixed and diffuse inflammatory infiltrate (I). Irregular presence of collagen fibers (T). Areas of cement resorption (arrow). (H&E stain 40X)

B – Magnification of the previous figure (circle), showing bone resorption with osteoclasts (arrow). (H&E stain 100X[15])

Because 5.25% sodium hypochlorite is a highly concentrated solution and consequently an irritant to periapical tissues, its use must be limited to the temporary working length (TWL). The TWL is obtained by means of diagnostic radiographs, by diminishing the apparent tooth length by about 2 to 3 mm for safety, since we still do not know the real tooth length (RTL). After working length determination and obtaining the RTL, sodium hypochlorite solution diluted to 2.5% (Labarraque solution) must be used with the purpose of neutralizing the toxic/septic content of the **apical five millimeters**. At this concentration, the solution is considered biologically compatible with the periapical tissues in cases of necropulpectomies II, because they present a defense granulomatous tissue, which is the periapical reaction. In these cases, neutralization must be performed by using the foramen apical instrument (FAI) to the real tooth length (RTL) with the purpose of performing foramen debridement.

After foramen debridement and while the apical stop is being made (a critical time in biological endodontics) the Labarraque solution continues to be used until the conclusion of biomechanical preparation.

In spite of not completely detoxifying the endotoxins, the concentrated sodium hypochlorite solution (5.25% – USP) continues to be the irrigation solution of choice worldwide for the operative stage that precedes biomechanical preparation of the root canal in cases of necropulpectomies II.

Note: Because of the high concentration of the sodium hypochlorite solution indicated by us, 5.25%, its use must be limited to the temporary working length (TWL). For the same reason, this solution **must never be injected in the root canal**, but taken applied slowly without excessively pressing the plunger of the syringe. This procedure must be performed with the index finger and not with the thumb. Thus, we limit the action of the product inside the root canal and without the risk of extravasating it into the periapical region. The interaction between the high concentration of sodium hypochlorite solution and the living or necrotic organic tissues occurs rapidly, releasing nascent chloride and oxygen in an effervescent and energetic manner. In the periapical region, this effervescence is responsible for the occurrence of emphysemas.

Case Report of Emphysema granted by Dr. Ruth Fuentes de Serme–o M.D.S., Prof. Dr. Henry W. Herrera, endodontist, and Helen de Herrera M.D.S., San Salvador, El Salvador

The patient Concepción López de Sanchez, a 65-year-old housewife, from San Salvador, El Salvador – San Jacinto, sought emergency treatment at the "Hospital 1º de Maio", San Salvador, for treatment on August 15th, 2006.

By means of a case history, a diagnosis of emphysema, as a result of a large **accidental extravasation** of 5% sodium hypochlorite solution into the periapical region, was made. The accident occurred in a private practice during root canal treatment of tooth 1.3 (right maxillary canine).

The patient who suffered from medication-induced hepatic cirrhosis, diabetes mellitus type 2 and controlled hypertension, while in hospital, was administered 500 mg amoxicillin (antibiotic prophylaxis) every 8 hours.

Clinically, the patient presented with ecchymosis and facial edema (emphysema), which developed from the right hemifacial region, to the neck, making it difficult for her to open her right eye. Clinical examination revealed slight pain on palpation of the affected region, pain on percussion and mobility (class 2) of #1.3, (Figs. 2.XVII-11A-G).

A periapical radiograph revealed a slight thickening of the apical periodontal ligament.

After diagnosis, the patient was referred to the Maxillofacial Surgery Department of the hospital for systemic evaluation. After detailed examination, therapy was recommended to control her systemic problems and the patient was discharged on August 30th, and advised to continue with root canal treatment.

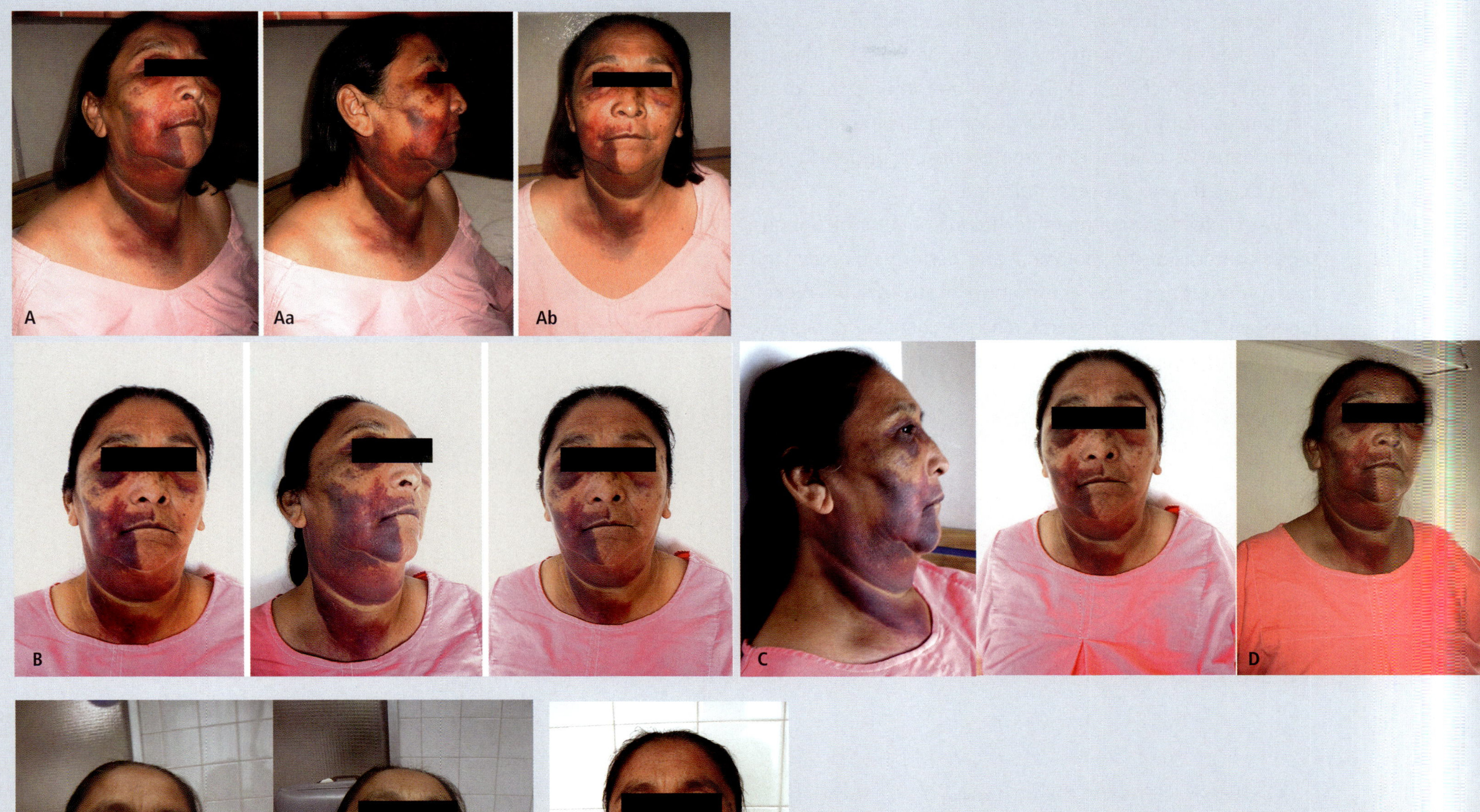

FIGS. 2.XVII-11A-G

A, Aa and Ab – Clinical view of patient C.L.S. (San Salvador – El Salvador), showing ecchymosis and emphysema, 48 hours after operative incident in which 5% sodium hypochlorite was accidentally extruded into the periapical region of tooth 1.3, which was undergoing endodontic treatment.
B – Clinical view: 3 days after operative incidence.
C – Clinical view: 4 days after incidence.
D – Clinical view: 5 days after incidence,
E – Clinical view: 15 days after incidence.
F – Clinical view: 30 days after incidence.
G – Clinical view: 55 days after incidence.

Note: Considering that sodium hypochlorite, even with a concentration of 5.25%, only partially neutralizes the endotoxins, it is important that the practitioner has sufficient technical skills when performing this procedure, to prevent toxic substances from inadvertently reaching the periapical region, thereby avoiding post-operative pain and/or acute chronic periapical abscesses, which Samuel Seltzer called Fenix abscesses (*flare-up*).

We prefer the treatment technique that simultaneously neutralize the toxic/septic contents of the root canal and performs biomechanical preparation. Among these techniques, we recommend motor-driven nickel/titanium instruments (Chapter 2.X – Rotary systems) and mechanical/manual techniques (*see* Chapters 2.I and 2.IV), which apply the crown/apex principle without pressure.

References

1. Assed S, Ito IY, Leonardo MR, Silva LAB, Lopatin D.E. Anaerobic microrganisms in root canal of human teeth with chronic apical periodontitis detected by immunofluorescent. Endod Dent Traumatol, v.12, p.66-69, 1996.
2. Dahlén G, Magnusson BC, Moller A. Histological and histochemical study of the influence of lipopolysaccharide extracted from Fusobacterium nucleatum on the periapical tissues in the monkey Macaca fasciculoris. Archs Oral Biol, v.26, p.591-8, 1981.
3. Goerig AC, Michelich RJ, Schultz HH. Instrumentation of root canals in molar using the step down technique. J. Endod., v.8, n.12, p.550-557, 1982.
4. Leonardo MR, Silva RAB, Assed S, Nelson Filho P. Importance of bacterial endotoxin (LPS) in endodontics. J. Appl. Oral Sci., v.12, n.2, p.93-98, 2004.
5. Marshall FJ, Pappin JA. A crown-down pressureless preparation root canal enlargement technique (Manual). Oregon Health Sciences University. Portland, Oregon-E.U.A., 1980.
6. Mattison GD, Haddix JE, Kehoc JC, Progulske-Fox A. The effect of Eikenella corrodeus endotoxin on periapical bone. J Endod, v.13, p.559-565, 1987.
7. Nelson Filho P. Efeito da endotoxina (LPS), associada ou não ao hidróxido de cálcio, sobre os tecidos apicais e periapicais de dentes de cães (avaliação histopatológica). Tese (doutorado em Odontopediatria). Faculdade de Odontologia de Araraquara – Unesp, 2000.
8. Nelson Filho P, Leonardo MR, Silva LAB, Assed S. Radiographic evaluation of the effect of endotoxin (LPS) plus calcium hydroxide on apical and periapical tissues of dogs. J Endod, v.28, p.644-646, 2002.
9. Pitts DL, Williams BL, Morton Jr TH. Investigation of role of endotoxin in periapical inflammations. J Endod, v.8, p.10-18, 1982.
10. Salgado AAM, Campielo IT, Oliveira Filho RM, Leonardo MR. Desobturação de canal radicular em caso de agudização de lesão periapical crônica (abscesso Fênix). J. Brasil. Endod., v.15, p.291-294, 2003.
11. Silva LAB, Leonardo MR, Assed S, Tanomaru Filho M. Histological study of the effect of some irrigant solution on bacterial endotoxin in dogs. Braz Dent J, v.15, n.2, p.109-114, 2004.
12. Silva LAB, Nelson Filho P, Leonardo MR, Rossi MA, Pansani CA. Effect of calcium hydroxide on bacterial endotoxin in vivo. J Endod, v.28, p.94, 98, 2002.
13. Siqueira Júnior R. In.(?) PRC methodology as a valuable tool for identification of endodontic pathogens. J Dent, v.31, p.333-339, 2003.
14. Sundqvist G. Ecology of the root canal flora. J Endod, v.18, p.427-430, 1992.
15. Tanomaru JMG, Leonardo MR, Tanomaru Filho M, Bonetti Filho I, Silva LAB. Effect of different irrigation solutions and calcium hydroxide on bacterial LPS. J Endod, v.36, p.7320739, 2003.

2.XVIII

Ergonomics with the use of the operating and surgical microscope in Endodontics

Carlos Garcia Puente
Juan Saavedra

"That which cannot be seen, cannot be treated" (KIM[25])

Most

endodontic procedures demand a high degree of precision, and take place in small, poorly illuminated working areas and success depends on the practitionerís tactile sense, dexterity, imagination and perseverance, as coronal openings are approximately 1 cm^2, and access to root canals vary from 3 mm in diameter in central incisors to 0.06 mm in molars.

Mostly, dentists base their endodontic work on radiographs, which serve as a guide to create an image of the anatomy of the root canal, although tactile sense, with certain limitations, also allow one to approximate a complex clinical reality.

Endodontists usually boast that they are capable of doing a large part of their work blind, due to the fact that "there is nothing to see". In reality, there is a great deal to see, if one has the suitable instruments and training (Fig. 2.XVIII-1).

"That which cannot be seen, cannot be treated". Those are the words of Dr. Syngcuk Kim[25], of the University of Pennsylvania – USA, one of the pioneers in microscopy and microsurgery, and are evidence of the problems we face on a daily basis. A microscope that can magnify and illuminate the operating field, allows treatment to be performed in a detailed and precise manner and helps solving cases that were difficult to treat in the past.

Light + Magnification = EXCELLENCE

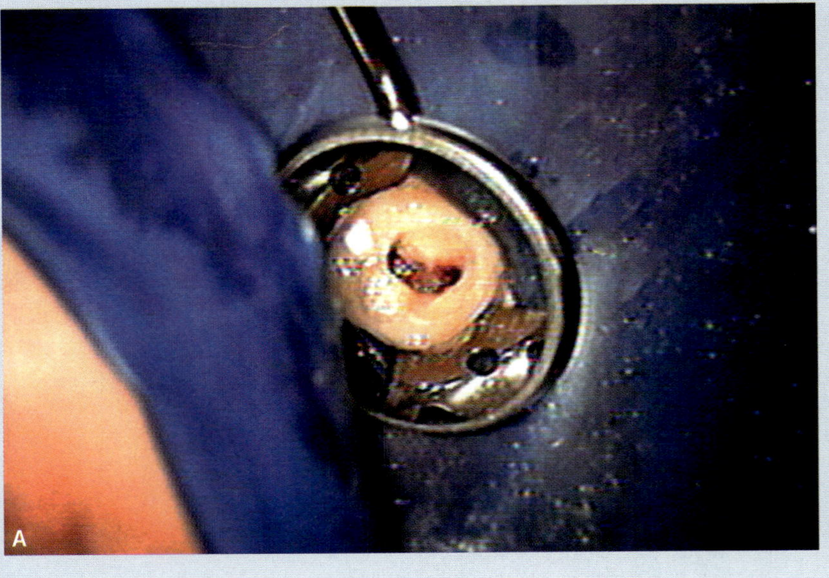

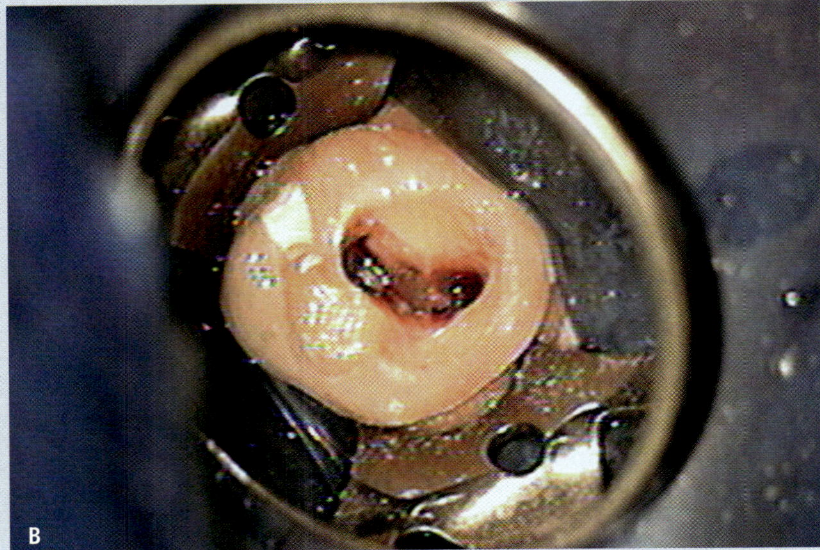

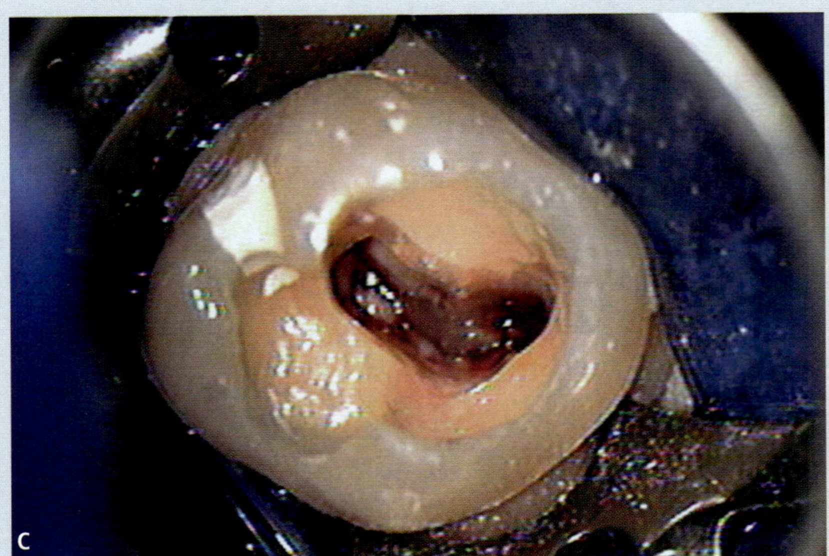

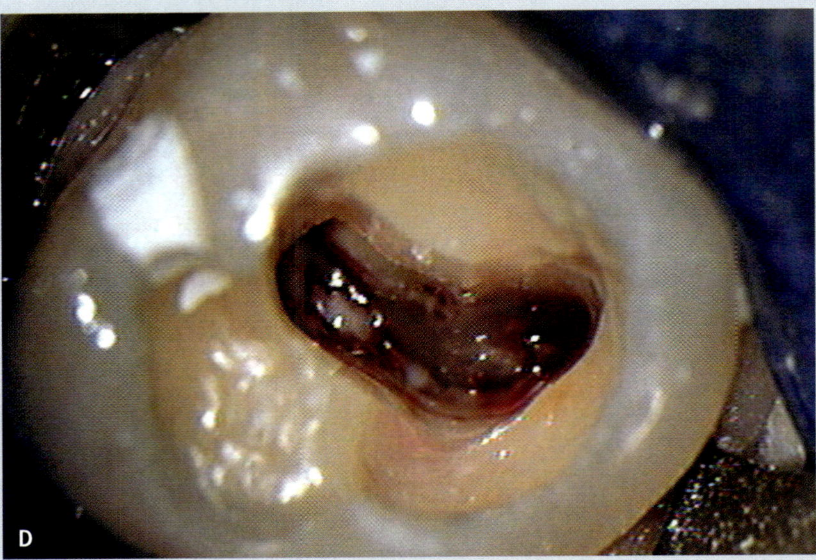

FIGS. 2.XVIII-1A-E

Images obtained with the OM:
A – 3.4x Magnification.
B – 5.1x Magnification.
C – 8.5x Magnification.
D – 13.6x Magnification.
E – 21.25x Magnification.

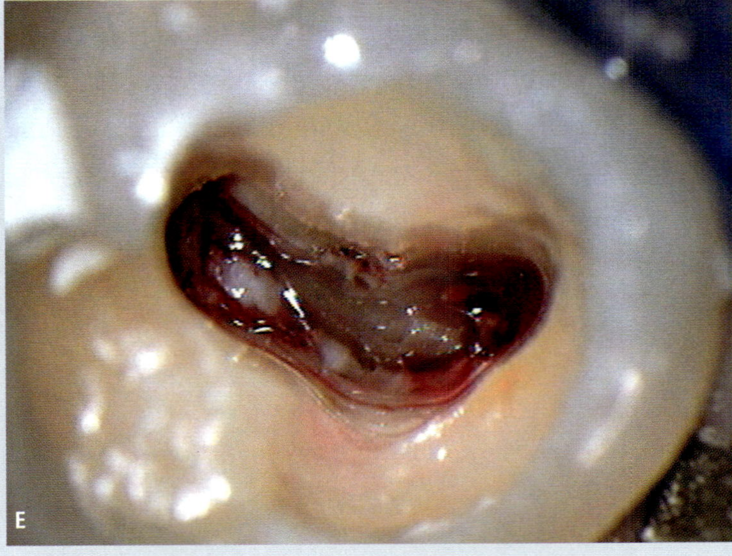

With the introduction of the microscope in endodontics it was called the surgical microscope (SM), since its use was restricted to peri-radicular surgery. At present it is used during various clinical stages in endodontics and is known as the clinical microscope (CLM) or operating microscope (OM).

Its use in conventional endodontics has made it safer and has promoted minimally invasive dentistry, as it allows access preparations free of obstructions, easy location of all root canals, enlarging the therapeutic field for the most precise solution of problems such as perforations, location of calcified canals, removal of fractured instruments, posts, or silver cones, detection of cracks (fissures), fractures and apical surgical procedures. Its use has now been extended to periodontics[27], implant dentistry[31,37], dentistry[4] and prosthodontics.

If the knowledge of dental anatomy and tactile skills of the endodontist are combined with adequate technological support, the end result is highly predictable and increases the level of care the patient receives considerably. The advantages of using the OM are magnification and illumination of the operating field, the possibility of documenting the procedures, improvement in ergonomic postures and consequently, increase in the quality of the entire endodontic therapy[42].

The operator feels motivated to use higher magnification in endodontics when, for the first time, he/she sees magnified areas that are difficult or impossible to see with the naked eye. Errors in removal of caries lesions can be detected during the preparation stage of the treatment and easily prevented.

Thus, we can sate that the operating microscope, ultrasound, electronic apex locators, mechanical debridement systems and thermoplastic and adhesive filling techniques have revolutionized endodontics.

Acquisition of an OM must be considered as a serious and responsible investment. Factors such as cost, installation of the equipment in the dental office, optic quality, technical service and the possibility of expansion with documentation systems for photography and video must be taken into account. It is also necessary to consider the cost of instruments especially designed for procedures with the OM, in addition to equipment such as cabinets, ultrasound units and points, and the need for training courses, as one cannot dispense with the inevitable training during the learning stage. In the United States and Europe, microscopic dentistry plays an increasingly important role.

In this chapter, in addition to a description of the possibilities of the OM for routine use and the establishment of the ergonomic principles of its use, the intention is also to motivate the dentist, and particularly the specialist in endodontics, to use it in the majority of his/her clinical procedures.

Microdentistry can be defined as the refinement of dental operative techniques, in which precision increases with the use of optical magnification[15]. At present, any irregularity in the straight portion of the root canal, even when it is in the more apical portion, can easily be seen, approached and treated, using different instruments in conjunction with the OM. With the use of the microscope, tactile sense corroborates the visual gains[33], and the more complex the procedure to be performed, the more justified will be the magnification[31].

The two challenges presently facing endodontists are to elect the advances that bring the greatest benefit to clinical practice, and progress in the learning curve in order to make the technology truly useful and advantageous in daily practice.

Therefore, we can conclude, as Kim[25] did: "whoever sees best works best".

HISTORY

The interest in "seeing more and better" has been demonstrated in dentistry by the use of loupes and headlamps. For many years dentists have been using loupes with 2.5X magnification to aid in dental operative procedures.

The OM began to be integrated into the medical specialty as early as 1957. Ear surgeons were the first to use microscopes and preferred them rather than loupes, because of advantages such as wider surgical field, variable magnification, greater depth of field and coaxial lighting[17]. It was not long before its use was extended to other areas, such as ophthalmology, neurosurgery, plastic surgery and microsurgery in general, in which it is widely used today.

The first publication about the use of the OM in dentistry, by Baumann[3] (an otorhinolaryngologist and dentist) appeared in 1977. Since the end of the 1970s, European and American dentists and endodontists, among them Ducamin & Boussens[18], Apotheker & Jako[1], Selden[45], Belizzi & Loushine[5], Pecora & Andreana[39], Carr[11], among others, have found interesting applications for the OM for daily use, both in endodontics and surgery, magnifying and illuminating their operating fields to resolve cases easily, reliably and predictably, which would have been impossible without a microscope.

The first author to describe the use of the OM in periapical surgery was Carr[10,11], in 1992. Carr, Pecora & Andrena[39] and Rubinstein & Kim[41] were the pillars of strength in the development and use of the OM in surgical procedures. They were followed by Ruddle[42] and others who studied in depth clinical microscopy, and developed techniques and instruments for microendodontics[16]. The use of the OM has been universally standardized and has expanded, as evidenced by the presence of microscopy societies that now exist in numerous countries[47,50].

Given the proliferation of microscopes in the 1990s, numerous theoretical and practical courses are presented to facilitate the understanding of OMs and train professionals in its use. The importance acquired by the OM has led the American Dental Association (ADA) to include it in the standard programs of the Commission on Dental Accreditation (CODA). Thus, at a meeting of directors of post-graduate programs, during the Congress of the American Association of Endodontists (AAE) in Chicago in 1995, it was decided to make it mandatory to teach OM techniques in all graduate programs in Endodontics, effective in1998, in compliance with *The Standards for Advanced Specialty Education Programs in Endodontics* in the United States[44].

COMPONENTS OF THE OM

One of the features of the OM is its versatility, the possibility of making modifications and/or adding accessories to its basic configuration.

A basic configuration includes the following:

- 5 magnification stages
- 10X oculars.
- Objective of 200 or 250 mm.
- Halogen light source.

The most commonly used accessories are:

- Tiltable binoculars.
- *Beam splitter* 50/50 (various, for image documentation).
- Photographic and/or video camera.
- Motorized *Zoom*.
- Second auxiliary ocular.
- Xenon lamp source of illumination.

All OMs do not have the same features nor are they identically manufactured. Some designs provide greater flexibility, meeting various requirements of the dentist, who commonly schedules and prepares quadrants or a complete arch in a single session. The endodontist works in a smaller operating field.

The features of an OM for endodontics are the following (Fig. 2.XVIII-2):

1. Excellent optics.
2. Abundant illumination.
3. Easy handling and flexibility.
4. Tiltable binoculars to improve the operator's posture and comfort.
5. Stability to reduce microtremors and movements.
6. Filters to prevent the polymerization of photosensitive restorative materials.

As the configuration of the OM varies per manufacturer, as well as the accessories that can be included, there are fundamental components, namely:

- Stator components.
- Magnification system.
- Oculars.
- Objective.
- Lighting system.

Stator components

Stator is the name given to the mechanical components that allows the OM to be mounted so that it is fixed to the ceiling, a wall or a mobile stand. The latter allows it to be moved. The majority of users prefer to attach it to the ceiling or a wall, since this reduces pendulum movement and increases ergonomics.

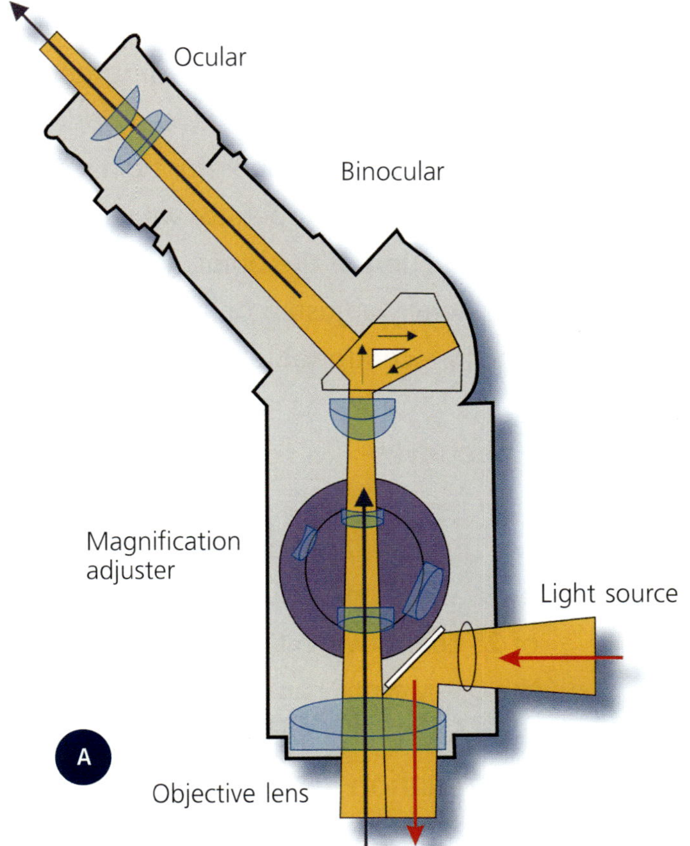

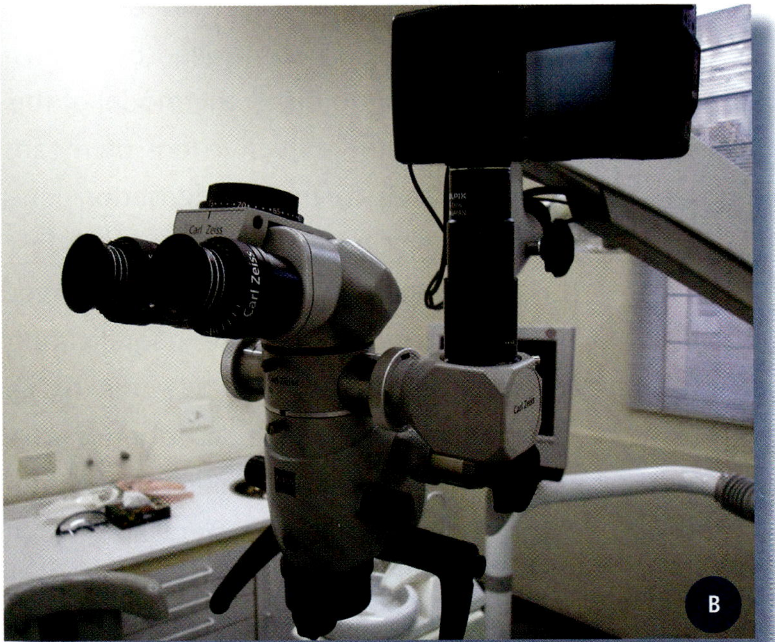

FIGS. 2.XVIII-2A-B

A – Diagram showing how an OM works.
B – Typical configuration of an OM, including a photographic camera and digital video.

Oculars

These are two lenses mounted in tubes (binoculars) through which the operator looks. The oculars generally have dioptic adjustments, in dioptic values of -5 and +5, and serve to accommodate the operator's individual eyesight condition? On the outside is a rubber ring, which is removed if the operator wears glasses. There are oculars with power of x6.3; x10; x12.5; x16; x20. The function of the binoculars is to support the oculars and provide interpupillar distance, which is generally adjusted on a scale (Fig. 2.XVIII-3). They can be fixed at 45° or be tiltable, which allows for more comfortable ergonomic positions (Fig. 2.XVIII-4).

Objectives

These are a set of lenses with focal lengths that range from 100 to 400 mm. A 400 mm objective focuses on a distance of 40 cm. The one most frequently used is 250 mm, which allows a distance of 25 cm between the objective and the working plane. This distance provides sufficient space for the operator to handle the instruments and work comfortably.

Illumination

Illumination is provided by a halogen lamp of at least 150 W, which intensity can be adjusted, and is controlled by means of a rheostat and cooled by air. The light source location varies depending on the model of the OM. In the current models the light is conducted from the source to the objective lens by means of fiber optics.

Thanks to the condensation lens, the light is reflected in a series of prisms and reaches the operating (surgical) field through the objective. The return path of the light, which reflects the image of what it being observed, once again crosses the objective, passing through the lenses for adjusting the magnification of the binoculars, and reaches the operator's eyes as two separate luminous bands – it is this separation that produces the stereoscopic effect that allows the clinician to have an optimum quality of vision (Fig. 2.XVIII-5).

The OM has coaxial lighting; that is, parallel to the line of vision, which allows the operator to observe an operating (surgical) field without shadows. The parallel light enables the operator's eyes to remain at rest, as if observing infinity, which helps performing prolonged observations without eye fatigue.

When a beam splitter for image documentation is incorporated, the quantity of light reaching the operator's eyes is diminished.

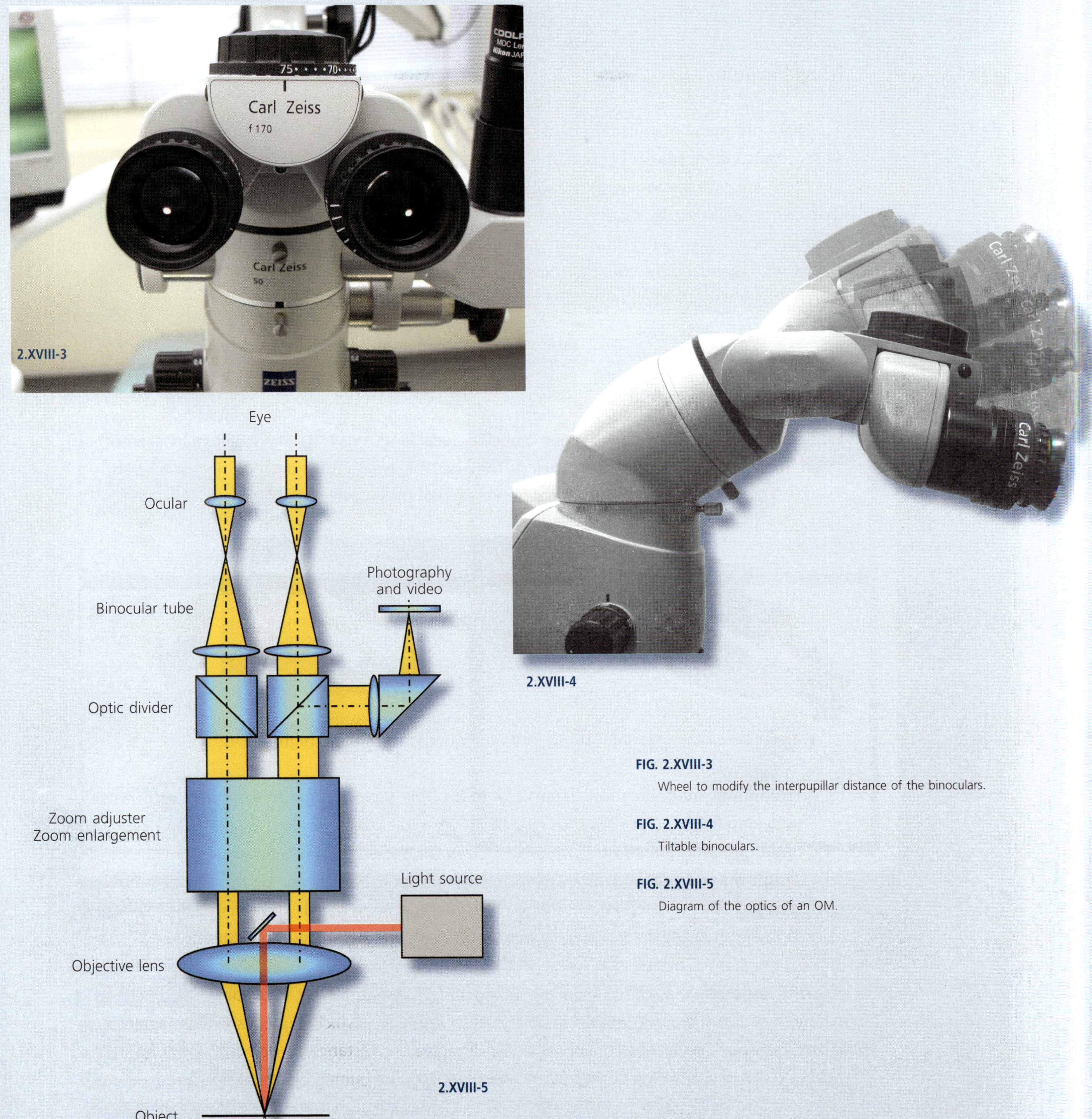

FIG. 2.XVIII-3
Wheel to modify the interpupillar distance of the binoculars.

FIG. 2.XVIII-4
Tiltable binoculars.

FIG. 2.XVIII-5
Diagram of the optics of an OM.

Magnification

There are many manufacturers of OM, but in general, they all have a stable fixation device, stereoscopic vision, coaxial lighting and variable magnifications.

There are simple models that have three fixed magnifications and standardized movements that can be adjusted by friction brakes, and complete models that have progressive motorized zoom capabilities, with full movement and a magnetic stabilizer. Many OMs have magnification in stages, with manual or motorized adjustments, and control pedals.

The total magnification of the OM can be calculated by using the following formula[24]:

$$\text{TOTAL MAGNIFICATION} = \frac{\text{Binocular focal length x Ocular manipulation factor x Magnification Factor}}{\text{Objective focal length}}$$

For example, for an OM with mean binocular focal length of 170 mm, objective focal length of 250 mm and a 12.5x magnification factor of the oculars, with a magnification ring of 5 levels (0.4, 0.6, 1.0, 1.6 and 2.5), the real magnification for each of these levels would be:

MAGNIFICATION FACTOR	TOTAL MAGNIFICATION
0.4	3.40x
0.6	5.10x
1.0	8.50x
1.6	13.60x
2.5	21.25x

We can classify the magnifications into minimum, medium and high.

- **Minimum magnification:** From 2.5x to 8x. This serves to guide the operator in a wide working field;
- **Medium magnification:** From 8x to 16x, which is used for precision work;
- **High magnification:** From 16x up to the maximum, which can be from 32x to 40x. This magnification is used for observing more subtle, refined details, however, at the expense of the depth of the field. Generally one works at medium and low magnifications.

Carr[10] reported that the human eye is capable of distinguishing two points separated by a minimum of 200 microns (0.2 mm), an ability called resolution, which improves when magnification and illumination are increased. Lenses of 2x diminish the distance of points recognized at 100 microns (0.1 mm); lenses of 4x, improve the resolution of the human eye to 50 microns (0.05 mm).

DEGREE OF MAGNIFICATION, RESOLUTION (mm)

MAGNIFICATION SYSTEM	DEGREE OF MAGNIFICATION	RESOLUTION (MICRONS)	RESOLUTION (mm)
Human eye	0x	200	0.2
Simple Lenses (loupes)	1.5x	133.33	0.133
Lenses (low magnification loupes)	2.5x	80	0.08
Lenses (medium magnification loupes)	4.0x	50	0.05
Probe	0x	36	0.036
Microscope – low magnification	6.4x	31	0.031
Microscope – medium magnification	10x	20	0.02
Microscope – high magnification	20x	10	0.01

Dentists need to distinguish details that are beyond the resolution of the human eye, such as early caries lesions, defects of the cavo surface ridge, evaluation of the coronal margin and microfissures, which are difficult to diagnose without an increase in natural visual capacity. Various studies have shown that a skilled clinician, using a sharp pointed explorer, can detect points separated by 36 microns.

DIFFERENCES BETWEEN LENSES (LOUPES) AND MICROSCOPES

FEATURES	LOUPES (LENSES)	MICROSCOPES
Power	3x on an average	Between 3x and 30x
Number of magnifications	Generally one	Mean of 5 (3x, 6x, 9x, 12x and 20x)
Weight:	Heavy (with 5x magnification)	Without weight
Cost	Low	High
illumination	Without illumination (can be incorporated)	Fiber optic in the system in coaxial form (in the same axis of vision)
Documentation	Does not allow it	Photography and video

Documentation

In addition to offering illumination and image magnification, the OM allows clinical documentation, by means of obtaining and storing (filing) of images recorded during the surgical operative procedures. Previously traditional 35 mm reflex photographic cameras were used, which required a *flash* because the light was insufficient to expose the films. At present, digital cameras are used, which surpass the previous cameras because of their high luminosity, operability, size and weight. Although they are unable to equal the quality of a 35 mm photograph, there are reflex digital cameras of 10 and 12 megapixels on the market.

Digital cameras for photos also have video outputs that allow connection to monitors on which the image of the OM can be observed (Fig. 2.XVIII-6). For greater sharpness when taking photographs, microscopy users suggest to use the monitor for focusing, as its size offers better possibilities than the much small monitor of the photographic camera or video. The monitor is very useful, since it allows the operator to observe clinical procedures without the need to use the oculars, which facilitates communication with the patient. Furthermore, the assistant can also watch the procedures on an auxiliary monitor and see them in more detail. Carr[9] (San Diego, USA) uses 3 monitors (Fig. 2.XVIII-7).

1. One to enable the patient to follow the treatment.
2. One for the assistant.
3. And one for the operator.

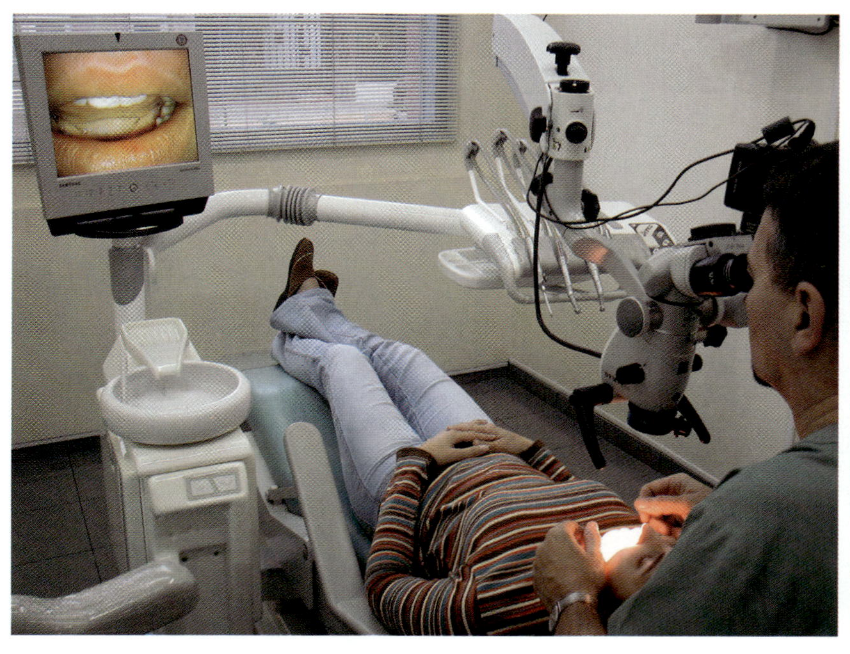

FIG. 2.XVIII-6

Digital photography camera with video output connected to an external monitor.

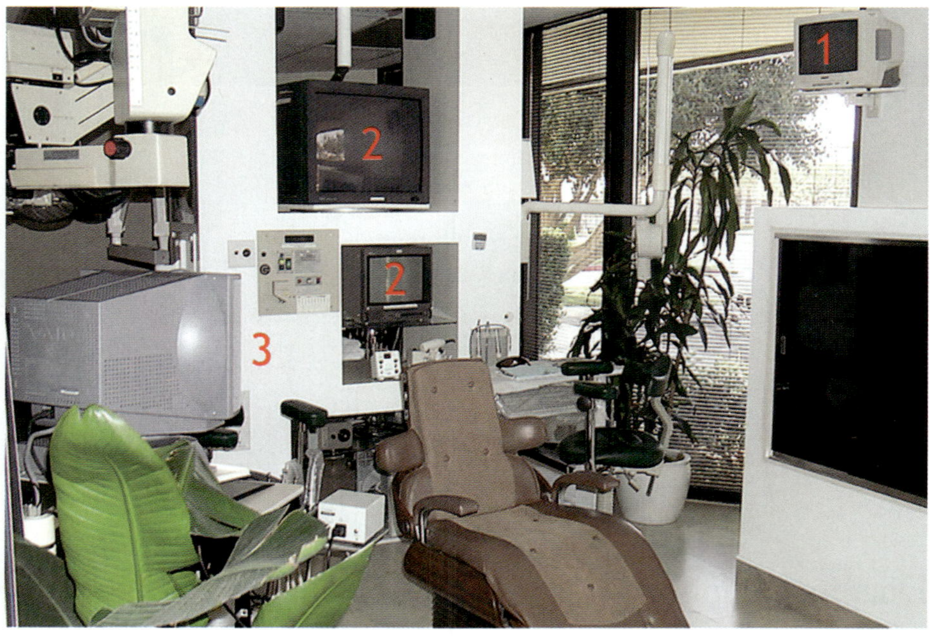

FIG. 2.XVIII-7

Projection on a monitor makes it easier for the operator and assistant. This also enables the patient to follow the procedures.

The capability of the OM to document procedures is useful for documentation for legal and insurance purposes, for teaching and allows for better communication with colleagues. The information that is used for transmission can be accompanied by illustrative photographs. Software has specifically been developed for filing and managing the images generated by the OM and for other functions, such as TDO.

To avoid external accessories (beam splitters and video cameras) some newer OMs incorporated them into the housing that contains the objective. This reduces the weight of the head and improves moving the OM in the desired position. An example is the OMI PICO ZEISS.

When selecting a microscope several requirements need to be considered, such as the procedures that will be performed (meeting the real demand for magnification), the time available for training and allowance for the necessary learning curve, the location of the OM in the operatory, and the cost/benefit ratio[27]. Further points to consider are the technical specifications of the equipment, such as the type of light (halogen or xenon), magnification possibilities, selection of manual or motorized magnification, whether to acquiring a fixed or tiltable binocular, options for documentation by means of a photographic camera and/or video, wall, ceiling or floor bases, as well as the warranty that is offered and technical maintenance.

The learning curve of the OM is long and requires the operator to master the correct coordination of hands, eyes and mind. In addition to become familiar with the OM, the clinician must study and practice techniques that are specifically designed when using endodontic microinstruments.

USE OF THE OPERATING MICROSCOPE IN ENDODONTICS

The dentist can improve his/her technical and diagnostic skills with magnification, therefore, the trend is to incorporate higher magnification and consistent illumination of the operating field [18,21], making it possible to observe details that are of interest thus improving treatment procedures[8]. Some examples are:

- Endodontic diagnosis (with special emphasis on cracks (fissures) and fractures);
- Coronal opening and management of anatomic variations;
- Location and approach to calcified root canals;
- Perforations;
- Removal of fractured instruments and/or obstructions in root canals;
- Endodontic retreatments;
- Peri-radicular surgical procedures.

The OM is particularly useful in the following clinical situations:

- Endodontic diagnosis.
- Non-surgical endodontics
- Peri-radicular surgery.

ENDODONTIC DIAGNOSIS

There are different procedures that can and must be used to make a correct diagnosis. With the OM, clinical diagnosis is performed with greater precision, as it allows perfect visualization of microleakage, recurrent caries and defective restoration margins[33], in addition to detecting cracked teeth (fissures) and fractures (Figs. 2.XVIII-8 to 2.XVIII-10).

FIG. 2.XVIII-8

There are situations in which a patient experiences acute pain and a radiograph shows no visible abnormalities. The result of diagnostic tests suggested a "cracked tooth syndrome" in the mandibular right second molar.

FIG. 2.XVIII-9

After removing the restoration, note the presence of a fissure line that runs from the distal marginal ridge to the mesial and lingual portions. In this case there was no need to use dyes (21.3x magnification).

FIG. 2.XVIII-10

With the OM, the trajectory of the fissure line could be determined, allowing an evaluation the structures involved, and the extent in an apical direction.

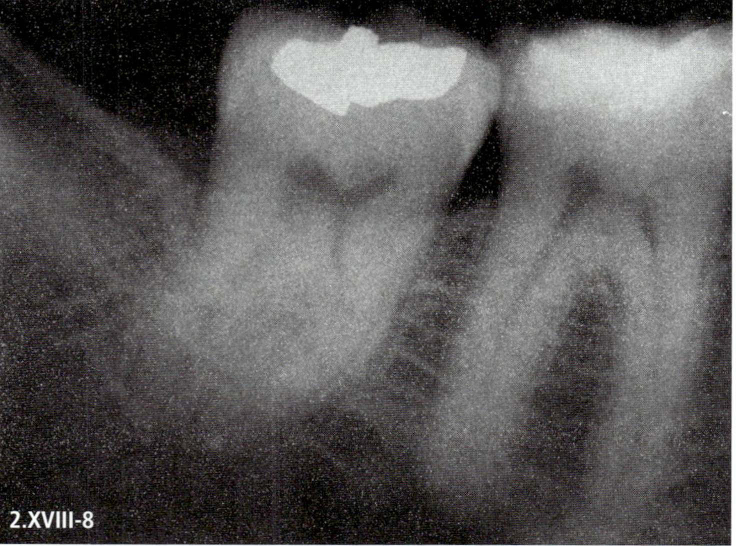
2.XVIII-8

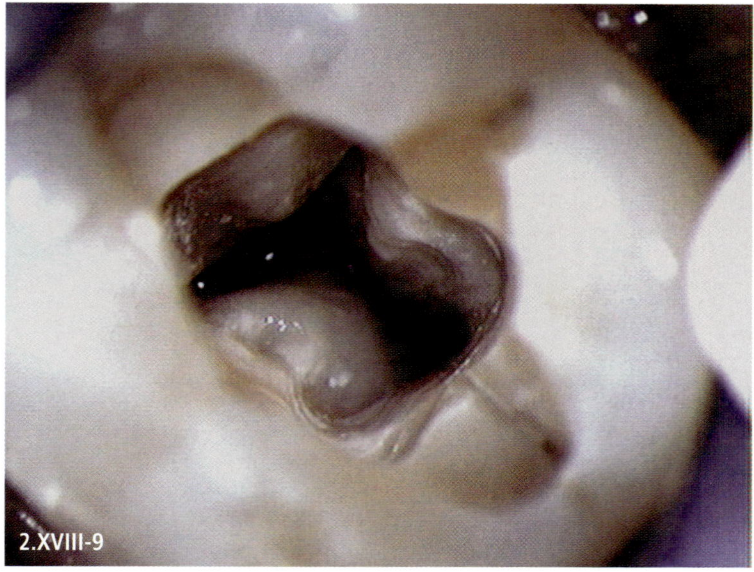
2.XVIII-9

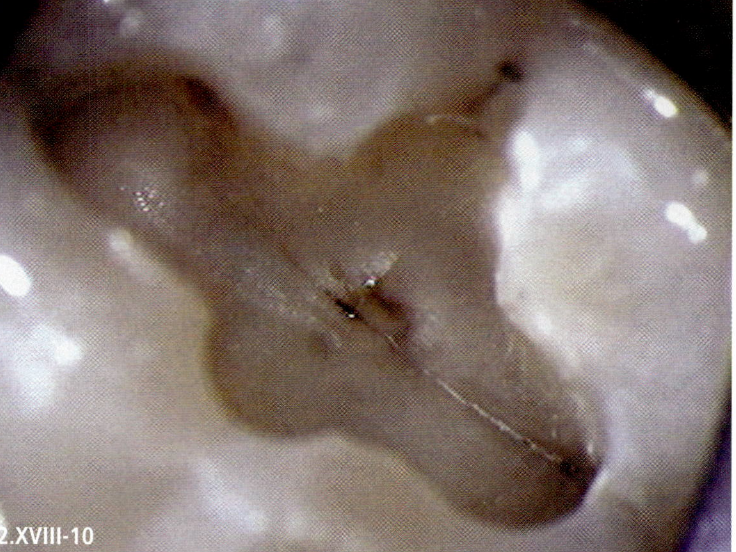
2.XVIII-10

Diagnosis of Vertical Cracks (Fissures) and Fractures

The cracked tooth syndrome, associated with incomplete fracture of the tooth[2], is difficult to diagnose and presents frustrating signs and symptoms. Although periodontal probing, radiographic examination and masticatory tests with the *Tooth Slooth* help with the diagnosis, cracks or fissures only become visible with the OM and dyes, such as methylene blue[2,28].

A methodical microscopic examination and an understanding of the types of fissure, can help the clinician arrive at a correct diagnosis. Although it is possible to treat the majority of coronal fissures with a restoration that protects the cusps, cracked roots compromise the prognosis of the tooth and its viability in the oral cavity. When located under extensive coronal restorations it may cause serious complications that are impossible to treat[11]. Once the restoration has been removed, it is necessary to evaluate the extent of the crown fissure. To do this, the gingival tissue must be carefully retracted, in order to visualize the root surface below the crown margin, drying the root surface lightly with air from a triple syringe that is fitted with a Stropko device, allowing fissures to be detected using the light of the microscope. In many cases, the fissures are the size of a human hair and cannot be seen without the help of the OM. The procedure is minimally invasive and avoids surgery, in which the practitioner has to raise a surgical flap during an exploratory diagnostic procedure[11,23,52].

After removing the coronal restoration, and using methylene blue dye, a thin colored line can be observed, which reveal the presence if a crack or fissure. Vertical fractures become evident using the same technique. Using the OM will prevent wasting time with treatments that have no possibility of being successful[33]. Fissures can also be present in caries-free teeth and/or restorations, making diagnosis more difficult (Figs. 2.XVIII-11 to 2.XVIII-16).

In patients without periodontal disease, the presence of a deep pocket suggests a dehiscency related to a vertical fracture (Figs. 2.XVIII-17 and 2.XVIII-18). If this is the result of occlusal factors, the lines appear on the occluding surface in an apical direction.

When treating these cases, the OM is used at intermediate and maximum magnifications. First the restoration and then gutta-percha from the root canal is removed close to the probing zone. It is recommended to use dyes with low surface tension (methylene blue, caries detectors, basic fuchsin, among others) that penetrate into the fissure lines and highlight them. To that end, the dye is put into the cavity and allowed to act for one minute, followed by abundant water irrigation. After air drying one can observe at a magnification between 14 and 18x the fissure and/or fracture lines, which would otherwise remain undetected (Fig. 2.XVIII-19).

When excessive pressure is exerted with the use of spreaders and/or vertical condensers during the gutta-percha compaction, fractures may be caused, starting at the apex and extending to the cervix. If bone loss results from the crack, extraction of the tooth is indicated. When examining the tooth after extraction, the vertical fracture can be found originating at the apex and running in a cervical direction (Fig. 2.XVIII-20).

FIG. 2.XVIII-11

The patient complained of intense and spontaneous pain in the maxillary right molars area. A radiograph offered no details that led to a precise diagnosis. Note the absence of caries and restorations.

FIG. 2.XVIII-12

After diagnostic tests, the maxillary right first molar was determined to be responsible for the problem (21.3x magnification).

FIG. 2.XVIII-13

The methylene blue penetrated into the fissures, clearly showing them. An area of wear from traumatic occlusion on the mesio-lingual cusp is noted, from which a thin line emerges, which joins the intercuspal central fissure.

FIG. 2.XVIII-14

Image at 21.3x magnification, showing evidence of the lingual area of the coronal opening. Note the fissure line in a coronal-apical direction, close to the pulp.

FIG. 2.XVIII-15

According to the text.

FIG. 2.XVIII-16

According to the text.

2.XVIII-11

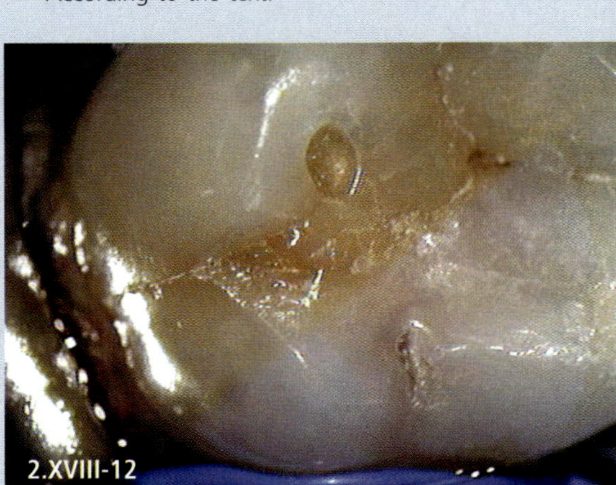
2.XVIII-12

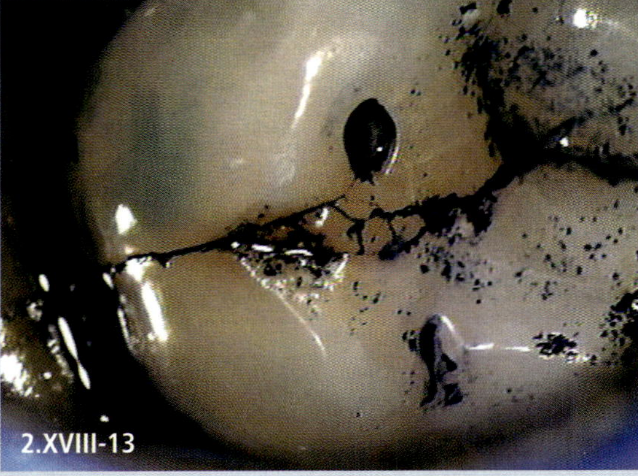
2.XVIII-13

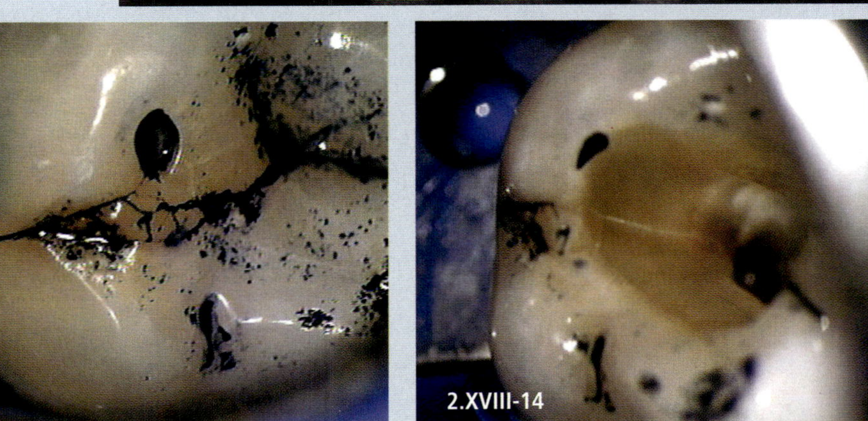
2.XVIII-14

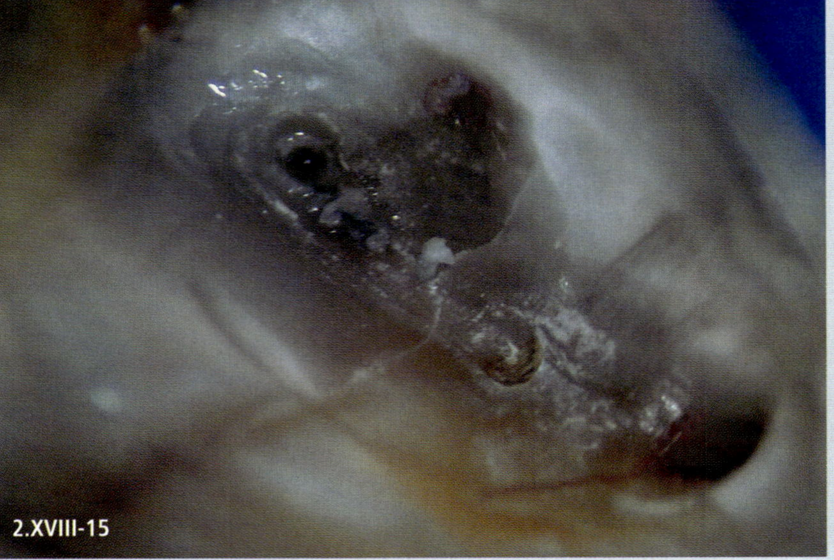
2.XVIII-15

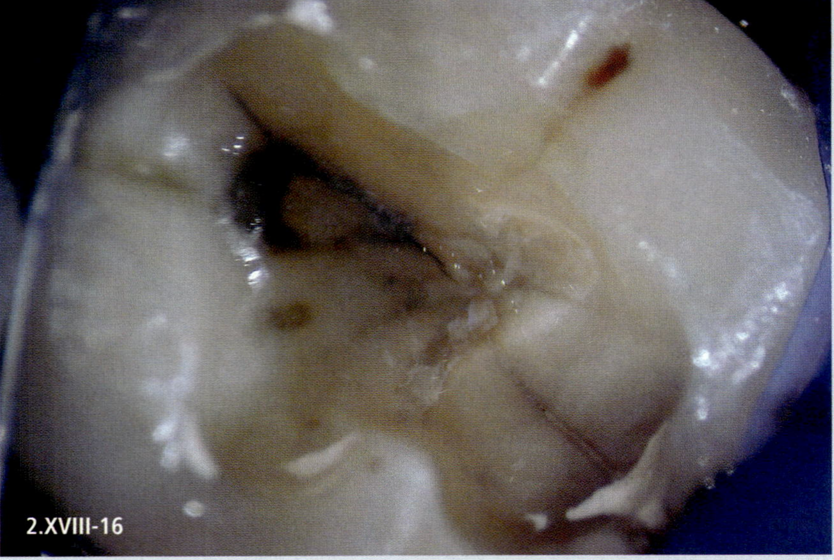
2.XVIII-16

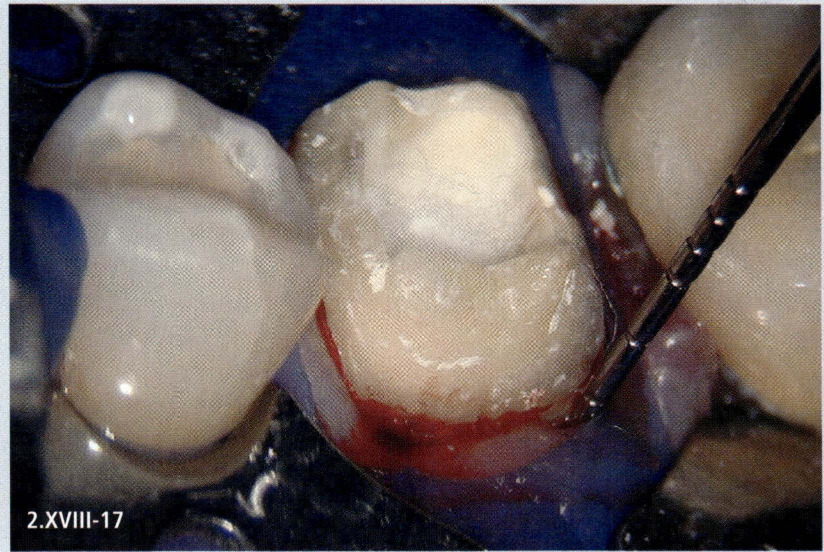
2.XVIII-17

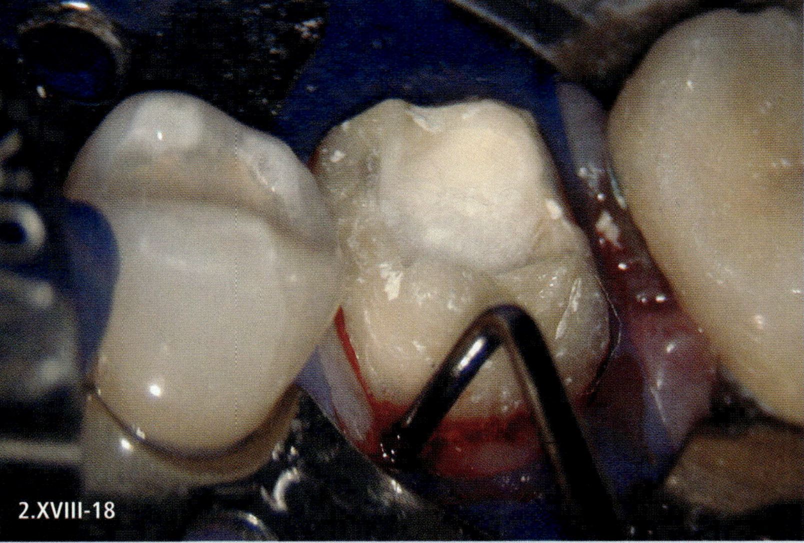
2.XVIII-18

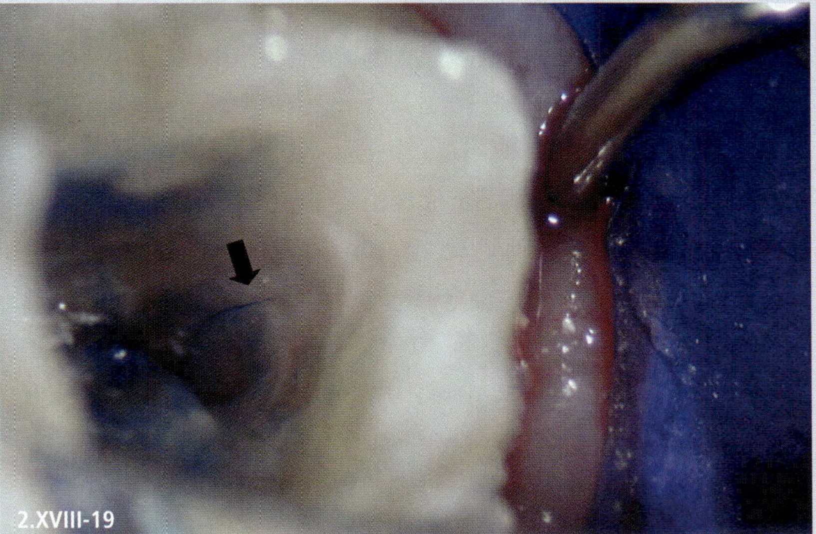
2.XVIII-19

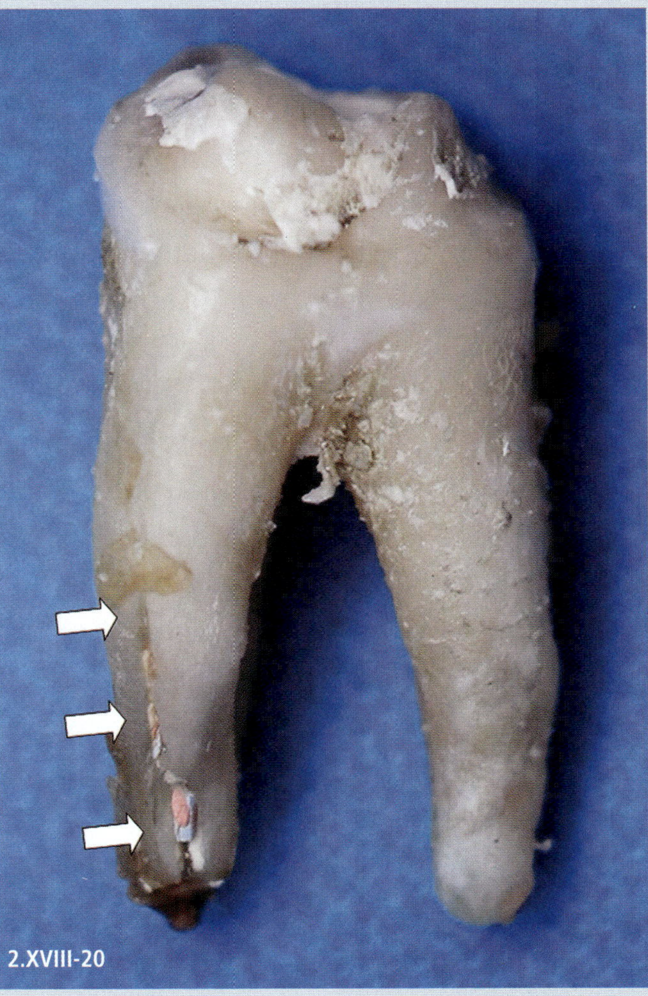
2.XVIII-20

FIG. 2.XVIII-17
Normal periodontal probing.

FIG. 2.XVIII-18
Normal periodontal probing.

FIG. 2.XVIII-19
Probing a deep periodontal pocket that coincides with a longitudinal crack.

FIG. 2.XVIII-20
A cracked root originating at the apex.

NON SURGICAL ENDODONTICS

Coronal opening, analysis of the pulp chamber floor, and access to the root canal

Coronal opening consists of complete removal of the pulp chamber roof and location of the root canal openings. When performed with the OM, the procedure respects the original anatomy of the tooth and is more precise.

Help from the OM is of immeasurable value during the location of the root canal openings, because it allows observation of subtle changes in the color of dentin, textures, shadows and contrasts on the pulp chamber floor with greater accuracy.

Provided the pulp chamber floor is not altered, it will reveal a "map", traced by thin dark lines that connect the root canal openings, which will guide the clinician as to their location. The practitioner must always respect the pulp chamber floor and interpret the information it offers. This stage can be performed at a magnification of 6x, increasing it to higher magnifications in order to complete the findings[7,24,52].

The above-mentioned dark lines result from the changes in orientation of the dentinal tubules and the concomitant alteration in the refraction of light. The pulp chamber floor is always centralized in the tooth and has a darker color than its walls. Therefore, when lighter colors are observed on the pulp chamber floor, the practitioner must suspect the presence of reparative dentin and/or calcifications which, after removal, allow the canals to be located. These can be situated where the floor joins the pulp chamber walls[16].

In a case of medially calcified pulp chambers, the pulp nodules or dystrophic calcifications can be easily detected and eliminated[11] with ultrasonic tips used in periodontics, or tips designed for this purpose: Diamond Ball (designed by Gary Carr), ProVetra points (Dentsply/Maillefer), Buc points 1 and 2 (Obtura Spartan and/or by SybronEndo). These tips, activated by ultrasound at maximum power, and used with smooth brush stroke movements, eliminate the secondary dentin deposited at the entrance of the root canals. During this operative procedure the floor should not be touched, thus preserving its original anatomy, which will serve as a guide for the procedure. For this stage, intermediate levels of magnification are used (12 – 16x). Some authors have mentioned statistics that show an increase in the rate of locating and approaching root canals when using the OM in their daily practices

De Carvalho & Zuolo[15] showed that when using magnification between 8 and 13x, they observed an increase of 7.8% in locating the entrances of canals in maxillary first and second molars. Coutinho *et al*. evaluated 108 molars and found 2 mesio-buccal canals in 58 teeth. Of the remaining 50, evaluated with the OM, 2 mesio-buccal canals were found in 37 teeth. When they analyzed the remaining 13 teeth in the laboratory, they observed 3 with 2 mesio-buccal canals that were not detected without magnification and also not with the OM. They concluded that 97.2% of the studied teeth presented 2 mesio-buccal canals and the OM was able to locate 90.7%. Stropko[49] performed endodontic treatments in 1,732 maxillary molars over a period of 8 years, and was able to locate 2 mesio-buccal root canals in 73.2% in first molars, in 50.7% in second molars and in only 20%, in third molars. The author also mentioned that with more experience, and routine use of the OM, he was able to locate 2 root canals in 93.0% of cases with first molars and in 60%, in maxillary second molars.

Endodontic treatment in teeth that present anatomic variations is a challenge to the clinician, since the anatomic references routinely used in normal teeth do not apply in these cases. Radiographs taken at different angles and detailing the anatomy of the clinical crown of the tooth to be treated are most useful, but having the OM available allows one to visualize the pulp chamber floor and identify the isthmus and bifurcations, as well as recognize and treat aspects specifically pertaining to the individual anatomy of these teeth.

Bóveda *et al.*[6] reported a case of an invaginated maxillary lateral incisor (*dens-in-dente*), with a C-shaped root canal, treated with the OM, and demonstrated its great usefulness by improving visualization of the complex anatomy and operator's performance, by helping him/her to recognize the colors and textures of dentin that allowed a more precise treatment. Girsch & Mcclammy[20] and Jung[23], among other authors, reported their experience in the treatment of cases of *dens invaginatus* with the use of the OM, and agreed that the OM is fundamental for treating root canals conservatively and successfully.

Location and treatment of calcified root canals

Although one cannot ignore the impact of public health policies with regard to water fluoridation, as well as educating the population in maintaining their teeth, the fact is that with the increase in the population's mean life expectancy, there is a growing number of adults and elderly persons with teeth who, for a long time, have been at risk of developing caries, receiving multiple restorations, and develop periodontal problems, etc. These conditions, as well as the physiological process of dentin apposition, have resulted in an increase in number of teeth with calcified root canals the endodontist has to deal with on a routine basis.

The OM is very useful for locating and preparing canals obliterated by the deposition of amorphous dentin, calcified degenerations (dystrophic calcifications) at different levels of root canals[4,22,27]. The calcifications always originate in a crown/apex direction which, in principle, allows one to grind away the calcified dentin at the cervical level, with the aim of advancing apically with a small diameter stainless steel instrument, promoting root canal cleaning and shaping.

To do this the operator must place the patient into position and ask him/her to move as little as possible. The OM is then placed over the patient, selecting a medium level of magnification. In case of calcification of the pulp chamber or cervical third of the canal, the magnification is increased. If the calcification is located more apically, removal will be performed with the use of ultrasonic diamond tips, which active part has a diameter that corresponds to the size of the canal area to be prepared, using maximum power without irrigation, so as not to lose visual control of the working area.

Of importance here is to observe the subtle changes in the color of dentin. When tertiary dentin deposition has taken place the dentinal tubules in this area are organized in a distinct fashion and when this occurs in the root canal, the calcified dentin acquires a darker color when it is illuminated with coaxial light of the OM. This allows the operator to determine the location of the canal.

Physiological dentin apposition occurs on both the roof and floor of the pulp chamber as well as the walls, diminishing the space and hiding the entrance openings of the canals. In Figure 2.XVIII-21 in the middle portion, from the buccal towards the lingual, in both the mesial and distal portions, one clearly observes the presence of dentin that must be removed.

While controlling the OM, and using ultrasonic diamond tips, removal is performed by carefully removing the dentin to widen the coronal opening and coronal access, at all times at the expense of the mesial and distal walls. A line is observed on the pulp chamber floor, which clearly indicates the existence of an isthmus between the mesio-buccal and mesio-lingual canals (Fig. 2.XVIII-22).

In general it is possible to observe the entrance of the mesio-lingual canal, or MB2, without necessarily being able to approach it at this time. For better access, better access must be prepared in a crown-apex direction, with a small diameter stainless steel instrument, proceeding with dilation and shaping of the canal (Fig. 2.XVIII-23).

This is followed by removal of all remaining dentin, so as to leave the pulp chamber clean to approach the root canals and allow the operator to work in an appropriate manner (Fig. 2.XVIII-24).

Appropriate coronal access opening allows the observation of two root canals (Fig. 2.XVIII-25).

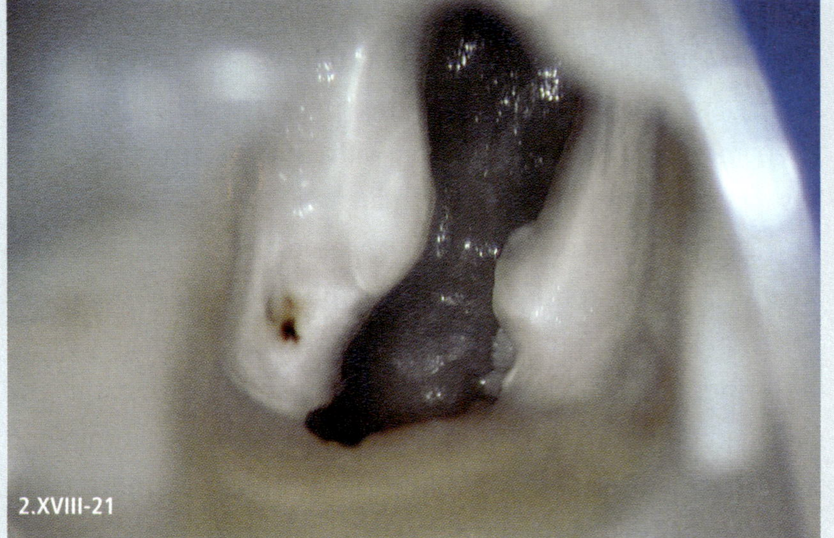
2.XVIII-21

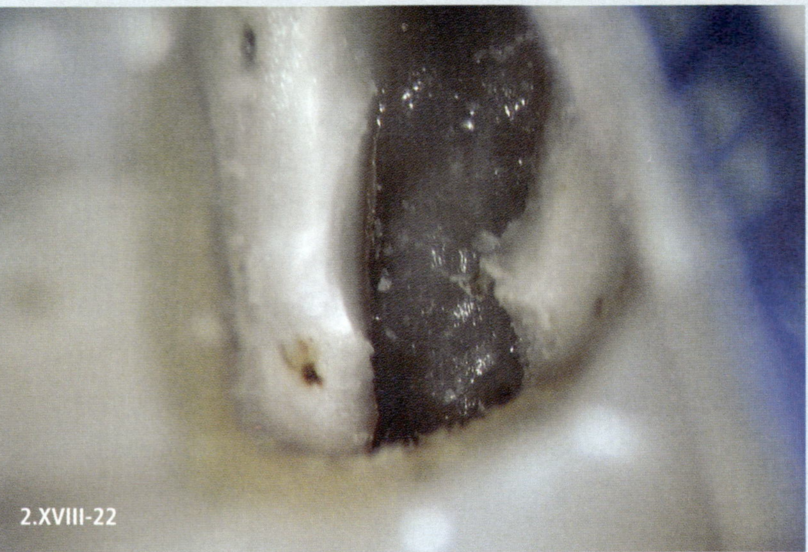
2.XVIII-22

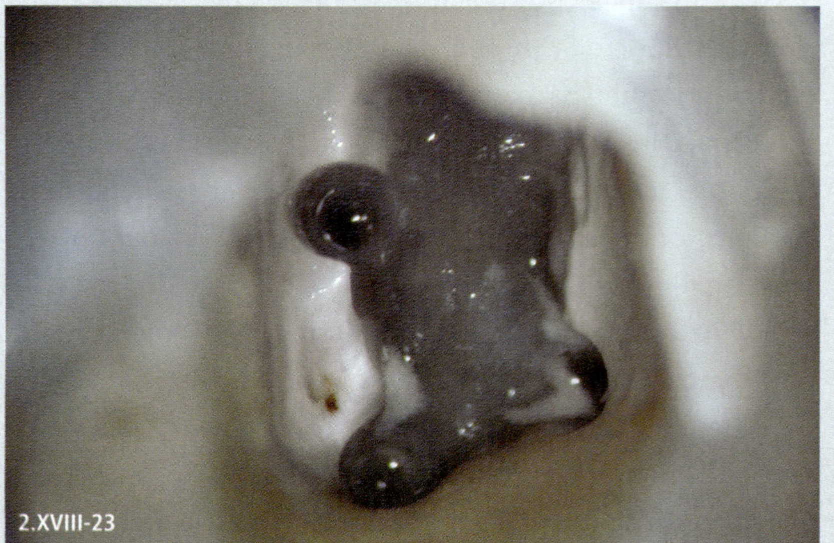
2.XVIII-23

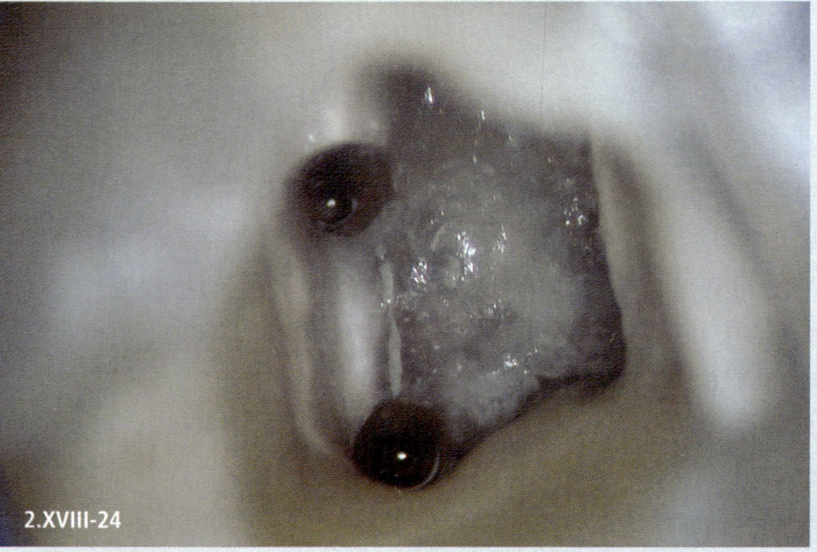
2.XVIII-24

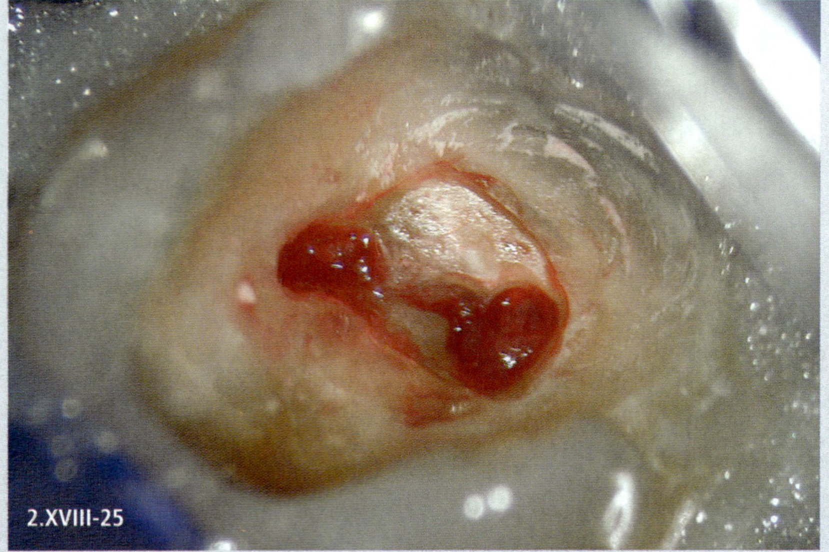
2.XVIII-25

FIG. 2.XVIII-21
According to the text.

FIG. 2.XVIII-22
According to the text.

FIG. 2.XVIII-23
According to the text.

FIG. 2.XVIII-24
According to the text.

FIG. 2.XVIII-25
Coronal opening, in which one observes two root canals.

Preparation with a diamond ball-shaped ultrasonic tip (Gary Carr), to remove dystrophic calcifications in the pulp chamber (Fig. 2.XVIII-26).

The pulp chamber is subtly widened in a mesio-distal direction, to allow better vision of the working field and direct access to the canals (Fig. 2.XVIII-27).

The disto-buccal canal is submitted to endodontic exploration followed by cleaning, shaping and filling (Figs. 2.XVIII-28, 2.XVIII-29, 2.XVIII-30, 2.XVIII-31, 2.XVIII-32 and 2.XVIII-33).

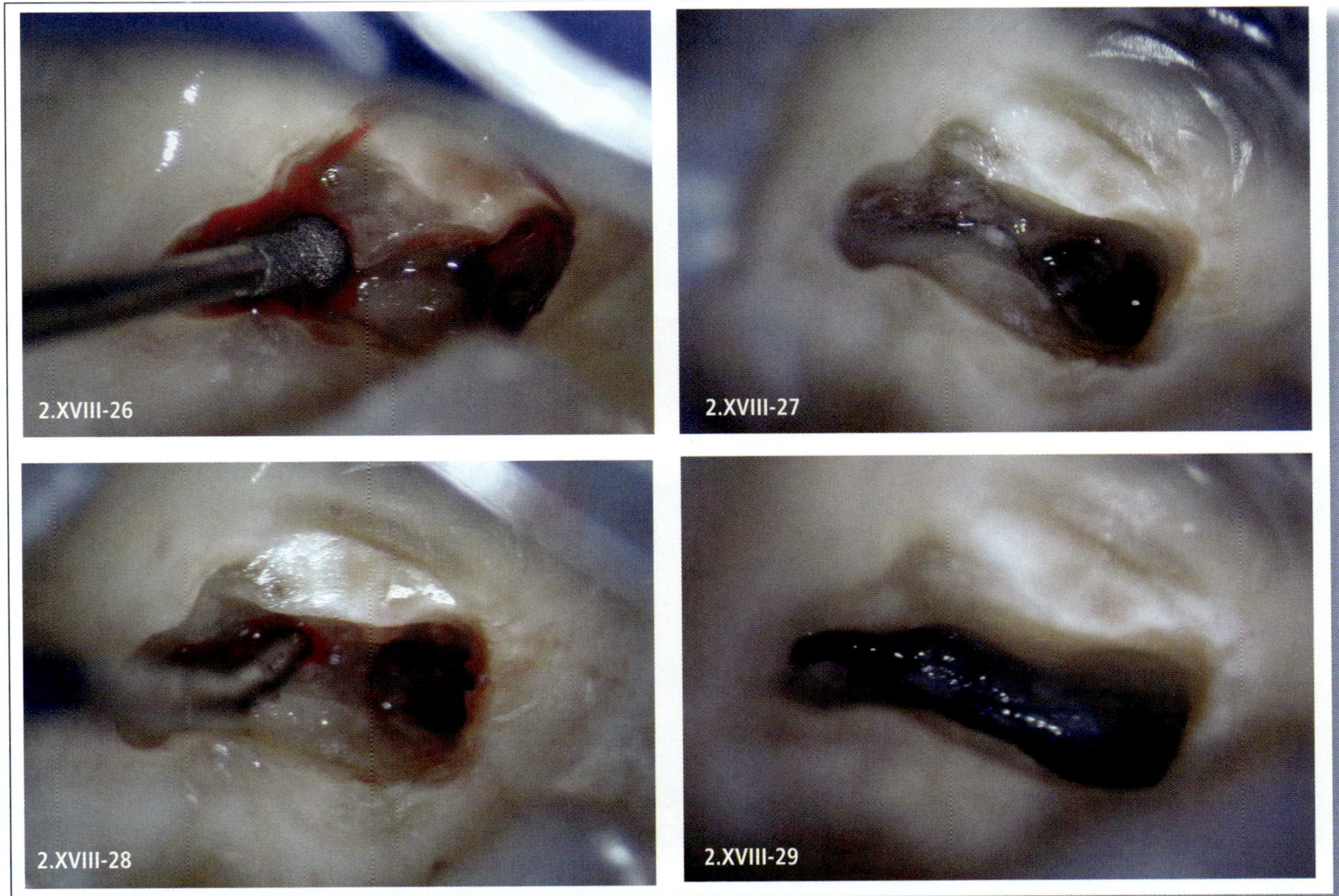

FIG. 2.XVIII-26

Grinding with a Diamond Ball ultrasonic tip (Gary Carr), to remove dystrophic calcifications in the pulp chamber.

FIG. 2.XVIII-27

The pulp chamber is subtly widened in a mesio-distal direction, to allow for better vision of the operating field and direct access to the canals.

FIG. 2.XVIII-28

According to the text.

FIG. 2.XVIII-29

According to the text.

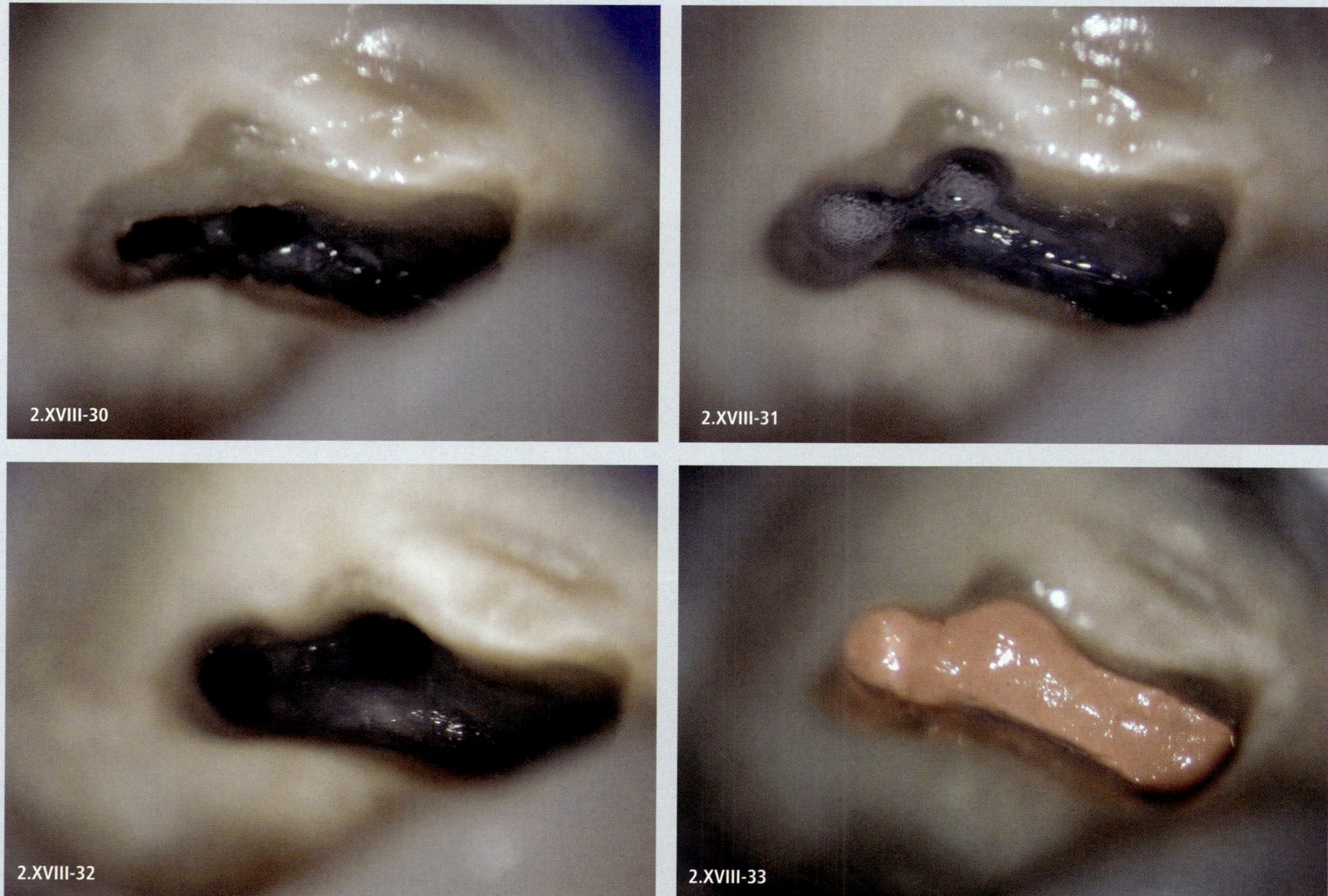

FIG. 2.XVIII-30
According to the text.

FIG. 2.XVIII-31
According to the text.

FIG. 2.XVIII-32
According to the text.

FIG. 2.XVIII-33
According to the text.

In the radiograph of Fig. 2.XVIII-34A, note a maxillary left second molar, with mesial calcified anatomy.

Meticulous analysis of the pulp chamber floor shows a "map", in which the line of the floor is divided in a lingual and mesial and distal portion (Fig. 2.XVIII-34B – white arrows), which necessitates reshaping of the coronal access opening.

Thanks to the magnification of the microscope two canals were located and accessed in the lingual area, drastically changing the shape of the coronal access opening that was initially performed (Fig. 2.XVIII-34C), thus allowing the root canals to be cleaned shaped and filled (Fig. 2.XVIII-34D).

Final radiograph (Fig. 2.XVIII-34D) showing evidence of four canals located and filled.

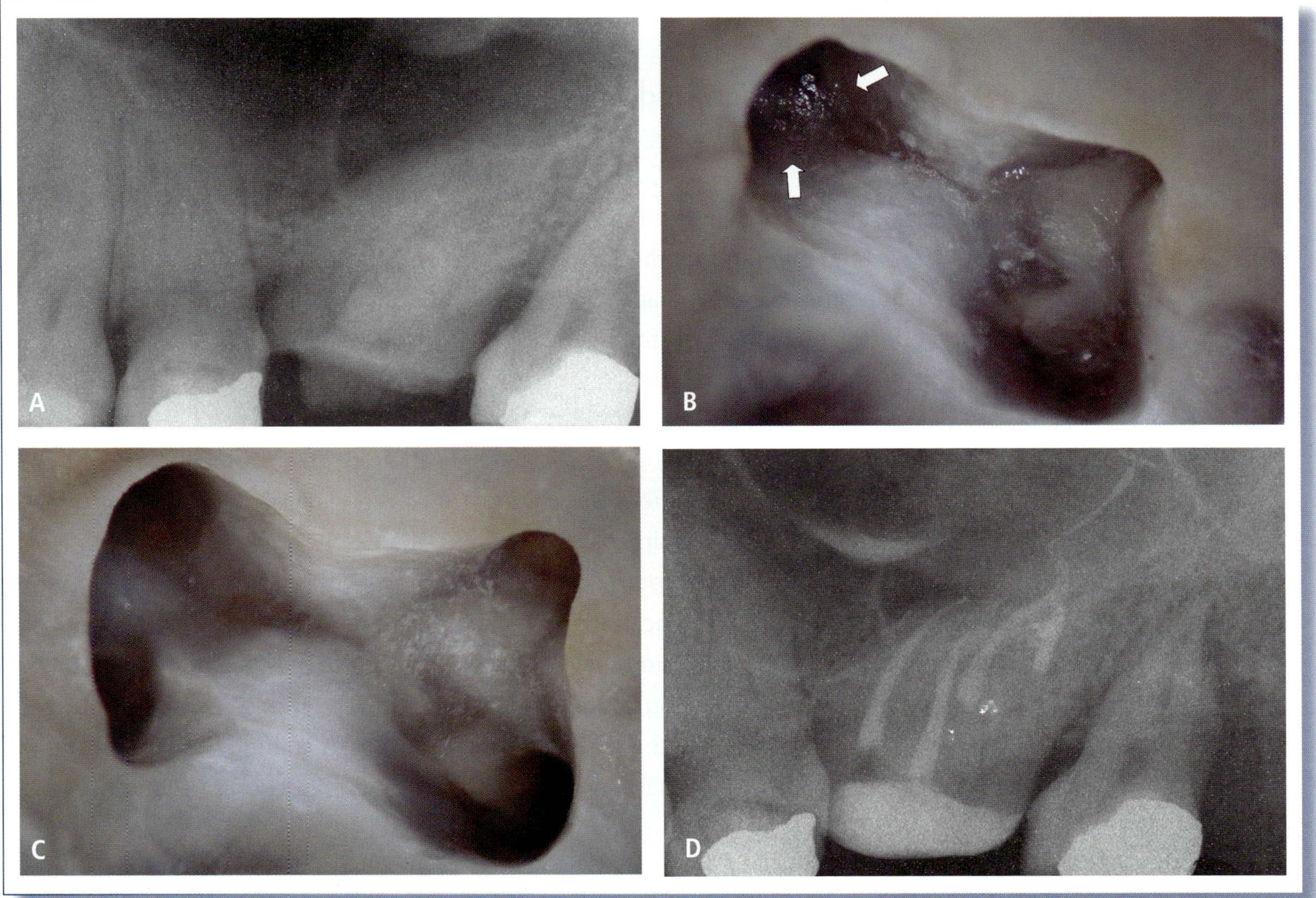

FIGS. 2.XVIII-34A-D

A – Radiograph, showing evidence of maxillary left second molar with medially calcified anatomy.
B – Map of pulp chamber floor.
C – Coronal opening.
D – Final radiograph, showing evidence of four filled root canals.

An image at 21x magnification (Fig. 2.XVIII-35A) shows evidence of normal location of the root canal entrances. Note the clarity and simplicity with which a clinician, guided by the information offered by the pulp chamber floor, can locate the entry of the second mesio-buccal canal (Fig. 2.XVIII-35B), in order to explore it afterwards with a pre-curved, small diameter stainless steel instrument that penetrates into the canal from the disto-lingual area (Fig. 2.XVIII-35C), then clean, shape and fill the root canals (Figs. 2.XVIII-35D-F).

In Figure 2.XVIII-36A note that the detailed analysis of the pulp chamber floor under coaxial light with magnification by the microscope, offers very valuable information for locating the root canal entrances. Note how the pattern of the lines on the floor guides the operator to locate the three entrances of the main root canals in the mesio-buccal root (MB1, MB2 and MB3). This is followed by shaping the access opening, cleaning and shaping of the canals (Figs. 2.XVIII-36B-C).

How to deal with calcifications and anatomic anomalies of the pulp chamber and root canals

Calcifications in the pulp chamber make endodontic treatment difficult. Dense calcifications inside the root canals, at different depths (Fig. 2.XVIII-37A) may contraindicate the treatment.

Access to calcified root canals is made easier with the use of the OM with the additional help of ultrasound and irrigation solutions, for instance sodium hypochlorite. This treatment promotes more conservative and precise canal preparation, avoiding unnecessary grinding of dentin and/or perforations.

Access to a calcified root canal begins with recognition of the problem before starting treatment. Radiographs taken at different angulations offer the clinician important information about the height of the roof of the pulp chamber, its size, the extent and density of calcification, and whether there is still space in the pulp chamber. With the OM, it is possible to distinguish the various shapes and colors of the calcifications, making it easier to locate the calcified root canals (Figs. 2.XVIII-38A-B). The dentin that surrounds the root canal entrance may be darker, and may have more pigmented points interconnecting various canals in a spatial relationship[45]. It is important to grind in the correct directions and to the correct depths, and not to change the floor of the pulp chamber, which can be construed as a "map" that guides us in the direction of the orifices of the root canals.

Under coaxial light of the OM, one is able to distinguish the difference in color between primary and calcified dentin.

Grinding of selective areas can be accomplished with ultrasonic tips (Satelec ET40, ET-40D, ProUltraEndo 3, 4 e 5) exclusively in the area in which there is evidence of color contrast. Other tips that are useful for removing calcifications are those developed by Gary Carr (Slim-Jim SJ-4, VT-4,

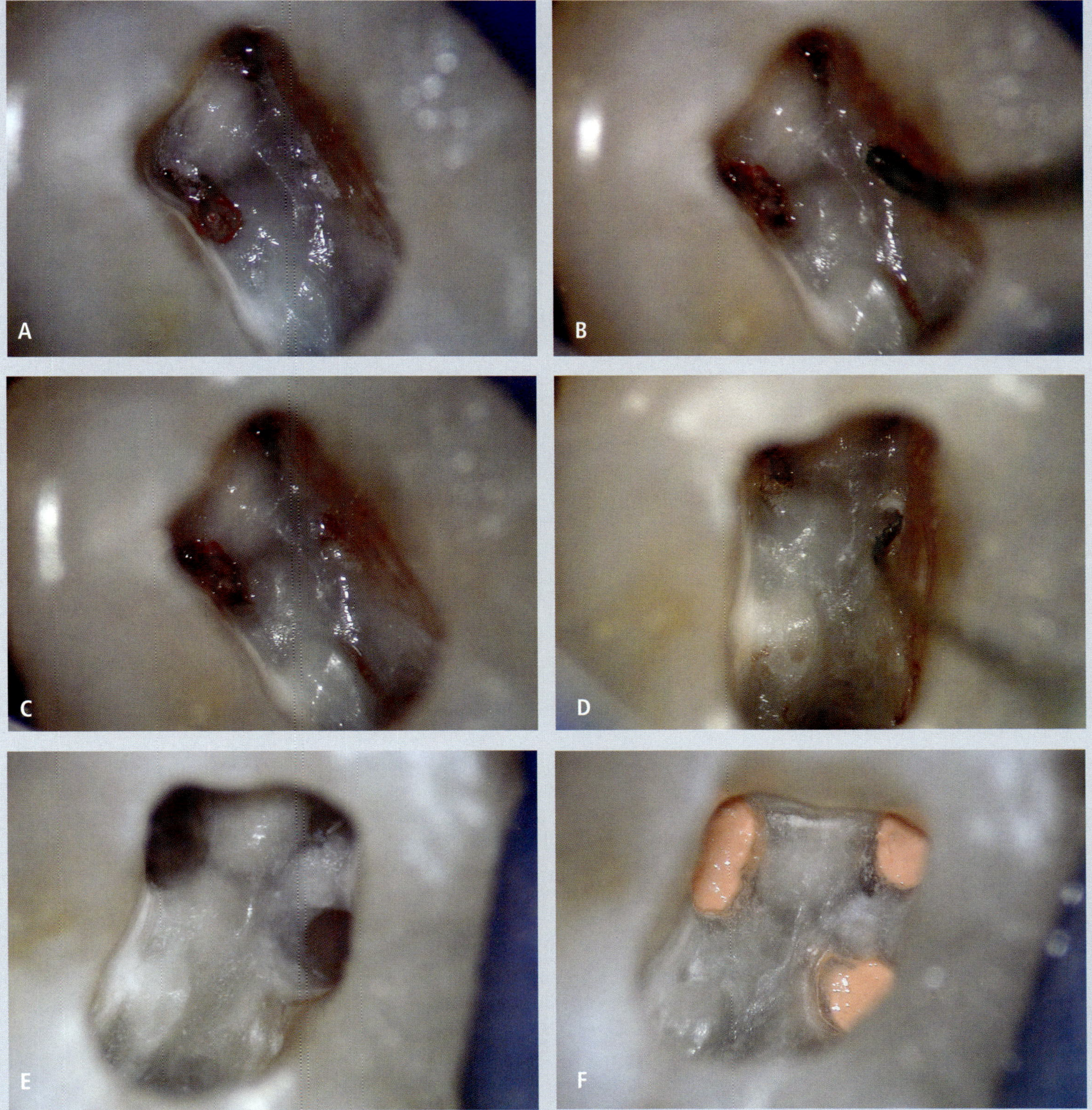

FIGS. 2.XVIII-35A-E

A – 21x magnification, showing normal location of root canal openings.
B-F – According to the text.

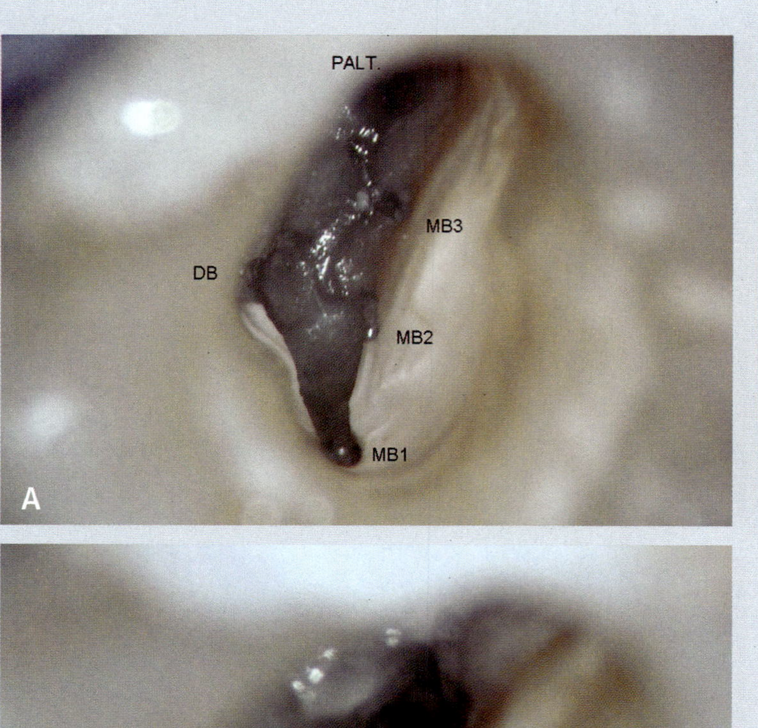

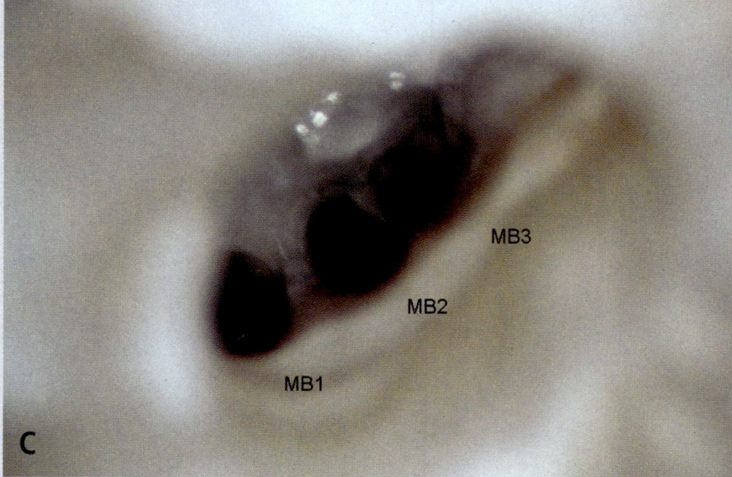

FIGS. 2.XVIII-36A-C

A-C – According to the text.

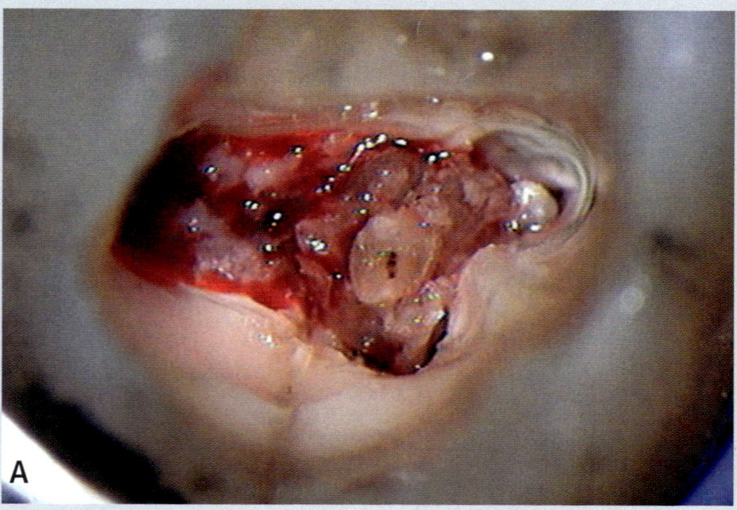

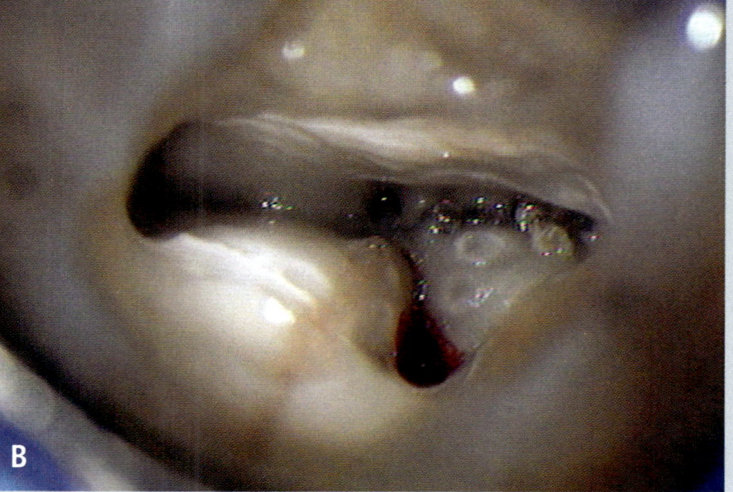

FIGS. 2.XVIII-37A-B

A – Maxillary second molar. Access to the root canals is obliterated by the presence of calcifications in the pulp chamber.
B – Clinical aspect after the use of ultrasound.

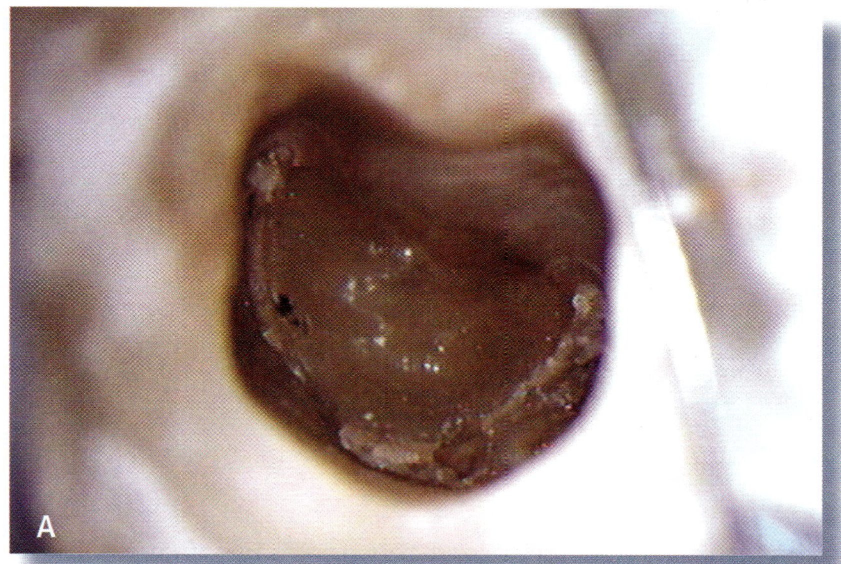

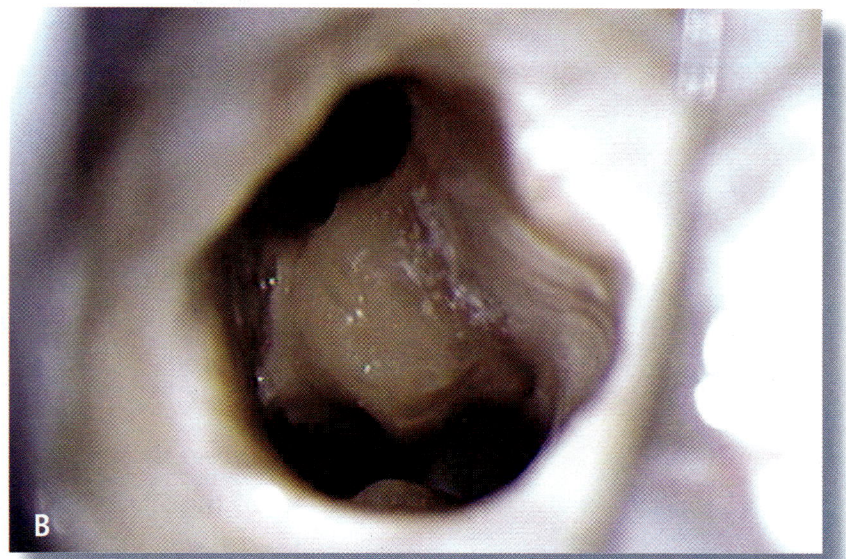

FIGS. 2.XVIII-38A-B

A – View at 21.3x magnification of C-shaped root canal, in a mandibular second molar. The surrounding calcifications appear in a different color due to the coaxial light of the microscope. Note the canal with darker projections in the pulp chamber floor.
B – Once the most coronal calcifications were removed with the use of sodium hypochlorite solution, the differences between the pulp chamber floor and the canal entrances can be observed, making it easier to identify them.

Troughing tip, Ball Diamond tip, CT-4 and CT-4D), which have a high resistance to wear and fracture.

When using these tips it is necessary to avoid wide movements; only the tip should be moved in a crown-apex direction, activating it for short periods (15 seconds) and allowing time for cooling, since irrigation is not recommended. An increase in temperature may result in irreversible damage to the supporting structures. Used in this manner, the ultrasonic tip removes dentin, pulverizing it by cavitation. The working area must be thoroughly washed with 5.25% sodium hypochlorite. When using this irrigation solution, it may be possible to observe bubbles in the solution at the calcified canal entrance. This is due to its action of dissolving tissues, which will help recognizing the true location of the canal entrance. This is followed by drying by aspiration. The use of absolute alcohol can also be recommended.

An adjustment of the microfocus of the microscope should be made to observe the ground surface in detail before trying to penetrate the center of the calcified zone with an explorer with a very sharp point. When the explorer becomes stuck, continue using a stainless steel instrument, such as a type K file No. 10, and attempt to place it at the point where the explorer became stuck, seeking to displace it, carefully, moving in an apical direction, while rotating (clockwise and counter-clockwise) the instrument which is held between thumb and index fingers. When the instrument penetrates into the canal it undergoes considerable stress. For that reason, it should be discarded after use and replaced with a new one to prevent it from fracturing inside the canal. On the other hand, if the tip of the endodontic explorer is stuck in the canal entrance, it makes no sense to try to enter it with a type K file. In this case, the grinding step with ultrasonic tips should be repeated, remembering that since we are moving in an apical direction, these points must be thinner, so as to not to perforate the root.

The area must be copiously irrigated with a 5.25% sodium hypochlorite solution to remove dentin debris. This step will also make the different colors and texture of the surrounding dentin more evident. Under the OM, the sodium hypochlorite solution can show an "effervescence" or "bubbling" in the area of the calcified canal entrance, or that of an additional canal, due to its tissue-dissolving effect on the organic tissues[35] (Fig. 2.XVIII-39).

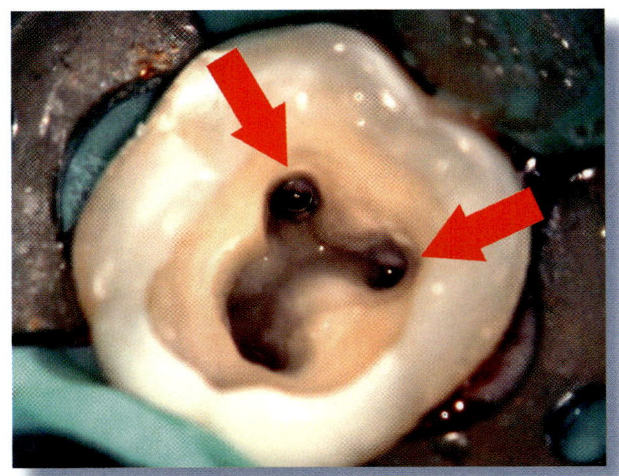

FIG. 2.XVIII-39

The arrows show "bubbling" due to the action of the sodium hypochlorite solution.

In some cases, placement of methylene blue and transillumination may help to locate extra or calcified canals. Another resource is the use of fluorescein, a solution that assumes a greenish color when it comes into contact with connective tissues and is exposed to blue light. This technique is very helpful when attempts are made to locate a calcified canal[28].

The OM increases the possibility of detecting and locating root canal orifices, and therefore, greatly increases the predictability of successful treatment (Figs. 2.XVIII-40A-C).

According to Buchanan[7], nine out of ten calcified root canals can be located with the use of the OM.

Ling *et al.*[29] recorded a percentage of 88.1% success in the treatment of root canals obstructed by calcification.

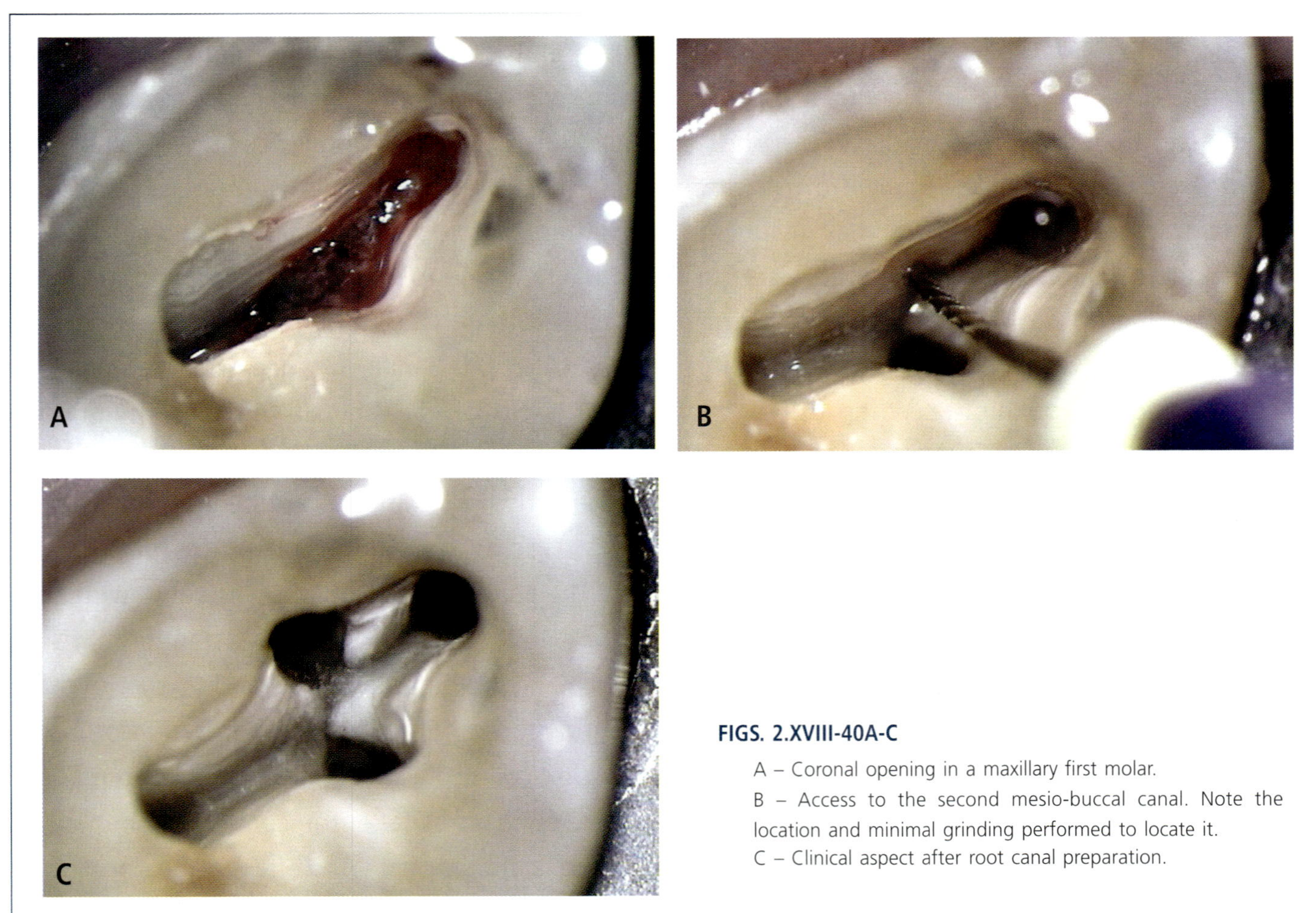

FIGS. 2.XVIII-40A-C

A – Coronal opening in a maxillary first molar.
B – Access to the second mesio-buccal canal. Note the location and minimal grinding performed to locate it.
C – Clinical aspect after root canal preparation.

Yoshioka *et al.*[52] concluded that the OM is more effective than surgical loupes for detecting root canal orifices.

Buhrley *et al.*[8] reported a study conducted on 312 cases, in which the location of two root canals in the mesio-buccal root in maxillary first and second molars was 57.4% when using an OM, 55.3%, with loupes, and without any type of magnification, only 18.2%. The frequency of locating the two canals only in maxillary first molars was 71.1% with a microscope, 62.5% with loupes and only 17.2% without any type of magnification.

De Carvalho & Zuolo[15] reported an increase of 7.8% in the number of canals located in maxillary first molars with magnification between 8 – 13x.

Gorduysus *et al.*[21] confirmed that the second mesio-buccal canal can be located in 80% of maxillary molars when the OM is used, although they detected the opening of a possible canal in 96% of the 45 maxillary first and second molars they studied.

Maggiore *et al.*[30] reported a case in which they located the root canals of a maxillary first molar using between 16x and 25x magnification.

Schwarze *et al.* recorded that out of 100 maxillary molars studied, they were able to locate two mesio-buccal canals in 63 molars. Only 26 of these canals (41.3%) were located with a loupe at 2x magnification, while in 5% they located two mesio-buccal canals (43.7%) with the OM at 8x magnification.

Stropko[49] reported a total of 1,732 maxillary molars treated in the course of 8 years (1,096 maxillary first molars, 611 maxillary second molars and 25 maxillary third molars). The author located the second mesio-buccal canal in 802 maxillary first molars (50.7%) and in 5 maxillary third molars (20%). However, after gaining more experience through routine use of the OM, he reported another study, in which in 93.0% of first molars the second mesio-buccal canal was located and in 60.4% of maxillary second molars.

Yoshioka *et al.*[52] studied the effectiveness of vision without magnification, with the OM and with surgical loupes and found statistically significant differences among the 3 methods, concluding that the OM was the most effective.

Bóveda *et al.*[6] reported a root canal treatment in a maxillary lateral incisor (*dens invaginatus*) with the use of the OM, already mentioned at the beginning of this chapter.

Root canal treatment of teeth with anatomic anomalies is a veritable challenge, since the anatomic parameters are related to normal teeth. The OM allows the clinician to make a precise analysis of the case, evaluating, recognizing and treating aspects intrinsic to dental anatomy (Figs. 2.XVIII-41 and 2.XVIII-42A-D).

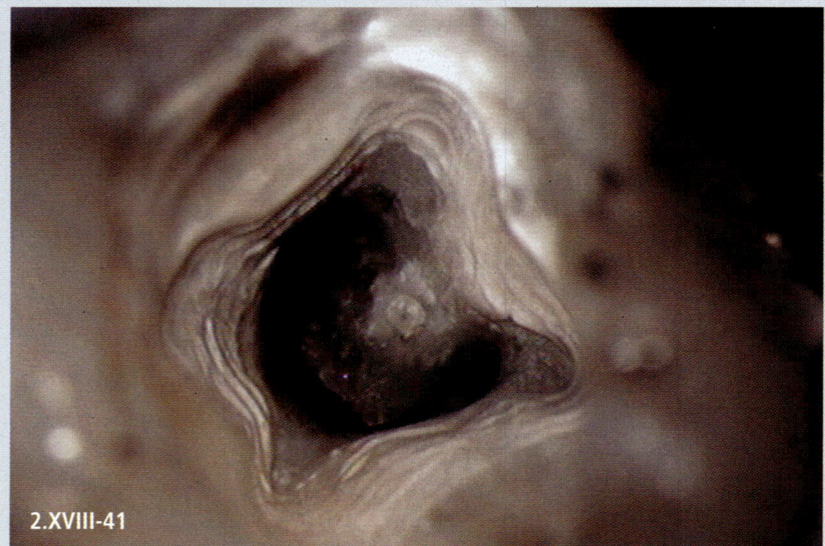

FIG. 2.XVIII-41

C-shaped root canal in a mandibular second molar (21.3x magnification).

FIGS. 2.XVIII-42A-D

A – Radiographic evaluation that suggests that the maxillary second molar had normal anatomy.
B – Coronal opening, under the OM, reveals an atypical pulp chamber.
C – After the removal of coronal pulp, note the presence of a second mesiovestibular canal (MB2) and an extra opening between the disto-buccal and lingual canals.
D – Final radiograph, showing five filled main root canals.

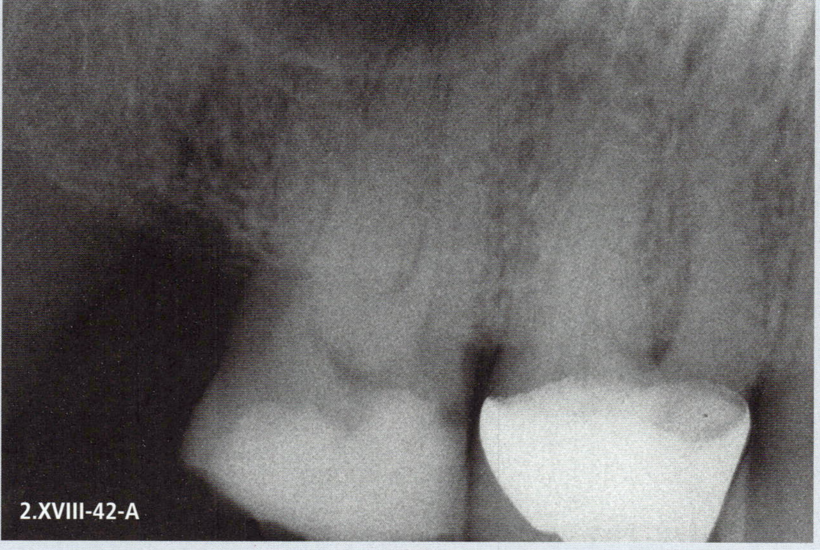

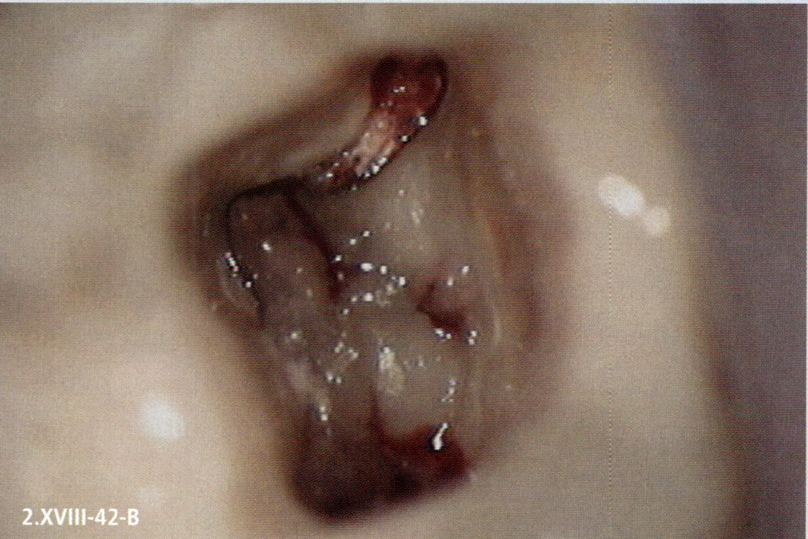

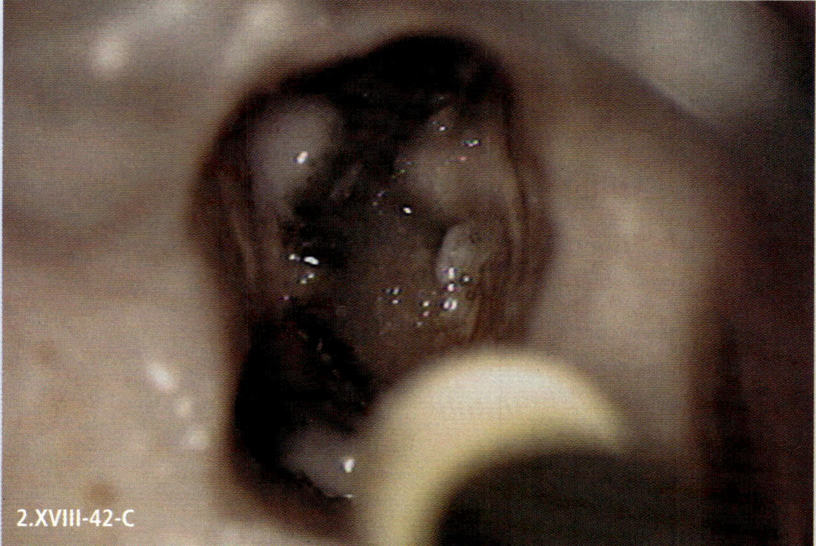

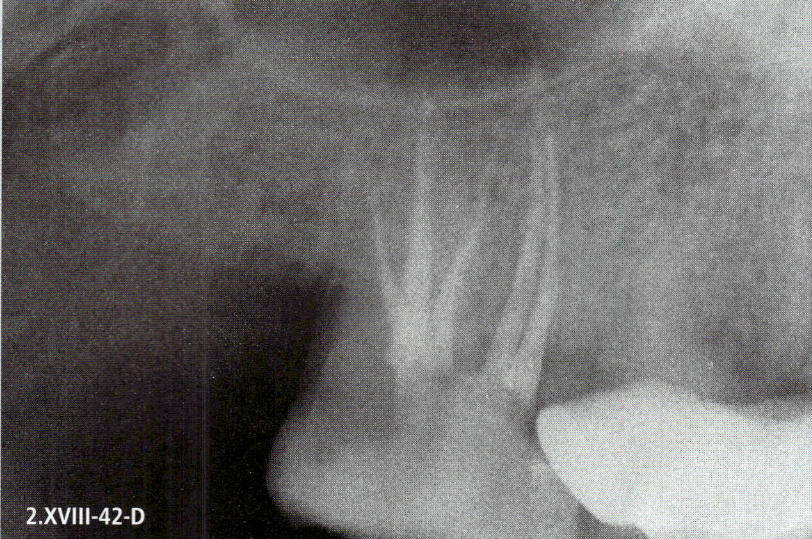

A resource to consider for locating calcified root canals in the most cervical portion is the use of fluorescein[2,28], which is applied to the connective tissues of the pulpal space of the calcified canal, and should remain there for 1 minute. It then has to be thoroughly washed with physiological saline and after drying, illumination with a blue light gives the tissues located in the calcified canal a greenish color, which can easily be observed with an OM. (Figs. 2.XVIII-43, 2.XVIII-44 and 2.XVIII-45).

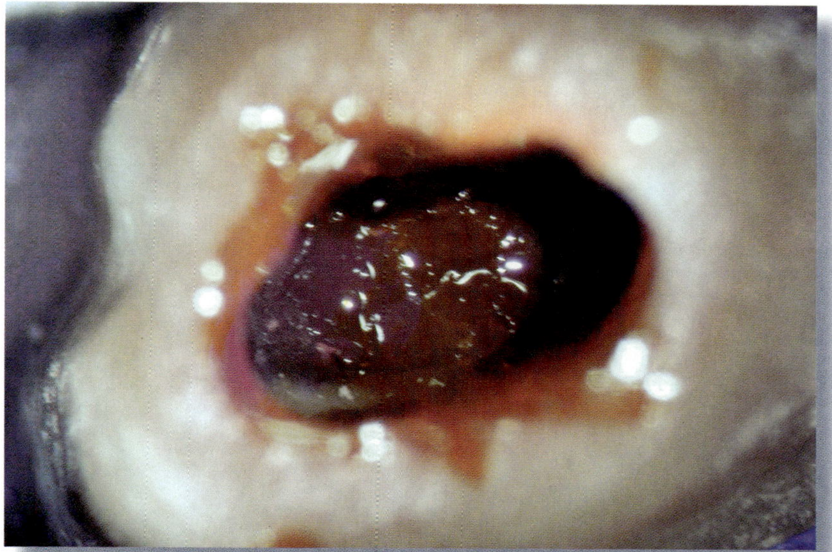

FIG. 2.XVIII-43
According to the text.

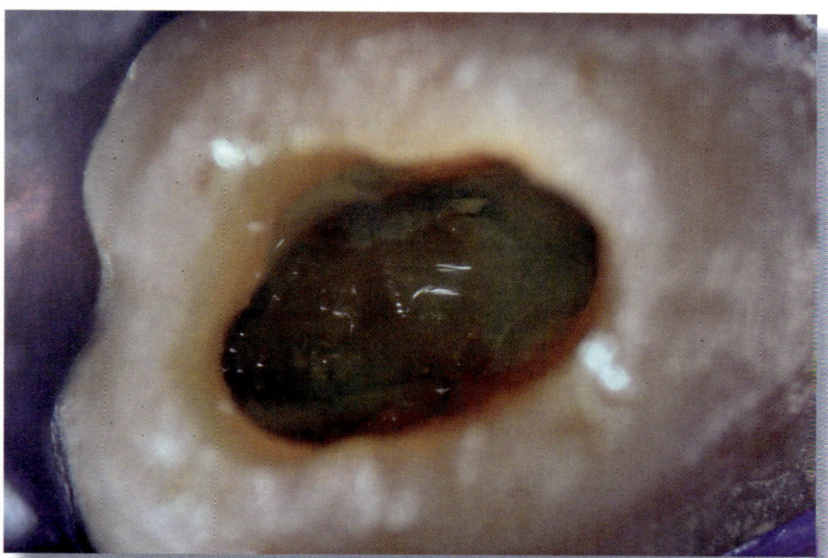

FIG. 2.XVIII-44
According to the text.

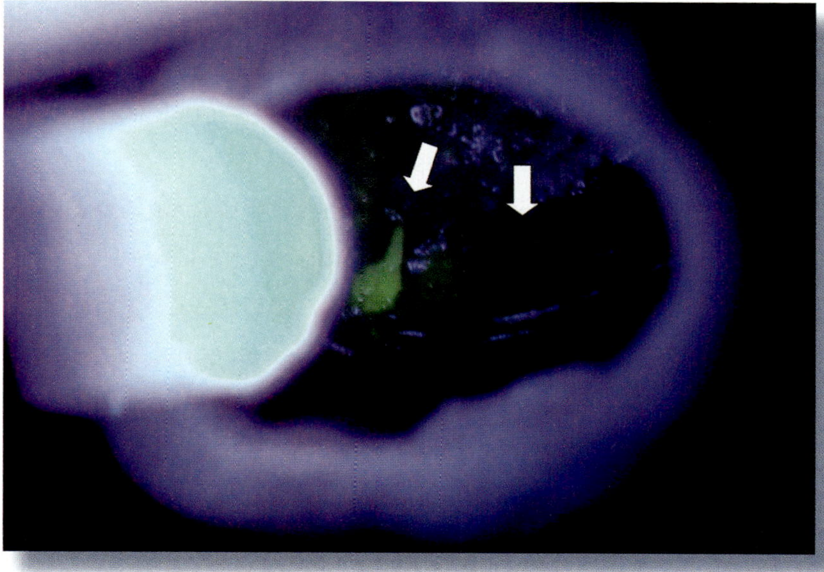

FIG. 2.XVIII-45
According to the text.

Using the OM to Remove Posts and Fractured Instruments

The OM and ultrasound enable a safer removal of posts and fractured instruments that obstruct root canals and prevent the perfect cleaning and shaping of the root canal system. This changes the ideal treatment of a case. The fractured instrument may be located in the direct line of vision; that is, before a curvature, or beyond. The use of nickel-titanium instruments in daily endodontic practice has resulted in an increase in the incidence of fracture[41,51]. Usually, a practitioner removes fractured instruments while relying on his/her tactile sense, intuition and with the help of a radiograph, without being in full control of the procedure.

When faced with a fractured instrument, the possibility of removal should be based on the following factors:

- The type of instrument that fractured (stainless steel or nickel titanium).
- The length of the fractured instrument.
- Location of the fragment in the root canal.
- The relationship between the diameter of the instrument and the diameter and shape of the canal.
- Adaptation of the fragment to the root canal walls.

Although there are a large number of techniques available, fractured instruments can be removed with the use of the OM, ultrasonic instrumentation and methods using microtubes which, when combined, give rise to microsonic techniques that increase the probability of safe removal[36,42,43,51]. Some studies have reported a success rate of 76.9% in cases in which fractured instruments were removing using the above mentioned techniques[29].

First a clinical and radiographic evaluation of the coronal opening has to be made. A first attempt in removing the fragment should be to by-pass it with another instrument of a smaller diameter and apical taper. If this fails more complicated techniques have to be used.

First the amount of magnification should be determined according to the location of the fragment in the root canal, taking into account that at higher magnifications one loses depth of field and one sees a darker working zone. If the fragment is in the apical third, the magnification required will be higher, demanding greater precision and modification of the canal walls. It is advisable to place cotton pellets in the openings of the other canals to prevent the fractured piece from inadvertently falling into them, as has happened on occasion (Figs. 2.XVIII-46A-C).

In all cases, it is necessary to create a straight line access to the fragment, starting by improving the coronal access opening by grinding the dentin as much as is necessary to obtain an unobstructed view of the root canal entrance.

FIGS. 2.XVIII-46A-C

View at 21.3x magnification of a fractured instrument in a mesiobuccal canal at the middle third of the root. The use of ultrasound driven instruments allows the fragment to be displaced. It is prudent to place cotton pellets in the other canals, as the fragment conceivably could be displaced and lodged into another canal, as shown in Figure C.

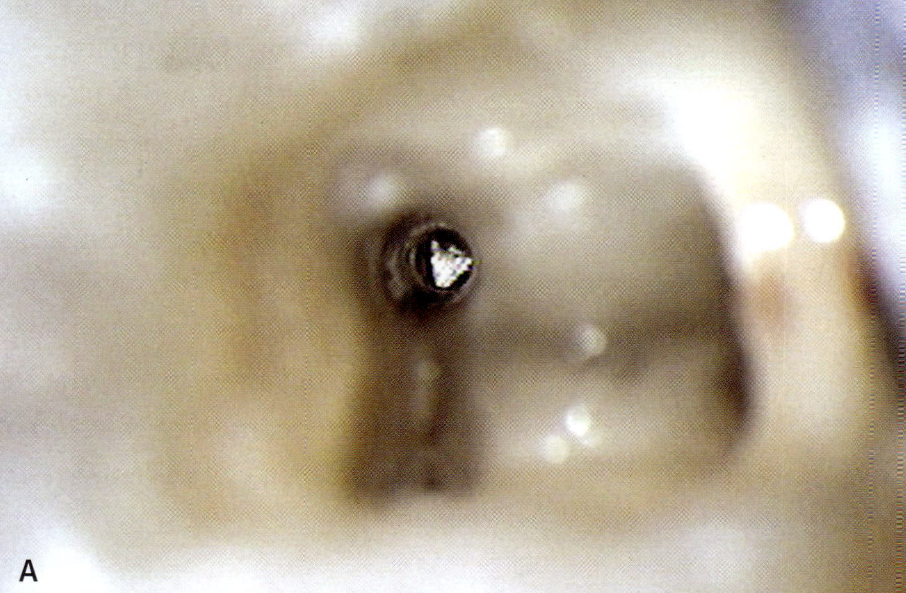

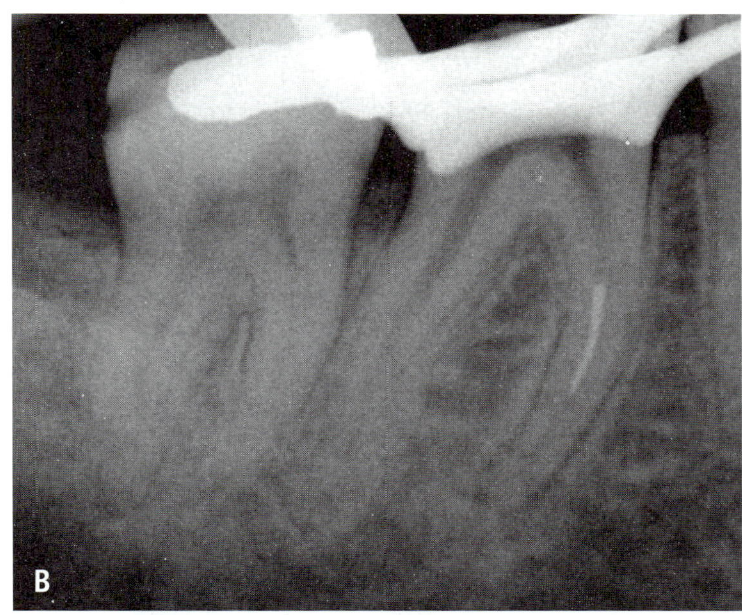

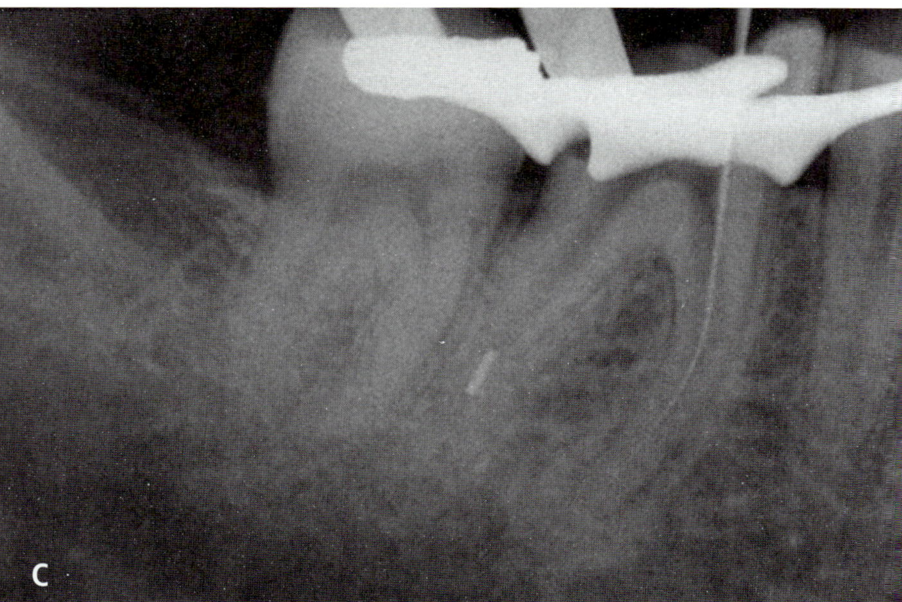

This is followed by carefully establishing straight line access to the root canal opening (anticurvature) endeavoring not to perform lateral wear beyond that which would correspond to shaping without the fractured instrument. Access can be made with modified Gates Glidden drills[43], cutting the active part of the bur perpendicular to its long axis at the height of the middle portion (Fig. 2.XVIII-47). Thus, a platform is created on the most coronal part of the fractured instrument, increasing visibility and access to the obstruction.

A selection of ultrasonic tips is then made after analyzing the diameter of the canal and the depth of the fractured instrument.

ProUltra Endo 3, 4 and 5 ultrasonic tips made of stainless steel and coated with zirconium nitrite can be used. They increase the cutting action, are more durable and more efficient, and safer to use as they are less aggressive than diamond coated tips. When the root is long, and the fragment is at the apex, ProUltra 6, 7 and 8 points are used (previously known as CPR 6, 7 and 8) (Fig. 2.XVIII-48), made of titanium. These tips are longer and thinner, allowing access to areas with little space.

Ultrasonic tips must be used at low power, intermittently, and without irrigation to avoid an increase in temperature of the supporting structures of the tooth. The operator must maintain constant microscopic visual contact with the working area in order to control the reduction (Figs. 2.XVIII-49A-E).

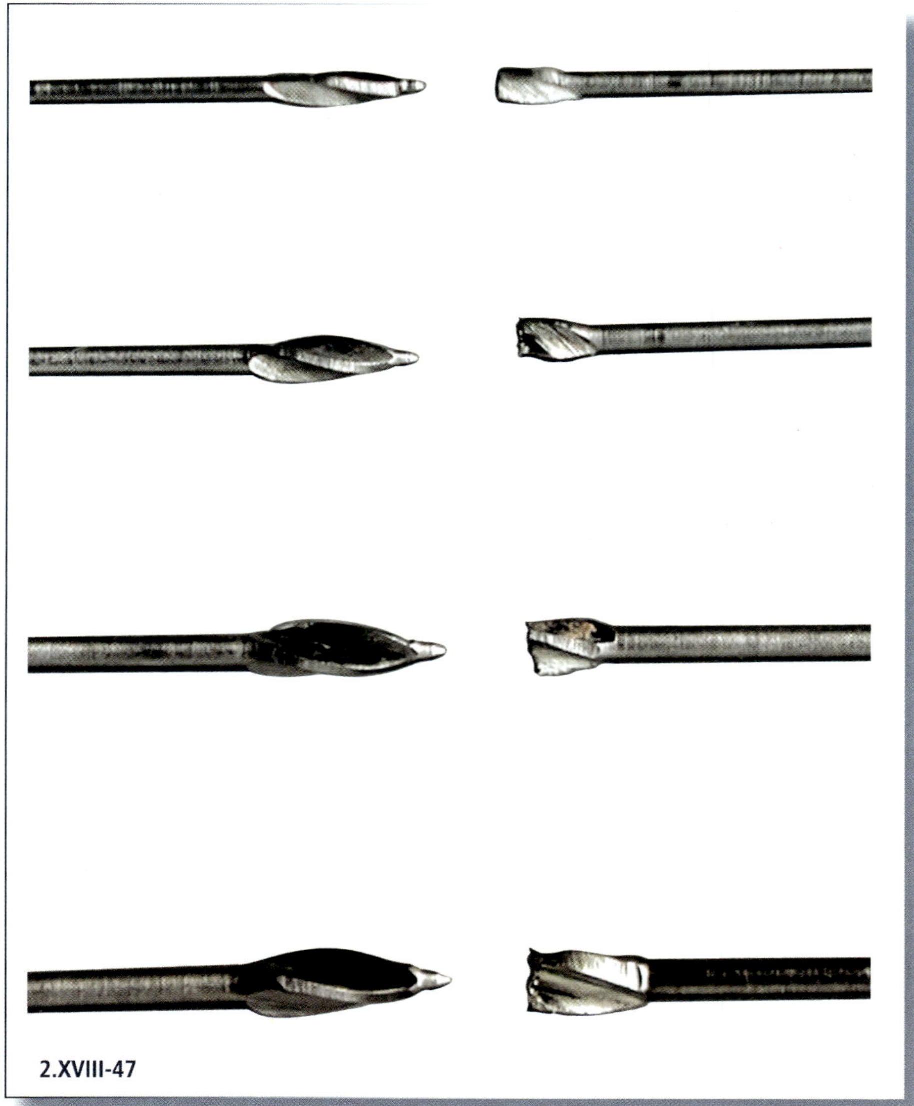

2.XVIII-47

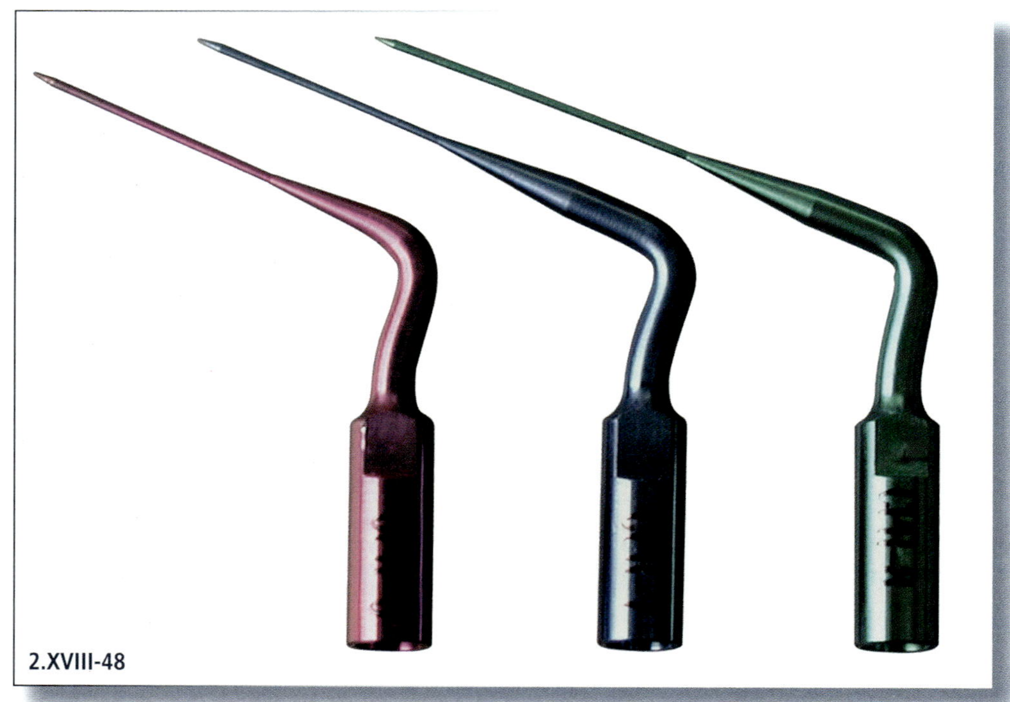

2.XVIII-48

FIG. 2.XVIII-47

Gates Glidden drills modified by a cutting of its active part.

FIG. 2.XVIII-48

Ultrasound tips CPR 6, 7 and 8, now denominated Endo ProUltra 6, 7 and 8.

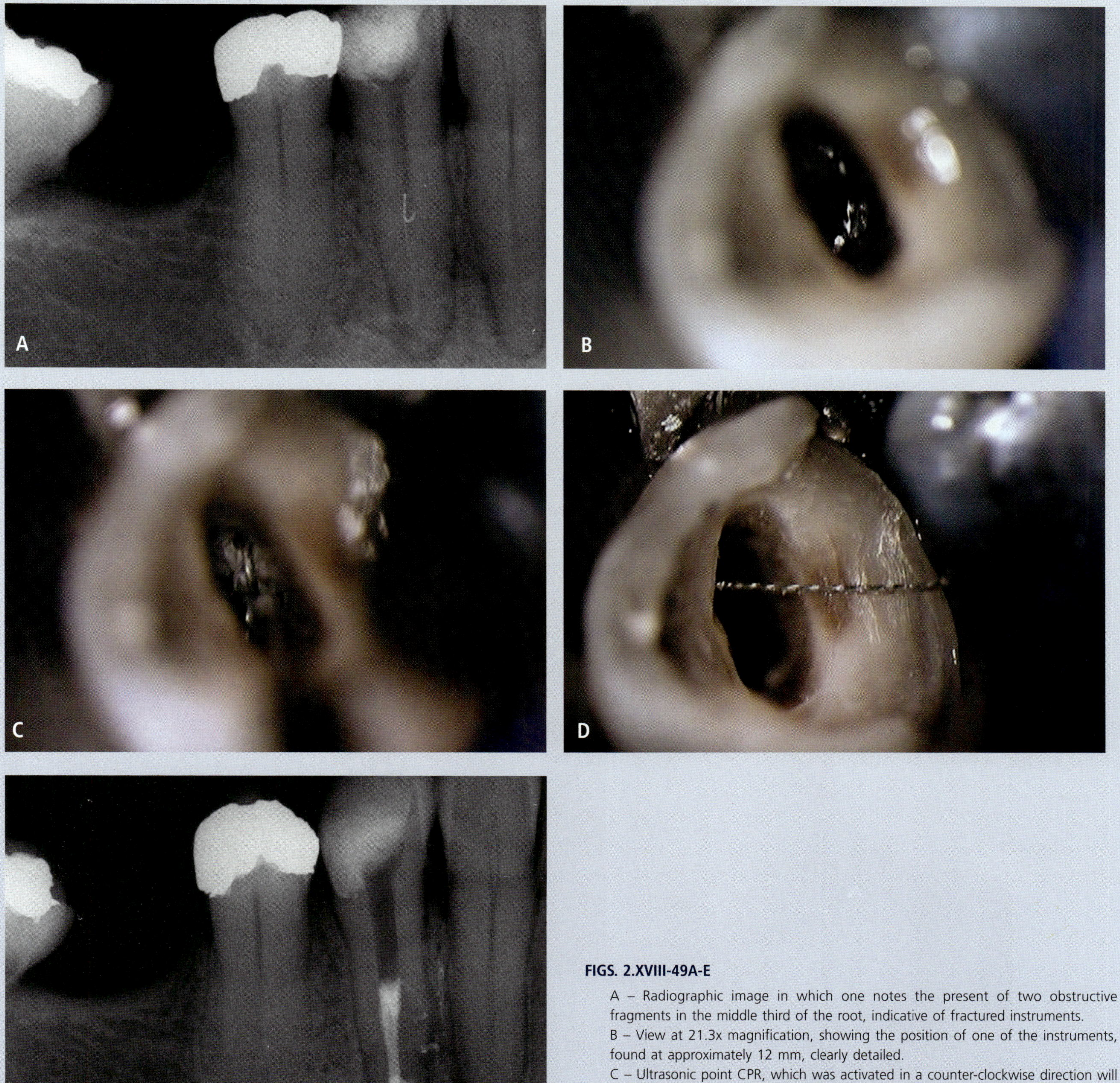

FIGS. 2.XVIII-49A-E

A – Radiographic image in which one notes the present of two obstructive fragments in the middle third of the root, indicative of fractured instruments.
B – View at 21.3x magnification, showing the position of one of the instruments, found at approximately 12 mm, clearly detailed.
C – Ultrasonic point CPR, which was activated in a counter-clockwise direction will remove dentin circumferentially around the instrument.
D – Ultrasonic cavitation helps to displace the instrument which may jump from the canal.
E – Final radiograph.

The ultrasonic tip will remove dentin peripheral to the obstruction, activating it in a counter-clockwise direction, thus exposing a few millimeters of the fragment. At that point an attempt should be made to dislodge it with an endodontic explorer with a very sharp point.

Once the fragment has been loosened, one must try to remove it with irrigation and suction, using a Hedström file, or activating it with an ultrasonic CT4 tip, with irrigation.

It is also possible to remove metal obstructions using the OM and ultrasonic SO4 points (Satelet, Merignace – France), grinding the fragment without changing the dentin that surrounds the obstruction[40].

Access to a fractured instrument can also be created with an ultrasonic ET-20D or E-40D tip (Satelet – France) taken up to the fragment.

Another useful device in combination with the OM is the IRS (*Instrument Removal System – Dentsply-Tulsa Oklahoma*) (Fig. 2.XVIII-50A), a "microtube" created for mechanically holding the fractured instrument, which is an alternative when the fractured instrument cannot be removed with the use of ultrasonic tips[43]. It has two components: A plastic handle (red or black, according to the diameter), and a hollow metal extension with a small opening on one side, close to the end of the microtube. The end part has a 45° bevel. The other part is a solid microcylinder, with an counter clockwise thread, which is introduced inside the microtube (Figs. 2.XVIII-50A-B).

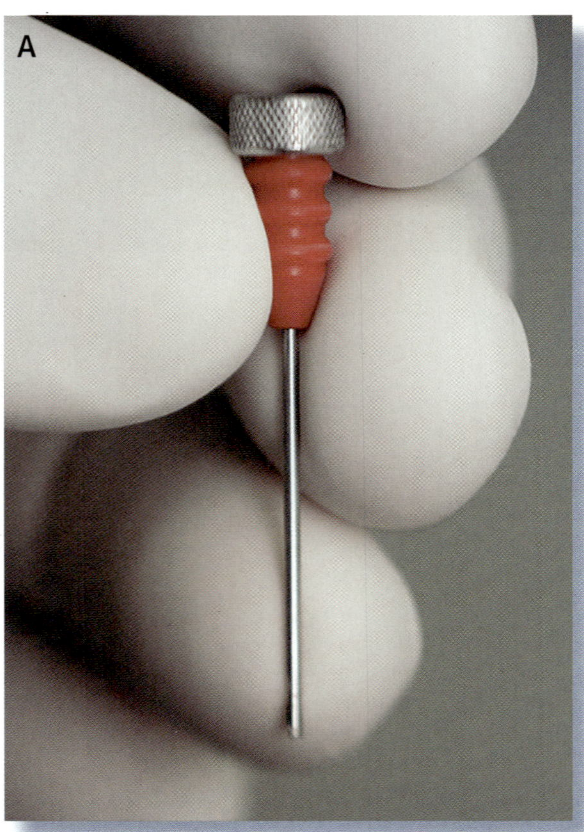

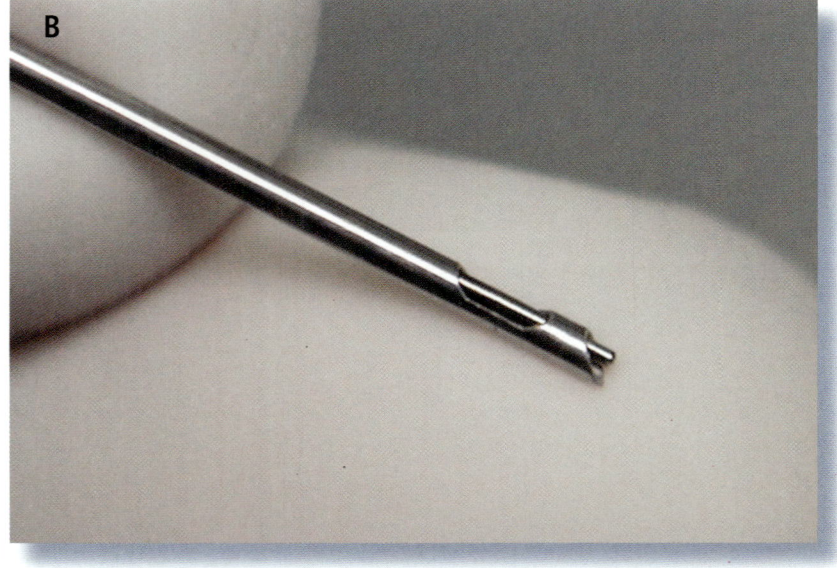

FIGS. 2.XVIII-50A-B

A – IRS System (*Instrumental Removal System*).

B – Detail of the shape of the point introduced into the root canal to lock the coronal portion of the fragment.

The instrument with the black handle resembles a 19 gauge needle (1.0 mm in diameter) and must be used in the two thirds coronal portion of root canals. The instrument with the red handle resembles a 21 gauge needle (0.80 mm in diameter), and allows one to work in more constricted and apical areas. Once the microtube has been selected according to the diameter of the fractured instrument and the depth at which it is located, it will be taken passively up to the coronal portion of the fragment, in such a way that it will be lodged inside the microtube (Fig. 2.XVIIII-50C).

After this the microcylinder will be taken into the microtube and threaded in a counter clockwise direction, so that it fits into the coronal portion of the fractured instrument at the end of the microtube (Fig. 2.XVIIII-51A). Next, one firmly proceeds with removing the IRS, together with the fragment (Fig. 2.XVIIII-51B).

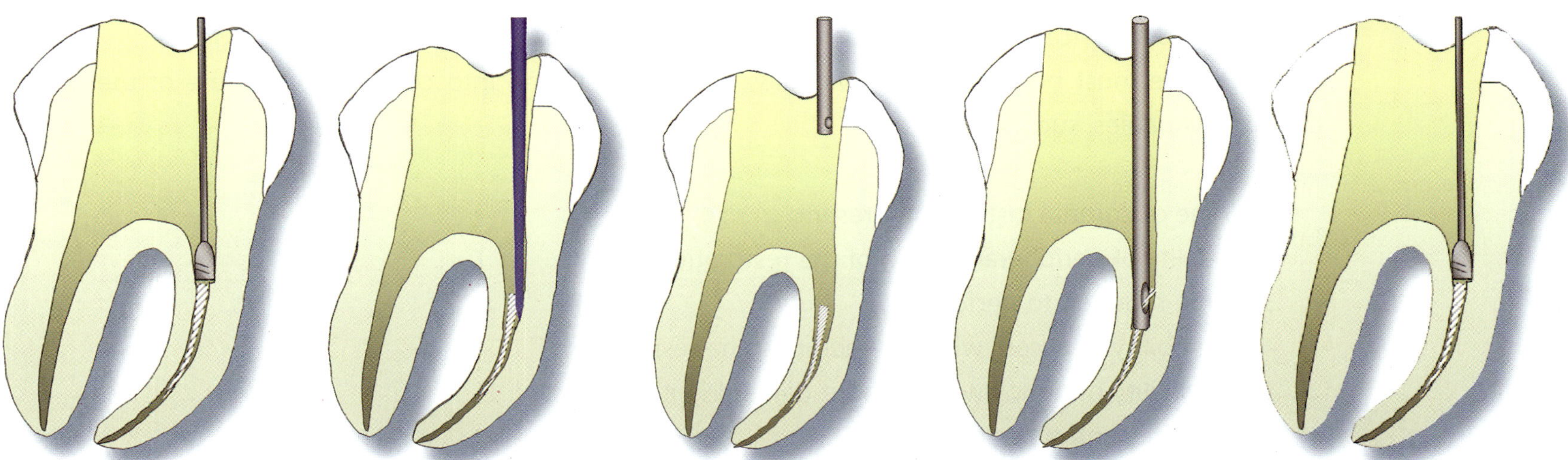

FIG. 2.XVIII-50C

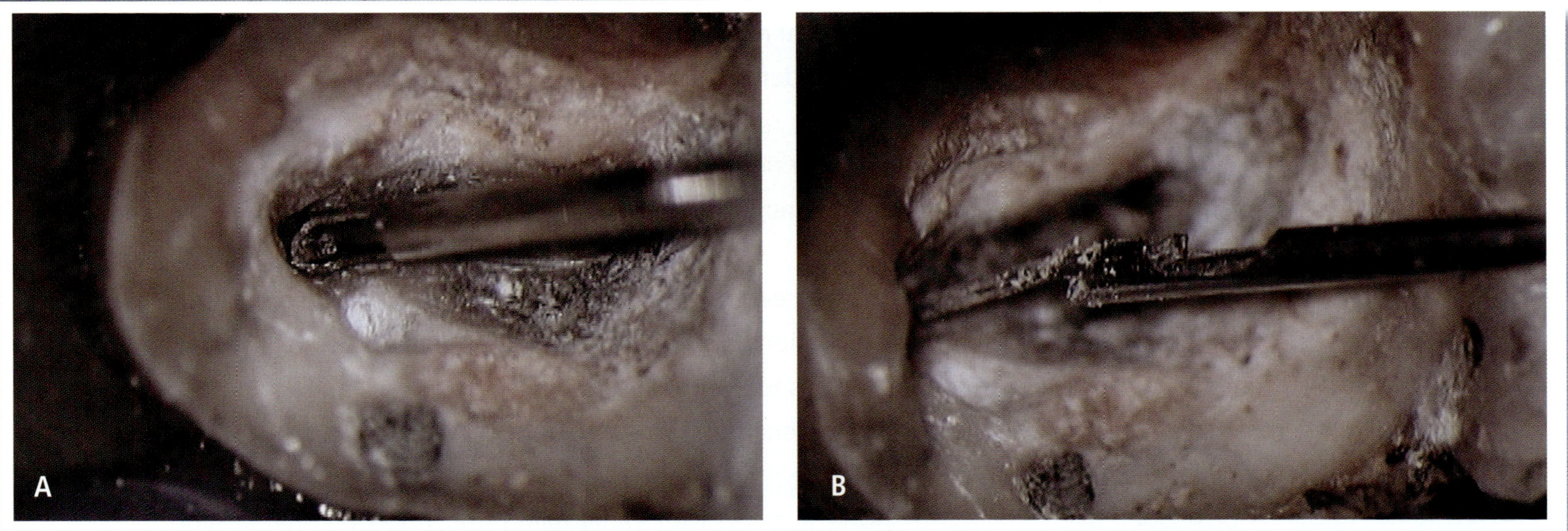

FIGS. 2.XVIII-51A-B

A – the microtube of the IRS, which slides until the coronal portion of the fragment in the lingual canal is put into its lateral opening. This is followed by placing the microcylinder in the microtube, threading it in a counter-clockwise direction, until one feels the fragment stick.
B – The IRS is subtly removed, and together with it, the fragment.

Another possibility is to use the Masseran kit, which has a larger space in the microtube. These alternatives, associated with ultrasound and the OM result in operating procedures that are effective for removing obstructions[38].

Retreatments

When faced with an endodontic failure, it is always necessary to evaluate the possibility of removing the existing filling, in order to access the apical third of the root canal through the crown of the tooth. Using an OM allows for a more conservative approach, minimizing the loss of tooth structure and significantly reducing the number of cases indicated for peri-radicular surgery[39].

Each case must be analyzed individually, particularly taking into consideration some of the common variables, such as:

1. Type of coronal restoration present;
2. Quality of peripheral sealing of the restoration;
3. Time required to perform it;
4. Possibility of access without fracturing the restoration;
5. Possibility of removing it without damaging it;
6. Presence and types of posts;
7. Root canal filling material;
8. Obstruction as a result of fractured instruments;
9. Untreated root canals;
10. Possibility of post-treatment coronal restoration;
11. Strategic value of the tooth in the dental arch.

In Figure 2.XVIII-52A note a mandibular right first molar with partial root canal fillings and some thickening of the apical periodontal ligament, as well as recurrent caries in the mandibular right second molar.

When removing the amalgam and proceeding with the coronal access opening one cannot see the root canal entrances under magnification (Fig. 2.XVIII-52B).

After preparation of straight line access to the canals openings, they are cleaned and the gutta-percha remnants from the previous treatment are removed. During a second session, the root canal system was filled (Fig. 2.XVIII-52C).

A post-operative radiograph shows a dense root canal filling and good coronal sealing (Fig. 2.XVIII-52D).

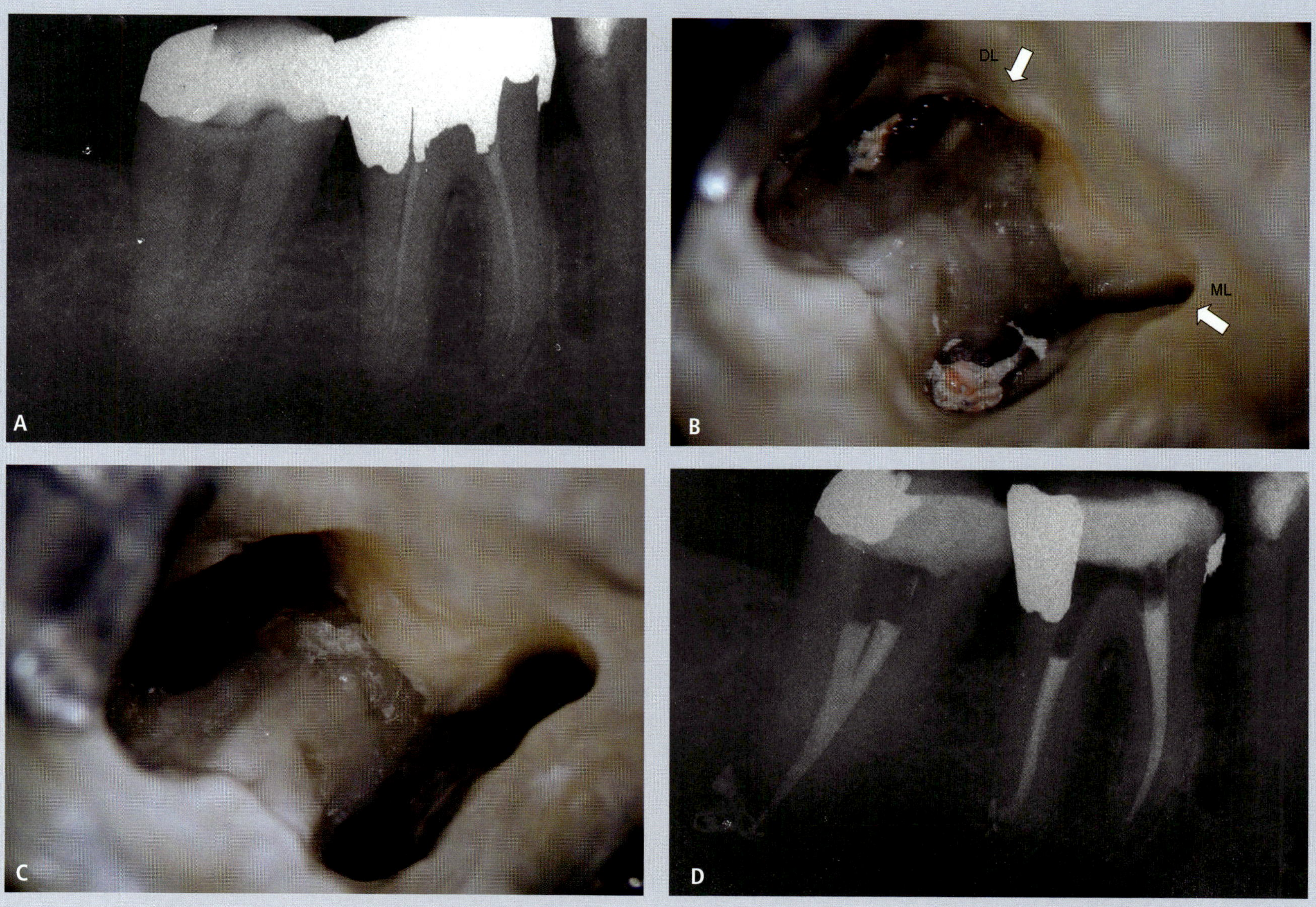

FIGS. 2.XVIII-52A-D

A-D – According to the text.

Repairing Perforations

Perforations are artificial communications between the interior of the root canal system and the oral cavity. They are frequently of iatrogenic origin, occurring during the stage of coronal access preparation, when locating calcified root canals, when preparing space for posts or during shaping in high risk areas of the root. In some cases perforations are pathological, occurring as a result of internal or external resorption.

When faced with a perforation, the operator must evaluate the possibility of sealing the perforation before the operative procedure, take into consideration whether the tooth can be restored or not.

The prognosis of every perforation will depend on the following considerations:

- Size;
- Aseptic conditions under which the accident occurred;
- The time elapsed since the perforation occurred up to the time treatment began;
- The presence of prior periodontal disease[8].

The practitioner must locate the level of the perforation and arrive at a prognosis. If the perforation is close to the crest of the alveolar bone (at the epithelium attachment), the treatment will be critical, due to the risk of bacterial contamination from the gingival sulcus, which may also create a periodontal defect. In general perforations located below the bone crest have a good prognosis.

The selection of the sealing material is based on the location of the perforation, below or above the crest of the bone. Sealing must be done immediately, or at a minimum calcium hydroxide has to be placed, for example Calen, to avoid microbial contamination, promote healing and prevent invagination of the granulation tissue into the interior of the root canal[3,46].

Magnification and illumination are tools of incalculable value when gaining access for treatment of perforations.

Although the principles of treatment of perforations with or without the use of a microscope are the same[51], the use of an OM resource will allow a more rapid location of the communication and a more detailed assessment of the severity of the lesion, thus facilitating hemostasis and preventing further damage of the perforation. Another option that is available and very helpful is the placement of a matrix[24,41].

To manage perforations with the OM, high magnification should be used almost throughout the entire procedure[41]. The amount of magnification is directly related to the location of the perforation. If it is located in the floor of the pulp chamber or in the cervical portion of the root, it is recommended to use medium magnification. If it is more apically, higher magnification is recommended, as a consequence of which light in the working area is diminished. In each case, with the use of endodontic microinstruments, a sealing material is transported and can be placed in the perforation with precision, allowing precise removal of excess material so that the perforation margins are clean and well-defined (Figs. 2.XVIII-53A-H and 2.XVIII-54A-F).

The material that is selected must offer excellent sealing qualities, be dimensionally stable after setting, and induce healing, or at least not affect the surrounding tissues. According to the type of material selected, it may be necessary to use barriers, against which the sealing material can be condensed, and which will have to possess hemostatic properties allowing the sealing material to set without contamination.

Treatment of a perforated tooth begins with periodontal probing. Then the reason for the perforation should be determined in order to correct the errors of coronal access opening and root canal location, by means of radiographs at various angles, to decide and evaluate the height and position (supra or infra-osseus) of the perforation. It is also necessary to evaluate the amount of affected tooth structure, in order to decide whether or not the tooth can be restored. Treatment

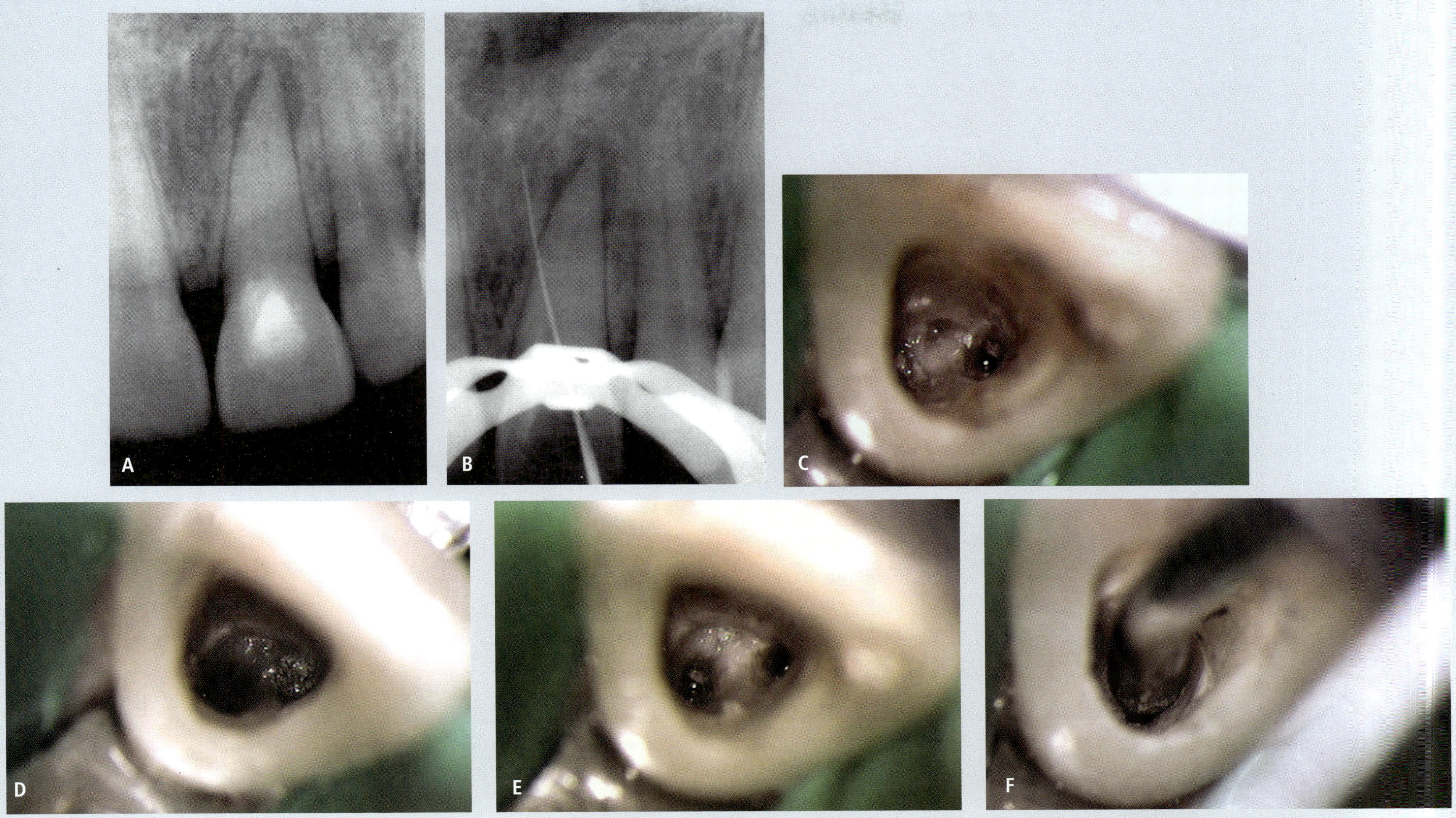

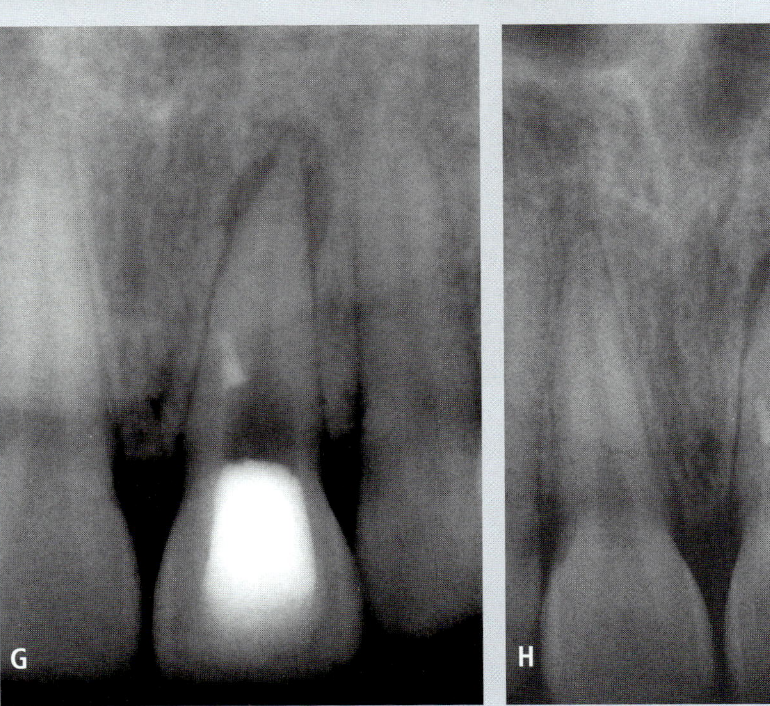

FIGS. 2.XVIII-53A-H

A – Radiographic evaluation shows evidence of a severely calcified root canal system.
B – To corroborate, observe a perforation at the level of the middle third of the root.
C – Image at 21.3x magnification, in which the perforation is noted.
D – Correction of the coronal opening, as a result of the changes in color between sclerotic and sound dentin, located at the main entrance of the canal.
E – Perforation is sealed with MTA placed with a Dovgan Carrier microtransporter.
F – Microinstruments allow great precision in perforation sealing procedures.
G – Post-operative radiograph of sealed perforation.
H – Final radiograph of completed case.

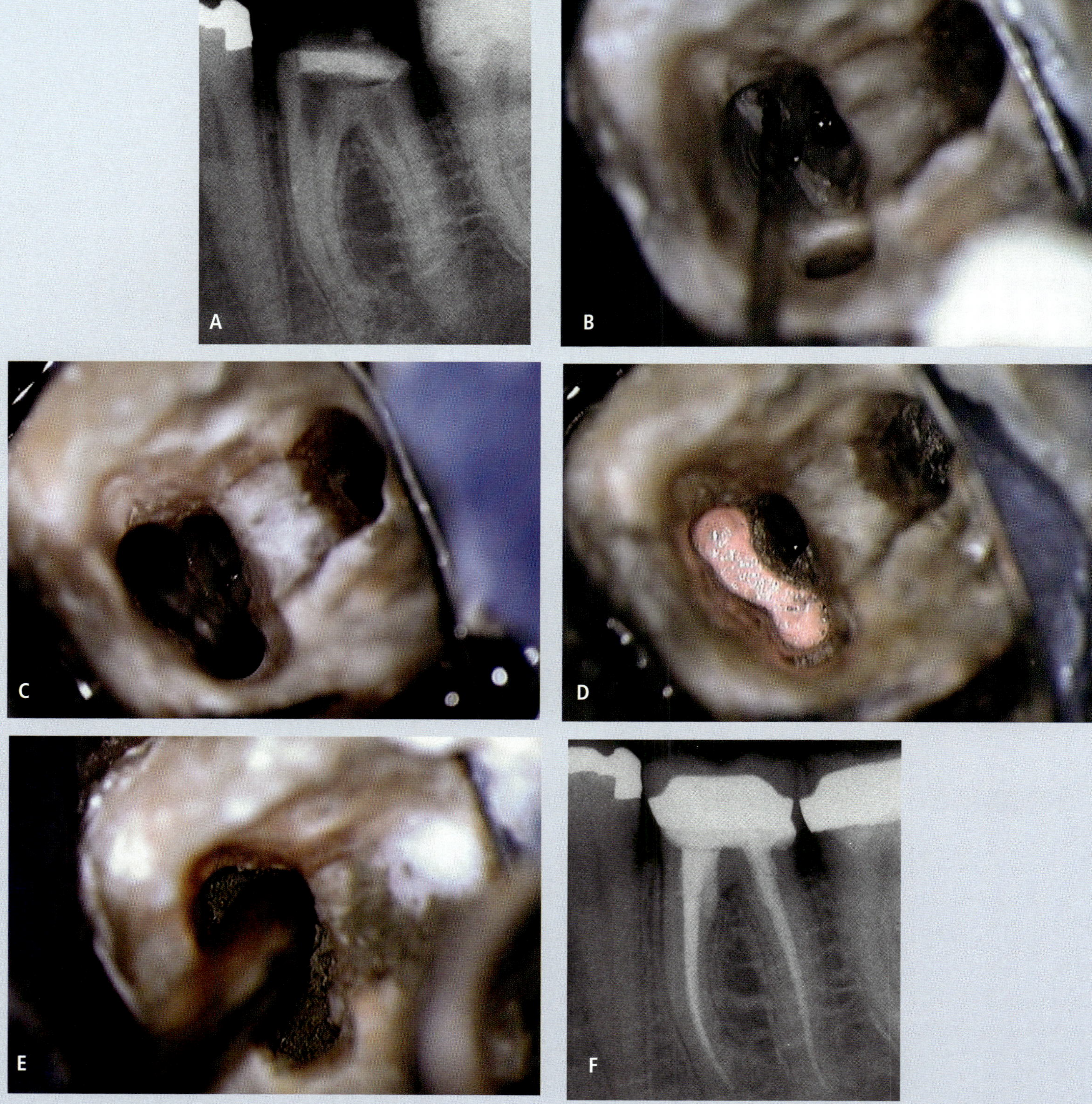

FIGS. 2.XVIII-54A-F

A – Radiographic evaluation shows the unsupported mesial coronal portion at the level of the furcation.
B – View at 21.3x magnification; note the communication with the periodontium. The difference in tonality of the dentin guides the operator when using the OM.
C – Root canal system cleaning and shaping.
D – Endodontic filling was performed below the perforation area.
E – Placement of MTA facilitated with the use of the OM.
F – Post-operative follow-up radiograph after 14 months. Note the close contact of the perforation sealing material and favorable response of the periodontium.

then begins by irrigation with a sodium hypochlorite solution to remove granulation tissue from the perforation. Some clinicians prefer to use chlorhexidine for antisepsis of the perforated area.

In Figure 2.XVIII-55A presents a mandibular first premolar with a calcified root canal system. While performing coronal opening there was a lateral distal deviation in an apical direction, as a result of an error during the operative procedure (Figs. 2.XVIII-55B-C). Figure 2.XVIII-55D shows the considerable reduction and deviation made by the operator in an attempt to locate the root canal.

During the treatment of severely calcified root canals, the operator must use endodontic instruments very carefully, as they tend undergo fatigue from the stress to which they are submitted during use.

In the clinical case of Figures 2.XVIII-55E and F, note a small diameter instrument fractured in the middle third when an attempt was made to move it in the apical direction.

Under magnification and with the use of illumination it was possible to save the root and establish working length with the help of a radiograph (Fig. 2.XVIII-55G).

The perforation was sealed with MTA and the pulp chamber filled with a glass ionomer (Figs. 2.XVIII-55H-K).

PERI-RADICULAR SURGERY

The OM is indispensable for improving surgical dexterity with respect to management of both hard and soft tissues. Light and visibility are always critical factors during any surgical procedure. One of the most frequent causes that contributes to failure in peri-radicular surgery is the inability to see small details of the operative field. The OM contributes to better control over apical surgical procedures, such as: osteotomy, apical curettage, apicectomy, root surface examination, apical cavity preparation and filling, later examination of the surgical area and documenting the case. It can be used continually during all the stages of peri-radicular surgery, allowing healthy tissue to be differentiated from pathological tissue and facilitating complete removal of the lesion, while healthy structures are protected. One can also visualize anatomical land marks, such as the maxillary sinus, mental nerve and orifice for microsuture 6-0 or 7-0[26] (Figs. 2.XVIII-56A-G).

The use of the OM improves root surface inspection, with high magnification and illumination, and makes it easy to locate anatomical details such as the isthmus, accessory and lateral canals, apical transport, quality of the root canal filling and a previous apicectomy, which will allow one to understand the reason for failure.

The location of the canalicular isthmus has frequently been overlooked, and when located, it was difficult to prepare. Currently, with the help of a surgical microscope and microsurgical equipment, practitioners have a better view of the root surface and are able to identify the isthmus and prepare it more precisely using an ultrasonic tip. Recognition and preparation of the canalicular

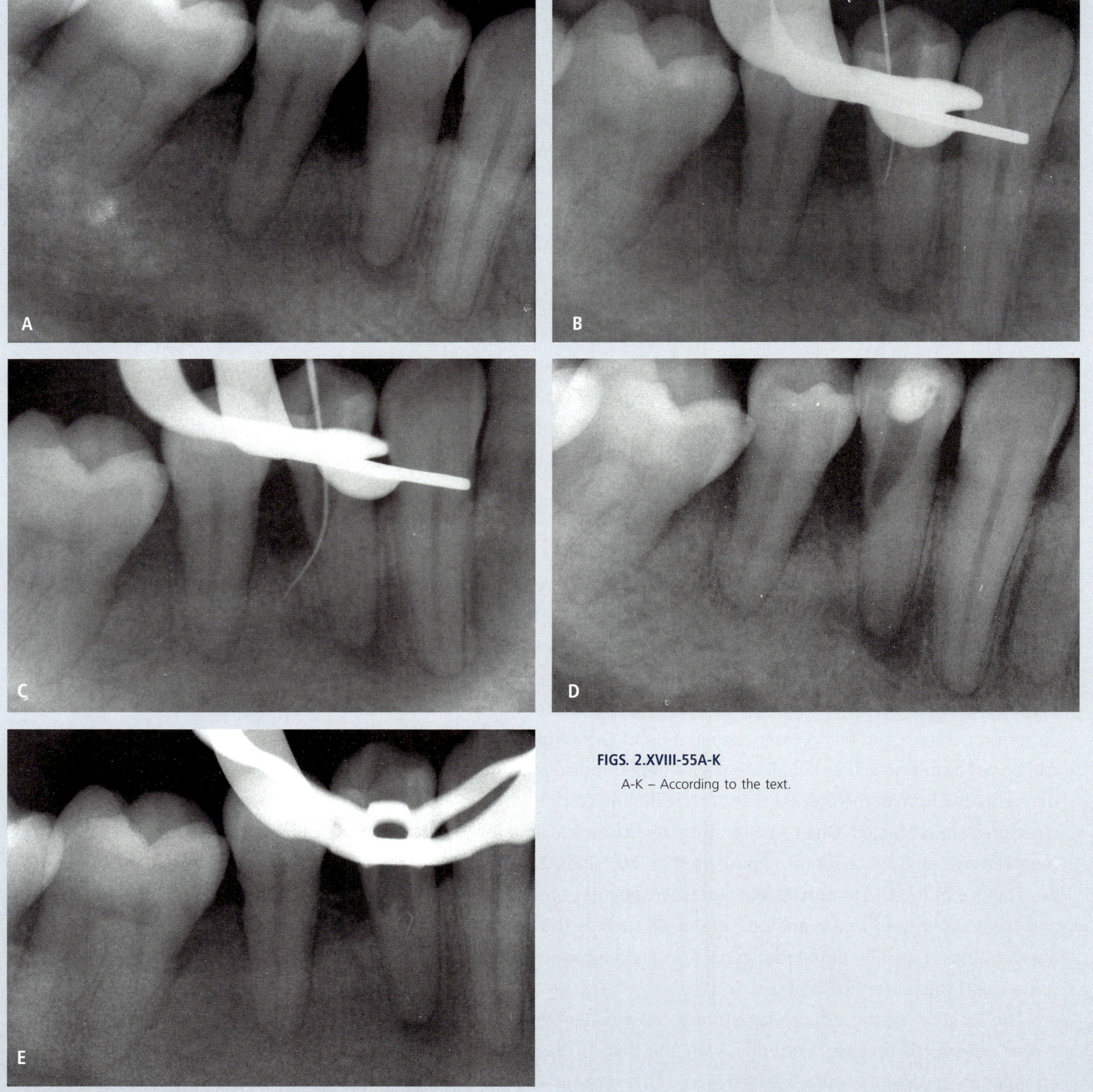

FIGS. 2.XVIII-55A-K

A-K – According to the text.

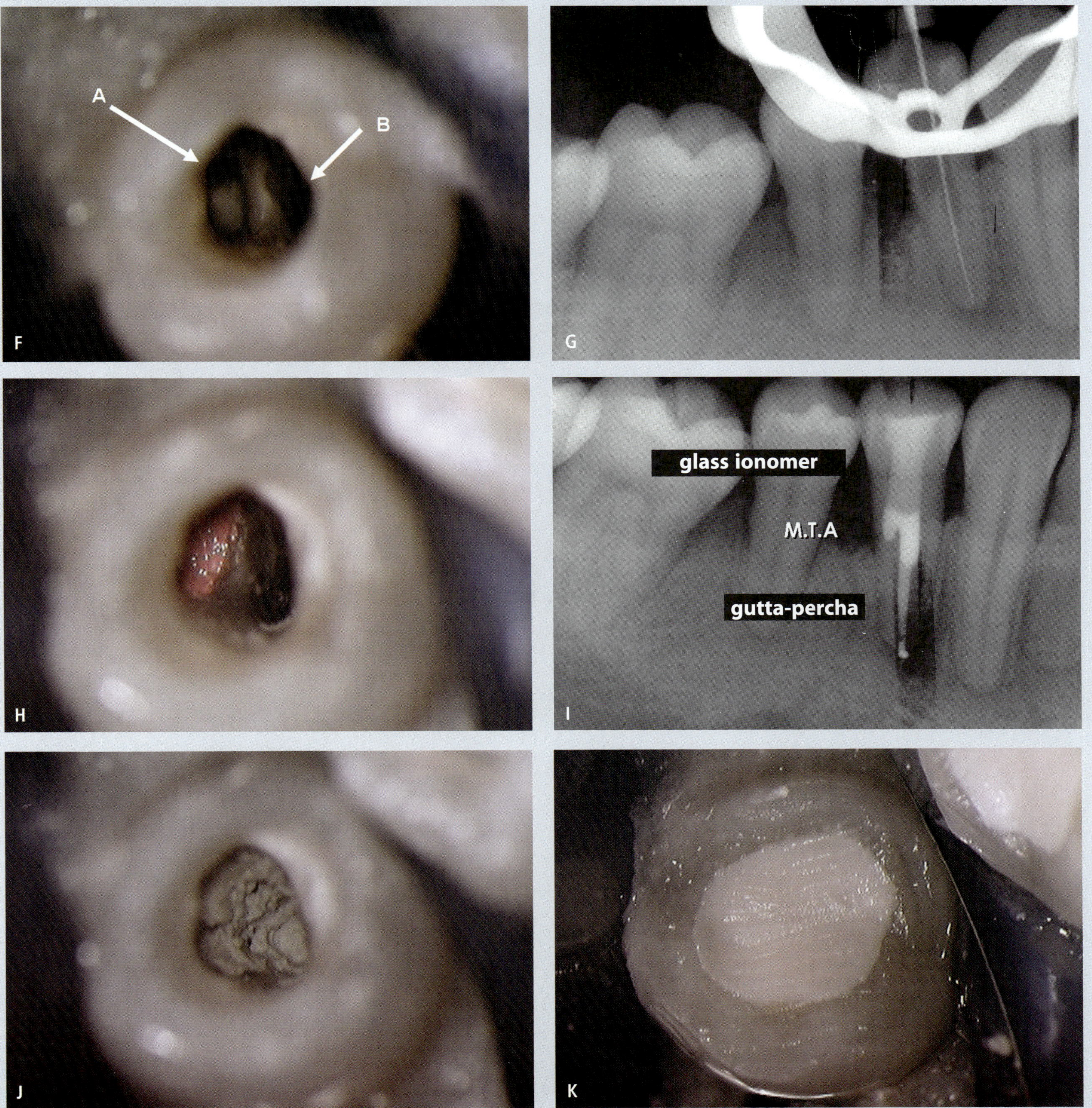
A
B
F
G
glass ionomer
M.T.A
gutta-percha
H
I
J
K

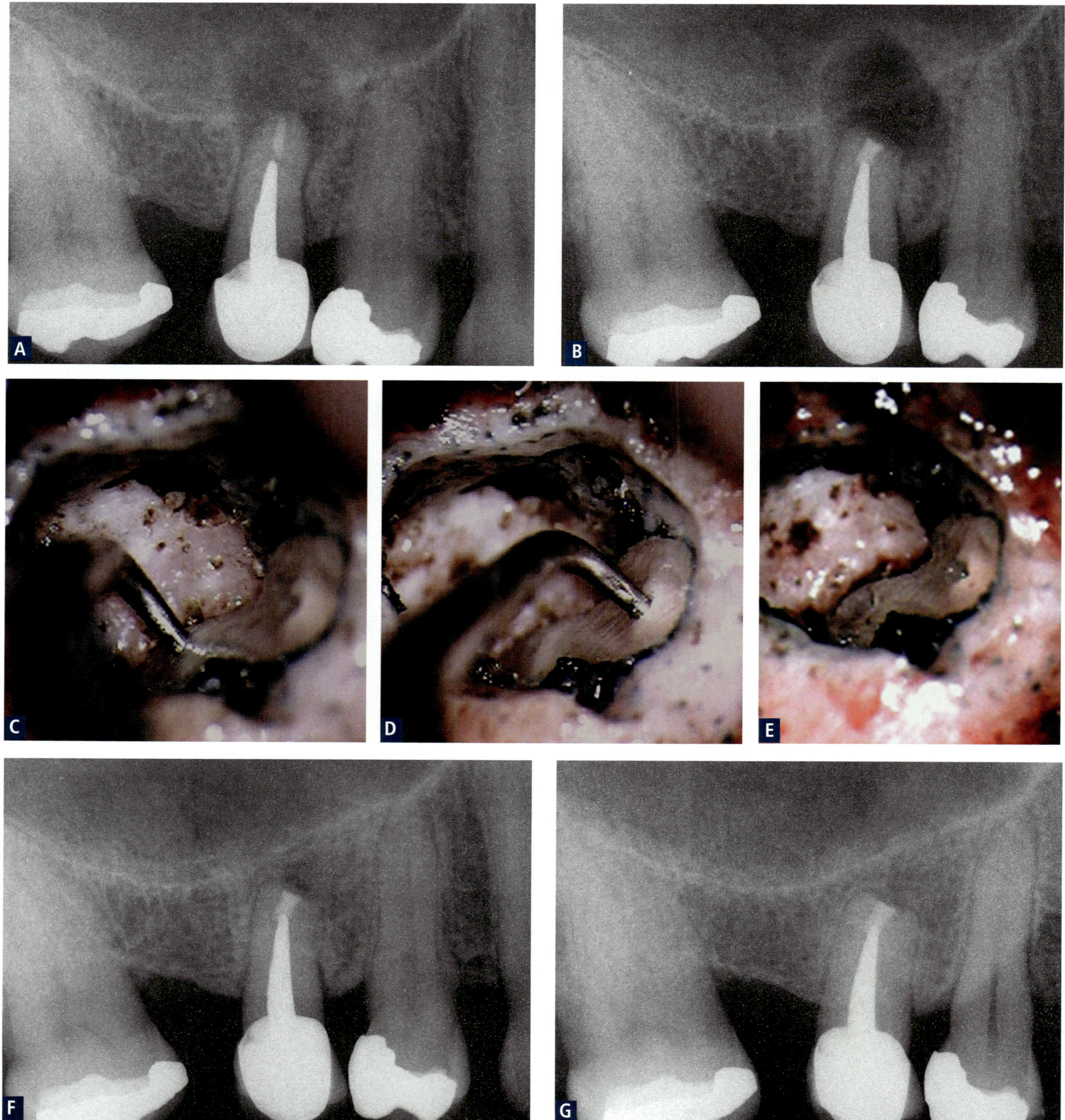

FIGS. 2.XVIII-56A-G

A – Radiograph for diagnosis. Note the circumscribed radiolucent periapical lesion and tooth restored with crown and post.

B – Radiographic image of the immediate post-operative period; as a result of the initial size of coronal destruction, coronal opening was wide.

C, D and E – Images at 21.3x magnification, in which one sees the apical preparation with and ultrasonic instrument. Methylene blue helps to identify the canals and periodontal ligament.

F – Follow-up radiograph taken at 6 months.

G – Follow-up radiograph taken after 1 year. Note the complete repair of the periapical region.

isthmus is a factor that improves the success rate in peri-radicular surgery evaluations of posterior teeth. It has also made it easier to better evaluate the cavity preparation for later retrofilling.

For these cases 8-10x magnification is recommended, to differentiate the root from the bone, and a high magnification (between 16-25x) to identify the cause of failure, examine the excised surface and evaluate the apical cavity and its filling.

As occurs in re-treatments, incorporation of the surgical microscope has improved instrumentation and the techniques especially prepared for microsurgery (Figs. 2.XVIII-57 to 2.XVIII-60), making it less traumatic.

The surgical microscope is extremely useful for the management of soft tissues. It is not imperative, but in the anterior regions, where there are relevant esthetic demands, it facilitates the incision and lifting of the surgical flap[18]. Incisions are made with microsurgical scalpel blades (Fig. 2.XVIII-57), which make the procedure more precise, allowing the flap to be replace without producing scars in the area[13].

Similarly, improvement in ultrasonic tips has revolutionized surgical procedures (Figs. 2.XVIII-59A-B), enabling smaller surgical access and osteotomies, creating more conservative apical preparations that are in the same long axis as the tooth, and providing a simple preparation of the isthmus. These apical preparations can be observed, evaluated and corrected with the use of surgical micromirrors, so that apical surgery is performed at a high level of excellence, with faster and more predictable healing[11].

Some authors[39] have reported a lower incidence of post-operative pain and faster recovery from peri-radicular surgeries performed with the surgical microscope. Due to being less invasive, the surgical procedure produces less displacement, tension and compression of the surgical flap, reducing tissue damage, inflammation and pain[33].

Rubistein & Kim[41], after one year, obtained 96.8% repair of the peri-radicular surgeries performed with the surgical microscope, using super-EBA as a retrofilling material. A follow-up 5 -d 7 years later showed that out of a total of 59 roots evaluated, 54 (91.5%) remained repaired, while 5 (8.5%) showed evidence of apical disorganization.

The main reason for failure in peri-radicular surgery is related to inadequate apical preparation. The operator must prepare the canals and the isthmus in order to ensure successful surgery. This demands that the operator has broad knowledge of root anatomy, the use of ultrasound activated instruments designed for this purpose, and in many cases, magnification.

There are also "special instruments" with particular handles for locating canals, made in such a way that they do not hamper vision while operating the OM (Fig. 2.XVIII-61).

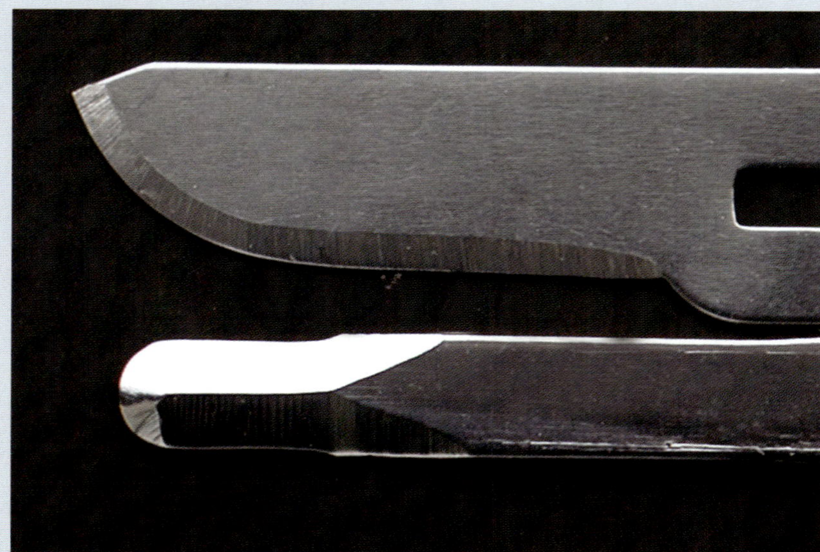

FIG. 2.XVIII-57
Conventional scalpel blade No.15 (above) and microscalpel blade (below).

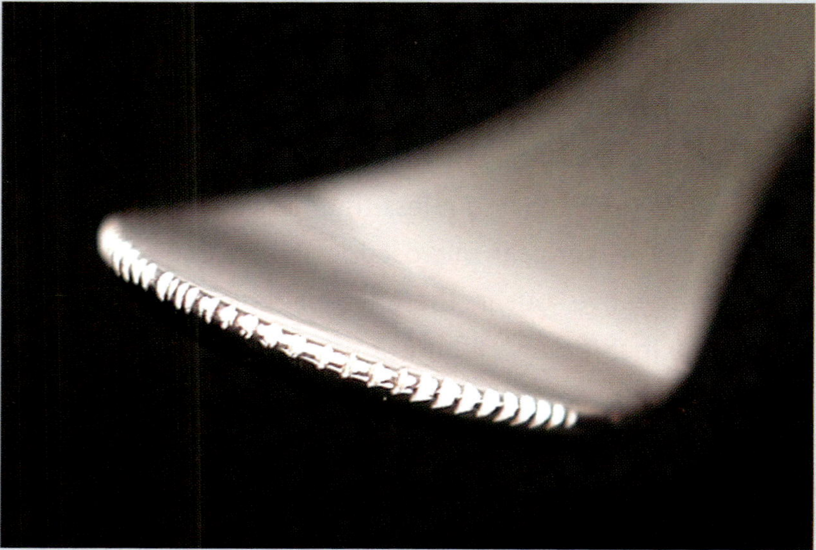

FIG. 2.XVIII-58
The present retractors have serrated surfaces that allow better support on bone structures.

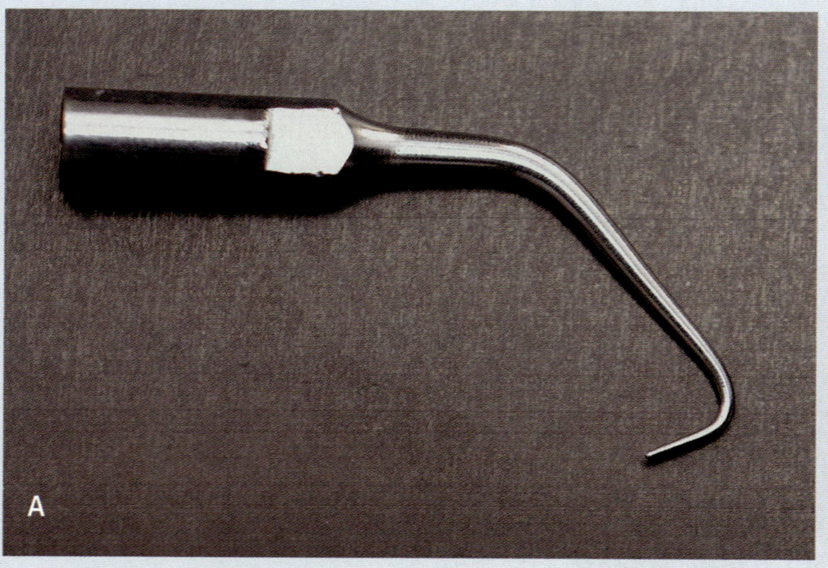

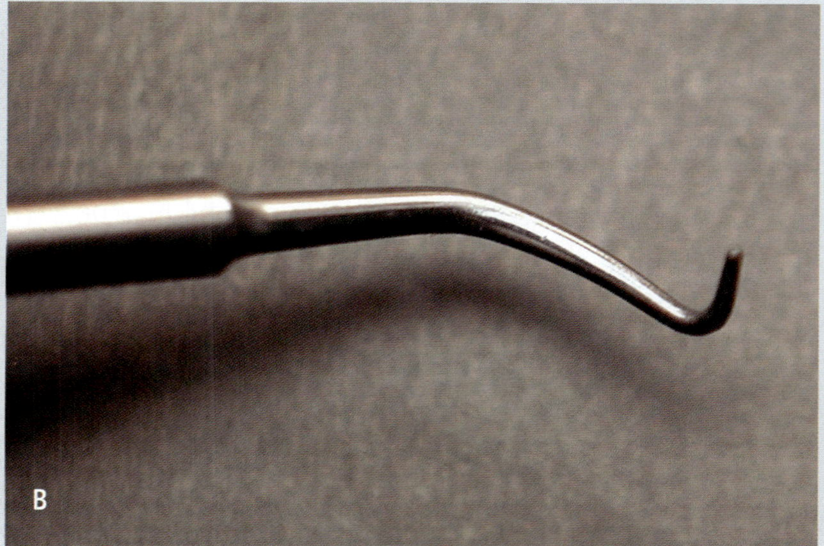

FIGS. 2.XVIII-59A-B
Ultrasonic tips designed for preparing apical cavities.

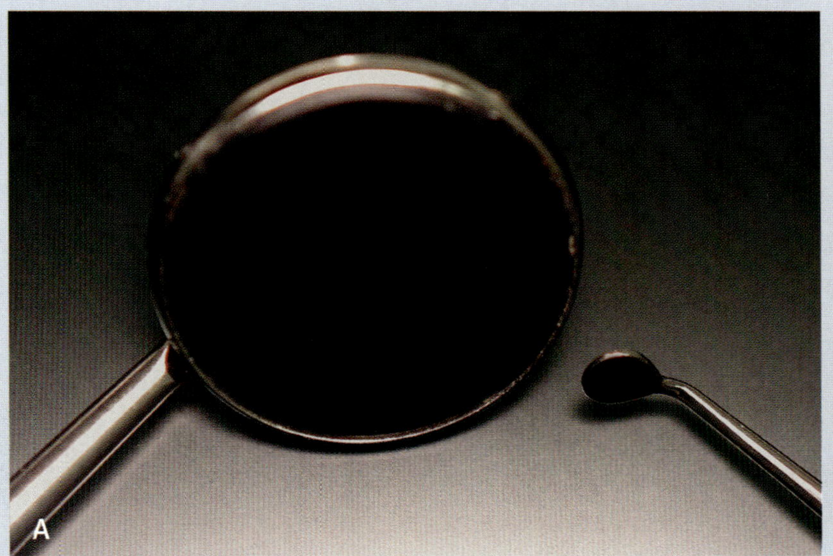

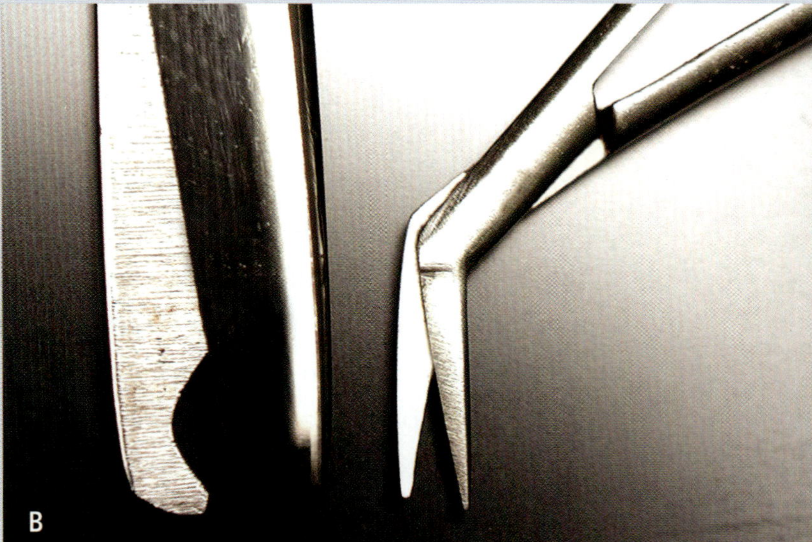

FIGS. 2.XVIII-60A-B

The use of the OM demands the creation of instruments that adapt to a new form of work.
A – Comparison between the sizes of conventional buccal mirrors and micromirrors.
B – Scissors for removing suture threads.

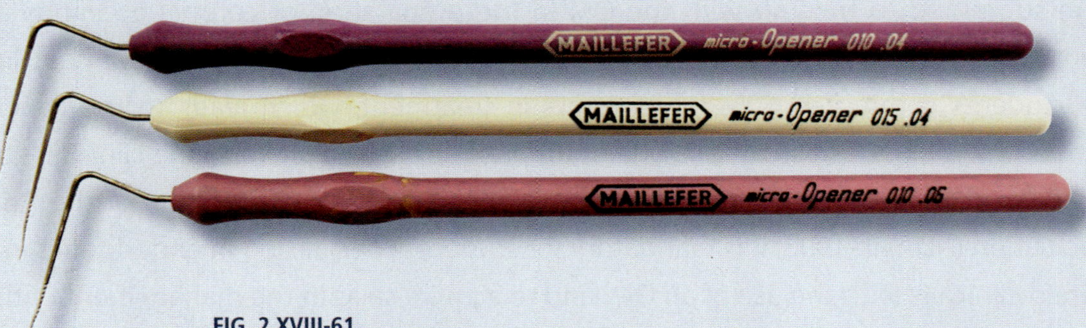

FIG. 2.XVIII-61

Special instruments for locating the apex.

ERGONOMICS

"The major problem of the Operating Microscope (OM) is ergonomics."
"The OM needs to be ergonomic in order to be used."
"The OM forces the practitioner to work in an ergonomic manner."[9]

The dentist is frequently faced with the problem of incorporating the OM into his/her clinical routine. This may happen due to a lack of knowledge or training, or because the dental office is not conveniently suited for the installation of the OM. We must bear in mind that this is a new piece of equipment with in addition auxiliaries, such as monitors, image receiving systems, ultrasound, and specific instruments. Therefore it requires its own ergonomics.

The introduction of the microscope in the dental office was a great revolution that included many ergonomic changes[4]. When starting working with the OM, the practitioner must not take his/her eyes off the binoculars, or hands off the operating field. For many, the value of magnification in dentistry brings ergonomic benefits, by diminishing the working time and eliminating the need to adopt adverse postures that place the head out of a position of balance on the center of the spinal column. In response to this type of posture, the neck and shoulder muscles contract to stabilize the head by the weight of gravity, worsening muscular problems. If these bad postural habits are not corrected, degeneration of the spinal disks and hernias may occur[15,20,39,43,49].

There is an apparent improvement in the motor skills of practitioners that begin using the OM, due to an increase in visual acuity[7,12,18,21,50]. It has been reported that post graduate dental students acquired valuable clinical endodontic skills, improving their performance, when they were submitted to training with the OM in the preparation of coronal openings and root canal identification[35]. Preliminary studies have shown that thanks to the improvement in visual acuity, the students committed 50% fewer errors in treatment, which leads to the conclusion that by increasing visibility, one increases operating precision, irrespective of the clinician's age or physical condition [21,39,43]. As decided by the Commission on Dental Accreditation of the American Dental Association (ADA) in 1998, it is mandatory for students specializing in endodontics in the USA to be trained clinically with the use of an OM, and to acquire skills in the management of the instruments associated with the OM, and to have knowledge about all the aspects of its use in endodontic therapy[1,11,21,41,44].

Control of blood, saliva, quantity of light, focus, vibrations of the equipment (OM), movements of the patient, direction of light, position of the chair, etc., are essential, individually or in combination, in determining success.

The present concept is not to move the OM around the patient, but to move the patient, the mirror, etc., and stabilize the OM[34]. For small movements, it is convenient for the operator to move the patient's head slightly, by displacing the chair or headrest with his/her legs (Fig. 2.XVIII-62).

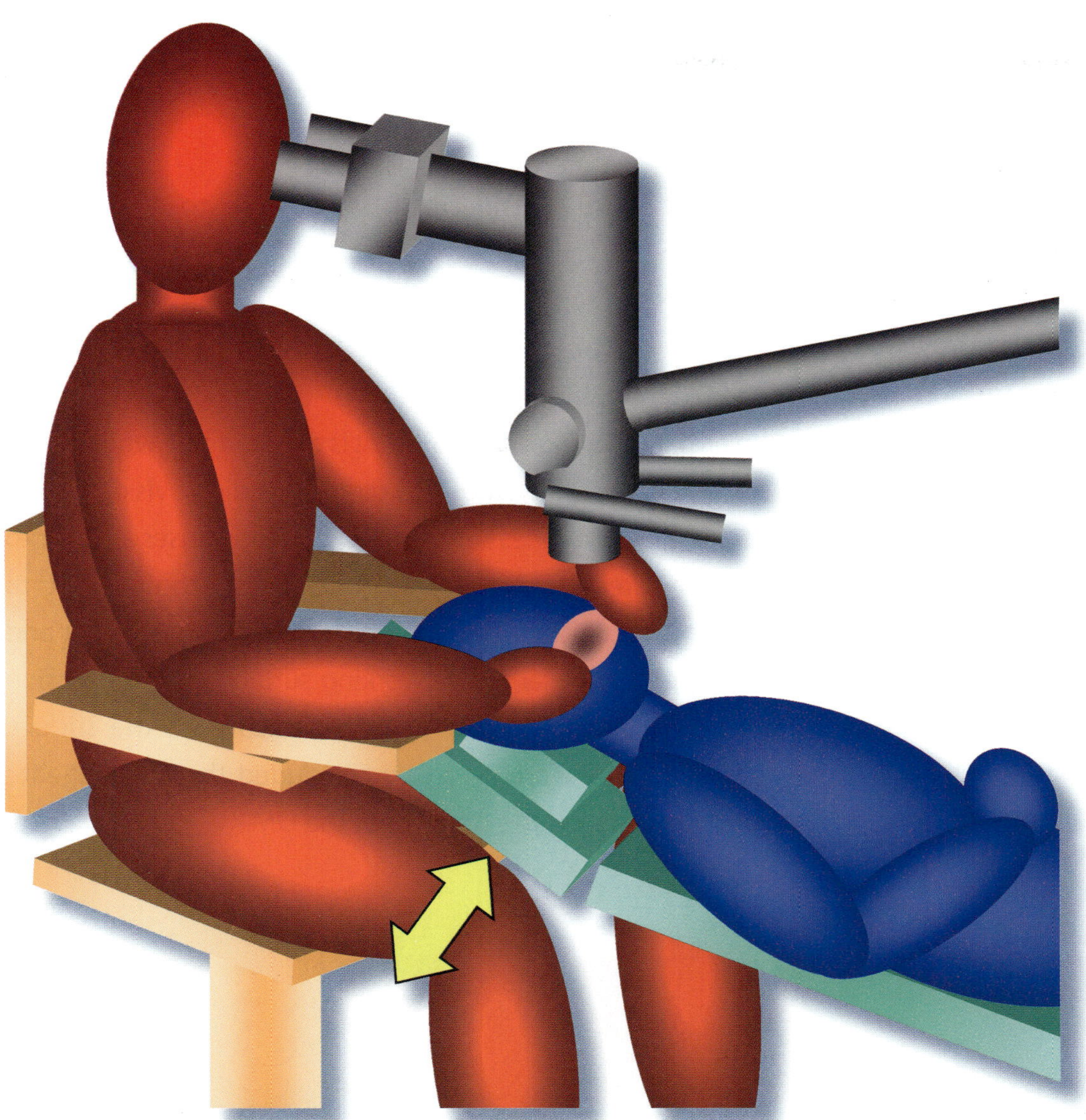

FIG. 2.XVIII-62

Operator's working position; he/she can slightly change the focus by displacing the patient's chair with his/her leg.

Frequent changes in the head of the OM, patient and mirror are necessary and predictable. It is critical for the operator to have the skill and training to move into new areas of magnification easily and quickly.

SUGGESTIONS

1. Find a position with which you feel comfortable and works well;
2. Do not start at the highest magnification;
3. Do not move the OM around the patient;
4. Raise the patient a little, so that he/she sits in a more vertical position. This allows the OM to have a view perpendicular to the occlusal plane;
5. Listen to and learn from colleagues that use the OM in daily practice, and not from those that simply fix it to the wall of the office as decoration.

WORKING POSITIONS

An optimum working position for the operator results in balance between the patient's head, dental chair, operating microscope, chair, lighting, assistant and control of accessories.

The patient's head must remain in the center of the headrest, for his/her comfort and allow for necessary movements. For high precision procedures, for example, in apical microsurgery, it is advisable to help the patient fixing his/her head with a neck pillow such as used for traveling. The neck muscles must not become tense, to avoid fatigue (Fig. 2.XVIII-63).

It has been demonstrated that it is more convenient to reposition the patient's head, or change his/her posture to facilitate a view of the working area, than to move the OM. That way the operator can maintain the ideal position and posture throughout the operative procedure.

Dentists have the tendency to suffer from muscle pain in the neck, shoulders and in the lower part of the back[32]. An angle of inclination of the head exceeding 25° increases the practitioners propensity to develop pain in the neck and back. To prevent this, it is important for the operator to maintain an erect posture. Here the use of tiltable binoculars becomes significant, as they allow the head to be kept in a neutral position, which meets the ergonomic demands.

THE PATIENT'S POSITION

With the use of the OM it is possible to examine an object at numerous magnifications, while the use of intra-oral mirrors provide visual access comparable with that of an endoscope, but without vision at any angle. This is the wonder of magnification.

In ergonomics, an essential point is to determine whether the practitioner will be working with direct or indirect vision, as the position of the OM varies substantially when one uses a mirror to focus on the area to be treated. In general it is recommended to work with direct vision: The operator must always be erect and the light perpendicular to the working surface. If indirect vision is necessary, the light must be perpendicular to the surface of the mirror. Therefore it can be concluded that the patient's position depends on the position of the OM.

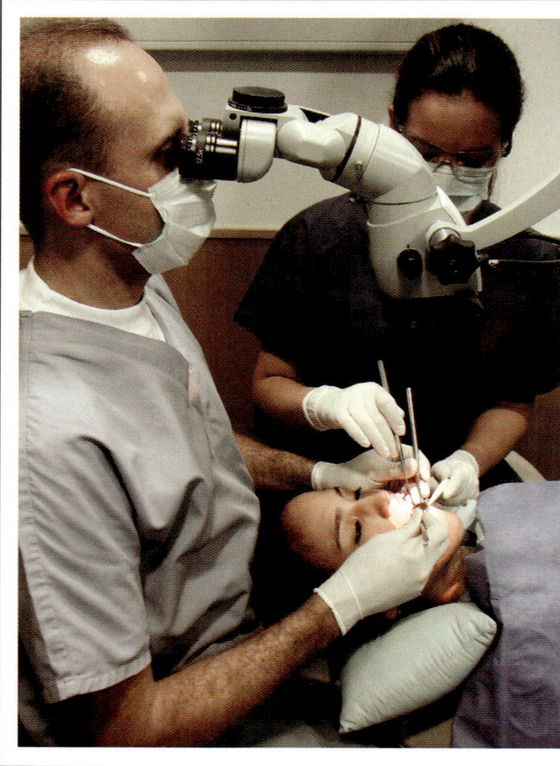

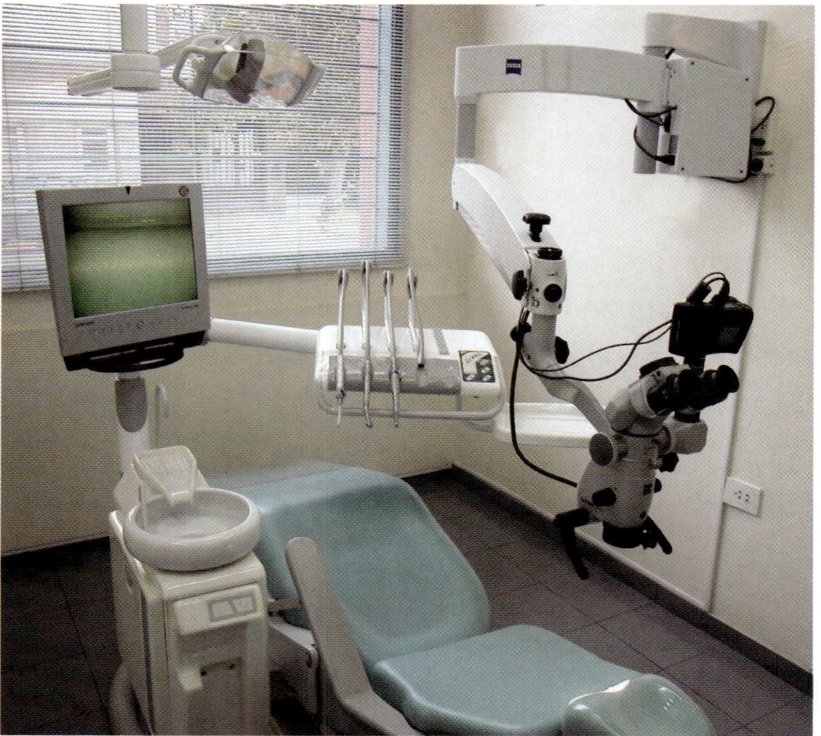

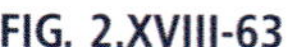

FIG. 2.XVIII-63
Pillow to support the patient's head in a fixed position.

FIG. 2.XVIII-64
Fixed, wall-mounted OM.

POSITION OF THE OPERATING MICROSCOPE

The OM, as well as the X-ray machine, must be placed in the dental office in a location that allows convenient and quick access, and does not interfere with traffic or with the operating area.

The **mobile model of OM** has a base that allows it to be moved. It is useful in clinics, in which the equipment has to be moved from one dental operatory to the other, and in teaching centers. In the dental office, however, it takes up a great deal of space and hampers the movement of the operator, assistant and patient.

The **fixed OM** can be attached to the wall, but the best option is **fixation to the ceiling**. In the latter position, the OM support must be positioned exactly over the dental spittoon. This position will give it the greatest stability and limit back and forth movements to a great extent. To sum up, the location must allow the operator to use one hand only to position it quickly and in a single maneuver (Fig. 2.XVIII-64).

The arms of the OM have ball bearings to allow for movement in three dimensions. By adjusting or loosening them, the mobility of the arms and articulations is fixed. It is important to obtain a balance between mobility and fixation, with exact adjustment of the washers that fix the rollers. Adjustments during operative procedures must be avoided, as this causes loss of time and concentration.

THE OPERATOR'S POSITION

The position of the operator and patient is similar to the one using for viewing without the use of the OM. Usually, the operator will be in position between 9 and 12 hours (Figs. 2.XVIII-65A-B).

With the use of the OM, the distance between the operator and patient is greater, and therefore, allows a more ergonomic position.

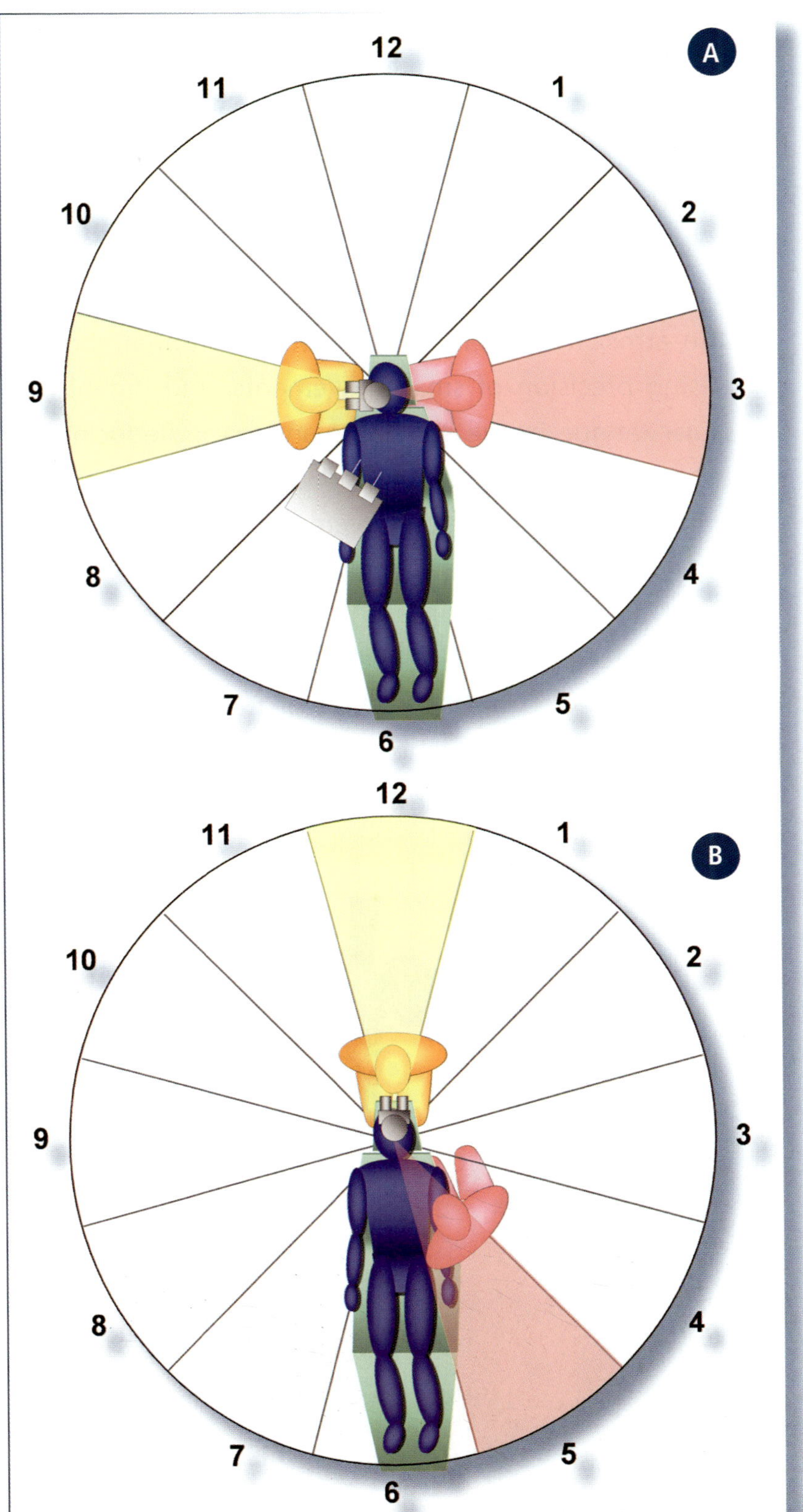

FIGS. 2.XVIII-65A-B

Diagram of location of operator and assistant in relation to the patient, analogous to a watch.
A – Operator at 9 hours.
B – Operator at 12 hours.

If it is in accordance with the general rules of ergonomics, the use of the OM practically forces the operator to adopt a correct position. The operator should be seated on an adjustable stool, with his/her thighs parallel to the floor, feet separated and completely supported, so that the groups of long muscles are maintained in equilibrium and at rest.

There are special stools with movable lateral supports for the arms, which can be used for additional support, increasing precision of small movements, and diminishing muscular fatigue in the shoulders and back. Reducing the distance between the arm support and the operating field will increase the precision of movements (Figs. 2.XVIII-66A-B).

The working area must at all times be at the level of the elbow, or slightly below it.

When one works with indirect vision and if for any reason the image reflected on the surface of the intra oral mirror is compromised (by fogging over or when using a high speed hand piece), the assistant could use a triple syringe to maintain a constant flow of air on the mirror, thus allowing for a clear view.

THE ASSISTANT'S POSITION

The OM can have an accessory ocular so that the assistant observes the same operating field as the practitioner and thus can participate in the operative procedures. When using an OM, one practically loses peripheral vision, therefore it is important for the assistant to be precise and efficient when transferring the instruments and material(s) to the operator.

Currently, with the use of monitors, the assistant can observe the details of the operating field on the monitor, in addition to also having a general view. In this case, it is not necessary to use the ocular, which will avoid movements of the OM and lessens the risk of losing balance and stability.

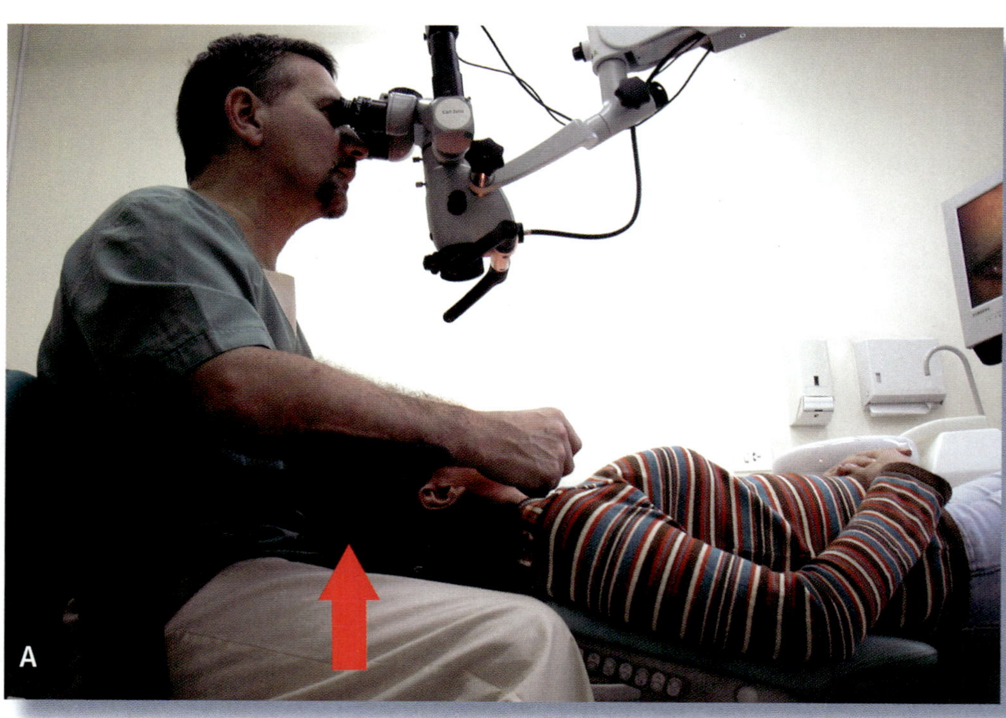

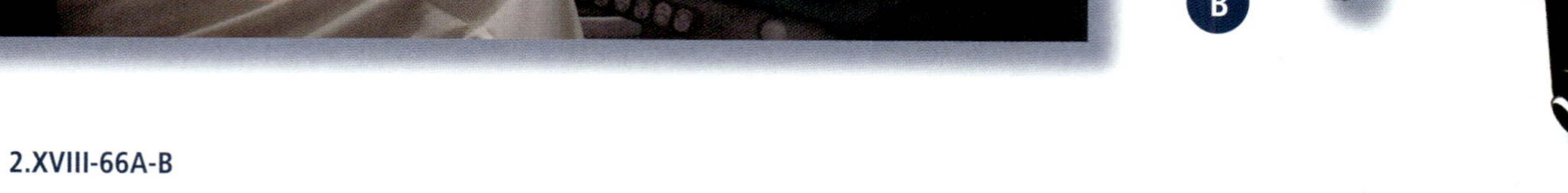

FIGS. 2.XVIII-66A-B

A-B – Special operator chair with arm support, allowing for extra stability.

PROTOCOL FOR USE OF THE OM

After installing the OM, it is necessary to organize a protocol for its use. This means determining specific procedures, according to the clinical requirements, however, all the operative steps performed with the OM must follow a basic working protocol[13]:

- Operator's position – The working position varies between 9 and 12 hours.
- Patient's position (superior or inferior maxillary).
- Position of the OM.
- Adjustment of the interpupillar distance.
- Precise position of the patient.
- General focus.
- Fine Focus.
- Assistant's position.
- Check the cameras (photographic or video) and monitors.
- Beginning of operative procedures.

The operator should not take his/her eyes from the binoculars and keep his/her hands in operating field, therefore the instruments and material must be taken to him/her in the position in which they will be used. If the operator performs these procedures, his/her eyes will not have to go through the process of refocusing.

In non surgical endodontics, only one assistant will be sufficient. However, in cases of peri-radicular surgery, a first assistant is required to maintain control over suction and another, who will supply instruments and materials.

LEARNING CURVE

Incorporation of the OM into the endodontist's daily activities must be adapted to individual requirements. Learning must begin with observation, followed by limited operative procedures, such as coronal cleaning and polishing, until skill and comfort are obtained. It is advised to increase the complexity of the clinical procedures slowly. Initial preparations can be performed under low magnification, to observe a broader field with greater depth of field. Detailed examination should be done at high magnifications.

Since it requires time to learn how to use the OM in complicated cases in which it is indispensable, it is necessary to start with the easy cases. An alternative approach that reduces the clinical learning curve is to participate training in practical multidisciplinary courses.

From the foregoing it can be concluded that the OM an instrument of immense importance in endodontic practice. Further development will allow the use of magnification to be incorporated into daily endodontic practice.

SUPERIOR MAXILLARY POSITION

The patient must be inclined with the chin slightly lifted. The light of the OM must be directed on the mirror and be reflected to illuminate the working area (Fig. 2.XVIII-67). The mirror must be placed at a distance that allows the head of the handpiece to be positioned in the operating field without obstructing the operator's vision. It is recommended to use low magnification to locate the working area at the angle of orientation. Once the image has been focused, one can take the OM to a higher magnification, if desired.

When the ideal position has been established, it is possible to change the areas of vision and focus simply by moving the buccal mirror (Fig. 2.XVIII-67).

INFERIOR MAXILLARY POSITION

Lower anterior teeth can be easily observed with the OM in the position of 12 hours (Fig. 2.XVIII-68).

A direct view of an incise preparation will provide the operator with a general orientation of the preparation of the tooth. Indirect vision by means of the mirror allows exact lingual or buccal orientation. In the same way, one can directly or indirectly obtain a lingual or buccal view of the premolars or molars using the mirror (Fig. 2.XVIII-68).

The OM can be directed in a line perpendicular to the buccal surfaces of the teeth. The position that offers the greatest difficulty is the occlusal view of the molars, as it will be necessary to use a handpiece with a small head, so as not to block the operator's view (Figs. 2.XVIII-69A-D).

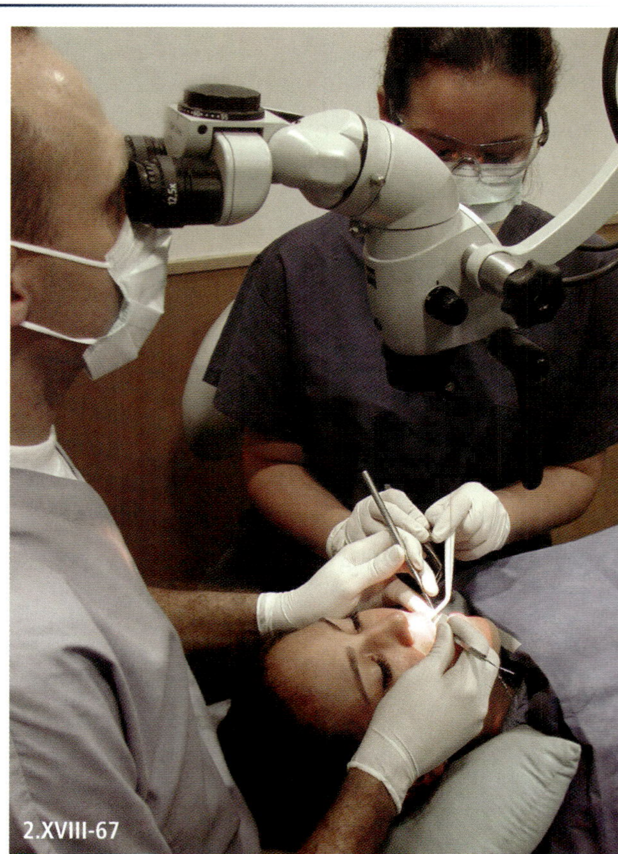

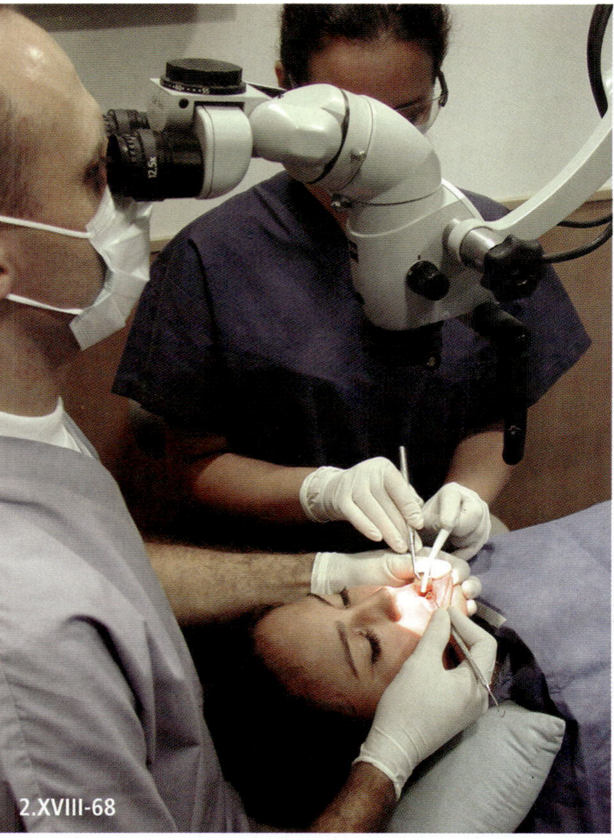

FIG. 2.XVIII-67

Operator at 12 hours, observing the superior maxillary position.

FIG. 2.XVIII-68

Operator at 12 hours, observing the inferior maxillary position.

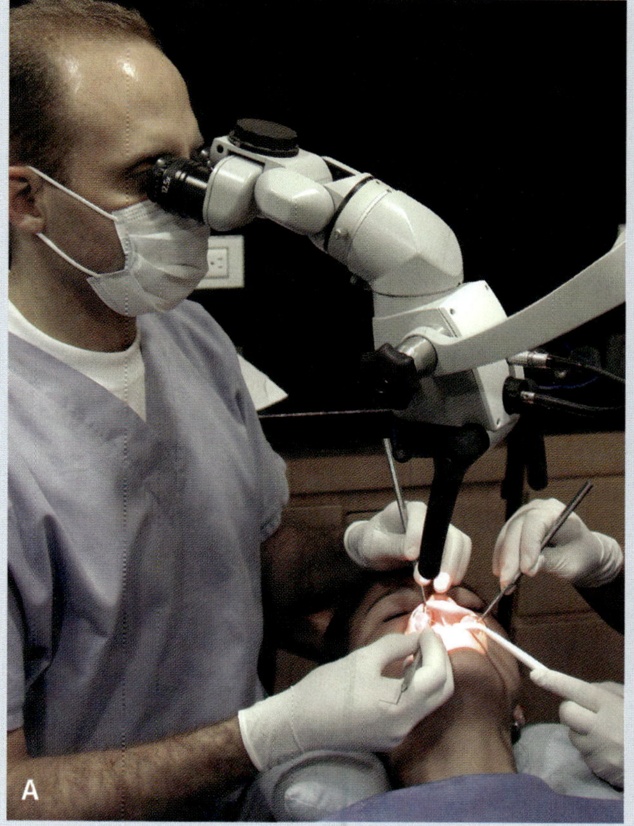

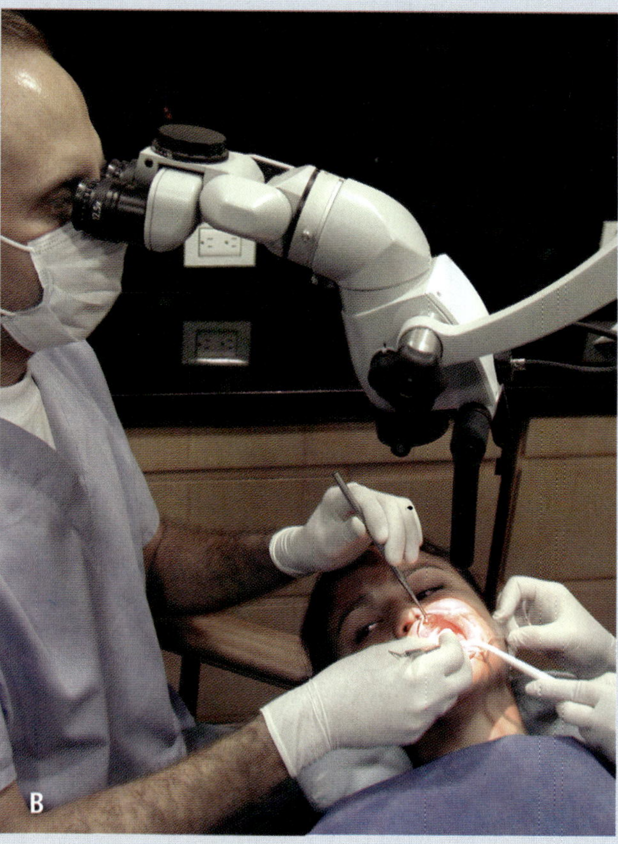

FIGS. 2.XVIII-69A-D

Working positions recommended for:
A – Right superior maxillary position.
B – Left superior maxillary position.
C – Left inferior maxillary position.
D – Mandibular (anterior) position.

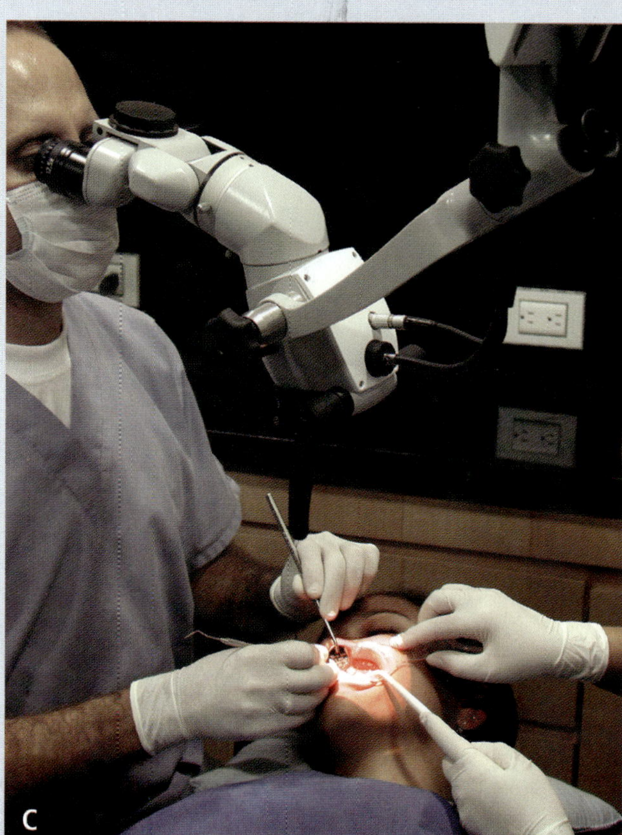

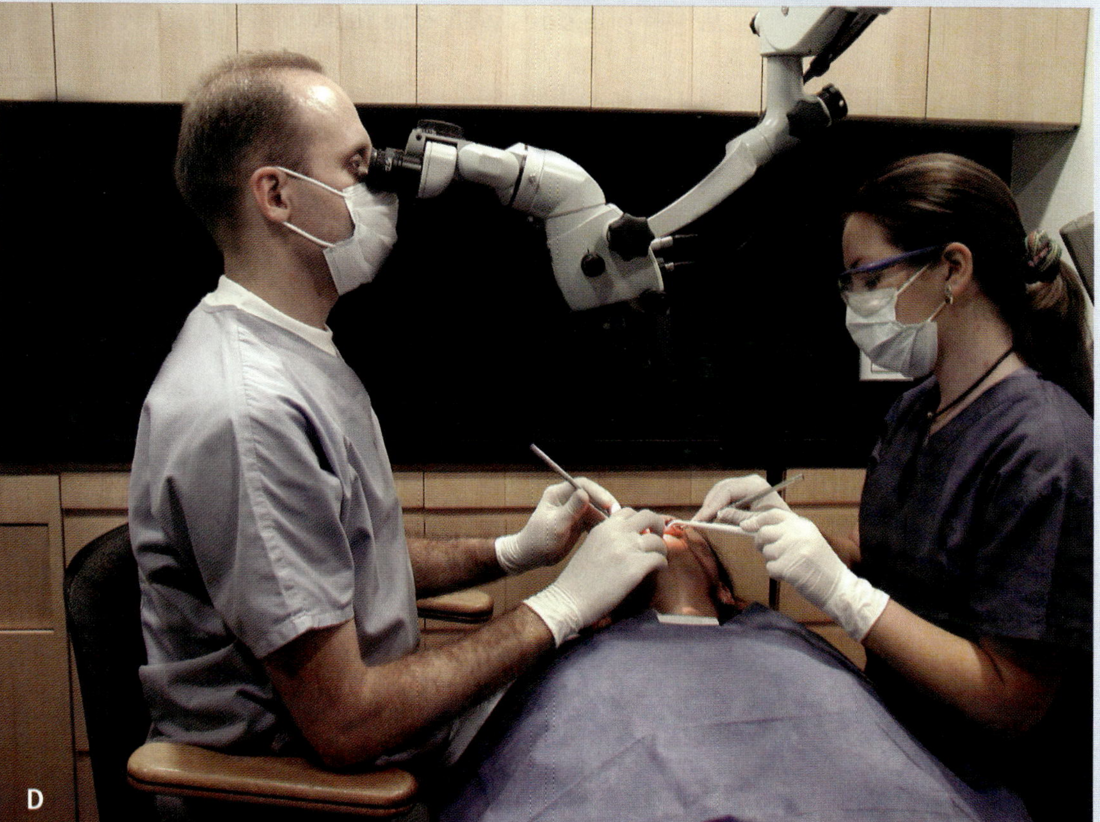

CONCLUSIONS

At present, thanks to the OM, difficult cases can be treated with a high degree of predictability and clinical success. The use of the OM does not change the operator's endodontic techniques, but offers him/her greater precision of use.

With the OM, more precise clinical diagnoses and more effective and conservative treatment can be performed.

Although the economic burden of an OM is considerable, the pursuit of professional excellence justifies the purchase, therefore one must not expect an immediate economic return.

Once the learning curve has is no longer an issue, the practitioner notably improves the quality of clinical procedures and enables himself/herself to resolve situations for which there would be no solution without the OM.

It is Prof. Arnaldo Castelucci's opinion[13] that "within a short period of time, the OM will be part of the general equipment of a dental office, as is the X-ray machine today".

According to Dr. David Clark[14] (President of the Academy of Microscopy – USA), the microscope is not only another dental instrument, it is a vehicle that can transport the clinician to a place. A place where diagnosis is definitive and treatment is precise".

"When one sees well, one does well;

When one does well, one feels well[49]".

References

1. Apotheker H, Jako GJ. A microscope for use in dentristy. J Microsurg, v.3, p.3-7, 1981.
2. Barnett F. Diagnosis dilemmas and decisions: Incompletely fractured teeth. Oral Health, July 2002.
3. Baumann RR. How may the dentist benefit from the operating microscope. Quint Int, v.5, p.17-18, 1977.
4. Behle C. Photography and the operating microscope in dentistry. J Calf Den Assoc, v.29, p.765-771, 2001.
5. Bellizi R, Loushine R. Adjuncts to posterior endodontic surgery. J Endod, v.16, p.604-606, 1990.
6. Bóveda C, Fajardo M, Millán B. Root canal treatment of an invaginated maxillary root lateral incisor with a C-shaped canal. Quintessence Int, v.30, p.707-711, 1999.
7. Buchanan S. The art of endodontics. Clinical monographs (access & negociation). J Endod.
8. Buhrley LJ, Barrows MJ, Begole EA. Effect of magnification on locating MB2 canal in maxillary molars. J Endod, v.28, n.4, p.324-327, 2002.
9. Carr G. Comunicação pessoal, 2004.
10. Carr G. Microscopes in endodontics. J Calif Dent Assoc, v.20, p.55-61, 1992.
11. Carr G. Microscopes in endodontics. J Endod, v.11, p.55-61, 1999.
12. Carr, G. Surgical Endodontics. In. Cohen, S.; Burns, R.C. (eds): Pathways of the Pulp, 1996, Mosby, St. Louis.
13. Castellucci, A. Magnification in Endodontics: The use of operating microscope. Endodontic Practice, p.29-36, Sep. 2003.
14. Clark, D.J. Definitive diagnosis of early enamel and dentin cracks based on microscopic evaluation. J. Esthet. Restor. Dent., v.15, p.391-401, 2003.
15. De Carvalho, M.C.; Zuolo, M.L. Orifice locating with a microscope. J. Endod., v.26, p.532-534, 2000.
16. De Souza Filho, F.J.; Texeira, F.B. Usos del microscopio en Endodoncia, Biología y Técnica. Elio Pereira Lopez e Jose Siqueira, MEDSI: Rio de Janeiro, p. 633, 1999.
17. Dohlman GF. Carl Olof Nylen and the birth of the Otomicroscope and Microsurgery. Arch Otolaryngology, p.161-165, Dec. 1969.
18. Ducamin JP, Boussens J. Surgical microscope in dentristy. Rev Odontostomatol, v.8, p.293-298, 1979.
19. Flanders DH. New techniques for removing separated root canal instruments. N. Y. State Den. J., v.62, p.30-32, 1996.
20. Girsch WJ, Mcclammy TV. Microscopic removal of dens invaginatus. J Endod, v.28, p.336-339, 2002.
21. Gorduysus MO, Gorduysus M, Friedman S. Operating microscope improves negotiation of second mesiobuccal canals in maxillary molars. J Endod, v.11, p.683-686, 2001.
22. Hulsman M. The removal of silver cones and fractured instruments using the canal finder system. J Endod, v.16, p.596-600, 1990.
23. Jung M. Endodontic treatment of dens invaginatus type III with three root canals and open apical foramen. Int Endod J, v.37, p.205-213, 2004.
24. Khayat BG. The use of magnification in endodontic therapy: the operating microscope. Pract Perodont Aesthet, v.10, n.1, p.137, 1998.
25. Kim S. Microscopios en Endodoncia en Clínicas Odontológicas de Norteamérica. Mc Graw Hill, 1997.
26. Kim S, Pecora G, Rubnistein RA. Color Atlas of Microsurgery in endodontics. W.B.Saunders Company, 2001.
27. Kleinert HE, Kasden ML. Salvage of Devascularized Upper Extremities Including Studies of Small Vessel Anastomoses. Clin Orthop, v.29, p.29-38, 1963.
28. Koch K. The Microscope: Its Effect on Your Practice. Den. Clin. North Am, v.41, p.625, 1997.
29. Ling JQ, Wei X, Gao Y. Evaluation of the use of dental operating microscope and ultrasonic instruments in the management of blocked canals. Zhonghua Kou Qiang Yi Xue Za Zhi, v.38, n.5, p.324-326, Sep. 2003 (Abstract).
30. Maggiore F, Jou YT, Kim S. A six canal maxillary molar: case report. Int Endod J, v.35, n.5, p.486-491, 2002.
31. Malt RA. Replantation of Severed Arms. JAMA, v.189, n.10, p.716-722, 1964.
32. Mangharam J, Mcglothan JD. Ergonomics and dentistry. In. MURPHY, D. ed. Ergonomics and the Dental Care Worker. Am Public Health Assoc, Washington DC, p.25-81, 1998.
33. Mounce R. Surgical microscopes in endodontics: the quantum leap. Den. Today, v.12, p.88-91, 1993
34. Murgel C. Conferência em: Roots Summit 3. LA, 2003.
35. Nallapati S. Three-canal maxillary premolar teeth: a common clinical reality. Endod Pract J, p.22-27, Sep 2003.
36. Nehme W. Elimination of intracanal obstructions by abrasion using an operational microscope and Ultrasonics. J Endod, v.27, p.365, 2001.
37. O'Brien BM. Clinical Implantation of Digits. Plast Reconstr Surg, v.52, n.5, p.490-502, 1973.
38. Okiji T. Modified usage of the Masseran kit for removing intracanal broken instruments. J Endod, v.29, p.466-467, 2003.
39. Pecora G, Andreana S. Use of dental operating microscope in endodontic surgery. Oral Surg Oral Med Oral Pathol, v.75, p.751-758, 1993.
40. Rosemberg D. Endodontic retreatment: Part One. Endod Pract J, p.15-20, Sep. 2003.
41. Rubinstein R, Kim S. Clinical success of endodontic surgery with the operating microscope using Super EBA as root-end filling materia. J Endod, 1997.
42. Ruddle CJ. Endodontic perforation repair: using the surgical microscope. Dent Today, p.49-53, 1994.
43. Ruddle CJ. Non-Surgical Endodontic Retreatment. CDA Journal, v.25, n.11, p.769-799, 1997.
44. Selden H. The Dental-Operating Microscope and its slow acceptance. J Endod, v.28, p.206-207, 2002.
45. Selden HS. The role of a dental microscope in improved nonsurgical treatment of calcified canals. Oral Surg Oral Med Oral Pahol, v.68, p.93-98, 1989.

46. Seltzer S. Endodontology. Biological consideration in endodontic procedures. Mc Graw Hill, Philadelphia, p.319-320, 1971.

47. Shanelec DA. Current trends in soft tissue. J Calif Dent Assoc, v.19, p.57-60, 1991.

48. Stropko JJ. Comunicação pessoal, 2003.

49. Stropko JJ. Canal morphology of maxillary molars: clinical observations of canal configurations. J Endod, v.25, p.446-450, 1999.

50. Tibbetts LS, Shanelec DA. An overview of periodontal microsurgery. Curr Opinion Periodontal, v.1, p.187-193, 1994.

51. Ward JR. The use of an ultrasonic technique to remove a fractured rotary nickel-titanium instrument from the apical third of a curved root canal. Aust Endod J, v.29, p.25-30, 2003.

52. Yoshioka T, Kobayashi C, Suda H. Detection rate of root canal orifices with a microscope. J Endod, v.28, p.452-453, 2002.

2.XIX

Oscillating Debridement

AET System
(Anatomic Endodontic Technology)
Endo-Eze

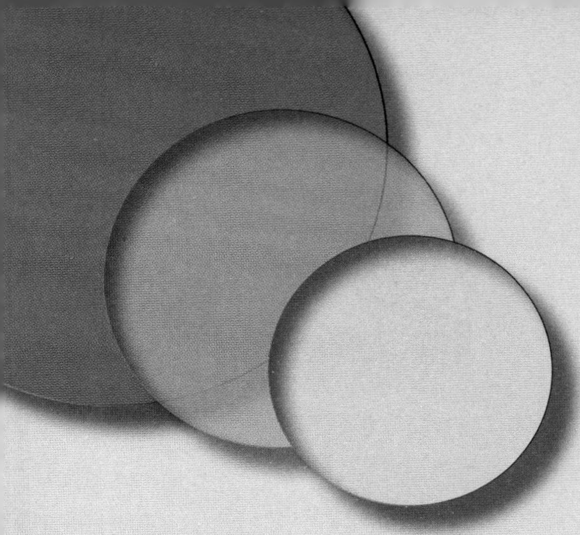

Renato de Toledo Leonardo
Fábio Luiz Camargo Villela Berbert

The terms cleaning and shaping (Schilder[11]), established in Endodontics worldwide, show the importance of biomechanical preparation. When endodontic treatment is divided into operating stages, biomechanical preparation corresponds to the stage at which irrigation/suction/inundation with irrigant solutions and instruments are used to prepare root canals[7].

Usually, manual, oscillatory, rotary and/or ultrasound instruments are used. Rotary instrumentation is characterized by promoting only root canal widening. Since the majority of the root canals have a flattened shape (Wu *et al.*[12]), widening alone, even when performed in an accentuated way, does not allow the instruments to act on all the root canal walls, thus compromising effective mechanical cleaning. On the other hand, effective widening allows the irrigant solution to act in areas where the rotary instrument did not act, promoting cleaning[8]. Ultrasound is also used for root canal debridement. However, with this technique, irrigation is more effective for cleaning the root canal system.

Even today, mechanical and manual debridement is the only one that has characteristics that allow the majority of the problems faced by the dentists to be solved[2], particularly if associated with other techniques or systems (oscillatory, rotary and/or ultrasound).

With oscillatory debridement, particularly when instruments with a diameter smaller than 0.15 mm D_1 (thinner than a standardized file No. 15) are used, one acts mechanically in all the areas of the root canal, and also avoids widening with excessive dentin removal[3]. For greater effectiveness, irrigation needs to be performed with smaller diameter needles[10].

Oscillatory debridement can be performed with different systems and files. In this chapter, the Endo-Eze system, Anatomic Endodontic Technology (AET) will be described, which was created by Francesco Rittano, Italy, and developed by Ultradent[4].

This type of debridement, which uses motor-driven stainless steel files, has been known since the 1960s, because in the last century, the Giromatic[6] system was already using conventional type K instruments adapted to a handpiece that fluctuated at 90°. As the type K instruments are made of stainless steel and have a constant taper (0.02 mm/mm), oscillating at 90° inside the root canal, instruments with a diameter greater than 0.20 mm D_1 offer risk of creating steps, deformations, deviations and may even fracture the root[5].

The Endo-Eze system is comprised of a counter-angle with reduction of 4:1, which oscillates the instruments at only 30° (Fig. 2. XIX-1).

In this system, there are only three instruments (Fig. 2. XIX-2), with diameters and tapers of 0.10 mm–0.025 mm/mm, 0.13 mm-0.045 mm/mm and 0.13 mm-0.060 mm/mm, respectively (Fig. 2. XIX-3).

Taking into consideration that the majority of root canals are oval or flattened, particularly in the middle and cervical thirds, by using instruments with diminutive diameter, it is possible to reach all the root canal walls.

The instruments offered by Endo-Eze System are modified type K files, with an active part of 16 mm and variable spiral angle, quadrangular cross-section, inactive and pre-curvable tips (Figs. 2.XIX-4, 2.XIX-5, 2.XIX-6, 2.XIX-7 and 2.XIX-8). In the proximities of the tip, the spiral angle exceeds the 60 degrees, allowing few points of contact with the root canal, making it difficult for the instrument to become locked in the canal, and diminishing wear. Although angles wider than 60° diminish its flexibility, it must be emphasized that these instruments

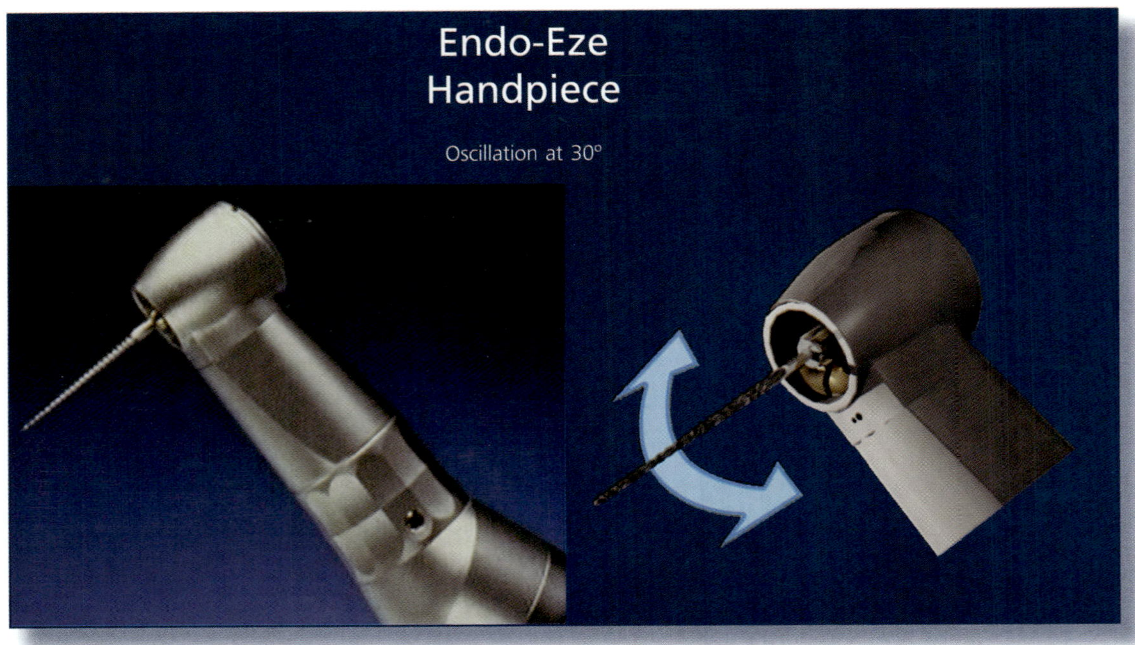

FIG. 2.XIX-1
Endo-Eze system handpiece.

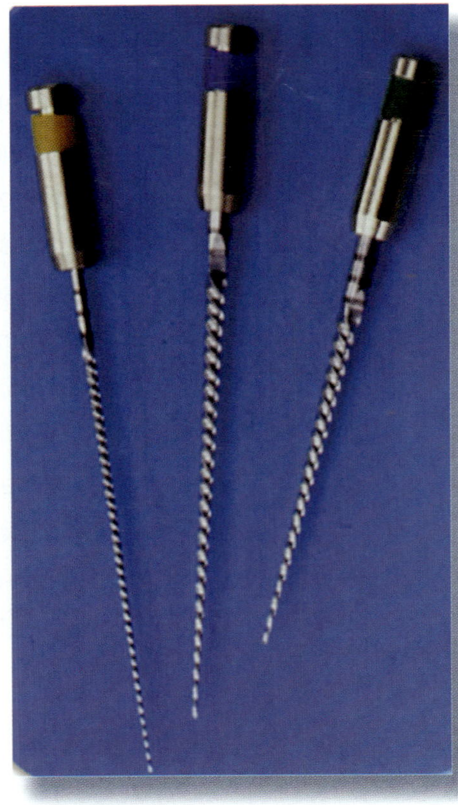

FIG. 2.XIX-2
Endo-Eze oscillatory instruments.

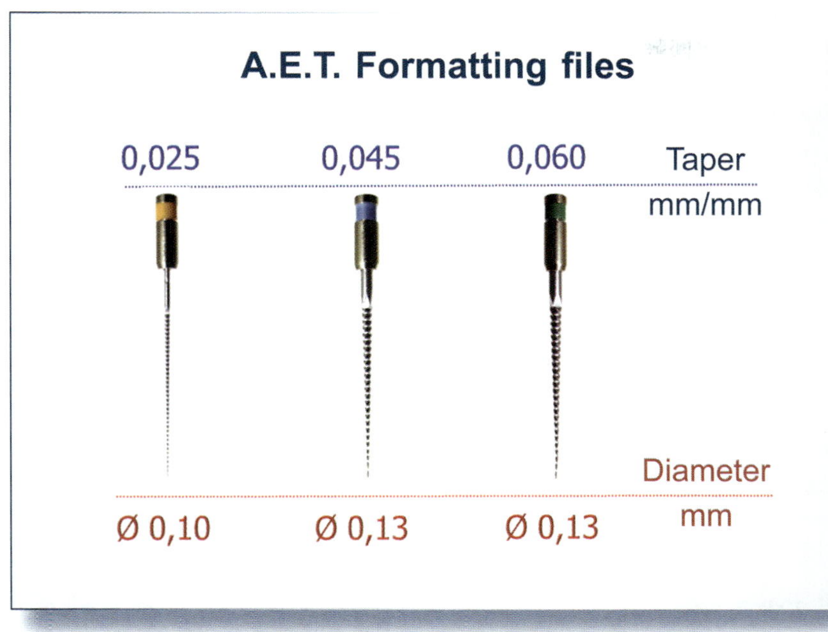

FIG. 2.XIX-3
Formatting files with their respective diameters and tapers.

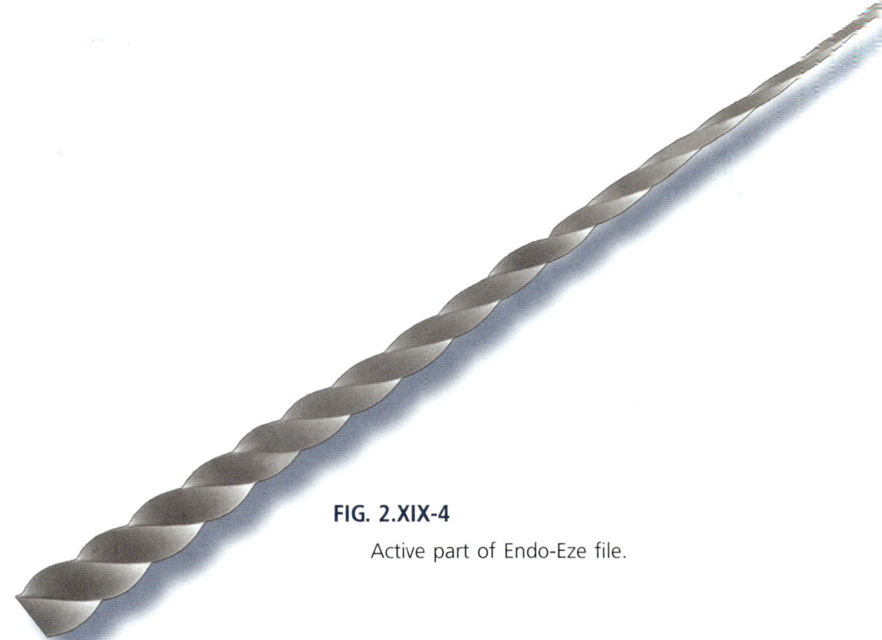

FIG. 2.XIX-4
Active part of Endo-Eze file.

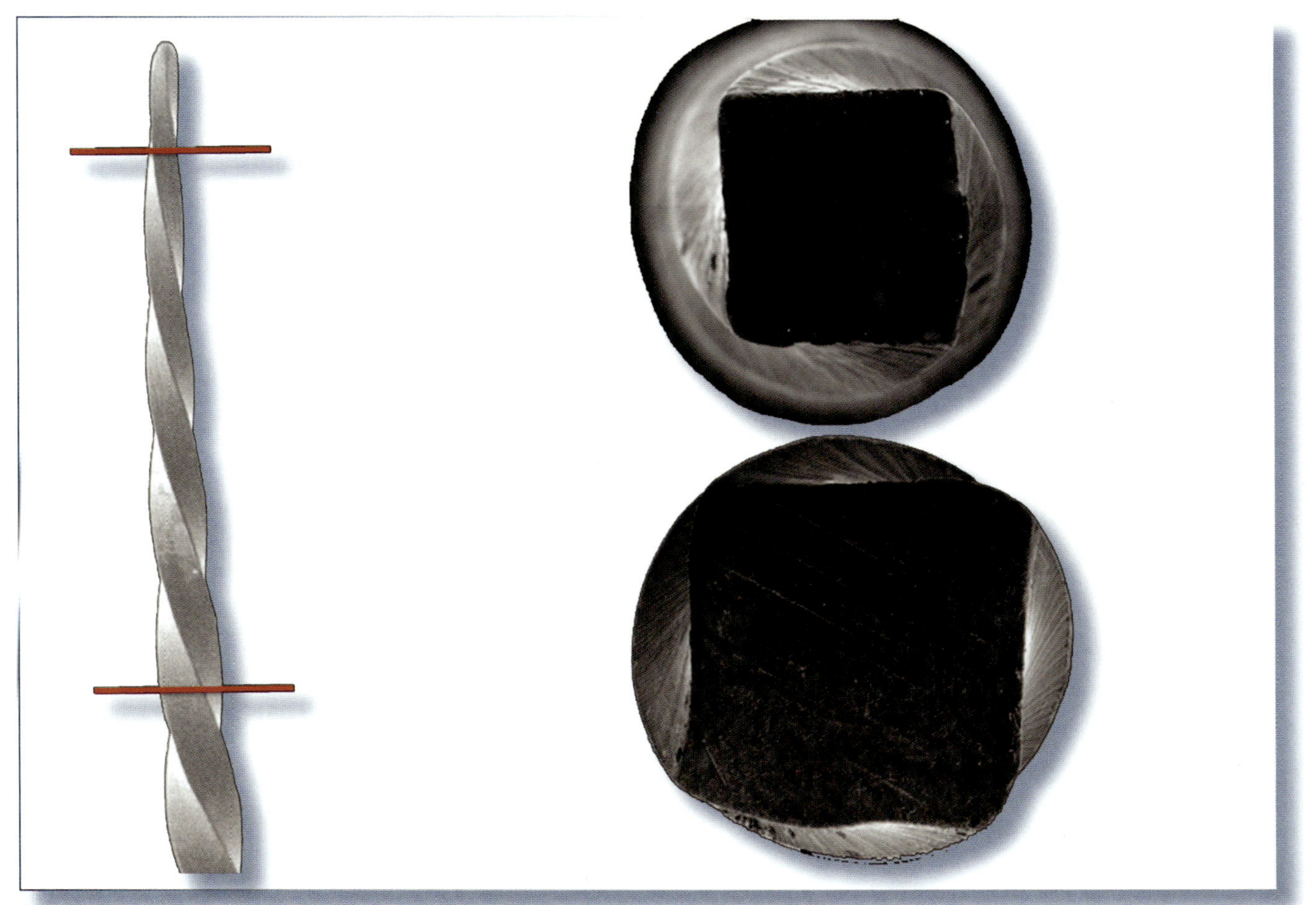

FIG. 2.XIX-5
Endo-Eze instrument presents a quadrangular cross-section. (By courtesy of Prof. Carlos Garcia Puente)

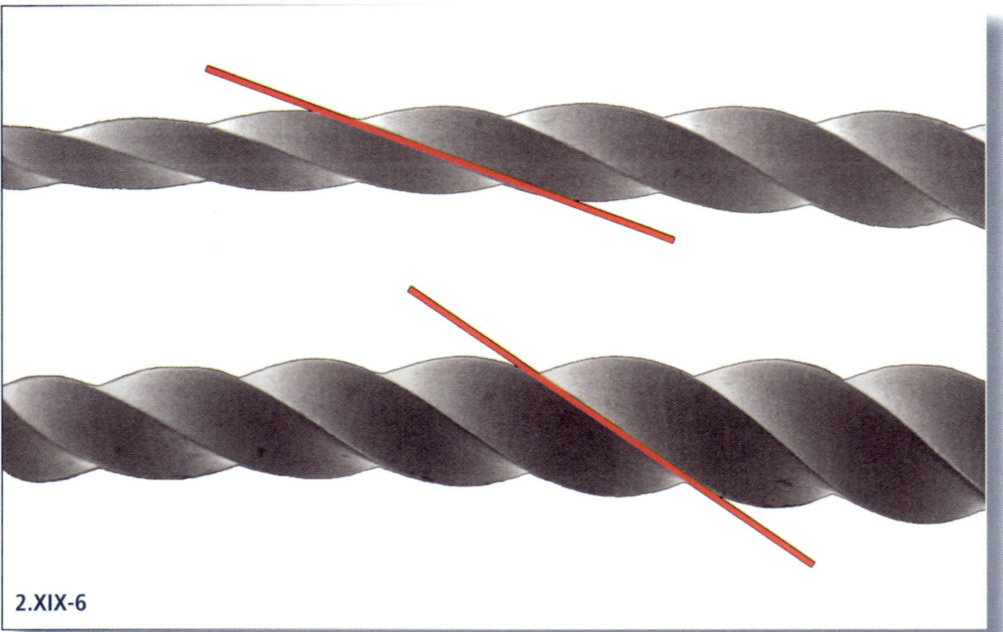

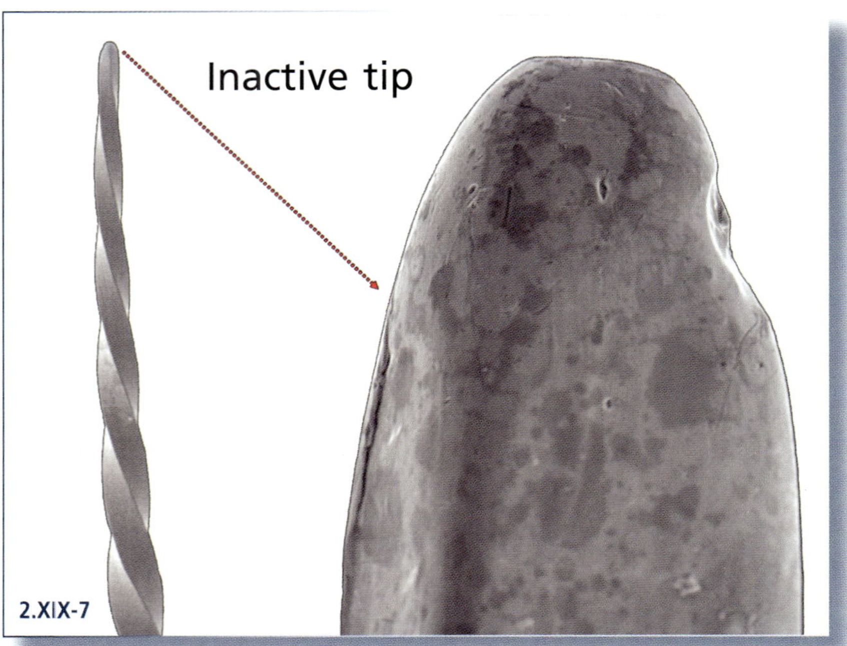

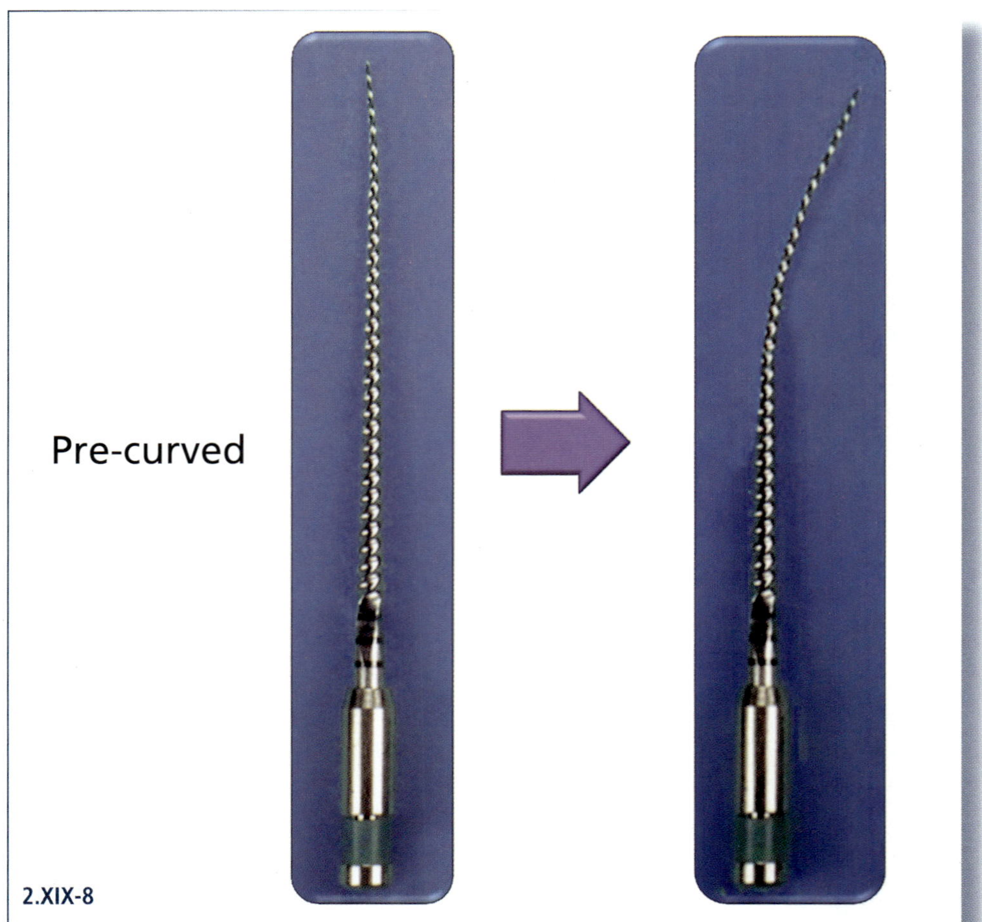

FIG. 2.XIX-6

Different spiral angles in the different portions of the instrument.

FIG. 2.XIX-7

Close-up view of the inactive tip.

FIG. 2.XIX-8

Endo-Eze instrument is made of stainless steel, therefore it is pre-curved.

loss is compensated by the diminutive diameter, particularly in the proximities of the tip. Thus, although made of stainless steel, these instruments with diameters that are similar to those of the type K file No 10, have accentuated flexibility and can be used in curved root canals with curvature angles of up to 60° or radii greater than 5 mm (Fig. 2.XIX-9). Whereas, from the cervical third to the middle third, the spiral angle is smaller than 30°, characterizing an active part with a large surface and greater number points of contact, high cutting efficiency and high flexibility, compensated by having greater metal mass in these areas with consequent loss of flexibility, but anatomic cases in which the curves are found in the cervical third are rare.

To make an analogy, we verified that oscillatory debridement is no more than manual instrumentation, with modified instruments but with greater speed and efficacy of action against the dentinal walls.

In the 1980s, when Morgan & Montgomery[9] proposed the crown/apex preparation of the root canal, they predicted a revolution in Endodontics. Working from the coronal portion with instruments going from larger to smaller diameter, a small area of the active part of the file acted on the root canal. With little strength in the instrument and a small contact area, pressure and efficacy increased. In apex/crown debridement, the 16 millimeters of the active part of conventional instruments acted on the 16 mm of the root canals. A large contact area between the instrument and root canal dissipates the force applied to the instrument, diminishing pressure and efficacy. In the crown/apex as well as the apex/crown preparation, instruments with the same taper are used, with only the diameter of the active tip varying. To increase efficacy of apex/crown preparation it is necessary to change the taper

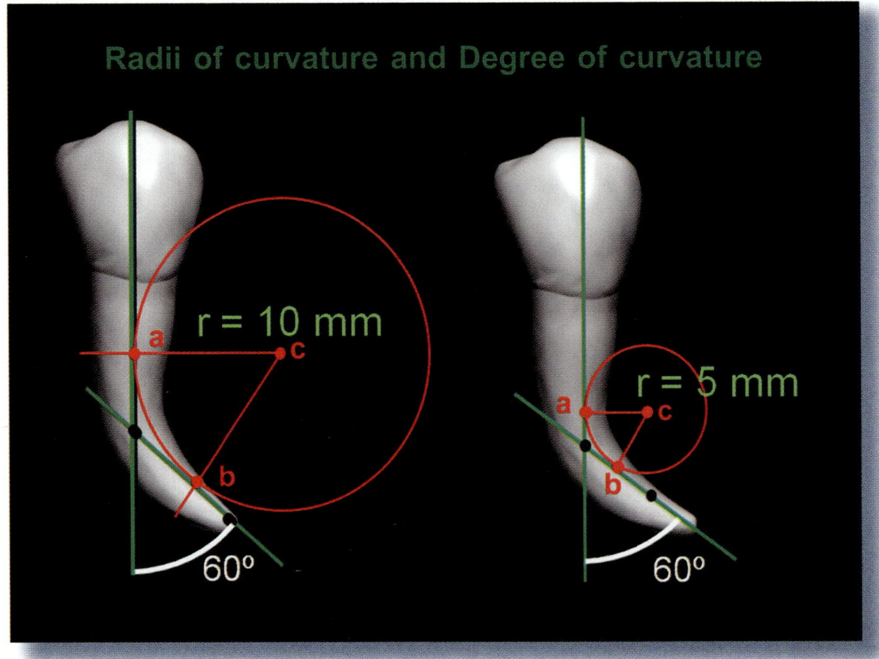

FIG. 2.XIX-9
Diagrammatic representation of two teeth at the same degree of root curvature, but with two different radii of curvature.

of the instruments, to keep the initial diameter and to increase speed of the instrument movement. These objects are attained with the Endo-Eze system, since the three instruments have very similar diameters, 0.10 mm and 0.13 mm, and different tapers (Figs. 2. XIX-10 and 2. XIX-11).

Since the handpiece (counter angle) (*push button*) used has a reduction of 4:1 (Fig. 2. XIX-12) and mean speed of a micromotor is about 12.000 rpm, the root canal is debrided at approximately 3.000 rpm. Such speed could cause fatigue in any stainless steel instrument, but with an oscillatory angle of only 30°, fatigue is significantly reduced and risk of fracture is close to zero.

With a small oscillation angle (30°), the performance of these instruments on the root canal walls can seem to be insufficient, but their quadrangular cross-section, allows them to act on a larger area of the root canal, which compensates for the small oscillation. They are made of stainless steel with an inactive tip that allows pre-curving, avoiding the creation of deviations or steps, although it is unlikely that a No 10 instrument would create such problems[1,13].

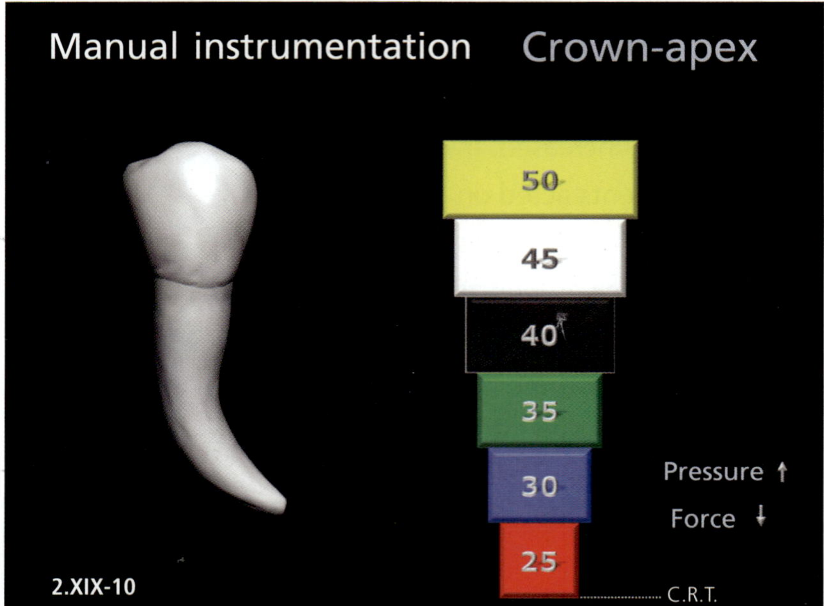

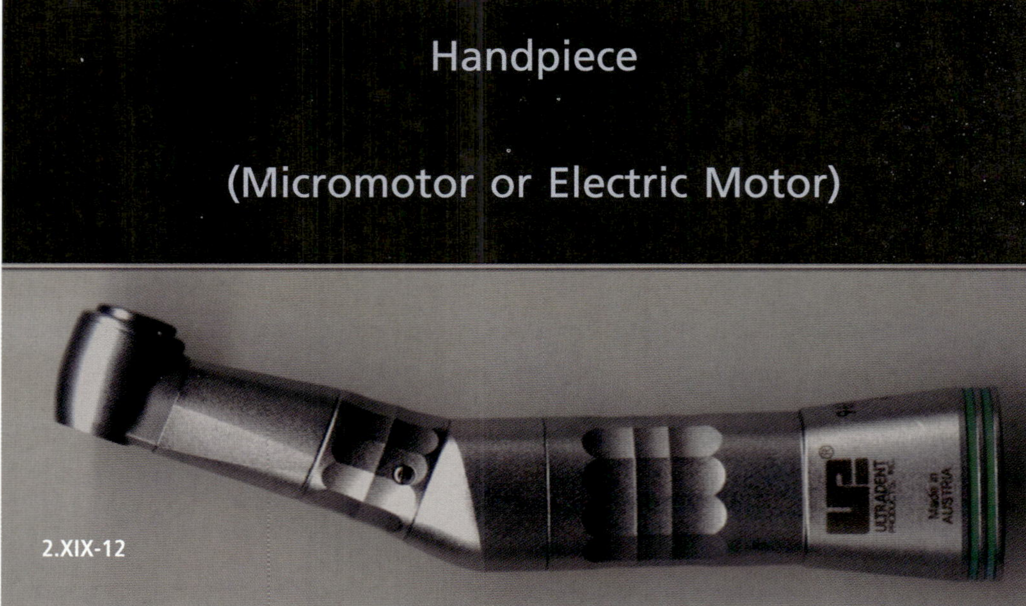

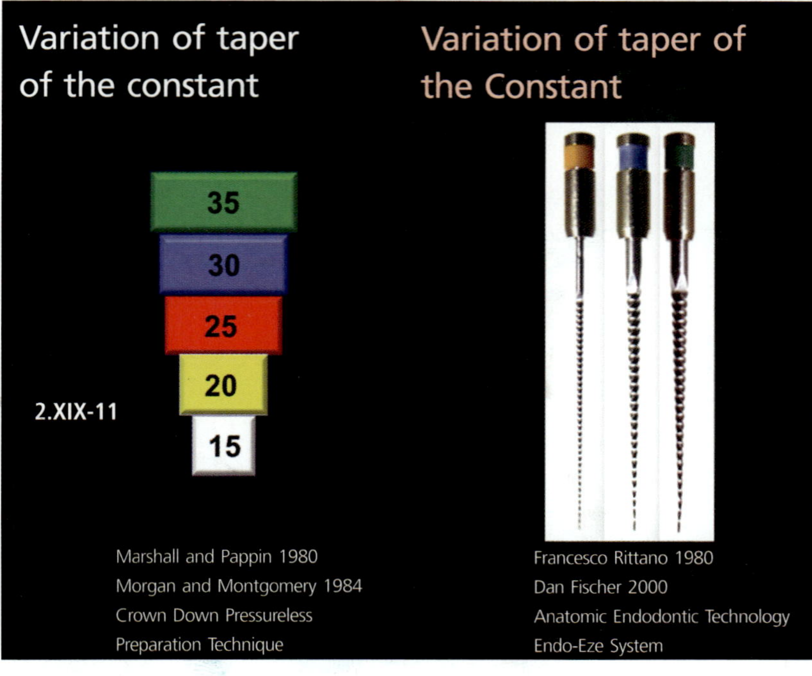

FIG. 2.XIX-10

In the crown/apex preparation, the diameter of the instrument varies and taper is maintained.

FIG. 2.XIX-11

In the Endo-Eze system, the variation in the instrument diameter is small, all that changes is the taper.

FIG. 2.XIX-12

Endo-Eze system handpiece, adjustable to micromotor or electric motor.

SEQUENCE OF USE

After determining the clinical and periapical radiography diagnosis (Fig. 2. XIX-13), coronal opening is performed under conditions of absolute isolation, (Figs. 2.XIX-14 and 2.XIX-15) and compensatory wear is performed with tapered-trunk cutters (Fig. 2.XIX-16). After this, real working length must be determined with electronic foramen locators, and confirmed by radiography for odontometry.

Depending on the diagnosis, teeth with pulp vitality or pulp necrosis, with or without periapical lesion, the manual instrument must be inserted into the root canal with catheterization in the cases of live pulp or progressive crown/apex emptying and neutralization, in the cases of necrotic pulp. For the treatment of teeth with live pulp (biopulpectomy), the instrumentation limit (Fig. 2.XIX-17) or real working length (RWL) is 1.0 mm short of the radiographic apex (Fig. 2.XIX-18). For the treatment of teeth with pulp

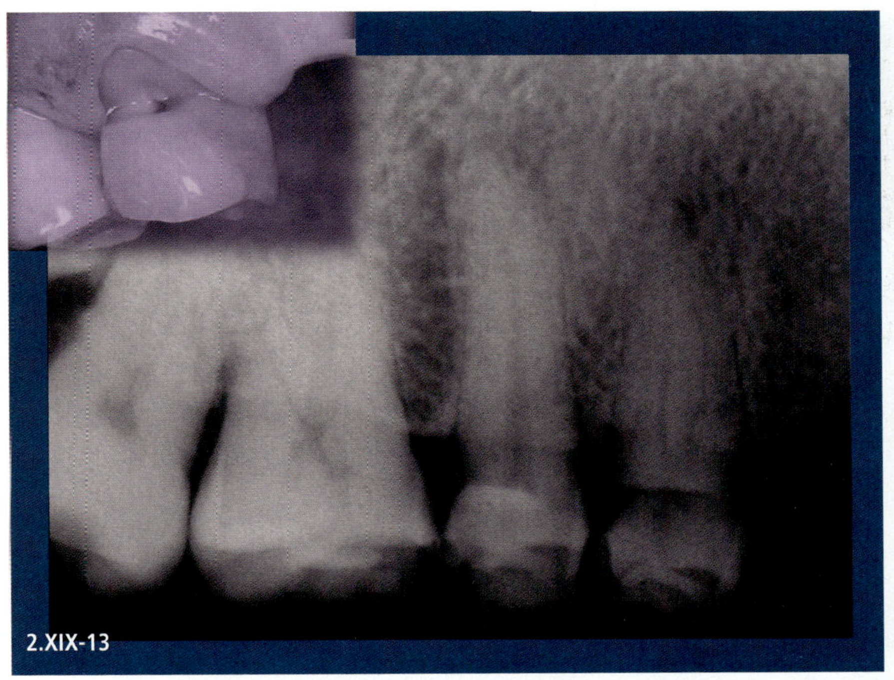

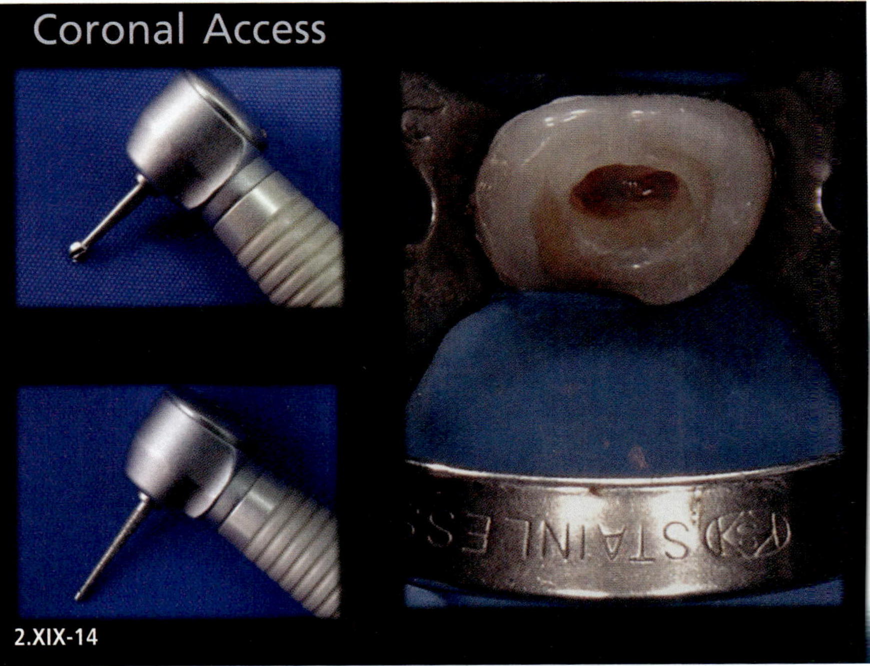

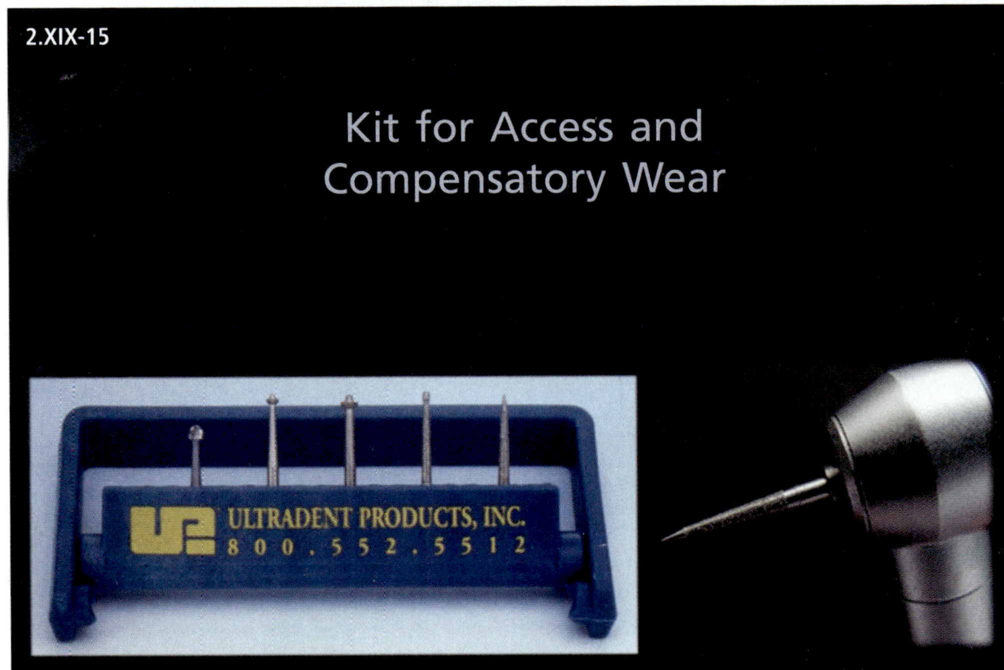

FIG. 2.XIX-13

periapical radiograph of maxillary pre-molar. Clinical case, by courtesy of Santiago Massi and Norberto Batista de Faria Júnior.

FIG. 2.XIX-14

Isolated premolar with coronal opening made with spherical and tapered trunk burs.

FIG. 2.XIX-15

Kit of burs for coronal opening and compensatory wear.

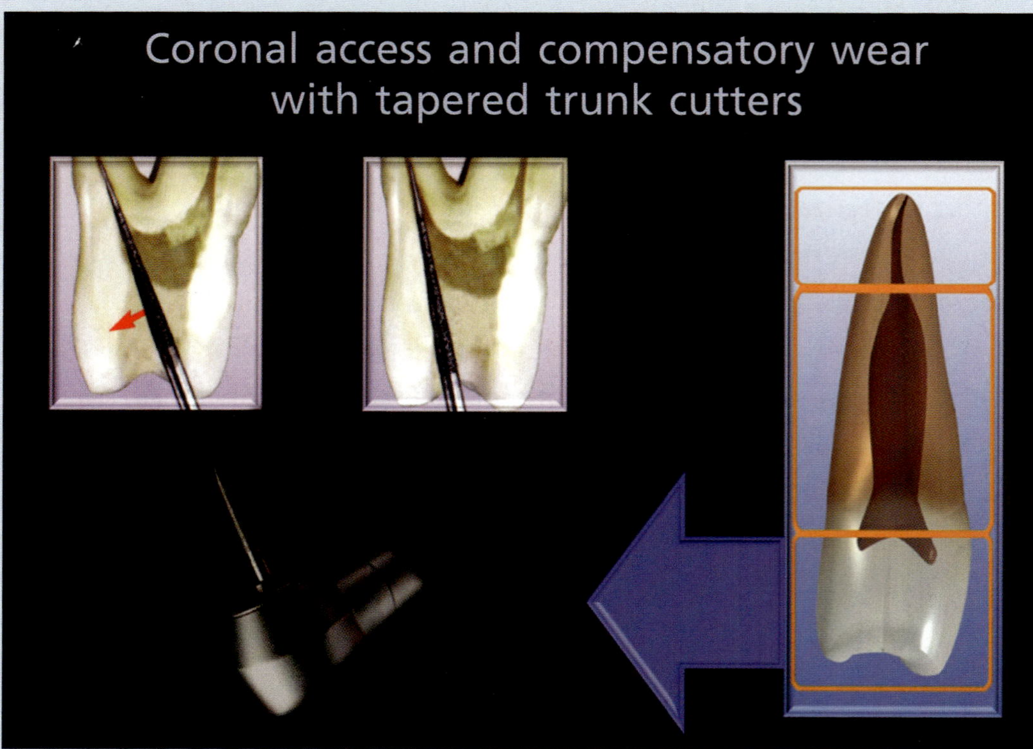

FIG. 2.XIX-16

Compensatory wear with tapered trunk cutters.

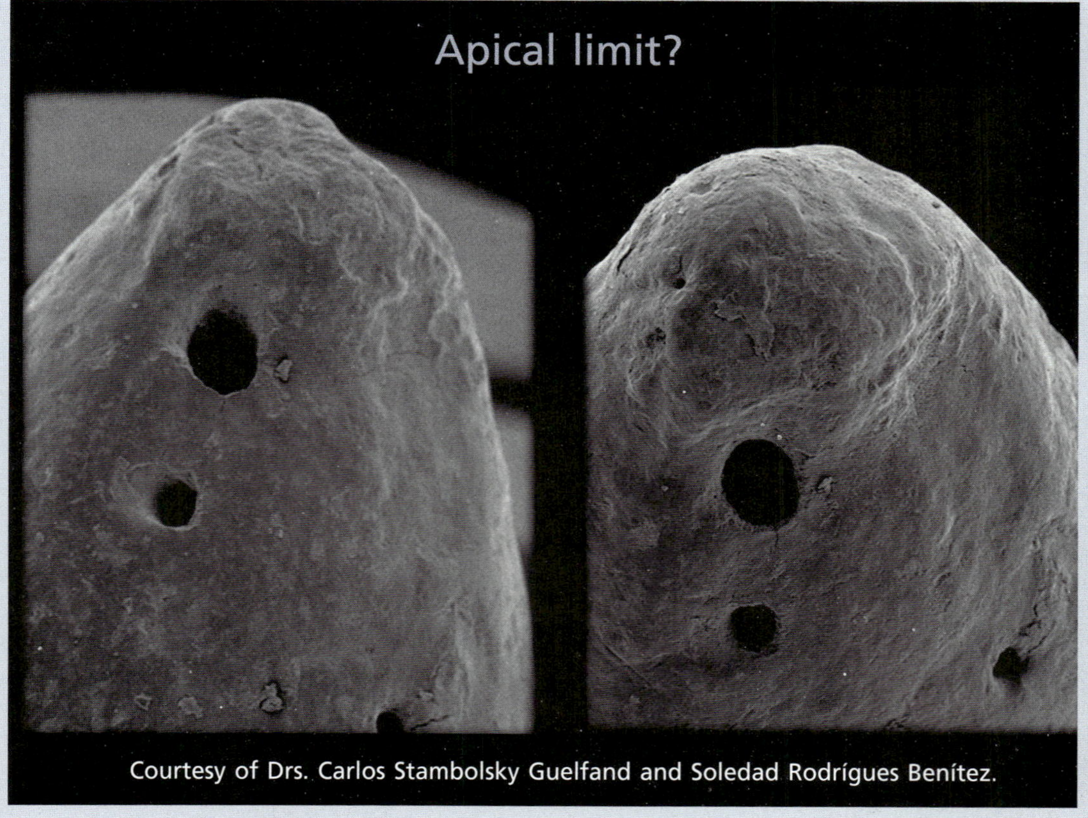

FIG. 2.XIX-17

Different anatomies and apical foramen position of vital pulp tooth. Apical limit? Courtesy of Drs. Carlos Stambolsky Guelfand and Soledad Rodrígues Benítez.

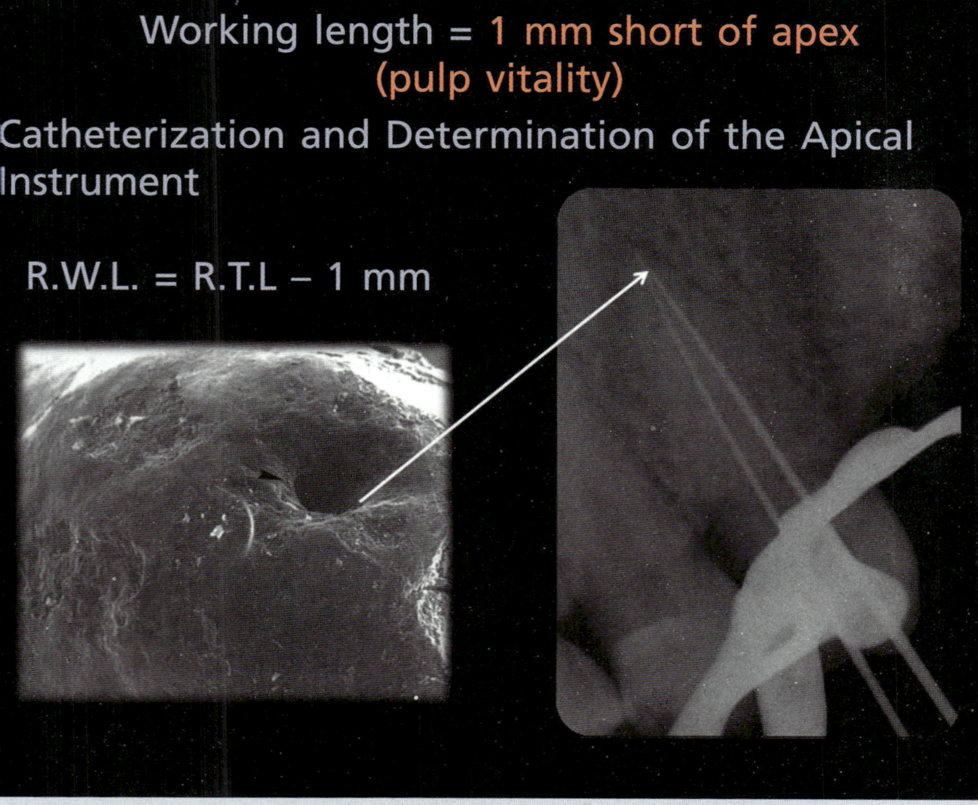

FIG. 2.XIX-18

For teeth with pulp vitality, the debridement limit with the Endo-Eze system is 1 mm short of the radiographic apex.

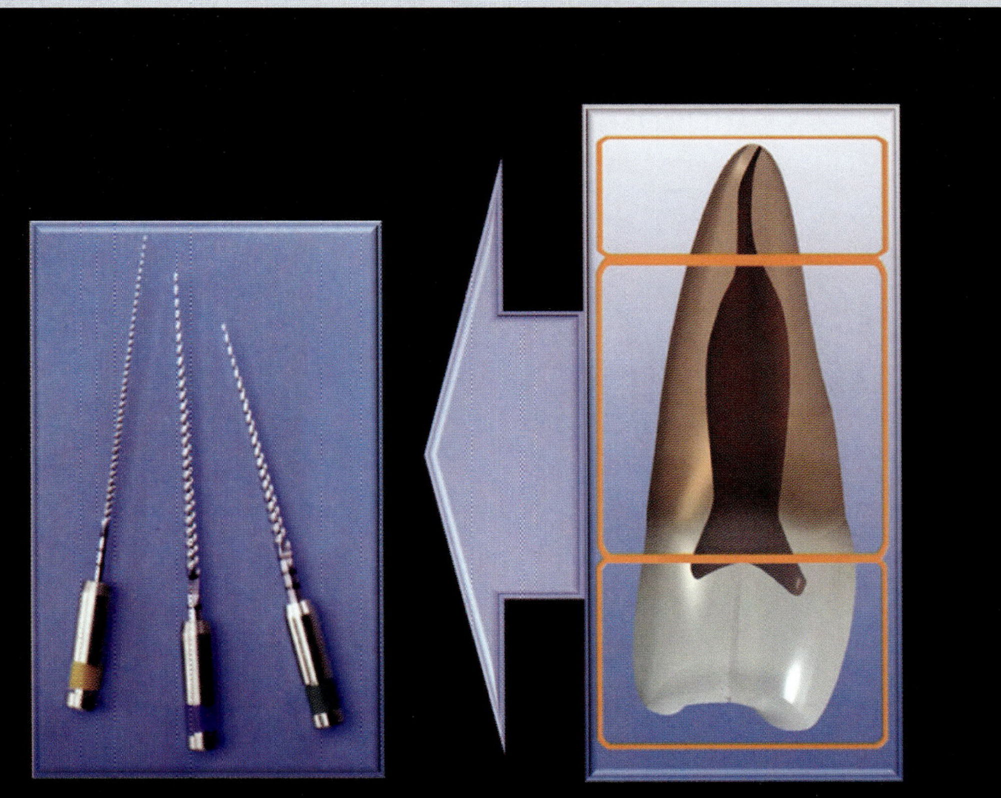

FIG. 2.XIX-22
Debridement of cervical and middle thirds.

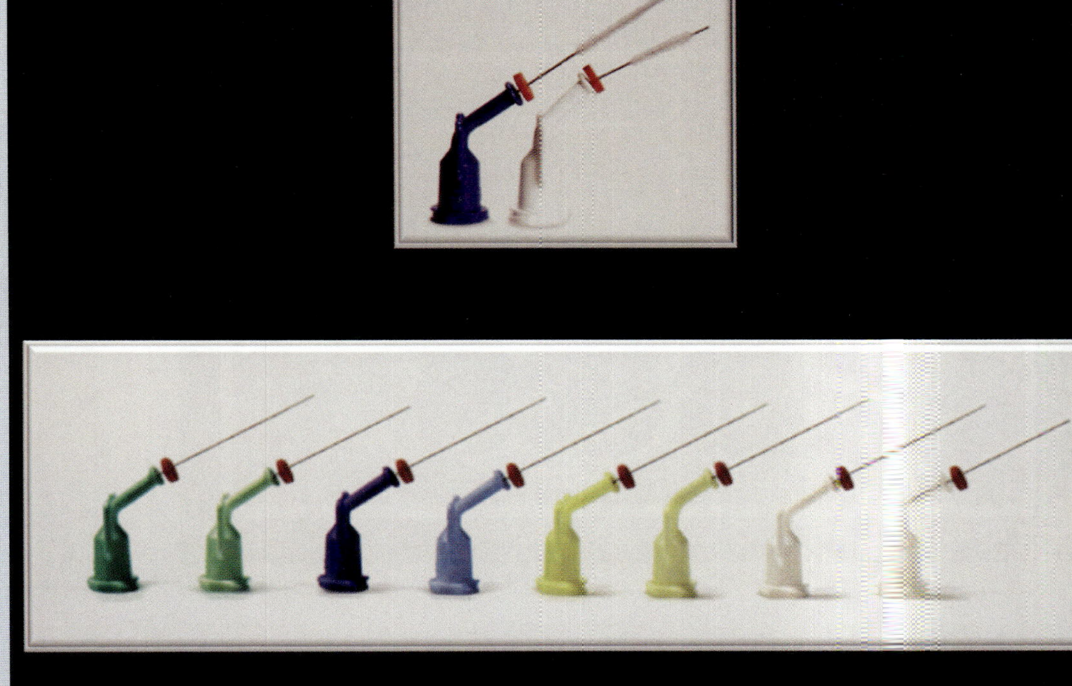

FIG. 2.XIX-23
Navi-tip needles of several lengths.

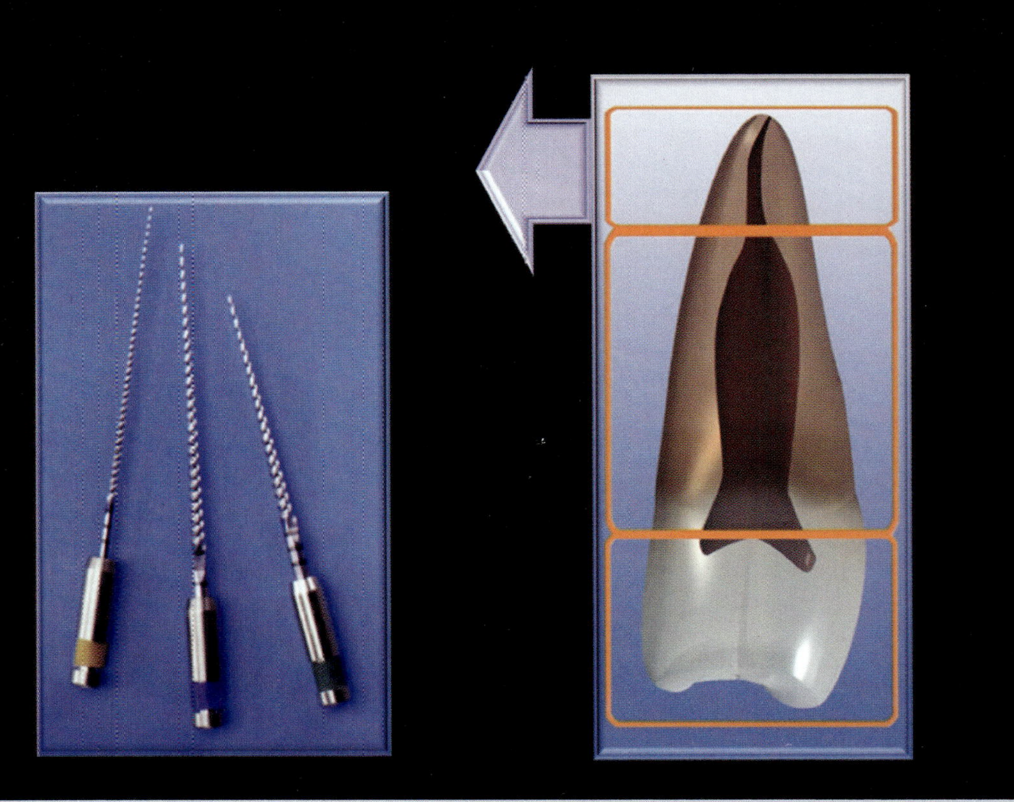

FIG. 2.XIX-24
Debridement of apical third.

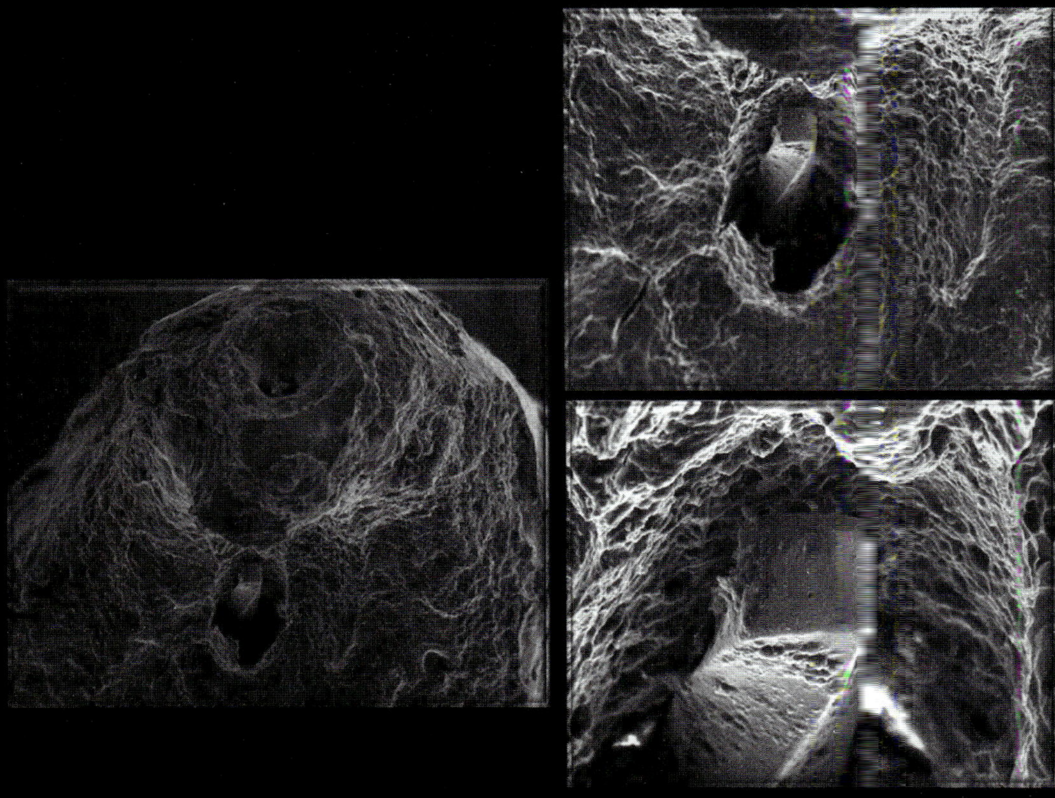

FIG. 2.XIX-25
Apical preparation 1 mm short of the tooth length.

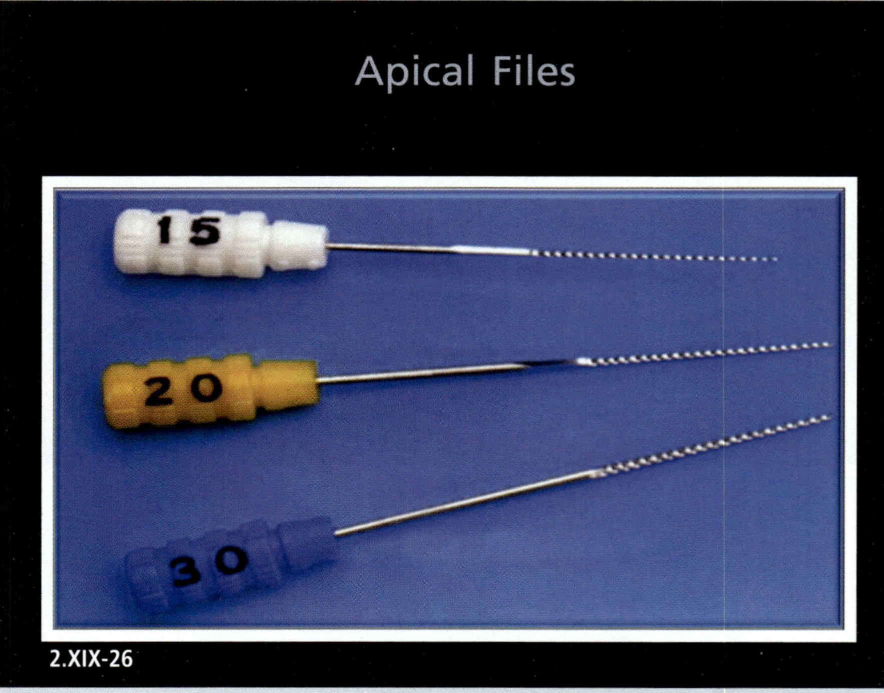

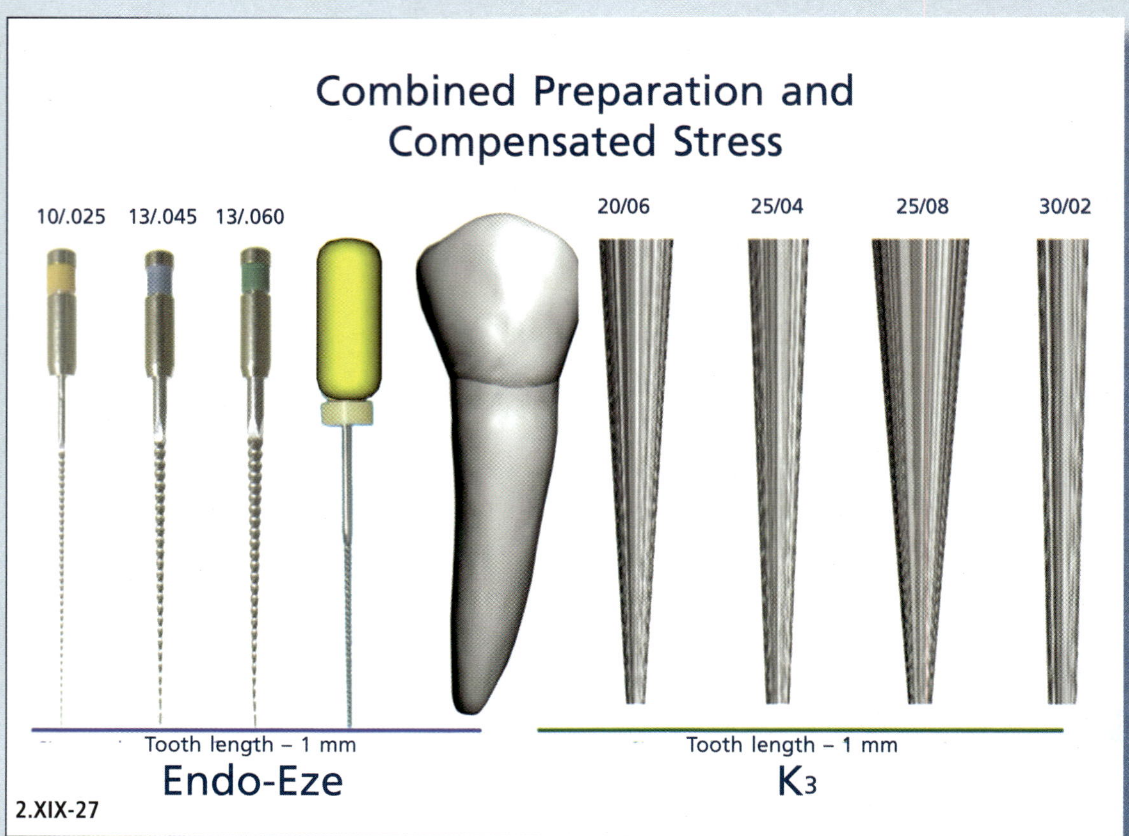

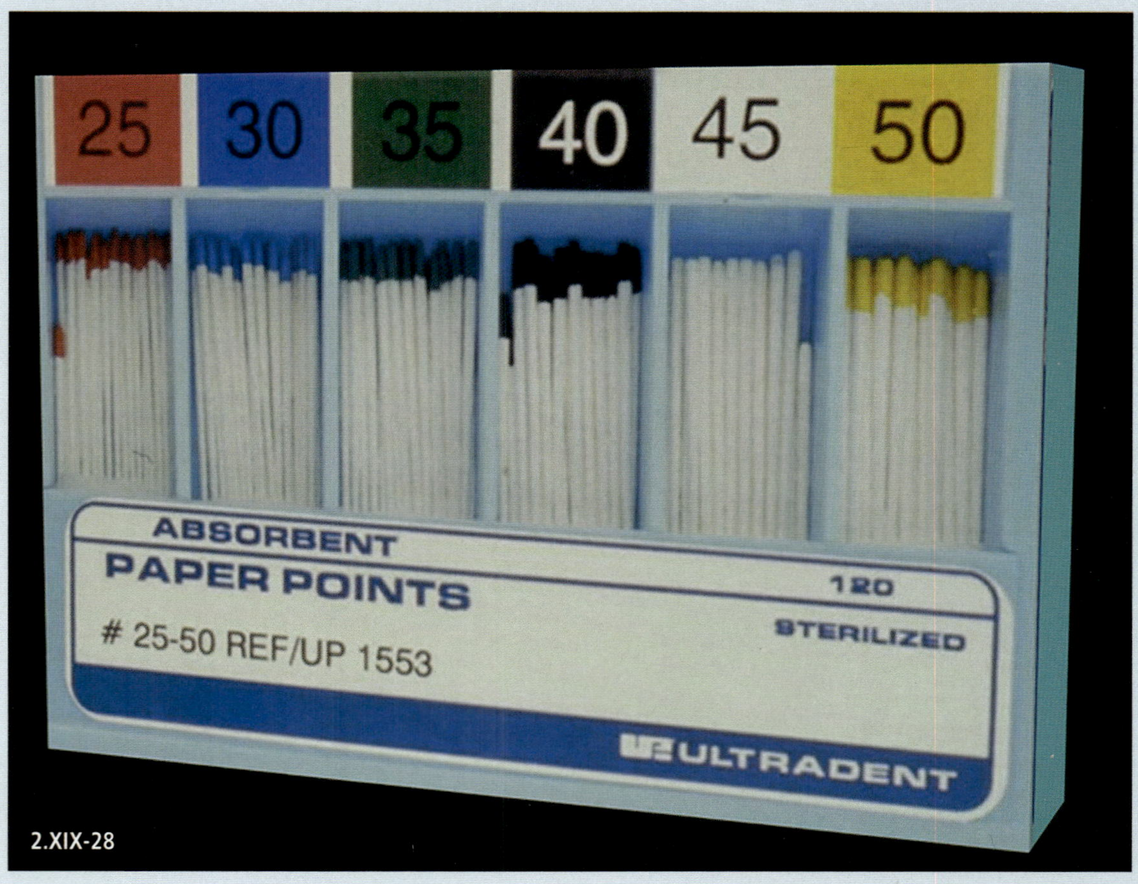

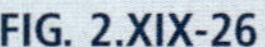

FIG. 2.XIX-26
Apical files for making apical preparation.

FIG. 2.XIX-27
Preparation combined with compensated stress.

FIG. 2.XIX-28
Sterile absorbent paper points.

References

1. Balseca GMA. Avaliação macroscópica do preparo apical de canais radiculares curvos pela instrumentação manual rotatória e mecanizada rotatória e oscilatória utilizando o sistema Protaper Universal. Araraquara, 2008. 133p. Tese (doutorado em Endodontia) – Faculdade de Odontologia, Universidade Estadual Paulista.
2. Bonetti Filho i, Esberard RM, Leonardo RT. Microscopic evaluation of three endodontic files pre and post instrumentation. J Endod, v.24, n.7, p.461-464, 1998.
3. Camargo JMP. Estudo comparativo do preparo do canal radicular de dentes artificiais utilizando diferentes técnicas automatizadas de instrumentação. Araraquara, 2004. 190p. Tese (doutorado em Endodontia) – Faculdade de Odontologia, Universidade Estadual Paulista.
4. Fischer D. Root canal preparation with Endo-Eze AET: changes in root canal shape assessed by micro-computed tomography. Int Endod J, v.38, n.7, p.456-464, 2005.
5. Frank AL. An evaluation of the Giromatic endodontic handpiece. Oral Surg, Oral Med Oral Pathol, v.24, n.3, p.419-421, 1967.
6. Hennicke A. Experiences with "Giromatic". Dent Dienst, v.18, n.4, p.19, 1966.
7. Leonardo MR. Endodontia: tratamento de canais radiculares – princípios técnicos e biológicos. 1.ª ed. São Paulo: Artes Médicas, 2005. v.2. 1.491p.
8. Leonardo MR, Leonardo RT. Endodontia: sistemas rotatórios: nova era no tratamento de canais radiculares. São Paulo: Artes Médicas, 2001. 400p.
9. Morgan LF, Montgomery S. An evaluation of the crown-down pressureless technique. J Endod, v.10, n.10, p.491-498, 1984.
10. Pappen FG, Souza EM, Giardino L, Leonardo RT, Leonardo MR, Ito IY. Antimicrobial activity of new solutions used in endodontic therapy. G Italiano Endo, v.20, n.4, p.211-214, 2006.
11. Schilder H. Cleaning and shaping the root canal. Dent Clin North Am, v.18, n.2, p.269-296, 1974.
12. Wu M, R'oris A, Barkis D, Wesslink P. Prevalence and extent of long oval canals in the apical third. Oral Surg Oral Méd, Oral Pathol, Oral Radiol & Endod, v.89, n.6, p.730-743, 2000.
13. Zanin FP. Avaliação in vitro de três diferentes técnicas de instrumentação quanto ao deslocamento do canal radicular. Araraquara, 2006. 110p. Dissertação (mestrado em Endodontia) – Faculdade de Odontologia, Universidade Estadual Paulista.

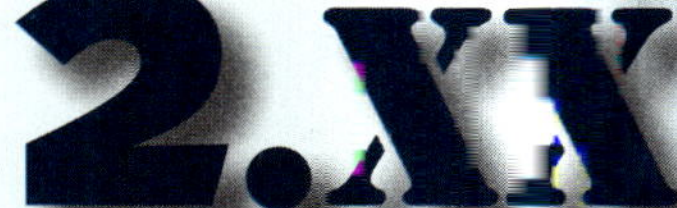

ADO System
(Apical Delivered Obturation)
EndoREZ

Renato de Toledo Leonardo
Cornelis Pameijer
Marco Aurélio Gagliardi Borges

Considering that root canal fillings using the monoblock concept[23], that is, filling starts from the apex and moves coronally, using adhesive materials, already form part of a range of options for root canal system fillings, we discuss in this chapter the ADO (Apical Delivered Obturation) EndoREZ* system, which consists of a resin-based filling material with dual polymerization properties[7,9].

One of the main factors for successful endodontic treatment is the prevention of microorganisms and toxins leaking into the root canal system[4,17], which is obtained by three-dimensional filling[20]. Inadequate filling of this system is the main factor for failure. Hence the development of the innovative filling technique with the monoblock concept, in which the filling material bonds to dentin and root canal core material, thus preventing leakage[6,12,13,22].

Because it is a hydrophilic material, the Endo-Rez system requires a well-controlled technique when filling the root canal. After instrumentation, the root canal must be abundantly irrigated (5 ml) with a 2% chlorhexidine solution (Concepsis*) (Fig. 2.XX-1). In addition to its residual antiseptic effect, chlorhexidine has a low surface tension (26 mj x m^2), which makes penetration into the dentinal tubules more effective, while interacting with collagen[3,8,16]. After this procedure, the root canal system must be irrigated and flooded with a 10% citric acid* solution (Fig. 2.XX-2) or 18% EDTA* solution (Fig. 2.XX-3) for 4 minutes. Both the EDTA and the citric acid play a fundamental role in removing the smear layer, a residual layer created during root canal instrumentation. These solutions, without or with the use of ultrasound, the latter being more effective, eliminate the smear layer from the root canal[5]. After removal, the dentinal tubules are opened, thus allowing for the deep penetration of hydrophillic filling materials (Figs. 2.XX-4A-B).

* Ultradent Products Inc. South Jordan – Utah, USA.

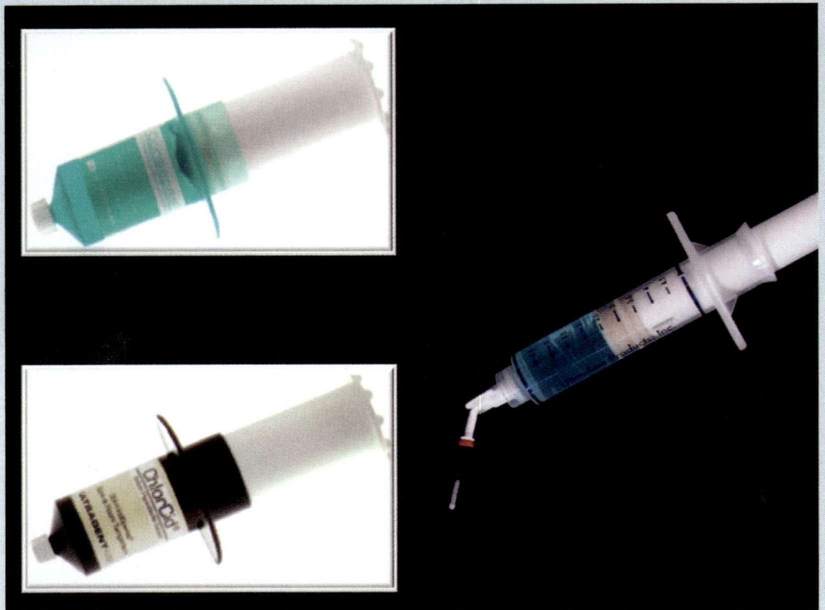

FIG. 2.XX-1
2% Chlorhexidine solution (Concepsis)*.

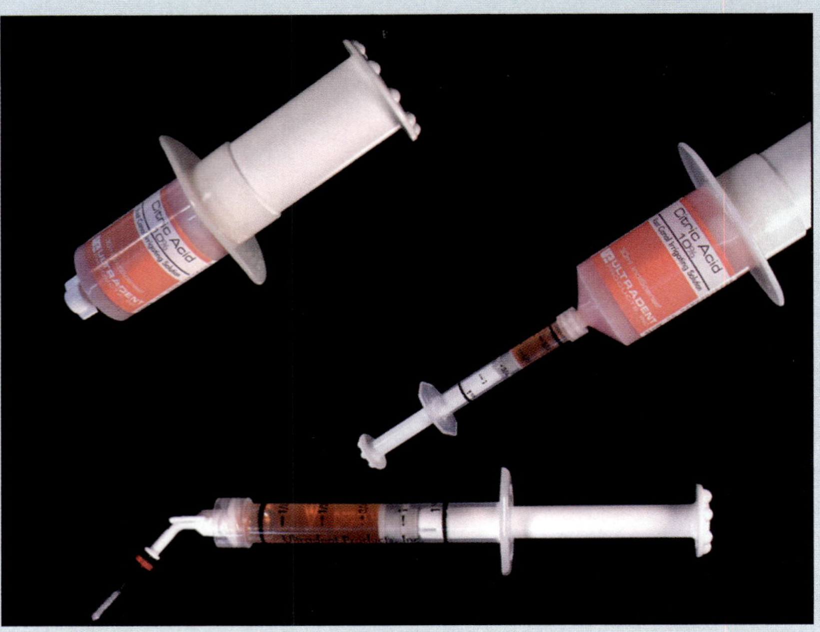

FIG. 2.XX-2
10% Citric acid solution*.

FIG. 2.XX-3
18% EDTA solution*.

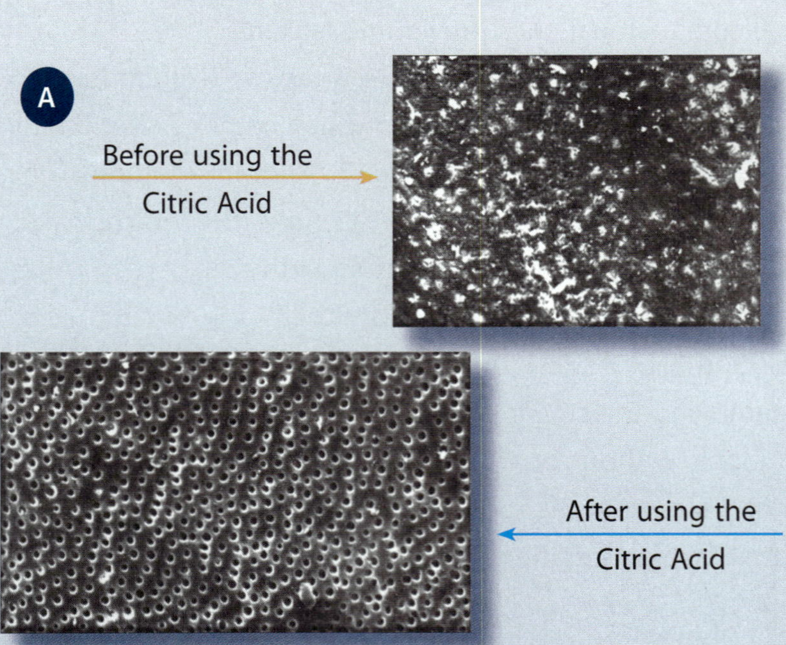

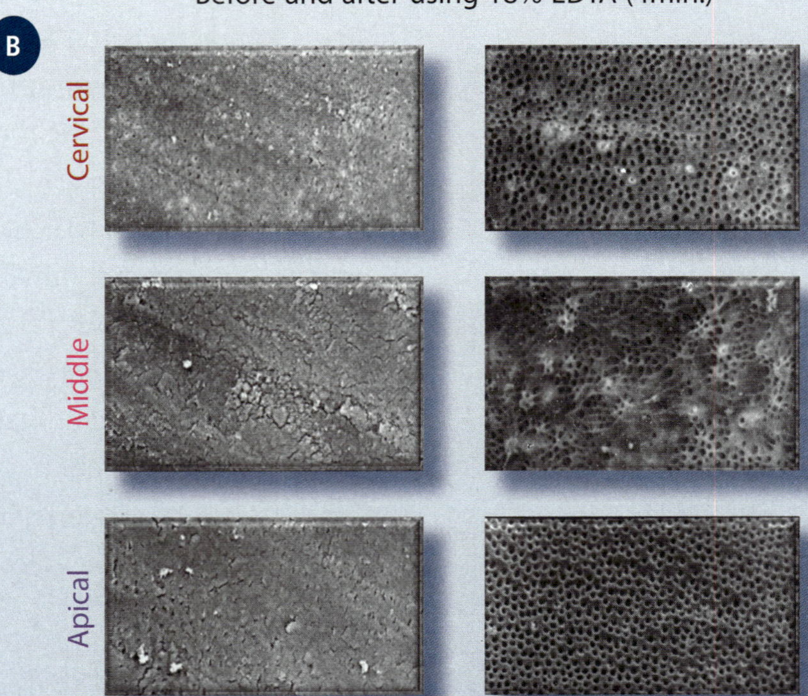

FIGS. 2.XX-4A-B
Removal of the smear layer with EDTA or citric acid.

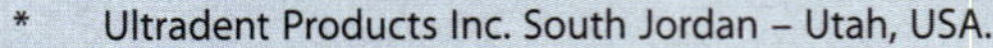

* Ultradent Products Inc. South Jordan – Utah, USA.

To remove EDTA or citric acid, 10 ml of distilled water or a 0.9% saline solution (physiological saline) is used to irrigate the area to prepare the root canal system to receive the hydrophilic filling material (Fig. 2.XX-5).

By using aspirator tips (Capillary Tip*) (Fig. 2.XX-6), the root canal is dried and the procedure is complemented only with one paper point that has a diameter compatible with that of the preparation* (Fig. 2.XX-7). To take advantage of the hydrophilic properties of the sealer the root canal has to remain moist at the time of filling. A moist root canal can be accomplished by making sure that the tip of the paper point used for drying, upon withdrawal, appears moist for at least 3-4 mm. At that time, in the absence of an exudate or pain, the root canal system will be ready to receive the ADO EndoREZ*. As with any other root canal filling material, EndoReEZ must meet the ideal physical-chemical and biological requirements[1,14], that is:

- be biocompatible;
- have low cytotoxicity;
- bond to dentin, points and coronal restorative materials;
- have higher radiopacity than dentin;
- have a working time longer than 30 minutes;
- be in a fluid state at the time of insertion;
- promote three-dimensional sealing of the root canal system;
- it must not shrink after setting or polymerization.

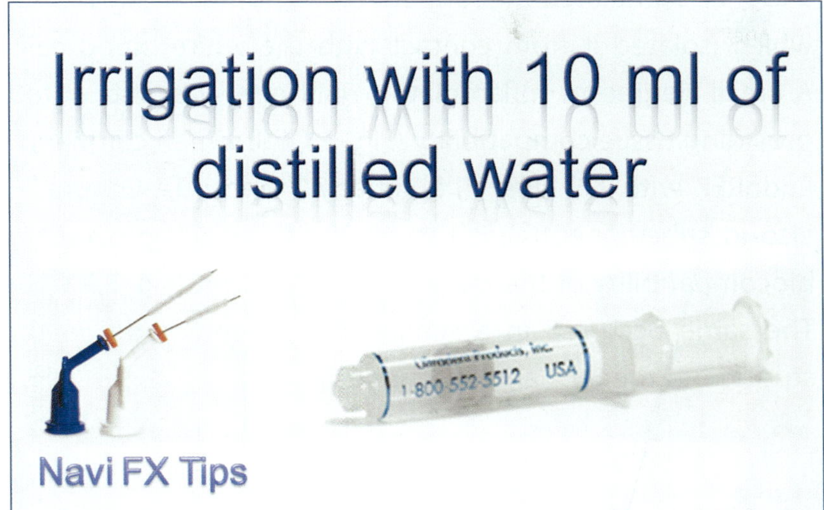

FIG. 2.XX-5
Ultradent syringe* and Navi FX* needles for irrigation.

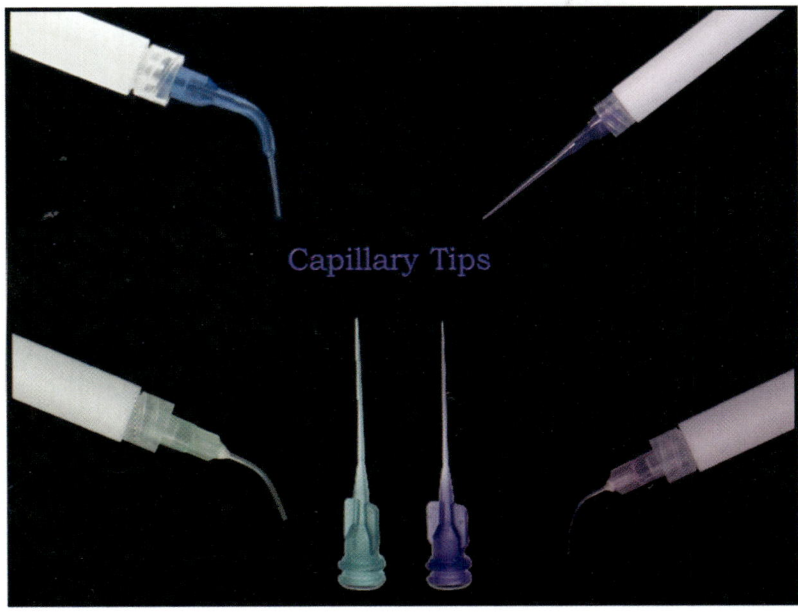

FIG. 2.XX-6
Capillary aspiration tips*.

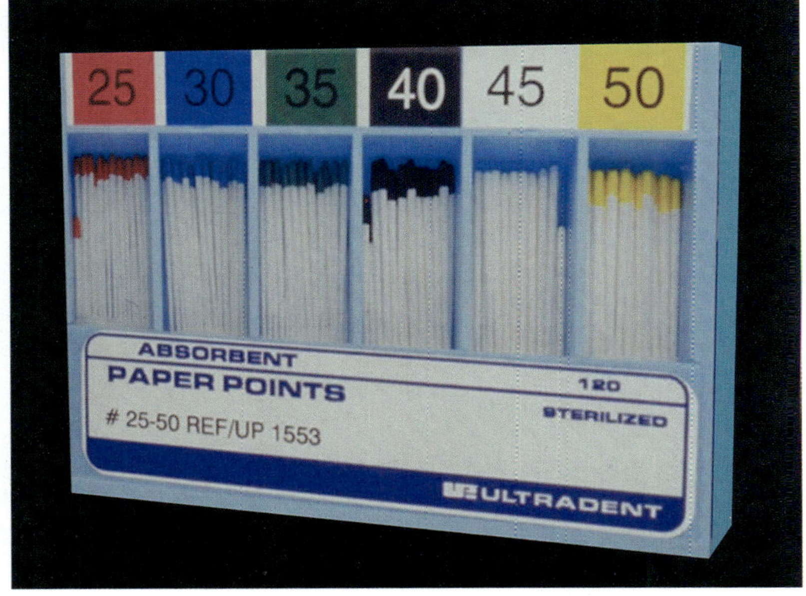

FIG. 2.XX-7
Paper points*.

* Ultradent Products Inc. South Jordan – Utah, USA.

The ADO EndoREZ* system comes in a double barrel auto mixing syringe and is composed of urethane dimethacrylate-based dual-cure resin (chemical and light polymerizable), with in addition barium sulphate, zinc oxide and pigments (Fig. 2.XX-8). The system is complemented by resin-coated gutta-percha cones.

In the EndoREZ system, the master and auxiliary gutta-percha cones are industrially coated with resin. The coating is firstly created by reacting with one of the isocyanate groups of diisocyanate with the hydroxyl group of a polybutadiene, since the latter bonds to the hydrophobic polyisoprene of the gutta-percha cones. The following step consists of the graft of the hydrophilic methacrylate functional group to another isocyanate of diisocyanate group, producing the gutta-percha cone coating that bonds to the hydrophilic[22] methacrylate-based Endo-Rez cement[22]. In this system, no adhesive is used and three-dimensional sealing depends on the hydrophilic cement penetrating into the dentinal tubules and lateral canals after the passive removal of the smear layer[18].

With regard to biocompatibility, when compared with Sealapex** and Endo-Fill*** in subcutaneous rat tissues, after 7 and 50 days in contact with connective tissue, the EndoREZ stimulated the formation of a fibrous tissue barrier, which isolated it from contact with the white blood cells. A small degree of inflammatory infiltrate was also noted, providing tissue compatibility (Fig. 2.XX-9). When comparing EndoREZ with AH Plus***, Epiphany**** and MTA-Obtura*****, also in subcutaneous rat tissues, Ykedy et al.[24] proved the biocompatibility of the material after 90 days. (Fig. 2.XX-10). The same occurred in a similar assessment model in the studies of Zmener[25] and Zmener et al.[26].

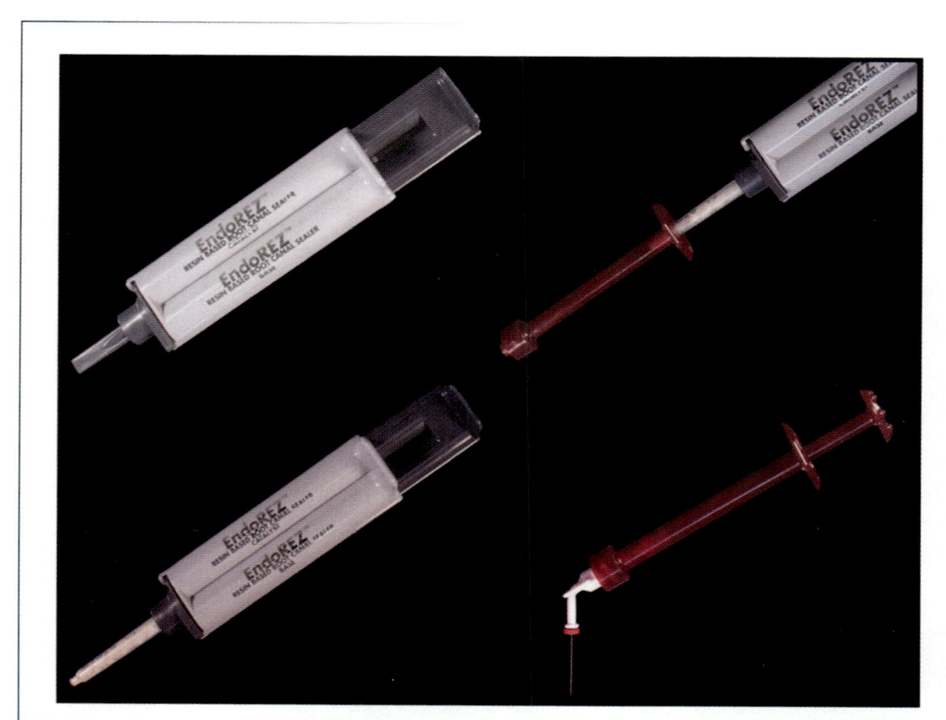

FIG. 2.XX-8
ADO EndoREZ syringe*.

* Ultradent Products Inc. South Jordan – Utah, USA.
** Sybron Endo – Orange Ca, USA.
*** Dentsply do Brasil (Petrópolis, RJ, Brazil).
**** Pentron Clinical Technologies – Wallingford, CT, USA.
***** Ângelus Indústria de Produtos Odontológicos – Londrina, PA, Brazil.

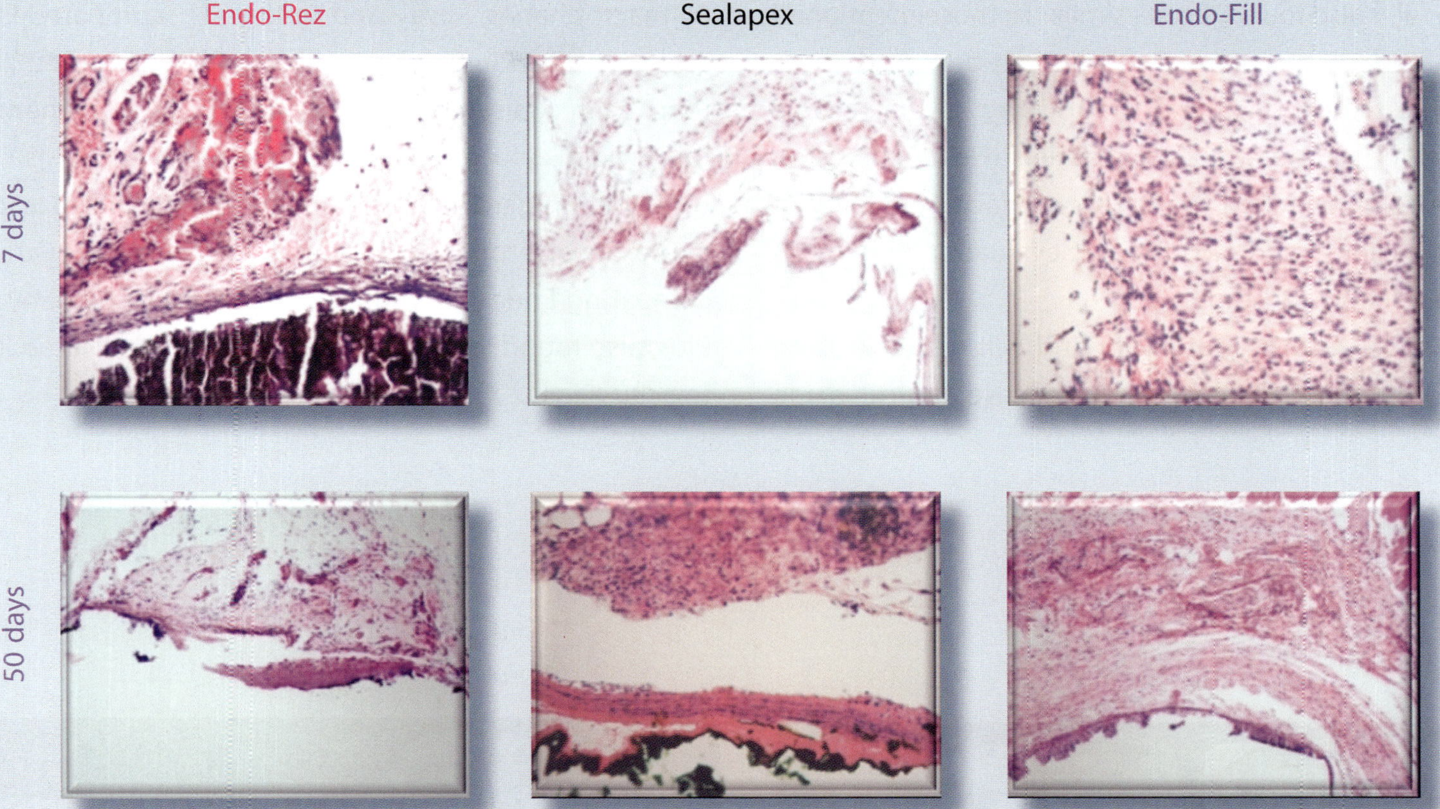

FIG. 2.XX-9

Evaluation of the tissue tolerance to different endodontic cements after 7 and 50 days in rat subcutaneous tissue.

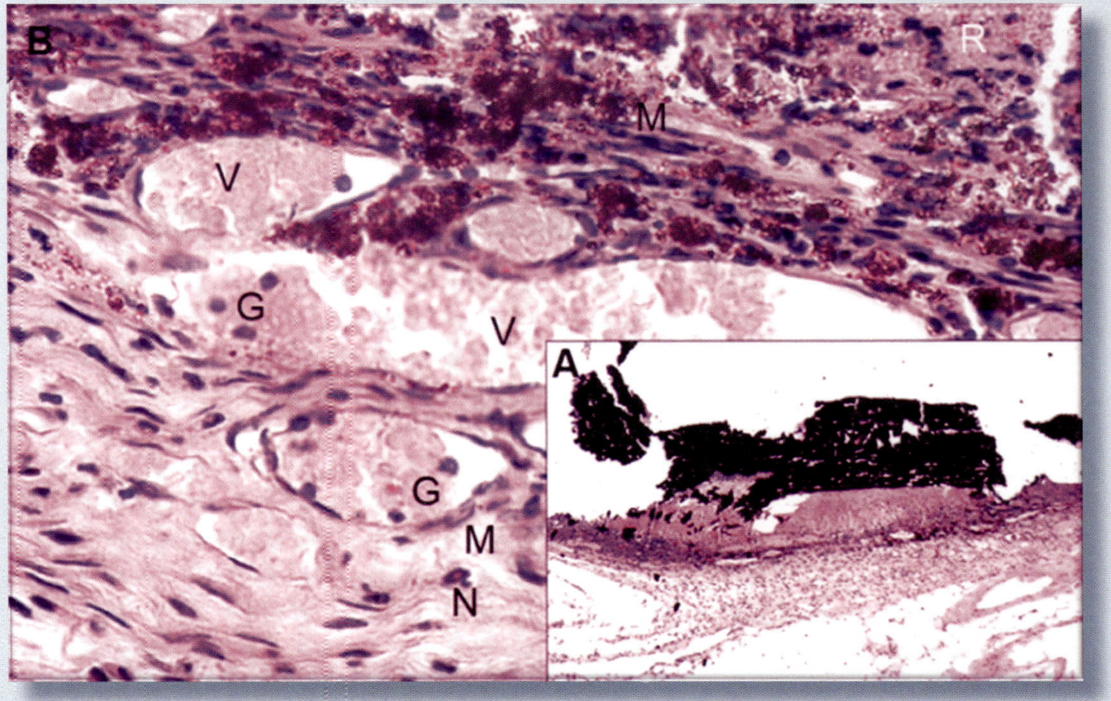

FIG. 2.XX-10

EndoREZ (90 days).

A – Fine layer of necrosis on thin reactional tissue with juxtaposed cement.

B – Connective tissue with a few inflammatory cells, dispersed filling material, phagocytized by macrophages.

V – Moderate ingestion.

G – Leukocyte.

M – Macrophages.

N – Neutrophils.

Louw et al.[15] also found results similar to those mentioned above. The periapical region of sub human primates [Papio Ursinus Ursinus (baboons)] appears to offer a very reliable study model for testing endodontic sealers (Fig. 2.XX-11).

Zmener et al.[27] verified the excellent biocompatibility of EndoREZ in a clinical and radiographic evaluation in humans in a two-year follow up study.

With respect to the cytotoxicity and cell viability, using the MTT tests with fibroblasts and the release of nitric oxide by macrophages, Silva[19] and Gutierrez[10], compared EndoREZ sealer with AH Plus*, Epiphany**, Intrafill***, Endomethasone****, Peru Balm (Bálsamo do Peru) and Polifil***** cements. They found low cytotoxicity values for EndoREZ (Figs. 2.XX-12 A-E). With regard to cell viability and the release of nitric oxide, Interferon and tumor necrosis factor, Gutierrez[11], comparing Endo-Rez with Sealapex, Polifil, Epiphany and AH Plus, also found low release values, which indicated little cell toxicity (Figs. 2.XX-13 A-D).

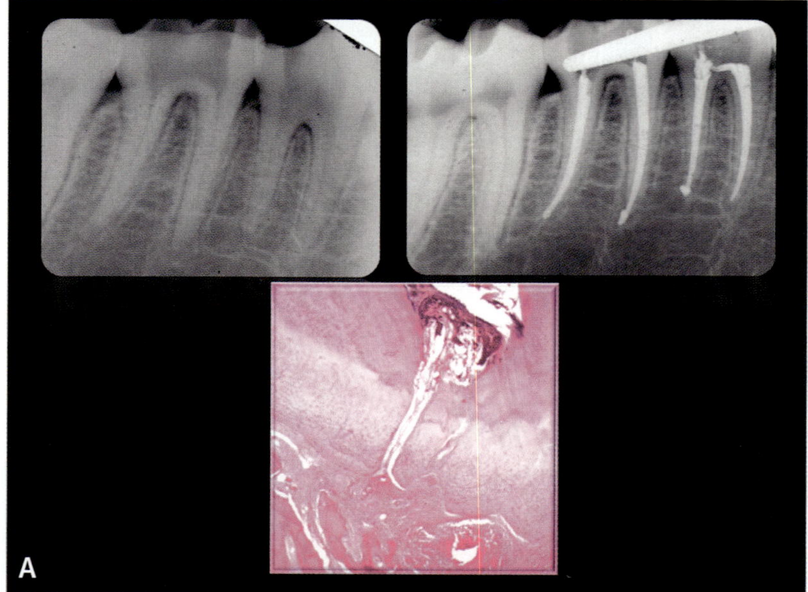

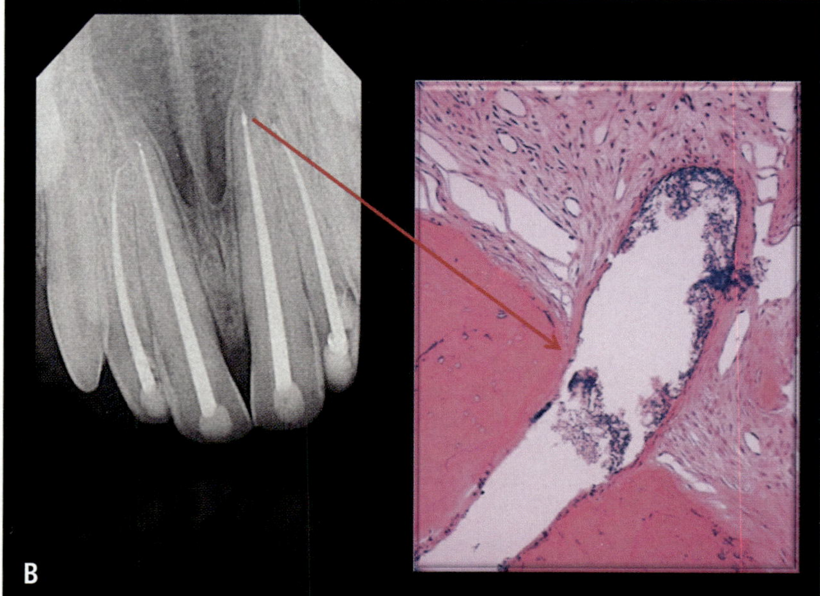

FIGS. 2.XX-11A-B

Periapical region of baboon teeth showing evidence of good tissue tolerance.

* Dentsply do Brasil (Petrópolis, RJ, Brazil).
** Pentron Clinical Technologies – Wallingford, CT, USA.
*** S.S.White, RJ, Brazil.
**** Saint Maur – France.
***** Araraquara, SP, Brazil.

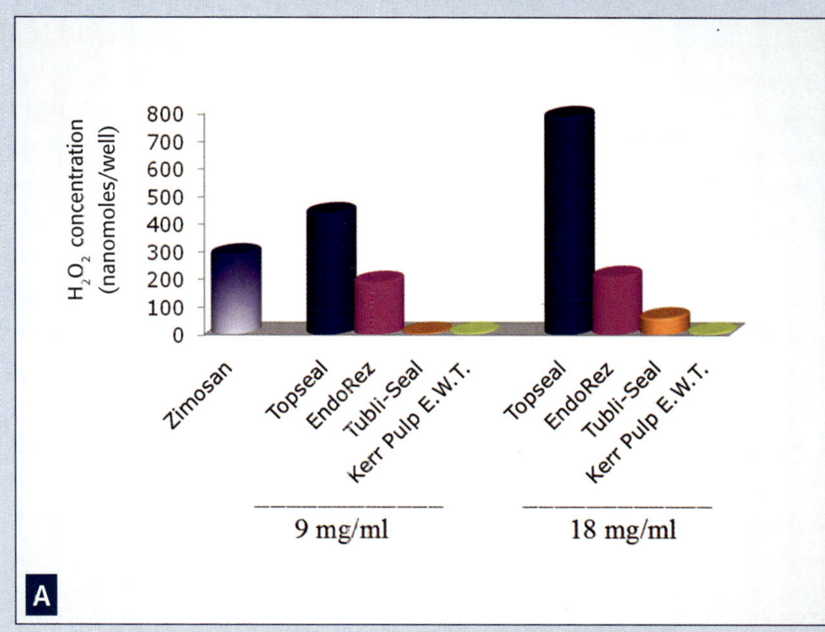

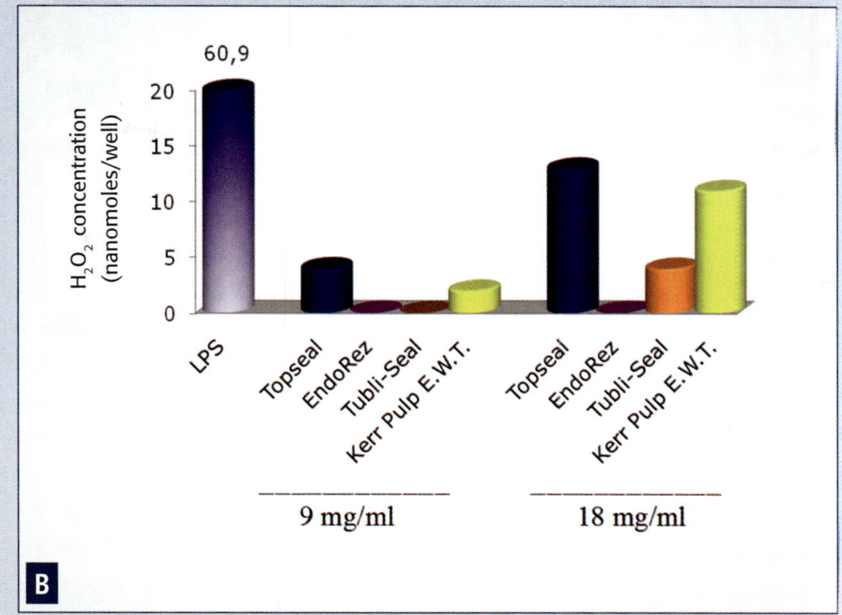

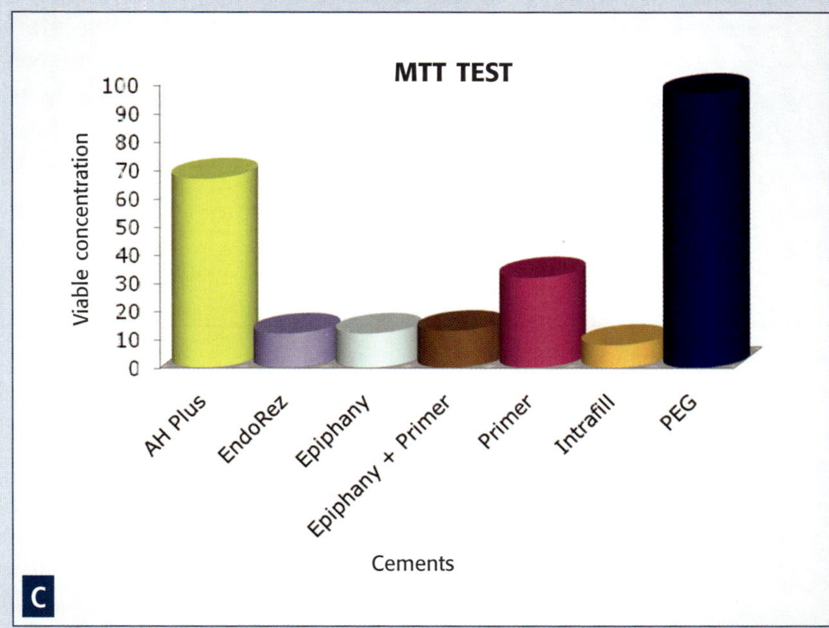

FIGS. 2.XX-12A-E

Nitric oxide, hydrogen peroxide release from concentration determined by MTT test.

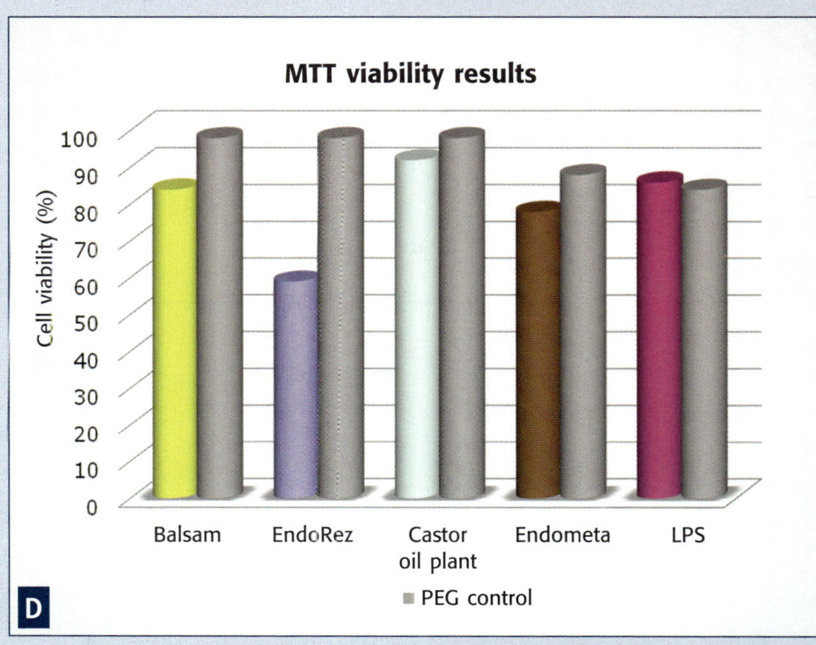

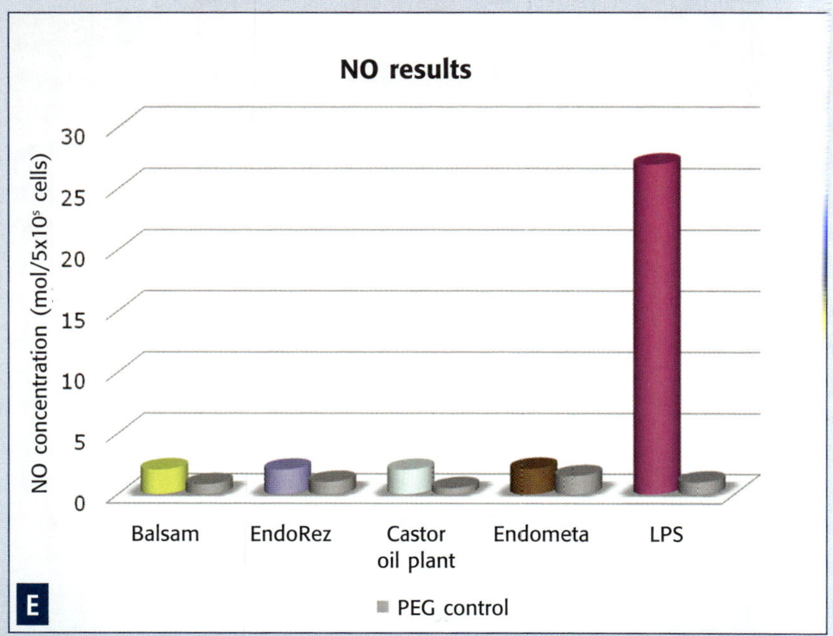

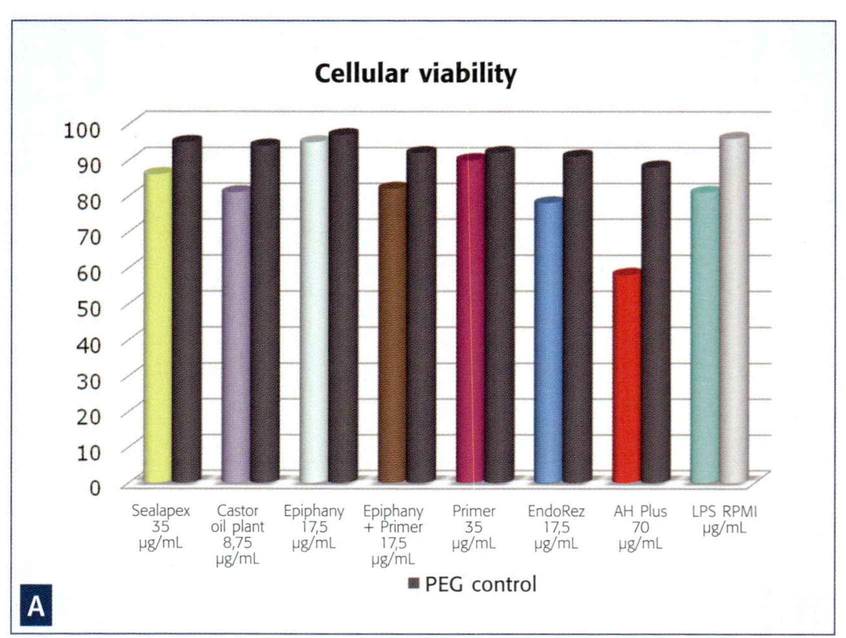

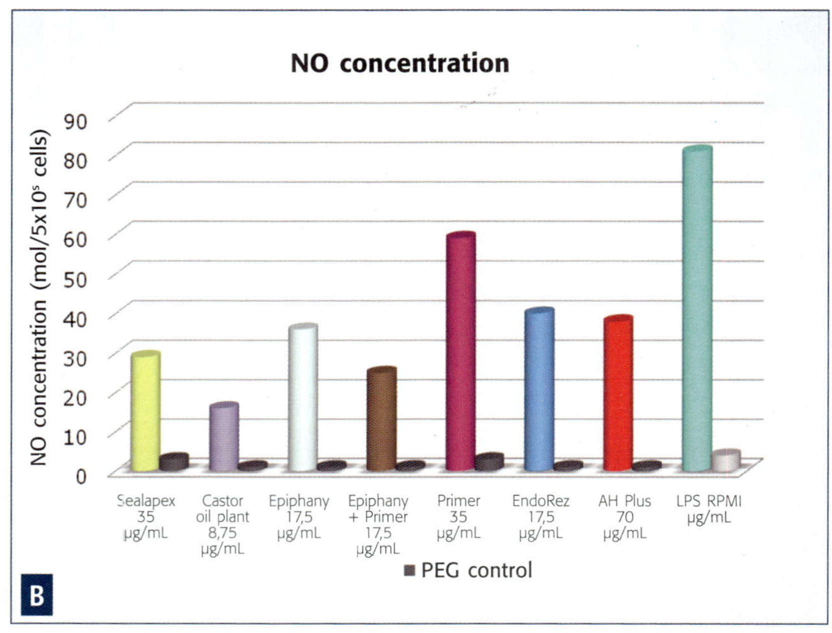

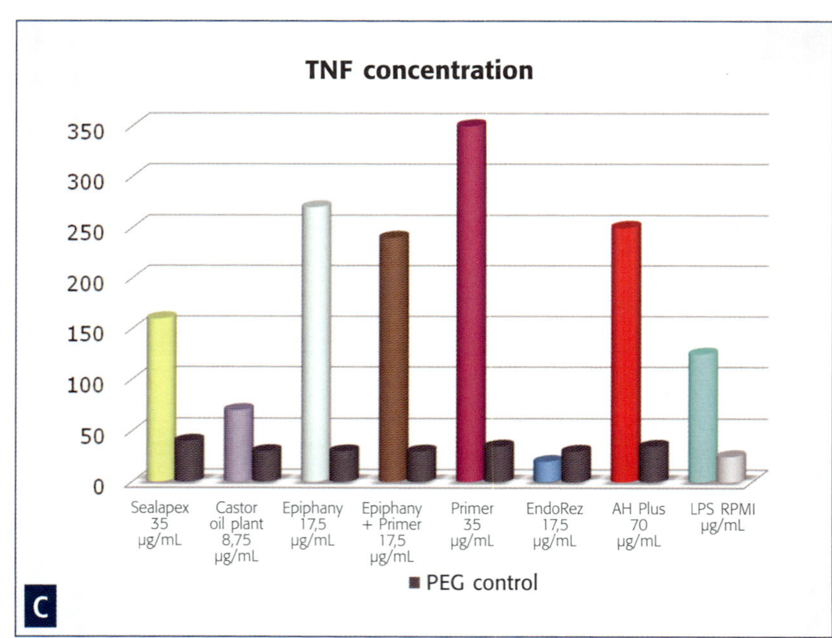

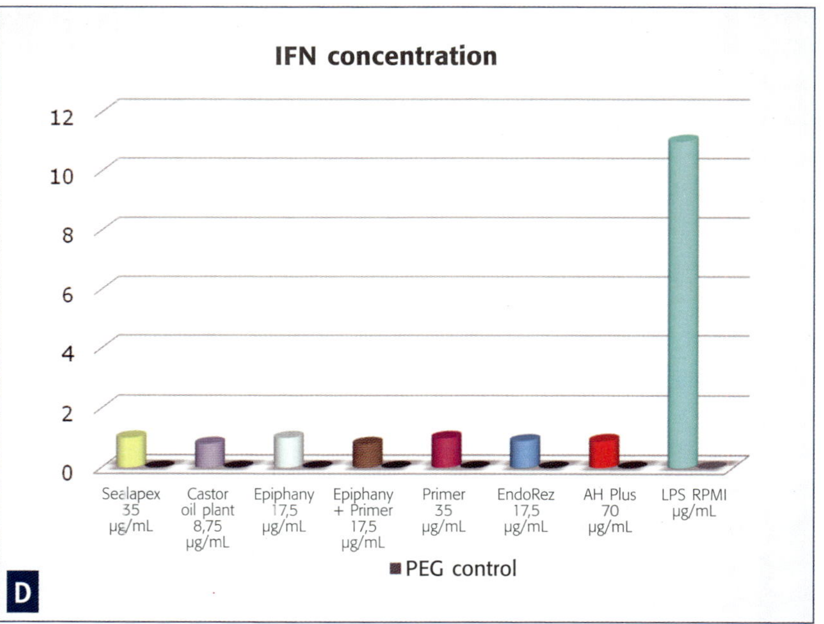

FIGS. 2.XX-13A-D

Release of nitric oxide, tumor necrosis factor, interferon from the viability determined by the MTT test.

When aiming at a monoblock filling concept, it is imperative that root canal filling materials have minimal shrinkage upon setting and polymerization, in addition to promoting excellent three-dimensional sealing. Thus, methodologies that involve dye leakage are used to assess sealing. To that end extracted single rooted teeth were used filled by active condensation. The outside was then coated with an impermeable material (sticky wax, or nail polish), while the apical foramen and 2 mm surrounding the opening remained exposed. Thus apical leakage could be determined with the use of Rodamine B stain. When EndoREZ was compared with AH Plus and Epiphany, Bobadilha[2] observed minimal leakage for the three materials (Figs. 2.XX-14A-B).

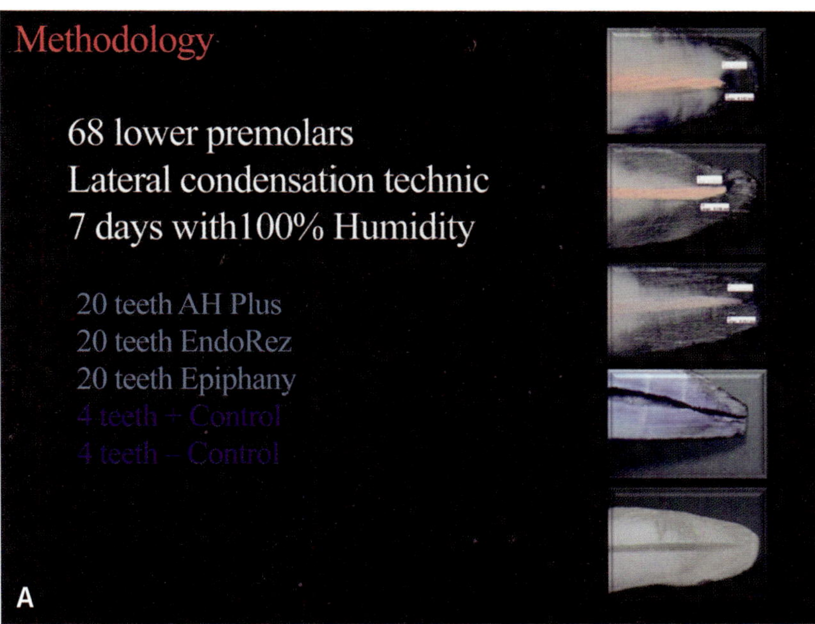

B Results

GROUP	X	S^2	SD	n
AH PLUS	0.373	0.35	0.186	20
EPIPHANY	0.412	0.42	0.205	20
ENDOREZ	0.404	0.41	0.202	20

X = Arithmetic Mean (mm)
S^2 = Variation
SD = Standard Deviation
n = Number of elements

FIGS. 2.XX-14A-B
Apical marginal leakage.

Paul et al.[18] filled the root canals of extracted human teeth with the ADO Endo-Rez system. After 7 days at 100% humidity, the teeth were dissolved in 30% hydrochloric acid for 30 hours, followed by 2.5% sodium hypochlorite for 10 minutes. Field Emission Scanning Electron Microscopy yielded images (Fig. 2.XX-15) that showed penetration of the EndoREZ sealer into the dentinal tubules to distances of more than 1000 µm. This leads us to conclude that, with this amount of penetration into de root canal system, leakage will unlikely occur in either a crown-apex and apex-crown direction (Figs. 2.XX-16A-C) The radiopacity of EndoREZ was tested by Tanomaru Filho et al.[21] (2006), by digital radiography.

FIGS. 2.XX-15

Field Emission Scanning Electron micrograph showing evidence of the EndoREZ sealer penetrating deep into the dentinal tubules.

Endo Rez 25 Endo Rez 27 Endo Rez 29
Endo Rez 24 Endo Rez 26 Endo Rez 28

Composition picture of six laterally compressed images.

Endo-Rez root canal filling with hair-like resin tag bundles.

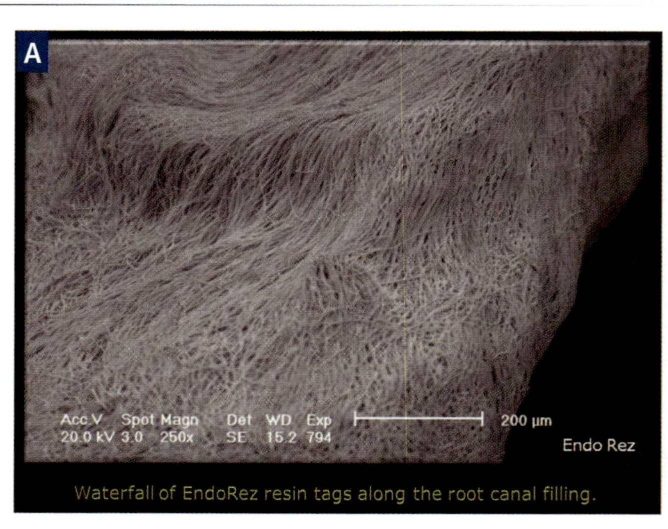

Waterfall of EndoRez resin tags along the root canal filling.

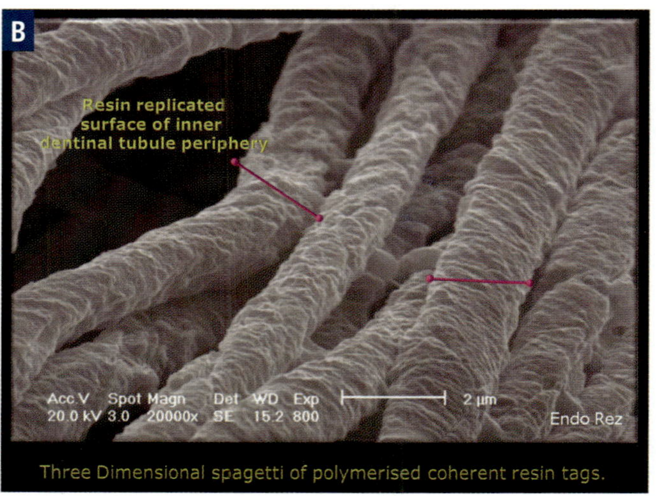

Three Dimensional spagetti of polymerised coherent resin tags.

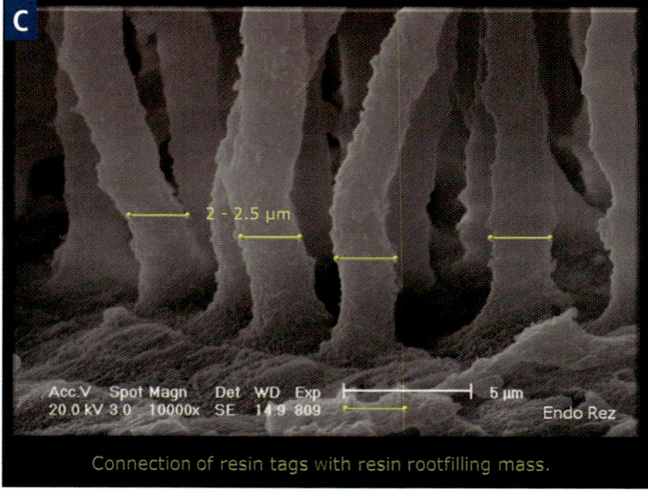

Connection of resin tags with resin rootfilling mass.

FIGS. 2.XX-16A-C

A – EndoREZ tags penetrating into the dentinal tubules.
B – Intertubular penetration.
C – Intertubular penetration.

EndoREZ, AH Plus, Intrafill, Roeko Seal and Epiphany all showed good radiopacity properties (Fig. 2.XX-17). One of the major advantages of the ADO EndoREZ, is the ease of the technique. The sealer comes in a double barrel syringe consisting of base and catalyst. When applying light pressure on the plunger, base and catalyst are mixed in the auto mixing tip. A small amount of what is extruded should be discarded to ensure properly mixed material. A skini syringe fitted with a Navi-Tip delivery needle is then back filled. Only half a syringe is needed to fill a tooth (Fig. 2.XX-18). The adaptation of the master resin coated gutta-percha cone(s) (Fig. 2.XX-19), has to be radiographically tested at 1 mm from the radiographic apex, following which it or they are removed. The Navi-Tip is then introduced 2-3 mm from the apex and the sealer is slowly extruded from the skini syringe, filling the root canal(s) in a coronal direction. While filling, the Navi-Tip is slowly moved out of the root canal. When the sealer can be seen in the canal opening, the master cone is inserted gradually until it is 1 mm short of the radiographic apex. Auxiliary cones dipped in an accelerator

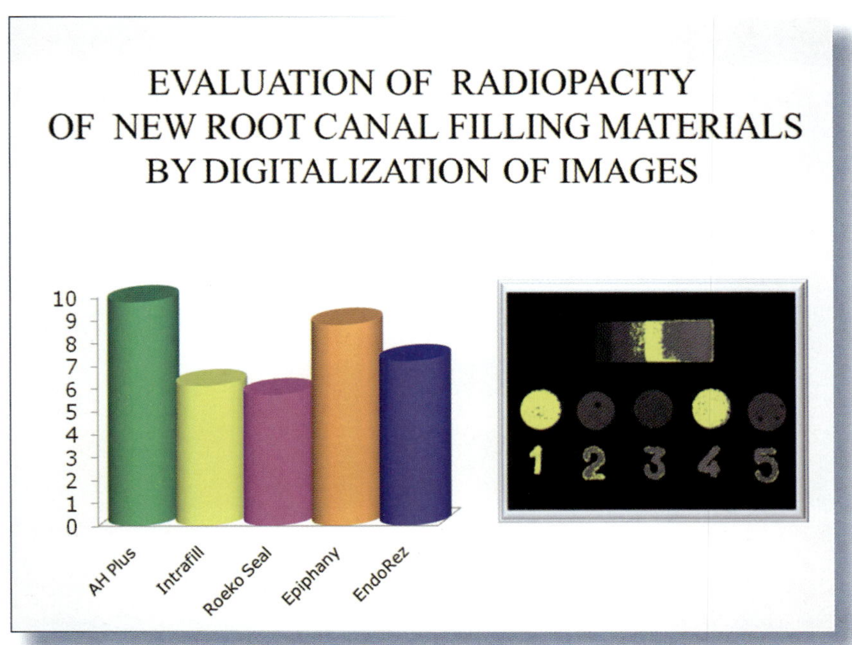

FIG. 2.XX-17

EndoREZ radiopacity in comparison with AH Plus, Intrafill, RoekoSeal and Epiphany cements.

* Ultradent Products Inc. South Jordan – Utah, USA.

may be harpooned adjacent to the master cone. This accelerates setting of the sealer and reduces polymerization shrinkage (Fig. 2.XX-20). Finally a radiograph is needed to verify a satisfactory root canal filling (Fig. 2.XX-21).

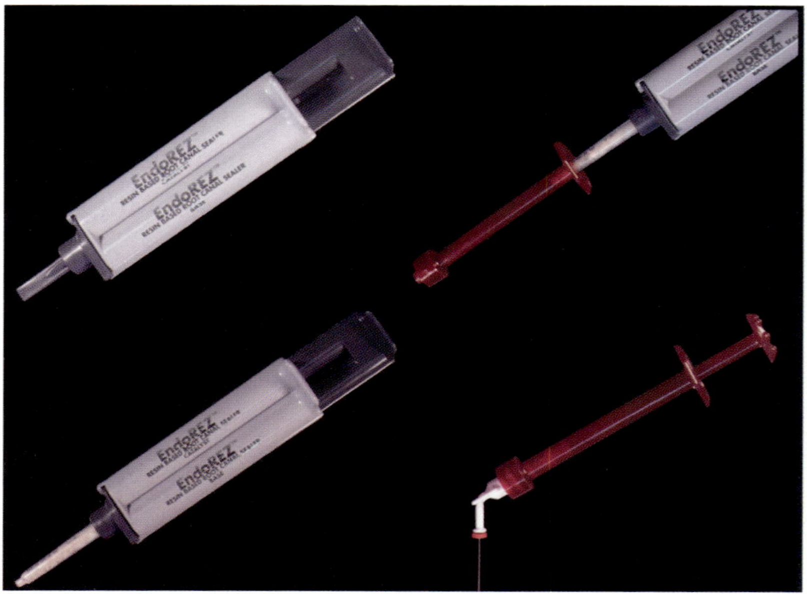

FIG. 2.XX-18

EndoREZ System.

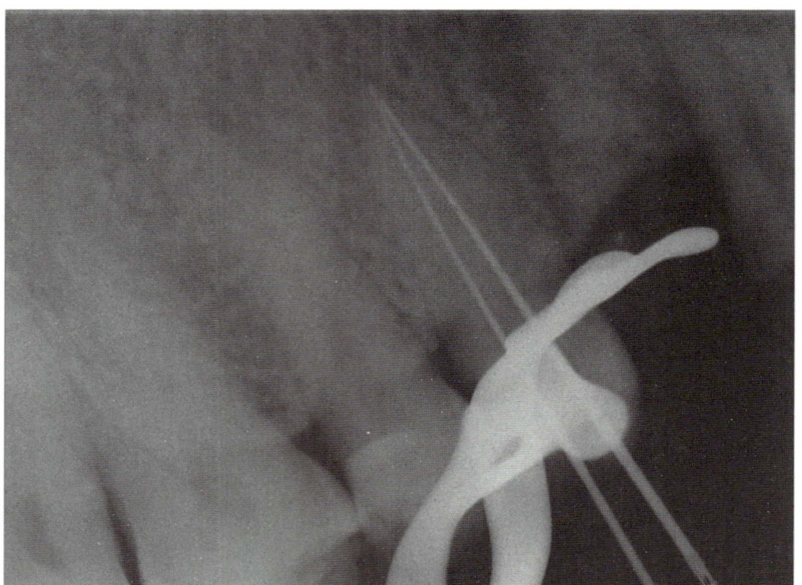

FIG. 2.XX-19

Radiographic testing of the resin coated gutta-percha cones.

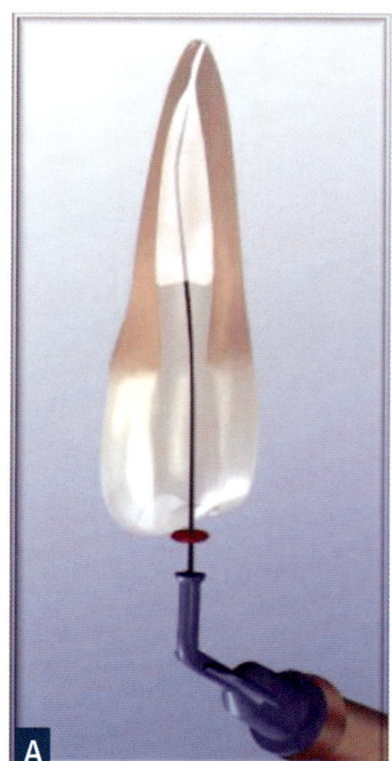

B

FIGS. 2.XX-20A-B

A – Root canal filled with EndoREZ.
B – Auxiliary cones passively placed.

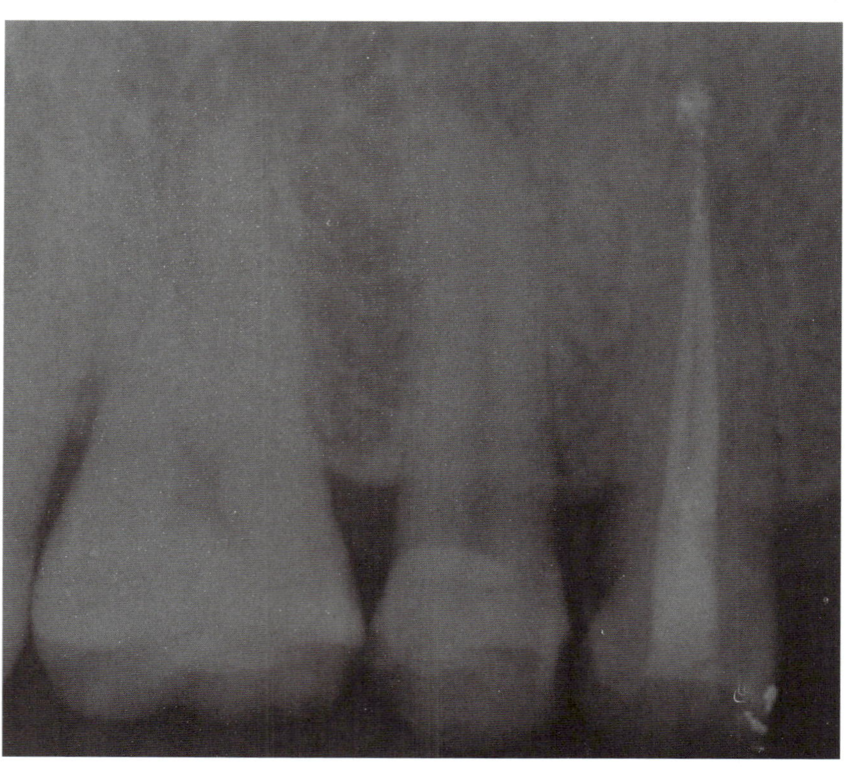

FIG. 2.XX-21

Radiographic testing of the resin coated cone.

With a heated instrument, the coronal excess is cut (Fig. 2.XX-22). As it is a dual-cure sealer, (it sets chemically and when exposed to visible light), light polymerization for 20 seconds will accelerate the coronal ± 2 mm polymerization (Fig. 2.XX-23), allowing an immediate continuation of the restorative phase. When in contact with the sealer, a dentin adhesive and a resin composite can be used or PermaFlo purple* (in case of temporary coronal restoration), to finish the restoration (Figs. 2.XX-24A-B). They will bond to the oxygen inhibited layer of the EndoREZ sealer.

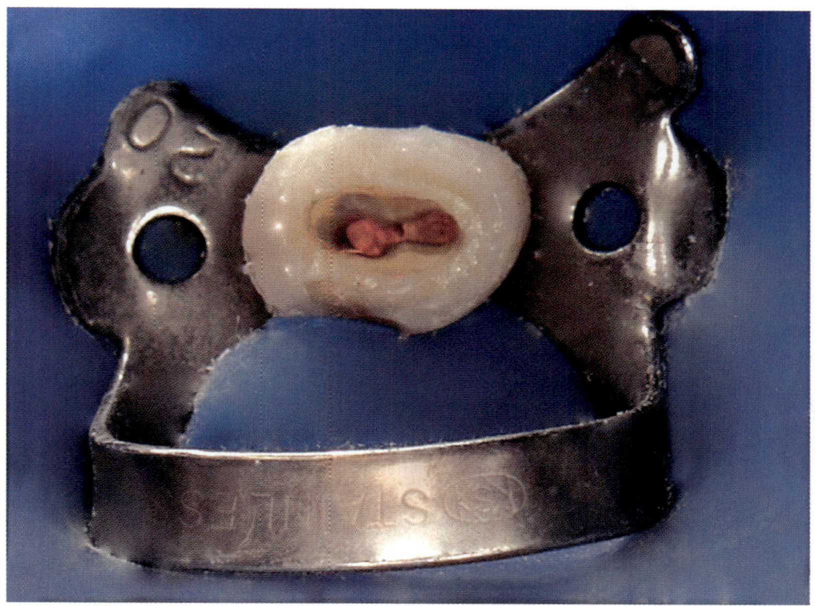

FIG. 2.XX-22

Appearance of the root fill after cutting the resin coated gutta-percha cones.

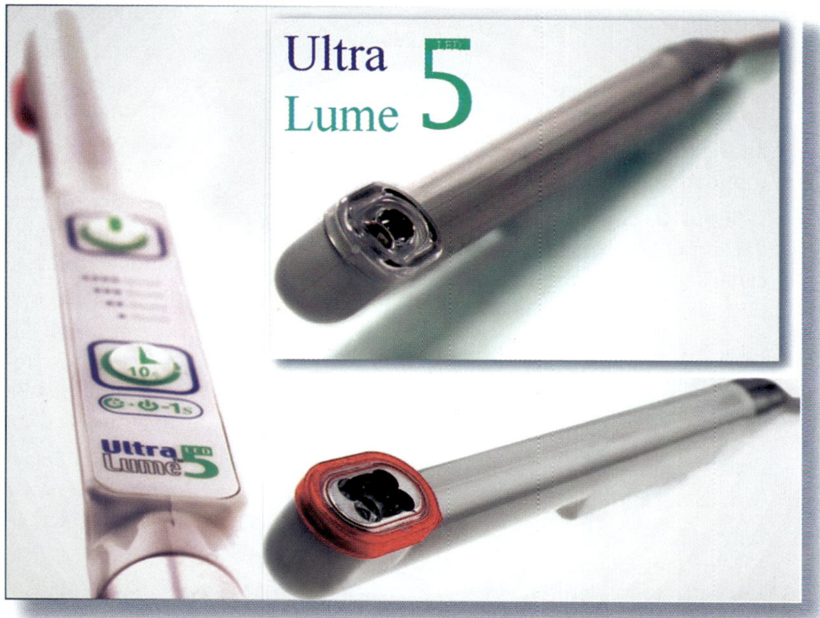

FIG. 2.XX-23

Light Polymerization*

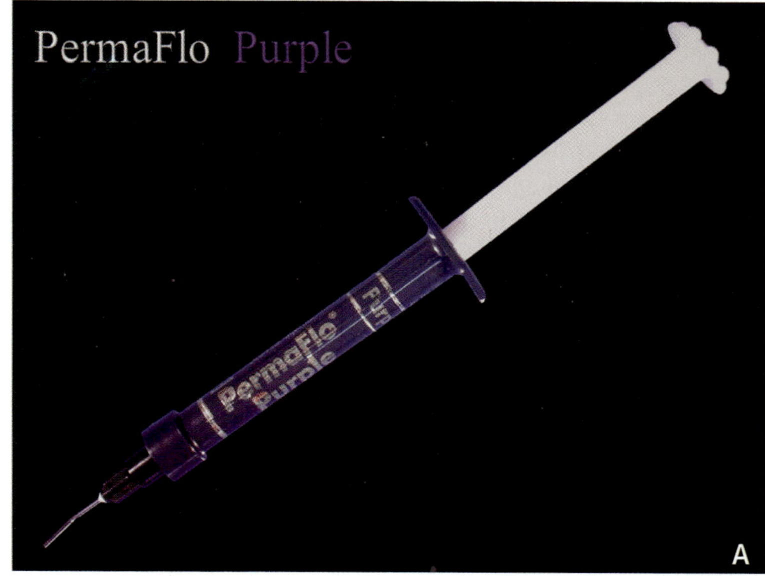

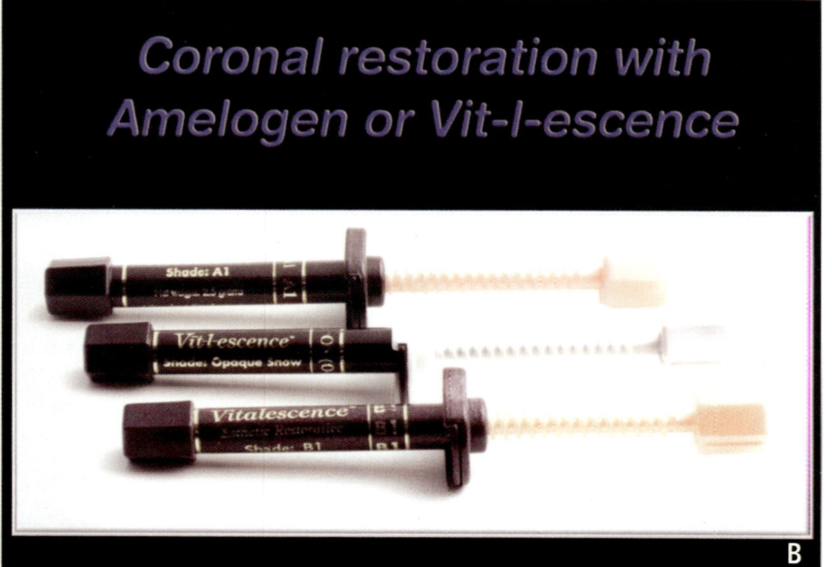

FIGS. 2.XX-24A-B

A – PermaFlo Purple.
B – Amelogen and Vit-l-escence resin composite.

* Ultradent Products Inc. South Jordan – Utah-USA.

References

1. Ansi/Ada and ISA. Biompatibility Protocol, 2004.
2. Bobadilha CG. Analysis of the sealing ability of different resin sealers. Guadalajara, p.187,2005. Dissertação (mestrado em Endodontia) – Faculdade de Odontologia, Universidade de Guadalajara, México.
3. Bui TB, Baumgartner JC, Mitchell JC. Evaluation of the interaction between sidum hypochlorite and chlorhexidine gluconate and its effect on root dentin. J Endod, v.34,n.2,p.181-185,2008.
4. De-Deus G, Coutinho-Filho T, Reis C, Murad C, Paciornik S. Polymicrobial leakage of four root canal sealers at two different thicknesses. J Endod, v.32,n.10,p.998-1.001,2006.
5. De-Deus G, Reis C, Fidel S, Fidel RA, Paciornik S. longitudinal and quantitative evaluation of dentin demineralization when subjected to EDTA, EDTAC, and citric acid: a co-site digital optical microscopy study. Oral Surg Oral Med Oral Pathol Oral Radiol Endod, v.105,n.3,p.391-397,2008.
6. Donne CL, Floris G, Bassareo A, Cotti E. Studio in vitro di un cemento endodontico di ultima generazione. Giorn. It. Conser., v.6,n.2,p.77-84,2008.
7. Doyle MD, Loushine RJ, Agee KA, Gillespie WT, Weller RN, Pashley DH, Tay FR. Improving the performance of EndoRez root canal sealer with a dual-cured two-step self-etch adhesive. I.(??) Adhesive strength to dentin. J Endod, v.32,n.8,p.766-770,2006.
8. Ferraz CC, Gomes BP, Zaia AA, Teixeira FB, Souza-Filho FJ. Comparative study of the antimicrobial efficacy of chlorhexidine solution and sodium hypochlorite as endodontic irrigants. Braz Dent J, v.18,n.4,p.294-298,2007.
9. Gillespie WT, Loushine RJ, Weller RN, Mazzoni A, Doyle MD, Waller JL, Pashley DH, Tay FR. Improving the performance of EndoRez root canal sealer with a dual-cured two-step self-etch adhesive. II. Apical and coronal seal. J Endod, v.32,n.8,p.771-775,2006.
10. Gutierrez JCR. Avaliação da citotoxicidade de materiais obturadores de canais radiculares quanto à liberação de óxido nítrico em culturas de macrófagos peritoneais de camundongos. Araraquara, 2004. 120p. Dissertação (mestrado em Endodontia) – Faculdade de Odontologia de Araraquara, Universidade Estadual Paulista.
11. Gutierrez JCR. Avaliação da citotoxicidade de materiais obturadores de canais radiculares: influência na liberação de fator de necrose tumoral-alfa, interferon-gama e óxido nítrico em cultura de células murinas. Araraquara, 2006. Tese (doutorado em Endodontia) – Faculdade de Odontologia de Araraquara, Universidade Estadual Paulista.
12. Hiraishi N, Loushine RJ, Vano M, Chieffi N, Weller RN, Ferrari M, Pashley DH, Tay FR. Is an oxygen inhibited layer required for bonding of resin-coated gutta-percha ato a methacrylate-based root canal sealer? J Endod, v.32,n.5,p.429-433,2006.
13. Kazemi RB, Safavi KE, Pameijer CH. Sealing properties of a new injectable root canal filling material [abstract]. IADR, Goteborg, p.2386,2003.
14. Leonardo MR, Flores DS, Silva FWGP, Leonardo RT, Silva LAB. A comparison study of periapical repair in dog's teeth using RoekoSeal and AH Plus Root Canal Sealers: a histopathological evaluation. J Endod, v.34,p.822-825,2008.
15. Louw NP, Pameijer CH, Norval G. Histopathological evaluation of root canal sealer in subhuman primates [abstract]. J Dent Res, v.80,p.1.019,2001.
16. Mohammadi Z, Shahriari S. Residual antibacterial activity of chlorhexidine and MTAD in human root dentin in vitro. J Oral Sci, v.50,n.1,p.63-67,2008.
17. Oruçoglu H, Sengun A, Yilmaz N. Apical leakage of resin based root canal sealers with a new computerized fluid filtration meter. J Endod, v.31,n.12,p.886-890,2005.
18. Paul PL, Van Meer Beek B, Bergans L, Moisiadis P. Environmental and normal Fé-SEM, evaluation of Endo-Rez leakage inside dentinal tubules. (Sent to publication).
19. Silva PT. Avaliação da citotoxicidade de cimentos endodônticos em relação aos reativos intermediários do oxigênio e nitrogênio em culturas de macrófagos peritoneais de camundongos. Araraquara, 2004. 168p. Tese (doutorado em Endodontia) – Faculdade de Odontologia de Araraquara, Universidade Estadual Paulista.
20. Silva Neto UX, Moraes IG, Westphalen VP, Menezes R, Carneiro E, Fariniuk LF. Leakage of 4 resin-based root-canal sealers used with a single-cone technique. Oral Surg Oral Med Oral Pathol Oral Radiol Endod, v.104,n.2,p.e-73-57,2007.
21. Tanomaru Filho M, Jorge EG, Tanomaru JMG, Gonçalves M. Radiopacity evaluation of new root canal filling materials by digitalization of images. J Endod, v.33,p.249-252,2007.
22. Tay FR, Loushine RJ, Monticelli F, Weller RN, Breschi L, Ferrari M, Pashley DH. Effectiveness of resin-coated gutta-percha cones and a dual-cured, hydrophilic methacrylate resin-based sealer in obturating root canals. J Endod, v.31,n.9,p.659-664,2005.
23. Tay FR, Pashley DH. Monoblocks in root canals: a hypothetical or a tangible goal. J Endod, v.33,n.4,p.391-398,2007.
24. Ykeda F, Spin Neto R, Bonetti Filho I, Ramalho LTO. Histometric biocompatibility evaluation of four root-canal sealers (AH Plus, Epiphany, Endo-Rez and MTA-Obtura) implanted into rat´s subcutaneous tissue. (Sent to publication.)
25. Zmener O. Tissue response to a new methacrilate-based root canal sealer: preliminary observations in the subcutaneous connective tissue of rats. J Endod, v.30,p.348-351,2004.
26. Zmener O, Banegas G, Pameijer CH. Bone tissue response to a methacrylate-based endodontic sealer: a histological and histometric study. J Endod, v.31,p.457-459,2005.
27. Zmener O, Pameijer CH. Clinical and radiographic evaluation of a resin-based root canal sealer. Am J Dent, v.17, p.19-22, 2004.

2.XXI

Bacterial Endocarditis Prevention (Recent recommendations from the American Dental Association)

Ricardo M. Oliveira-Filho

The recommendations for the prevention of infectious endocarditis (IE), in force since its last version, in 1997[2], were reviewed by the American Heart Association (AHA) in the first months of 2007[1]. With regard to Dentistry, the protocols were endorsed by the American Dental Association (ADA) and made available in electronic media by the *Journal of the American Dental Association* in July 2007[4].

The review was based on the analysis of the relevant literature about the relationships between the procedures that cause bacteremia and IE; in vitro susceptibility of the most common microorganisms that cause IE; the results of prophylaxis studies involving animal models of experimental endocarditis and retrospective and prospective studies with respect to IE prevention.

The main alterations introduced in the recommendations are the following:

1. The commission concluded that only an extremely small number of cases of IE could be effectively avoided by the use of antibiotic prophylaxis in dental procedures, *even if this prophylactic therapy were 100% efficient*.
2. Prophylactic measures for IE in dental procedures are recommended only for patients with cardiac conditions associated with higher risk of severe consequences of the occurrence of IE.
3. For patients in such conditions, prophylaxis is recommended in all dental procedures that involve manipulation of gingival tissue or the periapical region, or perforation of the oral mucosa.
4. Prophylaxis is not recommended when based only on the increased possibility of the occurrence of IE.

The first document issued by the AHA, which drew attention to the need to prevent IE, was published in the magazine *Circulation*, in 1955[3]. Since then, there have been another eight AHA publications with updates of prophylactic protocols (Table 2.XXI-1).

By decreasing the number of patients eligible for IE prophylaxis, the commission understands that the new guidelines touch on expectations that are to a great extent tied to "established" practices. On the other hand, the commission considers that it reduces complaints with regard to the misuse of prophylactic protocols, and lastly, expects to encourage prospective studies about IE prophylaxis.

The commission acknowledges that the diminishment of cases for IE prophylaxis may cause concern, both to patients in whom the protocol was previously applied, as well as to the health professionals, who assumed it to be the correct intervention in cases in which its application is at present no longer recommended.

The following arguments must guide the critical study of the new alterations:

- It is more probable that infectious endocarditis (IE) results from frequent exposure to bacteremias associated with common daily activities, than bacteremias caused by dental, gastrointestinal or genitourinary procedures.
- Prophylaxis may avoid (if it really does), an extremely low number of cases of IE in patients who are submitted to dental, gastrointestinal or genitourinary procedures.
- The risk of side effects associated with antibiotics exceeds the benefit of prophylactic measures.
- The maintenance of optimum conditions of oral hygiene and health may reduce the incidence of bacteremias coming from common daily activities, and is even more important in reducing the risk of IE than the use of prophylactic antibiotics.

Table 2.XXI-1 – Examples of the development of nine antibiotic protocols for IE prevention, recommended by the American Heart Association (AHA), from 1955 to 1997, in dental and respiratory tract procedures[1]

YEAR	PRIMARY PROTOCOLS FOR DENTAL PROCEDURES
1955	600.000 U of penicillin in aqueous solution, IM, and 600.000 U of procaine penicillin in oil with 2% aluminum monostearate, IM, 30 minutes before the procedure.
1965	On the day of procedure: 600.000 U procaine penicillin supplemented by 600.000 U crystalline penicillin, IM, 1 or 2 hours before the procedure. For two days after procedure: 600.000 U procaine penicillin, IM, once a day.
1977	1.000.000 U crystalline penicillin in aqueous solution, mixed with 600.000 U penicillin G-procaine, IM, 30 minutes and 1 hour before the procedure. After this, V 500 mg penicillin, V.O, every two hours, eight doses in total.
1990	Amoxicillin 3 g oral, 1 hour before the procedure. After this, 1.5 g Amoxicillin, oral, 6 hours after the procedure.

Abbreviations: IE = infectious endocarditis; IM = intramuscular; U = units; O = oral dose
Notes: In the original publications, the word "penicillin' is used as synonymous of "G penicillin" (more usual in Brazil), also known as benzilpenicillin.
V penicillin, mentioned in the 1977 protocol is fenoximetil penicillin.

Indeed, up to now, no controlled, randomized, multicentric and double blinded study with placebo has yet been conducted to assess the efficacy of IE prophylaxis in patients who are submitted to dental, gastrointestinal or genitourinary procedures. Furthermore, there is no published datum that precisely and reliably determines the absolute risk of the occurrence of IE resulting from a dental procedure.

In any event, it is acknowledged that certain cardiac conditions present real risk for the occurrence of endocarditis after a procedure and these are shown in Chart 2.XXI-1.

Dental procedures that require prophylaxis in the cardiac conditions listed below, are all those which involve manipulation of gingival tissue, or the periapical region, or perforation of the oral mucosa. The following procedures and eventualities *do not* require prophylactic measures: Routine injections of local anesthetics in non-infected tissues; placement of dentures or removable orthodontic appliances; adjustment of orthodontic appliances; loss of deciduous teeth and bleeding due to traumatic lesion in the lips or oral mucosa.

The prophylactic protocols for these dental procedures are presented in Table 2.XXI-2.

As regards myocardial revascularization surgery (mammary artery or saphenous vein grafts) there are no evidences that there is risk of infection in the long term. Thus, there is no need for antibiotic prophylaxis in patients who undergo this type of surgery. Equally, it is not recommended for patients with arterial stents. With regard to heart transplant, there are insufficient data to consistently justify the prophylactic protocol. However, such patients at under risk of valve dysfunction, especially during the episodes of rejection. Due to the high risk of severe consequences if there is occurrence of IE in these cases, the use of prophylaxis protocol is recommendable, even though it efficacy has not yet been well established.

Chart 2.XXI-1

CARDIAC CONDITIONS ASSOCIATED WITH HIGH RISK OF ADVERSE CONSEQUENCES DUE TO ENDOCARDITIS DENTAL POST-INTERVENTION IN WHICH PROPHYLAXIS IS RECOMMENDED
Artificial heart valve
Previous history of infectious endocarditis
Congenital heart disease (CHD)*: - Non-repaired cyanotic CHD - Repaired CHD with prosthetic material or equipment surgically placed or by catheterization, during the first six months after intervention** - Repaired CCD with residual defects at the site or near the site of the prosthetic material or equipment (which inhibit endothelization)
Heart transplant in patients who developed heart valve pathology.

Observations:

* Except on stated conditions *it is not recommended antibiotic prophylaxy for no other kind of CHD.*

** Prophylaxy recommended in these cases because prosthetic material epithelization (endothelization) takes about six months from intervention to complete.

Table 2.XXI-2 – Prophylactic protocols for dental procedures: *Single dose, 30 to 60 minutes before procedure*[1]

SITUATION	AGENT	ADULTS	CHILDREN
Oral	Amoxicillin	2 grams	50 mg/kg of body weight
Incapable of taking medication orally	Amoxicillin or Cefazolin or Ceftriaxon	2 g IM or IV* 1 g IM or IV	50 mg/kg IM or IV 50 mg/kg IM or IV
Allergic to penicillin	Cephalexine** or Clindamycin or Azytromicine or Clarithromycin	2 g 600 mg 500 mg	50 mg/kg 20 mg/kg 15 mg/kg
Allergic to penicillin or incapable of taking medication orally	Cefazolin or CeftriaxonÜ or Clindamycin	1 g IM or IV 600 mg IM or IV	50 mg/kg IM or IV 20 mg/kg IM or IV

Notes:

* IM = intramuscular; IV = intravenous.

** Or another oral cephalosporin of the first or second generation, in doses equivalent to those for adults cr children.

† Cephalosporins must not be used in patients with history of anaphylaxis, angioedema or urticaria after penicillins.

References

1. American College of Cardiology and American Heart Association Task Force on Practice Guidelines. Manual for ACC/AHA guideline writing committees: Methodologies and policies from the ACC/AHA Task Force on Practice Guidelines. Disponível em http://circ.ahajournals.org/manual/. Acessado em 2/5/2007.
2. Dajani AS, Taubert KA, Wilson W *et al*. Prevention of bacterial endocarditis: recommendations by the American Heart Association. *J Amer Med Assoc*, v.277,p.1.794-1.801,1997.
3. Jones TD, Baumgartner L, Bellows MT *et al*. Prevention of rheumatic fever and bacterial endocarditis through control of streptococcal infections. *Circulation*, v.11,p.317-320,1955.
4. Wilson W, Taubert KA, Gewitz M *et al*. Prevention of infective endocarditis: Guidelines from the American Heart Association. *J Am Dent Assoc*, v.138,p.739-760, June 2007. Disponível em http://jada.ada.org. Acessado em 25/6/2007.

2.XXII

Pain Control in Endodontics (Analgesic and anti-inflammatory medications)

Ricardo M. Oliveira-Filho

Although we all know what "pain" means, it is difficult to define it precisely. The following concept is useful in drawing attention to two important aspects:

Pain is an unpleasant psychophysical (that is, sensorial and emotional) experience associated with real or potential tissue lesion.

The first aspect concerns the provocative pain stimulus (*nociceptive stimulus*), which may be real (that is, with lesion) or only potential (that is, pain may occur without stimulus or true lesion), and this is a very frequent finding in the dental ambulatory – patients who inform they feel pain at a time when the professional merely approaches the oral structures with an the instrument. The second aspect is that the painful sensation, as does any other sensorial experience, involves well-defined objective phenomena (pain transmission pathways, number of action potentials generated, frequency of signal generation, etc.), along with subjective and emotional repercussions, which depend on innumerable factors whose assessment is almost always imprecise (previous experiences, personality, etc.). This interpretive "emotional side" is linked to the word "affective", which technically designates the set of psychological repercussions of sensorial experience.

In this context, although with a considerable margin of imprecision, pains may be classified as *minor affective pains and major affective pains*, as shown in Chart 2.XXII-1. Although the location of the lesion (that is, the embryonic origin of the affected organ) defines the type of pain reasonably well, the dental element presents a notable exception (although not the only one), due to its complex embryonic formation: *low intensity toothaches are minor affective pains, but high intensity toothaches become major affective pains.*

Both aspects have relevant therapeutic repercussions.

Chart 2.XXII-1 – Classification of pain according to *affectivity* and some distinctive characteristics

TYPE	LOCATION OF ORIGIN	REPERCUSSIONS
Minor affective pain	Superficial structures; lining epithelia; structure originating in the ectodermic component of embryonic development	Slight psychological disturbances; small neurovegetative variations (CF, BP and RF); *reactive* behavioral alterations
Major affective pain	Deep structures; hollow viscera; structures originating in the mesio and endodermic components of embryonic development	Severe psychological disturbances; extensive neurovegetative variations (increase or significant loss of CF, BP, and/or RF, involuntary emission of urine/feces, syncope; *aversive* behavioral alterations.

Abbreviations: CF – cardiac frequency; BP – blood pressure; RF – respiratory frequency

As regards the subjective nature of painful experience, the technical approach to the patient (conditioning) is relevant, along with the possible use of anxiolytic medication (group of benzodiazepines, e.g.: Diazepam). To control the objective aspect of pain, the drugs used are the **common analgesics** (for minor affective pains), **opiate analgesics** (for major affective pains) and **anti-inflammatory medications** (for minor affective pains). A discussion about other complementary medications used in specific pain (-algia) conditions (for example, *atypical odontalgia,* which responds to tricyclic antidepressants used alone or in association with phenotiazinic compounds) is outside the scope of this book[4].

COMMON ANALGESICS

This class of medications has other denominations such as minor analgesics, non-opiate analgesics, non-narcotic analgesics or antipyretic analgesics. These drugs belong to three chemical categories, each of them with only representative available in Brazil at present: **Salicylates** (aspirin or acetylsalicylic acid), **p-aminophenols** (paracetamol or acetaminophen), and **pyrazolonic medications** (dipyrone or methylmelubrin).

In normal doses, the analgesic efficiency of these three drugs may be considered equivalent[8]. As their clinical efficiency is similar, selection of the medication is ruled by other criteria: relative toxicity, different pharmacokinetics (that interfere in the therapeutic scheme), professional's experience, previous positive responses experienced by the patient, and finally, cost. Considering these criteria and bearing in mind that this class of drugs must be used for low-intensity pain, as they are not useful for more significant pains, the order of priority for selecting them is: paracetamol – aspirin – dipyrone.

It is important to note the recognized involvement of acetylsalicylic acid in the occurrence of Reye's syndrome. The first case associating the syndrome with salicylates in children with previous viral disease (particularly influenza and chicken pox) dates back to 1980. In the four following years, 1.003 cases were reported to US Centers for Disease Control, which caused the warning about the occurrence. Also described as "fatty liver with encephalopathy", the syndrome was only reported in children up to the age of 15. Typical signs are: vomiting, signs of progressive damage of the central nervous system, signs of hepatic lesion (without icterus) and hypoglycemia. The mortality rate is high (around 50%). Thus, aspirin is contra-indicated as an analgesic-antipyretic medication for any case of fever of viral origin in patients under 15 years of age.

Chart 2.XXII-2 shows a comparative summary of some of the essential characteristics of the analgesic-antipyretic medications available.

Chart 2.XXII-2 – Selected characteristics of commonly used analgesic-antipyretic medications

COMPOSITION	THERAPEUTIC USES	USUAL RECOMMENDED DOSE	MAIN ADVERSE EFFECTS	COMMENTS
Aspirin	analgesic-antipyretic anti-platelet aggregator	500 mg up to 4 times/day 100–200 mg/day	Coagulation time, hypersensitivity reactions.	The increase in dose (up to 6g/day) manifests an anti-inflammatory effect, but there is significant increase in adverse effects.
Paracetamol	analgesic-antipyretic	500–750 mg up to 3 times/day	Potential fatal hepatotoxicity in acute overdose. Important nephrotoxicity in very prolonged use of usual doses.	Without any appreciable anti-inflammatory effect.
Dipyrone	analgesic-antipyretic	500 mg up to 3 times/day	In rare susceptible individuals, possibility of agranulocytosis.	Without any appreciable anti-inflammatory effect.

Several types of association are available nowadays, involving analgesic-antipyretic medications. The main medications (for analgesic purposes) are as follows:

Type 1. *Among analgesics of distinct groups* (for example, acetylsalicylic acid with paracetamol), there is no conclusive evidence of real synergism (potentiation), but only simple synergism (addition) of effects. The disadvantage is the broad spectrum of adverse effects.

Type 2. *With anti-inflammatory medications* (e.g. paracetamol with ibuprofen), the clinical result is not clearly superior to the use of the anti-inflammatory drug alone, with the disadvantage of increasing the spectrum of adverse effects.

Type 3. *With opiates* (e.g. paracetamol with codeine or tramadol), the association is justifiable, because there is clear synergism of potentiation and significant increase in the clinical effect.

Type 4. *With antimuscarinic (antispasmodic effect) and anti-histaminic H_1 drugs (sedative effect)* (e.g. adiphenine and promethazine with dipyrone), there is an increased effect in comparison with the pure analgesic, but with clear interference in the alert state and motor coordination.

Among these associations, since those of Type 4 may also bring real clinical benefit, those of Type 3 are probably more efficient and conceptually more indicated in odontalgias peculiar to endodontic clinical practice.

NON-STEROIDAL ANTI-INFLAMMATORY DRUGS (NSAIDS)

Although pain relief with the use of these drugs frequently results from the anti-inflammatory action, the NSAIDs have intrinsic analgesic and antipyretic effects. Although a more extensive discussion about the action mechanism of NSAIDs is beyond the scope of this chapter, it is worth mentioning that the inhibition of prostaglandin synthesis plays a central role in this particular instance.

Differently from the steroidal anti-inflammatory drugs (hydrocortisone, dexamethasone, triamcinolone, betametasone, etc.), the NSAIDs inhibit the first enzyme in the prostaglandin synthesis pathway – prostaglandin G/H synthase – also known as cyclooxygenase (COX). This enzyme converts the arachidonic acid into unstable intermediates and leads to the production of thromboxane A_2 and a variety of prostaglandins (PGs), among which PGE_2 and PGI_2, which have a relevant role in pain perception. There are two isoforms of

COX, one which is constitutively expressed in the majority of cells with more physiological purposes (called COX-1), and the other expressed "on demand" with specific regulation and whose products interfere in the physiopathologic reactions (called COX-2)[6].

Although this view a oversimplified and misleading – because the stimulus of COX-1 does not always correspond exclusively to physiological situations, and equally, COX-2 does not always fulfill only pathologic purposes; and furthermore, because there are situations in which both work coordinately[7] – this created the idea that NSAIDs that "selectively" inhibit the isoform COX-2 (the so-called coxib) are therapeutically ideal.

While in reality the *coxibs* – that is, the preferential COX-2 inhibitors – really have an anti-inflammatory effect, coexisting with little gastric aggressiveness (differently from the COX-1 inhibitors), their severe adverse effects within the scope of cardiac, renal and brain microcirculation caused the withdrawal of several compounds from the market. Due to the uncertain (and eventually unfavorable) risk/balance coxibs present[5], their prescription must always be surrounded by the precaution to use the smallest effective doses for the shortest possible period.

Chart 2.XXII-3 summarizes comparatively some essential characteristics of the non-steroidal analgesic-antipyretic medications available, with emphasis on its use as analgesics.

Finally, in Brazil there are some preparations available, in which there has been an endeavor to improve the antialgic effect of NSAIDs with the addition of an analgesic. In two of them NSAID is diclofenac (one in association with paracetamol and another with codeine), and in the other one it is ibuprofen (in association with paracetamol). Between these two types of association, the most efficient one is with the opiate codeine, which significantly potentiates the analgesic effect of diclofenac (see above).

OPIATE ANALGESICS

The term *opiate* is applied to any endogenous or exogenous (synthetic or natural) substance that produces similar effects to those of morphine. These effects must be capable of being blocked by antagonists such as naloxone. The much older term opiate is usually linked to drugs derived from opium.

In spite of having some peripheral participation, the analgesic action of the opiates is fundamentally at central level on particular receptors (essentially μ, σ and κ). From this, an extensive range of side effects are derived from this class of drugs at the central nervous system level – mood changes, convulsive effect, endocrinal effects, myosis, respiratory depression, nausea and vomiting and dependence.

In the therapeutic context, it is worth noting the alteration that opiates bring to pain perception. The extremely powerful analgesic effect of these medications occurs without loss of consciousness. Furthermore, not only the pain sensation that is altered, but the associated affective responses (anxiety, fear, panic and suffering) are also reduced[2].

Chart 2.XXII-3 – Selected characteristics of non-steroidal anti-inflammatory drugs (NSAIDs) used for analgesic purposes[1]

COMPOSITION	USUAL RECOMMENDED DOSE*	MAIN ADVERSE EFFECTS AND WARNINGS**	COMMENTS
1. ACETIC ACID DERIVATIVES			
Mephanemic acid	Attack: 500 mg Maintenance: 250 mg up to 4 times/day	GI effects in approx. 25% of patients. About 5% of patients develop elevation (reversible) of transaminases. Potentially significant diarrhea. Watch out for symptoms of hemolytic anemia.	Seems to have inhibitory action on the $PGF_2\alpha$ receptors in the uterus, which would be responsible for its effect on dysmenorrhea. It has good analgesic effect.
Cetorolac	< 65 years: Attack: 20 mg and then 10 mg up to 4 times/day > 65 years: Attack: 10 mg and then 10 mg up to 4 times/day	Sleepiness, dizziness/vertigo, cephalgia, abdominal pain/ discomfort (GI), dyspepsia, nausea, pain in the injection site.	Cetorolac is more analgesic than anti-inflammatory. In any age group, total daily dose must not exceed 40 mg. There is injectable formula.
Diclofenac	50 mg 3 times/day or 75 mg 2 times/day	GI effects in approx. 20% of patients; around 5% abandon use for this reason. In 5 -15% of patients there may be discrete elevation of transaminases. Effects on CNS, skin rash, allergic reactions.	The coated pills must not be taken by <14 aged patients. It must not be used by children and women who are breastfeeding. Good balance of COX-1/COX-2 inhibition.
Etodolac	200-400 mg 3 to 4 times/day	Abdominal colic, dyspepsia, flatulence, diarrhea, nausea, dizziness, headache, weakness.	Single oral dose (200–400 mg) provides post-operative analgesia for 6-8 hours. The drug must not be used by patients <15 years of age.
Indomethacin	25 mg 2 to 3 times/day	From 3 to 50% of the patients: Frontal migraine, neutropenia, thrombocytopenia. Complaints of GI discomfort are common. Around 20% of patients interrupt therapy.	Strong COX-1 block. Intolerance limits dose to be administered; [illegible] to 40 times stronger than aspirin.
2. PROPIONIC ACID DERIVATIVES			
Ketoprofen	25 mg 3 to 4 times/day	Around 30% of patients show adverse effects (in general modest GI). There may be increase of plasmatic creatinine.	There is a formula in drops (1mg/drop) for pediatric use: From 1 to 7 years, 1 drop/kg of weight up to 3 times/day from 7 to 11 years, 25 drops up to 3 times/day. In general well tolerated.
Ibuprofen	200-400 mg up to 6 times/day	Mainly skin rash, tinnitus, cephalgia, effect on GIT (5-15% of patients), exacerbation of allergic reactions.	There is a pediatric formula (maximum dose: 40 mg/kg/day). Discrete elimination by milk, reason why it may be used, with caution, by breastfeeding women.
Naprcxen	Up to 1.000 mg/day from 2-4 intakes	In elderly patients there is greater risk of renal damage. Effects on CNS (dizziness, cephalgia, fatigue, depression, ototoxicity). There are (rare) reports of hematological disturbances.	It has prolonged elimination half-life (approx. 14 hours). In general, well tolerated.
3. ENOLIC ACID DERIVATIVES			
Meloxicam	7.5–15 mg/day	In low doses (7.5 mg/day) gastric irritation is lower than that caused by piroxicam (20mg/day).	Long half-life (15-20 hours). It has a certain specificity to COX-2, especially in low doses.
Piroxicam	20 mg/day	Usually well tolerated, although 20% of patients may experience adverse effects (in general in GIT).	Long half-life (45-50 hours).
Tenoxicam	20 mg/day (single daily dose). For post-operative pain, 40 mg once/day for 5 days	Nausea, gastralgia, prurience/urticaria, dizziness/vertigo. Exacerbation of asthma/rhinitis symptoms.	There is an injectable formula (freeze/dried powder for reconstitution).

(*) The mentioned doses prioritize the analgesic doses; in some cases the anti-inflammatory doses are higher.

(**) In general, the adverse effects are modest, rare and benign with short-term use (up to 1 week) of the recommended doses.

Abbreviations: COX = cyclooxigenase; GI = gastrointestinal; CNS = central nervous system; IM = intramuscular; IV = intravenous; GIT = gastrointestinal tract

Chart 2.XXII-3 – Selected characteristics of non-steroidal anti-inflammatory drugs (NSAIDs) used for analgesic purposes[1] *(continuation)*

COMPOSITION	USUAL RECOMMENDED DOSE*	MAIN ADVERSE EFFECTS AND WARNINGS**	COMMENTS
4. SULFONANILIDE			
Nimesulide	50-100 mg up to 2 times/day	Adverse effect in general discrete on TGI. Urticaria/prurience, dark urine, diarrhea, cephalgia, sleepiness/dizziness, can interfere with the capacity of driving or operating machines.	There is a pediatric formula (>3 years): The recommendation is to use this medication after meals. Good COX-2 selectivity. The β-cyclodextrine derivate has faster absorption.
5. SELECTIVE COX-2 INHIBITORS ("COXIBES")*			
Celecoxib	100 mg up to 2 times/day	Possible risk of thrombosis and hypertension; avoid use in patients prone to cardiovascular/cerebrovascular events.	There are no conclusive data about the superiority of this agent over the other NSAIDs as regards adverse effects on the GIT.
Etoricoxib	120 mg/day	Dizziness, low edema, weakness/tiredness, hypertension, GI discomfort, cephalgia, severe allergic/cutaneous episodes, aphthous stomatitis.	Must not be used in children. Contra-indicated when there is history of cardiovascular/cerebrovascular events, in pregnancy and breastfeeding.
Parecoxib	40 mg (single dose IM or IV) or 20-40 mg up to 2 times/days for not more than 7 days	hypotension, lombalgia, dizziness, constipation, agitation, insomnia, nausea, vomiting, hypersensitivity reactions, toxic epidermal necrolysis.	Only injectable form (IM/IV) is available for adults (>18 years). It is a pro-drug (after administration it is quickly transformed into valdecoxib).

(*) The mentioned doses prioritize the analgesic doses; in some cases the anti-inflammatory doses are higher.
(**) In general, the adverse effects are modest, rare and benign with short-term use (up to 1 week) of the recommended doses.
(***) The drugs whose sales in Brazil have been suspended at present are not shown.
Abbreviations: COX = cyclooxygenase; GI = gastrointestinal; CNS = central nervous system; IM = intramuscular; IV = intravenous; GIT = gastrointestinal tract

These drugs must be prescribed with a specially controlled prescription (white, two copies).

In endodontic practice, post-operative pain control will be reasonably short, which significantly reduces the most worrying adverse effects with this group of drugs: respiratory depression and tolerance/dependence. Furthermore, the most recent generation of drugs have less potential of causing these effects and must be part of the endodontist's therapeutic arsenal of analgesic medications. Nevertheless, it is essential for the clinician to warn the patient of the absolute necessity not to use any other central nervous system depressor (e.g. alcohol) during treatment with opiates.

Chart 2.XXII-4 summarizes some of the characteristics of the selected opiate drugs.

Chart 2.XXII-4 – Characteristics of selected opiate analgesics[3,9]

COMPOSITION	USUAL RECOMMENDED DOSE*	MAIN ADVERSE EFFECTS AND WARNINGS**	COMMENTS
Codeine	30-50 mg 1 or 2 times/day***	Abdominal discomfort, constipation, anorexia, cephalgia, sleepiness.	As with any other opiate, it is necessary to warn against alcohol consumption while using this drug.
Tramadol	50-100 mg 1 to 2 times/day (daily maximum dose: 400 mg)	Dizziness, nausea. Incidence of cephalgia and constipation tend to less than with codeine.	Elderly patients (>75 years) may require a reduction of approx. 20% of dose. Only adult use.
Oxycodone	10 mg 1 to 2 times/day	Constipation, nausea, sleepiness, vertigo, vomiting, prurience, cephalgia, dry mouth. Orthostatic hypotension.	Oxycodone has potential for abuse similar to that of morphine. Adult and pediatric use.
Methadone	20-30 mg/day	hypotension, sedation, nausea, perspiration, apnea. Cardio-respiratory depression. The drug has long half-life.	There is preparation for parenteral use.

(*) For any opiate, the dose must be adjusted depending on the severity of pain and clinical response. The dose must be the lowest effective analgesic dose.

(**) If the patient is under treatment with medications with action on the CNS (e.g. anti-histaminics H_1, hypnotics/sedatives, etc), the assistant doctor must be consulted as regards a possible medication interaction, before the dentist prescribes an opiate.

(***) There are preparations with 7.5 or 30 mg of codeine in association with paracetamol or 50 mg of codeine in association with diclofenac. Maximum daily dose of codeine allowed to be taken orally is 150 mg.

References

1. Burke A, Smyth E, FitzGerald GA. Analgesic-antipyretic agents; pharmacotherapy of gout. In: Brunton LL, Lazo JS, Parker KL. (eds.): Goodman & Gilman's. The Pharmacological Basis of Therapeutics, 11th ed. McGraw Hill, 2006, p. 675–680.
2. Cury Y, Oliveira-Filho RM, DeLucia R. Opióides. In: DeLucia R, Oliveira-Filho RM, Planeta CS, Gallaci M, Avellar MCW. (eds.): Farmacologia Integrada, 3.ª ed. Revinter, 2007, p.267–281.
3. Ferreira MBC, Hidalgo MPL, Caumo W. Analgésicos opióides. In: Wannmacher L, Ferreira MBC. (Eds.). Farmacologia Clínica para Dentistas, 3.ª ed. Guanabara-Koogan, 2007, p.214–230.
4. Melis M. et al. Atypical odontalgia: a review of the literature. Headache, v.43, p.1.060–1.074, 2003.
5. Melnikova I. Future of COX2 inhibitors. Nature Rev, v.4, p.453–454, 2005.
6. Simmons DL, Botting RM, Hla T. Cyclooxygenase isozymes: the biology of prostaglandin synthesis and inhibition. Pharmacol Rev, v.56, p.387–437, 2004.
7. Smith WL, Langenbach R. Why there are two cyclooxygenase isozymes. J Clin Invest, v.107, p.1491–1495, 2001.
8. Wannmacher L. Analgésicos não-opióides. In: Wannmacher L, Ferreira MBC. (Eds.). Farmacologia Clínica para Dentistas, 3.ª ed. Guanabara-Koogan, 2007, p 205–213.
9. Wells BG. Distúrbios neurológicos. Tratamento da dor. In: Wells BG, DiPiro JT, Schwinghammer TL, Hamilton CW. (Eds.). Manual de Farmacoterapia, 6.ª ed. McGraw Hill 2007, p.569–582.

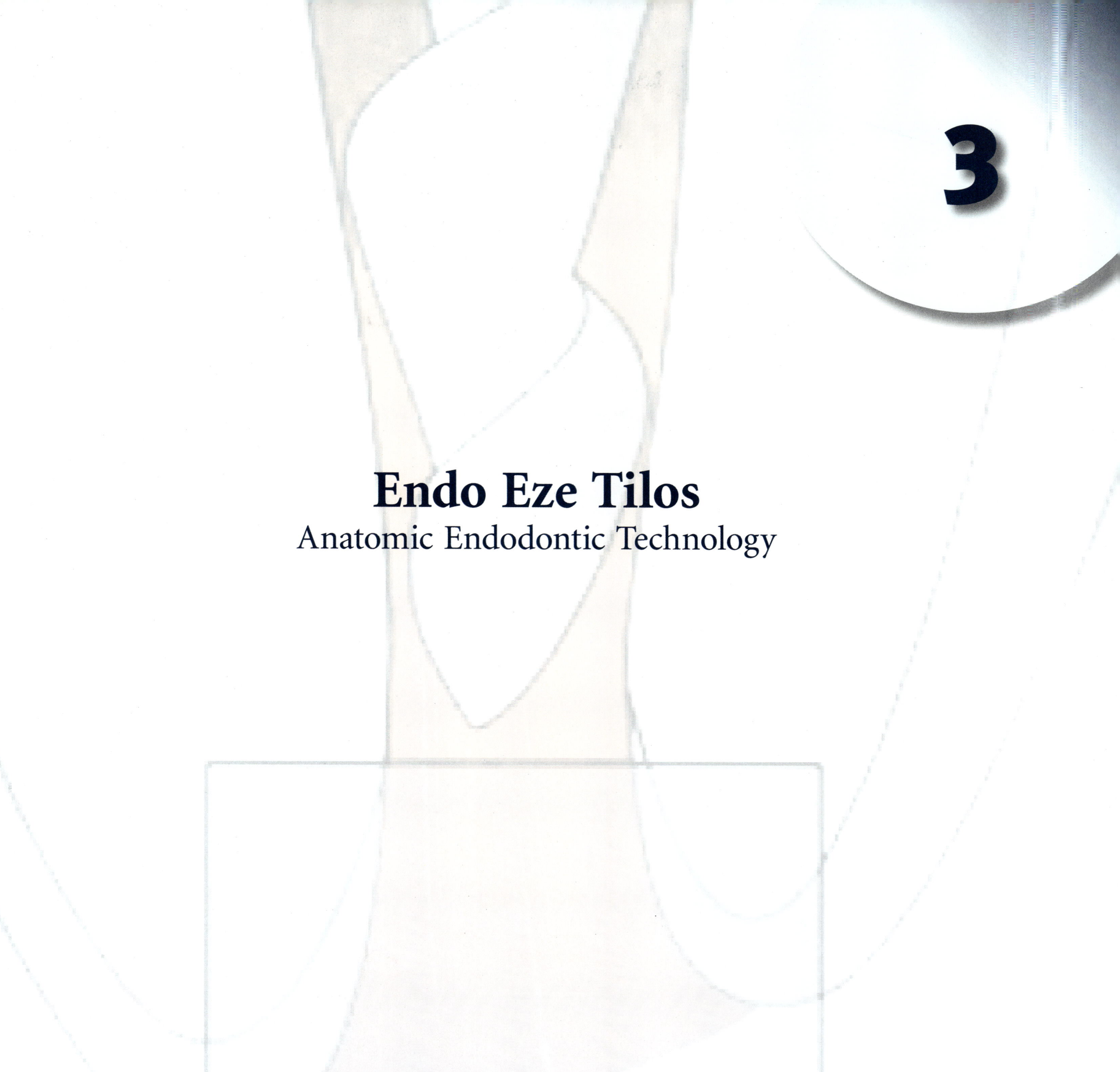

3

Endo Eze Tilos

Anatomic Endodontic Technology

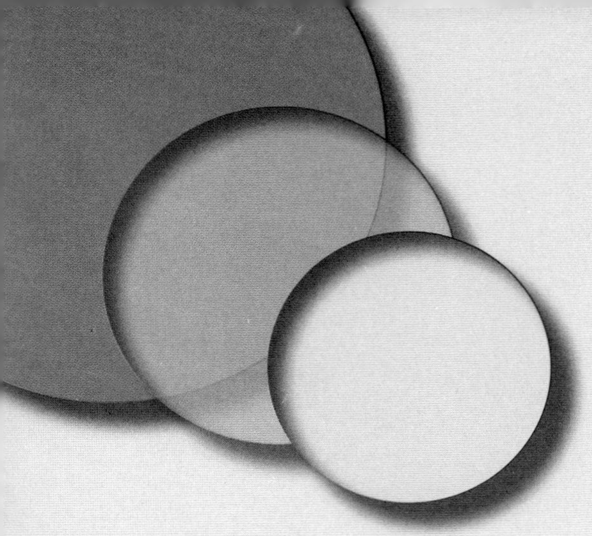

Renato de Toledo Leonardo
Renato Miotto Palo
Richard D. Tuttle

The critical factors determining the outcome of Endodontic treatment include the diagnosis of pre-operative root canal infection, the eradication of microorganisms, the preparation of the root canal space, the preservation of remaining tooth structure, and the maintenance of the "status quo" enhanced by the protective effect of coronal restoration[1]. In order for these factors to be effective, paradigms such as diagnosis, the correct understanding and knowledge of the inner root canal space, biomechanical preparation (cleaning and shaping), use of temporary dressings between appointments when required, obturation of the root canal, and coronal restoration should be respected.

Concurrently and/or after the process of pulpal inflammation and necrosis, the space corresponding to the main root canal, formerly occupied by the root pulp, suffers an invasion of microorganisms. Over time and with the decrease in oxygen supply, the entire root canal system suffers contamination and, depending on local and systemic factors, bacterial biofilm can form on the apex causing damage to the apical periodontal structures[2]. Because these microorganisms and by-products are an etiological factor in the development of periradicular lesions/periodontitis, the eradication of these microorganisms and by-products is essential for the repair process. Initially, this process depends on the thorough biomechanical preparation and disinfection of the root canal system.

As the importance of an effective biomechanical preparation becomes more apparent, the concern for knowing and understanding the internal anatomical configuration of the root canal is drawing more and more attention. Given the advancement of imaging technology today verses the one dimensional x-ray images of the past, it is now easy to understand how the root canal system has traditionally been perceived. Clinical and radiographic follow-up is used in order to assess the quality of endodontic treatment, including the evaluation of the longitudinal success. However this traditional radiographic image gives us only a bi-dimensional view of the root canal inner space. With today's newer 3-dimensional imaging equipment, the tools are available that show that the internal anatomy does not follow the external and the canals are not conical in shape.

The main objective of the biomechanical preparation is to clean and shape the root canal, facilitating obturation[3]. The biomechanical preparation is the one stage of endodontic treatment with greatest relevance, because it determines and reflects the effectiveness of all subsequent procedures[4]. This stage includes mechanical cleaning, creating space for the insertion of needles and irrigating solutions and medicines, and the creation of optimal geometry of the root canal for proper obturation[5]. It's by means of the biomechanical preparation that one attempts to form the tapered and uniform root canal shape. However this goal is not often realistic in cases where the root canals are not round, but instead have a flattened or oval shape. When endodontically treating a tooth, it is important to keep in mind that the root canal will rarely have the conical form and circular base as often assumed and will more likely have a flattened or ribbon shaped anatomy, especially in the coronal and middle third [6-8].

Today's newest instrumentation systems create a tapered shape in the root canals, reproducing the profile of the file. When first developed, the shaping instruments and systems were aimed at the removal of cervical interferences of the root canals. It is these negative interferences in the endondontic procedure that required the creation of numerous instruments in order to prepare that part of the canal. A second concern is the curvature of the root canals within the preparation. This concern lead to the development of NITI, a flexible metallic alloy instruments with a variable taper for optimizing the root canal preparation.

Unfortunately, a critical point of concern with the NiTi alloy instrument is that of instrument fracture. However, the question is not only *why* the instruments fail, but *how* they fail and *where* they bind within the root canal before failing. This may be answered in part by examining the problematic "V Zone."

The problematic "V Zone" is the root canal area with extreme flattening and that is not visible in the x-rays images because of the buccal-lingual orientation (Figs. 3.1A-C). It is common to find a flattened root with 2 canals (MB and ML) sharing the same foramen. This is treated as a two root canals situation but becomes a single root canal after the final instrumentation is complete (Fig. 3.2). This made it necessary to develop new instruments with a focus on the preparation of the root canals entrance (cervical third) and exit (apical third).

The present concern is how would it be half the way. How can it be that in one root a root canal may divide in two, or two canals may merge in one foramen? The answer is due to severe flattenings or problematic "V Zones". That's the region where instruments get stuck and fracture.

An important point is that if we analyze the troubled "V Zones" areas, they are more commonly found in the medium third of the root canals. However, this is the region where we find the beginning of the curved areas (as given by x-ray images). This is why we understand the nonsense of the new preparation systems, since in the curved region we must use the flexible and resistant instruments, even where we have the troubled "V Zones". In order to prepare the troubled "V Zone" areas, one must have instruments that may be forced against the flattened areas without the risk of fracture. That

CRITICAL "V" ZONE

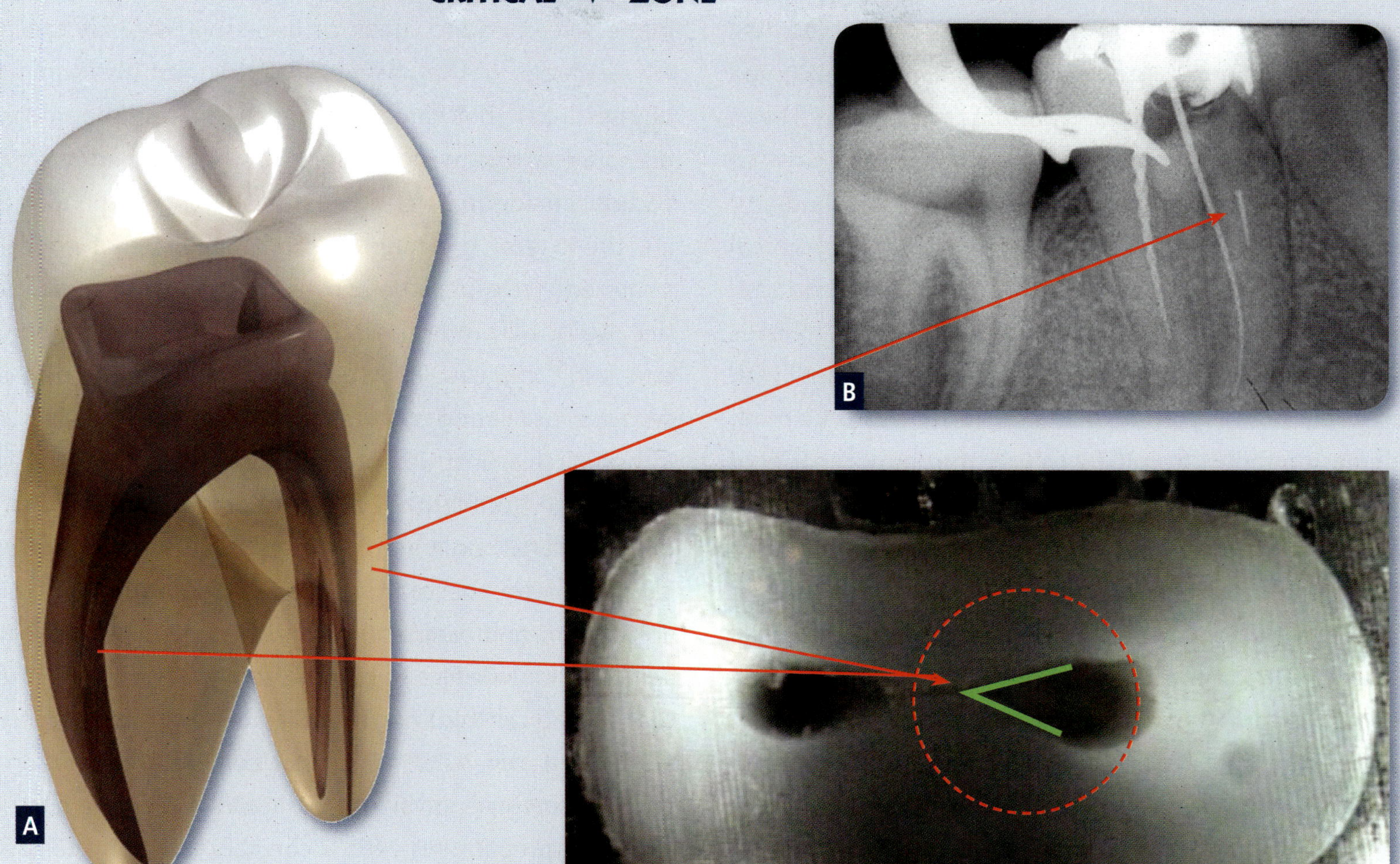

FIGS. 3.1A-C
Citical V Zone.

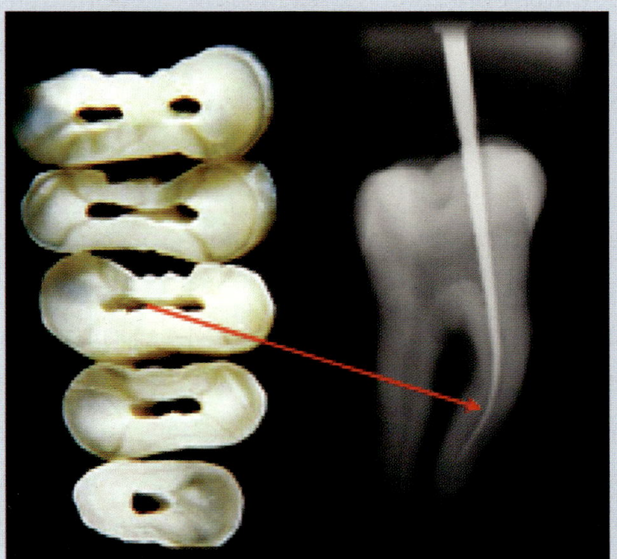

FIG. 3.2
Root root canals and only one exit.

being said, if we possess stainless steel instruments (which may be forced against the troubled "V Zones") with a small diameter active point (in order to allow flexibility in the curved region), varying taper (to work as a interference remover of irregularities of the inner walls) we may use it at low risk at the troubled "V Zones". Based on these anatomical findings, the oscillating instrumentation system A.E.T. (Anatomical Endodontic Technology) EndoEze by Ultradent Products, Inc. presents itself as a solution. The A.E.T. system uses stainless steel instruments, similar to the K type files, with a small initial active portion diameter (0.10 and 0.13 mm), with increasing tapers from 0.02 to 0.06 mm/mm, capable of reaching across all areas of root canals walls, whether they be round, oval or flattened[9]. Moved by the hand-piece coupled to the micromotor with a reduction of 4:1, these instruments have oscillatory kinematics of 30 degrees. Due to the small diameter at the tip of the active portion, they are very flexible and permit instrumentation without deviations, especially in curved root canals[10]. Furthermore, due to the small diameter, it does not produce an excessive enlargement. This fact avoids the indication of obturation techniques that require excessive enlargement of the cervical and middle third, as the active lateral condensation technique or the techniques of thermoplastic gutta-percha.

Since 1992, the interest in rotary instruments of nickel titanium has been growing and represents a revolution in endodontic therapy[11]. The kinematics of the rotary instruments, their super elasticity and self-centering properties such super-elasticity and self-centering properties result in a non-selective circular cutting action along the walls of the root canal[5]. Therefore, rather than creating an anatomical enlargement, the increased taper realizes a canal that has the same shape as the instrument, resulting in a cone-shaped enlargement with a circular base[12]. As previously mentioned, this is not the original shape of typical root canals, which are generally flat, but are more circular in the apical third, or 3-4 mm below the Cement-Dentin Junction[13]. Therefore, the concept of preparing flattened canals is dangerous and ineffective, creating areas of excessive wear at the points where dentin is thin, or areas of risk, and also reminiscent of the areas that remain untouched after biomechanical preparation, due to the existence of the troubled "V Zones". In addition, inadequate cleaning and shaping of the root canals are the one of the major reason for failure of endodontic treatment[14]. Despite these considerations, the benefits with the use of NiTi rotary instruments are generally predictable and result in a circularly shaped apex[15]. Compared to rotary systems, oscillating systems with stainless-steel files result in non-circular instrumentation, allowing them to be forced against the troubled "V Zones", according to the anatomy of the root canal. Only an oscillating stainless steel instrument can negotiate these anatomical configurations, reach the apical third and tune and gauge them to a diameter that is sufficient for NiTi files to be used safely[16]. However it's known that the apical third of pre-molars when instrumented with an AET system results in a circular, centered preparation, with a final diameter equivalent to 0.40 mm[12]. Moreover, to obtain an apical preparation with a conical diameter and taper to promote an ideal obturation, for both lateral condensation and/or thermoplastic techniques, NiTi rotary instruments should be used to facilitate this preparation[17].

More frequent and important than the anatomical considerations and incomplete cleaning – another factor of great concern, with regard to rotary instrumentation with NiTi files are fractures of the instrument. Over the years, it has become increasingly clear that rotary NiTi instruments are vulnerable to separation[16]. The characteristics of metal, especially bending and super-elasticity of this alloy, plus the new designs of the active part, seemed to solve the problems in shaping or preparation, specifically curved canals, avoiding the formation of steps, ledges, deviations etc...[18]. Even with the industry's commitment to offer the widest range of instruments of NiTi, with the most diverse designs of the active portion, they have not yet managed to avoid more of the same frequent fractures[19]. The continued need for K-files associated to rotary NiTi instrumentation confirms the inability of these files to create a safe preparation[16]. Unfortunately there is no reliable evidence, concrete or circulated, to predict and prevent such accidents. NiTi instruments may fracture without previous visible deformation. So the visual inspection is not a safe method to assess their conditions of operability[20]. One of the principal features of rotary instrumentation is the speed of instrumentation. This invariably results in increased stress which can lead the instruments to ultimate fatigue and consequent fracture. In fact the speed of the endodontic treatment does not depend on the speed of the intrumentation, but the proper planning and the ergonomic involvement of all endodontic procedures. Most existing information regarding the correct use of these instruments comes from the manufacturers or "opinion leaders" trying to convince professions to use a single kit, consisting of a few instruments (3 to 6 files) to be used in all clinical situations. Moreover, the information from the studies and researches is difficult to extrapolate to clinical conditions. In addition, the rules relating to existing standards do not reflect the clinical situations and dynamics relating to rotary instruments[21]. Thus, the clinical effect the rotary instrumentation of root canals based on uncertainties and unknowns that invariably lead to fracture of the instrument. This is the most frequent and feared accident when using NiTi rotary instruments. This would surprise the clinician, who in his eagerness to improve the quality of biomechanical preparation, stands before a difficult and sometimes impossible task, which is to remove a broken instrument from the root canal[22]. Moreover, manufacturers have built a set of rules that must be employed to use these instruments more safely. The limitations and requirements of safe usage have been imposed upon the dentist as their responsibility. If fracture ensues, it is invariably something that the dentist has not done correctly. This may in fact, be true, but what is missing is greater reality that states all these limitations and requirements to prevent separation[16]. It is no wonder that before a clinician instruments any canal with a rotary file, it is essential to build it with and hand instruments or oscillating hand pieces, which commonly create a "glide pathway" or a paved road, which is nothing but a prior instrumentation which removes all interferences – cervical, middle, and apical – allowing more flexible NiTi instruments to act with less stress, with an almost free tip preparation, reducing the risk of getting stuck on the walls of the canal and becoming fractured[23]. Complete mastering of this technique is of the utmost importance, and all the morphological characteristics of the root canal and the instrument itself, in order to avoid excessive fatigue of the instruments. Of course, this increase in technology requires increased knowledge of instrumentation with NiTi rotary instruments.

Based on this information and facts, we present a technique of cleaning and shaping, technologically possible and biologically appropriate, which exemplifies effectively the best scenario for preparing the root canals, easy to apply and used in a safe manner (reliable), profitable and predictable in most cases and clinical situations, regardless of anatomical variations and pathological conditions, while promoting the achievement of better results with fewer risks and costs. This concept of hybridizing systems and metals alloys combines the best of each system in terms of cleaning and shaping with less likelihood of errors during the biomechanical preparation, and the results are safe and predictable. The high flexibility of NiTi instruments allows adequate preparation of the apical portion of the root canal, even in the presence of severe and significant curvatures. Enlargement and the preparation of the coronary and middle thirds promoted by AET stainless steel instrument system allow NiTi instruments to reach through the apical areas of the root canal previously instrumented, and without coronal and middle third interferences, reducing the risk of getting engaged on the walls and curvatures of the root canal (especially the middle third), reducing stress, fracture, deviations and deformations of the canal. With the instruments of the AET System, it is possible to simultaneously negotiate the root canal and eliminate all interferences, while at the same time creating a straight line access of the first two thirds of the root canal, regardless of diameter, morphology or length. These instruments, in performing the pre and mid-cervical enlargement, replace the familiar "openers" of NiTi with initial diameters and excessive tapers used in the crown/down pressureless techniques and promote indiscriminate wear. Hybridization also includes change of kinematics, not only alloys. NiTi instruments need not necessarily be used in rotational kinematics. The Endo-Eze AET Handpiece System permits the use of any NiTi instrument. However, instead of rotating, with this handpiece, the NiTi instruments oscillate 30 degrees, promoting preparation with the same effectiveness when rotated[24]. This hybridization (NiTi oscillating) allows NiTi instruments to be used safely in any portion of the root canal without risk of having the tip fractured. This greatly reduces the risk of torsional and even flexural fractures. It should be noted, however, that before oscillating NitTi instruments in the root canal, it is recommended that the cervical and middle interference has been previously eliminated or reduced with the use of stainless steel instruments from the AET system. Thus, with the cervical and middle thirds straightened, it is possible to make apical preparations more effective, broad, facilitating irrigation and subsequent cleaning, and the placement or tug back with gutta-percha with larger diameters.

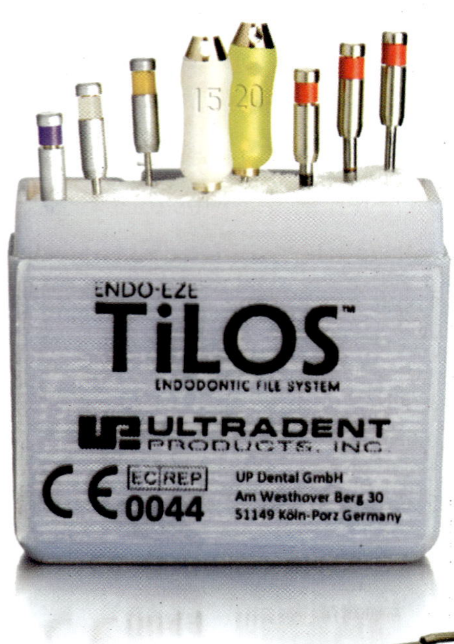

FIG. 3.3
Tilos System.

Developed by Ultradent, the Tilos System (Fig. 3.3) brings all of these developments together, or in other words; the right metal, in the correct area of the root canal, acting at exactly the right moment. It consists of three stainless-steel shaping files, all part of the Endo-Eze A.E.T system available in yellow, red, and blue files, with their respective diameters of the active portion and taper .10, .13, and 13 mm (diameter) and 0.020, 0.030 and 0.040 mm/mm (taper), two hand K-type stainless steel files, numbers 15 and 20, and supplemented by three NiTi files with a active portion diameter of 0.25 mm and tapers 0.08, 0.04, and 0.02 mm/mm. The following sequence (Fig. 3.4) indicates the use of the hand instrument K-file #15 for the catheterization, negotiation of the root canal and determination of tooth length (with x-ray or electronic apex locator). Having reached the length of the tooth, instrumentation is initiated. Sometimes, in canals with extreme atresia or curves, this step must be performed with hand instruments of smaller diameter, such as K-type files #10, 08. In large root canals this task can be performed with instruments of larger diameter, such as K-type files #20 or #25. The important thing is to observe and record is the first of these instruments which reached the tooth length, the anatomic diameter, and met resistance. This instrument is called the Apical Instrument (A.I.). When the case in question is a tooth with pulp necrosis, the catheterization and negotiation should be made by thirds – always thoroughly irrigating the root canal with sodium hypochlorite. After this first step, mechanical oscillating instrumentation starts with the use of Endo-Eze handpiece and shaping files yellow and red; 0.10 and 0.13 mm, respectively, to 0.02 and 0.03 mm/mm to 3 millimeters short of the tooth length. Follow with the mechanical use of the blue shaping file, 0.13 diameter and 0.004 mm/mm taper, to 6 mm short of the tooth length.

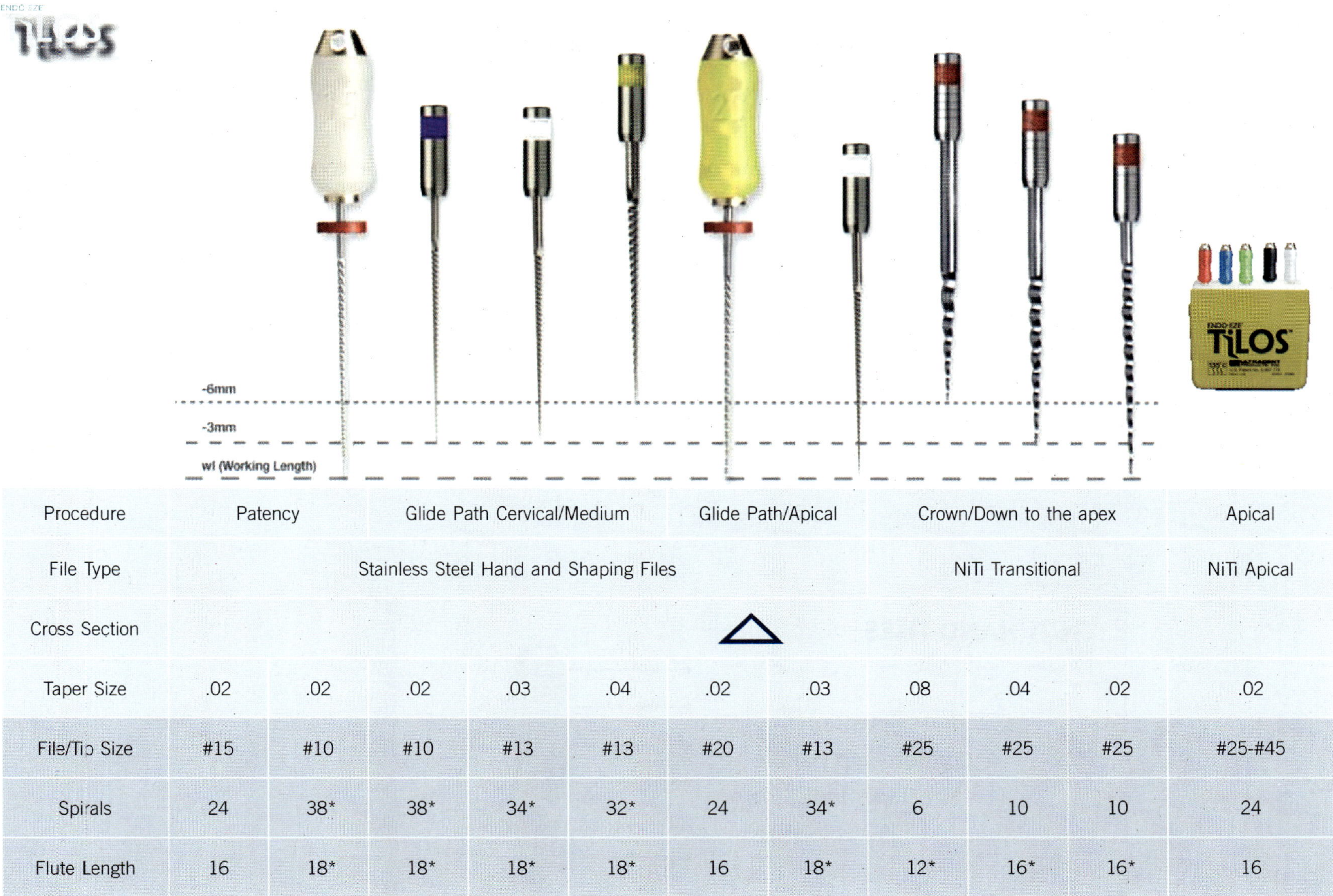

Procedure	Patency		Glide Path Cervical/Medium			Glide Path/Apical		Crown/Down to the apex			Apical
File Type	Stainless Steel Hand and Shaping Files							NiTi Transitional			NiTi Apical
Cross Section											
Taper Size	.02	.02	.02	.03	.04	.02	.03	.08	.04	.02	.02
File/Tip Size	#15	#10	#10	#13	#13	#20	#13	#25	#25	#25	#25-#45
Spirals	24	38*	38*	34*	32*	24	34*	6	10	10	24
Flute Length	16	18*	18*	18*	18*	16	18*	12*	16*	16*	16

* Number of spiral and flute lengths will change based on the file length. These are 24 mm-27 mm.

FIG. 3.4

Clinical sequence.

The kinematics of these files is the circular and perimetral motion – brushing with force against the entire length of the walls. Follow the change of each instrument, irrigation must be performed with 5ml of irrigant solution. By carrying out this initial preparation, all the interferences of coronary and middle thirds were eliminated. In this way, we easily reach the apex. In order for this to happen safely, we recommend the use of pre-curved stainless steel hand files that with catheterization must reach the tooth length, and then promote the instrumentation of the root canal. This is followed by using the white file, 0.03 to the working length to maintain the glide path. This justifies the interference removal and the transformation of the troubled "V Zones" in safe "U Zones", entirely cleaning the path towards the apical third and diminishing the risk of fracture, not to mention that one may use NITI instruments with a smaller risk to prepare the apical area. From this moment on, with the same oscillating handpiece, we instrument the root canal with #25 NiTi files and tapers 0.08, 0.04 and 0.02 mm/mm, respectively, in the cinematic crown-apex pressure less motion until the tooth length is reached. Depending on the anatomy, this result can occur with file 0.08 or 0.04 or in atresia and curved canals with the #25 NiTi file 0.02. As was identified at the beginning of the treatment, now you can use the apical instrument (A.I.) as a reference because the apical preparation should be done with NiTi hand files up to 5 numbers beyond the AI. For example, if the AI were a #15 instrument, instrument the apical portion with NiTi hand files until #40.In this case,Apical instruments manufactured by Ultradent in NiTI can be used (Fig. 3.5) available from # 25 to 45.

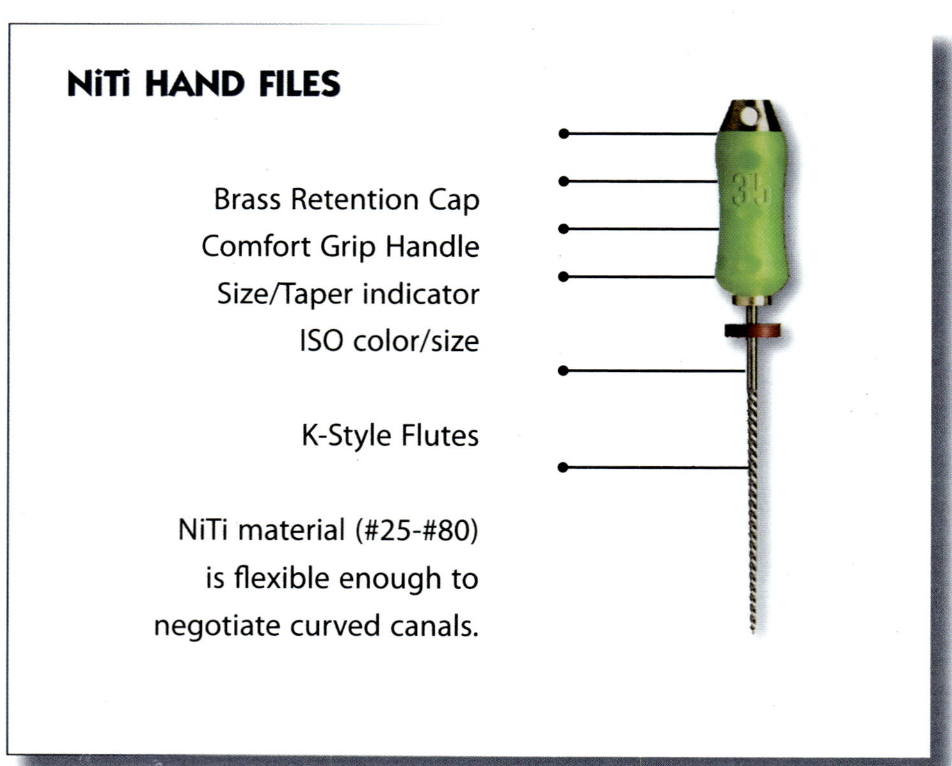

FIG. 3.5

Apical hand instrument.

References

1. Saito D, Leonardo RT, Rodrigues JL, Tsai SM, Höfling JF, Gonçalves RB Identification of bacteria in endodontic infections by sequence analysis of 16S rDNA clone libraries. J Med Microb. 2006; 55 (Pt 1): 101-7.
2. Leonardo MR, da Silva LA, Tanomaru Filho M, Bonifácio KC, Ito IY. In vitro evaluation of antimicrobial activity of sealers and pastes used in endodontics. J Endod. 2000; 26: 391-4.
3. European Society of Endodontology. Quality guidelines for endodontic treatment consensus report of the European Society of Endodontology. Int Endod J. 2006; 39: 921-30.
4. Leonardo MR, Flores DS, de Paula e Silva FW, de Toledo Leonardo R, da Silva LA. A comparison study of periapical repair in dogs' teeth using RoekoSeal and AH plus root canal sealers: a histopathological evaluation. J Endod. 2008; 34: 822-5. Epub 2008 May 16.
5. Peters OA. Current challenges and concepts in the preparation of root canal systems: a review. J Endod. 2004; 30: 559-65.
6. Kerekes K, Tronstad L. Morphometric observations on root canals of human anterior teeth. J Endod. 1977a; 3: 24-9.
7. Kerekes K, Tronstad L. Morphometric observations on root canals of human premolars. J Endod. 1977b; 3: 74-9.
8. Kerekes K, Tronstad L. Morphometric observations on root canals of human molars. J Endod. 1977c; 3: 114-8.
9. Fischer D. Root canal preparation with Endo-Eze AET: changes in root canal shape assessed by micro-computed tomography. Int Endod J. 2005; 38: 456-64.
10. Riitano F. Anatomic Endodontic Technology (AET) – a crown-down root canal preparation technique: basic concepts, operative procedure and instruments. Int Endod J. 2005; 38: 575-87.
11. Cheung GS, Liu CS. A retrospective study of endodontic treatment outcome between nickel-titanium rotary and stainless steel hand filing techniques. J Endod. 2009; 35: 938-43.
12. Grande NM, Plotino G, Butti A, Messina F, Pameijer CH, Somma F. Crosssectional analysis of root canals prepared with NiTi rotary instruments and stainless steel reciprocating files. Oral Surg Oral Med Oral Pathol Oral Radiol Endod. 2007a; 103: 120-6.
13. Bellucci C, Perrini N. A study on the thickness of radicular dentin and cementumin anterior and premolar teeth. Int Endod J. 2002; 35: 594-606.
14. Wu M, R'oris A, Barkis D, Wesselink PR. Prevalence and extent of long oval canals in the apical third. Oral Surg Oral Med Oral Pathol. 2000; 89: 739-43.
15. Success and failure in endodontics: an online study guide. JOE Editorial Board. J Endod. 2008; 34: e1-6.
16. Musikant BL. One good system beats two bad. Indian Dentist Research and Review. June 2009, p. 18-21.
17. Leoni D, Grande NM, Plotino G, Pecci R, Plasschaert A, Somma F. A preliminary micro-computed tomographic analysis of apical enlargement obtained using Mtwo NiTi rotary apical files. Int Endod J. 2007; 40: 994.
18. Al-Sudani D, Al-Shahrani S. A comparison of the canal centering ability of ProFile, K3, and RaCe Nickel Titanium rotary systems. J Endod. 2006; 32: 1198-201. Epub 2006 Oct 19.
19. Glossen CR, Haller RH, Dove SB, del Rio CE. A comparison of root canal preparations using Ni-Ti hand, Ni-Ti engine-driven, and K-Flex endodontic instruments. J Endod. 1995; 21: 146-51.
20. Câmara AS, de Castro Martins R, Viana AC, de Toledo Leonardo R, Buono VT, de Azevedo Bahia MG. Flexibility and torsional strength of ProTaper and ProTaper Universal rotary instruments assessed by mechanical tests. J Endod. 2009; 35: 113-6.
21. Alapati SB, Brantley WA, Svec TA, Powers JM, Nusstein JM, Daehn GS. SEM observations of nickel-titanium rotary endodontic instruments that fractured during clinical Use. J Endod. 2005; 31: 40-3.
22. McSpadden JT. Mastering Endodontic Instrumentation, 1ed, Cloudland Institute: Chattanooga; 2007. p. 105-23.
23. Vieira EP, França EC, Martins RC, Buono VT, Bahia MG. Influence of multiple clinical use on fatigue resistance of ProTaper rotary nickel-titanium instruments. Int Endod J. 2008; 41: 163-72. Epub 2007 Nov 12.
24. Soares JA, Leonardo RT. Root canal treatment of three-rooted maxillary first and second premolars-a case report. Int Endod J. 2003; 36: 705-10.
25. Aguirre GM, Pappen FG, Gutierrez JCR, Nogueira I, Bonetti Filho I, Puenta, CG et al. Effectiveness of root canal rotary and/or oscillatory preparation techniques in flattened root canals. Acta Odont Venez. 2007; 45: 1-8.
26. Palo, RM, Paradella TC, Faria R, Valera MC, Araujo MAM. Avaliação do desgaste das paredes internas de canais radiculares de molares. Rev Assoc Paul Cirurg Dent. 2006; 60: 375-8.